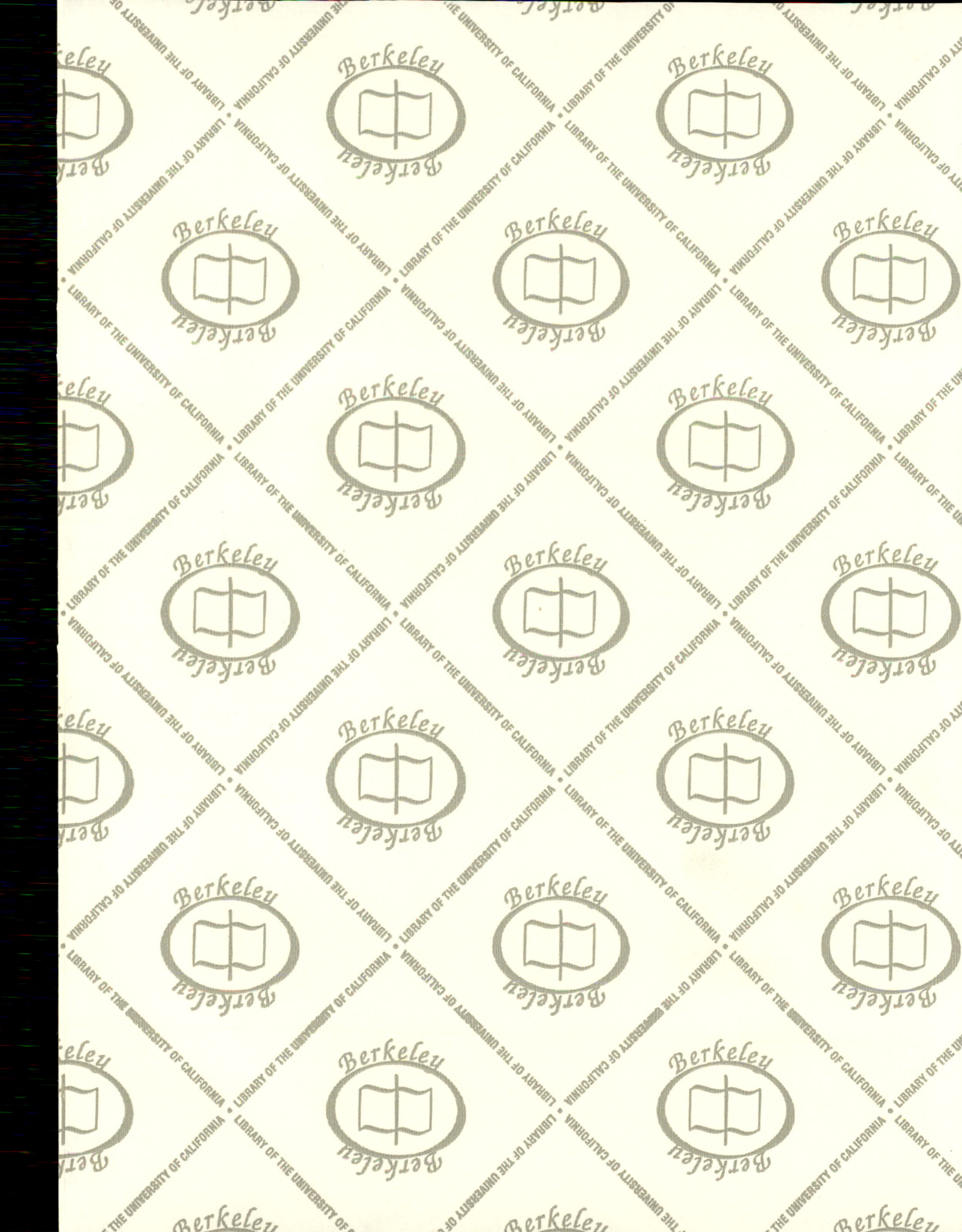

PRIMARY CARE OF THE GLAUCOMAS

PRIMARY CARE OF THE GLAUCOMAS

SECOND EDITION

Editors

MURRAY FINGERET, O.D.

Associate Clinical Professor
College of Optometry
State University of New York
Chief, Optometry Section
VA New York Harbor Health Care System
Brooklyn, New York

THOMAS L. LEWIS, O.D., Ph.D.

Professor and President
Pennsylvania College of Optometry
Philadelphia, Pennsylvania

Illustrations by
Stephanie P. Schilling
Lori A. Messenger

McGRAW-HILL
Medical Publishing Division

New York St. Louis San Francisco Auckland Bogotá Caracas Lisbon London Madrid
Mexico City Milan Montreal New Delhi San Juan Singapore Sydney Tokyo Toronto

McGraw-Hill

A Division of The McGraw-Hill Companies

PRIMARY CARE OF THE GLAUCOMAS
Second Edition

1 2 3 4 5 6 7 8 9 0 QPKQPK 0 9 8 7 6 5 4 3 2 1 0

ISBN   0-8385-8158-7

This book was set in Palatino by Progressive Information Technologies.
The editors were Sally Barhydt, Catherine Wenz, and Muza Navrozov.
The production supervisor was Rohnda Barnes.
The index was prepared by Alexandra Nickerson.
Quebecor Printing Kingsport was printer and binder.

This book is printed on recycled, acid-free paper.

Library of Congress Cataloging-in-Publication Data

Primary care of the glaucomas / edited by Murray Fingeret, Thomas L. Lewis; with 33 contributors.—2nd ed.
   p. ; cm.
  Includes bibliographical references and index.
  ISBN 0-8385-8158-7
  1. Glaucoma. 2. Optometrists. I. Fingeret, Murray. II. Lewis, Thomas L.
  [DNLM: 1. Glaucoma—diagnosis. 2. Glaucoma—therapy. WW 290
P9515 2000]
RE871.P75 2000
617.7'41—dc21
                                  99-087835

To
Janet and Stuart Fingeret and Blanche Fingeret Pindus
and
Harriet, Tracy, and Heather Lewis
for their love and support

and to those with glaucoma, who will benefit from
the knowledge gained by doctors from this book

Contents

Part I

BASIC UNDERSTANDING

Part III
TREATMENT AND MANAGEMENT

Part IV
TYPES OF GLAUCOMA

Contributors*

P. JUHANI AIRAKSINEN, M.D., Ph.D. [13]
Professor and Head
Department of Ophthalmology
University of Oulu
Oulu, Finland

PETER ÅSMAN, M.D., Ph.D. [15]
Associate Professor
Department of Ophthalmology
Malmo University Hospital
Malmo, Sweden

HOWARD S. BARNEBEY, M.D. [12, 23]
Associate Professor
Department of Ophthalmology
University of Washington School of Medicine
Seattle, Washington

G. RICHARD BENNETT, M.S., O.D. [11]
Associate Professor
Pennsylvania College of Optometry
Philadelphia, Pennsylvania

MICHAEL A. CHAGLASIAN, O.D. [17]
Associate Professor
Illinois College of Optometry
Chicago, Illinois
Chief, Center for Advanced Ophthalmic Care
Illinois Eye Institute
Chicago, Illinois

CONNIE L. CHRONISTER, O.D. [5]
Associate Professor
Pennsylvania College of Optometry
Philadelphia, Pennsylvania

HAK SUNG CHUNG, M.D., Ph.D. [6]
Department of Ophthalmology
Indiana University School of Medicine
Indianapolis, Indiana

EVAN BENJAMIN DREYER, M.D., Ph.D. [8]
Associate Professor
Department of Ophthalmology
University of Pennsylvania
Scheie Eye Institute
Philadelphia, Pennsylvania

KRISTINE A. ERICKSON, O.D., Ph.D. [20]
Associate Professor
Department of Ophthalmology
Boston University School of Medicine
Assistant Professor of Optometry
New England College of Optometry
Boston, Massachusetts

DAVID EVANS, Ph.D. [7]
Research Assistant Professor
School of Optometry
University of Alabama at Birmingham
Birmingham, Alabama

ROBERT D. FECHTNER, M.D. [25]
Associate Professor
Director, Glaucoma Service
Department of Ophthalmology
UMDNJ-New Jersey Medical School
Newark, New Jersey

MURRAY FINGERET, O.D. [19, 21, 28, 31]
Associate Clinical Professor
State University of New York, College of Optometry
New York, New York
Chief, Optometry Section
VA New York Harbor Health Care System
Brooklyn, New York

JOHN G. FLANAGAN, Ph.D., M.C.OPTOM. [14]
Professor, School of Optometry
University of Waterloo
Waterloo, Ontario, Canada
Professor, Department of Ophthalmology
University of Toronto
Toronto, Ontario, Canada
Director, The Glaucoma Research Unit
The Toronto Western Hospital Research Institute
Toronto, Ontario, Canada

*Numbers in brackets refer to chapter(s) written or cowritten by the contributor.

THOMAS F. FREDDO, O.D., Ph.D. [3]
Professor of Ophthalmology, Pathology, and Anatomy
Senior Consultant in Ophthalmic Pathology
Boston University School of Medicine
Boston, Massachusetts
Professor of Optometry
New England College of Optometry
Boston, Massachusetts

HANNA J. GARZOZI, M.D. [6]
Professor and Chairman
Department of Ophthalmology
Central Emek Hospital
Afula, Israel

DAVID S. GREENFIELD, M.D. [30]
Assistant Professor of Clinical Ophthalmology
Department of Ophthalmology
Bascom Palmer Eye Institute
University of Miami School of Medicine
Miami, Florida

ALON HARRIS, M.S., Ph.D. [6]
Letzter Professor of Ophthalmology
Professor of Physiology and Biophysics
Director, Glaucoma Research and Diagnostic Center
Indiana University School of Medicine
Indianapolis, Indiana

HIROSHI ISHIKAWA, M.D. [29]
Assistant Professor of Ophthalmology
New York Medical College
Valhalla, New York
Director, Ocular Imaging Center
The New York Eye and Ear Infirmary
New York, New York

CHRIS A. JOHNSON, Ph.D. [18]
Director of Diagnostic Research
Discoveries in Sight
Devers Eye Institute
Legacy Health Systems
Portland, Oregon

LARRY KAGEMANN, M.S., B.M.E. [6]
Biomedical Engineer
Glaucoma Research and Diagnostic Center
Indiana University School of Medicine
Indianapolis, Indiana

JOANNE KLOPFER CARR, O.D., M.PH. [2]
Associate Professor of Optometry and Community Health
Pennsylvania College of Optometry
Philadelphia, Pennsylvania

PETER LALLE, O.D. [10,16]
Adjunct Assistant Professor
Pennsylvania College of Optometry
Philadelphia, Pennsylvania
Chief, Optometry Section
Department of Veterans Medical Center
Baltimore, Maryland

PAUL J. LAMA, M.D. [25]
Assistant Professor
Glaucoma Service
VMDNJ New Jersey Medical School
Department of Ophthalmology
Newark, NJ

THOMAS L. LEWIS, O.D., Ph.D. [1, 4, 5, 19]
Professor and President
Pennsylvania College of Optometry
Philadelphia, Pennsylvania

JEFFREY M. LIEBMANN, M.D. [26, 27, 29]
Professor of Clinical Ophthalmology
New York Medical College
Valhalla, New York
Associate Director, Glaucoma Service
The New York Eye and Ear Infirmary
New York, New York

LORI R. REMINICK, O.D. [9]
Director, Optometric Residency Program
Department of Veterans Affairs,
New York Harbor Health Care System,
Brooklyn, New York
Adjunct Assistant Clinical Professor
State University of New York College of Optometry
New York, New York

ROBERT RITCH, M.D. [26, 27, 29]
Professor of Clinical Ophthalmology
New York Medical College
Valhalla, New York
Chief, Glaucoma Service
Surgeon Director
The New York Eye and Ear Infirmary
New York, New York

ALAN L. ROBIN, M.D. [31]
Professor of Ophthalmology
University of Maryland School of Medicine
Baltimore, Maryland
Associate Professor of Ophthalmology
Johns Hopkins University School of Medicine
Associate Professor of International health
Johns Hopkins University School of Hygiene and Public
    Health
Baltimore, Maryland

ALISON SCHROEDER [20]
Department of Ophthalmology
Boston University School of Medicine
Boston, Massachusetts

PAIT TEESALU, M.D., Ph.D. [13]
Director, Department of Ophthalmology
University of Tartu
Tartu, Estonia

J. JAMES THIMONS, O.D. [28]
Ophthalmic Consultants of Connecticut
Fairfield, Connecticut

ELLIOT B. WERNER, M.D. [22, 24]
Clinical Professor of Ophthalmology
Medical College of Pennsylvania/
      Hahnemann University School of Medicine
Glaucoma Consultant
Co-Director, Glaucoma Service
Pennsylvania College of Optometry
Philadelphia, Pennsylvania

KATHY C. YANG-WILLIAMS, O.D. [12, 23]
Formerly Glaucoma Fellow
Specialty Eyecare Centre
Seattle, Washington
TLC Northwest Eye
Seattle, Washington

JOAN TANABE WING, O.D. [4]
Associate Professor
Pennsylvania College of Optometry
Philadelphia, Pennsylvania

Foreword

Glaucoma is a disease that can result in both functional vision loss and total blindness. To minimize the devastating consequences of undiagnosed and/or poorly managed glaucoma, a "cast of thousands" of highly skilled and dedicated physicians within optometry and ophthalmology must be assembled to effectively meet such a clinical challenge.

In this completely revised and updated second edition of "Primary Care of the Glaucomas", Dr. Murray Fingeret and Dr. Tom Lewis have achieved a new milestone in glaucoma education: a collaborative, comprehensive textbook written by multiple teams of expert optometrists and glaucoma subspecialists.

From the mundane to the complex, this text provides a comprehensive understanding of the pathogenesis and management of the glaucomas. Concepts of pressure-dependent and non-pressure-dependent optic neuropathy are discussed, as well as bloodflow and neuroprotective cascades, including apoptotic axonal death. The critical new role of genetics in the early detection of glaucoma is beautifully presented.

New technology for evaluating the retinal nerve fiber layer and imaging the optic nerve and nerve fiber layer are reviewed in detail with emphasis on their roles in clinical practice. Advances in visual field quantification are thoroughly discussed with an indepth presentation of the Humphrey and Octopus perimeters and their software programs. Interpretation and new developments in perimetry highlight the critical role of visual field assessment in the diagnosis and treatment of glaucoma. The section on diagnosis is capped with a comprehensive presentation of a clinical approach to the early identification of the disease.

The treatment and management of glaucoma cover the entire spectrum—from basic pharmacology of medications through medical, laser, and surgical management. The latest techniques and clinical trials are presented with the goal of relating the information to the primary care of the glaucomas. An exciting look into the future of glaucoma treatment and management creates food for thought for all of us who deal with caring for patients with glaucoma each and every day.

This text ends with a presentation of the most common secondary (pigmentary, exfoliation) and angle-closure glaucomas. The final chapter, glaucoma case studies, allows the reader the opportunity to immediately apply all that they have mastered from their "journey through glaucoma".

In short, this text can well equip the astute reader in both the academic and clinical aspects of caring for patients with glaucoma. It is our fervent hope ophthalmologists and optometrists will use this exemplary text to enhance their knowledge base so that a common goal of preventing vision loss from the glaucomas can be realized.

On behalf of the physicians and their patients who will ultimately benefit from the sharing of knowledge in this text, we take this special opportunity to thank Dr. Fingeret and Dr. Lewis and their team of world-class colleagues for their time, sacrifice, and dedication to bringing this clinical masterpiece to the eye care professions.

RANDALL THOMAS, O.D., M.P.H
Concord, North Carolina
Adjunct Assistant Clinical Professor
State University of New York College of Optometry,
New York, New York
Pennsylvania College of Optometry, Philadelphia, Pennsylvania
Pacific University College of Optometry, Forest Grove, Oregon

RON MELTON, O.D.
Charlotte, North Carolina
Adjunct Assistant Clinical Professor
State University of New York College of Optometry,
New York, New York
Pennsylvania College of Optometry, Philadelphia, Pennsylvania
Pacific University College of Optometry, Forest Grove, Oregon

Preface

The idea for developing a textbook dedicated solely to glaucoma intended for optometrists was born in 1990. It took several years to bring the initial project to fruition, with the publication in 1993 of *Primary Care of the Glaucomas.* At that time the concept of a book dedicated to glaucoma written for optometrists was unusual. Questions included whether sufficient interest would exist for a topic as specific as glaucoma and how should the book be developed.

The first edition was built around the core areas of anatomy, pharmacology and diagnostic techniques, since we felt that those were most important for optometrists becoming involved in the management of glaucoma. At the time, optometry's sophistication in the area of glaucoma was limited, as only a few states allowed optometrists the privilege of treating glaucoma. Since the publication of the first edition, the number of states with glaucoma therapeutic privileges has expanded dramatically. Optometrists have become more comfortable in the care of individuals with ocular hypertension and glaucoma, and a paradigm shift has occurred. No longer do optometrists equate glaucoma with co-management, but recognize the condition as another in the spectrum of care O.D.s can provide. Having become more sophisticated in the management of glaucoma, optometrists have led us to reexamine the scope and nature of the second edition of *Primary Care of the Glaucomas.*

We realized early in planning for the second edition that we needed to expand our roster of authors to enlist individuals who have been leaders in glaucoma research as well as clinicians. We believe that optometrists will embrace a text written in part by experts who have performed the research that is impacting patient care. It is with pride that for our second edition, the author list has expanded to include individuals outside the optometric circle with expertise in many different areas of glaucoma: Robert Ritch, Juhani Airkensenen, Jeffrey Liebmann, Alan Robin, Robert Fechtner, Elliott Werner, David Greenfield, Chris Johnson, Evan Dreyer, Kristine Erickson, Howard Barnebey, Alon Harris, David Evans, John Flanagan, Pait Teesalu, and Peter Asman. Their names are familiar to many that peruse the literature, as they are all frequent contributors to the world's glaucoma literature. With so many new contributors, the second edition has become a "new text" rather than simply a revision.

Writing a new edition to an established book can be a challenge. Luckily in the area of glaucoma there is an abundance of new information. Since the first edition was published, the medical armamentarium has expanded to include topical prostaglandins, topical carbonic anhydrase inhibitors, new alpha agonists, and combinations with beta-blockers and carbonic anhydrase inhibitors. The concept of blood flow was in its infancy, and the term *neuroprotection* was not being discussed in relationship to glaucoma management when the first edition was developed. Genetics was rarely spoken about in reference to glaucoma, and the surgical options were limited. Finally, with the new cadre of medications, reduced dosing schedules with fewer side effects have become common and our management philosophies have evolved to incorporate these changing principles.

With regards to diagnosis, the optic nerve imaging instruments were in development and not commercially available when our first edition hit the shelves, and emerging diagnostic modalities like short-wavelength automated perimetry (SWAP), frequency doubling perimetry (FDP), and optical coherence tomography (OCT) were limited to a few research sites. Now a range of new diagnostic instruments such as these are emerging that may allow us to better detect and track changes to the optic nerve, nerve fiber layer, or visual field. While these instruments have not evolved to the point where they can be used alone to diagnose glaucoma, they often provide valuable information that complements other parts of the diagnostic puzzle, helping us when confronted with difficult management decisions.

With all the high-tech advances, the focus of *Primary Care of the Glaucomas, Second Edition,* is still primary care. We have limited the content of the book to topics that are most commonly encountered by practicing optometrists. More comprehensive textbooks on glaucoma exist, such as Robert Ritch's *The Glaucomas,* which are inclusive of all surgical approaches. Rather we have concentrated on areas that we feel are most appropriate for optometrists. This edition is built similar to the first, with the initial chapters related to epidemiology, anatomy and physiology, laying the framework followed by sections on diagnosis, treatment, and the different forms of glaucoma. The final chapter of the book examines the management of various cases.

It is our hope that this text will serve as a " silent colleague" whose guidance alongside you in the examining room will provide support and aid in many difficult and challenging decisions that confront all clinicians involved in the care of individuals with glaucoma.

MURRAY FINGERET
THOMAS L. LEWIS

Acknowledgments

In a book such as this, many individuals play a role either in helping with research, writing, typing, copying or in the many other tasks involved. For all who have helped in some way, we thank you.

In particular we would like to thank V. Michael Patella, Craig Percy, Lou Catania, Sally Barhydt, Muza Navrozov, Rohnda Barnes, Kellyann Dignam, Karen Fleigelmann, Rodney Gutner, Jeffrey Liebmann, Lisa Lonie, Lori Reminick, Robert Ritch, Leo Semes, Edward Smith, Stan Teplick, and Marian Weber for all their help and support.

Part I

BASIC UNDERSTANDING

Chapter 1

DEFINITION AND CLASSIFICATION OF GLAUCOMA

Thomas L. Lewis

Glaucoma is not a single clinical entity. It comprises a group of ocular diseases with various etiologies that ultimately result in a rather consistent optic neuropathy. Glaucomas are diseases in which the person's optic nerve becomes damaged, resulting in histopathological changes in this tissue. These changes eventually lead to a loss of visual function. It is important to realize that there exist various forms of glaucoma. From a clinical perspective, a generic diagnosis of glaucoma is inadequate to develop a proper management plan for the patient. A differential diagnosis, indicating the specific type of glaucoma, is necessary to predict the course and prognosis of the disease and to ensure appropriate and timely treatment.

CLASSIFICATION

Since glaucoma is a group of diseases with varying clinical presentations, prognoses, morbidity, treatment, and management, a system to properly classify these diseases is important. Various classifications have been proposed. These classification systems are based on (1) etiology, (2) mechanics, and (3) age of onset (i.e., infantile, juvenile, and adult). I have chosen a classification system with both an etiological and mechanical basis. This type of classification system

seems to make the most sense clinically. The terminology used can assist the doctor in the proper diagnosis and management of glaucoma patients.

OPEN- VERSUS CLOSED-ANGLE GLAUCOMA

Glaucomas can be divided into *open-* or *closed-angle* types. This relates to the gonioscopic appearance of the anterior chamber angle (Fig. 1–1). In open-angle glaucomas, the rise in intraocular pressure, if it occurs, is not due to a mechanical obstruction of the angle by the iris. In closed-angle glaucomas, the outflow of aqueous is obstructed by the root of the iris. This obstruction can be associated with pupillary block or can occur without pupillary block.

Both open- and closed-angle glaucomas can result from underlying primary, secondary, or developmental etiologies. *Primary* glaucomas are not associated with any other apparent ocular or systemic disorder. In primary open-angle glaucoma, the obstruction to aqueous outflow apparently occurs at a submicroscopic and/or biochemical level in the outflow pathways. These alterations are not visible on gonioscopic evaluation (Fig. 1–1). In primary closed-angle glaucoma, a pupillary block or plateau iris

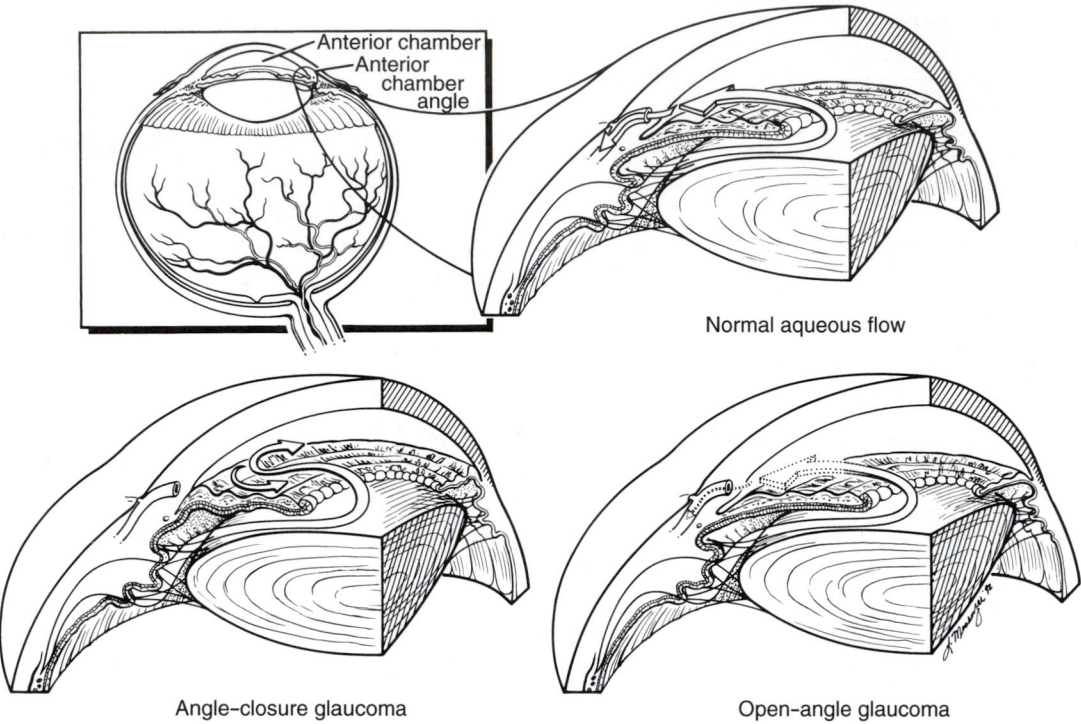

Anterior chamber
Anterior chamber angle

Normal aqueous flow

Angle–closure glaucoma

Open–angle glaucoma

Figure 1–1. Representation of the differences in aqueous flow and the configuration of the anterior chamber angle between open- and closed-angle glaucoma.

forces the iris into the anterior chamber angle, obstructing aqueous outflow (Table 1–1). Primary glaucomas are usually genetically based and bilateral in their clinical presentation.

Secondary glaucomas are caused by a variety of ocular and/or systemic disorders that cause a decrease in aqueous outflow, leading to either open- or closed-angle glaucoma. The obstruction of aqueous outflow in secondary open-angle glaucomas can occur by membrane formation over the anterior chamber angle; physical blockage of the trabecular meshwork by pigment, debris, or anatomical changes within the trabeculae; or changes in Schlemm's canal or the episcleral venous system (Table 1–2). Secondary closed-

angle glaucomas are most easily divided into anterior forms, in which the iris is *pulled* into the angle by the contraction of structures in the angle, and posterior forms, in which the iris is *pushed* forward into the angle either from increased pressure due to a pupillary block or from pressure built up behind the iris from a space-occupying change within the eye (Table 1–3). Secondary glaucomas can be inherited or acquired and may be either unilateral or bilateral in their clinical presentation.

TABLE 1–1. PRIMARY GLAUCOMAS

Open-Angle
High tension
Normal (low tension)

Closed-Angle
With pupillary block
Prodromal
Subacute
Acute
Chronic
Without pupillary block
Plateau iris

TABLE 1–2. SECONDARY OPEN-ANGLE GLAUCOMAS

Pigmentary
Exfoliation syndrome
Neovascular
Posttraumatic
Epithelial downgrowth
Fibrous ingrowth
Fuchs' endothelial dystrophy
Inflammation-induced
Tumor-induced
Lens-induced
Intraocular hemorrhage-induced
Retinal detachment
Following intraocular surgery
Following an increase in episcleral venous pressure

TABLE 1–3. SECONDARY CLOSED-ANGLE GLAUCOMAS

With Pupillary Block
  Miotic-induced
  Lens-induced—swollen, ectopic
  Synechiae to lens, vitreous, lens implant
  Spherophakia

Without Pupillary Block
  Anterior (Pulling)
    Neovascular
    Fibrous ingrowth
    Iridocorneal endothelial syndrome
    Posttraumatic
    Inflammation-induced

  Posterior (Pushing)
    Central retinal vein occlusion
    Iris or ciliary body cyst
    Ciliary block
    Tumor-induced
    Inflammation-induced
    Choroidal detachment
    Suprachoroidal hemorrhage
    Following panretinal photocoagulation
    Following scleral buckling

TABLE 1-4. DEVELOPMENTAL GLAUCOMAS

Primary
  Primary congenital (infantile)

Secondary
  Retinopathy of prematurity
  Posttraumatic
  Tumor-related
  Inflammation-induced

Associated with Congenital Anomalies or Syndromes
  Aniridia
  Sturge-Weber syndrome
  Neurofibromatosis
  Marfan's syndrome
  Pierre Robin syndrome
  Homocystinuria
  Goniodysgenesis
  Lowe's syndrome
  Microcornea
  Microspherophakia
  Rubella
  Chromosomal abnormalities
  Persistent hyperplastic primary vitreous

Developmental glaucomas are due to abnormalities in the anterior chamber angle, occurring during gestation, which result in a decrease in aqueous outflow. Most forms of developmental glaucomas are secondary; however, primary developmental glaucomas can occur (Table 1–4).

Whereas most forms of glaucoma are *chronic*, on rare occasions certain patients with closed-angle glaucoma can present with an acute form of the disease. A certain percentage of glaucoma patients will have a mixed-mechanism glaucoma, which is a combination of both open- and closed-angle glaucomas. The type of glaucoma in a given patient may change over time. This is important to keep in mind, since it influences the treatment plan for that patient.

Recent evidence indicates that a significant percentage of glaucoma patients have an intraocular pressure (IOP) at or below 21 mmHg at the time of initial diagnosis.[1] Some of these patients with *normal-tension* glaucoma will never have an IOP above 21 mmHg.[1] Even though patients with normal-tension glaucoma seem to have a pressure-dependent component to their glaucoma, evidence is increasing that there may be a pressure-independent component in many individuals with primary open-angle glaucoma.[1,2]

Tables 1–1 through 1–4 present a comprehensive but not exhaustive classification system for glaucoma. This textbook concentrates on primary open-angle glaucoma, since it is the most common form of glaucoma seen in optometric practices. Primary closed-angle and secondary glaucomas are also presented. Developmental glaucomas are not discussed in detail because of the infrequency with which they are seen by optometrists.

CONCLUSION

All classification systems are arbitrary. Some cases do not fit neatly into one category. Remember, however, that the classification of glaucoma can be critical to its proper treatment. A specific diagnosis should differentiate open-angle from closed-angle and primary from secondary; if possible, it should also identify the specific disorder causing the secondary glaucoma.

REFERENCES

1. Sommer A, Tielsch JM, Katz J, Quigley HA, et al. Relationship between intraocular pressure and primary open-angle glaucoma among white and black Americans. The Baltimore Eye Survey. *Arch Ophthalmol.* 1991;109:1090–1095.
2. Mitchell P, Smith W, Attebok K, Healey PR. Prevalence of open-angle glaucoma in Australia. The Blue Mountain Eye Study. *Ophthalmology.* 1996;103:1661–1669.

Chapter 2

EPIDEMIOLOGY OF GLAUCOMA

Joanne Klopfer Carr

Epidemiology is a fundamental science that evaluates the distribution and determinants of disease occurrence in human populations.[1] In the past decades, significant steps have been made in our understanding of the epidemiology of glaucoma.[2] These developments have resulted from increased compilation of data as well as several major studies being performed in the United States and other parts of the world. As our understanding of the epidemiology of glaucoma evolves, it becomes more important for practitioners to become familiar with the results of these studies and to utilize the insights of epidemiology in clinical practice.

Epidemiology offers a valuable alternative perspective from which to view the diagnosis of disease, especially glaucoma. The knowledge gained from epidemiological studies can provide the practitioner with a foundation to facilitate the diagnosis and management of disease. In addition, since the science of epidemiology is based on a probabilistic approach to disease, it can aid the practitioner in communicating with patients in the current health care environment. Owing in large part to strong economic forces, the primary purchasers of medical care now use probabilistic population-based measures to assess the effectiveness of medical interventions.[3] Practitioners need to be familiar with these assumptions and the strategies of current health programs. A change to consumer-oriented medicine also requires doctors to inform patients about an intervention's risk and effectiveness, both of which are based on epidemiological evidence.

This chapter reviews the essentials of our evolving understanding of the epidemiology of glaucoma and discusses the implications of this understanding for clinical practice. The focus is on adult-onset, primary open-angle glaucoma, a leading cause of blindness whose etiology remains unknown.

TOTAL PREVALENCE OF GLAUCOMA

Prevalence is defined as the proportion of a population that has a disease at a particular point in time. A landmark population-based glaucoma prevalence survey was conducted on 5308 noninstitutionalized persons aged 40 years or older in East Baltimore during 1985–1988.[4] Cases of primary open-angle glaucoma (POAG) in the Baltimore Eye Survey were identified based on ophthalmoscopic and/or visual-field evidence of glaucomatous optic nerve damage. Unlike in previous prevalence surveys,[5-7] intraocular pressure was not a criterion for glaucoma diagnosis. The Baltimore Eye Survey finding of 132 "definite" cases of POAG and 29 "probable" POAG cases has been extrapolated to determine the prevalence or "burden" of glaucoma in the United States. A total of 1.3 million definite cases and an additional 0.3 million probable cases of glaucoma have been projected using 1985 census data. Quigley and Vitale examined glaucoma prevalence studies with strong epidemiological study design features and estimated that 2.47 million people will have open-angle glaucoma in the year 2000.[8] The estimated 2 to 3 million cases of glaucoma among Americans 40 years of age or older is often used as an introductory statement for describing the prevalence of glaucoma in the United States.[9-11] Almost 67 million people worldwide will have open-angle glaucoma by the year 2000, making glaucoma the second leading cause of vision loss.[12]

SUBGROUP PREVALENCES

Subgroup analysis by age, gender, and racial or ethnic group can provide essential information about the patterns of distribution of disease in the population.

Age
Every population-based study has shown a strong increase in the prevalence of glaucoma with increasing age.[13] Results from the largest population studies show 4 to 10 times greater prevalence in the oldest age groups compared to persons in their forties.[4,5,14,15]

Ethnic Group
Differences in glaucoma prevalence among ethnic or racial groups are an important part of the epidemiology of glaucoma. Large differences in the prevalence of glaucoma have been found worldwide (Fig. 2–1 and Table 2–1). The Framingham Eye Study is a well-known source of information on the prevalence of eye disease in Caucasian U.S. residents over 52 years of age. Prevalence rates for glaucoma in the Framingham population ranged from 1.2 to 2.1 per hundred population.[16] Eighteen European and U.S. population-based studies were evaluated for an overall estimated average glaucoma prevalence of 2.42 per hundred population for both Europeans and U.S. residents of European ancestry over 40 years of age.[12] Studies from Blue Mountains and Melbourne, Australia, showed prevalences of 2.4 and 1.7 per hundred population, respectively. The higher Blue Mountains prevalence could be explained by the inclusion of only people aged 49 years or older.[17,18]

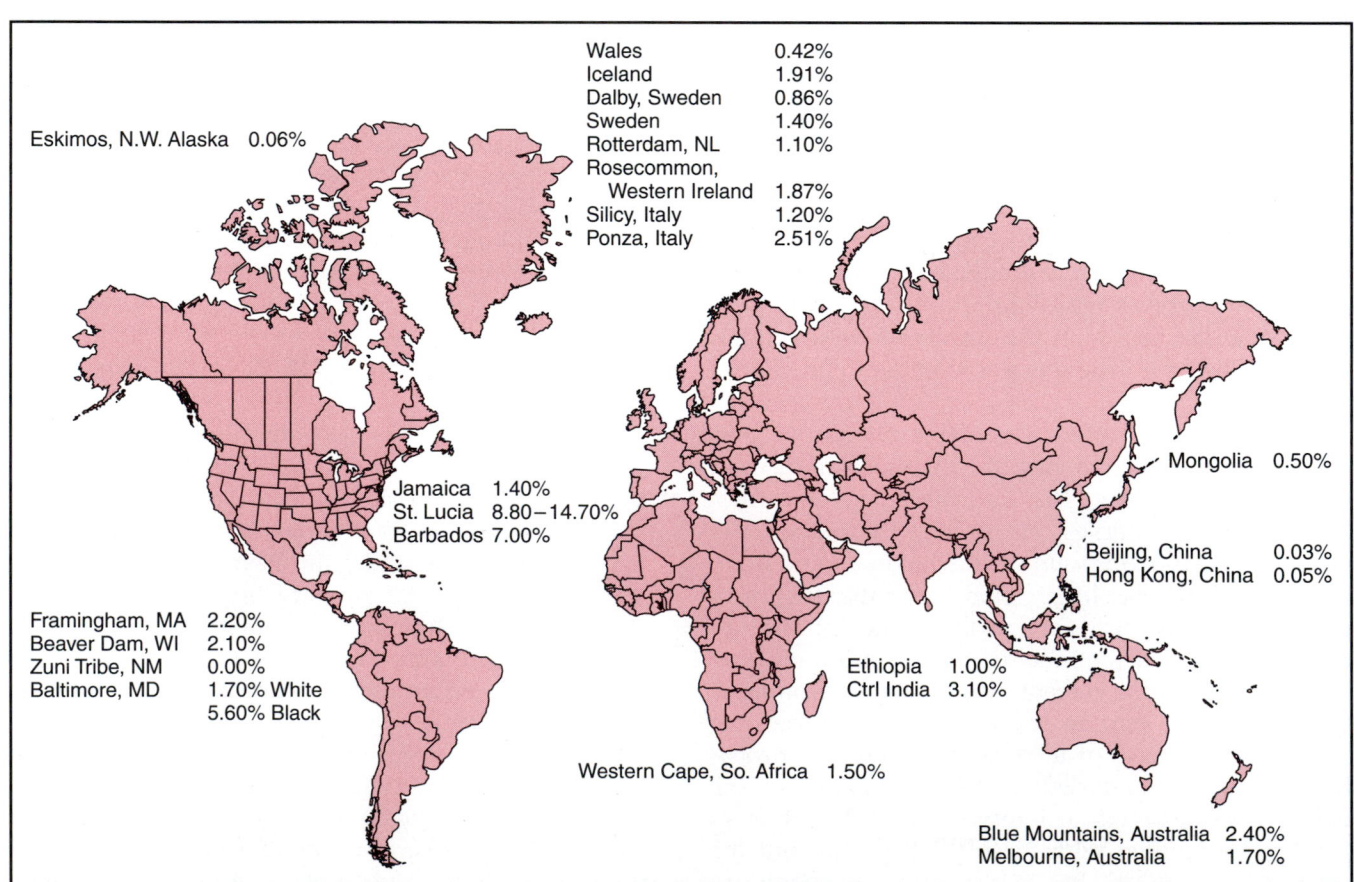

Figure 2–1. Reported prevalence of open-angle glaucoma. Note that the population and survey approaches may vary. See Table 2–1.

TABLE 2–1. REPORTED PREVALENCE OF OPEN-ANGLE GLAUCOMA IN SELECTED POPULATIONS

Source	Criteria for Defining OAG	Number	Age Range (years of age)	Estimated Prevalence (per 100)	Ethnicity	Dates of Study
Africa						
Western Cape, South Africa [27]	Optic nerve appearance consistent with visual field loss	1,194	40 and older	1.50	Southeast Asian and southern African	1992
Ethiopia [77]	IOP and optic nerve assessment	7,423	40 and older	1.00	African	1994–1995
Americas						
NW Alaska [25]	Glaucomatous field defects in presence of elevated IOP or optic disc cupping	1,686	15 and older	0.06	Eskimo	1985
Framingham, MA [14]	Visual-field loss	2,631	52–85	2.20	White Americans	1980
Beaver Dam, WI [15]	At least two of the following: visual-field loss, optic disc cupping, elevated IOP	4,926	43–84	2.10	White Americans	1991
Zuñi Tribe, NM [26]	IOP, optic nerve damage, and visual-field loss	119	40 and older	0.00	Zuni Indians	1976–1977
Baltimore, MD [4]	Visual-field loss and/or glaucomatous ON damage (definite)	2,913	40 and older	1.29	White Americans	1991
Baltimore, MD [4]	Visual field loss and/or glaucomatous ON damage (definite)	2,395	40 and older	4.74	Black Americans	1991
Asia						
Maharashtra, India [78]	Clinical "findings"	903	50–89	3.1	Indian	1990–1991
Hovsgol, Mongolia [24]	Visual-field defect and optic nerve damage	942	40 and older	0.50	Asian	1995
Beijing, China [22]	Any three of the following: OP > 24 mm, optic nerve assessment, visual-field loss, water provocative, aqueous outflow	10,414	10 and older	0.03	Chinese	1987
Hong Kong, China [23]	Any two of the following: visual-field loss, IOP > 21 mm, optic disc cupping or asymmetry	355	40 and older	5.10	Chinese	Mid-1990s
Australia						
Blue Mountains, Australia [17]	Visual-field defects, optic disc changes	3,241	49–97	2.4	White Australians	1992–1994
Melbourne, Australia [18]	Consensus of experts who reviewed visual-field defects, IOP, enlarged and/or asymmetric cupping, and nerve fiber defects	3,265	40–98	1.7	White Australians or Europeans and 1.5% Vietnamese	1994
Caribbean						
Jamaica [79]	Concurrent cupping of the optic disc and visual-field loss	574	35 and older	1.40	Black Jamaicans	1969
St. Lucia [21]	Visual-field loss and/or severe optic disc cupping	1,679	30 and older	8.80–14.70	Black St. Lucians	1989
Barbados [20]	Visual-field loss and/or glaucomatous ON damage	4,314	40–84	7.00	Black Barbadians	1994
Europe						
Wales, Great Britain [5]	Concurrent cupping of the optic disc and visual-field loss (fields were done on only 1/3 of sample)	4,231	40–75	0.42	White Welsh	1966

(Continued)

TABLE 2–1. *(Continued)*   REPORTED PREVALENCE OF OPEN-ANGLE GLAUCOMA IN SELECTED POPULATIONS

Source	Criteria for Defining OAG	Number	Age Range (years of age)	Estimated Prevalence (per 100)	Ethnicity	Dates of Study
Iceland[80]	Pharmacy and physician records of glaucoma treatment or hospital records indicating glaucoma surgery	—	50 and older	1.91	White Icelandic	1986
Dalby, Sweden[30]	Concurrent visual-field loss and glaucomatous ON cupping	1,511	55–69	0.86	White Swedish	1981
Rotterdam, NL[32]	Glaucomatous visual-field loss plus either optic disc cupping or asymmetry or IOP > 21 mmHg	3,062	55 and older	1.10	White Dutch	1994
County Roscommon, Ireland[81]	At least two of: IOP > 21 mmHg, glaucomatous ON damage, or visual-field loss	2,186	50 and older	1.87	White Irish	1988–1990
Ponzo, Italy[82]	Panel consensus on glaucomatous visual-field defect with one of following: IOP > 20, large or asymmetric C/D	1,034	40 and older	2.5	Italian	1986–1988
Sicily, Italy[83]	Glaucomatous visual-field loss with IOP > 21 mmHg and/or glaucomatous ON findings	1,062	40–99	1.2	Italian	1995

Key: OAG, open-angle glaucoma; IOP, intraocular pressure; ON, optic nerve.

Persons of West African ancestry in the United States and the Caribbean area have significantly higher prevalences of glaucoma than people of European ancestry. The Baltimore Eye Survey showed higher prevalences of glaucoma among African Americans compared to Caucasians at every age.[4] Moreover, glaucoma began at around age 40 in African Americans compared to approximately age 60 in Caucasians, with a consistent increasing linear trend with age (Fig. 2–2). Overall, African Americans had a 4.7 times higher prevalence of glaucoma than their Caucasian neighbors in East Baltimore. Blindness from glaucoma was found to begin 10 years earlier among African Americans.[19] The population-based design of the Baltimore Eye Survey permits these findings to be extrapolated to other multiracial urban populations in the United States.

Similar differences among ethnic subgroups have been reported in the Barbados Eye Study. The prevalence of glaucoma by self-reported ethnic groups was 7.0 per hundred population in "blacks," 3.3 per hundred population in those of "mixed race," and 0.8 per hundred population in "white or other" Barbadian citizens over 40 years of age. When suspected glaucoma cases were combined with definite cases, the overall estimated prevalence of glaucoma was 10.8 per hundred population in Barbados.[20] An earlier study in St. Lucia showed a 8.8 to 14.7 per hundred population glaucoma prevalence for the African-derived population over 30 years of age.[21]

The high glaucoma prevalences found in Caribbean populations contrast sharply with the low

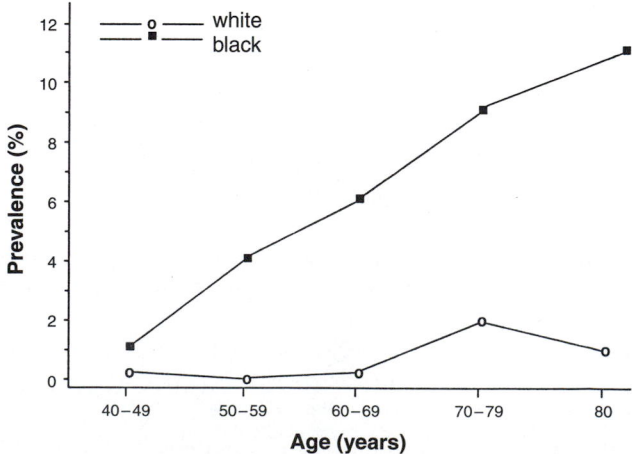

Figure 2–2. The prevalence of primary open-angle glaucoma (POAG) increases with age in East Baltimore, 1985–1988. Note the higher prevalence of POAG in the black population for each age group.

prevalences of open-angle glaucoma found in the Chinese and two indigenous U.S. populations. Prevalences of 0.03 to 0.05 per hundred population were found in Beijing and Hong Kong and 0.50 per hundred population in residents of northern Mongolia.[22-24] The prevalence of open-angle glaucoma among Northwest Alaskan Inuit (i.e., Eskimos) was 0.06 per hundred population[25]; it was 0.0 in a New Mexico Zuñi tribe.[26] It is interesting that the prevalence of glaucoma in a Western Cape South African group, with both Asian and African heritage, was reported to be 1.50 per hundred population.[27]

Available data suggest that there is a racial spectrum in the prevalence of glaucoma.[24] Open-angle glaucoma is believed to be rare among the Chinese and Inuit and more frequent among those of European ancestry. Both the Baltimore Eye Survey and the Barbados Eye Study found a higher prevalence of glaucoma among African descendants than among European descendants. Glaucoma is now the leading cause of blindness among African Americans in the United States.[28] Open-angle glaucoma is thought to be more "aggressive" among African Americans with an earlier onset and more rapid deterioration, despite lowered intraocular pressures.[29] A recommended age to begin screening for glaucoma among persons of African origins is 30 years; but in persons of European ancestry, it may be more efficient to anticipate glaucoma after 50 years of age.[12] Future population-based studies should provide insight into the intriguing differences noted in the prevalence of glaucoma between racial and/or ethnic groups.

Gender

Data on gender and the prevalence of glaucoma vary. A higher prevalence was found among females above age 55 than among males above age 65 in Dalby, Sweden.[30] Further analysis showed less significant gender differences after the age of 75 years.[31] The Framingham,[14] Barbados,[20] and Rotterdam[32] studies showed a higher prevalence of glaucoma among males. No association with gender was found in Wales,[5] Baltimore,[4] Beaver Dam, Wisconsin,[15] or the Collaborative Glaucoma Study.[33] The authors of the Rotterdam study propose that the small number of persons found with glaucoma could have accounted for the higher male prevalence in their study. Tielsch suggests that small samples of definite glaucoma cases could account for a higher prevalence of glaucoma among either males or females in some studies. Many large population-based studies do not show a difference in male/female prevalence, and gender is unlikely to be a factor in the occurrence of open-angle glaucoma.[4]

OCULAR FINDINGS

Intraocular Pressure

There is a strong relation between increased intraocular pressure (IOP) and glaucoma even when IOP is not a diagnostic criterion.[14,15,20,33-35] Elevated IOP is one of the strongest predictors of glaucoma. However, a significant proportion of persons with elevated IOP do not develop glaucomatous optic neuropathy.[34] Conversely, patients with low or "normal" IOPs can have undetected glaucoma.[5,14,35] The use of IOP as a sole criterion for glaucoma screening or diagnosis is strongly discouraged.[36,37] Other ocular examination findings must be considered as well.

Optic Disc

The appearance of the optic nerve head and cup-to-disc asymmetry have been used to identify groups in the population with a high risk for glaucomatous optic nerve damage. These optic nerve changes may represent markers of damage and are useful in determining progression of glaucoma.[13] However, it is important to recognize that there is no specific cup-to-disc ratio or degree of cup asymmetry between the two eyes that can serve as a reliable cutoff to diagnose glaucoma accurately.[37,38]

Nerve Fiber Layer

Determination of the degree of loss of the nerve fiber layer has been championed as an excellent technique to identify patients with early glaucomatous nerve damage, since defects in the nerve fiber layer precede loss of visual field. In a 10-year incidence study of an ethnically mixed population, 88% of defects in the nerve fiber layer were present when loss of visual field first occurred. These same defects were infrequent among normal subjects. Defects in the nerve fiber layer were noted in 60% of the eyes with open-angle glaucoma approximately 6 years before loss of visual field was found.[39] Unfortunately, the sensitivity of routine nerve fiber layer analysis is offset by the volume of data generalized in measuring nerve fiber thickness. Further developments in this area are anticipated.[13]

Myopia

Myopia has been reported to be related to higher levels of IOP,[40] but there does not appear to be a direct relationship with increased risk of developing POAG.[41] Clinical studies have shown that myopia above 3 diopters is associated with open-angle glaucoma in individuals under 35 years of age.[42] Selected records of open-angle glaucoma patients in the Collaborative Glaucoma Study showed four times as many myopic patients above 1 diopter than in a similar age-matched sample of the U.S. population.[43]

Conclusions regarding myopia from clinic-based or selected case studies must be tempered by the fact that persons with refractive error are more likely to seek eye care. Individuals who go more frequently for eye examinations are therefore more likely to be diagnosed with glaucoma.[13] Further population-based studies may elucidate the strength of the relationship between myopia and open-angle glaucoma. The Blue Mountain Eye Study among Australians 49 years of age and older showed that myopes had a two- to threefold increased risk of glaucoma compared with non-myopes. This risk was found to be independent of other glaucoma risk factors and IOP.[44]

SYSTEMIC HEALTH

Diabetes

Although complications of diabetes can produce secondary glaucoma, an association between diabetes and open-angle glaucoma is still unclear. The Framingham, Baltimore, Swedish, and Collaborative Glaucoma population-based prevalence studies showed no association between systemic diabetes and glaucoma.[4,14,30,33] However, a relationship between elevated IOP and diabetes was demonstrated in Framingham and other studies.[14,45,46] In addition, a positive association between systemic diabetes and glaucoma was found in 60 subjects in the Blue Mountains Study.[47]

A twofold increased risk of diabetes was found in persons with glaucoma in the Beaver Dam Study.[48] This difference from other population studies could be explained by the use of ophthalmic technicians who were not clinicians. The technicians were well trained for the procedures of the study but may not have been able to distinguish retinal complications of diabetes, which can produce false-positive visual-field changes similar to those of glaucoma.[13,48] More robust data from ongoing prospective studies should elucidate the relationship between systemic diabetes and open-angle glaucoma.

Systemic Hypertension

A positive association between increased IOP and high blood pressure has been found in several studies.[49–51] Whether the increase of IOP and concurrent increase in blood pressure are actually related to aging is not clear. Analysis of Framingham prevalence data has shown no association of either systolic or diastolic blood pressure with glaucomatous field defects.[50] More recent information from the Baltimore Eye Survey points to a complex relationship between glaucoma and systemic blood pressure. It appears that age modifies the effect of systemic hypertension in the development of glaucoma. East Baltimore Study residents with systemic hypertension who were below 60 years of age appeared to be protected from developing glaucoma, but those 70 years of age and older showed a positive association between systemic hypertension and glaucoma. This could be explained if elevated blood pressure results in increased perfusion early in the course of systemic hypertension. Later, blood flow to the optic nerve head could be reduced due to significant microvascular damage.[52] Additional large population studies that follow the effects of systemic hypertension with respect to the development of glaucoma are needed.

FAMILY HISTORY OF GLAUCOMA AND GENETICS

Intraocular pressure, cup-to-disc ratio, and facility of outflow have been found to be genetically determined.[53–55] Some studies suggest that 13 to 25% of patients with glaucoma have a positive family history of glaucoma.[56,57] Family history of glaucoma was found to be associated with glaucoma in the Barbados Eye Study.[58] In the Baltimore Eye Survey, family history of glaucoma was a strong predictor of glaucoma among the African-American population. In both the Caucasian and African-American populations in Baltimore, a stronger association with glaucoma was found with a sibling history of glaucoma compared to a parent, child, or other family member's history of glaucoma.[59] A glaucoma family aggregation study that used the Rotterdam Study participants showed a prevalence of 10.40% in siblings and 1.10% in the offspring of the group with glaucoma. The prevalence of glaucoma was found to be 0.70% in siblings and zero in the offspring of control participants with no glaucoma. It has been suggested that at least 1/6 of all glaucomas in the general population may be due to heredity.[60]

Several glaucoma genes have been identified recently, including loci for congenital, juvenile, and adult-onset glaucoma.[61,62] Wirtz and colleagues discovered an adult-onset glaucoma locus resulting from mutations in the same genes that cause developmental defects such as juvenile glaucoma and nail-patella syndrome. They suggest that transcription factors and possible effects of oxidative stress on genes could result in adult-onset open-angle glaucoma. Open-angle glaucoma has been identified as a heterogeneous group of diseases with at least six different loci that could result in the same phenotype or expression of glaucoma traits.[63] Lichter predicts that the classification of glaucoma will shift from phenotypic to genotypic emphasis in the future. DNA-based screening may be developed that will help identify some early forms of glaucoma.[64]

OCULAR HYPERTENSION

Ocular hypertension (OH) has been defined as an IOP greater than 21 mmHg without visual field defects, optic nerve damage, or anterior chamber angles abnormalities. Although an increase in IOP is associated with optic nerve changes and visual field defects, it is not axiomatic that patients with high IOP will develop POAG. Population studies have shown that the prevalence of IOP greater than 21 mmHg in persons over 40 years of age varies between 3 and 12.7 per hundred population.[17,35,65–69] Only 0.3 to 10% of ocular hypertensives will develop visual field defects. In a population-based study on the distribution of IOP measured with an applanation tonometer, Armaly found two statistically different groups. One subpopulation conformed to a normal Gaussian distribution, while another was biased toward higher IOPs.[66] Armaly's study has been used as evidence for documenting the existence of an ocular hypertensive subgroup within the normal population. While some investigators consider ocular hypertensives to be a separate population of individuals, with increased risk for developing POAG, others believe that high IOPs represent a physiological variant.

The risk for the development of POAG in patients with ocular hypertension cannot be ignored. Several studies following ocular hypertensive patients for years have found a high incidence of POAG development. One Swedish survey reported that 1.5% of ocular hypertensives developed POAG within a 5-year period.[70] This number rose to 10% after 10 years and 34% after 20 years.[70,71] The incidence of POAG that developed in "normotensive" patients during the entire 20-year time period was only 5 per hundred population.[72] In another large population study in Bedford, England, 3.23% of the ocular hypertensives developed POAG, compared to 0.52% of the normotensive population by the conclusion of the 7-year study period.[73] Epstein[74] reported a "conversion" rate of 5% per year in 54 patients with high IOP who were later diagnosed with POAG. This higher rate cannot be considered a true population-based incidence rate because only patients treated in a specialty hospital setting were examined.

Several researchers have described risk factors thought to be related to ocular hypertension. Armaly identified age, gender, and family history of glaucoma.[66] Case-control studies have pointed to hypertension, family history of glaucoma, myopia, absence of alcohol use, a history of nonocular surgery, and a history of high blood pressure.[75] Other factors thought to be associated with ocular hypertension are race or ethnic origin, cup-to-disc ratio, and diabetes.[76] It is important to note that several of these risk factors are based on anecdotal or clinical information and have not been substantiated in population-based epidemiological studies. Large, long-term studies are currently under way to determine the relative value of risk factors involved in the progression of ocular hypertension to open-angle glaucoma.

CONCLUSION

Epidemiological studies have led clinicians to a clearer understanding of glaucoma. To date, the highest prevalences of glaucoma have been found among persons of West African ancestry. A consistent increased prevalence of open-angle glaucoma has been found in all racial and ethnic groups as they advance in age. Many large population-based studies do not show a difference in the prevalence of glaucoma by gender. Elevated intraocular pressure is a strong predictor of glaucoma but should be considered along with evaluation of the optic nerve head and nerve fiber layer. Myopia is an intriguing factor that has been linked to open-angle glaucoma. The future results of longitudinal studies from Baltimore, Barbados, and Beaver Dam will yield population-based glaucoma incidence rates and should provide insight as to how myopia and/or systemic hypertension may be involved in the development of glaucoma. Research has confirmed an underlying genetic susceptibility for glaucoma but also revealed significant complexities and additional variants in the glaucoma picture that need to be solved.

ACKNOWLEDGMENT

This chapter is dedicated to Michael A. Carr.

REFERENCES

1. Greenberg RS, Daniels SR, Flanders WD, Eley JW, Boring JR. *Medical Epidemiology*, 2nd ed. Stamford, CT: Appleton & Lange; 1996.
2. Sommer A, Tielsch JM. Primary open-angle glaucoma: A clinical-epidemiologic perspective. In: Van Buskirk EM, Shields MB. *100 Years of Progress in Glaucoma*. Philadelphia: Lippincott-Raven, 1997:131–142.

3. Fox DM. Comment: Epidemiology and the new political economy of medicine. *Am J Public Health*. 1999;89: 493–496.

4. Tielsch JM, Sommer A, Katz J, Royall RM, et al. Racial variations in the prevalence of primary open angle glaucoma: The Baltimore Eye Survey. *JAMA*. 1991;266: 369–374.

5. Hollows FC, Graham PA. Intraocular pressure, glaucoma and glaucoma suspects in a defined population. *Br J Ophthalmol*. 1966;50:570–586.

6. Kini MM, Leibowitz HM, Colton T, Nickerson RJ, Ganley J, Dawber TR. Prevalence of senile cataract, diabetic retinopathy, senile macular degeneration, and openangle glaucoma in the Framingham Eye Study. *Am J Ophthalmol*. 1978;85:28–34.

7. Kahn HA, Milton RC. Revised Framingham Eye Study prevalence of glaucoma and diabetic retinopathy. *Am J Epidemiol*. 1980;111:769–776.

8. Quigley HA, Vitale S. Models of open-angle glaucoma prevalence and incidence in the United States. *Invest Ophthalmol Vis Sci*. 1997;38:83–91.

9. Potter JW. Understanding the risk factors for glaucoma. *Rev. Optom*. 1998;10(Suppl):7A–8A.

10. American Academy of Ophthalmology. *Primary Open-Angle Glaucoma: Preferred Practice Pattern*. San Francisco: American Academy of Ophthalmology; 1996.

11. Prevent Blindness America. Eye problems: Frequently asked questions about glaucoma. *www.preventblindness.org* 1999;1–3.

12. Quigley HA. Number of people with glaucoma worldwide. *Br J Ophthalmol*. 1996;80:389–393.

13. Tielsch JM. The epidemiology and control of open angle glaucoma, a population-based perspective. *Annu Rev Public Health*. 1996;17:121–136.

14. Leibowitz HM, Krueger DE, Maunder LR, et al. The Framingham Eye Study Monograph. *Surv Ophthalmol*. 1980;24(suppl): 335–610.

15. Klein BEK, Klein R, Sponsel WE, Franke T, et al. Prevalence of glaucoma: The Beaver Dam Eye Study. *Ophthalmology*. 1992;99:1499–1504.

16. Kahn HA, Milton RC. Revised Framingham Eye Study: Prevalence of glaucoma and diabetic retinopathy. *Am J Epidemiol*. 1989;111:769–776.

17. Mitchell P, Smith W, Attebo K, Healy PR. Prevalence of open angle glaucoma in Australia: The Blue Mountain Eye Study. *Ophthalmology*. 1996;103:1661–1669.

18. Wensar MD, McCarty CA, Stanislavsky YL, Livingston PM, Taylor HR. The prevalence of glaucoma in the Melbourne Visual Impairment Project. *Ophthalmology*. 1998; 105:733–739.

19. Sommer A, Tielsch JM, Katz J, Quigley H, et al. Racial differences in the cause-specific prevalence of blindness in east Baltimore. *N Engl J Med*. 1991;325: 1412–1417.

20. Leske MC, Connell AMS, Schachat AP, Hyman L. The Barbados Eye Study: Prevalence of open angle glaucoma. *Arch Ophthalmol*. 1994;112:821–829.

21. Mason RP, Kosoko O, Wilson MR, Martone JF, et al. National survey of the prevalence and risk factors of glaucoma in St. Lucia, West Indies: Part I. Prevalence findings. *Ophthalmology*. 1989;96:1363–1368.

22. Hu Z, Zhao ZL, Dong FT. An epidemiologic investigation of glaucoma in Beijing and Shun-yi County. *Chin J Ophthalmol*. 1989;25:115–118.

23. VanNewkirk MR. The Hong Kong Vision Study: A pilot assessment of visual impairment in adults. *Trans Am Ophthalmol Soc*. 1997;95:715–749.

24. Foster PJ, Jamyanjav B, Alsbirk PH, Munkhbayar D, et al. Glaucoma in Mongolia: A population-based survey in Hovsgol province, northern Mongolia. *Arch Ophthalmol*. 1996;114:1235–1241.

25. Arkell SM, Lightman DA, Sommer A, Taylor HR, et al. The prevalence of glaucoma among Eskimos of northwest Alaska. *Arch Ophthalmol*. 1987;105:482–485.

26. Kass MA, Zimmerman TJ, Alton E, Lemon L, Becker B. Intraocular pressure and glaucoma in the Zuñi Indians. *Arch Ophthalmol*. 1978;96:2212–2213.

27. Salmon JF, Mermoud A, Ivey A, Swanevelder A, Hoffman M. The prevalence of primary angle closure glaucoma and open angle glaucoma in Mamre, Western Cape, South Africa. *Arch Ophthalmol*. 1993;111:1263–1269.

28. Wison MR. Glaucoma in blacks: Where do we go from here? *JAMA*. 1989;261:281–282.

29. Wilson R, Richardson TM, Hertzmark E, Grant WM. Race as a risk factor for progressive glaucomatous damage. *Ann Ophthalmol*. 1985;17:653–659.

30. Bengtsson E. The prevalence of glaucoma. *Br J Ophthalmol*. 1981;65:46–49.

31. Bengtsson B. Aspects of the epidemiology of the chronic glaucoma. *Acta Ophthalmol*. 1981;146(suppl):1–48.

32. Dielemans I, Vingerlin JR, Wolfs RCW, Hofman A, et al. The prevalence of primary open-angle glaucoma in a population based study in the Netherlands. *Ophthalmology*. 1994;101:1851–1855.

33. Armaly MF, Krueger DE, Maunder L, Becker B, et al. Biostatistical analysis of the Collaborative Glaucoma Study: I. Summary report of the risk factors for glaucomatous visual field defects. *Arch Ophthalmol*. 1980; 98:2163–2171.

34. Armaly MF. Lessons to be learned from the Collaborative Glaucoma Study. *Surv Ophthalmol*. 1980;25:139–144.

35. Sommer A, Tielsch JM, Katz J, Quigley H, et al. Relationship between intraocular pressure and primary open angle glaucoma among white and black Americans: The Baltimore Eye Survey. *Arch Ophthalmol*. 1991; 109:1090–1095.

36. Eddy DM, Sanders LE, Eddy JF. The value of screening for glaucoma with tonometry. *Surv Ophthalmol*. 1983; 28:194–205.

37. Tielsch JM, Katz J, Singh K, Quigley H, et al. A population-based evaluation of glaucoma screening: The Baltimore Eye Survey. *Am J Epidemiol*. 1991;134:1102–1110.

38. Tielsch JM, Katz J, Quigley HA, Miller NR, Sommer A. Intraobserver and interobserver agreement in measurement of optic disc characteristics. *Ophthalmology*. 1988; 95:350–356.

39. Sommer A, Katz J, Quigley HA, Miller NR, et al. Clinically detectable nerve fiber atrophy precedes the onset of glaucomatous field loss. *Arch Ophthalmol*. 1991;109: 77–83.

40. David R, Zangwill L, Tessler Z, Yassur Y. The correlation between intraocular pressure and refractive status. *Arch Ophthalmol*. 1985;103:1812–1815.

41. Daubs JG, Crick RP. Effect of refractive error on the risk of ocular hypertension and glaucoma. *Trans Ophthalmol Soc UK*. 1981;101:121–126.

42. Lotufo D, Ritch R, Szmyd L, Burris JE. Juvenile glaucoma, race and refraction. *JAMA*. 1989;261:249–252.

43. Perkins ES, Phelps CD. Open angle glaucoma, ocular hypertension, low tension glaucoma and refraction. *Arch Ophthalmol*. 1982;100:1464–1467.

44. Mitchell P, Hourihan F, Sanbach J, Wang JJ. The relationship between glaucoma and myopia: The Blue Mountains Eye Study. *Ophthalmology*. 1999;106:2010–2015.

45. Quigley HA, Enger C, Katz J, Sommer A. Risk factors for the development of glaucomatous visual field loss in ocular hypertension. *Arch Ophthalmol*.1994;112:644–649.

46. Reynolds DC. Relative risk factors in chronic open angle glaucoma: An epidemiological study. *Am J Optom Physiol Optics*. 1977;54:116–120.

47. Mitchell P, Smith W, Chey T, Healey P. Open-angle glaucoma and diabetes: The Blue Mountains Eye Study, Australia. *Ophthalmology*. 1997;104:712–781.

48. Klein BEK, Klein R, Jensen SC. Open-angle glaucoma and older onset diabetes: The Beaver Dam Eye Study. *Ophthalmology*. 1994;101:1173–1177.

49. Klein BE, Klein R. Intraocular pressure and cardiovascular risk variables. *Arch Ophthalmol*. 1981;99:837–839.

50. Kahn HA, Leibowitz HM, Ganley JP, Kini MM, et al. The Framingham Eye Study: II. Association of ophthalmic pathology with single variables previously measured in the Framingham Heart Study. *Am J Epidemiol*. 1977;106: 33–41.

51. Leske MC, Podgor MJ. Intraocular pressure, cardiovascular risk variables, and visual field defects. *Am J Epidemiol*. 1983;118:280–287.

52. Tielsch JM, Katz J, Sommer A, Quigley HA, Javitt JC. Hypertension, perfusion pressure and primary open angle glaucoma: A population based assessment. *Arch Ophthalmol*. 1995;113:216–221.

53. Armaly MF. The genetic determination of ocular pressure in the normal eye. *Arch Ophthalmol*. 1967;78:187–192.

54. Armaly MF, Sayegh RE, The cup/disc ratio: The findings of tonometry and tonography in the normal eye. *Arch Ophthalmol*. 1969;82:191–196.

55. Armaly MF, Monstavicius BF, Sayegh RE. Ocular pressure and aqueous outflow facility in siblings. *Arch Ophthalmol*. 1968;80:354–360.

56. Becker B, Kolker AE, Roth FD. Glaucoma family study. *Am J Ophthalmol*. 1960;50:557–567.

57. Kellerman L, Posner A. The value of heredity in the detection and study of glaucoma. *Am J Ophthalmol*. 1955; 40:681–685.

58. Leske MC, Connell AMS, Wu S-Y, Hyman LG, Schachat AP. Risk factors for open-angle glaucoma: The Barbados Eye Study. *Arch Ophthalmol*. 1995;113:918–924.

59. Tielsch JM, Katz J, Sommer A, Quigley HA, Javitt JC. Family history and risk of primary open angle glaucoma: The Baltimore Eye Survey. *Arch Ophthalmol*. 1994;112:69–73.

60. Wolfs RCW, Klaver CCW, Ramrattan RS. Genetic risk of primary open-angle glaucoma: Population-based familial aggregation study. *Arch Ophthalmol*. 1998;116: 1640–1645.

61. Raymond V. Molecular genetics of the glaucomas: Mapping of the first five "GLC" loci. *Am J Hum Genet*. 1997; 60:272–277.

62. Stone EM, Fingert JH, Alward WLM, Nguyen TD, et al. Identification of a gene that causes primary open angle glaucoma. *Science*. 1997;275:668–670.

63. Wirtz MK, Samples JR, Rust K, Lie J, et al. GLCIF, a new primary open-angle glaucoma locus, maps to 7q35-q36. *Arch Ophthalmol*. 1999;117:237–241.

64. Lichter PR. Genetic clues to glaucoma's secrets: The Edward Jackson Memorial lecture: Part 2. *Am J Ophthalmol*. 1994;117:706–727.

65. Graham PA. Prevalence of glaucoma: Population surveys. *Trans Ophthalmol Soc UK*. 1978;98:288–289.

66. Armaly MF. On the distribution of applanation pressure. I. Statistical features and the effect of age, sex, and the family history of glaucoma. *Arch Ophthalmol*. 1965;73:11–18.

67. Bankes JLK, Perkins ES, Tsolakis S, Wright JE. Bedford glaucoma survey. *BMJ*. 1968;1:791–796.

68. Stromberg U. Ocular hypertension. *Acta Ophthalmol*. 1962;69(suppl):1–75.

69. David R, Zangwill L, Stone D, Yassur Y. Epidemiology of intraocular pressure in a population screened for glaucoma. *Br J Ophthalmol*. 1987;71:766–771.

70. Linner E, Stromberg U. Ocular hypertension: A five year study of the total population in a Swedish town, Skovde, Tutzing Castle. In: Leydhecker W. XXth International Congress of Ophthalmology. Glaucoma Tutzing Symposium (1966). Basel: Skarger AG; 1967:187–214.

71. Linner E. Ocular hypertension: I. The clinical course during ten years without therapy—aqueous humor dynamics. *Acta Ophthalmol*. 1976;54:707–720.

72. Lundberg L, Wettrell K, Linner E. Ocular hypertension. A twenty-year follow-up at Skovde. *Acta Ophthalmol (Copenh)*. 1985;63:473–474.

73. Perkins ES. The Bedford Glaucoma Survey. I. Long-term follow-up of borderline cases. *Br J Ophthalmol*. 1973;57: 179–185.

74. Epstein DL, Krug JH, Hertzmark E, Remis LL, Edelstein DJ. A long-term clinical trial of timolol therapy versus no treatment in the management of glaucoma suspects. *Ophthalmology*. 1989; 96:1460–1467.

75. Seddon JM, Schwartz B, Flowerdew G. Case-control study of ocular hypertension. *Arch Ophthalmol*. 1983; 101:891–894.

76. Kass MA, Hart WM, Gordon M, Miller JP. Risk factors favoring the development of glaucomatous visual field loss in ocular hypertension. *Surv Ophthalmol*. 1980; 25:155–162.

77. Zerihun N, Mabey D. Blindness and low vision in Jimma Zone, Ethiopia: Results of a population-based survey. Ophthal Epidemiol 1997; (1)4:19–26.

78. Singh MM, Murthy GVS, Venkatraman R, Rao SP, Nayar S. A study of ocular morbidity among elderly population in a rural area of Central India. *Indian J Ophthalmol.* 1997;45:61–65.

79. Wallace J, Lovell HG. Glaucoma and intraocular pressure in Jamaica. *Am J Ophthalmol.* 1969;67:93–100.

80. Viggoson G, Bjornsson G, Ingvason JG. The prevalence of open-angle glaucoma in Iceland. *Acta Ophthalmol.* 1986;64:138–141.

81. Coffey M, Reidy A, Wormald R, Wu XX, et al. Prevalence of glaucoma in the west of Ireland. *Br J Ophthalmol.* 1993;77:17–21.

82. Cedrone C, Culasso F, Cesareo M, Zapelloni A, et al. Prevalence of glaucoma in Ponza, Italy: A comparison with other studies. *Ophthal Epidemiol.* 1977;4:59–72.

83. Giuffre G, Giammanco R, Dardanoni G, Ponte F. Prevalence of glaucoma and distribution of intraocular pressure in a population: The Casteldaccia Eye Study. *Acta Ophthalmol Scand.* 1995;73:222–225.

Chapter 3

OCULAR ANATOMY AND PHYSIOLOGY RELATED TO AQUEOUS PRODUCTION AND OUTFLOW

Thomas F. Freddo

Central to an understanding of the glaucomas is an appreciation of the anatomy and physiology of the ciliary body and the aqueous outflow pathways as they relate to aqueous humor dynamics.

ANATOMY OF THE CILIARY BODY

The ciliary body, a portion of the anterior uvea, extends from the root of the iris to the ora serrata and is grossly subdivided into two portions, the pars plicata and the pars plana. Viewed from the posterior chamber, the pars plicata appears as a series of approximately 75 radially oriented, fin-like ciliary processes (Fig. 3–1). Most of these project approximately 1 mm into the posterior chamber and are termed *major processes*. The intervening minor processes are only one-third as high. The convoluted surface produced by the major processes in the pars plicata region serves to increase the area over which secretion of aqueous humor can occur. The lack of these surface specializations in the more posterior pars plana region of the ciliary body is consistent with

the generally accepted view that the pars plana plays little, or no role in aqueous production.

In sagittal sections, the ciliary body appears as shown in Fig. 3–2. Although not an obvious feature, the ciliary body, over most of its length, is separated from the sclera, by a potential space, the *supraciliary space*, which is continuous posteriorly with the suprachoroid. Having only minimal physical connections to the sclera, except at its anterior and posterior margins, the ciliary body is held against the outer wall of the eye primarily by intraocular pressure.

Most of the volume of the ciliary body is occupied by the ciliary muscle, a smooth muscle that is subdivided into three portions—longitudinal, radial, and circular—based on fiber orientation (Fig. 3–2). A loose connective tissue stroma is present between the muscle and the bilayered ciliary epithelium that lines the posterior chamber.

The two cell layers of the ciliary epithelium are named based upon their relative content of pigment. The layer closest to the ciliary body stroma is called the *pigmented ciliary epithelium* and that closest to the posterior chamber is called the *nonpigmented ciliary*

17

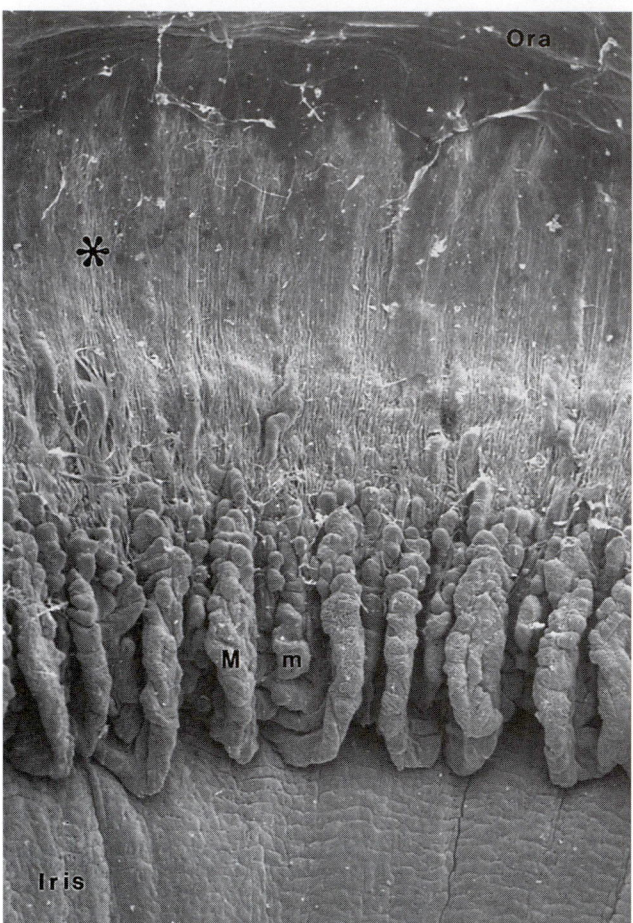

Figure 3–1. Scanning electron micrograph of the inner surface of the iris and ciliary body with the lens and zonules removed. The pars plicata region is distinguished from the more posterior pars plana region *(asterisk)* by the presence of major (M) and minor (m) ciliary processes. (62×) (Modified with permission from Morrison JC, Van Buskirk EM, Freddo T. Anatomy, microcirculation and ultrastructure of the ciliary body. In: Ritch R, Shields MB, Krupin T, eds. *The Glaucomas.* St. Louis: CV Mosby Co; 1989.)

epithelium (Fig. 3–2, inset). The pigmented ciliary epithelium is continuous with the posterior pigmented epithelium of the iris anteriorly and undergoes expansion at the ora serrata to become continuous with the neurosensory layers of the retina. All of the aforementioned layers are derived from the neuroectoderm of the optic vesicle, which invaginates upon itself during embryogenesis. As a consequence, the epithelia of the iris and the ciliary body are peculiarly arranged such that the two epithelial layers are attached to one another at their apical surfaces. Thus, the basal lamina of the pigmented ciliary epithelium fronts the ciliary body stroma and that of the nonpigmented layer faces the posterior chamber.

THE ROLE OF THE CILIARY BODY IN THE FORMATION OF AQUEOUS HUMOR

Aqueous humor is a clear, nutritive fluid, derived from a filtrate of plasma and secreted by the ciliary epithelium into the posterior chamber of the eye at a rate of approximately 2.5 μL/min. Under steady-state conditions, this rate of inflow, matched by an identical rate of outflow, will result in complete turnover of the aqueous humor approximately every 1 to 2 h. From the posterior chamber, the aqueous enters the anterior chamber of the eye through the pupil (Fig. 3–2), where it circulates in a convection current driven by the temperature difference between the warm iris and the cooler cornea. Rising posteriorly and falling anteriorly, the aqueous humor finally leaves the eye via one of various outflow pathways described further on. Along its route, aqueous provides for the metabolic needs of the avascular tissues of the ocular anterior segment. As a result, the chemical composition of the aqueous humor is continuously modified. Additional, potentially toxic modifications occur as a result of interaction with incoming light.[1] The production of aqueous humor is subject to diurnal variation, emphasizing the importance of recording the time of day at which pressure measurements are made. Pressure is generally highest in the early morning and lowest at night. Indeed, aqueous production is reduced sufficiently during sleep so that timolol, a beta blocker used to reduce aqueous production in glaucoma, has no additional measurable effect on the reduction of pressure during sleep.[2,3]

Correlating the anatomy with the physiology of aqueous humor formation, it is most convenient to describe the process in two steps: (1) elaboration of a plasma filtrate from which aqueous humor is derived, and (2) the formation of aqueous humor from this filtrate. Although these steps are not independent, the first is related primarily to the microvasculature of the ciliary body and the second, to the ciliary epithelium.

Elaboration of a Plasma Filtrate from the Microvasculature of the Ciliary Body

Filtration is a process whereby fluid is forced across a membrane by pressure. The volume of filtrate that crosses the membrane depends upon the pressure difference across the membrane and the surface area over which filtration can occur. The composition of the filtrate (e.g., water, ions, proteins) is determined largely by the size of the pores in the membrane—that is, by the permeability of the blood vessel wall. In the

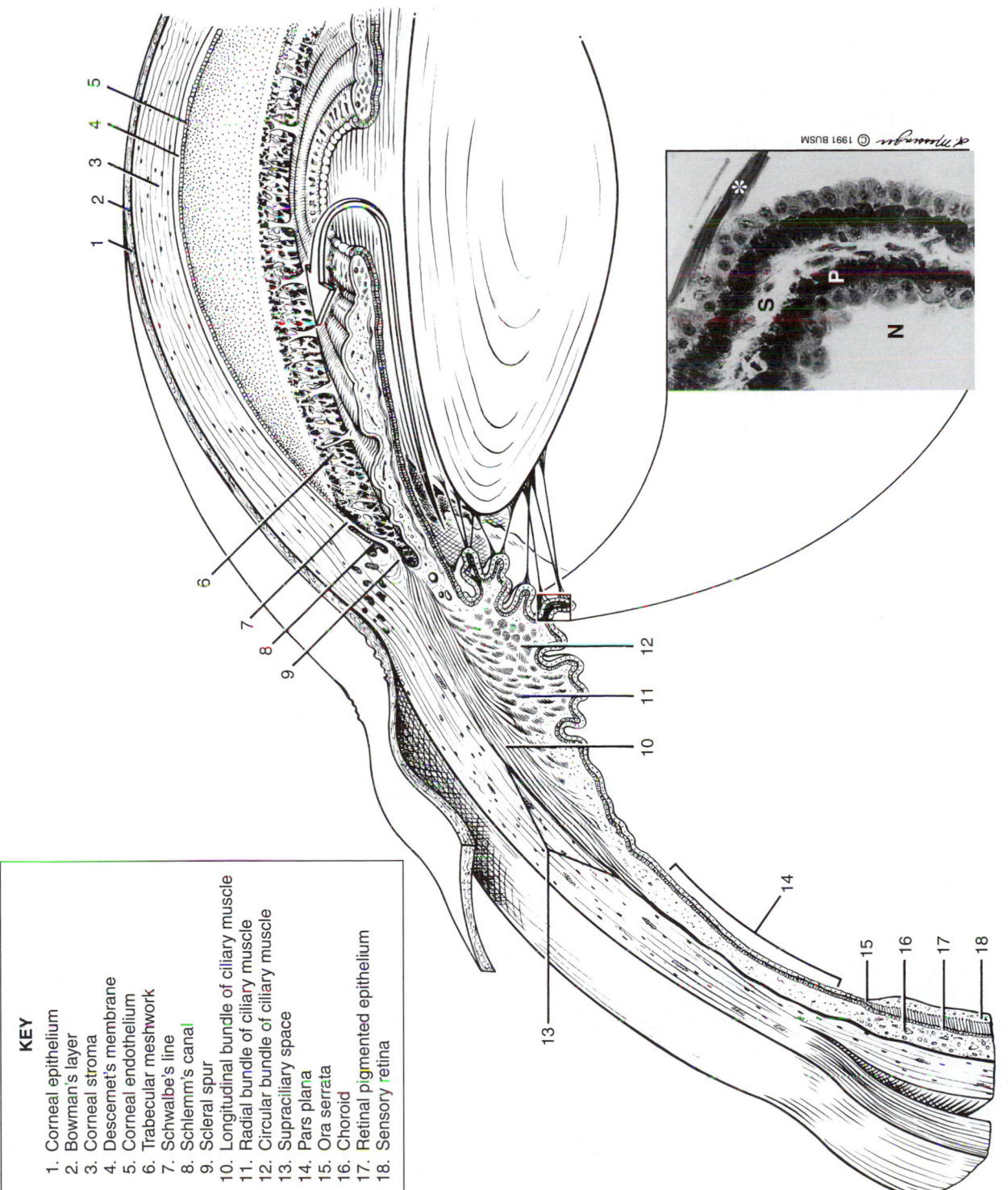

KEY

1. Corneal epithelium
2. Bowman's layer
3. Corneal stroma
4. Descemet's membrane
5. Corneal endothelium
6. Trabecular meshwork
7. Schwalbe's line
8. Schlemm's canal
9. Scleral spur
10. Longitudinal bundle of ciliary muscle
11. Radial bundle of ciliary muscle
12. Circular bundle of ciliary muscle
13. Supraciliary space
14. Pars plana
15. Ora serrata
16. Choroid
17. Retinal pigmented epithelium
18. Sensory retina

Figure 3–2. Diagram detailing the relationships between the ocular tissues of the anterior segment. The direction of aqueous flow is depicted by the arrow. Inset demonstrates the light microscopic appearance of a ciliary process showing the nonpigmented (N) and pigmented (P) ciliary epithelia, the ciliary body stroma (S), and a bundle of zonular fibers (*asterisk*). (318×)

ciliary body stroma, a filtrate of plasma is produced by filtration across the walls of its microvasculature.

The arterioles that serve the ciliary body stroma arise from the discontinuous major circle of the iris. Casts made of the ciliary body microvasculature of primate eyes have demonstrated that each major process is served by a set of anterior and posterior arterioles (Fig. 3–3).[4] The anterior arterioles supply the large-diameter capillaries near the crests of the processes while the posterior arterioles supply the smaller-caliber capillaries deep within each process. The direction of blood flow in both of these systems is from anterior to posterior, toward a network of choroidal veins (Fig. 3–4).

There is increasing anatomic and physiological evidence that blood flow in the ciliary body is regionalized and that these various regions respond differently to agents such as epinephrine.[5] Given the presence of adrenergic nerve endings associated with the ciliary body microvasculature, and the fact that blood flow in these vessels is reduced by sympathetic stimulation,[6–7] it is possible that controlled alterations in blood flow may occur that could, at various times, either enhance or reduce filtrate production.

The capillaries of the ciliary body stroma are lined by endothelial cells that are fenestrated and lack continuous tight junctions (Fig. 3–5). As can be demonstrated using tracers, such as horseradish peroxidase (HRP), for plasma protein leakage, the capillaries of the ciliary body stroma are very permeable to macromolecules as well as ions and fluid (Fig. 3–6). Not sur-

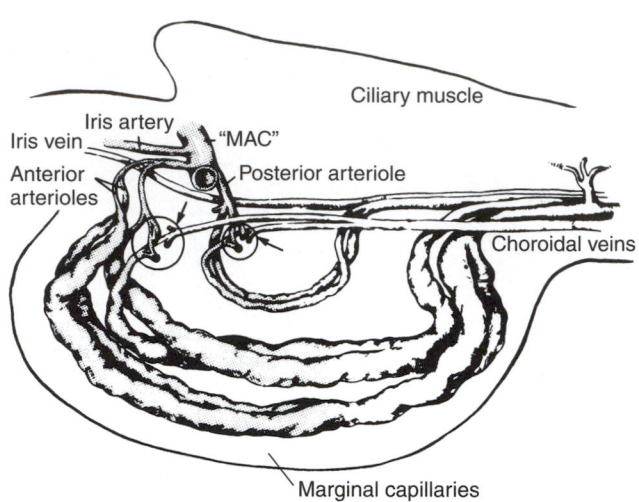

Figure 3–4. Diagrammatic representation of Fig. 3-3 demonstrating the system of anterior and posterior arterioles that enter each process, ultimately draining into a set of choroidal veins. (Reproduced with permission from Morrison JC, Van Buskirk EM, Freddo T. Anatomy, microcirculation and ultrastructure of the ciliary body. In: Ritch R, Shields MB, Krupin T, eds. *The Glaucomas.* St. Louis: CV Mosby Co; 1989.)

prisingly, these vessels are limited in their capacity to serve as a selective permeability barrier. The proteins entering the plasma filtrate in this manner contribute to the oncotic pressure of the ciliary body stroma.

The ions, fluid, and small molecules of the plasma filtrate are driven into the ciliary body stroma by the hydrostatic pressure within the capillaries of the ciliary processes.[8] The magnitude of the hydrostatic pressure is partly dependent on neuroregulatory and/or humoral influences on the microvasculature.

Countering the hydrostatic pressure within the vasculature is the interstitial fluid pressure of the ciliary body stroma, which increases with increasing intraocular pressure.[8] Because of this relationship, moderate elevations of intraocular pressure give rise to reductions in aqueous inflow and, after a time-delay, a decrease in intraocular pressure. The dynamics of this relationship are actually more complex, and the effect is insufficient to serve as a protective mechanism against the development of glaucoma.

There is, nonetheless, a clinical consequence of the relationship between intraocular pressure and inflow, but it has principally to do with measurements of aqueous outflow. Certain methods used to measure the facility of aqueous outflow, such as tonography and constant-pressure perfusion techniques, rely on elevating the intraocular pressure artificially. Aqueous outflow facility is then calculated from the rate of decrease in the elevated pressure over time.[9–10] Since reduction in aqueous production contributes to the

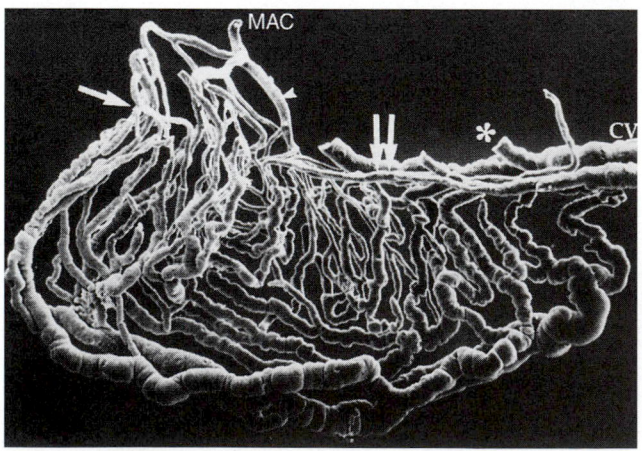

Figure 3–3. A cast of the vasculature within a single ciliary process. The major circle of the iris (MAC) gives rise to an anterior (*arrow*) and posterior (*arrowhead*) arteriole. Double arrow denotes choroidal vein (CV). Drainage from ciliary muscle to choroidal veins has been removed at asterisk. (110×) (Reproduced with permission from Morrison JC, Van Buskirk EM, Freddo T. Anatomy, microcirculation and ultrastructure of the ciliary body, In: Ritch R, Shields MB, Krupin T, eds. *The Glaucomas.* St. Louis: CV Mosby Co; 1989.)

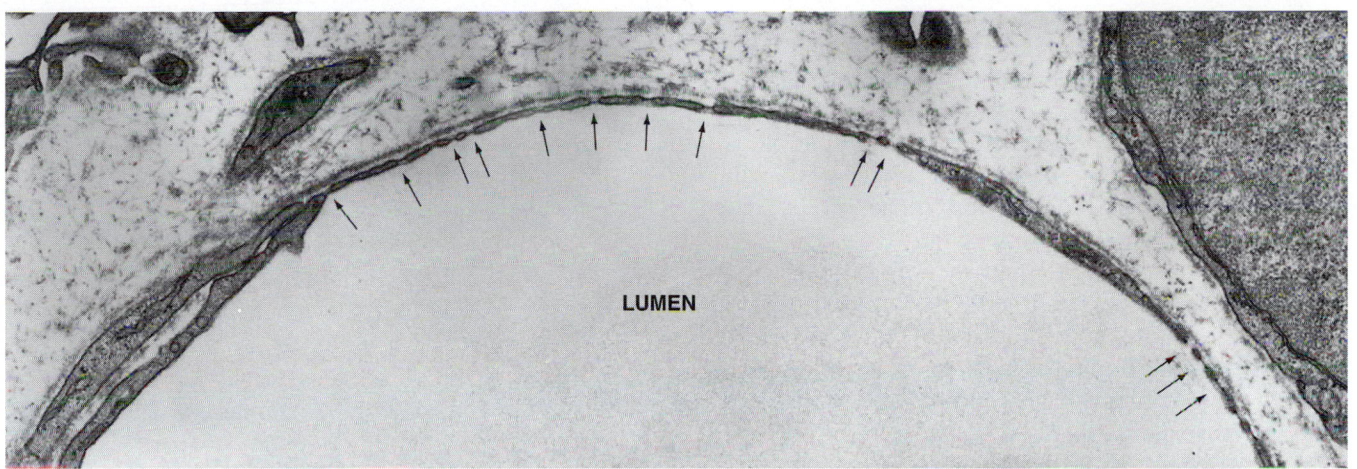

Figure 3–5. Transmission electron micrograph demonstrates the appearance of capillaries in the ciliary body stroma. Numerous fenestrations (*arrows*) are evident along the circumference of the vessel wall. (34,800×) (Modified with permission from Morrison JC, Van Buskirk EM, Freddo T. Anatomy, microcirculation and ultrastructure of the ciliary body. In: Ritch R, Shields MB, Krupin T, eds. *The Glaucomas.* St. Louis: CV Mosby Co; 1989.)

fall in intraocular pressure measured under these circumstances, the resulting outflow facility is proportionally increased. The proportion of total outflow facility resulting from the pressure-induced reduction in the production of aqueous is termed *pseudofacility.* Although early measurements suggested that pseudofacility might account for as much as 20% of total outflow facility,[11] improved methods suggest that pseudofacility probably accounts for only about 5 to 10% of the total.[12]

In summary, it appears that the dynamic equilibrium between the forces of the hydrostatic interstitial and intraocular pressures combined with the vascular tone and permeability characteristics of the ciliary body's microvasculature are the major factors determining the amount of filtrate available in the ciliary body stroma for aqueous production.

The Blood-Aqueous Barrier

In order for the aqueous humor secreted into the posterior chamber to have a composition different from that of the protein-laden filtrate in the ciliary body stroma, a selective permeability barrier must exist between the ciliary body stroma and the posterior chamber. Because aqueous humor in the anterior chamber freely permeates the stroma of the iris, a bar-

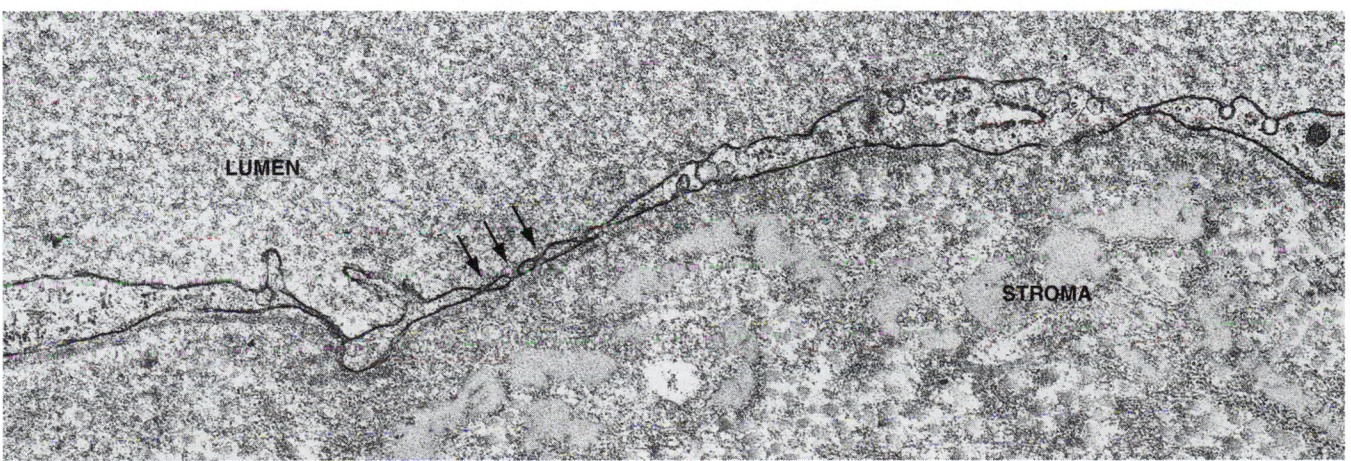

Figure 3–6. Transmission electron micrograph demonstrates that granular HRP reaction product leaks through fenestrations *(arrows)* into the surrounding ciliary body stroma. (40,800×) (Reproduced with permission from Morrison JC, Van Buskirk EM, Freddo T. Anatomy, microcirculation and ultrastructure of the ciliary body. In: Ritch R, Shields MB, Krupin T, eds. *The Glaucomas.* St. Louis: CV Mosby Co; 1989.)

rier to the leakage of plasma protein must also exist within the walls of iris's blood vessels. Several investigators have demonstrated that the morphologic equivalents of the blood-aqueous barrier to macromolecules are the zonulae occludens (tight junctions), which join the cell membranes of adjacent vascular endothelial cells of the iris and those of the nonpigmented ciliary epithelial cells.[13-15]

Unlike the microvasculature of the ciliary body stroma, the vessels of the iris do not leak plasma proteins or analogous macromolecular tracers such as HRP (Fig. 3–7). The reasons are twofold. The vessels of the iris are nonfenestrated and the endothelial cells of these vessels are joined by complex tight junctions that are relatively impermeable to macromolecules. In cross sections of the iris's vessels, tight junctions are recognized as a series of contact points between the membranes of adjacent endothelial cells (Fig. 3–8). Using the technique of freeze-fracture electron microscopy, the membranes of these cells can be cleaved to reveal the three-dimensional organization of their tight junctions. In freeze-fracture electron micrographs, the series of contact points observed in cross-sections is revealed in actuality to be a complex network of branching and anastomosing lines of contact between strands of particles (probably proteins) embedded within the membranes of the adjacent cells (Fig. 3–9). The relationship between these two views of tight junctions is shown in Fig. 3–10. This network

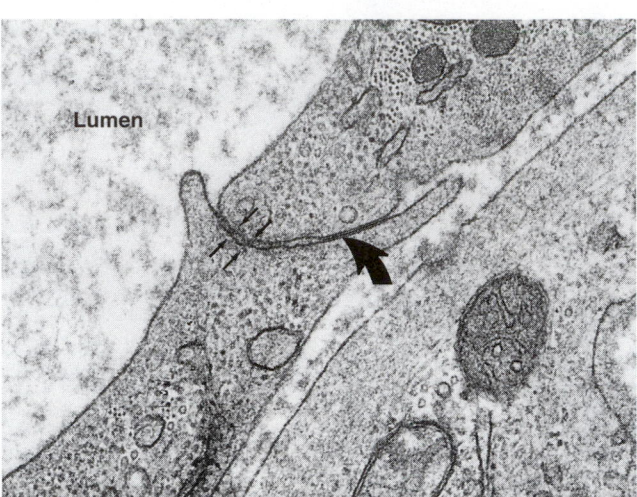

Figure 3–8. Transmission electron micrograph of an iris blood vessel demonstrating that the endothelial cells (E) are joined by tight junctions *(small arrows)* and gap junctions *(curved arrow)*. (40,000×).

of tight junctional strands serves to occlude the interendothelial cleft, preventing leakage of macromolecules from the bloodstream into the aqueous humor.

As mentioned, continuous tight junctions also constitute the morphologic equivalents of the blood-aqueous barrier in the ciliary body.[13-14] Following intravenous injection of HRP in primates, the tracer leaves the fenestrated capillaries of the ciliary processes, moving easily through the loose connective tissue of the ciliary body stroma to the bilayered ciliary epithelium. The tracer readily permeates the

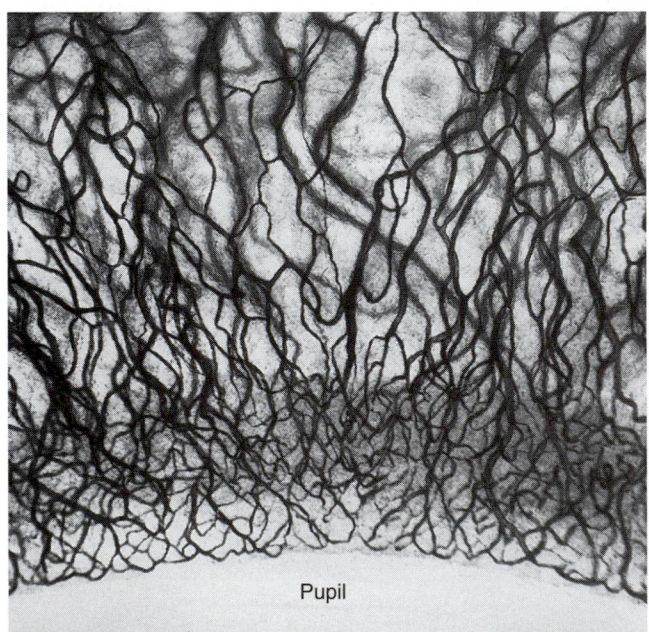

Figure 3–7. Whole-mount preparation of the iris vasculature demonstrating that the macromolecular tracer HRP is confined within the vessels. (38×).

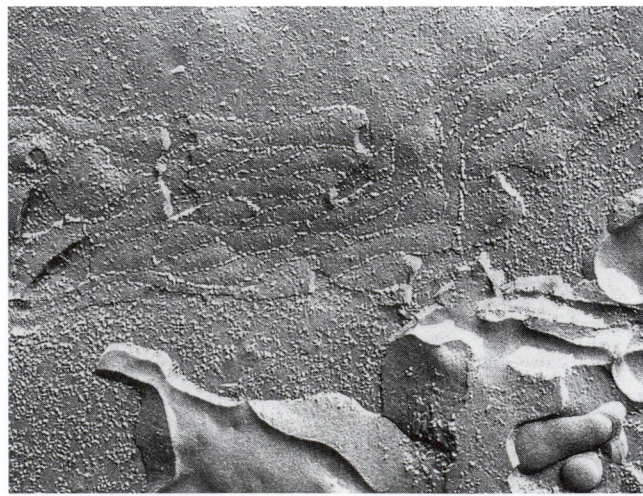

Figure 3–9. Freeze-fracture electron micrograph of iris vascular endothelial cells demonstrating the branching and anastomosing pattern of tight junctional strands that constitute the zonula occludens. (38,000×).

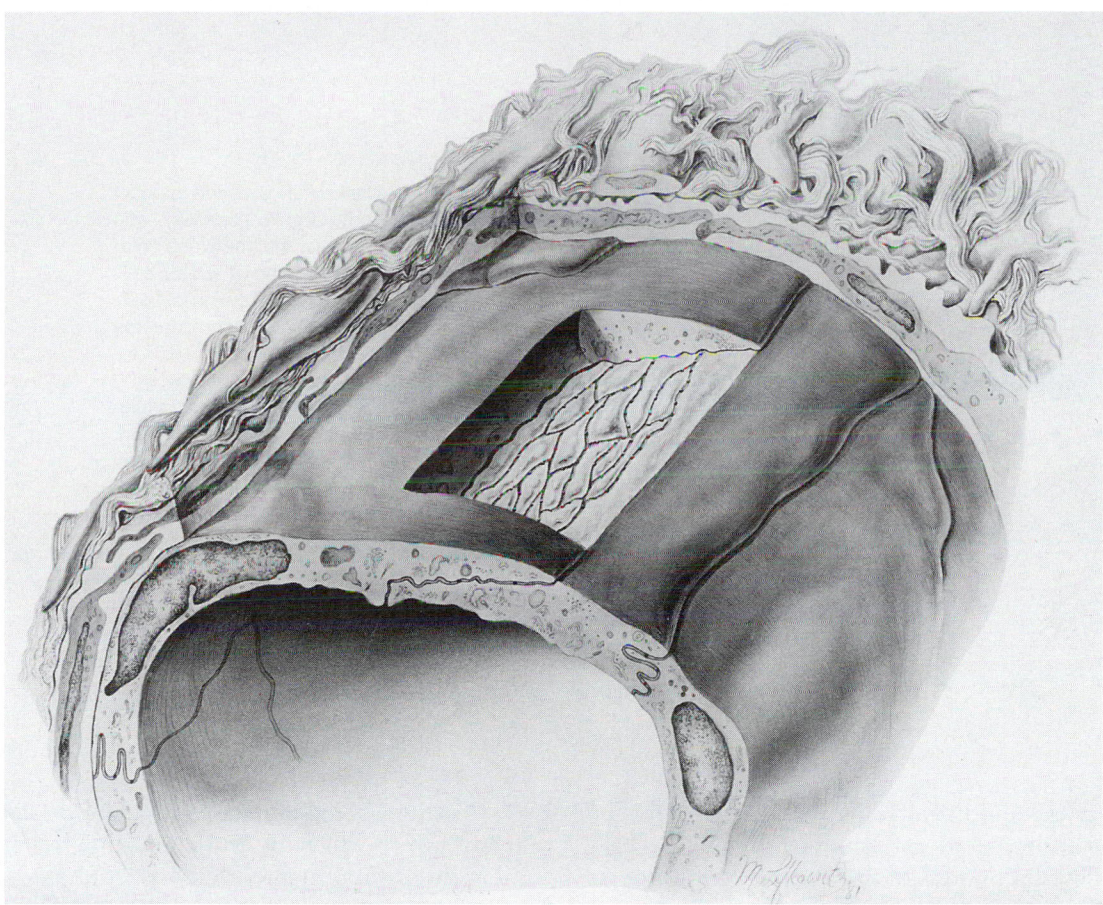

Figure 3–10. Diagrammatic representation of an iris blood vessel demonstrating the relationship between the sectioned and freeze-fracture appearances of the zonula occludens. (Reproduced with permission from Freddo T, Raviola G. *Invest Ophthalmol Vis Sci.* 1982;23:154.)

intercellular clefts between adjacent pigmented ciliary epithelial cells and between the adjoining apical surfaces of the pigmented and nonpigmented layers. However, further migration of the tracer toward the posterior chamber, between the cells of the non-pigmented layer, is blocked at their apico-lateral surfaces by the presence of tight junctions (Fig. 3–11). The appearances of these junctions, in both sectioned material and freeze-fracture, are shown for comparison (Fig. 3–11, inset, and Fig. 3–12).

Despite these epithelial and endothelial barriers, a small amount of plasma protein does enter the aqueous humor. The protein concentration in aqueous humor equals less than 1% of that in plasma,[8] but the route of entry for this protein has remained uncertain. Examining the anterior segment of the eye, it is clear that no anatomical barrier exists between the protein-laden ciliary body stroma and the anterior chamber along the gonioscopically visible ciliary body band. Recently, it has been shown that most of the plasma-derived protein present in aqueous humor actually enters the anterior chamber directly, diffusing from the ciliary body stroma via the root of the iris.[16–17] With this new information on the existence of an anterior protein pathway in the normal eye, studies are underway to determine whether this additional protein, added to the aqueous humor just as it enters the trabecular meshwork, may play a role in normal outflow resistance or the increased resistance that characterizes primary open-angle glaucoma.[18–20]

Formation of Aqueous Humor from the Plasma Filtrate by the Ciliary Epithelium

The formation of aqueous humor by the ciliary epithelium is dependent primarily upon two forces: hydrostatic pressure and the magnitude of the oncotic pressure gradient across the ciliary epithelium.

One of the most widely accepted models for the process of aqueous secretion was reviewed by Cole[8]

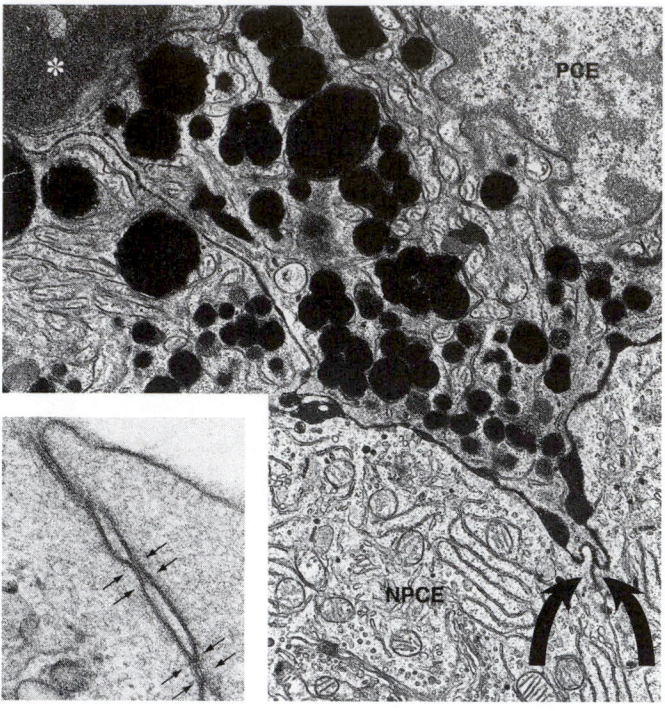

Figure 3–11. Black HRP reaction product fills the ciliary body stroma *(asterisk)*, and blackens the intercellular cleft between adjacent pigmented ciliary epithelial (PCE) cells as well as the area between the apical surface of the pigmented and nonpigmented layers (NPCE). Further diffusion of HRP toward the posterior chamber is blocked by tight junctions between adjacent nonpigmented epithelial cells (curved arrows). (19,000×). *INSET:* Higher magnification demonstrates the points of fusion *(arrows)* between membranes of adjacent nonpigmented ciliary epithelial cells that constitute the tight junction. (131,000×). (Reproduced with permission from Morrison JC, Van Buskirk EM, Freddo T. Anatomy, microcirculation and ultrastructure of the ciliary body. In: Ritch R, Shields MB, Krupin T, eds. *The Glaucomas.* St. Louis: CV Mosby Co; 1989.)

and represents a modification of the Diamond-Bossert model for standing gradient osmotic flow (Fig. 3–13).[21] More detailed discussions of this complex topic appear elsewhere.[22]

The process of aqueous secretion is clearly dependent upon ion movement from the ciliary body vasculature into the stroma and finally, across the ciliary epithelium. Recently, a Na+/K+/2Cl symport has been reported in the pigmented ciliary epithelium that appears to be the main exchanger delivering sodium, potassium, and chloride ions into the ciliary epithelium from the ciliary body stroma.[23-24] Once inside the pigmented ciliary epithelial cells, these ions are conveyed to the nonpigmented ciliary epithelial cells via gap junctions, which serve to couple the two cell layers electronically and metabolically into a functional syncytium.[25-26]

Sodium, bicarbonate, and chloride ions are actively transported into the intercellular clefts between adjacent nonpigmented ciliary epithelial cells. The presence of these solutes creates a standing osmotic gradient that draws water into the cleft. The tight junctions joining the apico-lateral surfaces of the nonpigmented cells, restrict aqueous flow at the apical end of the cleft, directing it toward the posterior chamber.

Although the evidence for active transport of ions by the ciliary epithelium is quite substantial, there remains some evidence that the movement of ions into the intercellular cleft may be enhanced by ultrafiltration. This is a process wherein dialysis (i.e., the separation of ions from an ion-protein mixture such as that existing in the ciliary body stroma) is augmented by application of a hydrostatic pressure. Both processes likely play roles in aqueous production, but secretion, in

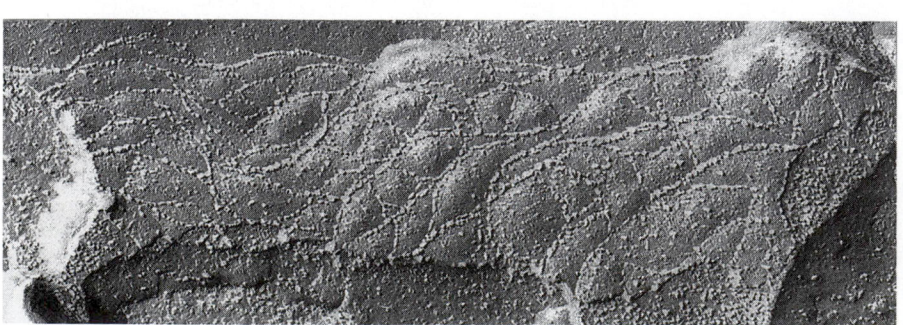

Figure 3–12. Freeze-fracture electron micrograph demonstrates the branching and anastomosing tight junctional strands of a zonula occludens between adjacent nonpigmented ciliary epithelial cells. (57,500×). (Reproduced with permission from Morrison JC, Van Buskirk EM, Freddo T. Anatomy, microcirculation and ultrastructure of the ciliary body. In: Ritch R, Shields MB, Krupin T, eds. *The Glaucomas.* St. Louis: CV Mosby Co; 1989.)

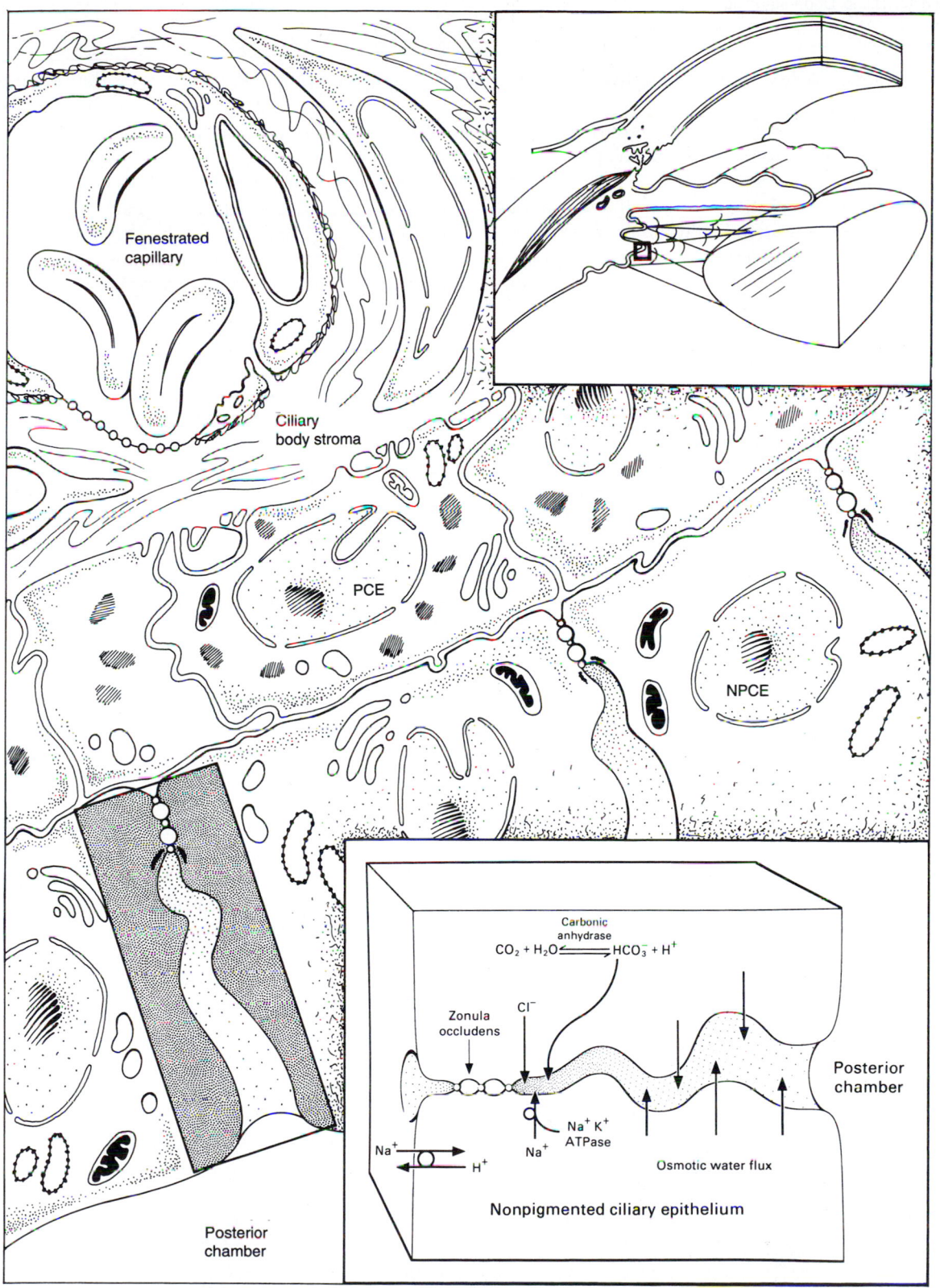

Figure 3–13. Diagrammatic representation of the portion of the bi-layered ciliary epithelium and underlying stroma with fenestrated capillaries that corresponds to the boxed area of the upper inset. The shaded area in the main figure corresponds to that shown in the lower inset depicting the major elements of the standing gradient model of aqueous flow. The role of the pigmented ciliary epithelium (PCE) has been neglected for simplicity. The gradient shown by stippling in the lower inset corresponds to the solute concentration along the intercellular cleft between adjacent nonpigmented ciliary epithelial (NPCE) cells. The normally narrow dimensions of the intercellular cleft ensure the hypertonicity required to maintain osmotic water flux and hence flow.

the form of metabolically-dependent active transport, plays the far greater role.[27]

Regardless of the mechanism that moves ions into the intercellular cleft, fluid in the apical part of the cleft must remain hypertonic to assure a continuous flow of water.[8] It is thus important that the volume of the cleft remain small to avoid dilution of solutes. The various types of adhering intercellular junctions present between ciliary epithelial cells ensure that the volume of the intercellular cleft does not expand significantly. Without interfering with aqueous flow, these adhering junctions join the cells at intervals along the entire length of the intercellular cleft. The most plentiful of these adhering junctions are desmosomes. In the ciliary epithelium, desmosomes exhibit a peculiar relationship with certain mitochondria in each of the cells being joined (Fig. 3–14). Although the functional importance of this relationship is unknown, it appears to occur only in epithelia that, like the ciliary epithelium, are secretory.[28]

Evidence Supporting the Model

Evidence for the dependency of aqueous secretion on oxidative metabolism comes from numerous studies demonstrating that metabolic inhibitors, reduction of oxygen tension, and hypothermia all reduce the rate of aqueous production.[27,29,30]

Na$^+$, K$^+$ ATPase

Evidence that ion transport is central to the process comes from studies that have localized sodium-potassium ATPase activity to the nonpigmented

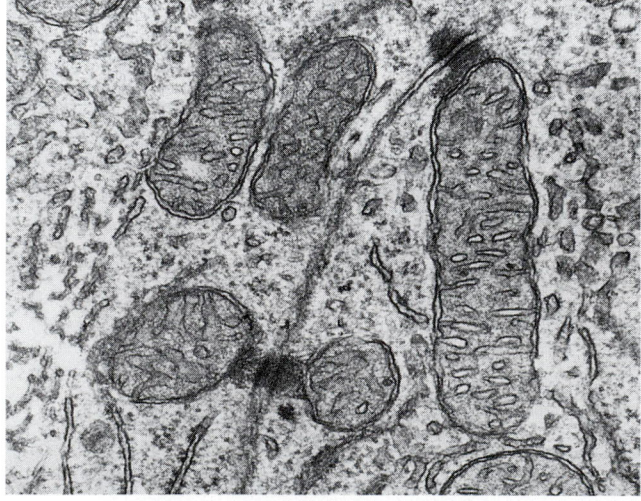

Figure 3–14. Mitochondria within adjacent nonpigmented ciliary epithelial cells are attached to desmosomal junctions that bridge the intercellular cleft. (46,170×) (Reproduced with permission from Freddo T. *Cell Tiss Res.* 1988;251:671.)

ciliary epithelium.[31] Additional evidence comes from documentation that inhibition of this enzyme with ouabain reduces aqueous secretion.[29]

Carbonic Anhydrase

Carbonic anhydrase also plays a significant role in the process of aqueous secretion by producing bicarbonate ions. This enzyme has also been histochemically localized to the pigmented and nonpigmented ciliary epithelium of the major ciliary processes.[32] Interestingly, this enzyme was not found associated with the nonpigmented ciliary epithelium in the valleys between the major ciliary processes or in the pars plana areas presumed not to be involved in aqueous production.

Carbonic anhydrase catalyzes the hydration of carbon dioxide to carbonic acid, leading to the subsequent liberation of hydrogen and bicarbonate ions according to the following equation:

$$H_2O_2 + CO_2 \longleftrightarrow H_2CO_3 \longleftrightarrow HCO_3^- + H^+$$

The roles of the ionic products of this reaction in the overall process of aqueous humor secretion remain uncertain and may vary by species. Inhibition of carbonic anhydrase decreases the entry not only of bicarbonate ions into the posterior chamber but also that of sodium ions.[33] Whether a direct linkage between sodium and bicarbonate transport exists remains unclear, however. One theory regarding the role played by bicarbonate ions in aqueous humor production maintains that HCO_3^- is transported in parallel with Na$^+$, primarily to maintain electroneutrality. Another states that, HCO_3^- movement may serve primarily to alter pH, optimizing sodium-potassium ATPase activity.[34]

Regardless of the specific mechanism of action, the well-known clinical utility of carbonic anhydrase inhibitors (CAIs) in the treatment of glaucoma illustrates the importance of this enzyme in aqueous secretion. In years past, only systemically administered CAIs were available. These carried unwanted side effects that complicated therapy, often resulting in noncompliance. More recently, a topical CAI (dorzolamide) has become available that has rapidly found acceptance in standard glaucoma therapy.[35–36]

Beta-Adrenergic Receptors

Although the direct relationship with the model outlined above is unclear, there is convincing evidence that the secretory activity of the ciliary epithelium is influenced by beta-adrenergic activity, probably mediated by the adenylyl cyclase, enzyme-receptor complex.

Beta-adrenergic receptors have been localized to the ciliary epithelium.[37] Stimulatory activation of these receptors initiates a signal-transduction cascade (Fig. 3–15) beginning with activation of an intramembranous G protein. G proteins are regulators of certain enzymes and ionic channels (Fig. 3–15). In the case of beta-adrenergic stimulation, the G protein activates the second messenger adenylyl cyclase, which has also been localized to the ciliary body.[38–39] Adenylyl cyclase increases cytoplasmic levels of cyclic AMP, leading to the phosphorylation of protein kinase A. How these events lead to the ultimate effect on aqueous humor inflow remains uncertain. The literature in this area is remarkably contradictory, even disregarding the added complexities that arise in trying to compare data obtained from different species.[40] Regardless of the molecular mechanisms at work, it does seem clear that beta-adrenergic antagonists such as timolol lead to reductions in both aqueous inflow and intraocular pressure.[41] Equally well established, if not well explained, is the belief that neither beta-adrenergic agonists nor antagonists demonstrate an outflow-mediated effect on intraocular pressure, despite the presence of beta-adrenergic receptors on cells within the trabecular outflow pathways.[42]

Alpha-Adrenergic Receptors

Alpha$_2$-adrenergic receptors are also present in the ciliary body.[43] They appear to be negatively coupled with adenylyl cyclase, and can block the elevations of cAMP levels induced by beta-agonists (Fig. 3–15).[42] A similar paradox to that described above for beta-adrenergic receptors exists here as well, for *both* alpha-adrenergic agonists and antagonists have been reported to lower intraocular pressure.[44] In the case of alpha$_2$ receptor–mediated agents, the sites of action appear to be different. Alpha$_2$-antagonists appear not to affect either inflow or trabecular outflow,[45] suggesting a possible uveoscleral mechanism. Alpha$_2$-agonists, on the other hand, appear to act on aqueous inflow without an apparent effect on outflow facility.[46] Additional effects, mediated through reduction in episcleral venous pressure or ciliary body vascular flow, have not been ruled out.[47] The first commercially available alpha agent, apraclonidine, was initially approved only for prophylactic use in preventing the acute elevations of intraocular pressure that often

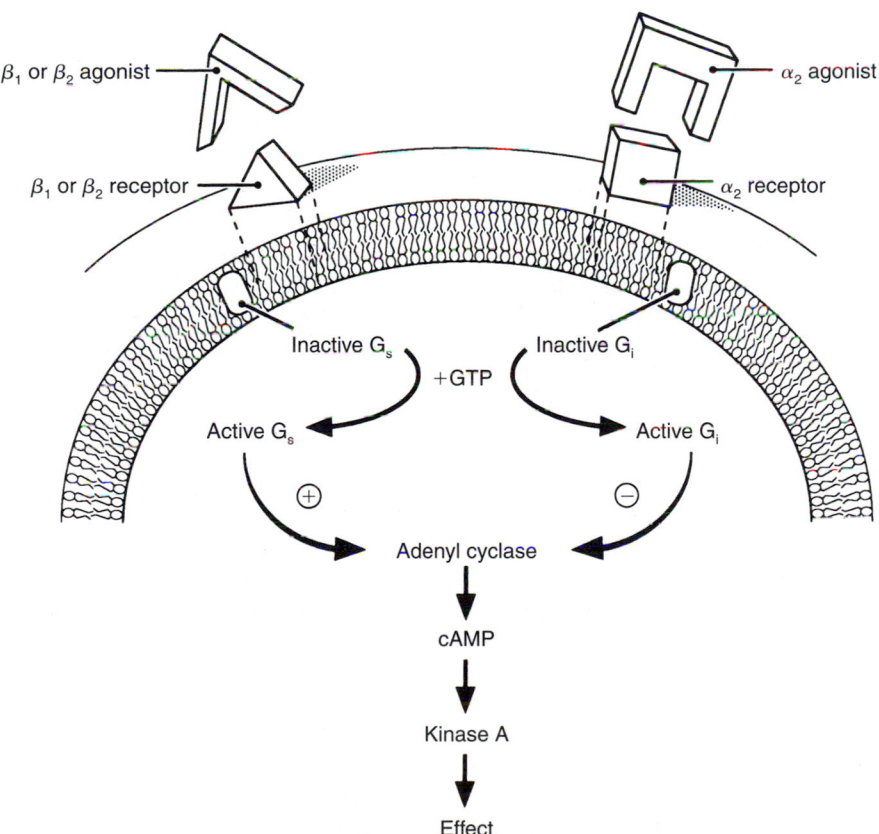

Figure 3–15. Diagrammatic representation of the signal transduction process which ensues after binding at beta$_1$-, beta$_2$-, and beta$_3$-adrenergic receptors. In each case, intramembranous activation of G protein occurs, which either increases or decreases levels of cyclic-AMP through alterations in adenyl cyclase activity.

follow argon laser trabeculoplasty.[48–49] The more recent and promising alpha agent brimonidine is now available for the management of glaucoma, adding a useful alternative for patients with contraindications to the use of beta blockers.

THE AQUEOUS OUTFLOW PATHWAYS

The major pathway for the outflow of aqueous humor is through the trabecular meshwork and canal of Schlemm into the venous system of the eye via a series of intrascleral collector channels and venous plexi. Three alternate pathways have also been identified that vary in their presumed importance to aqueous outflow from species to species. The most significant of these alternate routes is the uveoscleral pathway. Very minor additional contributions to outflow may occur via the vitreous body and the corneal stroma, but an earlier assumption that iris vessels might participate significantly in outflow has been refuted.[50] Of these pathways, only trabecular and uveoscleral outflow are considered here.

ANATOMY OF THE TRABECULAR MESHWORK

The trabecular meshwork is a triangular wedge of tissue encircling the anterior chamber, with its apex at the peripheral terminus of Descemet's membrane, called *Schwalbe's line*. From this anterior boundary, the meshwork expands as it bridges the irido-corneal angle of the eye, ending posteriorly by blending with the stromas of the both the iris and ciliary body (Fig. 3–16). Projecting like a shelf into the meshwork near its posterior margin is the scleral spur, which serves as a point of insertion for the longitudinal bundle of the ciliary muscle.

A portion of the meshwork lies wholly within a recess in the sclera termed the *internal scleral sulcus*. The limits of this sulcus are defined by an imaginary line drawn on a sagittal section of the meshwork from Schwalbe's line to the anterior tip of the scleral spur (Fig. 3–16). Within the confines of the sulcus are the corneoscleral and juxtacanalicular areas (also termed the *cribriform* areas) of the meshwork and the canal of Schlemm. The portion of the meshwork that is not confined within the sulcus and is most readily viewed gonioscopically is termed the *uveal meshwork*.

The importance of understanding the relationship between the views of the meshwork obtained from sagittal sections and those obtained gonioscopically

cannot be overemphasized. In Figs. 3–17 and 3–18 the macroscopic appearance of these structures—and corresponding diagrammatic representations as seen from both perspectives—can readily be compared. In addition, because the canal of Schlemm is filled with blood in Fig. 3–17, the relationship between the canal and the other angle structures is also evident. These macroscopic views should be compared with the goniophotograph of a normal open angle, as seen in Fig. 3–19. The principal landmarks evident in such a view of an open anterior chamber angle include, from superior to inferior: (1) Schwalbe's line (i.e., the peripheral terminus of Descemet's membrane), (2) the trabecular meshwork, (3) the scleral spur, and (4) the ciliary body band.

The Uveal and Corneoscleral Portions of the Meshwork

The uveal and corneoscleral portions of the trabecular meshwork have an approximately analogous structure. Both are composed of a series of trabeculae that delimit a system of aqueous flow channels. These channels become progressively smaller from the uveal to the corneoscleral meshwork.

The appearance of the uveal face of the trabecular meshwork as viewed under the scanning electron microscope is seen in Fig. 3–20. The cord-like trabecular beams seen in this view characterize only the innermost layers of the meshwork. The trabeculae of the corneoscleral meshwork have fewer, smaller openings that give them an appearance more like that of perforated sheets.

In microscopic sections, the uveal and corneoscleral trabeculae are each seen to be covered by a single layer of endothelial cells (Fig. 3–21). The cores of the beams and corneoscleral sheets are composed largely of various collagen subtypes and some elastic fibers, which have only recently been shown definitely to contain elastin.[51]

The intercellular junctions that join the trabecular endothelial cells include only gap junctions and short, discontinuous, tight junctional strands.[52] As such, aqueous humor readily permeates the cores of the trabecular beams, and there is little evidence to suggest that the trabeculae are continually being deturgesced by their endothelial cells in any manner similar to that observed in the cornea. It is therefore unlikely that trabecular endothelial cells could operate to regulate outflow by varying the thickness of the trabeculae and, indirectly, the dimensions of the outflow channels. There is, however, increasing interest in whether endothelial cells can alter their volume in a clinically significant and controlled fashion.[53,54]

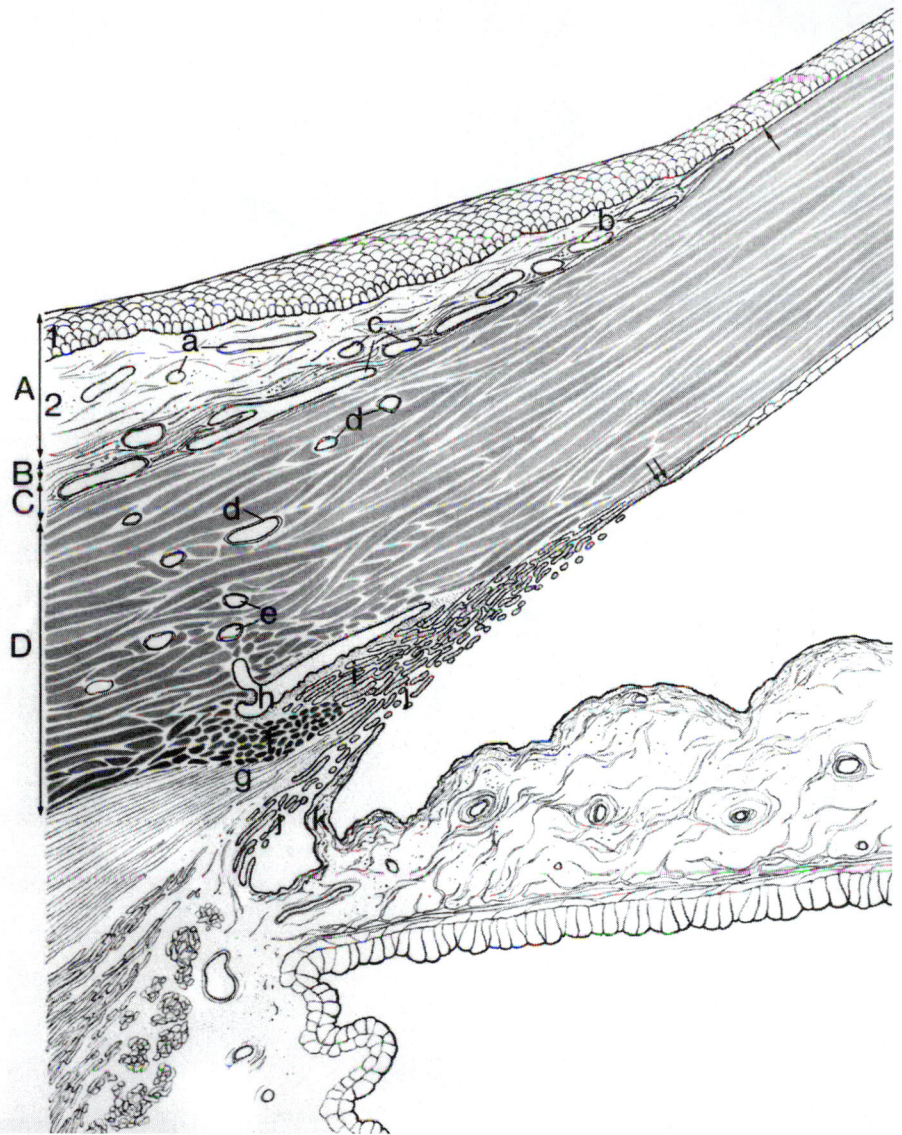

Figure 3–16. Drawing of the limbus to illustrate the structures evident by microscopic examination. The limbal conjunctiva (A) is formed by an epithelium (1) and an areolar connective tissue stroma (2). Tenon's capsule (B) forms an ill-defined connective tissue layer over the episclera (C). The limbal corneosclera occupies area (D). a, conjunctival vessels; b, corneal arcades; single arrow, terminus of Bowman's layer. The triangular tissue wedge of the trabecular meshwork (i) originates at Schwalbe's line *(double arrows)* and broadens posteriorly to become continuous with the root of the iris and the ciliary body. An iris process (k) extends from the iris surface to the trabecular meshwork. Entering the posterior margin of the trabecular meshwork is the scleral spur (f), to which tendons of the longitudinal bundle of the ciliary muscle (g) are attached. Aqueous passing through the trabecular meshwork enters the canal of Schlemm (h), deep scleral plexus (e), intrascleral plexus (d), and finally the episcleral vessels (c). (Reproduced with permission from Hogan M, Alvarado J, Weddell J. *Histology of the Human Eye.*, Philadelphia: WB Saunders Co; 1971.)

The endothelial cells of the trabecular meshwork are known to be phagocytic.[55,56] They are capable of ingesting both endogenous materials such as pigment[57,58] and exogenous particulates such as latex microspheres,[59] presumably for the purpose of keeping the trabecular outflow channels free of potentially obstructive debris. It appears, however, that this phagocytic capacity involves some long-term cost to the meshwork, for it is widely held that phagocytosis leads to detachment of endothelial cells from their beams and to their migration out of the eye.[55]

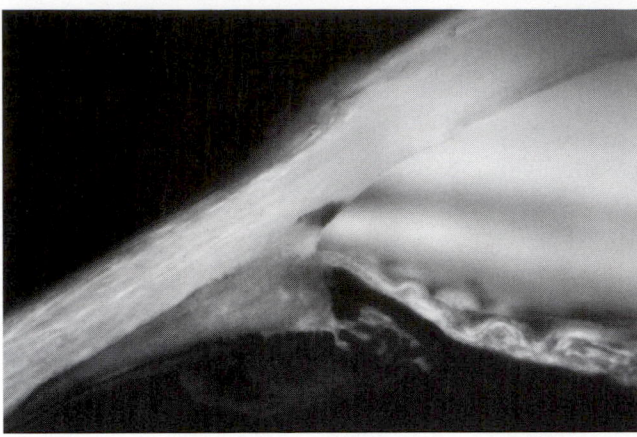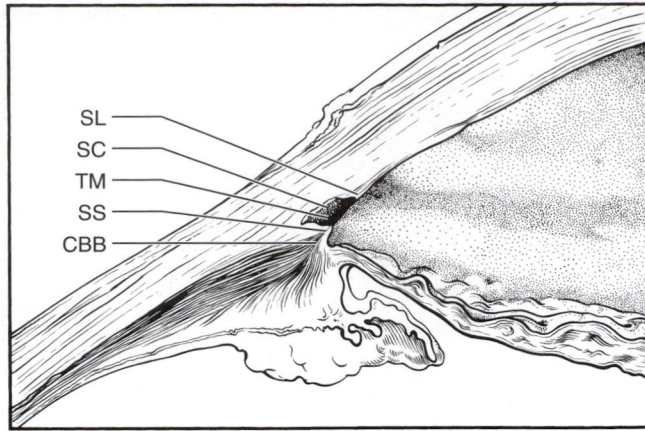

Figure 3–17. Macroscopic photograph and corresponding sketch identifying structures visible in a sagittal section of the normal anterior chamber angle. The anterior chamber is artifactually deepened due to posterior sagging of the iris following removal of the crystalline lens. *(See also Color Plate 1.)*

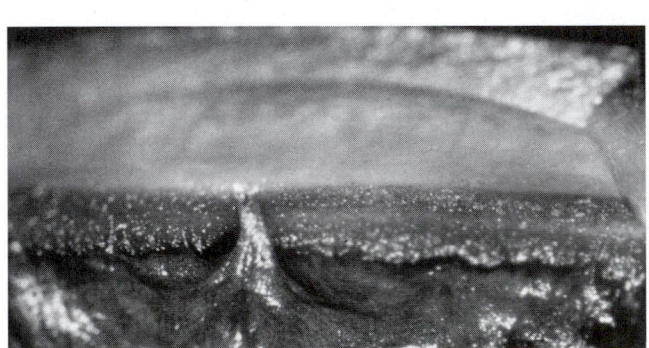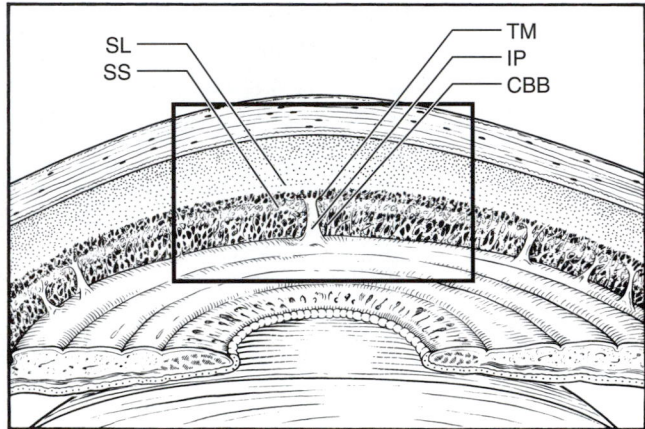

Figure 3–18. Macroscopic photograph and corresponding sketch of angle structures viewed from the perspective shown in the adjacent sketch. Schlemm's canal is filled with blood in this specimen, demonstrating its relationship to the other angle structures. An iris process is also shown. Compare the view of the angle structures in this figure with the corresponding sagittal view shown in Fig. 3-17. *(See also Color Plate 2.)*

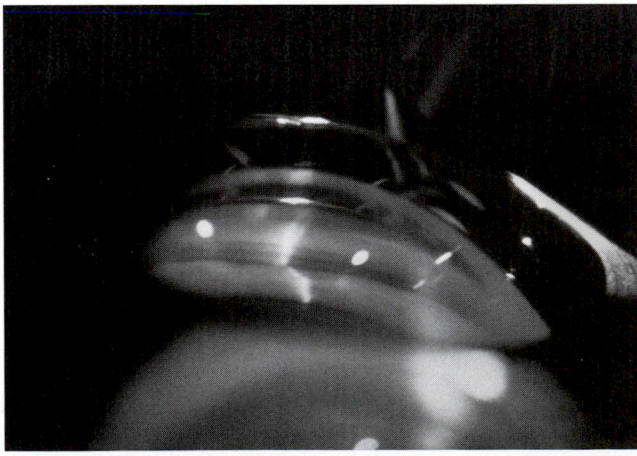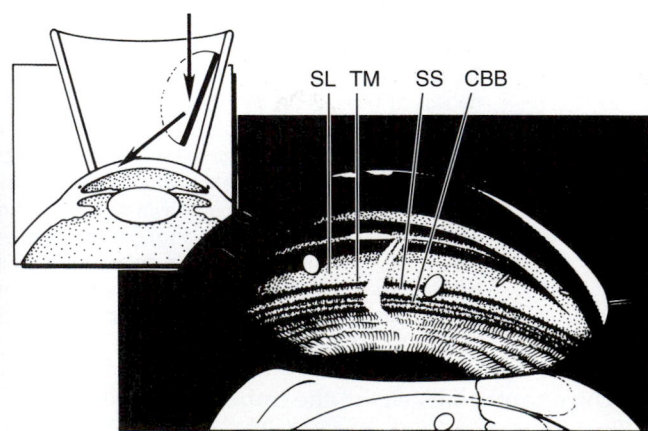

Figure 3–19. Goniophotograph of a normal open angle, and corresponding sketch representing a view analogous to that shown in Fig. 3-18. Inset in sketch depicts the placement of the gonioscope onto the cornea and the manner in which the angle structures are viewed. Key: SL = Schwalbe's line; SC = Schlemm's canal; TM = trabecular meshwork; SS = scleral spur; CBB = ciliary body band; IP = iris process. (Photograph courtesy of Rodney Gutner, O.D.) *(See also Color Plate 3.)*

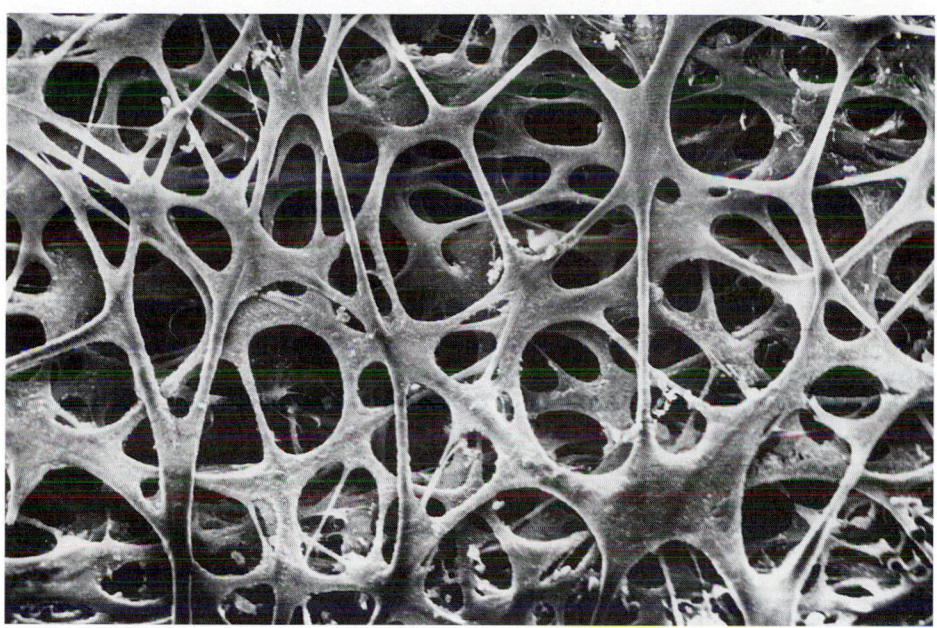

Figure 3–20. Scanning electron micrograph demonstrates the appearance of the uveal face of the trabecular meshwork as viewed from the anterior chamber. (504×). (Reproduced with permission from Freddo TF et al. *Invest Ophthalmol Vis Sci.* 1984;25:278.)

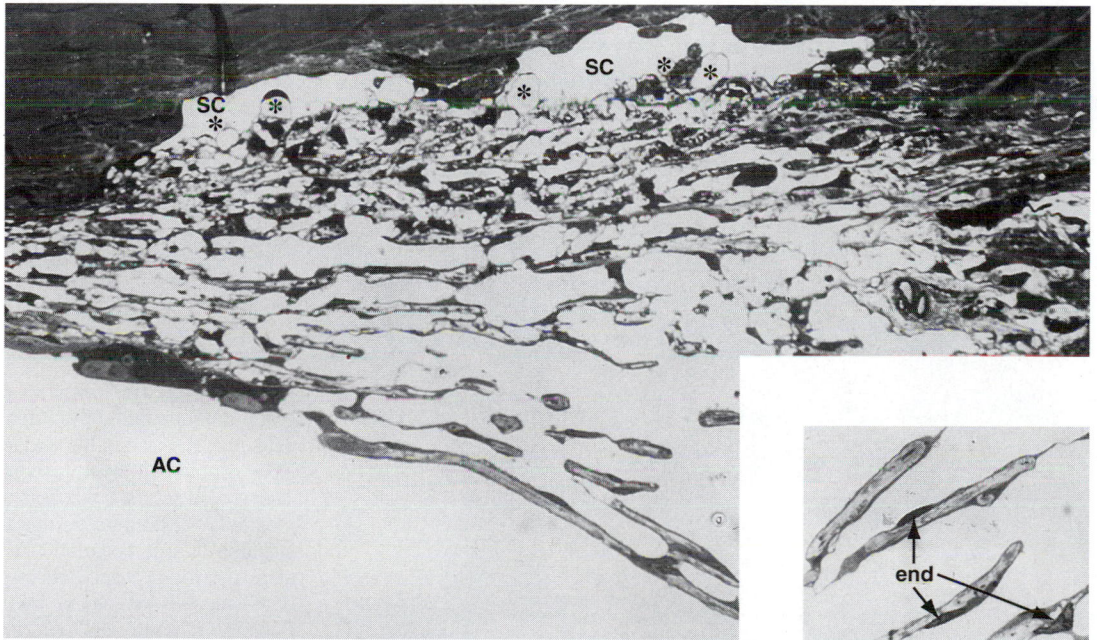

Figure 3–21. Light micrograph of the trabecular meshwork. Note that in this section Schlemm's canal (SC) is divided into two parallel channels. Outlines of giant vacuoles can be seen protruding into the lumen of the canal *(asterisks)*. AC, anterior chamber. (383×). *INSET:* Higher-magnification view of trabecular beams demonstrating the central core of connective tissue surrounded by slender trabecular endothelial (end) cells. (650×).

Given the limited capacity for cell division that is seen in the trabecular meshwork,[60] a progressive reduction in the number of trabecular endothelial cells is to be expected. These findings are consistent with the documented decrease in trabecular cell number seen with increasing age.[61-62] Whether this cell loss is a major factor leading to the development of glaucoma remains to be established.[63]

The Cribriform or Juxtacanalicular Meshwork

The type of cell found in the region of the meshwork between the innermost corneo-scleral trabecular beam and the inner wall of Schlemm's canal appears to be different from the endothelial cells that cover the trabeculae. They are more fibroblast-like and lack a basal lamina (Fig. 3–22).[64] The portion of the meshwork occupied by these cells, and the extracellular matrix with which they are associated, represents the cribriform or juxtacanalicular region of the trabecular meshwork (JCT). Forming an integral part of the extracellular matrix in this region is a plexus of elastic-like fibers. These fibers are connected both to a subclass of tendons from the longitudinal bundle of the ciliary muscle (discussed below) and to the basal surface of the endothelial cells that line the inner wall of Schlemm's canal. This anatomic system, called the *cribriform plexus*,[65] has the potential to effect alterations in the permeability of this region. Such changes are likely of clinical importance, for it is the cribriform region of the aqueous outflow system that is generally held to represent the principal site of normal aqueous outflow resistance.[66-67]

The Role of the Ciliary Muscle in Trabecular Outflow

Three types of tendons have been reported to extend from the tips of the muscle fibers of the ciliary muscle either into or through the trabecular meshwork (Fig. 3–23).[68] One of these is responsible for attaching the longitudinal bundle of the ciliary muscle to the scleral spur. As a result, contraction of the ciliary muscle—whether it occurs naturally as a part of accommodation or is induced pharmacologically using miotics such as pilocarpine—pulls on the scleral spur and in

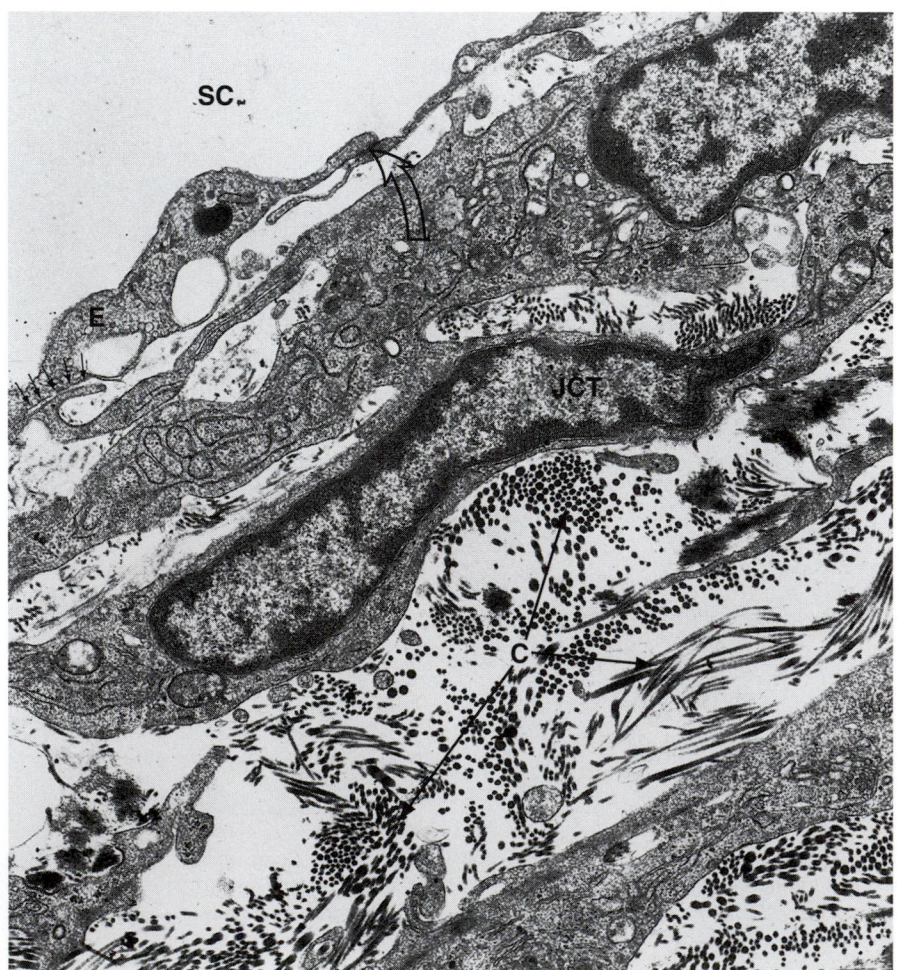

Figure 3–22. Transmission electron micrograph demonstrating the appearance of the cells predominant in the juxtacanalicular region of the trabecular meshwork (JCT). These cells lack a basal lamina and are enmeshed in a connective tissue matrix that includes fibrillar collagen (C). The relationship between these cells and the endothelial cells (E) lining the inner wall of Schlemm's canal (SC) is evident. Mushroom-like processes from JCT cells appear to contact the inner wall cells *(small arrows)*. An interendothelial cell junction between two inner-wall cells is also present *(curved arrow)*. (16,600×). (Courtesy of Haiyan Gong, M.D., Ph.D.)

this way serves to spread the trabecular sheets open, facilitating trabecular outflow.

A second type of tendon extends through the trabeculum, inserting into the peripheral corneal lamellae and having little apparent impact on outflow.

The third tendon type extends into the outermost corneoscleral trabeculae and also inserts within the cribriform region of the meshwork.

From these tendons, elastin-containing connecting fibrils (the cribriform plexus mentioned earlier) extend to the basal lamina of the endothelial cells lining the inner wall of Schlemm's canal (Fig. 3–24). Contraction of these fibers also likely contributes to increasing trabecular flow through the cribriform region of the meshwork.[68]

Underscoring the physiological importance of these various anatomic connections is the work of Kaufman and Bárány, who first demonstrated that surgical disinsertion of the ciliary muscle eliminates the outflow-enhancing effects of pilocarpine.[69] More recently, Kaufman et al. have begun to question whether the progressive loss of ciliary muscle tone that contributes to presbyopia,[70] and the age-related loss of responsiveness to pilocarpine demonstrated in the monkey eye[71] might also result in a diminished capacity to open up the meshwork, leading to a progressive accumulation of obstructive material and possibly glaucoma.[70–71]

The "Open" Spaces of the Trabecular Meshwork

It is always initially tempting to view the apparently ample "open" spaces seen in light or electron microscopic sections of the trabecular meshwork as though they represented an accurate depiction of the area available for aqueous flow. However, calculations of outflow resistance in the juxtacanalicular meshwork, using a mathematical model that assumed the "open" spaces to be real, have been shown to fall two orders of magnitude short of generally accepted values for outflow resistance.[72] Recently, however, the use of a new technique known as "quick-freeze/deep-etch" has permitted ultrastructural visualization of much more of this matrix. With this new technique, correlates between modelling predictions of outflow mechanics and morphometric data on the amounts of truly "open" space are rapidly improving.[73]

Even before quick-freeze/deep-etch methods allowed visualization of this additional material, it was evident from biochemical and some histochemical studies that a substantial fraction of the space that appeared empty in conventionally prepared electron micrographs of the juxtacanalicular region of the trabecular meshwork was filled by an extracellular matrix. The matrix is composed of proteoglycans, proteoglycan-associated and unassociated glycosaminoglycans (GAGs), proteins, and other moieties.[74]

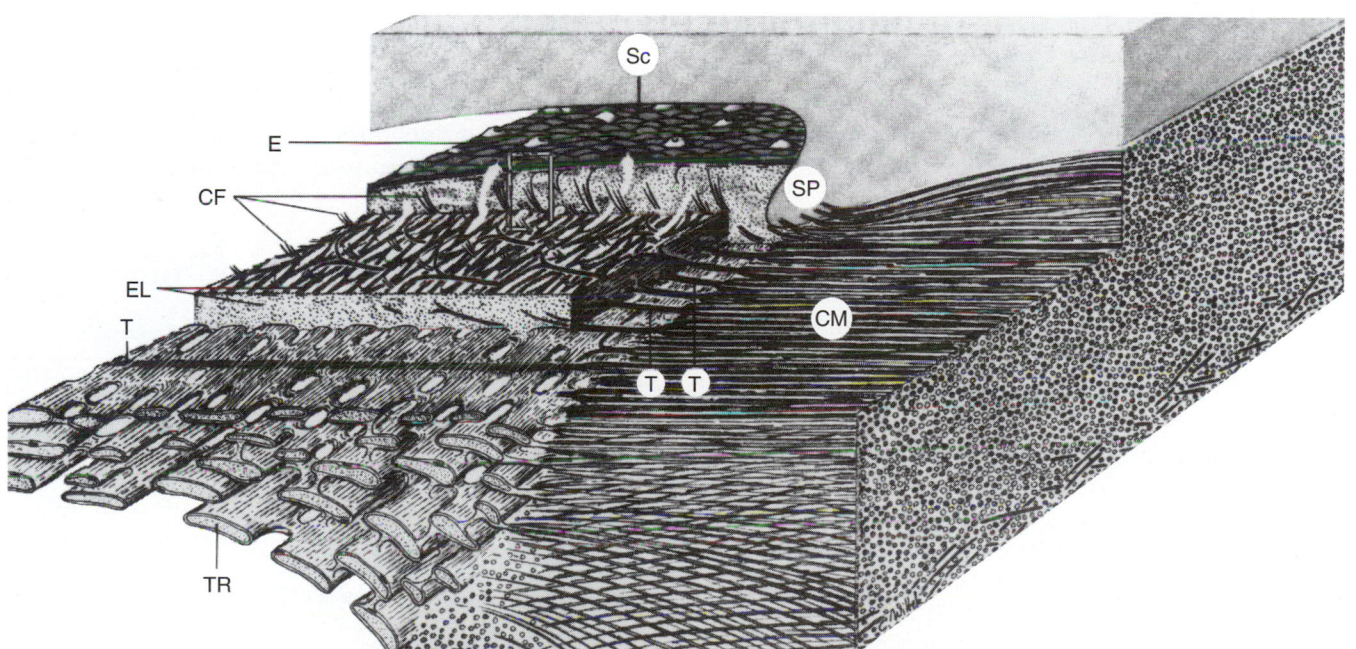

Figure 3–23. Anterior ciliary muscle tendons (T) and their connections with the trabecular meshwork. Tendons from the smooth muscle cells of the ciliary muscle (CM) extend to the scleral spur (SP), into the outermost corneoscleral trabeculae and into the juxtacanalicular region contributing to the cribriform plexus. Connecting fibrils (CF) extend from the plexus toward the endothelial cells (E) lining the inner wall of Schlemm's canal (Sc) (Reproduced courtesy of Rohen JW. *Ophthalmology.* 1983;90:758.

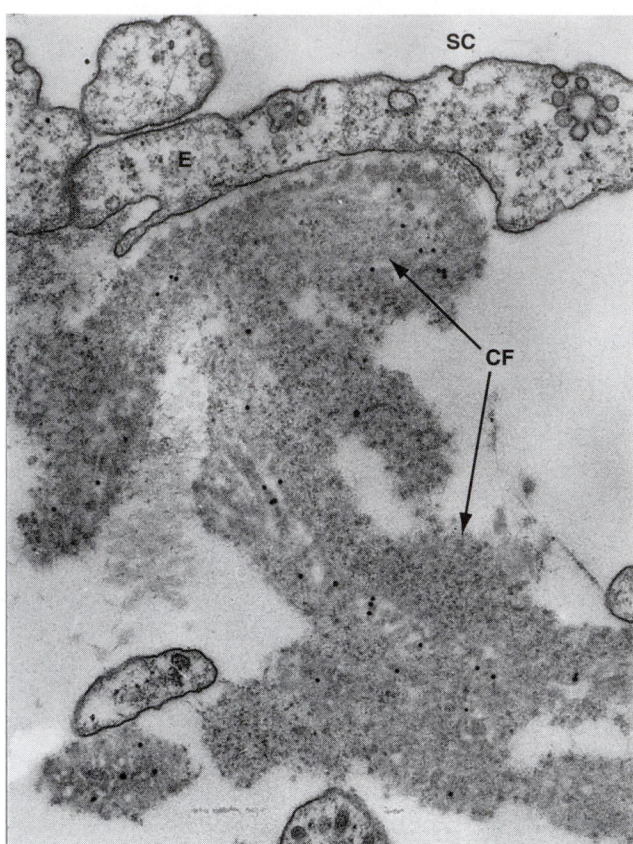

Figure 3–24. Transmission electron micrograph demonstrates the appearance of a connecting fibril (CF) corresponding to the area outlined in Fig. 3-23. These fibrils extend from the cribriform plexus to endothelial cells (E) of the inner wall of Schlemm's canal (SC). Small black dots represent colloidal gold particles localizing sites of antielastin antibody binding, confirming the presence of elastin in these fibers. (36,000×). (Reproduced with permission from Oxford University Press and Gong H, Trinkaus-Randall V, Freddo T *Curr Eye Res.* 1989;8:1071.)

Changes in the amount and distribution of these various constituents are generally felt to influence, or even regulate the passage of aqueous humor out of the eye.[75–77] Particularly interesting in this regard are the matrix metalloproteinases (MMPs) and their inhibitors. These proteins are used by an array of connective tissues to regulate synthesis and degradation of extracellular matrices. MMPs and their inhibitors are both made by the cells of the trabecular meshwork.[77–78] Whether a derangement of these regulatory systems represents an initiating event in the increased extracellular flow resistance that typifies glaucoma remains uncertain, but they are strong candidates.

Another more recently identified protein that may influence extracellular flow mechanics in the meshwork is a novel protein called TIGR (also known as myocilin). TIGR was first identified from trabecular cell cultures exposed to glucocorticoids (TIGR *trabecu-*

lar meshwork *inducible glucocorticoid response*).[79] This protein is an olfactomedin-related glycoprotein that is immunohistochemically localized to the inner portions of the trabecular meshwork and appears to exhibit increased expression in glaucoma.[80–81] It is still too soon to know how much of a role this protein might play in forms of glaucoma beyond that induced by steroids, but several recent studies have documented mutations in the TIGR gene that co-segregate with the presence of the disease.[82]

The Canal of Schlemm

The canal of Schlemm is a continuous, circumferentially oriented channel situated deep within the internal scleral sulcus. The lumen of Schlemm's canal is in direct continuity with the venous system of the eye. Despite this connection, blood is not usually seen in the canal unless intraocular pressure falls below that of episcleral venous pressure.

Transected and viewed by scanning electron microscopy, the canal usually appears slit-like and, at several points around the circumference of the eye, can be seen to divide into two parallel channels that rejoin one another after a short distance (Figs. 3–21 and 3–25). One side of the canal directly abuts the sclera and is termed its *outer wall*. The opposite side, which faces the trabecular meshwork, is formed by a continuous row of nonfenestrated endothelial cells and is termed the *inner wall* of Schlemm's canal.

Given that the inner wall is continuous, the issue of how aqueous humor crosses this wall has proven to be one of the most frustrating enigmas in attempts to understand the dynamics of aqueous outflow. There have traditionally been two schools of thought on the

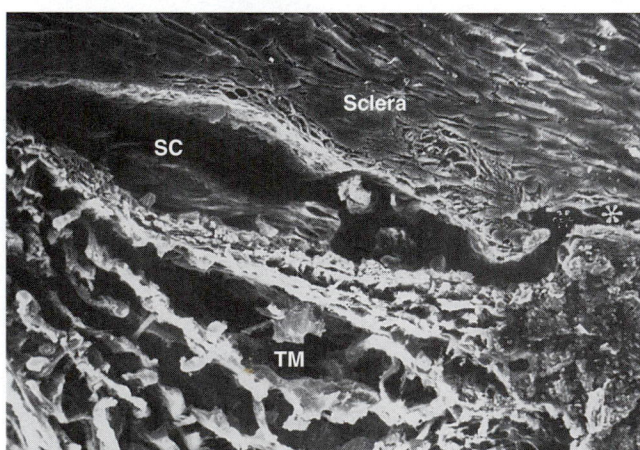

Figure 3–25. Scanning electron micrograph of transected trabecular meshwork (TM) and Schlemm's canal (SC) demonstrates the slit-like appearance of the canal, its relation to the sclera, and its continuity with an external collector channel *(asterisks)*. (304×).

subject of how aqueous humor crosses the inner wall of Schlemm's canal. One argues that the aqueous passes between the endothelial cells that form the inner wall and the other argues that the aqueous passes through the cells via specialized structures commonly referred to as *giant vacuoles*.

Ultrastructural studies, using the technique of freeze-fracture electron microscopy, have demonstrated that the endothelial cells of the inner wall are joined by two types of intercellular junctions, gap junctions and discontinuous tight junctions.[52] Unlike the continuous tight junctions of the blood vessels of the iris, the discontinuous tight junctions between the endothelial cells of the inner wall do not form an uninterrupted system of branching and anastomosing strands (Fig. 3–26). Instead, there are maze-like pathways through the junctions that have been termed *slit pores* (Fig. 3–27).[52] At first glance these pores would seem to offer a potentially significant conduit for aqueous flow. In her manuscript reporting the existence of slit pores, however, Raviola states that she went on to measure the dimensions of these pores and to calculate that they could not account for more than a small fraction of the aqueous humor that reaches the lumen of the canal. More recent studies, however, have demonstrated that under conditions of increased perfusion pressure, paracellular permeability increases, while the length of endothelial cell overlap and the complexity of the tight junctions decreases.[83–84] A reappraisal of the role of the paracellular pathway is in progress.

Current consensus favors the view that the inner wall of Schlemm's canal harbors only a minor portion of the outflow resistance measured in a normal eye.[85]

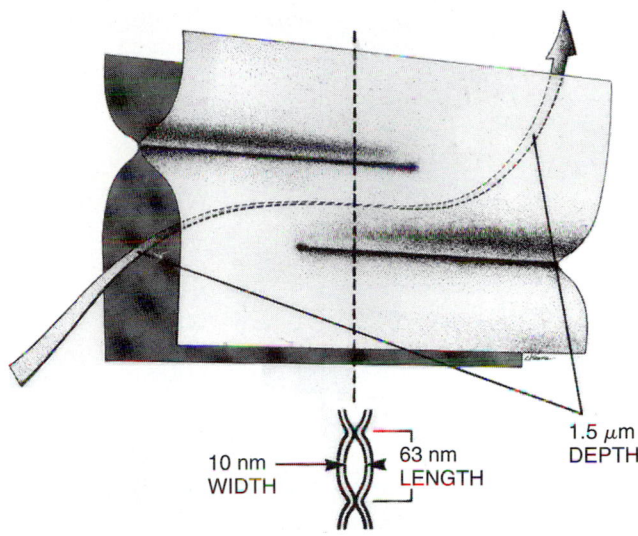

Figure 3–27. Diagrammatic representation of the freeze-fracture electron micrograph in Fig. 3-26 demonstrating the nature of the "slit-pores" between adjacent endothelial cells forming the inner wall of Schlemm's canal. (Reproduced with permission from: Raviola G, Raviola E. *Invest Ophthalmol Vis Sci.* 1981;21:52.)

A recent and novel theory termed *funneling* argues, however, that preferential pathways of flow exist in the juxtacanalicular meshwork in close proximity to the pores in the wall of Schlemm's canal.[86] If the funneling phenomenon can be proved to exist, then a larger role for the inner wall in outflow resistance would be possible.

Putting the issue of resistance aside, most authors would continue to agree that the bulk of aqueous flow across the inner wall of Schlemm's canal is carried by giant vacuoles. Giant vacuoles in the wall of Schlemm's canal are demonstrated in Fig. 3–28. These appear to represent distentions within or between inner-wall endothelial cells that are formed around an aliquot of aqueous humor.[87] This aliquot is then released into the lumen of Schlemm's canal through a small opening or pore that develops in the vacuolar wall.[88] As odd as these vacuoles initially appear, there is precedent for the existence of such structures in other tissues. Specifically, it has been found that similar vacuoles are present in the arachnoid villi of the meninges, surrounding the brain, where they are felt to play a role in the resorption of cerebrospinal fluid.[88–90]

Giant vacuole formation is not energy-dependent, but rather pressure-dependent. As intraocular pressure is increased, (within physiologically obtainable limits), the size of vacuoles in the inner wall of Schlemm's canal also increases.[89] Conversely, when intraocular pressure is reduced, as in paracentesis, the size of vacuoles is also reduced.[91–92] Specimens of

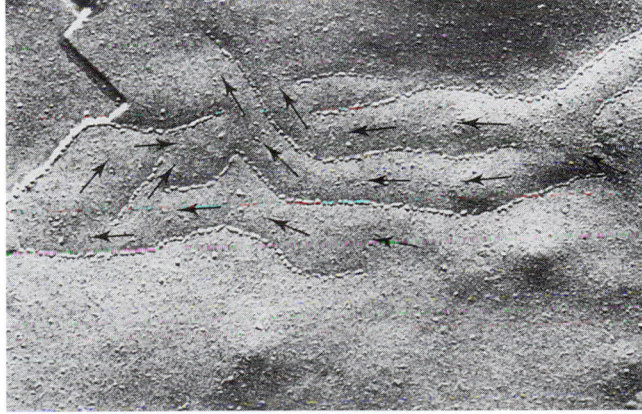

Figure 3–26. Freeze-fracture electron micrograph of the intercellular junctions between endothelial cells of the inner wall of Schlemm's canal. The tight junctional strands are discontinuous, providing a maze-like pathway through the junction as demonstrated by the arrows. (62,300×). (Reproduced with permission from Raviola G, Raviola E.: *Invest Ophthalmol Vis Sci.* 1981;21:52.)

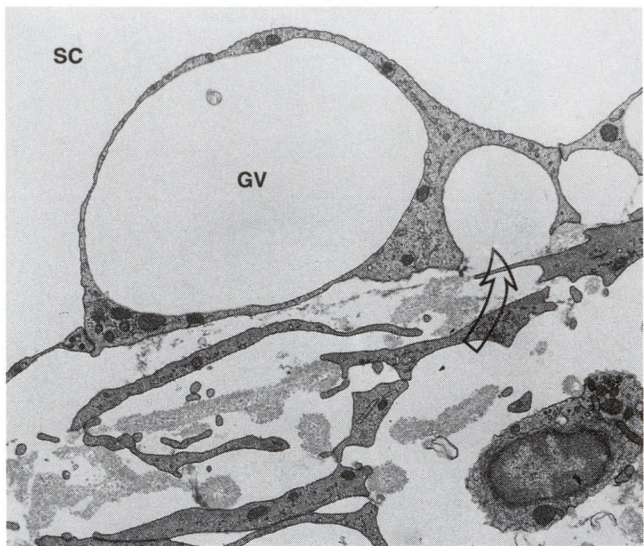

Figure 3–28. Transmission electron micrograph demonstrates a giant vacuole (GV) in the inner wall of Schlemm's canal (SC). Another vacuole is seen in the process of formation *(curved arrow).* (6,500×).

trabecular meshwork that are not under flow conditions while the tissue is being fixed for microscopic study commonly exhibit few if any vacuoles at all.

The Outflow Channels Beyond Schlemm's Canal

From the canal of Schlemm, aqueous humor is ultimately conducted to the venous system. In this regard,

it is important to appreciate that elevations of venous pressure can result in significant elevations of intraocular pressure. The pathways connecting the canal of Schlemm to the venous system of the episcleral venous plexus are depicted in Fig. 3–29. From the canal of Schlemm, aqueous passes into one of approximately 30 to 35 external collector channels (Figs. 3–25 and 3–29). These channels are unevenly distributed, with more on the nasal than on the temporal side of the eye. From the external collector channels, two separate pathways conduct the aqueous to the episcleral venous plexus. One pathway leads through an anastomotic system of deep and more superficial intrascleral plexi. The other is a more direct pathway to the venous system via a sparsely distributed set of aqueous veins. The aqueous veins, first described by Ascher, are identifiable clinically because there is a tendency for the aqueous and blood to resist immediate mixing and thus to be seen running in a laminar flow within these vessels.[93]

It appears that only about 20 to 25% of the normal resistance to aqueous outflow in the human or primate eye is attributable to the portions of the aqueous outflow system between Schlemm's canal and the venous system. There has been renewed interest in these channels, however, with identification of the contractile protein smooth muscle myosin in cells adjacent to collector channels in human eyes. The presence of contractile elements in this distal portion of the outflow system raises the tempting possibility

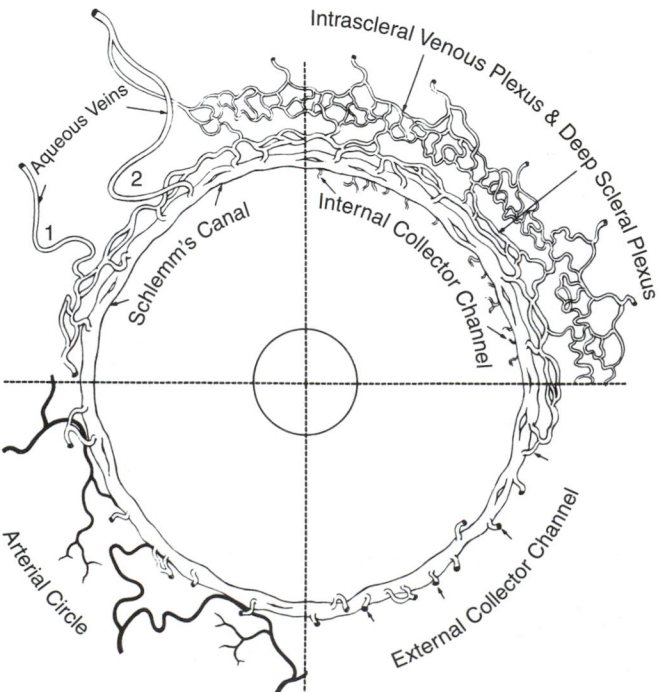

Figure 3–29. Diagrammatic representation of the distal portion of the aqueous outflow pathways from Schlemm's canal. External collector channels *(lower right);* Deep and intrascleral plexi *(upper right);* Aqueous veins (1 and 2) *(upper left).* (Reproduced with permission from Hogan M, Alvarado J, Weddell J. *Histology of the Human Eye.* Philadelphia: WB Saunders Co; 1971.)

that they are capable of altering channel dimensions and therefore aqueous outflow.[94]

Fluid Mechanics of Trabecular Outflow

From the discussion above, it is clear that a number of factors, influencing several anatomical sites and physiological processes, interrelate to account for aqueous flow and intraocular pressure. A general appreciation of these interrelationships, although substantially oversimplified, can be realized through an understanding of the equations developed by Goldmann, in which

$$\Delta P = P_i - P_e \quad \text{and} \quad F = C_{tm}(P_i - P_e)$$

where

P_i = intraocular pressure in millimeters of mercury
P_e = episcleral venous pressure in millimeters of mercury
F = aqueous flow in microliters per minute (at steady state, $F = F_{in} = F_{out}$)
C_{tm} = facility of trabecular outflow

This equation presumes that outflow of aqueous humor represents an entirely passive bulk flow down a pressure gradient from the anterior chamber to the venous system. It further assumes that *all* outflow is trabecular. Since, under steady-state conditions, the outflow facilities relating to pseudofacility and uveoscleral drainage are very low compared to trabecular flow, and the episcleral venous pressure is relatively stable, this equation represents a reasonable approximation of events affecting intraocular pressure in vivo. With the addition of a flow component for uveoscleral outflow (F_{us}) and insertion of typical values for the various parameters as illustrated by Kaufman,[95] the Goldmann equation takes on additional clinical relevance.

Assuming that

$$F_{in} = F_{out} = 2.5 \ \mu L/min$$
$$C_{tm} = 0.3 \ \mu L/min/mmHg$$
$$P_i = 16 \ mmHg$$
$$P_e = 9 \ mmHg$$
$$F_{us} = 0.4 \ \mu L/min$$

Then

$$F_{in} = F_{out} = C_{tm}(P_i - P_e) + F_{us}$$
$$2.5 = 2.5 = 0.3 \ (16 - 9) + 0.4$$

A Role for Aqueous Humor in Aqueous Outflow Resistance

Until recently, little attention has been paid to the possibility that aqueous humor might be an active contributor to its own resistance. Interestingly, how-

ever, when aqueous humor is passed through microporous filters having pore dimensions of 0.2 μm, significantly greater resistance is produced than occurs using either saline or plasma diluted to the same protein concentration as aqueous.[96] This effect was shown to be mediated through hydrophobic interactions with the pore wall.[97] The fact that perfusion of obstructed filters with GAG failed to relieve the obstruction, while perfusion with protease eliminated it, led to a presumption that proteins, or glycoproteins were involved in the process.[96]

Although the effects on nonphysiologic filters described above have not been confirmed in vivo, several hydrophobic moieties (i.e., collagen and elastin) are present in the juxtacanalicular trabecular (JCT) region. It may be the case that the outflow resistance in the JCT region results not simply from the nature of the extracellular matrix found here, but also from the way in which these matrix components interact with constituents of the aqueous humor.

Uveoscleral Outflow

When particulate tracers such as thorotrast or fluoresceinated dextrans are perfused into primate eyes under appropriate conditions, some of the tracer can be demonstrated to enter the uvea through the tissues of the chamber angle, migrating through the interstices of the ciliary muscle to reach first the supraciliary and finally the suprachoroidal space (Fig. 3–30).[98,99] From the suprachoroidal space of the uvea, the aqueous passes either through the sclera or its emissaria; hence the choice of the term *uveoscleral* for this pathway.

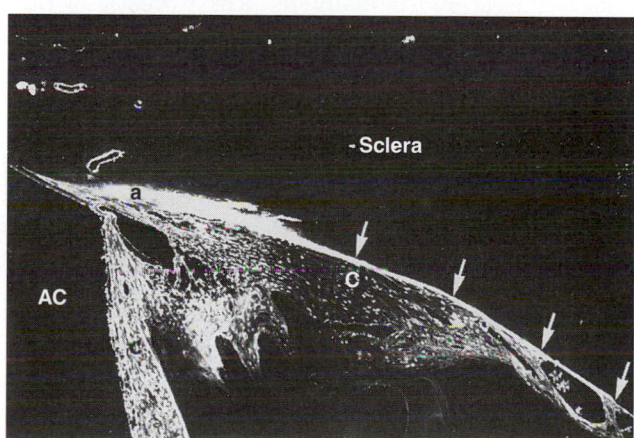

Figure 3–30. Light micrograph demonstrating the distribution of fluoresceinated dextran after intracameral perfusion into the anterior chamber (AC). The tracer has moved posteriorly into the angle tissues (a), including the ciliary muscle (b), and ultimately to the supraciliary and suprachoroidal spaces *(arrows)*. Tracer has also freely permeated the iris stroma (c). (38.5×). (Reproduced with permission from Tripathi R. *Exp Eye Res (suppl)*. 1977;25: 305.)

Uveoscleral outflow appears to be pressure-independent, representing a bulk flow rather than a diffusion-related phenomenon. The percentage of total aqueous outflow attributed to this pathway varies from species to species, but in human eyes, uveoscleral flow accounts for 10 to 20% of total outflow.[100]

Evidence of pressure-independence comes directly from measurements in which uveoscleral flow rates were statistically unchanged at normal and elevated intraocular pressures.[100] One exception to this otherwise general rule was found for markedly lower intraocular pressure around 2 mmHg. In this instance, uveoscleral outflow was demonstrated to decrease with decreasing pressure, although the mechanism remains unclear.[101]

Evidence that diffusion is not the primary driving force in uveoscleral outflow comes from several studies. It has been demonstrated that molecules having very different dimensions, and therefore presumably different diffusional characteristics, leave the anterior chamber at similar rates.[102] Furthermore, the rate of movement of macromolecular dextran from the suprachoroid to the anterior chamber is 200 times less than that in the opposite direction.[103] Clearly, if diffusion were the principal mechanism governing this movement, the rates would be essentially the same. Both of these results argue that another mechanism besides diffusion (i.e., bulk flow) underlies uveoscleral flow.

Because the uveoscleral outflow pathway involves the ciliary body, and specifically the intercellular spaces within the ciliary muscle, it should not be surprising that the state of contraction of the ciliary muscle can significantly alter the amount of uveoscleral flow. Although beneficial for trabecular flow, contraction of the ciliary muscle substantially reduces uveoscleral flow by compressing the intercellular spaces within the muscle that constitute the drainage pathway.[104]

Increasing effort is being directed at improving uveoscleral outflow as a means of reducing intraocular pressure in glaucoma. One of the most fruitful efforts has emerged from the studies of Bito, Camras, and others on the ocular effects of prostaglandins (PGs). PGs are a family of compounds derived from arachidonic acid, which were examined originally for their role in mediating intraocular inflammation.[105] More recently, however, attention has focused on certain subclasses of PGs that lowered intraocular pressure. Most promising initially was prostaglandin-$F_{2\alpha}$[106,107] and later PGA_2, which lowered intraocular pressure at lower doses than did $PGF_{2\alpha}$ and with less irritation.[108] Given that these agents altered neither aqueous inflow nor episcleral venous pressure sufficiently to account for their effect on intraocular pressure, it was presumed that PGs acted through enhancement of uveoscleral outflow.[109] Demonstra-

tion that the intraocular pressure-lowering effect of PGs could be blocked by pretreatment with pilocarpine (which blocks uveoscleral flow, as described earlier) clearly implicates uveoscleral outflow as the main site of action of PGs.[110] The results of this study would also suggest that pilocarpine and PGs could not be paired to enhance both trabecular and uveoscleral outflow simultaneously. But, clinical experience using the commercially available agent latanoprost (Xalatan) has thus far shown that these drugs can be addictive.[111,112] This finding clearly demonstrates the need for additional studies to provide us with a more complete understanding of uveoscleral outflow.

CONCLUSION

In summary, this chapter has presented merely an overview of the knowledge gained over the years regarding the production and drainage of aqueous humor and how these may relate to the glaucomas. Despite significant progress, our understanding of these complex processes and the mechanisms underlying many of the treatment regimens used in glaucoma management remains far from complete.

REFERENCES

1. Varma SD, Ets TK, Richards RD. Protection against superoxide radicals in rat lens. *Ophthalmol Res.* 1977;9:421.
2. Reiss GR et al. Aqueous humor flow during sleep. *Invest Ophthalmol Vis Sci.* 1984;25:776.
3. McCannel CA, Heinrich SR, Brubaker RF. Acetazolamide but not timolol lowers aqueous flow in sleeping humans. *Graefes Arch Clin Exp Ophthalmol.* 1992; 230:518.
4. Morrison J VanBuskirk EM. Ciliary process microvasculature of the primate eye. *Am J Ophthalmol.* 1984; 97:372.
5. Funk R, Rohen JW. Intraocular microendoscopy of the ciliary-process vasculature in albino rabbits: effects of vasoactive agents. *Exp Eye Res.* 1987;45:597.
6. Bill A. Autonomic nervous control of uveal blood flow. *Acta Physiol (Scand).* 1962;56:70.
7. Bill A. The protective role of ocular sympathetic vasomotor nerves in acute arterial hypertension. In: *Proceedings of the Ninth European Conference in Microcirculation.* Antwerp, Belgium: *Biblioteca Anatomica* 1977;16:30.
8. Cole DF. Secretion of aqueous humor. *Exp Eye Res(suppl).* 1977;25:161.
9. Brubaker RF. The measurement of pseudofacility and true facility by constant pressure perfusion in the normal rhesus monkey eye. *Invest Ophthalmol.* 1970;9:42.

10. Bill A, Bárány EH. Gross facility, facility of conventional routes, and pseudofacility of aqueous humor outflow in the cynomolgus monkeys: The reduction in aqueous humor formation rate caused by moderate increments in intraocular pressure. *Arch Ophthalmol.* 1966;75:665.

11. Kupfer C, Sanderson P. Determination of pseudofacility in the eye of man. *Arch Ophthalmol.* 1968;80:194.

12. Kaufman PL, Bill A, Bárány EH. Formation and drainage of aqueous humor following total iris removal and ciliary muscle disinsertion in the cynomolgus monkey. *Invest Ophthalmol Vis Sci.* 1977;16:226.

13. Raviola G, Raviola E. Intercellular junctions in the ciliary epithelium. *Invest Ophthalmol Vis Sci.* 1978;17:958.

14. Hirsch M, Mountcourrier P, Arguilliere P, Keller N. The structure of tight junctions in the ciliary epithelium. *Curr Eye Res.* 1985;4:493.

15. Freddo T, Raviola G. Freeze-fracture analysis of interendothelial junctions in the blood vessels of the iris in *Macaca mulatta. Invest Ophthalmol Vis Sci.* 1982; 23:154.

16. Freddo TF, Bartels SP, Barsotti MF, Kamm RD. The source of protein in the aqueous humor of the normal rabbit. *Invest Ophthalmol Vis Sci.* 1990;31:125.

17. Kolodny N, Freddo T, Lawrence B, Suarez C, Bartels SP. Contrast-enhanced MRI confirmation of an anterior protein pathway in the normal rabbit eye. *Invest Ophthalmol Vis Sci.* 1996;37:1602.

18. Russell P, Koretz J, Epstein DL. Is primary open angle glaucoma caused by small proteins? *Med Hypoth.* 1993;41:455.

19. Sit AJ, Gong H, Ritter N, Freddo TF, Kamm RD, Johnson M. The role of soluble proteins in generating aqueous outflow resistance in the bovine and human eye. *Exp Eye Res.* 1997;64:813.

20. Doss EW, Ward KA, Koretz JF. Investigation of the "fines" hypothesis of primary open-angle glaucoma: The possible role of alpha-crystallin. *Ophthalmol Res.* 1998;30:142.

21. Diamond JR, Bossert WH. Standing gradient osmotic flow: A mechanism for coupling of water and solute transport in epithelia. *J Gen Physiol.* 1967;50:2061.

22. Civan MM, ed.*The Eye's Aqueous Humor: From Secretion to Glaucoma.* San Diego: Academic Press; 1998.

23. Edelman JL, Sachs G, Adorante JS. Ion transport asymmetry and functional coupling in bovine pigmented and nonpigmented ciliary epithelial cells. *Am J Physiol.* 1994;266.C1210.

24. Xu JC et al. Molecular cloning and functional expression of the bumetanide-sensitive Na-K-Cl co-transporter. *Proc Nat Acad Sci USA.* 1994;91.2201.

25. Green K, Bountra C, Georgiou C, House R. An electrophysiological study of rabbit ciliary epithelium. *Invest Ophthalmol Vis Sci.* 1985;26:371.

26. Schutte M, Wolosin JM. Ca^{2+} mobilization and interlayer signal transfer in the heterocellular bilayered epithelium of the rabbit ciliary body. *J Physiol.* 1996;496 (pt 1):25–37.

27. Krupin T, Civan MM. Physiologic basis of aqueous humor formation. In: Ritch R, Shields MB, Krupin T, eds. *The Glaucomas, I,* 2nd ed. St. Louis: CV Mosby Co; 1989: chap 12.

28. Freddo T. Mitochondria attached to desmosomes in the ciliary epithelia of human, monkey and rabbit eyes. *Cell Tiss Res.* 1988;251:671.

29. Becker B. Ouabain and aqueous humor dynamics in the rabbit eye. *Invest Ophthalmol.* 1963;2:325.

30. Becker B. Hypothermia and aqueous humor dynamics of the rabbit eye. *Trans Am Ophthalmol Soc.* 1960;58:337.

31. Flügel C, Lütjen-Drecoll E. Presence and distribution of Na^+/K^+-ATPase in the ciliary epithelium of the rabbit. *Histochemistry.* 1988;88:613.

32. Lütjen-Drecoll E, Lönnerholm G, Eichorn M. Carbonic anhydrase distribution in the human and monkey eye by light and electron microscopy. *Graefes Arch Clin Exp Ophthalmol.* 1983;220:285.

33. Maren TH. The rates of movement of sodium, chloride and bicarbonate from plasma to posterior chamber: Effect of acetazolamide and relation to the treatment of glaucoma. *Invest Ophthalmol.* 1976;15:356.

34. Caprioli J. The ciliary epithelia and aqueous humor. In: Moses RA, Hart WM Jr, eds. *Adler's Physiology of the Eye,* 8th ed. St. Louis: CV Mosby Co; 1987;7:212.

35. Lippa EA et al. Dose-response and duration of action of dorzolamide, a topical carbonic anhydrase inhibitor. *Arch Ophthalmol.* 1992;110:495.

36. Podos SM, Serle JB. Topically active carbonic anhydrase inhibitors for glaucoma. *Arch Ophthalmol.* 1991; 109:38.

37. Lavah M, Melamed E, Dofna Z, Atlas D. Localization of ß-receptors in the anterior segment of the eye by a fluorescent analog of propranolol. *Invest Ophthalmol Vis Sci.*1978;17:645.

38. Tsukahara S, Maezawa N. Cytochemical localization of adenyl cyclase in the rabbit ciliary body. *Exp Eye Res.* 1978;26:99.

39. Nathanson JA. Adrenergic regulation of intraocular pressure: Identification of $beta_2$-adrenergic stimulated adenylate cyclase in ciliary process epithelium. *Proc Natl Acad Sci USA.* 1980;77:7421.

40. Brubaker RF, Gaasterland D. The effect of isoproterenol on aqueous humor formation in humans. *Invest Ophthalmol Vis Sci.* 1984;25:357.

41. Coakes RL, Brubaker RS. The mechanism of timolol in lowering intraocular pressure. *Arch Ophthalmol.* 1978;96:2045.

42. Mittag T. Adrenergic and dopaminergic drugs in glaucoma. In: Ritch R, Shields MB, Krupin T, eds.*The Glaucomas, I,* 2nd ed. St. Louis: CV Mosby Co; 1996: chap 67.

43. Mittag TW, Tormay A, Severin C, Podos SM. Alpha adrenergic antagonists: Correlation of the effect on intraocular pressure and on α_2-adrenergic receptor binding specificity in the rabbit eye. *Exp Eye Res.* 1985;40:591.

44. Mittag TW. Ocular effects of selective alpha-adrenergic agents: A new drug paradox? *Ann Ophthalmol.* 1983;15:201.

45. Serle JB, Stein AJ, Podos SM, Severin CH. Corynanthine and aqueous humor dynamics in rabbit and monkeys. *Arch Ophthalmol.* 1984;102:1385.

46. Gharagozolo NZ, Relf SJ, Brubaker RF. Aqueous flow is reduced by the α_2-adrenergic agonist, apraclonidine hydrochloride, (ALO 2145). *Ophthalmology*. 1988; 95:1217.

47. Abrahms DA et al. A limited comparison of apraclonidine's dose response in subjects with normal and increased intraocular pressure. *Am J Ophthalmol*. 1989; 108:230.

48. Brown RH et al. ALO 2145 reduces the IOP elevation after anterior segment surgery. *Ophthalmology*. 1988;95:378.

49. Robin AL et al. Effect of ALO-2145 on intraocular pressure following argon laser trabeculoplasty. *Arch Ophthalmol*. 1987;105:646.

50. Bill A. The role of iris blood vessels in aqueous humor dynamics. *Jpn J Ophthalmol*. 1974;18:30.

51. Gong H, Trinkaus-Randall V, Freddo T. Ultrastructural immunocytochemical localization of elastin in normal human trabecular meshwork. *Curr Eye Res*. 1989;8:1071.

52. Raviola G, Raviola E. Paracellular route of aqueous outflow in the trabecular meshwork and canal of Schlemm. *Invest Ophthalmol Vis Sci*. 1981;21:52.

53. O'Donnell ME, Brandt JD, Curry FR. Na-K-Cl co-transport regulates intracellular volume and monolayer permeability of trabecular meshwork cells. *Am J Physiol*. 1995;268(4 pt 1):C1067.

54. Freddo TF, Patterson MM, Scott DR, Epstein DL. Influence of sulfhydryl agents on aqueous outflow pathways in enucleated eyes. *Invest Ophthalmol Vis Sci*. 1984;25:278-285.

55. Rohen JW, van der Zypen E. The phagocytic activity of the trabecular meshwork endothelium: An electron microscope study of the vervet (*Cercopithecus æthiops*). *Graefes Arch Clin Exp Ophthalmol*. 1968;175:143,.

56. Grierson I, Lee WR. Erythrocyte phagocytosis in the human trabecular meshwork. *Br J Ophthalmol*. 1973;57:400.

57. Richardson TM, Hutchinson BT, Grant MW. The outflow tract in pigmentary glaucoma: A light and electron microscopic study. *Arch Ophthalmol*. 1977;95:1015.

58. Epstein DL, Freddo TF, Anderson PJ, Patterson MM, Bassett-Chu S. Experimental obstruction to aqueous outflow by pigment particles in living monkeys. *Invest Ophthalmol Vis Sci*. 1986;27:387.

59. Buller C, Johnson DH, Tschumper RC. Human trabecular meshwork phagocytosis: observations in an organ culture system. *Invest Ophthalmol Vis Sci*. 1990;31:2156.

60. Johnson DH. Do trabecular cells replicate? *Invest Ophthalmol Vis Sci(suppl)*. 1986;27:210.

61. Alvarado J, Murphy C, Polansky J , Juster R. Age-related changes in trabecular meshwork cellularity. *Invest Ophthalmol Vis Sci*. 1981;21:714.

62. Grierson I, Howes RC. Age-related depletion of the cell population in the human trabecular meshwork. *Eye*. 1987;1:204.

63. Alvarado J, Murphy C, Juster R. Trabecular meshwork cellularity in primary open angle glaucoma and nonglaucomatous normals. *Ophthalmology*.1984;91:564.

64. Lütjen-Drecoll E, Rohen JW. Morphology of aqueous outflow pathways in normal and glaucomatous eyes. In:, Ritch R, Shields MB, Krupin T, eds. *The Glaucomas, I*, 2nd ed. St. Louis: CV Mosby Co; 1996:chap 5.

65. Rohen JW, Futa R, Lütjen-Drecoll E. The fine structure of the cribriform meshwork in normal and glaucomatous eyes as seen in tangential sections. *Invest Ophthalmol Vis Sci*. 1981;21:574.

66. Lütjen-Drecoll E. Structural factors influencing outflow facility and its changeability under drugs: a study in *Macaca arctoides*. *Invest Ophthalmol*.1973;12:280.

67. Bill A, Svedbergh B. Scanning electron microscopic studies of the trabecular meshwork and the canal of Schlemm—An attempt to localize the main resistance to outflow of aqueous humor in man. *Acta Ophthalmol*. 1972;50:295.

68. Rohen JW, Lütjen E, Bárány EH. The relation between the ciliary muscle and the trabecular meshwork and its importance for the effect of miotics on aqueous outflow resistance: A study in two contrasting monkey species, *Macaca irus* and *Cercopithecus æethiops*. *Graefes Arch Clin Exp Ophthalmol*. 1967;172:23.

69. Kaufman PL, Bárány EH. Loss of acute pilocarpine effect on outflow facility following surgical disinsertion and retrodisplacement of the ciliary muscle from the scleral spur in cynomolgus monkey. *Invest Ophthalmol*. 1976;15:793.

70. Kaufman PL. Aging and aqueous humor dynamics. In: DiVincentis M, ed. *The Fundamental Aging Processes of the Eye*. Florence: Baccini and Chiappi; 1987:41.

71. Lütjen-Drecoll E, Tamm E, Kaufman PL. Age-related loss of morphologic responses to pilocarpine in rhesus monkey ciliary muscle. *Arch Ophthalmol*. 1988;106:1591.

72. Ethier CR, Kamm RD, Palaszewski BA, Johnson M, Richardson TM. Calculation of flow resistance in the juxtacanalicular meshwork. *Invest Ophthalmol Vis Sci*. 1986;27:1741.

73. Gong H, Brown K, Johnson M, Kamm RD, Freddo TF. Hydraulic conductivity of juxtacanalicular connective tissue using quick-freeze/deep-etch. *Invest Ophthalmol Vis Sci*. 1997;38(suppl):S564.

74. Acott TS, Westcott M, Passo MS, VanBuskirk EM. Trabecular meshwork glycosaminoglycans in human and cynomolgus monkey eye. *Invest Ophthalmol Vis Sci*. 1985;26:1320.

75. Bárány EH, Scotchbrook S. Influence of testicular hyaluronidase on the resistance to flow through the angle of the anterior chamber. *Acta Physiol (Scand)*. 1954;30:240.

76. Knepper PA, Farbman AI, Tesler AG. Aqueous outflow pathway glycosaminoglycans. *Exp Eye Res*. 1981; 32:265.

77. Alexander JP, Samples JR, VanBuskirk EM, Acott, TS. Expression of matrix metalloproteases and inhibitor by human trabecular meshwork. *Invest Ophthalmol Vis Sci*. 1991;32:172.

78. Acott TS, Wirtz MK. Biochemistry of aqueous outflow. In: Ritch R, Shields MB, Krupin T, eds.*The Glaucomas, I*, 2nd ed. St. Louis: CV Mosby Co; 1996: chap 13.

79. Nguyen TD, Chen P, Huang WD, Johnson D, Polansky JR. Gene structure and properties of TIGR, an olfactomedin-related glycoprotein cloned from glucocorticoid-induced trabecular meshwork cells. *J Biol Chem*. 1998;273:6341.

80. Lütjen-Drecoll E, May CA, Polansky JR, Johnson DH, Bloemendal H, Nguyen TD. Localization of the stress

proteins alpha B-crystallin and trabecular meshwork inducible glucocorticoid response protein in normal and glaucomatous trabecular meshwork. *Invest Ophthalmol Vis Sci.* 1998;39:517.

81. Polansky JR, et al. Cellular pharmacology and molecular biology of the trabecular meshwork inducible glucocorticoid response gene product. *Ophthalmologica.* 1997;211:126.

82. Wiggs JL, Allingham RR, Vollrath D, et al. Prevalence of mutations in TIGR/myocilin in patients with adult and juvenile primary open angle glaucoma. *Am J Hum Genet.* 1998;63:1549.

83. Epstein DL, Rohen JW. Morphology of the trabecular meshwork and inner-wall endothelium after cationized ferritin perfusion in the monkey eye. *Invest Ophthalmol Vis Sci.* 1991;32:610.

84. Ye W, Gong H, Sit A, Johnson M, Freddo TF. Interendothelial junctions in normal human Schlemm's canal respond to changes in pressure. *Invest Ophthalmol Vis Sci.* 1997;38:2460.

85. Meapea O, Bill A. Pressures in the juxtacanalicular tissue and Schlemm's canal in monkeys. *Exp Eye Res.* 1992;54:879.

86. Johnson M, Shapiro A, Ethier CR, and Kamm RD. Modulation of outflow resistance by the pores of the inner wall endothelium. *Invest Ophthalmol Vis Sci.* 1992; 33:1670.

87. Johnstone MA. Pressure-dependent changes in nuclei and the process origins of the endothelial cells lining Schlemm's canal. *Invest Ophthalmol Vis Sci.* 1979;18:44.

88. Tripathi BJ, Tripathi RC. Vacuolar transcellular channels as a drainage pathway for cerebrospinal fluid. *J Physiol (Lond).* 1974;239:195.

89. Tripathi RC. The functional morphology of the outflow systems of ocular and cerebrospinal fluids. *Exp Eye Res.* (suppl). 1977;25:65.

90. Gomez DG, Potts G. Effects of pressure on the arachnoid villus. *Exp Eye Res (suppl).* 1977;25:117.

91. Raviola G. Effects of paracentesis on the blood-aqueous barrier: An electron microscope study on *Macaca mulatta* using horseradish peroxidase as a tracer. *Invest Ophthalmol Vis Sci.* 1974;13:828.

92. Grierson I, Lee WR. Pressure-induced changes in the ultrastructure of the endothelium lining Schlemm's canal. *Am J Ophthalmol.* 1975;80:863.

93. Ascher KW. *The Aqueous Veins.* Springfield, IL: Charles C. Thomas;1961.

94. de Kater AW, Spurr-Michaud SJ, Gipson IK: Localization of smooth muscle myosin-containing cells in the aqueous outflow pathway. *Invest Ophthalmol Vis Sci.* 1990;31:347.

95. Kaufman PL. Pressure-dependent outflow. In: Ritch R, Shields MB, Krupin T, eds. *The Glaucomas, I.* St. Louis: CV Mosby Co;1989;9:220.

96. Johnson M, Ethier CR, Kamm RD, Grant WM, Epstein DL, Gaasterland D. The flow of aqueous humor through microporous filters. *Invest Ophthalmol Vis Sci.* 1986;27:92.

97. Ethier CR, Kamm RD, Palaszewski BA, Johnson M, Richardson TM. Calculations of flow resistance in the juxtacanalicular meshwork. *Invest Ophthalmol Vis Sci.* 1986;27:1741.

98. Bill A. The aqueous humor drainage mechanism in the cynomolgus monkey (*Macaca irus*) with evidence for unconventional routes. *Invest Ophthalmol.* 1965;4:911.

99. Tripathi RC. Uveoscleral drainage of aqueous humor. *Exp Eye Res (suppl).* 1977;25:305.

100. Bill A. Further studies on the influence of the intraocular pressure on aqueous humor dynamics in cynomolgus monkeys. *Invest Ophthalmol.* 1967; 6:364.

101. Toris CB, Pederson JE. Effect of intraocular pressure on uveoscleral outflow following cyclodialysis in the monkey eye using a fluorescent tracer. *Invest Ophthalmol Vis Sci.* 1985;26:1745.

102. Toris CB, Gregerson DS, Pederson JE. Uveoscleral outflow using different-sized fluorescent tracers in normal and inflamed eyes. *Exp Eye Res.* 1987;45:525.

103. Pederson JE, Toris CJ. Uveoscleral outflow: diffusion or flow? *Invest Ophthalmol Vis Sci.* 1987;28:1022.

104. Bill A. Uveoscleral drainage of aqueous humor in human eyes. *Exp Eye Res.* 1971;12:275.

105. Camras C. Prostaglandins. In: Ritch R, Shields MB, Krupin T, eds. *The Glaucomas, III,* 2nd ed. St. Louis: CV Mosby Co; 1996: chap 69.

106. Giuffre G. The effects of prostaglandin $F_2\alpha$ in the human eye. *Graefes Arch Clin Exp Ophthalmol.* 1985;222:139.

107. Villumsen J, Alm A. The effect of prostaglandin $F_2\alpha$ eye drops in open angle glaucoma. *Invest Ophthalmol Vis Sci.* 1987;28:266.

108. Bito LZ, Baroody RA, Miranda OC. Eicosanoids as a new class of ocular hypotensive agents: 1. The apparent therapeutic advantages of derived prostaglandins of the A and B as compared with the primary prostaglandins of the E, F and D type. *Exp Eye Res.* 1987;44:825.

109. Nilsson SFE, Stjernschantz J, Bill A. $PGF_2\alpha$ increases uveoscleral outflow. *Invest Ophthalmol Vis Sci* (suppl) 28:284, 1987.

110. Crawford K, Kaufman PL. Pilocarpine antagonizes prostaglandin $F_2\alpha$ induced ocular hypotension in monkeys. *Arch Ophthalmol* 105:1112, 1987.

111. Fristrom B, Nilsson SEG. Interaction of PhXA41, a new prostaglandin analogue, with pilocarpine. *Arch Ophthalmol* 111:662, 1993.

112. Villumsen J, Alm A. Effect of prostaglandin $F_2\alpha$ analogue PhXA41 in eyes treated with pilocarpine and timolol. *Invest Ophthalmol Vis Sci* 33(suppl): 1248,1992.

Chapter 4

ANATOMY AND PHYSIOLOGY OF THE OPTIC NERVE

Thomas L. Lewis
Joan Tanabe Wing

An understanding of the normal anatomy and physiology of the optic nerve is necessary to fully comprehend the histopathological changes that occur in this tissue due to abnormal levels of intraocular pressure. In addition, the clinician can better appreciate the clinical changes that appear in the optic nerve during the progression of glaucoma by having a strong foundation in the anatomy and physiology of this tissue. This chapter discusses the gross and microscopic anatomy and relevant physiology of the optic nerve, its blood supply, the process of axonal transport, and the clinical appearance and characteristics of the optic nerve and surrounding structures.

GROSS ANATOMY

The optic nerve is formed by ganglion cell axons and their accompanying glial cells. It extends from the retina through the posterior scleral foramen to the lateral geniculate body in the thalamus. The center of the optic nerve head is about 4 mm medial and 1 mm superior to the center of the macula. The optic nerve, for descriptive purposes, can be subdivided into various regions extending from its origin to the optic chiasm (Fig. 4–1). This chapter concentrates on the intraocular

and intraorbital portions, since they are most important to an understanding of glaucoma.

Intraocular Portion

The anterior limit of the intraocular portion of the optic nerve is the inner limiting membrane covering the optic nerve head, while the posterior limit is the back surface of the scleral lamina cribrosa (Fig. 4–2). The intraocular portion is subdivided into the surface nerve fiber layer—the prelaminar and laminar regions. Its length can vary but it is usually about 1 mm. The width of this portion of the optic nerve often increases from anterior to posterior, giving it a conical shape.

Intraorbital Portion

As the optic nerve extends beyond the posterior surface of the sclera and enters the orbit, several anatomical changes occur. The diameter of the nerve doubles compared to the intraocular portion, primarily owing to myelination of the ganglion cell axons and the covering of the nerve by meningeal sheaths (Fig. 4–2). The central retinal artery and vein run along the inferior lateral aspect of the nerve and pierce the meningeal sheaths to enter the nerve about 12 mm behind the eye (Fig. 4–3).

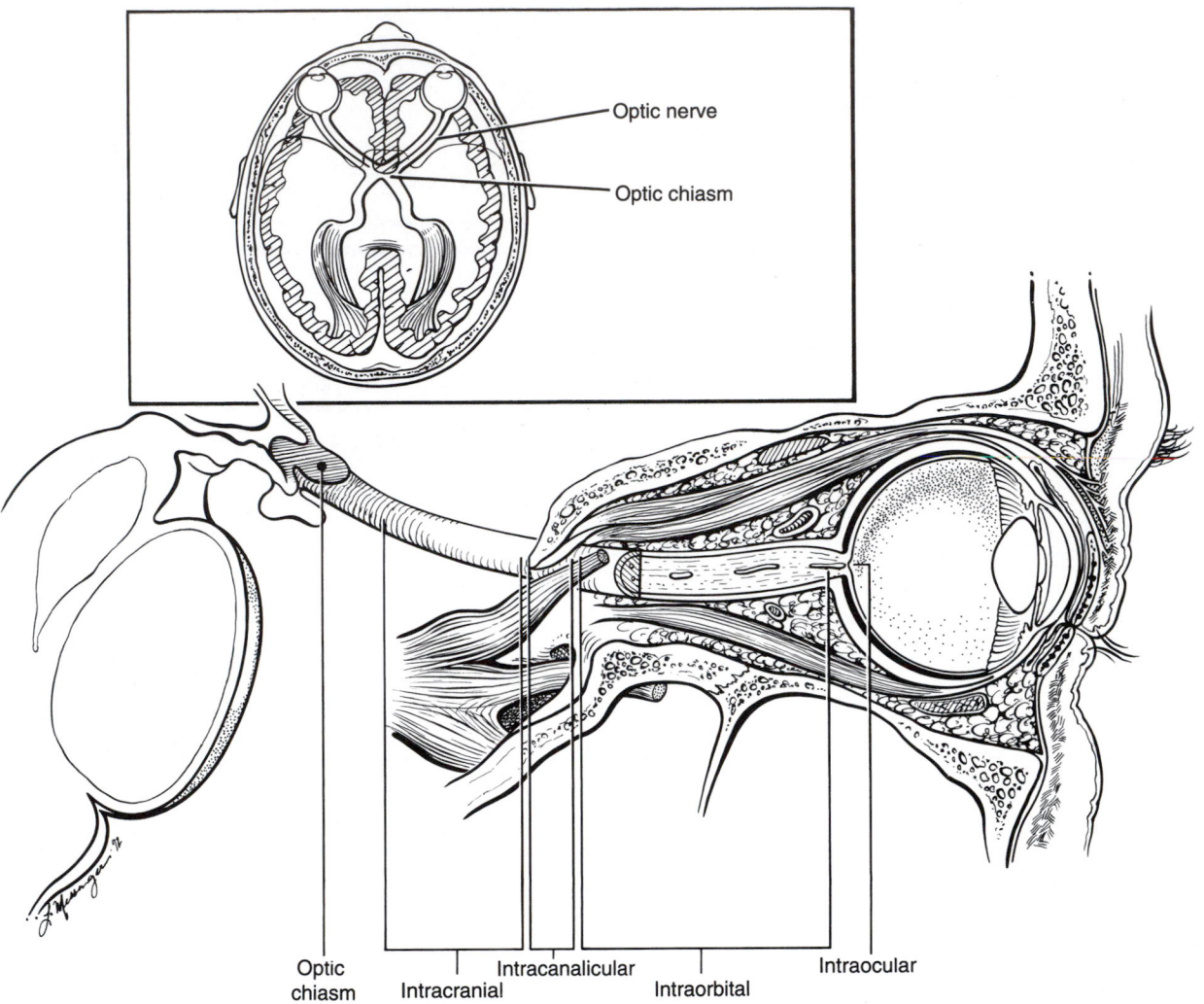

Figure 4–1. Schematic representation of the subdivisions of the optic nerve from its origin to the optic chiasm. Inset shows the intracranial course of the optic nerve to the lateral geniculate body.

MICROANATOMY

Intraocular Portion

Surface Nerve Fiber Layer

The nerve fiber layer of the retina comprises unmyelinated axons of retinal ganglion cells. It is supported by blood vessels and glial tissue that occupy about 5% of the volume of this layer.[1] The number of nerve fibers varies dramatically from individual to individual but is often estimated at about 1 million (700,000 to 1,250,000) per eye.[2-11] A possible reason for the great variability in the number of axons is the fact that, in mature adults, the number of axons results from an overproduction during the first half of gestation followed by elimination of approximately 70% of these fibers by the 16th through 30th weeks.[12] Elimi-

nation of axons occurs by apoptosis, a process of programmed cell death.[13] This type of developmental process can result in significant differences in the ultimate number of axons remaining in the adult eye.

There is debate as to whether or not a significant decrease in the number of ganglion cell axons occurs as a normal change of aging. Some studies have shown no loss of axons with age,[10,14] while others have shown a loss of axons ranging from approximately 500 to 5500 per year.[9,11,15] This becomes significant because most people who develop glaucoma are over the age of 60. If a larger number of axons are lost in the eyes of older individuals, they may be more susceptible to earlier loss of visual field from glaucoma, and the differentiation of a normal from an early glaucomatous nerve fiber layer and optic nerve may then be more difficult.[11]

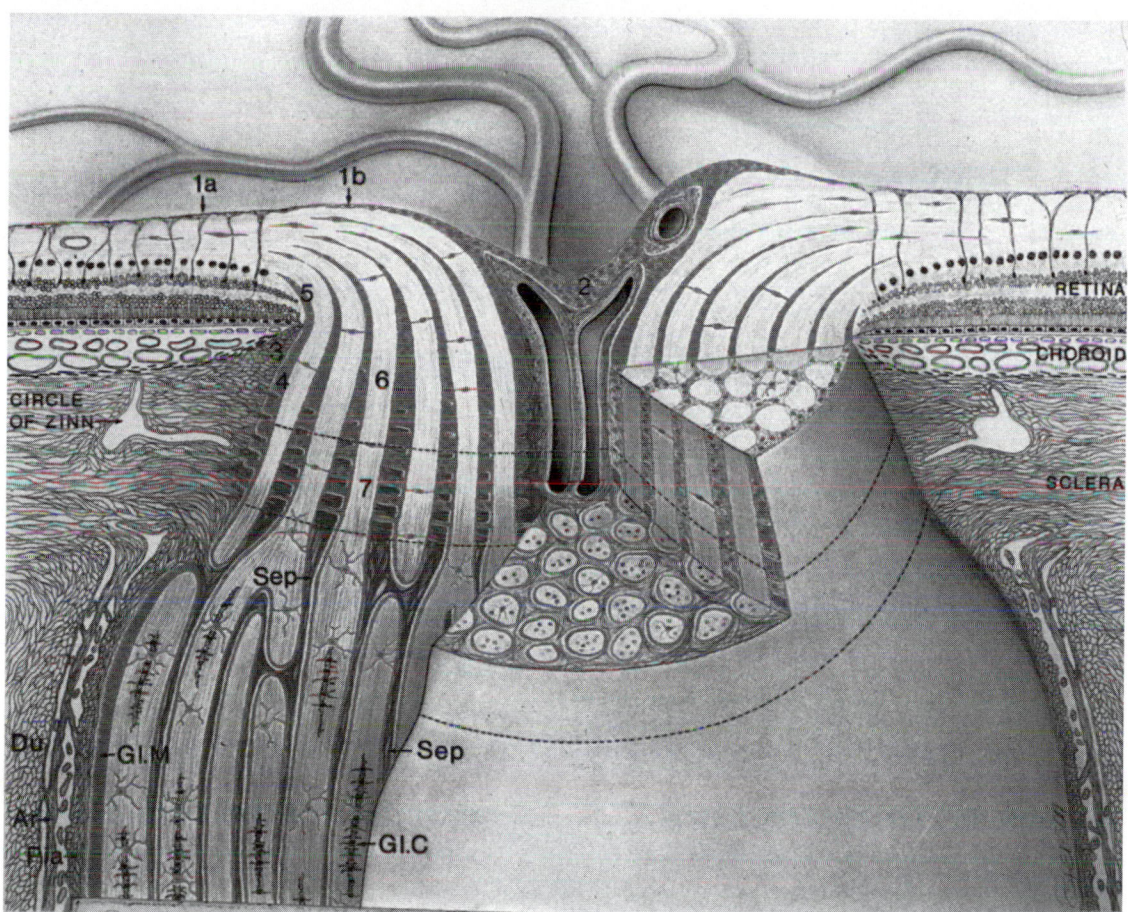

Figure 4-2. Three-dimensional drawing of the intraocular and part of the orbital optic nerve. The intraocular portion extends from the inner limiting membrane covering the optic nerve head to the back surface of the scleral lamina cribrosa. The nerve fibers of the retina (6) are separated into bundles by astrocytes. At the lamina cribrosa (*upper dotted line*), the nerve fascicles (7) and their surrounding astrocytes are separated from each other by the cribriform plate. At the external part of the lamina cribrosa (*lower dotted line*), the nerve fibers become myelinated and the diameter of the nerve doubles. Columns of oligodendrocytes (black and white cells) and a few astrocytes (red cells) can be seen within the the nerve fascicles. Other cells and regions include Muller cells (1a), internal limiting membrane of Elschnig (1b), central meniscus of Kuhnt (2), and border tissue of Elschnig (3). Astrocytes line the optic nerve canal (4) and glial tissue is found at the termination of the retina (5). Septal tissue (Sep), glial mantle (Gl.M), and the dura (Du), arachnoid (Ar), and pia mater (Pia) are shown. (Reproduced with permission from *Arch Ophthalmol.* 1969;82:506-530. Copyright 1969, American Medical Association.)

Ganglion cell axons converge on the optic nerve in an organized pattern (Fig. 4-4). Axons from the nasal, superior, and inferior retina have a relatively straight course. Axons arising in the temporal retina arc above or below the macular region and enter the superior temporal and inferior temporal portions of the optic nerve, respectively. Axons arising in the macular region pass directly to the temporal edge of the optic nerve, forming the papillomacular bundle.[16] Since the fovea is slightly inferior to the center of the optic nerve head, more axons enter the temporal side of the disc inferiorly than superiorly, making the neuroretinal rim slightly thicker inferiorly.[17] The density

of the axons is greatest in the papillomacular bundle; however, the greatest number of axons enter the superior and inferior poles of the optic nerve.

The ganglion cell axons arising in the temporal retina, arcing above or below the macular region, are known as *arcuate nerve bundles*. Ganglion cell axons, which are located in the temporal retina above an imaginary horizontal line passing through the macula, always enter the superior arcuate nerve fiber bundle, while axons located below this line always enter the inferior arcuate nerve fiber bundle. This creates the appearance of a horizontal raphe, temporal to the macula. This raphe is confined to temporal fibers

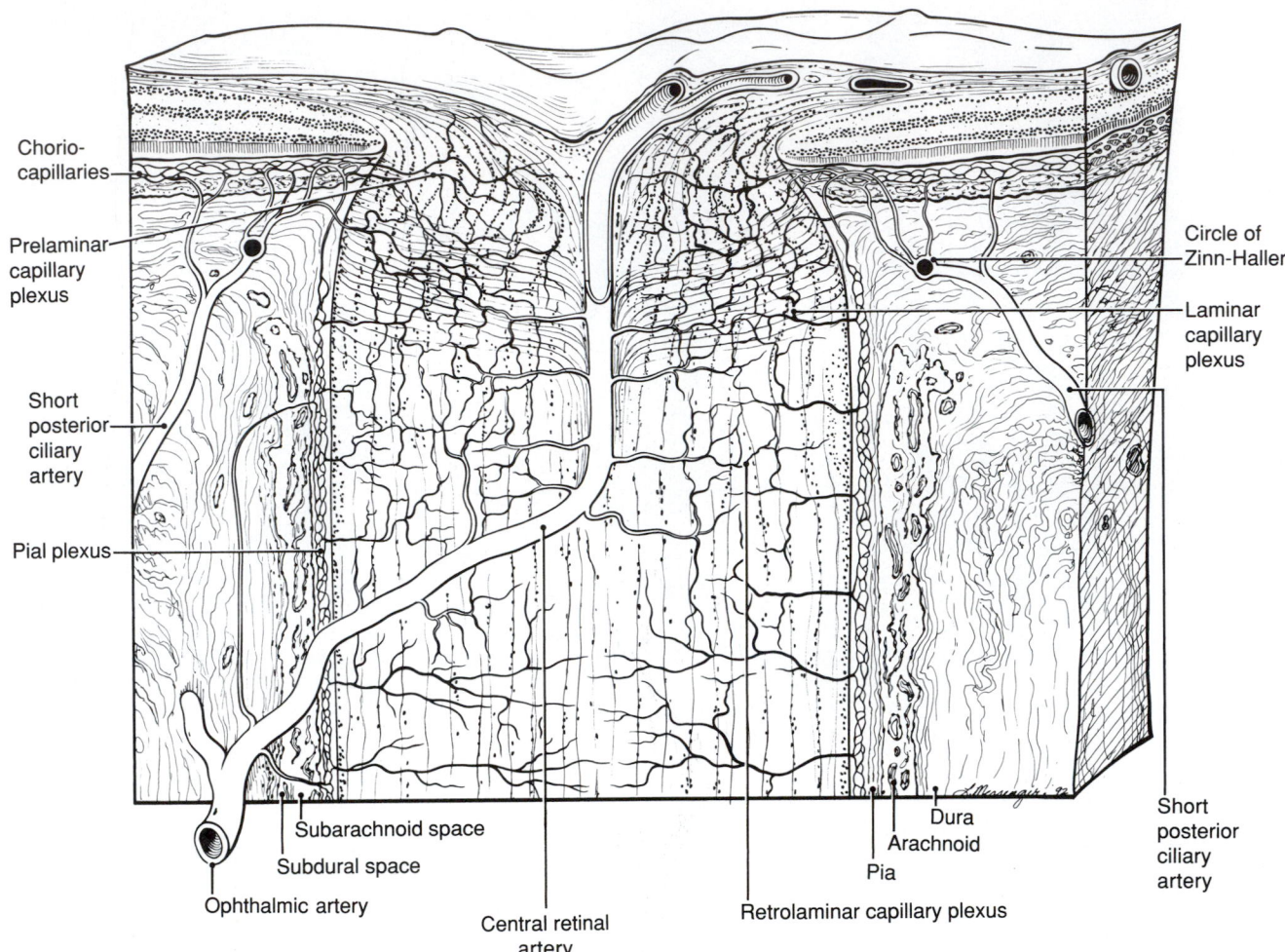

Chorio-
capillaries

Prelaminar
capillary
plexus

Short
posterior
ciliary
artery

Pial plexus

Circle of
Zinn-Haller

Laminar
capillary
plexus

Subarachnoid space

Subdural space

Ophthalmic artery

Central retinal
artery

Dura
Arachnoid

Pia

Retrolaminar capillary plexus

Short
posterior
ciliary
artery

Figure 4–3. Composite drawing of blood supply to the optic nerve. The central retinal artery, a branch of the ophthalmic artery, pierces the dura of the optic nerve. It sends branches to the central portion of the optic nerve and to the pial system of vessels. Transverse and longitudinal vessels emerge from the pia mater to supply the retrolaminar optic nerve. The laminar region receives its major centripetal blood supply from the circle of Zinn-Haller, which originates from the short posterior ciliary arteries. The prelaminar region is supplied by the short posterior ciliary arteries and by some centripetal branches from the peripapillary choroid. The nerve fiber layer receives its blood supply from branches of the central retinal artery and some choroidal vessels. Longitudinal capillary networks connect the laminar, prelaminar, and nerve fiber layer tissues.

making up the posterior pole region of the retina and does not include fibers arising from the temporal peripheral retina. Knowledge of the pattern created by the direction of ganglion cell axons from all parts of the retina is important in understanding the types of field defects seen in various types of retinal and optic nerve diseases, including glaucoma.

There is not only a topographical pattern to the axons of ganglion cells but also an organization relating to their depth within the nerve fiber layer based on the original location of the ganglion cell nucleus (see Fig. 4–4). Axons from the peripheral retina tend to run deeper in the nerve fiber layer and enter the outer edge of the neuroretinal rim of the optic nerve.

Axons from ganglion cells located closer to the posterior pole are more superficial in the nerve fiber layer and enter the optic nerve toward the inner edge of the neuroretinal rim.[16,18,19]

Ganglion cell axons can vary in thickness but average about 1 μm.[10,12] There may be a decrease in the density of axons of the optic nerve with age,[15] possibly due to a selective loss of thicker axons.[10]

Prelaminar Region of the Optic Nerve
The prelaminar region of the optic nerve is composed primarily of axons of ganglion cells along with their supporting glial tissue and blood vessels. It is located between the surface of the optic nerve

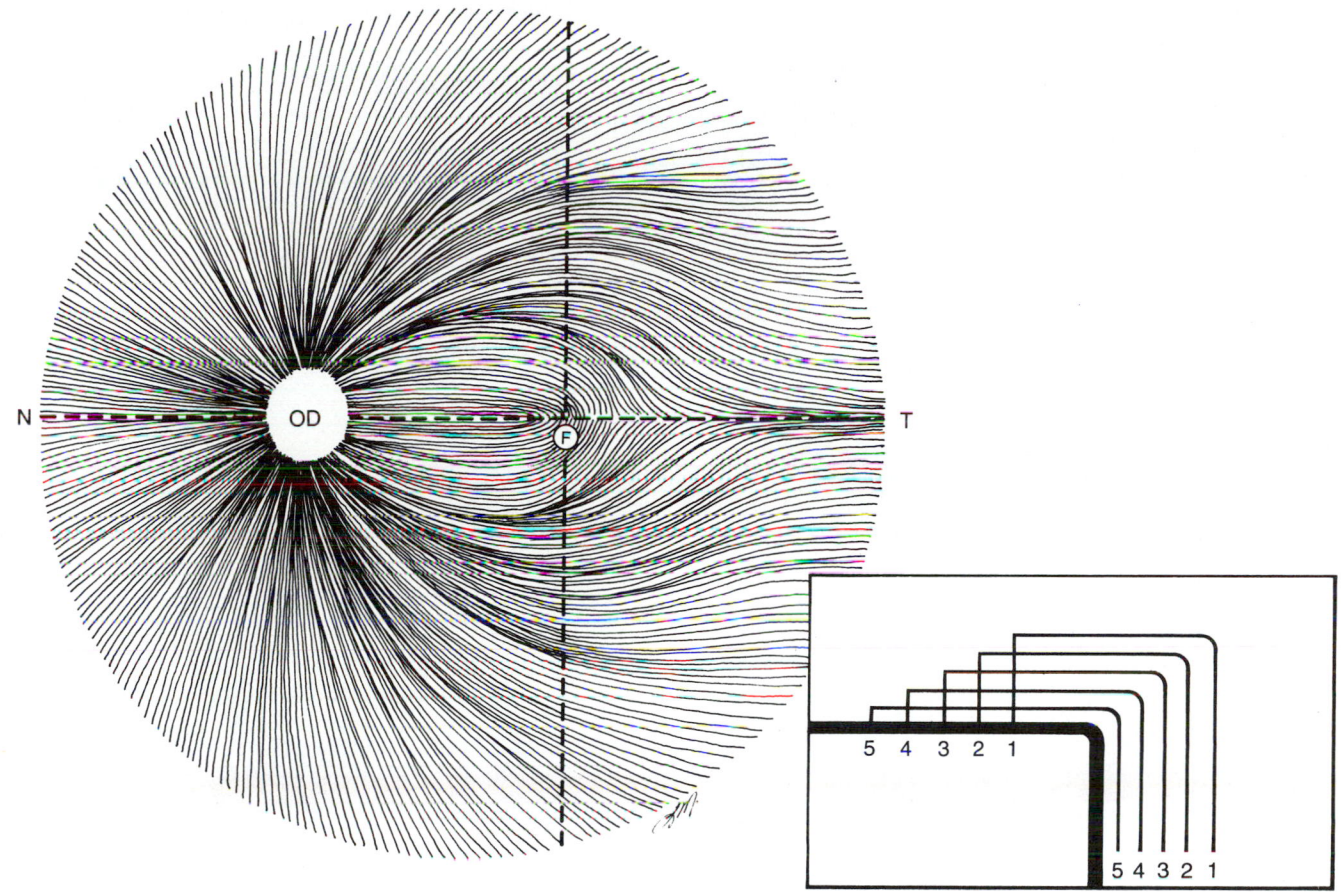

Figure 4–4. Drawing of the distribution of the retinal nerve fibers. Axons from the nasal, superior, and inferior retina have a relatively straight course. Axons arising in the temporal retina arc above or below the macular region. Axons from the macular region pass directly to the optic disc (OD) as the papillomacular bundle (P). Temporal to the fovea (F) is the horizontal raphe (R). N, nasal; T, temporal. *INSET:* Schematic drawing showing the relationship between ganglion cell axons in the retina and their position within the optic nerve. Axons from the peripheral retina run deeper in the nerve fiber layer and enter the outer edge of the neuroretinal rim. Axons originating closer to the posterior pole are more superficial in the nerve fiber layer and enter the optic nerve toward the inner edge of the neuroretinal rim. (Modified with permission from Hogan MJ, Alvarado JA, Weddell JE. *Histology of the Human Eye.* Philadelphia: WB Saunders; 1971:536.)

head and the anterior border of the scleral lamina cribrosa (Fig. 4–5).

The surface of the optic nerve, next to the vitreous, is covered by thin inner limiting membrane composed of glial cells and their accompanying basal lamina (see Fig. 4–5). At the edge of the optic nerve, this inner limiting membrane merges with the much thicker internal limiting membrane covering the surface of the retina. The outer edge of the prelaminar portion of the optic nerve is covered by a mantle of glial cells that abut against the retina, retinal pigment epithelium, and choroid (see Fig. 4–5).

As the approximately 1 million ganglion cell axons converge toward the optic nerve, they make a 90-degree turn to exit the eye through the posterior scleral foramen. As this turn is made, the axons become segregated into bundles or fasciculi by glial cells (Figs. 4–6 and 4–7; see Fig. 4–2). The exact number of fasciculi formed has been estimated from as few as several hundred to over a thousand.[16]

Glial cells, which are so apparent in the prelaminar region, are fibrous astrocytes. These cells make up about 50% of the volume of the prelaminar portion of the optic nerve[20] and participate in forming the inner limiting membrane covering the optic nerve as well as the thin mantle coat around the optic nerve and around and between the fasciculi or bundles of axons (see Figs. 4–2, 4–6, and 4–7). In a cross-section view of the prelaminar region, the fibrous astrocytes appear to surround the bundles of axons like tubes, both running perpendicular to the surface of the optic nerve head (see Figs. 4–6 and 4–7). These astro-

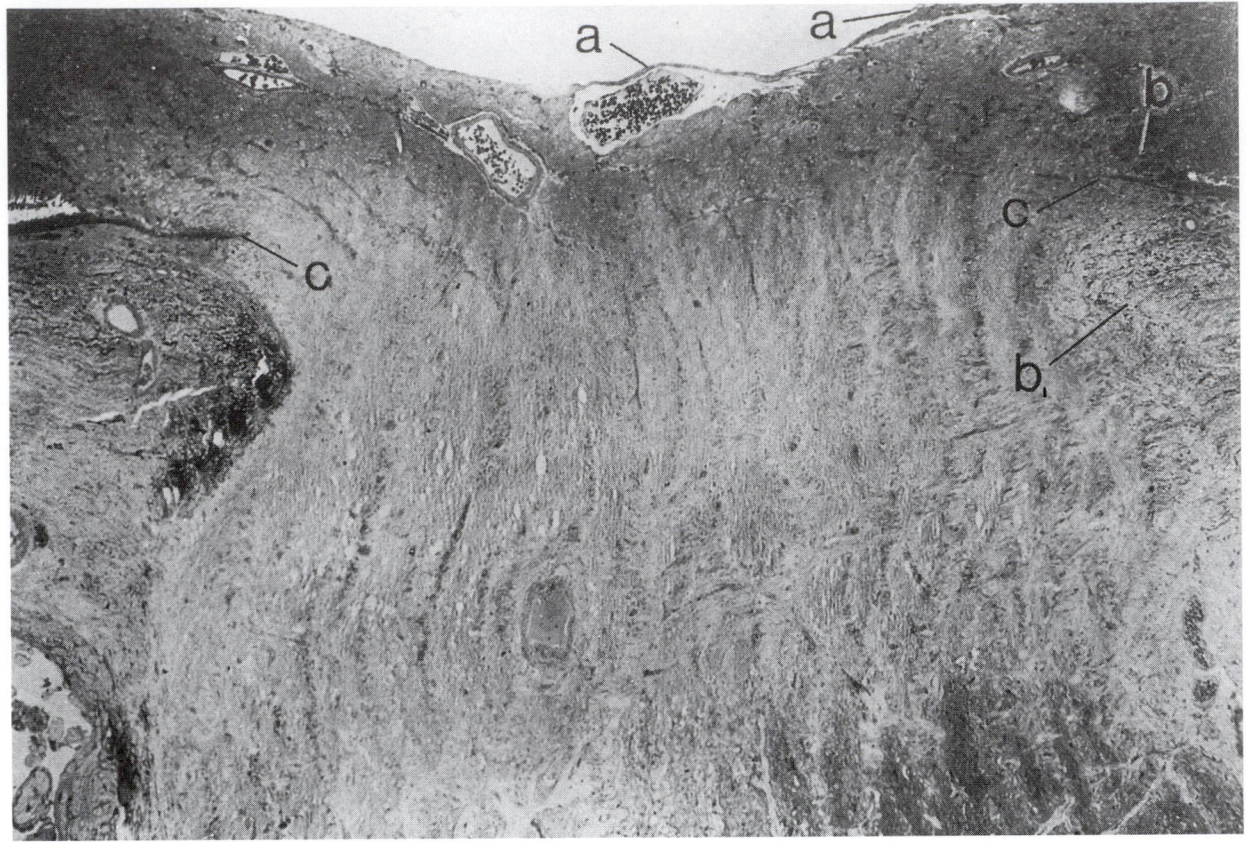

Figure 4–5. Light micrograph of the optic nerve near its anterior surface. The inner limiting membrane (a) is composed of glial tissue and forms the anterior border of the prelaminar optic nerve. A mantle of glial cells separates the nerve fiber layer from the adjacent retinal tissue (b) and the choroid (b₁). Bruch's membrane ends at (c). (Reproduced with permission from Hogan MJ, Alvarado JA, Weddell JE. *Histology of the Human Eye.* Philadelphia: WB Saunders; 1971:528.)

cytic tubes and their enclosed bundles of axons continue in this anatomic arrangement through the laminar and postlaminar regions of the optic nerve. Blood vessels supplying the nerve fiber bundles in this region are located in the glial septa found between the nerve fiber bundles (see Figs. 4–6 and 4–7).[20,21] Astrocytes often end as footplates on the blood vessels forming sheaths around them.

There is very little connective tissue in the form of collagen in the prelaminar region; that which is present is found as a thin covering around the blood vessels.[21] The blood vessels are made up of an endothelial cell lining that is continuous and nonfenestrated. The endothelial cells are connected by tight junctions (zonulae occludentes) and accompanied by pericytes and a basal lamina.[20,21]

The bundles of ganglion cell axons are confined to the outer portion of the prelaminar region of the optic nerve (see Fig. 4–2). This forms the neuroretinal rim seen clinically. The center of the prelaminar region does not contain axons but is occupied by additional fibrous astrocytes (see Fig. 4–2).

Laminar Region of the Optic Nerve

The lamina cribrosa, often called the *scleral lamina cribrosa*, represents a continuation of the inner two-thirds of the sclera across the posterior scleral foramen. It reinforces the posterior eye by forming scaffolding to support the nerve fiber bundles. The lamina cribrosa is made up of approximately 10 lamellae (sheets, trabeculae) of connective tissue,[22] which are separated from each other by fibrous astrocytes and fenestrated to allow for the passage of nerve fiber bundles carrying ganglion cell axons (see Figs. 4–2 and 4–7). The lamellae are anchored firmly at the periphery to the surrounding sclera, centrally to the connective tissue envelope of the central retinal vessels, and posteriorly to the septa of the retrolaminar optic nerve.[23, 24]

The anterior surface of the lamina cribrosa is shaped like a saddle, with the medial and temporal regions more anterior than the superior and inferior.[22,25] The center of the lamina cribrosa contains large openings for the passage of the central retinal artery and vein (Fig. 4–8). The central retinal vessels are surrounded by connective tissue and a layer of astrocytes and share a common adventitia at the level of the lamina cribrosa. Posteriorly, the lamellae become more prominent. The connective tissue septa from the postlaminar region of the optic nerve are attached to the posterior surface of the lamina cribrosa. The outer surface of the lamina cribrosa is separated from the sclera by a thin envelope of glial tissue.

The composition of the lamellae differs from that of the rest of the sclera. Each lamella is composed of a core of elastin fibers, a network of filamentous basement membranes, and sparse, patchy areas of type III collagen.[26] In addition, type IV collagen is distributed in the margin of the cribriform plates.[27,28] Capillaries supplying the lamina cribrosa are found within these sheets of connective tissue. They are similar to blood vessels in the prelaminar region with a continuous endothelial cell lining with tight junctions and pericytes (see Fig. 4–11). The lamellae are coated on both sides with collagen, laminin, and fibrous astrocytes.

Collagen fibrils are found in small amounts in the anterior lamina cribrosa, usually limited to the area surrounding blood vessels. In contrast, collagen fibers are a prominent feature of the posterior (scleral) portion.[29] The combination of elastin and collagen provides tensile strength and allows that region of the eye to resist distortion and potentially recover its original shape if compressed.[26,28]

The lamellae contain approximately 200 to 600 fenestra or pores.[22] A wide variation is noted in the diameter of the pores, ranging from 10 to 250 μm (Fig. 4-9; see Fig. 4–8).[22,29,30] The pores are greater in number and

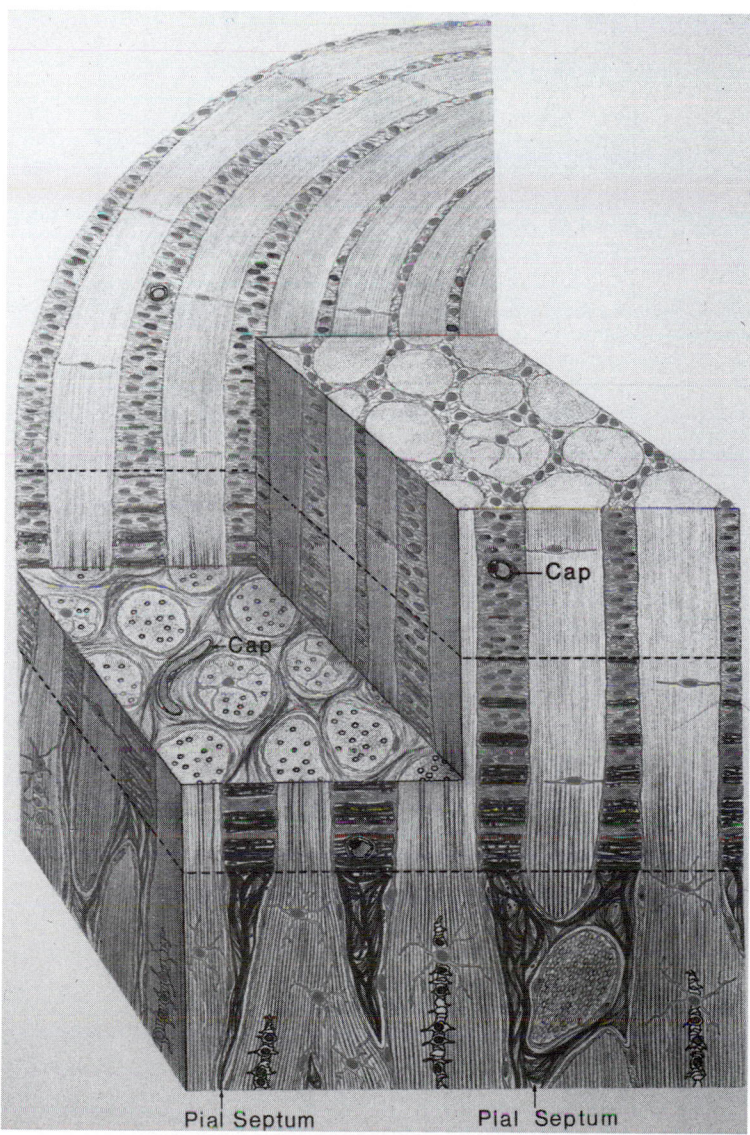

Figure 4–6. Detailed view of the prelaminar, laminar, and post laminar optic nerve. Astrocytes separate the nerve fibers into bundles. Capillaries (Cap) are seen within these astrocytic columns. The lamina cribrosa is present between the dotted lines. The connective tissue of the lamina cribrosa is continuous posteriorly with the pial septa. Nerve fibers become myelinated in the postlaminar region. (Reproduced with permission from *Arch Ophthalmol.* 1969; 82:800–814. Copyright 1969, American Medical Association.)

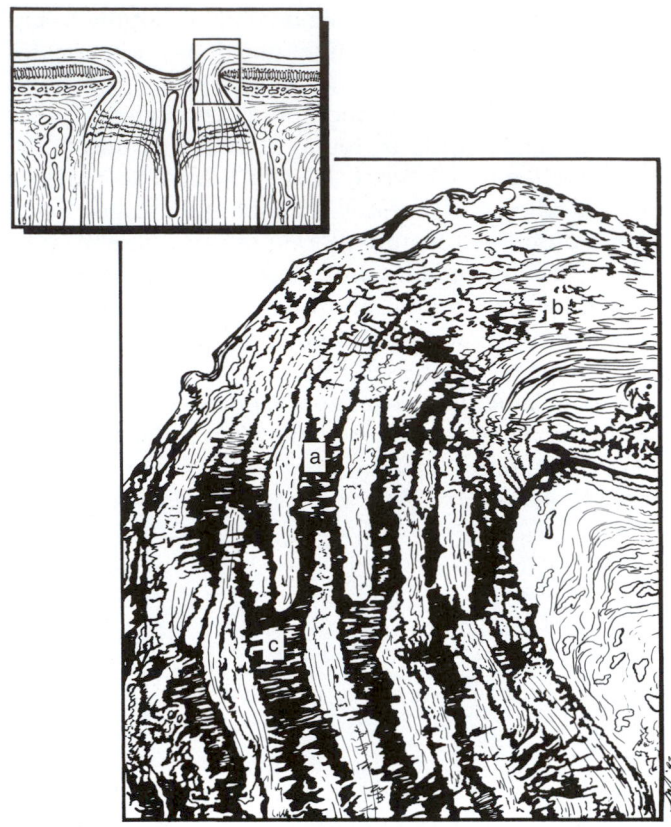

Figure 4–7. Drawing of the prelaminar portion of the optic nerve. Glial columns (a) arrange the ganglion cell axons (b) into bundles. The lamina cribrosa (c) is fenestrated to allow the nerve fiber bundles to exit the eye. (Modified with permission from Hogan MJ, Alvarado JA, Weddell JE. *Histology of the Human Eye.* Philadelphia: WB Saunders; 1971:540.)

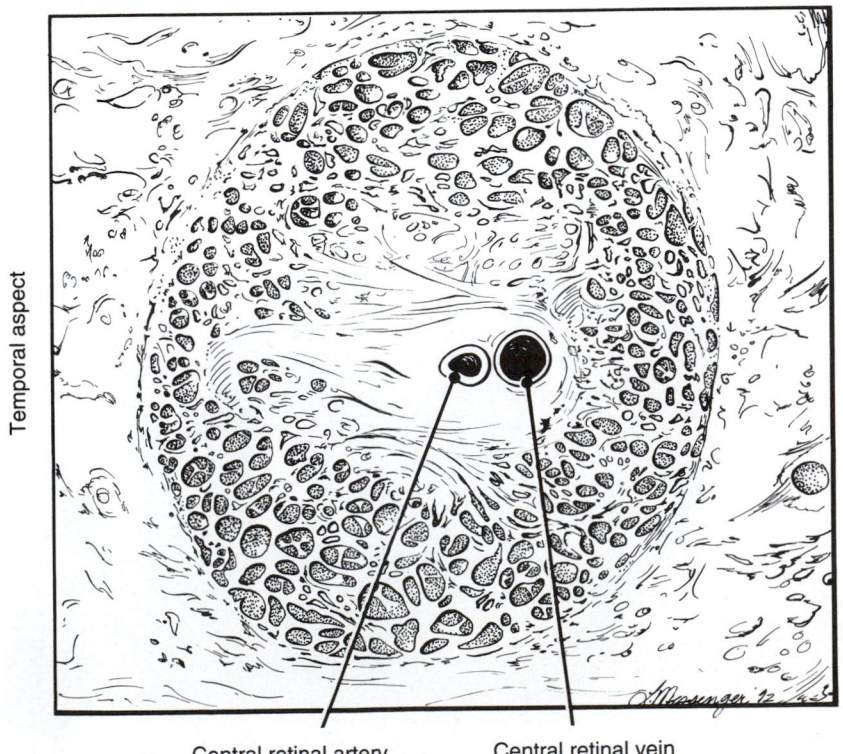

Temporal aspect

Nasal aspect

Central retinal artery   Central retinal vein

Figure 4–8. Drawing of the cross-sectional view of the lamina cribrosa shows the central retinal artery and vein. Pore size is larger in the superior and inferior region than in the nasal or temporal region.

larger in size in the lamellae located more anteriorly. Although some pores appear to branch and divide, creating a labyrinth, pores through which a specific bundle of ganglion cell axons pass are generally aligned in successive lamellae (see Figs. 4–8 and 4–9).

Pores in the superior and inferior poles of each lamella are larger and less supported by surrounding connective tissue than in the nasal or temporal regions[22,25,31] (see Fig. 4–8). Also, there is increased complexity of axonal channels superiorly and inferiorly. This may make these areas more susceptible to distortion from an increase in intraocular pressure.[22,32,33]

There does not appear to be a decrease in the number of pores with age. However, the proportion of the optic nerve occupied by pores does decrease with age, probably due to a loss of ganglion cell axons. The space created by a loss of axons is usually filled with connective tissue.[22,28,34]

The pores in each lamella are lined by fibrous astrocytes. Nuclei of the astrocytes are arranged around the edges of the pores but can also be found in the center of the larger pores. Processes extending from the astrocytes form the borders of the pores. In addition, similar astrocytic processes extend across the pores, creating an intricate meshwork that separates the axons of the optic nerve into bundles of varying size. In the posterior portion of the lamina cribrosa, astrocytic processes, surrounded by basement membrane, are embedded within the collagenous lamellae.[29] The close association between axons, astrocytic processes, and lamellae emphasizes the role of astrocytes and their meshwork in the mechanical and metabolic support of optic nerve axons.[29]

Intraorbital (Postlaminar) Portion

Posterior to the scleral lamina cribrosa, the optic nerve leaves the eye and becomes intraorbital. The axons of the ganglion cells become myelinated, and meningeal sheaths cover the surface of the optic nerve (see Fig. 4–2). At the optic foramen, the meninges are continuous with the intracranial meningeal covering of the nerve. Anteriorly, the connective tissue components of the meninges blend with the outer layers of the sclera. The outer meningeal coat, the dura mater, is composed of dense connective tissue and fibroblasts, with mesothelial cells (meningothelium) lining its inner surface (Fig. 4–10). Collagen and elastic tissue is prominent in the dura mater.[35] Beneath the dura is a potential subdural space separating the dura mater from the arachnoid (see Fig. 4–10).[35] The arachnoid consists of several layers of meningothelial cells and a network of collagen bundles and some elastic fibers. The subarachnoid space is located between the inner surface of the arachnoid and the outer surface of the pia mater (see Fig. 4–10). Within the subarachnoid space is cerebrospinal fluid and trabeculae or columns of collagen that connect the pia mater to the arachnoid. These trabeculae contain blood vessels and are covered by

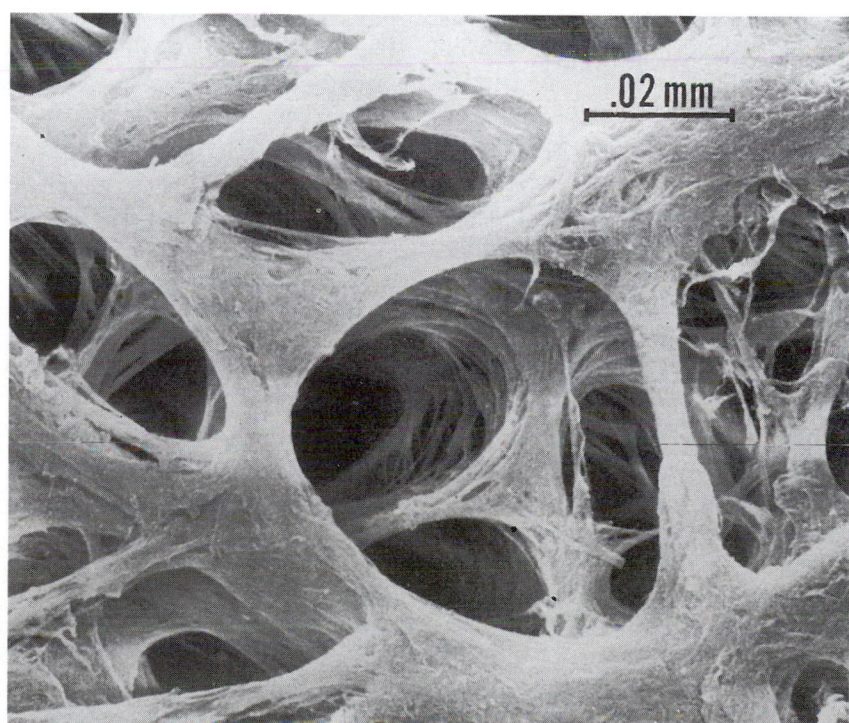

Figure 4–9. Scanning electron micrograph shows enlarged cross-sectional view of the lamina cribrosa. The lamellae of connective tissue contain fenestrations or pores to allow for the passage of nerve fiber bundles. (Reproduced with permission from Emery JM, Landis D, Paton D, Bonisk M, Craig JM. The lamina cribrosa in normal and glaucomatous human eyes. *Trans Am Acad Ophthalmol Otolaryngol.* 1974;78:290–297.)

.02 mm

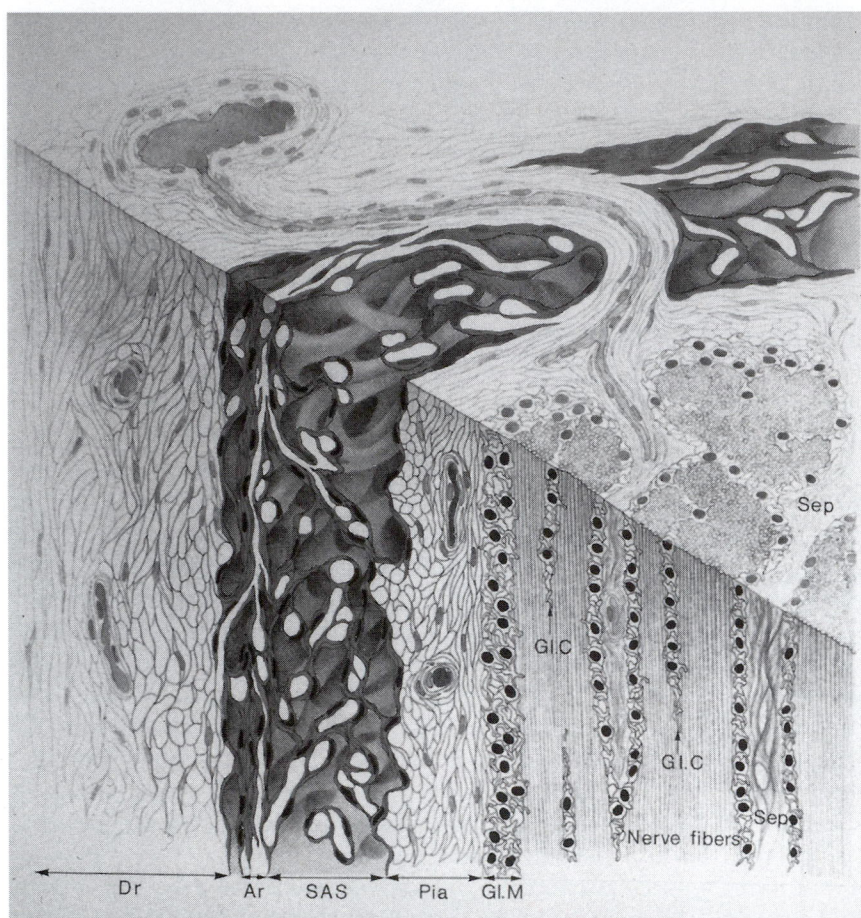

Figure 4–10. Photograph of vaginal sheaths of optic nerve, showing relationship between dura mater (Dr), arachnoid mater (Ar), subarachnoid space (SAS), and pia mater (Pia). Meningothelial cells contribute to the arachnoid mater and form linings for the dura mater, arachnoid trabeculae, and pia mater. The inner surface of the pia mater is separated from the intraorbital portion of the optic nerve by a layer of fibrous astrocytes, forming the glial mantle (Gl.M) and glial columns (Gl.C). Elements from the pia mater form the pial septae (sep), which enclose the axonal bundles. The septae originate in the posterior lamina cribrosa, continue through the orbital and intracanalicular portions, and end in the intracranial portion of the optic nerve. (Reproduced with permission from Anderson DR. Ultrastructure of meningeal sheaths. *Arch Ophthalmol.* 1969;82:659–674. Copyright 1969, American Medical Association.)

meningothelium. In fact, the entire subarachnoid space is lined by meningothelial cells (Fig. 4–10).[35]

The innermost component of the meninges is the pia mater. It is mostly connective tissue with some elastic fibers, and its outer surface is covered by meningothelium (see Fig. 4–10). The pia mater is highly vascularized, containing capillaries with continuous, nonfenestrated endothelial cells. The inner surface of the pia mater is separated from the intraorbital portion of the optic nerve by a layer of fibrous astrocytes (see Fig. 4–10).

From the under surface of the pia mater, connective tissue extends inward to form longitudinal septa, which additionally separate ganglion cell axons into bundles (see Fig. 4–2). Each bundle is still surrounded by fibrous astrocytes, as was true in the prelaminar and laminar regions (see Fig. 4–10). The pial septa, in addition to separating the nerve fiber bundles, also provide a pathway for blood vessels and nerves into the substance of the intraorbital portion of the optic nerve (see Figs. 4–2 and 4–10). The septa are attached to the pia mater, to the connective tissue that surrounds the central retinal vessels lo-cated centrally within the optic nerve, and to the posterior surface of the scleral lamina cribrosa.[23,24]

Meningothelial cells, which are so prominent within the meninges, resemble fibroblasts in their structure and function and are held together at many locations by desmosomes and some tight junctions.[35] A second type of glial cell, oligodendroglia, is also found in the intraorbital portion of the optic nerve and is responsible for the formation of myelin.

BLOOD SUPPLY

An understanding of the blood supply to the optic nerve is extremely important because ischemia from vascular insufficiency is considered a likely contributing factor to the damage occurring from glaucoma.[23,24,32,36,37]

There is tremendous interindividual variation in the blood supply to each specific portion of the optic nerve.[23,24,36,37] Not even both eyes in the same patient have similar vascular patterns. Therefore it is difficult to draw precise conclusions regarding the anatomic pattern and subsequent physiological impact that might result from the compression of a specific vessel in a given individual.

The blood supply to the optic nerve comes from one to five posterior ciliary arteries and the central retinal artery arising from the ophthalmic artery (see Fig. 4–3). Usually, two to three posterior ciliary arteries are distributed on the medial or lateral side of the optic nerve. The posterior ciliary arteries form both long and short posterior ciliary arteries. Each posterior ciliary artery is an end-artery system, supplying a specific territory of tissue with no anastomoses between vessels.[37,38] A watershed area is thus created at the outer edges of the territory supplied by adjacent posterior ciliary arteries and their major branches (Fig. 4–11). The watershed region for an individual with a medial and lateral posterior ciliary artery may be found anywhere between the nasal edge of the optic nerve and the fovea (see Fig. 4–11).[23,24,37,38] This individual variation may influence the relative susceptibility of the optic nerve to potential damage from an increase in intraocular pressure.

Nerve Fiber Layer

The nerve fiber layer is supplied by branches of the central retinal artery (see Fig. 4–3), with venous drainage

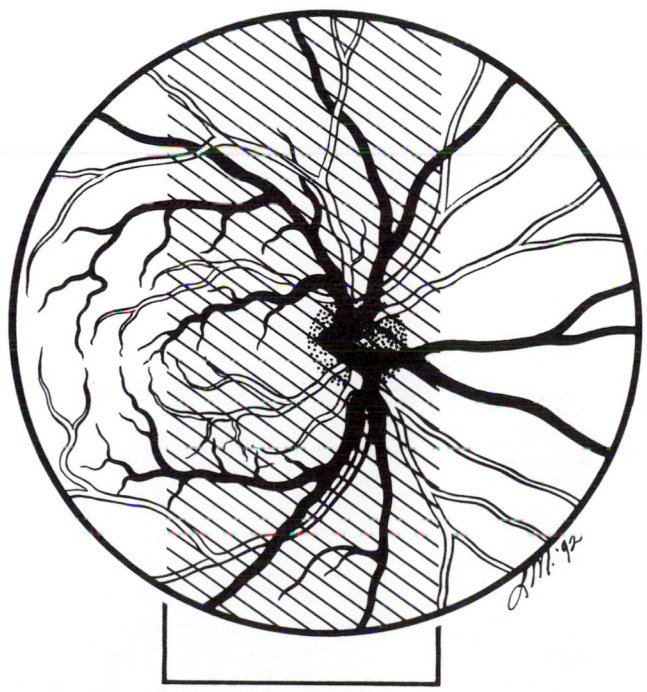

Figure 4–11. Drawing of the vasculature of the posterior pole. The shaded region represents the potential watershed area for an individual with a medial and lateral posterior ciliary artery.

Watershed zone

into the central retinal vein. There is a continuous capillary network from the level of the surface nerve fiber layer back through the postlaminar region of the optic nerve (see Fig. 4–3).[23,24] Capillaries on the surface of the optic nerve are also continuous with those in the peripapillary retina.[23,24,39,40] Some choroidal vessels may contribute to the blood supply of the nerve fiber layer, especially on the temporal side of the optic nerve head (see Fig. 4–3).[23,24] If these are large in diameter, a cilioretinal vessel becomes apparent.[36]

Prelaminar Portion

The prelaminar portion of the optic nerve receives its blood supply from centripetal branches of the peripapillary choroid (see Fig. 4–3).[23,24] These branches arise from short posterior ciliary arteries and have a segmental (sectoral) distribution.[23,24,36] No anastomoses exist between vessels supplying the optic nerve and the choriocapillaris at this level. Longitudinal capillary networks connect the tissues of the laminar, prelaminar, and nerve fiber layers[23,24,40] (see Fig. 4–3). The peripapillary choriocapillaris and central retinal artery play no role in the blood supply to this area.[23,24] The temporal portion of the prelaminar region may be more vascularized than other areas.[36] Capillaries from the prelaminar region drain into the central retinal vein or through the choroid into vortex veins.

Laminar Portion

The laminar region contains both a centripetal (transverse) system of vessels located within the lamellae and a longitudinal system of capillaries interconnecting the various regions of the optic nerve[23,24,36,40,41] (see Fig. 4–3). Although some centripetal vessels arise from pia mater arterioles, the major centripetal supply is from the circle of Zinn-Haller (see Figs. 4–2 and 4–3). This vascular complex is formed by an anastomosis within the sclera, just outside the optic nerve, of branches of adjacent short posterior ciliary arteries. In most individuals, this vascular circle is incomplete.

The central retinal artery does not contribute appreciably to the blood supply in the prelaminar or laminar regions.[23,24] The venous drainage of the lamina cribrosa is primarily into the central retinal vein.

Intraorbital (Postlaminar) Region

Blood supply to the postlaminar region is more complex than in other portions of the optic nerve (see Fig. 4-3). It consists of one network of vessels supplying the periphery of the nerve and another supplying the central or axial portion.[40] The peripheral portion is supplied by branches from the pia mater's vascular plexus. This plexus is formed by branches from muscular arteries, the ophthalmic artery, and recurrent branches from the peripapillary choroid and the circle of Zinn-Haller (see Fig. 4–3). These vessels enter the substance of the optic nerve through the pial septa. They anastomose freely within this portion of the optic nerve and extend forward as a continuous capillary network to more anterior regions of the optic nerve.[23,24]

The central retinal artery contributes small branches to the central or axial portion of the postlaminar region of the optic nerve (see Fig. 4–3).[23,24] Venous drainage from the postlaminar region is into the central retinal vein.

In summary, there are both centripetal (transverse) and longitudinal blood vessel systems in all portions of the optic nerve. Short posterior ciliary arteries contribute to some extent to the blood supply of all portions of the optic nerve, whereas the branches of the central retinal arteries supply only the nerve fiber layer and the axial portion of the postlaminar region. The longitudinal system of blood supply is continuous from the postlaminar region through to the nerve fiber layer.[23,24]

PHYSIOLOGY OF THE OPTIC NERVE

Axonal Transport

An increase in intraocular pressure can ultimately damage the axons of the ganglion cells, leading to clinically visible changes in the optic nerve and surrounding nerve fiber layer of the retina. As discussed in Chapter 5, on the etiology and pathophysiology of glaucoma, damage to ganglion cell axons appears to occur at the level of the scleral lamina cribrosa by a blockage of axonal transport.[1,22,32] Therefore, in order to provide a more complete picture of glaucoma, the concept of axonal transport must be discussed.

Cells throughout the body must be able to transport material within their cytoplasm to all areas of the cell. This becomes especially important in cells such as nerve cells, with long cytoplasmic extensions. The axon of a neuron is the cytoplasmic extension from the cell body that usually transmits impulses through synapses to other neurons or effector tissues (Fig. 4–12). Axons of neurons can be extremely long; for example, some

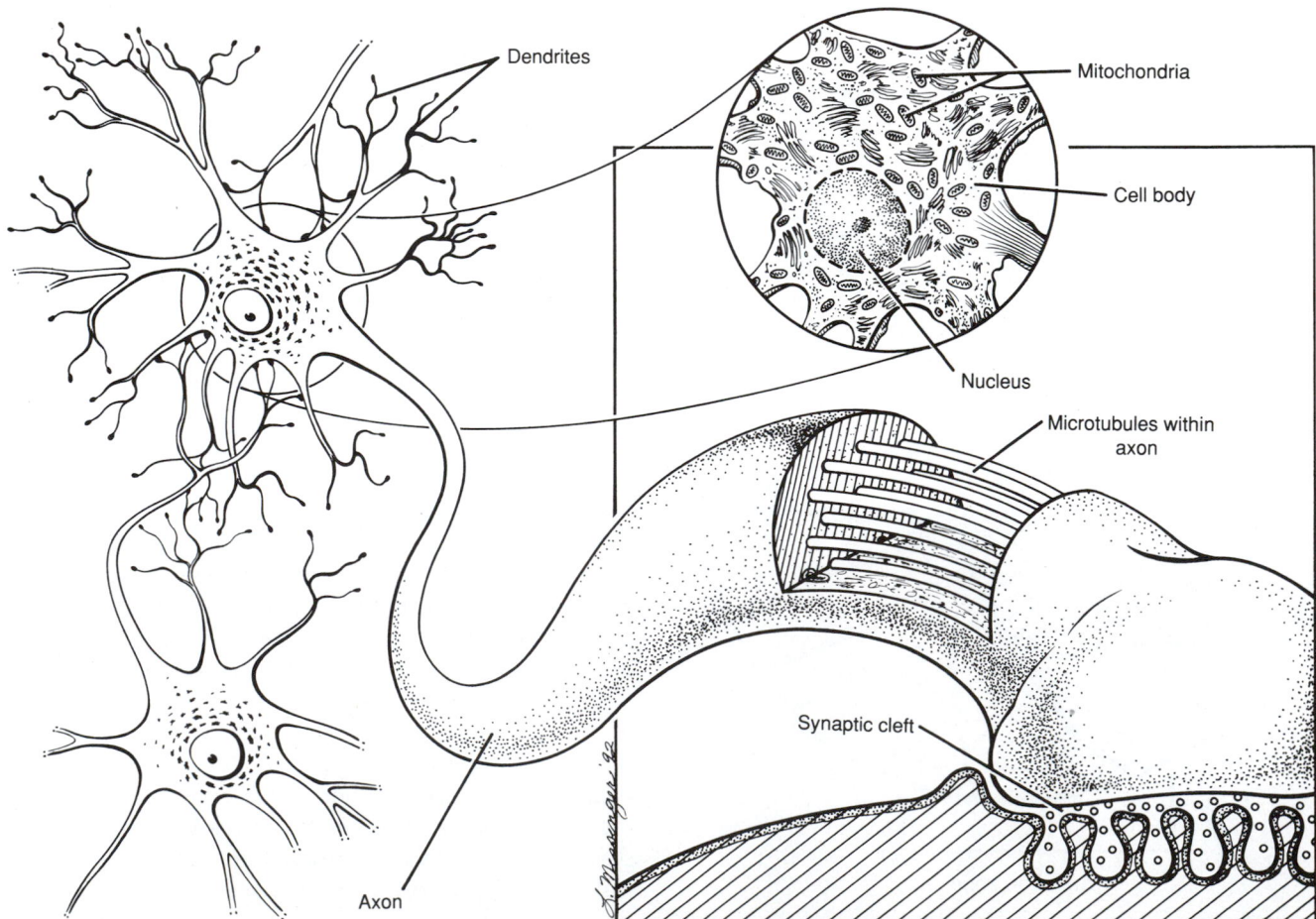

Figure 4–12. Schematic drawing showing the main components of a neuron. Axons contain microtubules and can synapse with effector tissues or other neurons. Inset shows the cell body of the neuron with its mitochondria and nucleus.

nerve cells located in the lumbar region of the spine send axons down as far as the foot. The difficulty in moving intracellular material along the axon is that the axonal extension does not contain many of the organelles found within the cytoplasm of the cell body. Axons of neurons, including those of the ganglion cell of the retina, contain only mitochondria, smooth endoplasmic reticulum, fine filaments (6 to 7 nm), and microtubules (20 to 25 nm) (see Fig. 4–12).[16,21] Consequently, intracellular substances and material necessary to sustain the axon and supply its synapse must be transported from the manufacturing source in the cell body down the axon to the synaptic junction. Conversely, by-products of metabolism from the axon must be transported back to the nerve cell body for digestion and, in some cases, removal from the nerve cell.

The process of moving material back and forth is known as *axonal transport*. It is an energy-dependent process that is essential for the survival of the axon and therefore of the nerve cell. Material moving from the nerve cell to the synaptic end of the axon is considered axonal transport in an anterograde (orthograde) direction. Anterograde axonal transport can occur slowly (0.5 to 3 mm per day)[42] or quickly (200 to 1000 mm per day).[43] Slow anterograde axonal transport is believed to occur through peristaltic action of the axon's cell membrane. It primarily serves the function of maintaining and assisting in the growth of the axon. Fast anterograde axonal transport uses the microtubular elements within the axon as "railroad tracks" to move material from the cell body to supply the synaptic end.

Retrograde axonal transport moves material from the synapse back to the cell body at a rate of approximately 50 to 250 mm per day.[43] It also uses microtubules as conduits.

Clearly, microtubules play an essential role in both orthograde and retrograde axonal transport. Compression of an axon resulting in crushing, distorting, or bending of the microtubules can result in the blockage of axonal transport and ultimately death of the nerve cell. Since axonal transport is an energy-dependent process, an adequate supply of oxygen is also essential to maintain the transport systems. A reduction in blood supply to the nerve cell or any portion of the axon to a level that results in ischemia can also block axonal transport and lead to death of the nerve cell.

Therefore, blockage of axonal transport can occur through mechanical compression of the axon, which disrupts the microtubules, or by a reduction in blood supply, which reduces the availability of the energy necessary to maintain these transport systems. Glaucoma, ocular hypotony, and papilledema are some examples of ocular conditions that may have the blockage of axonal transport as their pathophysiological basis.

Ganglion Cell Types

There is an increasing use of electrodiagnostic testing, including contrast sensitivity tests, pattern electroretinography, and testing of visual evoked potentials for the early diagnosis of glaucoma. To understand the psychophysical changes observed in glaucoma, it is necessary to appreciate how the visual system functions.

Retinal ganglion cells can be categorized into a variety of classes based on anatomical, physiological, or psychophysical criteria (Table 4–1). The different functional properties of these classes of ganglion cells are preserved throughout the visual pathway from the retina to the primary visual cortex and extrastriate regions. Although there is probably some overlap in functional characteristics and a mixing of the pathways at higher visual centers, parallel pathways do exist for visual processing.

P System

The P-ganglion cells represent 80%[44] of the ganglion cells of the retina and are concentrated primarily in the fovea.[45] They are small in size, becoming larger toward the periphery of the retina.[46] These cells project to the parvocellular layers (3 through 6) of the dorsolateral geniculate nucleus (dLGN).[47] Through thinly myelinated axons, the parvocellular layers of the dLGN project primarily to layer 4C beta of the visual cortex and on to layers II and III.[46,47] From here, connections are made with a variety of areas including the caudal portion of the inferior temporal cortex.

TABLE 4–1. COMPARISON OF P-GANGLION CELLS AND M-GANGLION CELLS

	P-System	M-System
Ganglion cell population	80%	10%
Projection to lateral geniculate nucleus	Parvocellular layers	Magnocellular layers
Distribution	Fovea	Throughout retina
Size	Small	Large
Myelination	Thin	Thick
Conduction velocity	Slow	Fast
Receptive field	Small	Large
Type of stimuli	Sustained	Transient
Spatial frequency	High	Low
Function	Central visual acuity	Location of visual stimulus
	Color vision	Gross figure-to-ground configuration
		High temporal resolution

M System

The M-ganglion cells make up 10% of the ganglion cells and are distributed evenly through the retina.[46] They have large cell bodies and axons and they increase in size toward the periphery of the retina. These cells project to the magnocellular layers (1 and 2) of the dLGN.[47] The magnocellular layers project through thickly myelinated axons primarily to layer 4C alpha and on to area 3 of the visual cortex.[46,47] From here, connections are made to a variety of extrastriate areas including the posterior parietal cortex.

Physiological Responses

The P system contains cells with smaller receptive fields than the M system. The M system responds best to luminance changes that extend across larger areas of the retina. P cells respond primarily to sustained stimuli, while the M cells respond primarily in a transient manner when a light is turned on or off.[46,48,49] Although there is considerable overlap in the spatial characteristics of the two parallel systems, the M system responds best to lower spatial frequency and also mediates contrast thresholds at lower and intermediate spatial frequency. It has a 10 times higher contrast sensitivity than the P system through many spatial frequencies.[50] Because of the larger axons, the M system conducts impulses more quickly than the P system, and also responds more briskly, with a shorter visual latency. Combining these two facts and a superior temporal sensitivity, the M system is most likely involved with high temporal resolution or critical luminance flicker fusion.[46,51]

The P system responds best to higher spatial frequencies and poorly to higher temporal frequencies; it is therefore believed to be the system involved with central visual acuity.[46] It does not respond at scotopic and low mesopic levels.[48] The P system is involved, however, in color vision, with 90% of the cells in the P system possessing chromatic opponency.[49]

It seems that the M-cell pathway is most responsive to coarse visual form that is modulated or moving at a fast rate and thereby provides gross information of the figure-to-ground configuration and location of a visual stimulus. This information serves to guide the processing of the P-cell pathway by generating positional information for foveation. The P system, then, determines the color and detail of the visual stimulus.[46] There is significant histological, physiological, and psychophysical evidence pointing to the early involvement of the M-cell pathway in glaucoma.[46,52] Damage to larger axons[52,53] and changes in pattern electroretinograms and pattern visual evoked potentials found in glaucoma are all consistent with M-cell involvement and decrease of low-to-

middle spatial frequencies of contrast sensitivity.[54,55] The largest of the P cells constituting the blue cone system may be destroyed in glaucoma earlier than smaller P cells.[52] This may help explain the color vision loss of the blue-green or blue-yellow hues that occurs in some glaucoma patients.[56]

CLINICAL APPEARANCE OF THE NORMAL OPTIC NERVE AND SURROUNDING TISSUE

The interpretation of subtle changes in the optic nerve is critical to the early diagnosis of glaucoma. In order to appreciate these early changes, it is essential to understand the normal appearance of the optic nerve and surrounding tissue. Unfortunately, it is sometimes difficult to differentiate normal from abnormal optic nerves clinically. This is due in large part to the tremendous variation that occurs in the tissue of the optic nerve and therefore in the clinical presentation of the structure. In describing the clinical appearance of the optic nerve and surrounding tissue, it is necessary to discuss the optic disc, the neuroretinal rim, the cup, the parapapillary tissue, and the retinal nerve fiber layer.

Optic Disc

The size of the optic disc is determined by the opening in the back of the eye, the posterior scleral foramen, through which the optic nerve exits the eye. The size of this opening varies greatly in healthy eyes, with a mean area of approximately 1.6 mm^2 but a range from 0.68 to 4.42 mm^2.[57] Therefore, there is a difference of about 6.5 times between the area of the smallest and that of the largest posterior scleral foramen in normal individuals.

The optic disc itself shows similar variation. The edge of the optic disc is usually defined clinically by a thin white rim, the peripapillary scleral ring, which represents a flange of sclera separating the choroid from the optic nerve head tissue. This scleral ring is sometimes obscured by the thick layer of nerve fibers that crosses over the edge of the optic disc. Various studies have shown the optic disc area to have a mean size of between 1.4 and 2.9 mm^2,[58-61] with a range of almost seven times from 0.8 to 5.5 mm^2.[58,59, 62] The size of the optic disc may be greater in African Americans,[63] but it does not seem to correlate with the axial length of the eye, age, or refractive error, except for high myopia.[58,63] Some studies suggest that disc size does not vary between women and men.[62] Others have found a larger disc size in men.[63] In whites, excluding highly myopic patients, the susceptibility to glaucoma may be independent of optic disc size.[64] Most individuals have an optic disc that is slightly oval in a vertical dimension.[62,63] The mean horizontal diameter of the optic disc is between 1.6 and 1.8 mm, and the mean vertical diameter between 1.7 and 2.0 mm.[58–60,63] African Americans tend to have a slightly more vertical optic disc.[63] The shape of the optic disc is not correlated with age, sex, right or left eye, or body weight and height.[62] Additionally, in considering individuals with less than 8D of myopia, the shape of the optic disc does not appear to increase the susceptibility to glaucoma. Assessment of the disc shape, as a single feature, is not markedly important in the diagnosis of glaucoma.[62]

Neuroretinal Rim

The size of the neuroretinal rim is directly proportional to the size of the optic disc. Therefore, individuals with large discs tend to have larger neuroretinal rim areas.[60–62,63] For a given increase in the optic disc area, there can be up to a 50% increase in the rim area,[63] with the greatest effect in eyes with no disc cupping, less marked effect in eyes with a temporal flat sloping of the cup, and least effect in eyes with circular steep disc cupping.[62] The association between large rim area and large disc area is further correlated with increased numbers of optic nerve fibers and ganglion cells,[65] less nerve fiber crowding per square millimeter of disc area,[62] and a higher count and larger total area of lamina cribrosa pores.[33,62] There may also be a proportionate increase in glial tissue and capillaries; however, glia and capillaries make up only a small portion of the volume of the prelaminar optic nerve.

As was true in the case of the optic disc, there is also a significant range of variation in the neuroretinal rim area. The mean neuroretinal area in healthy eyes is between 1.2 and 2.2 mm^2,[58–61,66] increasing with the size of the optic disc.[65] The outer edge of the neuroretinal rim is defined by the edge of the optic disc, whereas the inner edge of the neuroretinal rim is defined by the outer edge of the cup portion of the optic nerve head.

The width of the neuroretinal rim depends on the number of ganglion cell axons entering the optic nerve at a given location. Because the fovea is slightly inferior to the center of the optic nerve head and because of the pattern of axons in the nerve fiber layer of the retina, the neuroretinal rim is normally widest in the inferior region, followed by the superior, nasal, and temporal regions.[58] Understanding that the width of the neuroretinal rim normally varies in different locations is critical to appreciating the earliest changes in this tissue in glaucoma.

The color of the neuroretinal rim when observed clinically is usually described as orangish- to yellow-ish-red. This coloration is due to the components found in the rim tissue (axons, blood vessels, glial tissue) as well as the anatomic arrangement of these components. Because the fasciculi of ganglion cell axons are wrapped in glial tubes and surrounded by capillaries, a fiberoptic effect between the fasciculi is created as light from an ophthalmoscope or a biomicroscope strikes the surface of the optic nerve head. Light reflects off of the scleral lamina cribrosa back between the bundles of axons, with an orangish-red color arising from the capillaries between the fasciculi. The variation in color of the rim tissue is due to the clarity of the media in front of the optic nerve head, the angle of exit of the optic nerve from the eye, and the anatomic variability in the components making up the rim tissue.

Pallor of the neuroretinal rim (whitening of the rim tissue) may be due to a decrease in the capillaries or blood flow between the fasciculi (ischemia), an increase in the amount of glial tissue in the optic nerve head (gliosis), or disruption of the precise arrangement of the components of the neuroretinal rim, thus eliminating the normal fiberoptic effect when the optic nerve head is illuminated. Pallor of the optic disc and especially of the neuroretinal rim is a typical sign of optic nerve damage. However, pallor of the neuroretinal rim is usually associated with nonglaucomatous optic neuropathy. The observation of a generalized pallor in a glaucomatous disc mainly results from the loss of neuroretinal rim tissue and its corresponding components.

Cup Portion of the Optic Nerve Head

The cup represents the concavity or area of excavation in the center of the optic nerve head. The cup varies greatly in normal individuals because there is a direct correlation between the size of the optic disc and the size and depth of the cup.[58,60–63,67] The size of both the optic disc and cup is genetically determined.[64] Clinically, the size of the cup is recorded as a ratio to the overall size of the optic disc in both the horizontal and vertical dimensions.

The cup is normally round or horizontally oval in shape.[58] In a study of over 1000 eyes, Carpel and Engstrom[68] found only 9% of cups to be shaped ovally and 90% of these oval cups to be slightly elongated in a horizontal dimension. The mean horizontal diameter of the cup is between 0.65 and 0.8 mm, whereas the mean vertical diameter is between 0.7 and 0.77 mm.[58,60] The mean area of the optic cup is between 0.6 and 0.7 mm^2.[58,61]

The cup-to-disc ratio shows significant variation when clinical studies of normal, healthy individuals are compared. This is due in part to the method of observation used in the study and the varying clinical criteria for defining the cup area. Direct ophthalmoscopy tends to result in a slightly smaller cup-to-disc ratio than a stereoscopic evaluation.[68] Cup-to-disc ratios in normal individuals can range from 0.00 to 0.9.[58] Much of the variability in cup size results from the physiological relation between the size of the cup and the size of the optic disc. In the Framingham Eye Study, the average cup-to-disc ratio was 0.28 ± 0.17.[69] In a study of 475 normal eyes, Jonas and associates[58] found the mean horizontal cup-to-disc ratio to be 0.39 ± 0.28 and the mean vertical cup-to-disc ratio to be 0.34 ± 0.25. Recent studies have shown a mean vertical cup-to-disc ratio of 0.43–0.44.[70,71] In general, the shape of the optic cup in normal eyes is horizontally oval, with the horizontal diameter about 8% longer than the vertical diameter.[62] The size of the cup area may be larger in African Americans.[63] There is debate as to whether the cup size changes with age. [58,68,71–76]

Parapapillary Chorioretinal Atrophy
Parapapillary chorioretinal atrophy has been described in terms of two zones. The central beta-zone is closer to the optic disc and is characterized by visible sclera and visible choroidal vessels. Histologically, this zone represents a complete loss of retinal pigment epithelium and an incomplete loss of adjacent photoreceptors.[77,78] The more peripheral alpha-zone is located between the beta-zone and the retina. It has the appearance of irregular hypopigmentation and hyperpigmentation. Histologically, it corresponds to pigmentary irregularities in the retinal pigment epithelium.[78]

Alpha- and beta- zones can be present in normal eyes, most frequently in the inferotemporal region of the disc. The alpha-zone is present in almost all normal eyes.[79] Similar findings occur developmentally ("tilted disc") or may be associated with the myopic scleral crescent as seen in the highly myopic eye. Parapapillary atrophy can change with time because of aging processes in the retinal pigment epithelium, retinal diseases, or acquired atrophy of the choroid or retinal pigment epithelium. Historically, changes in the parapapillary tissue have been described as occurring in some eyes with advanced glaucoma. Clinically, it has been described as more common in glaucomatous eyes with moderately elevated intraocular pressure, shallow disc cupping, and marked tessellated fundus.[80] Parapapillary atrophy does not occur as a result of nonglaucomatous optic neuropathy and is therefore useful in differentiating it from glaucomatous damage. However, atrophy is of secondary importance in the detection of glaucomatous optic nerve damage.

Nerve Fiber Layer
The retinal nerve fiber layer is best observed clinically by using red-free light. The brightness of the red-free light reflected off the nerve fiber layer is directly proportional to the thickness of the layer. The nerve fiber layer adjacent to the optic nerve head is relatively thicker superiorly and inferiorly by as much as 150 to 200 μm than it is nasally and temporally.[81]

When one observes the nerve fiber layer in the retina within two disc diameters of the optic disc, it will appear brightest and most visible in the inferior arcuate arcade, followed by the superior arcuate arcade, papillomacular bundle and finally, the nasal side of the optic nerve head.[82] There does not seem to be any difference normally between the appearance of the nerve fiber layer in the eyes of the same individual, nor is there a gender difference.[82]

A change in the brightness of the nerve fiber layer adjacent to the optic disc may be one of the earliest signs of glaucomatous damage. As axons of the ganglion cells of the retina are destroyed in glaucoma, the nerve fiber layer thins and becomes less bright.

Large Discs
Large optic discs are defined clinically as those having an optic cup area greater than 2.1 mm^2.[58] Large discs tend to be associated with large neuroretinal rim and cup areas. Physiological cupping greater than 0.6 was found in 91% of individuals with large optic discs but in only 25% of individuals with average or small discs.[83] Since the areas of the optic disc, neuroretinal rim, and optic cup do not change proportionately, there is no constant ratio between these three clinical variables.

One of the greatest clinical challenges in glaucoma is the differential diagnosis of a large physiological cup from an optic disc that has acquired a large cup due to damage from glaucoma. In a comparison of normal-sized optic cups, large physiological cups, and glaucomatous optic discs, Jonas and colleagues[84] found that individuals with large physiological cups had large, slightly vertical discs, normal neuroretinal rim areas and configurations, normal nerve fiber layers, no peripapillary chorioretinal atrophy, and slightly horizontal cups with a mean horizontal cup-to-disc ratio of 0.78. The glaucomatous group had normal-sized disc areas, decreased neuroretinal rim areas, abnormal rim configurations (narrowing of the inferior and superior neuroretinal rim), defects in the retinal nerve fiber layer, vertically oval optic cups, and significant variation in the size of the cup-to-disc ratio.[84]

CONCLUSION

An understanding of the anatomy and physiology of the optic nerve helps to explain the clinical appearance of this tissue as well as its histopathological and clinical changes in glaucoma. This allows the clinician to make an accurate and early differential diagnosis of the disease.

REFERENCES

1. Quigley HA. Early detection of glaucomatous damage: II. Changes in the appearance of the optic disc. *Surv Ophthalmol.* 1985;30:111–126.
2. Arey LB, Schaible AJ. The nerve-fiber composition of the optic nerve. *Anat Rec.* 1934;58(suppl):3.
3. Arey LB, Bickel WH. The number of nerve fibers in human optic nerve. *Anat Rec.* 1935;61(suppl):3.
4. Bruesch SR, Arey LB. An enumeration of myelinated and unmyelinated fibers in the optic nerve of vertebrates. *Anat Rec.* 1940;76(suppl):10.
5. Bruesch SR, Arey LB. The number of myelinated and unmyelinated fibers in the optic nerve of vertebrates. *J Comp Neurol.* 1942;77:631–665.
6. Kupfer C, Chumbley L, Downer JC. Quantitative histology of optic nerve, optic tract and lateral geniculate nucleus of man. *J Anat.* 1967;101:393–401.
7. Potts AM, Hodges D, Shelman CB, et al. Morphology of the primate optic nerve. I. Method and total fiber count. *Invest Ophthalmol.* 1972;11:980–988.
8. Quigley HA, Addicks EM, Green WR. Optic nerve damage in human glaucoma: III. Quantitative correlation of nerve fiber loss and visual field defect in glaucoma, ischemic neuropathy, papilledema and toxic neuropathy. *Arch Ophthalmol.* 1982;100:135–146.
9. Balazsi AG, Rootman J, Drance SM, et al. The effect of age on the nerve fiber population of the human optic nerve. *Am J Ophthalmol.* 1984;97:760–766.
10. Repka MX, Quigley HA. The effect of age on normal human optic nerve fiber number and diameter. *Ophthalmology.* 1989;96:26–32.
11. Jonas JB, Muller-Bergh JA, Schlotzer-Schrehardt UM, et al. Histomorphometry of the human optic nerve. *Invest Ophthalmol Vis Sci.* 1990;31:736–744.
12. Provis JM, van Driel D, Billson FA, et al. Human fetal optic nerve: Overproduction and elimination of retinal axons during development. *J Comp Neurol.* 1985;238:92–100.
13. Li Y, Schlamp CL, Nickells RW. Experimental induction of retinal ganglion cell death in adult mice. *Invest Ophthalmol Vis Sci.* 1999;40:1004–1008.
14. Kee C, Koo H, Ji Y, et al. Effect of optic disc or age on evaluation of optic disc variables. *Br J Ophthalmol.* 1997;81:1046–1049.
15. Dolman CL, McCormick AQ, Drance SM. Aging of the optic nerve. *Arch Ophthalmol.* 1980;98:2053–2058.
16. Hogan MJ, Alvarado JA, Weddell JE. *Histology of the Human Eye.* Philadelphia: W.B. Saunders; 1971:523–606.
17. Jonas JB, Nguyen NX, Naumann GOH. The retinal nerve fiber layer in normal eyes. *Ophthalmology.* 1989;96:627–632.
18. Radius RL, Anderson DR. The course of axons through the retinal and optic nerve head. *Arch Ophthalmol.* 1979;97:1154–1158.
19. Minkler DS. The organization of nerve fiber bundles in the primate optic nerve head. *Arch Ophthalmol.* 1980;98:1630–1636.
20. Anderson DR. Ultrastructure of human and monkey lamina cribrosa and optic nerve head. *Arch Ophthalmol.* 1969;82:800–814.
21. Anderson DR, Hoyt WF. Ultrastructure of intraorbital portion of human and monkey optic nerve. *Arch Ophthalmol.* 1969;82:506–530.
22. Quigley HA, Addicks EM. Regional differences in the structure of the lamina cribrosa and their relation to glaucomatous optic nerve damage. *Arch Ophthalmol.* 1981;99:137–143.
23. Hayreh SS. Blood supply of the optic nerve head. *Ophthalmologica.* 1996;210:285–295.
24. Hayreh SS. The optic nerve head circulation in health and disease. *Exp Eye Res.* 1995;61:259–272.
25. Dichtl A, Jonas JB, Naumann GOH. Course of the optic nerve fibers through the lamina cribrosa in human eyes. *Graefes Arch Clin Exp Ophthalmol.* 1996; 234:581–585.
26. Hernandez MR, Luo XX, Igoe BS, et al. Extracellular matrix of the human lamina cribrosa. *Am J Ophthalmol.* 1987;104:567–576.
27. Tamura Y, Konomi H, Sawada H, et al. Tissue distribution of type VIII collagen in human adult and fetal eyes. *Invest Ophthalmol Vis Sci.* 1991;32:2636–2644.
28. Hernandez MR, Luo XX, Andrzejewska W, et al. Age-related changes in the extracellular matrix of the human optic nerve head. *Am J Ophthalmol.* 1989;107:476–484.
29. Elkington AR, Inman CBE, Steart PV, et al. The structure of the lamina cribrosa of the human eye: An immunochemical and electron microscopical study. *Eye.* 1990;4: 42–57.
30. Emery JM, Landis D, Paton D, et al. The lamina cribrosa in normal and glaucomatous human eyes. *Trans Am Acad Ophthalmol Otolaryngol* 1974;78:OP-290–OP-297.
31. Radius RL. Regional specificity in anatomy at the lamina cribrosa. *Arch Ophthalmol.* 1981;99:478–480.
32. Radius RL. Anatomy of the optic nerve head and glaucomatous optic neuropathy. *Surv Ophthalmol.* 1987;32:35–44.
33. Jonas JB, Mardin CY, Schlotzer-Schrehardt U, et al. Morphometry of the human lamina cribrosa surface. *Invest Ophthalmol Vis Sci.* 1991;32:401–405.
34. Ogden TE, Duggan J, Danley K, et al. Morphometry of nerve fiber bundle pores in the optic nerve head of the human. *Exp Eye Res.* 1988;46:559–568.
35. Anderson DR. Ultrastructure of meningeal sheaths: Normal human and monkey optic nerves. *Arch Ophthalmol.* 1969;82:659–674.
36. Hayreh SS. Anatomy and physiology of the optic nerve head. *Trans Am Acad Ophthalmol Otolaryngol.* 1974; 78:240–251.
37. Hayreh SS. Interindividual variation in blood supply of the optic nerve head. *Doc Ophthalmol.* 1985;59:217–246.

38. Hayreh SS. Segmental nature of the choroidal vasculature. *Br J Ophthalmol.* 1975;59:631–648.

39. Anderson DR, Braverman S. Reevaluation of the optic disk vasculature. *Am J Ophthalmol.* 1976;82:165–174.

40. Lieberman MF, Maumenee AE, Green WR. Histologic studies of the vasculature of the anterior optic nerve. *Am J Ophthalmol.* 1976;82:405–423.

41. Fryczkowski AW, Grimson BS, Peiffer Jr RL. Scanning electron microscopy of vascular casts of the human scleral lamina cribrosa. *Intern Ophthalmol.* 1984;7:95–100.

42. Griffin JW, Watson DF. Axonal transport in neurological disease. *Ann Neurol.* 1988;23:3–13.

43. Yanoff M, Fine BS. *Ocular Pathology.* Philadelphia: JB Lippincott; 1989:486.

44. Perry VH, Oehler R, Cowley A. Retinal ganglion cells that project to the dorsal lateral geniculate nucleus in the macaque monkey. *Neuroscience.* 1984;12:1101–1123.

45. DeMonasterio PM. Properties of concentrically organized X- and Y-ganglion cells of the macaque retina. *J Neurophysiol.* 1978;41:1435–1449.

46. Bassi CJ, Lehmkuhle S. Clinical implications of parallel visual pathways. *J Am Optom Assoc.* 1990;61:98–110.

47. Kulikowski JJ. Terminology of P and M pathways. In: *Seeing Contour and Colour: Proceedings of the Third International Symposium of the Northern Eye Institute.* Oxford: Pergamon Press; 1989:11–17.

48. Kaplan E. The role of P and M systems: (A) Introductory remarks. In: *Seeing Contour and Colour: Proceedings of the Third International Symposium of the Northern Eye Institute.* Oxford: Pergamon Press; 1989:224–227.

49. Hubel DH, Livingstone MS. Segregation of form, colour, movement and depth processing: Anatomy and physiology. In: *Seeing Contour and Colour: Proceedings of the Third International Symposium of the Northern Eye Institute.* Oxford: Pergamon Press; 1989:116–119.

50. Kulikowski JJ. The role of P and M systems: (C) Psychophysical aspects. In: *Seeing Contour and Colour: Proceedings of the Third International Symposium of the Northern Eye Institute.* Oxford: Pergamon Press; 1989:232–237.

51. Merigan WH. Assessing the role of parallel pathways in primates. In: *Seeing Contour and Colour: Proceedings of the Third International Symposium of the Northern Eye Institute.* Oxford: Pergamon Press; 1989:198–206.

52. Glovinsky Y, Quigley HA, Dunkelberger GR. Retinal ganglion cell loss is size dependent in experimental glaucoma. *Invest Ophthalmol Vis Sci.* 1991;32:484–491.

53. Quigley HA, Sanchez RM, Dunkelberger GR, et al. Chronic glaucoma selectively damages large optic nerve fibers. *Invest Ophthalmol Vis Sci.* 1987;28:913–920.

54. Johnson MA, Drum BA, Quigley HA, et al. Pattern-evoked potentials and optic nerve fiber loss in monocular laser-induced glaucomatous primate eyes. *Invest Ophthalmol Vis Sci.* 1989;30:897–907

55. Marx MS, Podos SM, Bodis-Wollner I, et al. Flash and pattern electroretinograms in normal and laser-induced glaucomatous primate eyes. *Invest Ophthalmol Vis Sci.* 1989;27:378–386.

56. Airaksinen PJ, Lakowski R, Drance SM, et al. Color vision and retinal nerve fiber layer in early glaucoma. *Am J Ophthalmol.* 1986;101:208–213.

57. Jonas JB, Gusek GC, Guggenmoos-Holzmann I, et al. Size of the optic nerve scleral canal and comparison with intravital determination of optic disc dimensions. *Graefes Arch Clin Exp Ophthalmol.* 1988;226:213–215.

58. Jonas JB, Gusek GC, Naumann GOH. Optic disc, cup and neuroretinal rim size, configuration and correlations in normal eyes. *Invest Ophthalmol Vis Sci.* 1988;29:1151–1158.

59. Jonas JB, Gusek GC, Guggenmoos-Holzmann I, et al. Variability of the real dimensions of normal human optic discs. *Graefes Arch Clin Exp Ophthalmol.* 1988;226:332–336.

60. Britton RJ, Drance SM, Schulzer M, et al. The area of the neuroretinal rim of the optic nerve in normal eyes. *Am J Ophthalmol.* 1987;103:497–504.

61. Caprioli J, Miller JM. Optic disc rim area is related to disc size in normal subjects. *Arch Ophthalmol.* 1987;105;1683–1685.

62. Jonas JB, Budde WM, Panda-Jonas S. Ophthalmoscopic evaluation of the optic nerve head. *Surv Ophthalmol.* 1999;43:293–320.

63. Quigley HA, Brown AE, Morrison JD, et al. The size and shape of the optic disc in normal human eyes. *Arch Ophthalmol.* 1990;108:51–57.

64. Jonas JB, Fernandez MC, Naumann GOH. Correlation of the optic disc size to glaucoma susceptibility. *Ophthalmology.* 1991;98:675–680.

65. Quigley HA, Coleman AL, Dorman-Pease ME. Larger optic nerve heads have more nerve fibers in normal eyes. *Arch Ophthalmol.* 1991;109:1441–1443.

66. Jonas JB, Montgomery DMI. Determination of the neuroretinal rim area using the horizontal and vertical disc and cup diameters. *Graefes Arch Clin Exp Ophthalmol.* 1995;233:690–693.

67. Bengtsson B. The variation and covariation of cup and disc diameters. *Acta Ophthalmol (Copenh).* 1976;54:804–818.

68. Carpel EF, Engstrom PF. The normal cup-disc ratio. *Am J Ophthalmol.* 1981;91:588–597.

69. Liebowitz HM, Krueger DE, Maunder LR, et al. The Framingham Eye Study monograph. *Surv Ophthalmol.* 1980;24(suppl):335–610.

70. Healey PR, Mitchell P, Smith W, et al. Relationship between cup-disc ratio and optic disc diameter: The Blue Mountains Eye Study. *Aust N Z J Ophthalmol.* 1997;25(suppl 1):S99–S101.

71. Garway-Heath DF, Ruben ST, Viswanathan A, et al. Vertical cup/disc ratio in relation to optic disc size: Its value in the assessment of the glaucoma suspect. *Br J Ophthalmol.* 1998; 82:1118–1124.

72. Garway-Heath DF, Wollstein G, Hitchings RA. Aging changes of the optic nerve head in relation to open angle glaucoma. *Br J Ophthalmol.* 1997;81:840–845.

73. Pickard R. The alteration in size of the normal optic disc cup. *Br J Ophthalmol.* 1948;32:355–361.

74. Ford M, Sarwar M. Features of a clinically normal optic disc. *Br J Ophthalmol.* 1963;47:50–52.

75. Snydacker D. The normal optic disc: Ophthalmoscopic and photographic studies. *Am J Ophthalmol.* 1964;58:958–964.

76. Schwartz JT, Reuling FH, Garrison RJ. Acquired cupping of the optic nervehead in normotensive eyes. *Br J Ophthalmol.* 1975;59:216–222.

77. Fantes FE, Anderson DR. Clinical histologic correlation of human peripapillary anatomy. *Ophthalmology.* 1989; 96:20–25.

78. Kubota T, Jonas JB, Naumann GOH. Direct clinco-histological correlation of parapapillary chorioretinal atrophy. *Br J Ophthalmol.* 1993;77:103–106.

79. Jonas JB, Fernandez MC, Naumann GOH. Glaucomatous optic nerve atrophy in small discs with low cup-to-disc ratios. *Ophthalmology.* 1990;97:1211–1215.

80. Jonas JB, Fernandez MC, Naumann GOH. Glaucomatous parapapillary chorioretinal atrophy: Occurrence and correlations. *Arch Ophthalmol.* 1992;110:214–222.

81. Caprioli J. The contour of the juxtapapillary nerve fiber layer in glaucoma. *Ophthalmology.* 1990;97:358–366.

82. Jonas JB, Nguyen NX, Naumann GOH. The retinal nerve fiber layer in normal eyes. *Ophthalmology.* 1989;96: 627–632.

83. Maisel JM, Pearlstein CS, Adams WH, et al. Large optic disks in the Marshallese population. *Am J Ophthalmol.* 1989;107:145–150.

84. Jonas JB, Zach FM, Gusek G, et al. Pseudoglaucomatous physiologic large cups. *Am J Ophthalmol.* 1989;107: 137–144.

Chapter 5

ETIOLOGY AND PATHOPHYSIOLOGY OF PRIMARY OPEN-ANGLE GLAUCOMA

Thomas L. Lewis
Connie L. Chronister

Understanding the causes for the increase in intraocular pressure and the damage to the optic nerve that occurs in glaucoma helps explain the rationale for the proper diagnosis and treatment of these diseases. Unfortunately, definitive explanations of the etiology and histopathology of glaucoma are still not available. This chapter summarizes current research and clinical data and reviews the theories being proposed to explain the disease.

THE CAUSES OF ELEVATED INTRAOCULAR PRESSURE

With age, there is a progressive increase in the resistance to the outflow of aqueous humor along with a concurrent decrease in aqueous production. This can result in a slight increase in intraocular pressure. In a few individuals, an imbalance is created between the increased resistance to outflow and the decrease in aqueous production, resulting in a more significant rise in intraocular pressure. Of these individuals, those with susceptible optic nerves will develop an optic neuropathy from the elevated intraocular pressure, resulting in glaucoma.

In primary open-angle glaucoma (POAG), there is no apparent systemic or secondary condition contributing to the decrease in aqueous outflow. Although the exact etiology of the decreased outflow is not known, the most likely causes involve biochemical or histological changes in both the conventional outflow pathway (i.e., Schlemm's canal) and the uveoscleral pathway.[1-22]

The most direct method of uncovering the etiology of the glaucomatous changes in the anterior segment of the eye would be by comparing histological specimens from normal eyes with those from glaucomatous eyes of similar age.[2,4-9] Studies of tissue from glaucomatous eyes are hampered by changes that may result from treatment with drugs, lasers, or surgery rather than from the disease itself. Furthermore, most available specimens reflect late rather than early stages of the disease. Attempts to overcome these problems have led to the use of animal models, cell culture, organ culture, and model systems. Human trabecular meshwork tissue has been grown in cell culture and organ culture and used as monolayer filters to create research models.[1,3,23-28]

The results of ultrastructural and biochemical studies of both normal and glaucomatous human tissue have led to the conclusion that many of the pathological features associated with glaucoma are possibly exaggerated and accelerated changes that occur with age in all eyes (Table 5-1).[2,22,25,29]

TABLE 5–1. ANTERIOR CHAMBER CHANGES SEEN WITH AGING AND PRIMARY OPEN-ANGLE GLAUCOMA

Loss of trabecular endothelial cells
Pigment accumulation within trabecular endothelial cells
Thickening of trabecular lamellae
Fusion of trabecular lamellae
Thickening of scleral spur
Increase in extracellular (plaque) material in juxtacanalicular zone
Decrease in giant vacuoles along inner wall of Schlemm's canal

Not everyone agrees that glaucoma is associated with accelerated aging of the anterior chamber structures.[30] It is agreed, however, that an increase in resistance to outflow appears to be the primary cause of increase in intraocular pressure. Therefore, in discussing the etiology of POAG, it makes more sense to first describe the normal aging changes in the anterior chamber angle. A detailed explanation of the normal anatomy of the anterior chamber is found in Chapter 3.

Normal Aging Changes

1. A loss of trabecular endothelial cells. Alvarado and colleagues demonstrated that trabecular cellularity decreases rapidly during the first 2 years of life and continues to decline at a slower, linear rate for the next 98 years.[2] Between ages 20 and 80, there is an approximate 350,000-cell (47%) loss.[2] The loss of endothelial cells from the trabecular lamellae is greatest posteriorly and in the uveal meshwork and least in the juxtacanalicular zone.[2,22] This cell loss and the associated enlargement of the remaining cells on the trabeculae is similar to the aging changes occurring in the corneal endothelium.[2,31] The continuous loss of endothelial cells is accompanied by an increase in abnormal lattice (curly) collagen within the trabeculae and by swelling and lamellation of the basement membrane.[13,22]

2. An increase in the accumulation of pigment within the endothelial cells of the trabecular meshwork. At age 20, approximately 3% of the cells covering the trabeculae contain melanin within their cytoplasm.[22] By age 80, some 18% of the cells contain melanin.[22] The source of the melanin is most likely from the pigmented epithelial cells of the ciliary body and iris.[22]

3. Thickening of the trabecular lamellae. There is a 30% increase in the thickness of the trabeculae from age 20 to age 80.[22] This occurs primarily from an accumulation of material in the basement membrane of the endothelial cells and also the addition of extracellular material within the core of the trabecular beam.[22] It is possible that this thickening is a result of loss of the endothelial cell covering.[22]

4. Fusion of trabecular lamellae. This is most likely due to the loss of endothelial cells.[22,25]

5. Thickening of the scleral spur. This occurs as a result of hyalinization and/or atrophy of the ciliary muscle along with collapse and condensation of the uveal trabecular meshwork.[16,29]

6. Increase in extracellular (plaque) material in the juxtacanalicular zone. Some of the tendons of the longitudinal portion of the ciliary muscle are connected to a specific network of elastic-like fibers in the juxtacanalicular zone, which, in turn, are connected by fine fibrils to the basement membrane of the endothelial cells lining the inner wall of Schlemm's canal. These small "connecting fibrils" are oxytalan fibers.[1] Sheath material composed of fine fibrils embedded in a homogeneous matrix covers the anterior ciliary muscle tendons and continues over the elastic-like fibers in the juxtacanalicular zone.[1] With age, proteoglycan deposits accumulate as plaques within the sheaths covering the elastic-like fibers.[7] Ultimately, these plaques may form broad interlacing plates of extracellular deposits. Sheath-derived plaques have also been observed to accumulate with age in the outer wall of Schlemm's canal and in the tips of the longitudinal ciliary muscle tendons.[7,8]

7. A loss of the ability to form giant vacuoles along the inner wall of Schlemm's canal.[22]

8. A proliferation of endothelial cells forming the lining of Schlemm's canal into the lumen of the canal.[16]

GLAUCOMATOUS CHANGES

The increase in intraocular pressure in glaucoma may result from a variety of possible causes. In the late 1960s, it was proposed that elevated intraocular pressure was due to an increase in intrascleral venous pressure.[1,32] Such an increase would decrease the pressure head for aqueous outflow and cause intraocular pressure to rise.[1,32,33] Nesterov concluded that the greatest resistance to aqueous outflow in POAG was not in the intrascleral veins but in the juxtacanalicular tissue of the anterior chamber angle.[1,33] Thus, although an increase in intrascleral venous pressure could cause a rise in intraocular pressure, it may not be the most likely cause for the chronic pressure elevation found in POAG.

Canalicular blockage from a direct collapse of Schlemm's canal along its inner wall was another early idea as a cause for decreased aqueous outflow in glaucoma.[1,33] Moses and colleagues suggested that the collapse of Schlemm's canal was not the primary cause of increased intraocular pressure but secondary to a primary defect along the inner wall of the canal, leading to an increase in resistance to the outflow of aqueous.[1,34,35]

Endothelial Cell Alterations

The loss of endothelial cells from the trabecular meshwork, which occurs normally with age, may occur earlier and to a greater extent in individuals with POAG. The excessive loss of endothelial cells seen in glaucoma is not uniform but is greatest in the inner (uveal) meshwork.[2] On the other hand, the juxtacanalicular zone has a similar number of cells as in age-matched normal eyes.[2] Alvarado found fewer endothelial cells at a given age in glaucomatous eyes than in normal eyes, although the rate of decline in the two groups was similar.[2] Thus the age-cellularity curves for normal and glaucoma individuals are parallel.[2] Those that develop POAG seem to reach their "critical" level of cell loss sooner than normal people.[2]

The rapid and excessive decrease in cellularity seen in POAG may be due to a congenital defect resulting in fewer endothelial cells at birth.[2] An alternative explanation is that a critical depletion of trabecular endothelial cells occurs rapidly in adulthood as a result of a "glaucoma factor."[22] Grierson believed that excessive wear and tear on endothelial cells could be the glaucoma factor for certain individuals.[22] A recent study has shown that patients with glaucoma also have a lower corneal endothelial cell density than age-matched controls.[36]

Grierson and other investigators found that prolonged phagocytic activity by endothelial cells can cause injury and necrosis.[22,23,37] In contrast, a study by Matsumoto found that the phagocytic ability of the trabecular meshwork appears similar between eyes with POAG and normal eyes.[38] Other causes of cell loss could be nutritional insufficiencies or toxins in the aqueous, or excessive accumulation of intracellular pigment.[22]

The loss of endothelial cells results in a reparative response from the remaining cells similar to that which occurs from aging changes in the corneal endothelium.[2] The innermost trabeculae respond to the loss of endothelial cells by marked enlargement (hypertrophy) of the remaining cells in order to cover over the denuded areas.[2,25,29] These activated cells may extend across trabecular beams, partially covering the usually opened "aqueous channels" and creating a new and abnormal cellular lining across the inner surface of the meshwork.[2] This "membrane" may be what Fine and colleagues describe as an accretion and compactness of the uveal meshwork in glaucoma.[16] Chaudhry also observed marked alterations in the innermost trabeculae, although his coating substance, which resulted in a "pretrabecular membrane," could not be confirmed by other investigators.[2,39] The increased metabolic activity of the remaining endothelial cells may also produce excessive or unusual extracellular material, including glycosaminoglycans, fibronectin, basement membrane–like material, and abnormal lattice (curly) collagen.[5,10,13,14,27,29,40,41]

In the deeper layers of the meshwork (corneoscleral trabeculae), the remaining endothelial cells do not hypertrophy or activate. Instead, the denuded areas of the trabeculae remain bare (Fig. 5–1).[2] This results in swelling (thickening) and fusion of adjacent trabeculae.[2,22] The fusion is often focal, particularly posteriorly, near the scleral spur. As the endothelial cells drop off the trabeculae, they may flow downstream with the aqueous and lodge in the juxtacanalicular region.

To summarize, the net effect of an accelerated and excessive loss of endothelial cells in the trabecular meshwork of glaucomatous eyes is the formation of an abnormal cell lining along the inner surface of the meshwork, thickening and fusion of the trabeculae, an accumulation of the extracellular material, the formation of abnormal collagen, and the accumulation of cells in the juxtacanalicular tissue.

Plaque Formation

Sheath-derived plaque material, which apparently accumulates in several regions of the anterior chamber angle with age, is found in a greater concentration in age-matched glaucomatous eyes (Fig. 5–2).[10,14,22] Not only is the "sheath material" more excessive, but it is also qualitatively different in older eyes.[8] Sheath material has been noted in both treated and untreated cases of POAG.[42] This verifies that the material is not due to treatment but is related to the disease itself. In glaucoma, the sheath-derived plaques have more fibrils and are unevenly distributed (Fig. 5–3).[14] Their fibrillar components include type VI collagen and abnormal lattice collagen.[14] Along with an increase in other extracellular material, such as fibronectin, these changes can close off preferential aqueous outflow pathways (Fig. 5–4).[8,14] Gottanka noted that an increase in the severity of optic nerve damage in POAG is accompanied by an increase in the amount of sheath-derived plaque material in the meshwork.[43]

There is, however, evidence that POAG may not occur as a result of an accumulation of excessive material in the anterior chamber angle. Quigley did not

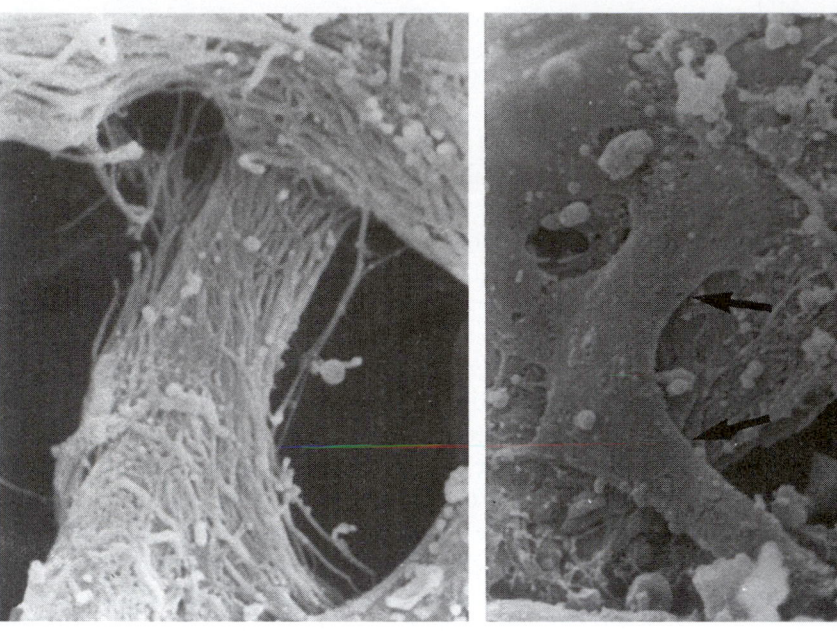

Figure 5–1. Scanning electron micrograph of trabeculae in "early" (*A*) and "late" (*B*) POAG. *A* shows the collagen core of a denuded trabeculae and *B* shows a migratory meshwork cell (*arrows*). (Original magnifications: *A*, ×6000; *B*, ×10,000.) (Reproduced with permission from Grierson I. What is open angle glaucoma? *Eye.* 1987;1:22.)

observe the obstruction of pores of the inner trabecular meshwork by extracellular material in trabeculectomy specimens of eyes with POAG.[11] DeCater was unable to find any correlation between the presence or absence of plaques and a reduction in aqueous outflow.[12] Lütjen-Drecoll, although finding sheath-derived plaque material, found no correlation between the amount of material and the level of intraocular pressure.[8]

Alvarado did find an increase in electron-dense material in the juxtacanalicular tissue with age.[4] However, in patients with POAG under the age of 40, the electron-dense material appeared to be similar in amount to that in age-matched normal eyes.[4] Older glaucoma patients had more electron-dense material than normal eyes, but the difference was not great enough to explain the decrease in aqueous outflow present in these individuals.[4]

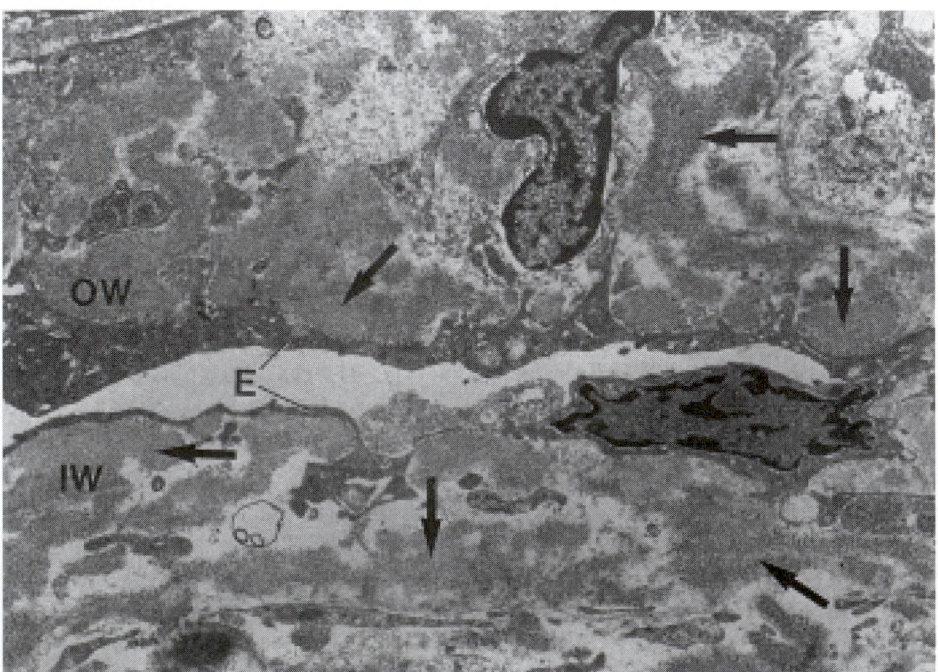

Figure 5–2. Electron micrograph of inner and outer wall of Schlemm's canal in cases of POAG. Sheath-derived plaque material (*arrows*); endothelium of Schlemm's canal (E); inner wall (IW); outer wall (OW). (Sagittal section, trabeculectomy specimen; original magnification: ×17,280.) (Reproduced with permission from Rohen JW, Lütjen-Drecoll E. Morphology of aqueous outflow pathways in normal and glaucomatous eyes. In: Ritch R, Shields MB, Krupin T, eds. *The Glaucomas.* St. Louis: CV Mosby Co, 1989:56.

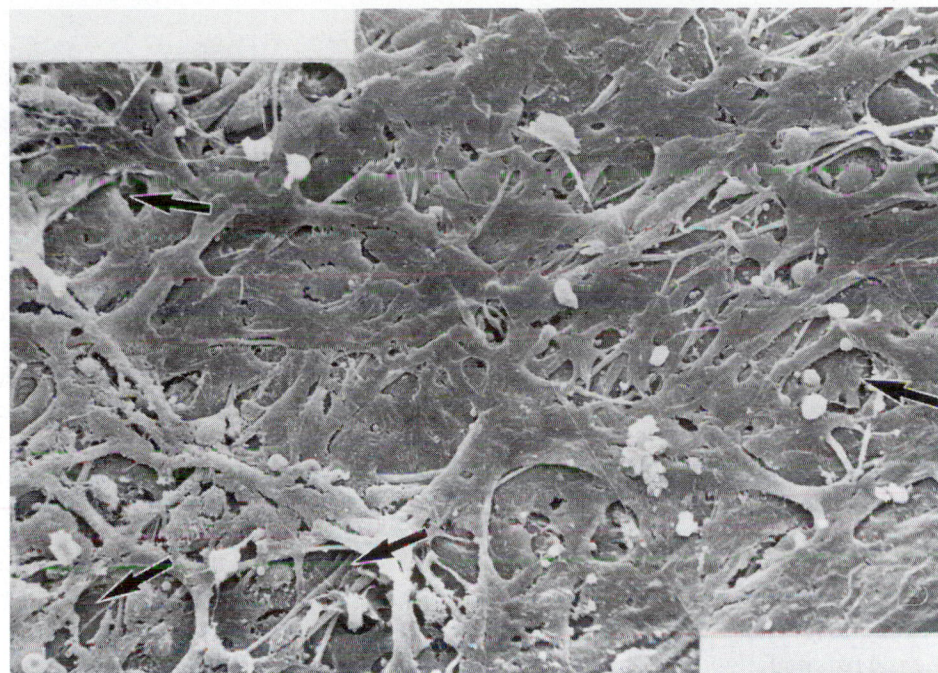

Figure 5–3. Scanning electron micrograph of uveal meshwork in case of POAG. Note the openings of uveal meshwork are partly closed by extracellular material along trabecular beams, still partly open (*arrows*). (Flat preparation, internal aspect; original magnification: ×500.) (Reproduced with permission from Rohen JW, Lütjen-Drecoll E. Morphology of aqueous outflow pathways in normal and glaucomatous eyes. In: Ritch R, Shields MB, Krupin T, eds. *The Glaucomas.* St. Louis: CV Mosby Co, 1989:56.)

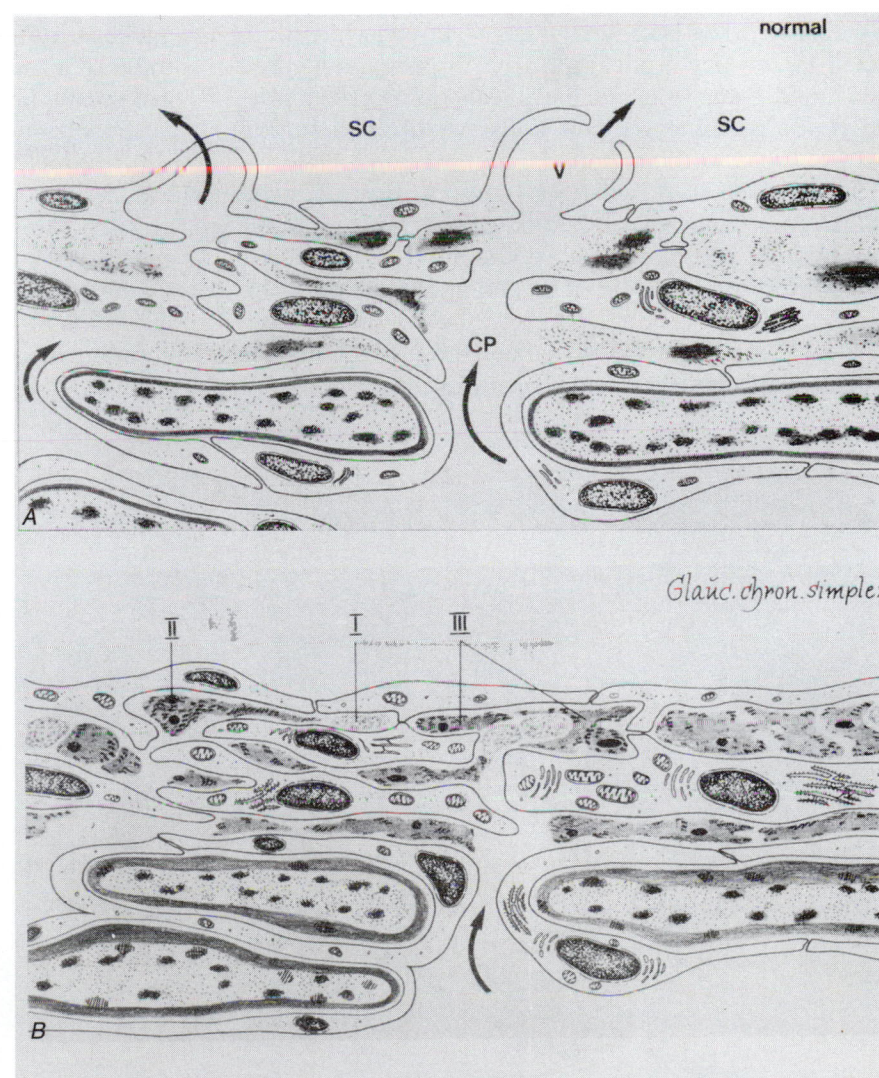

Figure 5–4. *A.* Schematic drawing of the normal ultrastructure of juxtacanalicular (cribriform) layer and inner wall of Schlemm's canal. Cribriform pathway (CP); normal aqueous outflow (*arrows*). *B.* Schematic drawing of accumulation of excess fibrillar or extracellular material (types I, II, and III) along juxtacanalicular tissue. The extracellular deposits blocking the juxtacanalicular tissue have been categorized: type I deposits are plaques; type II deposits are elastic-like fibers; type III deposits are sheath-material. Flow and partial blockade of aqueous outflow (*arrow*). (Reproduced with permission from Rohen JW. Why is intraocular pressure elevated in chronic simple glaucoma? *Ophthalmology.* 1983;90:759.)

Also, there was a tremendous variation in the amount of electron-dense material found in glaucomatous eyes, with no correlation between the amount of this material and the severity of the glaucoma.[4]

Decrease in Giant Vacuoles

Since 1971, Tripathi has proposed a role in the outflow of aqueous for the endothelial cells lining the inner wall of Schlemm's canal.[44] He believes that these cells form giant intracellular vacuoles that allow aqueous access to the lumen of the canal (Fig. 5–5).[44] In POAG, it is theorized that a decrease in sialic acid receptors on the endothelial cells reduces their ability to form giant vacuoles, thus decreasing the outflow of aqueous through Schlemm's canal.[9] Other studies have not found any difference in the quantity of giant vacuoles between normal and glaucomatous eyes.[15]

Histopathological studies of glaucomatous eyes have demonstrated that both pathways (Schlemm's canal and the uveoscleral pathway) are altered by the disease.[7,8,16] The earliest changes in POAG were localized to the uveal portion of the drainage angle and included compaction of the uveal meshwork, formation of a prominent scleral spur, hyalinization and/or atrophy of the ciliary muscle, and atrophy of the iris root.[7,16] Late-stage changes demonstrated marked atrophy of the uveal meshwork, ciliary muscle, and the root of the iris, along with obliteration of Schlemm's canal from proliferation of its endothelial lining.[7,16] Interestingly, the changes affecting the uveoscleral outflow of aqueous occurred before those involving the juxtacanalicular tissue and Schlemm's canal.[16]

Role of Aqueous Humor

Certain elements of the aqueous humor may affect outflow structures and increase resistance to outflow. Aqueous humor from glaucomatous eyes may have an increased level of transforming growth factor $\beta2$ (TGF$\beta2$).[45] TGF$\beta2$ has a role in promoting the synthesis and deposition of components of the extracellular matrix. Excess TGF$\beta2$ could possibly induce a buildup of excessive materials in the outflow apparatus and thus reduce outflow.[45] Other specific growth factors are released by trabecular meshwork cells and may play an important role within the microenvironment of the trabecular meshwork.[46] However, their role in the pathogenesis of glaucoma remains unclear.

Individuals with POAG have a decrease in collagenase activity and an increase in collagen synthesis when compared to a control group with cataracts.[47] An increase in collagen may contribute to excess deposition, with a loss of trabecular cells in POAG.[47] Alpha-crystallin from the lens cells released into the aqueous humor may play a role in obstruction of the trabecular meshwork.[48] Further studies are needed to investigate how substances released into the aqueous may contribute to reduced aqueous outflow.

In conclusion, the histopathological and biochemical changes occurring in the anterior chamber angle of patients with open-angle glaucoma have not been conclusively identified, quantified, or characterized. Current evidence would lead to the conclusion that glaucoma may be caused by an acceleration and exaggeration of normal aging changes occurring both in the uveoscleral outflow pathway and in the trabecular

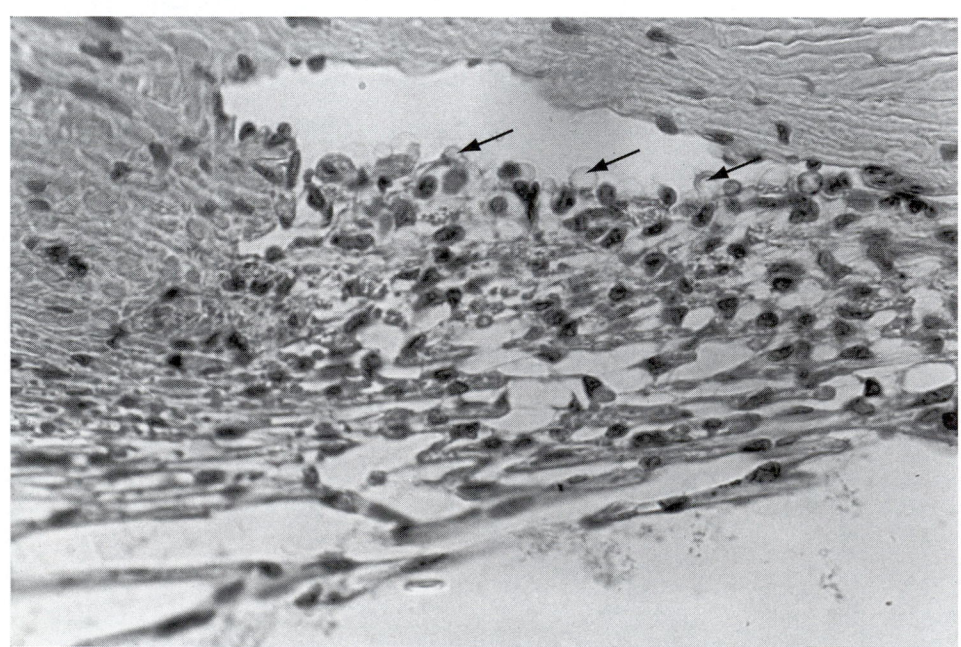

Figure 5–5. Light micrograph of adult monkey eye. The large lumen is Schlemm's canal. Note giant vacuoles (clear looking evaginations) along inner wall of Schlemm's canal. Inner wall is adjacent to trabecular meshwork. (Original magnification: ×400.) (Photograph by Chronister CL.)

meshwork, juxtacanalicular tissue, and Schlemm's canal (Fig. 5–6).

GLAUCOMATOUS CHANGES IN THE OPTIC NERVE

After a period of time, depending on the susceptibility of the optic nerve head, abnormal levels of intraocular pressure will cause damage to this tissue. Clinically, this is reflected as a loss of retinal nerve fiber layer, an increase in excavation of the surface of the optic nerve, and/or a loss of neuroretinal rim tissue.[49–52] The histopathological explanation of these changes is a destruction of the ganglion cell axons that transmit impulses from the retina to the thalamus.[53] The death of these nerve fibers is due to a blockage of axonal transport at the level of the scleral lamina cribrosa.[54,55]

The retrograde blockage of axonal transport leads to the loss of neurotrophic factors supplied to the ganglion cells from the lateral geniculate body.[56,57] A set of genes under control of these neurotrophic factors is turned on to generate a sequence of events that disposes of ganglion cells through apoptosis and phagocytosis in the absence of inflammation.[56,58] In apoptosis, the DNA of the ganglion cell is broken into fragments of specific size by endonuclease enzymes.[56,58] This process is genetically driven and represents a form of "cellular suicide" that differs from necrosis.[56] In addition to deprivation of neurotrophic factors, the stimuli for apoptosis in glaucoma may include excitotoxic injury initiated by ischemia.[59,60]

Early Glaucomatous Changes in the Optic Nerve

It seems that the earliest changes in the optic nerve tissue in POAG involve the following:

1. Compression, stretching, and remodeling (rearrangement) of the sheets of the scleral lamina cribrosa (Fig. 5–7).[52,61–63]
2. Posterior (outward) displacement of the laminar sheets.[61,64–66]
3. Distortion and/or enlargement of the laminar pores, which may progress to the point of laminar ectasia.[67,68] This may be due to a stretching of connective tissue elements or a rupture of smaller, less pliable connective tissue beams (Fig. 5–7).[50,61–63]
4. Transformation of type 1β astrocytes from a quiescent to a reactive state.[69,70]

- Increase in type VI collagen[71,72]
- Reactivation of elastin synthesis,[73] elastotic degeneration,[74] and curling of elastic fiber[75,76]
- Proliferation of basement membranes[71,77,78] and an increase in type IV collagen[70,71]

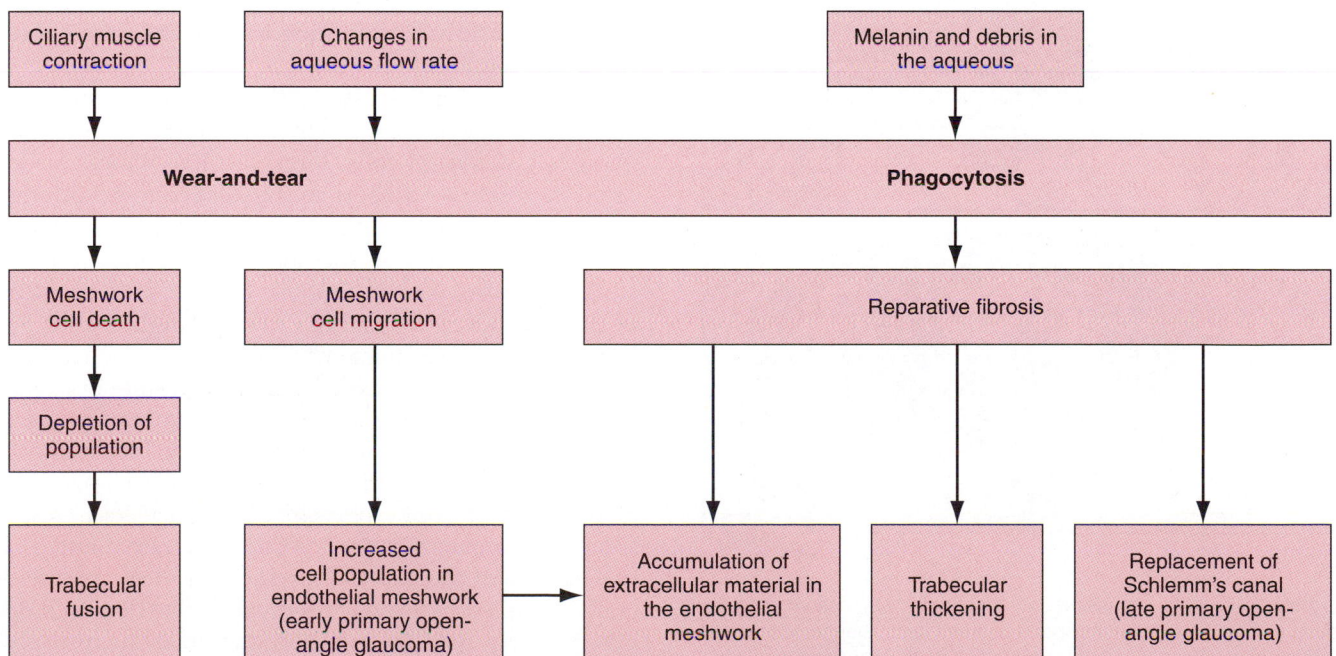

Figure 5–6. Flowchart indicating possible interrelationships of pathological events as seen in aging and POAG. (Reproduced with permission from Grierson I. What is open angle glaucoma? *Eye.* 1987;1:24.)

- Increased synthesis of TGFβ2.[79,80] TGFβ2 is a major modulator of wound healing[81] and an inducer of reactivation of astrocytes[82]
- Increased synthesis of tenascin[83] as a reaction to tissue trauma and in part due to high levels of TGFβ2[84] (Tenascin is found in the central nervous system at sites of wound healing and tissue remodeling.[85])

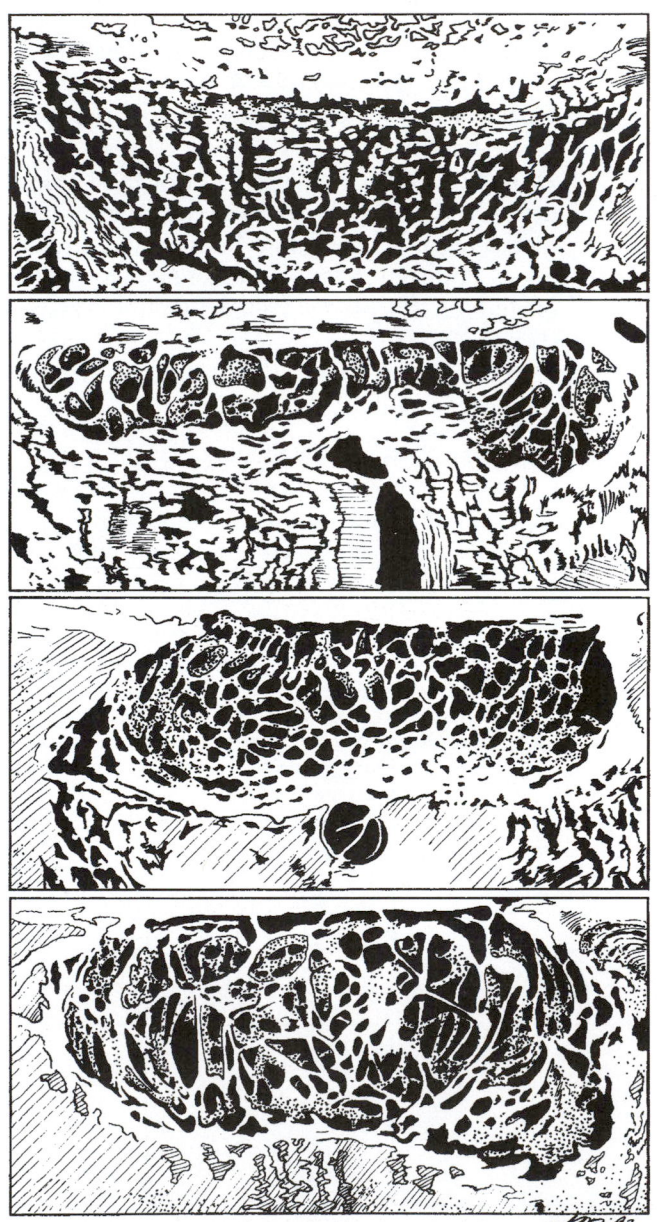

Figure 5–7. Artist rendition of digested optic nerve laminar sheets. This illustrates the posterolateral extension or backward bowing of the floor of the optic nerve head with glaucomatous damage. The top drawing represents a normal adult. The middle two represent moderate glaucomatous damage, and the bottom severe backward bowing secondary to glaucoma.

These abnormal deposits most likely result from type 1β astrocyte hyperplasia[69,86] and may represent an effort to heal the damaged tissue.[71,77]

5. Extensive remodeling of the laminar sheets and extracellular matrix.[69,71,72]

   - Disappearance of astrocytic columns in the prelaminar region and migration of astrocytes into nerve bundles in the lamina cribrosa[69]
   - Decrease in total collagen content[87]

6. Loss of compliance or increase in stiffness of the scleral lamina cribrosa.[77,88]
7. Absence of inflammation, significant participation of microglia, or scarring.[72]

Remodeling of the optic nerve head may be a primary or secondary response to factors such as abnormal intraocular pressure, ischemia, or loss of axons.[69,72] Once the initial injury to the nerve occurs, a cascade of events results in type 1β astrocyte reactivation and de-generative changes in the extracellular matrix of the lamina cribrosa.[72] This can lead to collapse of the laminar sheets. Remodeling of the extracellular matrix and reactivation of astrocytes represent the earliest and most dominant responses in the optic nerve in glaucoma. They are present in all stages of the disease,[69,72,83] creating an inhospitable environment for neuronal regrowth.[89] Individual age-related and/or racial differences may affect the lamina cribrosa, possibly contributing to and sustaining glaucomatous damage.[72,90]

The result of these early changes is a blockage of axonal transport, initially in the largest of the ganglion cell axons (M cells, large P cells), which are located in greatest numbers in the superior and inferior polar regions of the optic nerve.[57,58,91–93] Also, axons located peripherally in the nerve fiber bundles (fasciculi) are destroyed before those located in the middle of these bundles.[94] Although many ganglion cells are lost, few cones are affected.[95]

The blockage of axonal transport results in axonal swelling from the accumulation of membranous vesicles and mitochondria at the point of the blockage and cystic degeneration of the ganglion cells, causing a loss of tissue in the optic nerve.[54] This tissue loss creates some prelaminar thinning of the optic nerve and also hyperplasia of the glial cells, which fill in spaces previously occupied by axons and phagocytize dead cell debris.[52,71] They manufacture new materials such as glycosaminoglycans to fill in the spaces.[63,78,96] Cavernous degeneration in the optic nerve rarely occurs in glaucoma except in cases of very high intraocular pressure.[97]

Later Glaucomatous Changes in the Optic Nerve

In the advanced stages of glaucoma, other changes occur in the tissue of the optic nerve. These include additional compression of the scleral laminar sheets, causing a tripling of the surface area of the scleral lamina cribrosa; additional posterior (outward) displacement of the lamina;[66] and extension of the lamina out and under the choroid with greater than a 90-degree posterior rotation, creating a bean pot–shaped excavation (see Fig. 5–7).[52,62,64] This appears clinically as an undermining of the neuroretinal rim (Fig. 5–8).[64] There is a marked loss of elastin in the lamina bordering the surface of the optic nerve head.[71] Ultimately, there is backward bowing of the entire scleral lamina cribrosa.[61]

At no time during the glaucomatous process does the posterior scleral foramen enlarge. Also, there is no selective or disproportionate loss of glial tissue or blood vessels from the optic nerve.[61] Capillaries in the optic nerve are lost at a rate that maintains the usual ratio of capillaries to axons to glial cells (Table 5–2).[61]

Patterns of Optic Nerve Damage from Glaucoma

The damage occurring in the optic nerve can present in either a diffuse or focal pattern.[98] Diffuse damage is distributed uniformly over the surface of the optic nerve and scleral laminar sheets.[52,63,91] Some studies have held that diffuse damage is more likely to occur in patients with higher intraocular pressure or in younger individuals, therefore making it more of a barotrauma.[99–101] Glaucoma patients with diffuse optic nerve damage tend to present clinically with symmetrical enlargement of the optic cup or a symmetrical thinning of the neuroretinal rim, later onset of visual field loss, field loss presenting initially as a general depression of retinal sensitivity, and the possibility of abnormal responses to various psychophysical tests such as color vision, contrast sensitivity, and visual-evoked potentials.[102–105]

Damage in the optic nerve can also occur focally, primarily in a vertical hourglass-shaped area encompassing the superior and inferior poles of the optic nerve (see Fig. 5–8).[63] It is believed that the superior and inferior polar regions are more susceptible to damage because of the larger, less supported laminar pores in these regions.[51,67] The larger ganglion cell axons also pass through these regions.[51]

Focal damage of the optic nerve from glaucoma has been thought to be related more to vascular insufficiency than to elevated intraocular pressure.[99,101] Some studies have indicated that focal damage occurs more often in people with slightly elevated intraocular pressure and older individuals.[99–101,104]

Localized changes in the optic nerve are very specific for glaucoma. Patients present with vertical elongation of the optic cup, notching of the neuroretinal rim, earlier onset of visual field defects, and paracentral

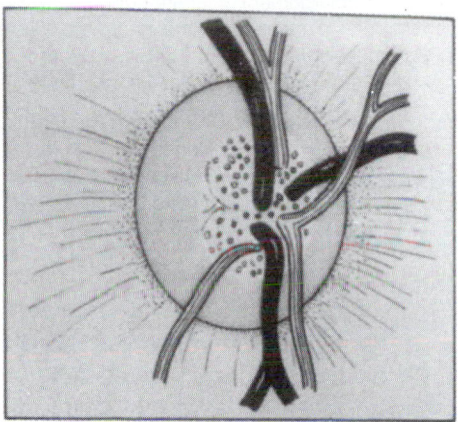
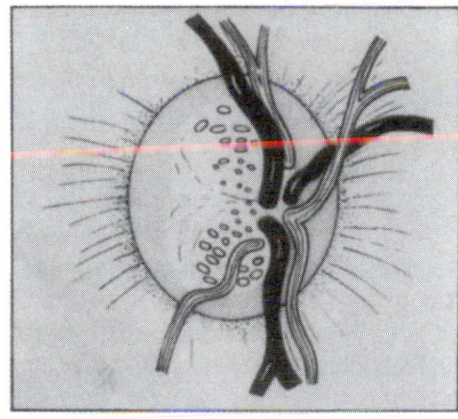
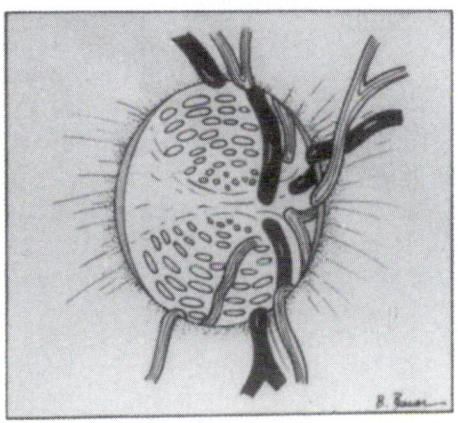

Figure 5–8. The clinical appearance of the optic nerve head as a function of increasing optic atrophy. Pores within the lamina cribrosa scleralis enlarge as glaucomatous nerve head damage progresses. (Reproduced with permission from Miller KM, Quigley HA. The clinical appearance of the lamina cribrosa as a function of the extent of glaucomatous optic nerve damage. *Ophthalmology.* 1988;95:135–138.)

TABLE 5-2. SUMMARY OF DAMAGE TO THE OPTIC NERVE HEAD

Early Glaucomatous Changes in the Optic Nerve
   Compression, stretching, and remodeling of laminar sheets
   Posterior displacement of scleral lamina cribrosa
   Distortion and/or enlargement of laminar pores
   Astrocyte hyperplasia and reactivation in the optic nerve
   Changes in composition of laminar tissue and extracellular matrix
   Loss of compliance of scleral lamina cribrosa

More Advanced Glaucomatous Changes in the Optic Nerve
   Additional compression of laminar sheets
   Additional posterior displacement of scleral lamina cribrosa
   Bean pot-shaped excavation of lamina
   Marked loss of elastin

---

scotomas or nasal steps as the earliest visual field changes. Patients with focal damage tend to be less likely to show changes on psychophysical testing.[104]

The Causes of Blockage of Axonal Transport

There is strong evidence that a blockage of axonal transport at the level of the scleral lamina cribrosa is the cause of optic nerve damage in glaucoma.[54,106-111] This blockage affects both the orthograde and the retrograde movement of material in the ganglion cell axons.[54,106-110] Retrograde blockage of axonal transport eliminates neurotrophic factors from the lateral geniculate body from reaching the retinal ganglion cell nuclei.[57,58] This is a major factor contributing to the apoptotic cell death that occurs in the ganglion cells during glaucomatous damage.[58] The degree of axonal transport blockage seems to be proportional to the level and duration of elevated intraocular pressure; however, using a variety of techniques involving animal model experiments, it has been demonstrated that even slightly elevated levels of intraocular pressure for short periods of time will inhibit axonal transport.[107,112-114] Short intervals of elevated intraocular pressure block axonal transport only in the most peripheral bundles of axons in the optic nerve.[115] A progressive increase in the intraocular pressure results in injury that extends both across and longitudinally along the axon bundles.[111]

A partial but chronic obstruction of axonal transport may exist normally at the level of the lamina cribrosa. This "physiological obstruction" affects unmyelinated axons and is most likely due to the pressure gradient across the lamina. It may help explain normal-tension glaucoma.[116]

Axonal transport is dependent on adequate blood supply to the ganglion cell axons as well as the presence of intact microtubules in the axons for the movement of material.[117] Any change that blocks the flow of blood to the axon[108,118] or mechanically damages the microtubules can result in a blockage of axoplasmic flow.[117]

As early as the mid-1800s, it was proposed that an elevation of intraocular pressure could cause the death of ganglion cells due to direct compression.[119] At about the same time, von Jaeger suggested that a vascular abnormality was the cause of glaucomatous damage.[120] Thus began a controversy that still exists today as to whether the cause of glaucomatous damage is mechanical or vascular. Since either could cause a block in axonal transport, both concepts are theoretically valid.[121] Most likely, the etiology of optic nerve damage in glaucoma is multifactorial, including mechanical, vascular, and other factors. Elevated intraocular pressure alone does not account for all POAG.[121]

In summary, abnormal levels of intraocular pressure can eventually cause compression of the scleral laminar sheets and distortion of the laminar pores. This may in part be due to remodeling of the optic nerve, causing degenerative changes in the extracellular matrix and reactivation of astrocytes. Backward displacement of the laminar sheets leads to excavation of the surface of the optic nerve. The combination of compressed sheets and distorted laminar pores can mechanically compress axons of the ganglion cells as they pass through this region and also compress the capillaries supplying the axons. Direct mechanical compression of the axons and/or a reduction in their blood supply can lead to a blockage of axonal transport. With time, this blockage leads to the apoptotic death of ganglion cells. Ganglion cell death results in a loss of tissue, causing additional cupping of the surface of the optic nerve, and also a loss of nerve fiber layer and pallor of the neuroretinal rim tissue. Cupping of the optic nerve head, dropout of the nerve fiber layer, and pallor of the neuroretinal rim are the classical changes on the nerve head seen clinically in glaucoma.

Mechanical Theory

The mechanical theory of glaucoma suggests that abnormal levels of intraocular pressure ultimately cause direct damage to the optic nerve, which alters the structure of this tissue. Elevated intraocular pressure can create an inside-outside push that compresses the laminar sheets and bows them outward, while it also increases tension on the scleral wall, which pulls on the rim of the posterior scleral foramen and disturbs the shape of the scleral lamina cribrosa (see Fig. 5-7).[88]

Compression of the sheets of the lamina cribrosa and distortion of the laminar pores, which have been observed histopathologically in glaucomatous eyes, could crimp or pinch the ganglion cell axons as they pass through this area, causing a blockage of axonal transport.[61,64] An alteration in the elastic characteristics of the lamina cribrosa resulting in an increased weakness or stiffness could lead to a permanent deformation.[52,61,88]

It is difficult to explain normal-tension glaucoma on the basis of the concepts expressed in the mechanical theory. If normal-tension glaucoma is not due to vascular insufficiency in the optic nerve, then the scleral lamina cribrosa must have some connective tissue abnormality or an unusual susceptibility to structural alterations even from "normal" levels of intraocular pressure.[122]

There is research evidence that does not support the mechanical theory as a cause of axonal transport blockage in glaucoma. Anderson and coworkers found that increases in intracranial pressure did not prevent the blockage of axonal transport when the intraocular pressure was concurrently increased.[123] They concluded that it may be more than a simple mechanical process that is involved in the obstruction of axoplasmic flow in glaucoma.[123] Radius and colleagues found no correlation between the location of axonal transport blockage and the cross-sectional area of nerve fiber bundles, the shape of the laminal pores, or the density of the interbundle septa.[124,125]

Vascular Theory

The vascular theory of glaucoma assumes that a decrease in blood flow in the scleral lamina cribrosa blocks axoplasmic flow by reducing the energy available to keep this system operational.[108,118,126] This is supported by evidence that areas of localized ischemia show localized blockage of rapid axonal transport.[117,127]

The basis for this theory is that a rise in intraocular pressure, even to levels commonly seen in POAG, causes a reduction in blood flow in intraocular vessels.[126,128] This is true in the choroid; but in the retina, autoregulatory mechanisms rapidly restore retinal blood flow in response to moderate rises in intraocular pressure or a decrease in blood pressure, thus preventing any tissue damage from ischemia.[117,126]

A key issue for the vascular theory is whether autoregulation of blood flow exists for blood vessels supplying the optic nerve.[117,129] The vascular theory assumes a lack of autoregulation in these vessels.[86,117,126,130–132] Even if autoregulation is normally present in blood vessels of the optic nerve, it may become abnormal in glaucoma.[121,133] Sossi and Anderson indicate that abnormal physiological conditions or age may lead to an impairment of autoregulation in vessels of the optic nerve, which can result in ischemia from elevated intraocular pressure.[134] Ab-

normal autoregulation may also exist in retinal blood vessels in glaucoma.[121,135,136]

There is histopathological, experimental, or clinical evidence to support the vascular theory of glaucoma.[86,126,137–145] Abnormal blood flow in the optic nerve, retinal and ophthalmic artery has been found to be abnormal in patients with POAG.[121] Histopathological studies have shown a severe reduction in the number and size of peripapillary choroidal vessels in glaucoma patients.[86,146,147] Henkind originally reported a selective atrophy of the radial peripapillary capillaries supplying the arcuate areas of the nerve fiber layer in glaucoma.[148,149] Later studies disproved these findings.[131,150] Occlusion of either the short posterior ciliary arteries or the central retinal artery can obstruct axonal transport.[151–154] Acute rises in intraocular pressure reduce the perfusion pressure in blood vessels in the optic nerve, which lowers metabolic activity in this tissue.[139] Hemodynamic differences in ophthalmic artery flow have been demonstrated between glaucoma patients and normal subjects.[155]

Many investigators have demonstrated, through fluorescein angiography, a decrease in intraocular blood flow as a result of elevated intraocular pressure.[117,145,156] Significant delays in circulation time have been shown in patients with most types of glaucoma.[117,145,156] Doppler studies have also shown a decrease in blood velocity in the optic nerve head and lamina cribrosa of patients with glaucoma.[128,157,158] Abnormalities in retinal blood flow have been detected in glaucoma.[136] Dramatic improvement in blood flow occurs in some individuals following an adequate lowering of intraocular pressure.[86] Poor filling of blood vessels in the prelaminar region of the optic nerve can also occur with a decrease in blood pressure when the difference between diastolic blood pressure and intraocular pressure is 10 mmHg or less.[86,159]

Fluorescein angiography has demonstrated not only a delay in filling of intraocular vessels, but also filling defects and leakage in glaucoma (Fig. 5–9).[86,145,160] Ischemia could induce focal endothelial damage to blood vessels, accounting for this leakage.[138] Laatikainen found peripapillary choroidal filling defects in 60% of glaucomatous eyes.[161]

The clinical presence of juxtapapillary choroidal atrophy in glaucoma patients may be an indicator of circumpapillary choroidal ischemia.[162,163] The presence of splinter or flame-shaped hemorrhages, frequently seen in glaucoma, suggests that damage to the optic nerve could be due to recurrent small, acute, focal ischemic lesions superimposed on chronic ischemia.[86,164]

The existence of normal-tension glaucoma points to a chronic vascular insufficiency as the cause of this

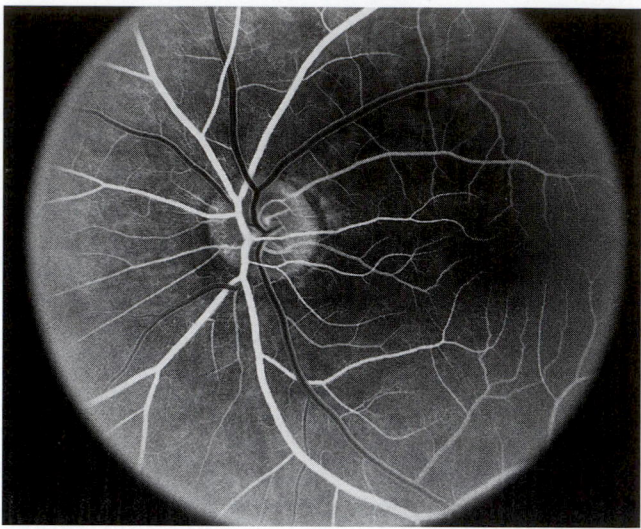

Figure 5–9. Fluorescein angiography of a patient with primary open-angle glaucoma. Note the large optic disc fluorescein filling defect involving the central portion of the disc from the superior to the inferior margin. (Reproduced with permission from Schwartz B. Nerve fiber layer and optic disc fluorescein defects in glaucoma and ocular hypertension. *Ophthalmology.* 1988;95:1227–1233.)

type of glaucoma.[165] Increased vasospastic activity is more prevalent in patients with normal-tension glaucoma.[166] Ischemic optic neuropathy can appear histopathologically and present clinically with changes in optic nerve and visual field similar to those of glaucoma.[132,137,167] A rise in intraocular pressure or lowering of systemic blood pressure can increase susceptibility to glaucoma, as well as cause progression in patients who already have the disease.[86,141] Nocturnal blood pressure decreases are more marked in glaucoma patients with progressive loss of visual fields.[168,169] A decrease in blood flow to the optic nerve can occur from local embolic disease, arteriosclerotic plaques in small arterioles, or carotid artery stenosis.[170,171] Anemia, diabetes mellitus, and migraine headaches are risk factors for glaucoma and support a vascular etiology.[86,147]

As was true for the mechanical theory, there may be an anatomic explanation applicable to the vascular theory with regard to the predilection of glaucoma to damage the superior and inferior polar regions of the optic nerve.[126] Hayreh proposes that these regions are often at the watershed of the blood supply to the optic nerve coming from the medial and lateral posterior ciliary arteries.[126,132,137,159] The watershed is the area furthest away from the source of blood and therefore the location with the lowest perfusion pressure.[126,137] Since there is no anastomosis between the medial and lateral posterior ciliary arteries, the polar regions of

the optic nerve are at greatest risk in ischemic disease processes.[126,137]

There is a significant body of knowledge that refutes the vascular theory of glaucoma.[131,150,172] No direct evidence exists for any vascular abnormality in glaucoma, nor is there anything to indicate that normal-tension glaucoma is due to chronic ischemia.[150] Histological studies have shown the presence of capillaries in the lamina cribrosa in glaucoma patients at all stages of the disease.[150] The percentage of capillaries remains remarkably constant in early and late glaucoma.[150] Other studies have shown that laminar blood flow does not decrease with an elevation of intraocular pressure, nor do glaucoma patients suffering a profound drop in blood pressure always show progressive loss of visual field.[172]

Ischemic blockage of axonal transport may not result in glaucomatous optic nerve damage. Ligation of the common carotid artery did not significantly affect the extent to which elevated intraocular pressure interrupted axonal transport.[173] Elevated intraocular pressure can experimentally block axonal transport even when maintaining a 100% Pa_{O_2} in the optic nerve tissue.[108]

The finding of fluorescein angiographic filling defects in glaucoma patients provides no direct support for the lack of adequate nutrition to axons. Fluorescein angiography allows viewing of blood vessels in the superficial optic nerve, but not in the scleral lamina cribrosa (Fig. 5–10).[150] Filling defects seen in glaucoma patients with angiography may simply represent a proportional loss of capillaries in advanced glaucoma and not areas of ischemia (see Fig. 5–9). Therefore, filling defects may be the result of tissue loss in the optic nerve and not its cause.[64,150]

Leakage of fluorescein into the optic nerve from the surrounding choroid is seen in normal individuals and may not represent a vascular abnormality of glaucoma.[145] However, the vasculature of the choroid does not share the tight junctions of the capillaries of the optic nerve. Therefore, a variety of vasoactive substances may enter the nerve head and affect the tissue. This may occur at a greater rate when discontinuities in the normal junction of choroid and the optic nerve, a crescent, occur. These crescents are more common in glaucoma.[57]

Leakage from capillaries in the scleral lamina cribrosa would not likely present on the retinal edge of the neuroretinal rim as splinter hemorrhages.[129] These flame-shaped hemorrhages may be an expression of abnormal forces acting on the walls of the capillaries in the optic nerve due to tissue loss, stretching, or rearrangement.[129]

Clearly, therefore, there remains significant debate regarding the cause of axonal transport blockage in

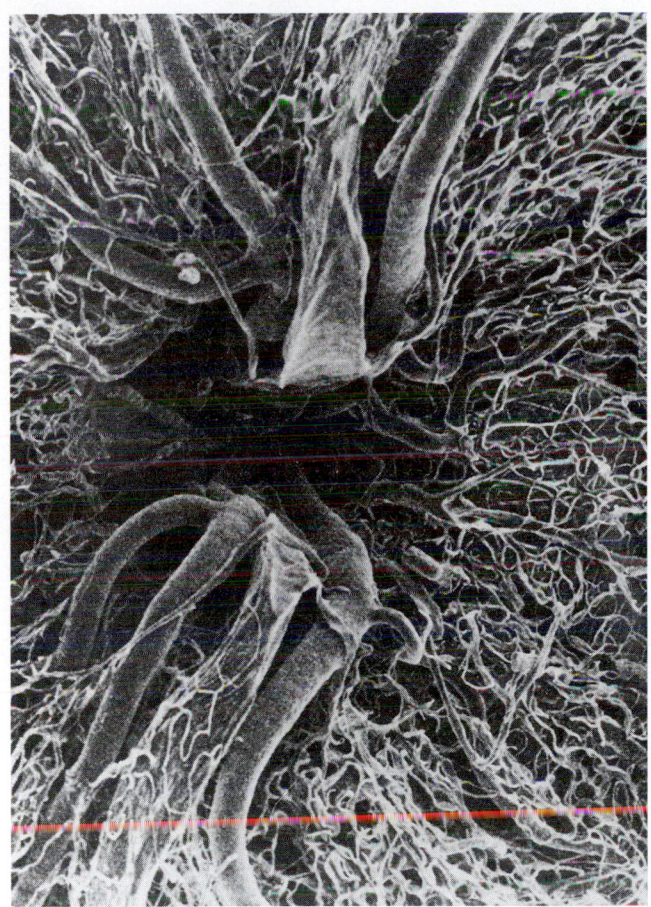

Figure 5–10. Vascular cast of optic nerve head viewed from vitreous side. Note the large number of capillaries, especially between vessels, that are poorly resolved in angiograms. Large veins are surrounded by capillaries and arteries appear to be bare. (Original magnification: ×90.) (Reprinted from *Am J Ophthalmol*, 93; Quigley HA, Hohman RM, Addicks EM, Quantitative study of optic nerve head capillaries in experimental optic disk pallor, 689–699, copyright 1982, with permission from Elsevier Science.)

glaucoma. More than likely, both mechanical and vascular factors contribute to this damage. In some patients, one is the primary cause and the other secondary.

CONCLUSION

Glaucoma represents a disease in which abnormal levels of intraocular pressure cause a chronic, gradual destruction of ganglion cell axons by the blockage of axonal transport at the level of the scleral lamina cribrosa. This blockage could be caused by a variety of contributing factors—mechanical, vascular, or biochemical. The individual contribution of these various factors to glaucomatous damage differs from patient to patient.

Some people with very low levels of intraocular pressure develop glaucomatous optic nerve damage,

whereas many individuals with elevated pressures do not. The real clinical dilemma is why an optic neuropathy from a certain level of intraocular pressure develops in some patients and not others. The answer lies in the varying susceptibility of the optic nerve, which is most likely explained by normal variations among individuals in the anatomy and physiology of this tissue. Variation could occur in the size and structural support of the pores in the scleral lamina; in the blood supply to this region, including the location of the short posterior ciliary arteries watershed zones; in the connective tissue framework of the laminar sheets; and in the composition of components of the extracellular matrix of the scleral lamina. These variations could explain the development of glaucomatous damage to the optic nerve.

An understanding of the etiology and pathophysiology of glaucoma is essential to an early differential diagnosis and appropriate management. Knowledge of the changes occurring in the optic nerve as a consequence of the glaucomatous process makes the early subtle changes in this tissue much easier to detect clinically.

REFERENCES

1. Rohen JW, Lütjen-Drecoll E. Morphology of aqueous outflow pathways in normal and glaucomatous eyes. In: Ritch R, Shields MB, Krupin T, eds. *The Glaucomas.* St. Louis: CV Mosby; 1989:41–74.
2. Alvarado J, Murphy C, Juster R. Trabecular meshwork cellularity in primary open-angle glaucoma and nonglaucomatous normals. *Ophthalmology.* 1984;91:564–579.
3. Rohen JW. Why is intraocular pressure elevated in chronic simple glaucoma? Anatomic considerations. *Ophthalmology.* 1983;90:758–768.
4. Alvarado JA, Yun AJ, Murphy CG. Juxtacanalicular tissue in primary open angle glaucoma and in nonglaucomatous normals. *Arch Ophthalmol.* 1986;104:1517–1528.
5. Rohen JW, Futa R, Lütjen-Drecoll E. The fine structure of the cribriform meshwork in normal and glaucomatous eyes as seen in tangential sections. *Invest Ophthalmol Vis Sci.* 1981;21:574–585.
6. Lütjen-Drecoll E, Futa R, Rohen J. Ultrahistochemical studies on tangential sections of the trabecular meshwork in normal and glaucomatous eyes. *Invest Ophthalmol Vis Sci.* 1981;21:563–573.
7. Lütjen-Drecoll E, Shimizu T, Rohrbach M, Rohen JW. Quantitative analysis of "plaque material" between ciliary muscle tips in normal and glaucomatous eyes. *Exp Eye Res.* 1986;42:457–465.
8. Lütjen-Drecoll E, Shimizu T, Rohrbach M, Rohen JW. Quantitative analysis of "plaque material" in the inner

and outer wall of Schlemm's canal in normal and glaucomatous eyes. *Exp Eye Res.* 1986;42:443–455.

9. Tripathi RC, Tripathi BJ, Spaeth GL. Localization of sialic acid moieties in the endothelial lining of Schlemm's canal in normal and glaucomatous eyes. *Exp Eye Res.* 1987;44:293–306.

10. Floyd BB, Cleveland PH, Worthen DM. Fibronectin in human trabecular drainage channels. *Invest Ophthalmol Vis Sci.* 1985;26:797–804.

11. Quigley HA, Addicks EM. Scanning electron microscopy of trabeculectomy specimens from eyes with open-angle glaucoma. *Am J Ophthalmol.* 1980;90: 854–857.

12. deKater AW, Melamed S, Epstein DL. Patterns of aqueous human outflow in glaucomatous and nonglaucomatous human eyes. *Arch Ophthalmol.* 1989;107:572–576.

13. Tawara A, Varner HH, Hollyfield JG. Distribution and characterization of sulfated proteoglycans in the human trabecular tissue. *Invest Ophthalmol Vis Sci.* 1989;30:2215–2231.

14. Lütjen-Drecoll E, Rittig M, Rauterberg J, Jander R, Mollenhuser J. Immunomicroscopical study of type VI collagen in the trabecular meshwork of normal and glaucomatous eyes. *Exp Eye Res.* 1989;48:139–147.

15. Fink AF, Felix MD, Fletcher RC. The electron microscopy of Schlemm's canal and adjacent structure in patients with glaucoma. *Trans Am Ophthalmol Soc.* 1972;70:82–102.

16. Fine BS, Yanoff MS, Stone R. A clinicopathologic study of four cases of primary open-angle glaucoma compared to normal eyes. *Am J Ophthalmol.* 1981;91: 88–105.

17. Rohen JW. Presence of matrix vesicles in the trabecular meshwork of glaucomatous eyes. *Graefes Arch Clin Exp Ophthalmol.* 1982;218:171–176.

18. Tripathi RC. Pathologic anatomy of the outflow pathways of aqueous humor in chronic simple glaucoma. *Exp Eye Res.* 1977;25(suppl):403–407.

19. Buller C, Johnson D. Segmental variability of the trabecular meshwork in normal and glaucomatous eyes. *Invest Ophthalmol Vis Sci.* 1994;35:3841–3851.

20. Quigley HA, Addicks EM. Scanning electron microscopy of trabeculectomy specimens from eyes with open-angle glaucoma. *Am J Ophthalmol.* 1980;90: 854–857.

21. Rohen JW, Witmer R. Electron microscopic studies on the trabecular meshwork in glaucoma simplex. V. *Graefes Arch Clin Exp Ophthalmol.* 1972;183:251–266.

22. Grierson I, Calthorpe CM. Characteristics of meshwork cells and age changes in the outflow system of the eye: Their relevance to primary open-angle glaucoma. In: Mills KB, ed. *Glaucoma: Proceedings of the Fourth International Symposium of the Northern Eye Institute.* Manchester, UK: Pergamon Press; 1988:12–31.

23. Shirato S, Murphy CG, Bloom E, Franse-Carman L, et al. Kinetics of phagocytosis in trabecular meshwork cells. *Invest Ophthalmol Vis Sci.* 1989;30:2499–2511.

24. Samuelson DA, Gum GG, Gelatt KN. Ultrastructural changes in the aqueous outflow apparatus of beagles with inherited glaucoma. *Invest Ophthalmol Vis Sci.* 1989;30:550–561.

25. Polansky JR, Wood IS, Maglio MT, Alvarado JA. Trabecular meshwork cell culture in glaucoma research: Evaluation of biological activity and structural properties of human trabecular cells in vitro. *Ophthalmology.* 1984;91:580–595.

26. Fei PF, Yue BY, Tso MOM. Effects of chondroitin sulfate on trabecular meshwork in rabbit eyes: An electron microscopic study. *Exp Eye Res.* 1984;39:583–594.

27. Yun AJ, Murphy CG, Polansky JR, Newsome DA, Alvarado JA. Proteins secreted by human trabecular cells. *Invest Ophthalmol Vis Sci.* 1989;30:2012–2022.

28. Murphy CG, Yun AJ, Newsome DA, Alvarado JA. Localization of extracellular proteins of the human trabecular meshwork by indirect immunofluorescence. *Am J Ophthalmol.* 1987;104:33–43.

29. Grierson I. What is open angle glaucoma? *Eye.* 1987;1:15–28.

30. Chapman SA, Bonshek RE, Stoddart RW, O'Donoghue E, Gooda II K, McLeod D. Glycans of trabecular meshwork in primary open angle glaucoma. *Br J Ophthalmol* 1996;80:435–444.

31. Alvarado J, Murphy C, Polansky J, Juster R. Age-related changes in trabecular meshwork cellularity. *Invest Ophthalmol Vis Sci.* 1981;21:714–727.

32. Larina IN. On intrascleral outflow channels in glaucoma. *Vestn Oftalmol.* 1967;2:18–23.

33. Nesterov AP. Role of the blockade of Schlemm's canal in pathogenesis of primary open-angle glaucoma. *Am J Ophthalmol.* 1970;70:691–696.

34. Moses RA, Grodzki WJ, Etheridge EL, Wilson CD. Schlemm's canal: The effect of intraocular pressure. *Invest Ophthalmol Vis Sci.* 1981;70:61–68.

35. Allingham RR, Dekater AW, Ethier CR. Schlemm's canal and primary open angle glaucoma: A correlation between Schlemm's canal dimensions and outflow facility. *Exp Eye Res.* 1996;62:101–109.

36. Gagnon MM, Boisjoly HM, Brunette I, Charest M, Amyot M. Corneal endothelial cell density in glaucoma. *Cornea.* 1997;16(3):314–318.

37. Johnson DH, Richardson TM, Epstein DL. Trabecular meshwork recovery after phagocytic challenge. *Curr Eye Res.* 1989;8:1121–1130.

38. Matsumoto Y, Johnson DH. Trabecular meshwork phagocytosis in glaucomatous eyes. *Ophthalmologica.* 1997;211:147–152.

39. Chaudhry HA, Dueker DK, Simmons RJ, Bellows R, Grant WM. Scanning electron microscopy of trabeculectomy specimens in open-angle glaucoma. *Am J Ophthalmol.* 1979;88:78–92.

40. Knepper PA, Goossens W, Huizd M, Palmberg PF. Glycosaminoglycans of the human trabecular meshwork in primary open-angle glaucoma. *Ophthalmol Vis Sci.* 1996;37:1360–1367.

41. Knepper PA, Goossens W, Palmberg PF. Glycosaminoglycans of the juxtacanalicular tissue in normal and primary open-angle glaucoma. *Invest Ophthalmol Vis Sci.* 1996;37:2414–2415.

42. Rohen JW, Lütjen-Drecoll E, Flügel C, Meyer M, Grierson I. Ultrastructure of the trabecular meshwork in

untreated cases of primary open-angle glaucoma (POAG). *Exp Eye Res.* 1993;56:683–692.

43. Gottanka J, Johnson DH, Martus P, Lütjen-Drecoll E. Severity of optic nerve damage in eyes with POAG is correlated with changes in the trabecular meshwork. *J Glaucoma.* 1997;6:123–132.

44. Tripathi RC. Mechanism of the aqueous outflow across the trabecular wall of Schlemm's canal. *Exp Eye Res.* 1971;11:116–121.

45. Tripathi R, Li J, Chan WFA, Tripathi BJ. Aqueous humor in glaucomatous eyes contains an increased level of TGF-B2. *Exp Eye Res.* 1994;59:723–728.

46. Wordinger RJ, Clark AF, Agarwal R, Lambert W, et al. Cultured human trabecular meshwork cells express functional growth factor receptors. *Invest Ophthalmol Vis Sci.* 1998;39:1575–1589.

47. Gonzalez-Avila G, Ginebra M, Havakawa T, Vadillo-Ortega F, et al. Collagen metabolism in human aqueous humor from primary open-angle glaucoma: Decreased degradation and increased biosynthesis play a role in its pathogenesis. *Arch Ophthalmol.* 1995;113:1319–1323.

48. Doss EW, Ward KA, Koretz JF. Investigation of the "fines" hypothesis of primary open-angle glaucoma: The possible role of alpha-crystallin. *Ophthalm Res.* 1998;30:142–156.

49. Iwata K, Kurosawa A, Sawaguchi S. Wedge-shaped retinal nerve fiber layer defects in experimental glaucoma: Preliminary report. *Graefes Arch Clin Exp Ophthalmol.* 1985;223:184–189.

50. Kitazawa K, Matsubara K. Optic disc changes in early glaucoma (summary). *Surv Ophthalmol.* 1989;37(suppl): 417–418.

51. Quigley HA, Sanchez RM, Dunkelberger GR, et al. Chronic glaucoma selectively damages large optic nerve fibers. *Invest Ophthalmol Vis Sci.* 1987;28:913–920.

52. Quigley HA. Reappraisal of the mechanisms of glaucomatous optic nerve damage. *Eye.* 1987;1:318–322.

53. Quigley HA. Glaucoma's optic nerve damage: Changing clinical perspectives. *Ann Ophthalmol.* 1982;14: 611–612.

54. Radius RL, Anderson DR. Rapid axonal transport in primate optic nerve: Distribution of pressure induced interruption. *Arch Ophthalmol.* 1981;99:650–654.

55. Minckler DS. Histology of optic nerve damage in ocular hypertension and early glaucoma. *Surv Ophthalmol.* 1989;33(suppl):401–402.

56. Quigley HA, Nickells RW, Kerrigan LA, Pease ME, et al. Retinal ganglion cell death in experimental glaucoma and after axotomy occurs by apoptosis. *Invest Ophthalmol Vis Sci.* 1995;36:774–786.

57. Quigley HA. Neuronal death in glaucoma. *Prog Retin Eye Res.* 1998;18:39–57.

58. Quigley HA. Ganglion cell death in glaucoma: Pathology recapitulates ontogeny. *Aust N Z J Ophthalmol.* 1995;23:85–91.

59. Dreyer EB, Zurakowski D, Shumer RA, Podos SM, Lipton MA. Elevated glutamate levels in the vitreous body of humans and monkeys with glaucoma. *Arch Ophthalmol.* 1996;114:299–305.

60. Nickells RW. Retinal ganglion cell death in glaucoma: The how, the why, and the maybe. *J Glaucoma.* 1996;5: 345–356.

61. Quigley HA, Hohman RM, Addicks EM, et al. Morphologic changes in the lamina cribrosa correlated with neural loss in open-angle glaucoma. *Am J Ophthalmol.* 1983;95:673–691.

62. Brooks DE, Samuelson DA, Gelatt KN, Smith PJ. Morphologic changes in the lamina cribrosa of beagles with primary open angle glaucoma. *Am J Vet Res.* 1989;50:936–941.

63. Quigley HA. The pathogenesis of optic nerve damage in glaucoma: Symposium on the laser in ophthalmology and glaucoma update. *Trans New Orleans Acad Ophthalmol.* 1985;111–128.

64. Quigley HA, Addicks EM, Green WR, Maumenee AE. Optic nerve damage in human glaucoma: II. The site of injury and susceptibility to damage. *Arch Ophthalmol.* 1981;99:635–649.

65. Burgoyne CF, Quigley HA, Thompson HW, Vitale S, Varma R. Early changes in optic disc compliance and surface position in experimental glaucoma. *Ophthalmology.* 1995;102:1800–1809.

66. Yan DB, Coloma FM, Metheetrairut A, Trope GE, et al. Deformation of the lamina cribrosa by elevated intraocular pressure. *Br J Ophthalmol.* 1994;78:643–648.

67. Miller KN, Quigley HA. The clinical appearance of the lamina cribrosa as a function of the extent of glaucomatous optic nerve damage. *Ophthalmology.* 1988;95: 135–138.

68. Fontana L, Bhandari A, Fitzke FW, Hitchings RA. In vivo morphometry of the lamina cribrosa and its relation to visual field loss in glaucoma. *Curr Eye Res.* 1998;17:363–369.

69. Varela HJ, Hernandez MR. Astrocyte responses in human optic nerve head with primary open-angle glaucoma. *J Glaucoma.* 1997;6:303–313.

70. Hernandez MR, Ye H, Roy S. Collagen type IV gene expression in human optic nerve heads with primary open angle glaucoma. *Exp Eye Res.* 1994;59:41–52.

71. Hernandez MR, Andrzejewska WM, Neufeld AH. Changes in the extracellular matrix of the human optic nerve head in primary open-angle glaucoma. *Am J Ophthalmol.* 1990;109:180–188.

72. Hernandez MR, Pena JDO. The optic nerve head in glaucomatous optic neuropathy. *Arch Ophthalmol.* 1997;115:389–395.

73. Hernandez MR, Yong J, Ye H. Activation of elastin mRNA expression in human optic nerve heads with primary open angle glaucoma. *J Glaucoma.* 1994;3: 214–225.

74. Hernandez MR. Ultrastructural immunocytochemical analysis of elastin fibers in primary open angle glaucoma. *Invest Ophthalmol Vis Sci.* 1992;33:2891–2903.

75. Quigley HA, Brown A, Dorman-Pease ME. Alterations in elastin of the optic nerve head in human and experimental glaucoma. *Br J Ophthalmol.* 1991;75:552–557.

76. Quigley HA, Pease ME, Thibault D. Change in the appearance of elastin in the lamina cribrosa of

glaucomatous optic nerve heads. *Graefes Arch Clin Exp Ophthalmol.* 1994;232:257–261.

77. Morrison JC, Dorman-Pease ME, Dunkelberger GR, Quigley HA. Optic nerve head extracellular matrix in primary optic atrophy and experimental glaucoma. *Arch Ophthalmol.* 1990;108:1020–1024.

78. Fukuchi T, Sawaguchi S, Hara H, Iwata K, et al. Ultrastructural changes in the lamina cribrosa in experimental monkey glaucoma. *Nippon Ganka Gakkai Zasshi.* 1995;99:1222–1229.

79. Taylor AW, Pena JDO, Hernandez MR. Cytokines produced by explanted human optic nerve heads of normal and glaucomatous eyes. *Invest Ophthalmol Vis Sci ARVO.* 1995;36(suppl):S607.

80. Tripathi BJ, Li T, Li J, Chalam KV, Tripathi RC. Upregulated expression of gamma-interferon and transforming growth factor β1 in the optic nerve head of glaucomatous eyes. *Invest Ophthalmol Vis Sci ARVO.* 1996;37 (suppl):S411.

81. O'Brien MF, Lenke LG, Lou J, Bridwell KH, Joyce ME. Astrocyte response and transforming growth factor beta localization in acute spinal cord injury. *Spine.* 1994;19:2321–2330.

82. Flanders KC, Lüdecke G, Renzig J, Hamm C, et al. Effect of TGF-bs and bFGF on astroglial cell growth and gene expression in vitro. *Mol Cell Neurosci.* 1993;4: 406–417.

83. Pena JDO, Varela HJ, Ricard CS, Hernandez MR. Enhanced tenascin expression associated with reactive astrocytes in human optic nerve heads with primary open angle glaucoma. *Exp Eye Res.* 1999;68:29–40.

84. Pena JDO, Taylor AW, Ricard CS, Vidal I, Hernandez MR. Transforming growth factor β isoforms in human optic nerve heads. *Br J Ophthalmol.* 1999;83:1–9.

85. Koukoulis GK, Gould VE, Bhattacharyya A, Gould JE, et al. Tenascin in normal, reactive, hyperplastic, and neoplastic tissues: Biologic and pathologic implications. *Hum Pathol.* 1991;22:636–643.

86. Minckler DS, Spaeth GL. Optic nerve damage in glaucoma. *Surv Ophthalmol.* 1981;26:128–148.

87. Quigley HA, Dorman-Pease ME, Brown AE. Quantitative study of collagen and elastin of the optic nerve head and sclera in human and experimental glaucoma. *Curr Eye Res.* 1991;10:877–888.

88. Zeimer RC, Ogura Y. The relationship between glaucomatous damage and optic nerve head mechanical compliance. *Arch Ophthalmol.* 1989;107:1232–1234.

89. Eddelston M, Mucke L. Molecular profile of reactive astrocytes: Implications for their role in neurological diseases. *Neuroscience.* 1993;54:15–36.

90. Hernandez MR, Ye H. Glaucoma: Changes in extracellular matrix in the optic nerve head. *Ann Med.* 1993;25:309–315.

91. Dandona L, Hendrickson A, Quigley HA. Selective effects of experimental glaucoma on axonal transport by retinal ganglion cells to the dorsal lateral geniculate nucleus. *Invest Ophthalmol Vis Sci.* 1991;32:1593–1599.

92. Quigley HA, Dunkelberger GR, Green WR. Chronic human glaucoma causing selective greater loss of large optic nerve fibers. *Ophthalmology.* 1988;95:357–363.

93. Chaturvedi N, Hedley-Whyte T, Dreyer EB. Lateral geniculate nucleus in glaucoma. *Am J Ophthalmol.* 1993;116:182–188.

94. Glovinsky Y, Quigley HA, Dunkelberger GR. Retinal ganglion cell loss is size dependent in experimental glaucoma. *Invest Ophthalmol Vis Sci.* 1991;32:484–491.

95. Wygnanski T, Desatnik H, Quigley HA, Glovinsky Y. Comparison of ganglion cell loss and cone loss in experimental glaucoma. *Am J Ophthalmol.* 1995;120: 184–189.

96. Schnabel J. Die Entwicklungsgeschichte der glaukomatosen Exkavation. *Z Augenheilkd.* 1905;14:1.

97. Quigley HA, Addicks EM, Green WR. Optic nerve damage in glaucoma: III. Quantitative correlation of nerve fiber loss and visual field defect in glaucoma, ischemic neuropathy, papilledema, and toxic neuropathy. *Arch Ophthalmol.* 1982;100:135–146.

98. Airaksinen PJ, Drance SM, Douglas GR, et al. Diffuse and localized nerve fiber loss in glaucoma. *Am J Ophthalmol.* 1984;98:566–571.

99. Glowazki A, Flammer J. Is there a difference between glaucoma patients with rather localized visual field damage and patients with more diffuse visual field damage? *Doc Ophthalmol Proc Ser.* 1987;49:317–320.

100. Chauhan BC, Drance SM. The influence of intraocular pressure on visual field damage in patients with normal-tension and high-tension glaucoma. *Invest Ophthalmol Vis Sci.* 1990;31:2367–2372.

101. Caprioli J, Spaeth GL. Comparison of visual field defects in the low-tension glaucomas with those in the high-tension glaucomas. *Am J Ophthalmol.* 1984;97: 730–737.

102. Drance SM. The early structural and functional disturbances of chronic open-angle glaucoma: Robert N. Shaffer Lecture. *Ophthalmology.* 1985;92:853–857.

103. Bodis-Wollner I. Electrophysiological and psychophysical testing of vision in glaucoma. *Surv Ophthalmol.* 1989;33(suppl):301–307.

104. Stamper RL. Psychophysical changes in glaucoma. *Surv Ophthalmol.* 1989;33(suppl):309–318.

105. Sommer A, Katz J, Quigley HA, et al. Clinically detectable nerve fiber atrophy precedes the onset of glaucomatous field loss. *Arch Ophthalmol.* 1991;109:77–83.

106. Sakugawa M, Chihara E. Blockage at two points of axonal transport in glaucomatous eyes. *Graefes Arch Clin Ophthalmol.* 1985;223:214–218.

107. Minckler DS, Tso MOM, Zimmerman LE. A light microscopic, autoradiographic study of axoplasmic transport in the optic nerve head during ocular hypotony, increased intraocular pressure and papilledema. *Am J Ophthalmol.* 1976;82:741–757.

108. Minckler DS, Bunt AH, Johanson GW. Orthograde and retrograde axoplasmic transport during acute ocular hypertension in the monkey. *Invest Ophthalmol Vis Sci.* 1977;16:426–441.

109. Lampert PW, Vogel MH, Zimmerman LE. Pathology of the optic nerve in experimental glaucoma. *Invest Ophthalmol Vis Sci.* 1968;7:199–213.

110. Elkington AR, Inman CBE, Steart PV, Weller RO. The structure of the lamina cribrosa of the human eye: An

immunocytochemical and electron microscopic study. *Eye.* 1990;4:42–57.

111. Minckler DS. Histology of optic nerve damage in ocular hypertension and early glaucoma. *Surv Ophthalmol.* 1989;33(suppl):401–402.

112. Radius RL. Distribution of pressure-induced fast axonal transport abnormalities in primate optic nerve: An audioradiographic study. *Arch Ophthalmol.* 1981;99: 1257–1263.

113. Minckler DS, Tso MOM. A light microscopic audioradiographic study of axoplasmic transport in the normal rhesus optic nerve head. *Am J Ophthalmol.* 1976;82:1–15.

114. Quigley HA, Anderson DR. The dynamics and location of axonal transport blockade by acute intraocular pressure elevation in primate optic nerve. *Invest Ophthalmol Vis Sci.* 1976;15:606–616.

115. Minckler DS, Ogden TE. Distribution of axonal transport injury in the lamina in experimental glaucoma in the monkey. In: Krieglstein GK, ed. *Glaucoma Update III.* Berlin: Springer-Verlag; 1987:27–35.

116. Holländer H, Makarov F, Stefani FH, Stone J. Evidence of constriction of optic nerve axons at the lamina cribrosa in the normotensive eye in humans and other mammals. *Ophthalm Res.* 1995;27:296–309.

117. Radius RL. Anatomy of the optic nerve head and glaucomatous optic neuropathy. *Surv Ophthalmol.* 1987;32: 35–44.

118. Sossi N, Anderson DR. Blockade of axonal transport in optic nerve induced by elevation of intraocular pressure: Effect of arterial hypertension induced by angiotensin I. *Arch Ophthalmol.* 1983;101:94–97.

119. Müller H. Anatomische Beitrage zur Ophthalmologie: Über Nerven-Veranderungen an der Eintrittsstelle des Sehnerven. *Arch Ophthalmol.* 1858;4:1.

120. von Jaeger E. Über Glaucom und seine Heilung durch Iridectomie. *Z Ges Aerzte Wien.* 1858;14:465–484.

121. Fechtner RD, Weinreb RN. Mechanisms of optic nerve damage in primary open angle glaucoma. *Surv Ophthalmol.* 1994;39:23–42.

122. Iwata K. Primary open angle glaucoma and low tension glaucoma—pathogenesis and mechanism of optic nerve damage. *Acta Soc Ophthalmol Jpn.* 1992;96: 1501–1531.

123. Anderson DR, Hendrickson AE. Failure of increased intracranial pressure to affect rapid axonal transport at the optic nerve head. *Invest Ophthalmol Vis Sci.* 1977; 16:423–426.

124. Radius RL, Bade B. Axonal transport interruption and anatomy at the lamina cribrosa. *Arch Ophthalmol.* 1982; 100:1661–1664.

125. Radius RL. Pressure-induced fast axonal transport abnormalities and the anatomy at the lamina cribrosa in primate eyes. *Invest Ophthalmol Vis Sci.* 1983;24: 343–346.

126. Hayreh SS. The pathogenesis of optic nerve lesions in glaucoma. Symposium: The optic disc in glaucoma. *Trans Am Acad Ophthalmol Otolaryngol.* 1976;81:197–213.

127. Ochs S. Local supply of energy to the fast axoplasmic transport mechanism. *Proc Natl Acad Sci USA.* 1971;68:1279–1282.

128. Grunmwald JE, Piltz J, Hariprasad SM, DuPont J. Optic nerve and choroidal circulation in glaucoma. *Invest Ophthalmol Vis Sci.* 1998;39:2329–2336.

129. Gasser P. Ocular vasospasm: A risk factor in the pathogenesis of low-tension glaucoma. *Int Ophthalmol.* 1989;13:281–290.

130. Neetens A. Autoregulation of the blood supply to the anterior optic nerve lamina cribrosa. *Trans Ophthalmol Soc UK.* 1977;97:168–176.

131. Maumene EA. Causes of optic nerve damage in glaucoma. *Ophthalmology.* 1983;90:741–752.

132. Hayreh SS. Pathogenesis of visual field defects: Role of the ciliary circulation. *Br J Ophthalmol.* 1970;54:289–311.

133. Ulrich WD, Ulrich C, Bohne BD. Deficient autoregulation and lengthening of the diffusion distance in the anterior optic nerve circulation in glaucoma: An electro-encephalo-dynamographic investigation. *Ophthalm Res.* 1986;18:253–259.

134. Sossi N, Anderson DR. Effect of elevated intraocular pressure on blood flow: Occurrence in the cat optic nerve head studied with iodantipyrine I 125. *Arch Ophthalmol.* 1983;101:98–101.

135. Anderson DR. Glaucoma, capillaries and pericytes: 1. Blood flow regulation. *Ophthalmologica.* 1996;210: 257–262.

136. Grunwald JE, Riva CE, Stone RA, Keates EU, Petrig BL. Retinal autoregulation in open angle glaucoma. *Ophthalmology.* 1984;91:1690–1694.

137. Hayreh SS. Interindividual variation in blood supply of the optic nerve head. *Doc Ophthalmol.* 1985;59: 217–246.

138. Brooks DE, Samuelson DA, Gelatt KK. Ultrastructural change in laminar optic nerve capillaries of beagles with primary open-angle glaucoma. *Am J Vet Res.* 1989;50: 929–935.

139. Novack RL, Stefánsson E, Hatchell DL. Intraocular pressure effects on optic nerve-head oxidative metabolism measured in vivo. *Graefes Arch Clin Exp Ophthalmol.* 1990;228:128–133.

140. Radius RL, Anderson DR. Breakdown of the normal optic nerve head blood-brain barrier following acute elevation of intraocular pressure in experimental animals. *Invest Ophthalmol Vis Sci.* 1980;19:244–255.

141. Yabionski M. An analysis of the "vascular hypothesis" concerning optic disc pathology in glaucoma. *Ann Ophthalmol.* 1979;11:67–69.

142. Sebag J, Thomas JV, Epstein DL, Grant WM. Optic disc cupping in anterior ischemic optic neuropathy resembles glaucomatous cupping. *Ophthalmology.* 1986;93:357–361.

143. Robert Y, Steiner D, Hendrickson P. Papillary circulation dynamics in glaucoma. *Graefes Arch Clin Exp Ophthalmol.* 1989;227:436–439.

144. Tuulonen A. Asymptomatic miniocclusions of the optic disc veins in glaucoma. *Arch Ophthalmol.* 1989;107: 1475–1480.

145. Nanba K, Schwartz B. Nerve fiber layer and optic disc fluorescein defects in glaucoma and ocular hypertension. *Ophthalmology.* 1988;95:1227–1233.

146. Jonas JB, Naumann GOH. Parapapillary retinal vessel diameter in normal and glaucomatous eyes: II.

Correlations. *Invest Ophthalmol Vis Sci.* 1989;30: 1604–1611.

147. Hayreh SS. Pathogenesis of optic nerve head changes in glaucoma. *Semin Ophthalmol.* 1986;1:1–13.

148. Henkind P, Alterman M. Radial peripapillary capillaries of the retina: II. Possible role in Bjerrum scotoma. *Br J Ophthalmol.* 1968;52:26–31.

149. Henkind P. Radial peripapillary capillaries of the retina: I. Anatomy: Human and comparative. *Br J Ophthalmol.* 1967;51:115–123.

150. Quigley HA, Hohman RM, Addicks EM. Quantitative study of optic nerve head capillaries in experimental optic disk pallor. *Am J Ophthalmol.* 1982;93:689–699.

151. Levy NS, Adams CK. Slow axonal protein transport and visual function following retinal and optic nerve ischemia. *Invest Ophthalmol Vis Sci.* 1975;14:91–97.

152. Levy NS. The effect of interruption of the short posterior ciliary arteries on slow axoplasmic transport and histology within the optic nerve of the rhesus monkey. *Invest Ophthalmol.* 1976;15:495–499.

153. Radius RL. Optic nerve fast axonal transport abnormalities in primates. Occurrence after short posterior ciliary artery occlusion. *Arch Ophthalmol.* 1980;98:2018–2022.

154. Radius RL, Anderson DR. Morphology of axonal transport abnormalities in primate eyes. *Br J Ophthalmol.* 1981;65:767–777.

155. Rojanapongpun P, Drance SM, Morrison BJ. Ophthalmic artery flow velocity in glaucomatous and normal subjects. *Br J Ophthalmol.* 1993;77:25–29.

156. Shaffer RN. Nerve fiber loss and disparity of disc and field changes in glaucoma: Symposium on the laser in ophthalmology and glaucoma update. *Trans New Orleans Acad Ophthalmol.* 1985;129–133.

157. Michelson G, Langhans MJ, Groh MJM. Perfusion of the juxtapapillary retina and the neuroretinal rim area in primary open angle glaucoma. *J Glaucoma.* 1996;5:91–98.

158. Nicolela MT, Hnik P, Drance SM. Scanning laser Doppler flowmeter study of retinal and optic disk blood flow in glaucomatous patients. *Am J Ophthalmol.* 1996;122:775–783.

159. Hayreh SS, Revie HS, Edwards J. Vasogenic origin of visual field defects and optic nerve changes in glaucoma. *Br J Ophthalmol.* 1970;54:461–472.

160. Schwartz B, Reiser JC, Fishbein SL. Fluorescein angiographic defects of the optic disc in glaucoma. *Arch Ophthalmol.* 1977;95:1961–1974.

161. Laatikainen L. Fluorescein angiographic studies of the peripapillary and perilimbal regions in simple, capsular and low tension glaucoma. *Acta Ophthalmol.* 1971;111(suppl):10–13.

162. Jonas JB, Nguyen XN, Gusek GC, Naumann GOH. Parapapillary chorioretinal atrophy in normal and glaucomatous eyes. *Invest Ophthalmol Vis Sci.* 1989;30: 908–918.

163. Jonas JB, Nguyen XN, Naumann GOH. Parapapillary retinal vessel diameter in normal and glaucomatous eyes: I. Morphometric data. *Invest Ophthalmol Vis Sci.* 1989;30:1599–1603.

164. Krakau T. Disc haemorrhages and the etiology of glaucoma. *Acta Ophthalmol.* 1989;67(suppl):31–33.

165. Carter CJ, Brooks DE, Doyle DL, Drance SM. Investigations into a vascular etiology for low-tension glaucoma. *Ophthalmology.* 1990;97:49–55.

166. Drance SM, Donglas GR, Wijsman K, Schulzer M, Britton RJ. Response of blood flow to warm and cold in normal and low-tension glaucoma patients. *Am J Ophthalmol.* 1988;105:35–39.

167. Sebag J, Thomas JV, Epstein DL, Grant WM. Optic disc cupping in arteritic anterior ischemic optic neuropathy resembles glaucomatous cupping. *Ophthalmology.* 1986;93:357–361.

168. Hayreh SS, Zimmerman MB, Padajsky P, Alward WL. The role of nocturnal hypotension in ocular and optic nerve ischemic disorders (abstract). *Invest Ophthalmol Vis Sci (suppl).* 1993;34:994.

169. Graham SL, Drance SM, Sijsman K, Douglas G, Mikelberg FS. Ambulatory blood pressure monitoring in glaucoma: The nocturnal dip. *Ophthalmology.* 1995;102:61–69.

170. Harrington DO. The Bjerrum scotoma. *Trans Am Ophthalmol Soc.* 1964;62:324–348.

171. Harrington DO. The pathogenesis of the glaucoma field. *Am J Ophthalmol.* 1959;47:177–185.

172. Quigley HA, Hohman RM, Sanchez R, Addicks EM. Optic nerve head blood flow in experimental glaucoma. *Arch Ophthalmol.* 1985;103:956–962.

173. Radius RL, Schwartz EL, Anderson DR. Failure of unilateral carotid artery ligation to affect pressure-induced interruption of rapid axonal transport in primate optic nerves. *Invest Ophthalmol Vis Sci.* 1980;19:153–157.

Chapter 6

THE MEASUREMENT OF BLOOD FLOW

Larry Kagemann, Alon Harris, Hak Sung Chung, Hanna J. Garzozi

There is a growing body of evidence that vascular pathologies may play an important role in the etiology of a number of ophthalmic afflictions. In diseases such as diabetic retinopathy, the vascular component is clear. In others, such as glaucoma and age-related macular degeneration, the role of altered hemodynamics is still debated, though it is finding support among clinicians.[1-5] The importance of measuring ocular blood flow, specifically in the posterior segment, is therefore increasing in all aspects of ophthalmic research and patient care. Ophthalmic disorders may lead to or result from deficits in ocular blood flow. Clinically, the assessment of ocular hemodynamics offers promise for detection, differentiation, and diagnosis of diseases. The severity of specific hemodynamic changes can be assessed to monitor disease progression. Further, assessment of ocular blood flow will allow clinicians to monitor the efficacy of treatment.

ANATOMY OF THE VASCULATURE OF THE OPTIC NERVE HEAD

The eye is a unique organ. It contains the most vascularized tissue in the body and its anatomy has been extensively studied.[6-17] Despite these efforts, the precise microvascular anatomy of the optic nerve head remains difficult to ascertain because of its complexity, size, and inaccessibility.

The ophthalmic artery supplies all blood flow into the eye, which is made up of the retinal and uveal systems. One to five posterior ciliary arteries (PCAs) supply the uveal system, which brings blood to the iris, ciliary body, and choroid. They emerge from the ophthalmic artery in the posterior orbit.[18-22] Short posterior ciliary arteries penetrate the sclera surrounding insertion of the optic nerve. These vessels supply the peripapillary choroid as well as the majority of the anterior optic nerve. Some short PCAs course, without branching, through the sclera directly into the choroid; others divide within the sclera to provide branches to both the choroid and the optic nerve. Often, a noncontinuous arterial circle exists within the perineural sclera, the circle of Zinn-Haller. This structure is formed by converging branches from the short posterior ciliary arteries.[23-28] The circle of Zinn-Haller provides blood for various regions of the anterior optic nerve, the peripapillary choroid, and the pial arterial system.

The retinal system is supplied by the central retinal artery (CRA) and sustains the inner retina. The CRA, itself a branch of the ophthalmic artery, penetrates the optic nerve approximately 12 mm behind the globe.[20,29-32] The CRA courses adjacent to the

81

central retinal vein through the center of the optic nerve, and then emerges from the optic nerve within the globe, where it branches into four major vessels.

The anterior optic nerve may be divided into four anatomic regions: the superficial nerve fiber layer, the pre-laminar region, the lamina cribrosa, and the retro-laminar region.[11,33,34] The superficial nerve fiber layer, the anterior-most region, is continuous with the nerve fiber layer of the retina and is the only nerve head structure visible by funduscopic examination. It is supplied by retinal arterioles arising from the branches of retinal arteries.[9,35] These small vessels originate in the surrounding nerve fiber layer and run toward the center of the optic nerve head. They have been referred to as *epipapillary vessels*.[36] The temporal nerve fiber layer may receive additional blood from a cilioretinal artery when this artery is present.[37] No direct choroidal or choriocapillaris contribution is observed in the superficial nerve fiber layer.

Immediately posterior to the nerve fiber layer is the pre-laminar region, which lies adjacent to the peripapillary choroid. In this region, ganglionic axons group into bundles for passage through the lamina cribrosa. The pre-laminar region is supplied primarily by branches of the short posterior ciliary arteries and by branches of the circle of Zinn-Haller,[38] though some investigators have observed a vascular contribution to the pre-laminar region from peripapillary choroidal arterioles.[6,14,39–42] The amount of choroidal contribution may be difficult to ascertain, as there are branches from both the circle of Zinn-Haller and from the short posterior ciliary arteries, which course through the choroid and ultimately supply the optic nerve in this region. These vessels do not originate in the choroid, but merely pass through it. The direct arterial supply to the pre-laminar region arising from the choroidal vasculature is minimal.[9,10, 43,44] This minimal contribution from the choroidal vasculature is limited to small arterioles. There is no vascular contribution from the choriocapillaris.

More posteriorly, the laminar region is continuous with the sclera and is composed of the lamina cribrosa, a structure consisting of fenestrated connective tissue, which allows the passage of neural axons through the scleral coat.[11,24,34,43,45] Like the pre-laminar region, the lamina cribrosa also receives its blood supply from branches of the short posterior ciliary arteries and branches of the circle of Zinn-Haller.[10,33,39,44] These precapillary branches perforate the outer lamina cribrosa before branching centrally and forming a capillary network throughout the fenestrated connective tissue. Larger vessels of the peripapillary choroid may contribute occasional small arterioles to the lamina cribrosa region.

Finally, the retro-laminar region lies posterior to the lamina cribrosa and, marked by the beginning of axonal myelination, is surrounded by the meninges of the central nervous system. The retro-laminar region has two blood supplies, from the CRA and the pial system. The pial system is an anastomosing network of capillaries located immediately within the pia mater. The pial system originates at the circle of Zinn-Haller and may also be fed directly by the short posterior ciliary arteries. Its branches extend into the optic nerve to nourish the axons.[6,10,12,39] The CRA may provide several small intraneural branches in the retro-laminar region.[7,10,42,46] Some of these branches anastomose with the pial system.

MEASUREMENT TECHNIQUES

Attempts to assess vascular aspects of the eye date back to the origins of ophthalmoscopy,[47] though in the last 25 years our ability to assess ocular circulation has evolved from a subjective description of visible vessels to direct quantitative measurement of ocular blood velocity and flow. Technological developments within the past two decades include color Doppler imaging, minimally invasive (no eye contact and a 22-gauge needle stick) angiography, and scanning laser Doppler flowmetry. The result has been an ever-increasing number of blood flow studies in clinical and experimental ophthalmic literature. It is important to realize that each method of assessing some portion of ocular hemodynamics is likely to have its own inherent limitations. Common safety concerns include the limits for retinal illumination[48] and orbital insonation.[7]

No single method can give us a complete description of ocular hemodynamics. It is impossible to obtain a measurement from a single hemodynamic assessment technique and extrapolate a complete and accurate understanding of ocular hemodynamics. Therefore, the relevance of any one hemodynamic measure must be considered within a greater context. This dilemma is best illustrated by the large amount of attention given to various reports of retinal hemodynamics in glaucoma. Although these reports are each valid, their interpretation must be performed in light of the fact that the anterior optic nerve, the primary location of neural damage in glaucoma, has a different vascular supply than the retina. The retinal circulation accounts for approximately 5 to 10% of total ocular blood flow. The relevance of retinal hemodynamic measures in glaucoma is not immediately clear. The techniques discussed below, when used in concert, provide a comprehensive examination of the ocular vasculature. Color Doppler imaging quantifies retrobulbar hemodynamics, scanning laser ophthalmoscope angiography examines choroidal vasculature, and scanning laser Doppler flowmetry quantifies retinal circulation.

Color Doppler Imaging

A-scan ultrasound is commonly used to measure the eye's axial length. B-scan ultrasound is used to produce gray-scale images of ocular structures. Color Doppler imaging (CDI) is an ultrasound technique that combines b-scan gray-scale imaging of tissue structure and color representation of blood velocity computed from Doppler-shifted reflections. By singling out an individual sound wave and using time of flight to isolate reflections from a single location, pulsed-Doppler measurement of blood flow velocities may be performed.[49]

CDI in the color imaging mode generates ultrasound power levels below the FDA limit of 17 mW/cm^2 for ocular ultrasound.[50] In the spectral analysis mode, during which blood flow velocity measurements are made, the required 77 mW/cm^2 exceeds FDA limits. This limit was conceived prior to the usage of CDI in the eye and was intended for a and b-scan techniques, which are older and simpler forms of ultrasound technology. The American Institute for Ultrasound in Medicine and the British Medical Ultrasound Society have since recommended a higher limit of 100 mW/cm^2. Much higher ultrasound intensities than are used in imaging studies (100 W/cm^2) are required to damage the choroid and lens of the rabbit's eye.[51] Innumerable ocular CDI examinations have been safely performed, and this methodology is used routinely at leading ophthalmic research centers throughout the world.

CDI is used to measure blood velocities in veins and arteries that drain and feed the eye. Current CDI analysis focuses primarily on velocities in arteries: specifically, the ophthalmic artery (OA), CRA, and short posterior ciliary arteries (PCAs) immediately behind the globe.[52] The specific PCAs of interest are those that feed the temporal and nasal sides of the optic nerve head (TSPCA and NSPCA, respectively). Blood velocities in these arteries are measured and displayed in real time. These waveforms can supply more information than one might immediately suspect. In this chapter we examine the interpretation of ophthalmic color Doppler ultrasound waveforms.

The CD Image

The CDI image consists of a gray-scale image of the globe with color-coded velocity data overlaid (Fig. 6–1). The direction of blood flow is used to color-code Doppler shifts. Blood flow away from the center of the body and toward the CDI probe is generally arterial and displayed in red; blood flow toward the center of the body and away from the probe is venous and displayed in blue. It is important that the technician performing the ultrasound exam have knowledge of both retrobulbar vascular anatomy and an understanding of the characteristic waveforms of the relevant arteries and veins. The central retinal artery and vein are in such proximity within the anterior optic nerve as to be measurable in a single reading. In Fig. 6-1, the waveform is made up of both vessels. The arterial waveform, located above the zero line, displays a pronounced peak systolic velocity as well as a distinct dichrotic notch. The vein lacks these features and displays a gently sinusoidal variation in blood velocity throughout the cardiac cycle.

Two blood velocity values are displayed on the CDI image: the peak systolic velocity (PSV) and the end-diastolic velocity (EDV). Accurate identification of these velocities depends on the skill and experience of the ultrasonographer. A horizontal line on the screen is placed on the PSV and a second line on the EDV. With this information, the CDI unit displays the velocity values and calculates Pourcelot's resistive index (RI)[51] as

$$RI = \frac{PSV - EDV}{PSV} \qquad (6-1)$$

RI is a dimensionless parameter ranging in value between 0 and 1. The value 0 represents completely

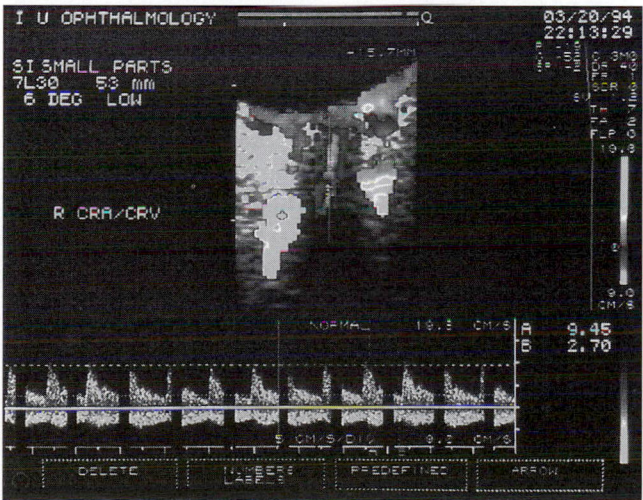

Figure 6–1. The CDI consists of a gray-scale structural image with color-coded velocity data overlaid. Peak systolic and eye-diastolic velocities are measured from the velocity waveform presented below the image.

non-pulsatile flow, with EDV equal to PSV, and 1 represents purely pulsatile flow, with velocity equal to zero during diastole.

CDI Reproducibility

Reproducibility of CDI measurements has been studied using a test/retest analysis.[53] In a recent study of 15 normal subjects, the coefficient of variation was determined for each of the measurement parameters PSV, EDV and RI in the OA, CRA, TPCA, and NPCA. The results are displayed in Table 6–1. Accurate, consistent positioning of the probe is essential for good reproducibility. In the CRA, radically different velocity measurements are obtained, depending upon whether one positions the measurement window anteriorly or posteriorly along the vessel, as reported by Dennis et al.[54] The CRA is unique among the ocular vessels in that it must become narrow in order to pass through the lamina cribrosa, and this is the area in which the CRA is measured in ocular hemodynamic exams. This high level of location-dependent variability is reflected in the reproducibility data for the CRA.

Interpretation of CDI Data

Several studies have been performed in which the clinical meaning of CDI data has been examined. A summary of their results is presented in Table 6–2. The first three studies in the table took the form of CDI examination of the retrobulbar circulation of eyes with specific diseases. CDI examination found absent or reduced orbital blood flow in patients with occlusion of the carotid artery.[55] In cases of carotid stenosis, the Doppler spectrum produced by turbulent flow in the area of the stenosis is broadened.[56] This is observed as an increase in PSV within the stenosis.[57]

In a study of the effect of surgery for decompression of the optic nerve sheath on blood flow within the orbital vessels, Flarety et al. observed an increase in PSV in the ophthalmic and central retinal arteries.[58] The authors concluded that their results reflect an increase in blood flow in the arteries in question arising from decreased resistance within the optic nerve. In a letter

to the editor of the journal that published this work, Hayreh suggested that post-operative edema was likely to have occurred.[59] This edema may compress vessels, resulting in increased PSV, as observed in vascular stenosis. It is thus not possible to state with certainty how the surgical procedure affected flow within the retrobulbar vessels on the basis of CDI evidence.

Pourcelot's resistive index is calculated from PSV and EDV as shown in Eq. (6–1). It has been shown in early animal studies that alterations in vascular resistance induced by quantified arterial stenosis proximal to the CDI measurement have little effect on RI. A proximal stenosis of approximately 86% is required to alter RI.[60] Similarly, the effect upon RI of vascular resistance distal to the point of CDI measurement has been examined in a number of studies. In these, it has been demonstrated that RI is sensitive to changes in vascular resistance when the resistance is distal to the measurement point.[59–62] There is consensus on this fact, based on animal, in vitro, and mathematical hemodynamic models. The in vivo models used in CDI studies were, however, constructed by altering resistance to flow in the renal, abdominal, aortic, femoral, and brachial arte-

TABLE 6–1. COEFFICIENTS OF VARIATION FOR EACH MEASUREMENT OF THE FOUR VESSELS MEASURED BY CDI

	PSV	EDV	RI
OA	5.1	9.6	1.7
CRA	5.3	17.9	4.6
TSPCA	11.6	8.8	7.6
NSPCA	12.0	14.2	4.9

TABLE 6–2. INTERPRETATIONS OF CDI MEASUREMENTS BASED ON A COMBINATION OF IN VITRO, IN VIVO, AND MATHEMATICAL MODELS AS WELL AS CLINICAL OBSERVATIONS

Condition	Interpretation
Carotid occlusion	Greatly reduced or absent flow in ocular vessels
Carotid stenosis	Broadening of Doppler spectra at the site
Carotid stenosis	Increased PSV
Post optic-nerve sheath decompression	Increased PSV in the OA and CRA; increased flow(?)
Post optic-nerve sheath decompression	Post-operative edema may induce vessel narrowing and decreased flow as in stenosis
Post optic-nerve sheath decompression	CDI results are inconclusive; caution needed in interpretation
Proximal stenosis	Proximal stenosis of 86% is required to alter RI distal to the point of measurement
Distal stenosis/ systemic and in vitro models	Increased RI
Increased IOP/in vivo ocular model	Increased RI in CRA and PCA but not the OA
Carbon dioxide-induced vasodilation	CDI cannot isolate the distal vessels that effect changes in RI

Key: CDI, color Doppler imaging; IOP, intraocular pressure; PSV, peak systolic velocity; OA, ophthalmic artery; CRA, central retinal artery; RI, resistive index; PCA, posterior ciliary artery.

rial beds. Although the evidence they furnish in support of the above generalization is very strong, none of these studies deals with the ocular vasculature specifically. Harris used scleral suction to increase intraocular pressure (IOP), thereby increasing resistance to blood flow into the eye as IOP rose above venous pressure.[63] RI in both the CRA and PCAs was found to be linearly dependent on IOP. Interestingly, the RI in the ophthalmic artery remained unaffected by IOP levels, which acutely exceeded 55 mm-Hg.[64] This suggests that blood flow may be shunted away from the eye by increased resistance to flow within the eye without affecting the hemodynamic behavior of the OA. Further, reductions in ophthalmic blood velocities, as observed in glaucoma and other diseases, may be due to factors other than increased IOP.

So what can be gleaned from the study of PSV and EDV in combination? The authors of a 1991 in vitro study were the first to hypothesize that simultaneous increase or decrease of both EDV and PSV reflects a rise or fall in total volumetric flow.[65] This view is supported by subsequent studies of renal hemodynamics in humans and of porcine renal obstruction.[66,67] Unlike the animal and in vitro studies of RI described above, this work has not been replicated in the human ocular circulation.

CDI Interpretation in a Study of Glaucomatous Eyes

It has long been proposed that vascular factors have a role in the etiology of glaucoma.

> . . . the glaucomatous cup is not purely a mechanical result . . ., but is in part at least, an atrophic condition which, though primarily due to pressure, includes vascular changes and impaired nutrition in the back of the disk and around its margin. . . .
> —Priestly Smith, 1879

If vasospasm is occurring in the ocular vessels in glaucoma, those vessels should have a higher RI than the corresponding vessels of healthy eyes.[68] Further, a potent vasodilator such as CO_2 should reduce RI in those vasospastic eyes. In a study by Harris et al., CDI was performed on the eyes of a group of normal-tension glaucoma (NTG) patients and healthy control subjects in the presence and the absence of elevated levels of CO_2.[68] Baseline measurements were obtained as the subjects breathed room air; CDI examination was repeated as they breathed room air with a small amount of CO_2 mixed in. The small amount usually between 2 and 3% was set so that the subjects' end-tidal CO_2 content was increased by 15% of the initial value; i.e., if a subject's end-tidal CO_2 content was 4%, it was raised to

4.6% in the experiment.[68] Baseline values for EDV were found to be lower in the ophthalmic arteries of glaucoma patients than in those of healthy subjects, and RI was found to be higher. It can be inferred from the high baseline OA RI in the glaucomatous group, and its susceptibility to reduction with a vasodilator, that some vessels in the orbit or eye of the NTG sufferers initially presented high resistance to blood flow. This high resistance was reduced by a vasodilator. CDI would not have been able to discriminate which distal vascular bed or beds were vasospastic at baseline, nor whether the OA itself was vasospastic at baseline. Nor could it have been used to identify in which distal vessels vasodilation occurred. Previously it was mentioned that OARI was not affected by changes in IOP,[67] though PCA and CRA RI were. This introduces the possibility that the changes in the glaucoma patients' OA RI may have been induced by distal vasodilatory changes in vessels other than the CRA and PCAs, such as the vessels which perfuse the ocular muscles.

CDI can be used to describe blood flow to the eye in terms of a set of well-defined parameters. It does not provide absolute measurements of flow, but with knowledge of the meaning of CDI readings, useful and reliable information regarding changes in volumetric flow and vascular resistance distal to the measurement point are obtainable. Yet some basic questions remain. With a 7.5-MHz probe, CDI is able to resolve structures 0.2 mm or larger, this being the amplitude of a single sound wave at that frequency.[69] In this light, how can researchers report on velocities within the PCAs when the largest PCAs have a diameter of approximately 0.18-mm?[46] The answer is that CDI indeed cannot *visualize* PCAs but that it can still be used to obtain useful information about them. CDI detects the influence that moving blood within the PCAs has upon the ultrasound wave. PCAs appear as single red or blue pixels on the CDI image. No vessel is visible, but the Doppler shift is measurable. This is analogous to our ability to see stars in the night sky. Just as our retinas are sensitive enough to detect starlight even though the stars are too small to be "seen" from this distance, the Doppler shift induced by PCAs is well within the sensitivity of the CDI, even though the vessels are too narrow to be delineated by the device. It is possible that PCA measurements include more than one vessel; clusters of PCAs ramify as they enter the posterior globe, and there is no way of knowing how many are encompassed within a measurement. This does not invalidate PCA measurements. Reproducibility of the readings is good, and whether a CDI reading measurement arises from one or several vessels, placing the sample window adjacent to structures of interest secures useful information about the PCAs supplying those structures. Can CDI be used to measure the same location on a vessel on different occasions? Yes, with angle correction. It is difficult for an operator using a hand-held probe to reproduce an earlier site of application with precision. The most important factor in reproducing velocity measurements of a vessel is the angle of the incident beam. The angle between the incident beam and the velocity vector of the moving blood affects the Doppler shift in the frequency of the reflected beam.[70] As long as the user takes the angle into account, the CDI measurement of velocity will be accurate. After angle correction, consistency in the appearance of the waveform can be used to ensure measurement of the same location within a vessel.

Color Doppler imaging is already being incorporated into ophthalmic clinical practice. It is too early in the evolution of other techniques to state with confidence which method or methods of investigating the hemodynamics of the eye will prove to be the most reliable and to furnish the most useful information. As our understanding of deficits in ocular blood flow in disease states grows, one or more existing or as yet undeveloped techniques for the assessment of blood flow in the human eye are likely to find widespread utilization. The prospects for the continued evolution of such technologies and for sustained growth in the body of knowledge that we obtain from their application appear bright, although successful use of CDI and allied methodologies will depend on a thorough understanding of the data they produce.

SCANNING LASER OPHTHALMOSCOPY

The macula and optic nerve head depend almost entirely on the choroidal blood flow. Choroidal anatomy and hemodynamics and the role of the choroid in the pathogenesis of several important ocular disorders—such as age-related macular degeneration, diabetic retinopathy, and glaucoma—remain poorly understood. Since Flower and Hochheimer first successfully performed indocyanine green (ICG) angiography in humans in the early 1970's,[71,72] clinicians and researchers have attempted to image the choroid with high resolution. Compared with sodium fluorescein dye, ICG dye is preferred for angiographic study of the choroid for several reasons. First, the near-infrared light used to excite ICG is much more efficient in its penetration of pigmented layers of the fundus than is the shorter wavelength used to excite fluorescein.[73] A second advantage is the tendency of ICG dye to bind to plasma proteins. Approximately 98% of the ICG dye is bound to plasma albumin.[74] Sodium fluorescein dye molecules are far less com-

pletely bound. As a result, ICG diffuses slowly out of the fenestrated choriocapillaris, in contrast to the rapid leakage of fluorescein dye, which prevents visualization of choroidal vascular details.

The recent introduction of the scanning laser ophthalmoscope (SLO) has brought quantitative angiography to new heights. This instrument overcomes many of the limitations of traditional photographic or video angiography. The SLO is a confocal laser device. Reflected light exits the eye through the pupil and must pass through a confocal aperture before reaching a solid-state detector. Scattered light and light reflected from sources outside of the focal plane is blocked by the confocal aperture. Overall retinal illumination is reduced and contrast is improved, since the laser beam illuminates only a single spot at any given moment. A timer image is added to the video image. The final image is recorded on a S-VHS video recorder. The resulting images are similar to those obtained with standard video angiography, but with improved spatial resolution and contrast.

SLO ICG angiography (ICGA) may be useful in the study of glaucoma. Because the blood supply for the optic nerve head comes in part from the choroidal circulation, choroidal circulatory insufficiency is another possible etiologic factor for glaucoma. Further, both the optic nerve head and the choroid are fed by the same PCAs. A deficit in choroidal hemodynamics may imply reduced blood flow to the optic nerve head. Recently, a study using ICGA with SLO showed that glaucomatous eyes have more peripapillary hypofluorescent area in late phase.[75] Although these morphological data are valuable, they do not quantify hemodynamic changes, an essential step in evaluating the autoregulation of ocular perfusion. Scanning-laser ICGA has also been used to investigate ocular hemodynamics. Several authors have attempted to quantify morphological and dynamic parameters in the choroidal circulation. In a recent pilot study done by the Glaucoma Research and Diagnostic Center, a new area dilution analysis technique for SLO ICGA demonstrated that NTG patients have peripapillary choroidal filling deficits compared to the filling patterns of normal eyes.[76] This new analysis software is based on the analysis of dye-dilution curves which have been studied, surprisingly since the 1920's. This approach can provide various new hemodynamic parameters for SLO-ICGA.

Dye-Dilution Techniques

Dye dilution is a technique in which a known amount of a dye is introduced into a vein of an animal or human; its passage is then observed at some point within the arterial system. The dye, or indicator, must be easily observable by whatever measurement technique is employed by the study.[77] The concentration of the indicator within the blood at the observation point is graphed over time, producing a dye-dilution curve. The technique was based on a principle proposed by Aldolf Fick, stating that the rate at which an indicator substance is delivered to an area by a moving fluid stream is equal to the product of the flow rate and the difference between the concentration of the indicator substance proximal and distal to the area. In hemodynamic studies in the 1920's, dye-dilution curves were used to estimate cardiac output in humans.[78] Phenol-tetroidphthalein sodium was quickly injected into an antecubital vein. Blood was then sampled from the femoral artery and samples were placed into collection tubes mounted on a rotating drum. The speed of the rotation was set so those individual samples were taken once per second. The concentration of the indicator was measured and plotted against time (Fig. 6–2).

Dye-Dilution Analysis

The dye-dilution curve in Fig. 6–2 can be used to calculate cardiac output. Interestingly, one of the earliest uses of ICG involved determination of cardiac output by this method in the 1950's. ICG was commercially available as Cardio-Green. [79] The dye-duration area, the time between first arterial appearance and the extrapolated zero concentration time, is then analyzed. (Fig. 6–2). Within that area, the average measured dye concentration is calculated. Using this average and the dye-duration time, cardiac output is computed. This relationship was confirmed experimentally in dogs by comparing it to that found by Fick's method. In Fick's method, oxygen consumption and oxygen concentration on the arterial and venous sides are measured. The total blood flow is then calculated as the ratio between oxygen consumption and the dif-

ference between arterial and venous oxygen concentration. This early work demonstrated the usefulness of dye-dilution techniques in hemodynamic research.

Dye-Dilution Analysis in Ophthalmology

In ophthalmology, dilution-curve techniques have been used to quantify retinal hemodynamics. Using computerized video analysis techniques, the concentration of a dye, fluorescein, is quantified by measuring the brightness of fluorescence from within the blood. Although blood flow is not derived as above, velocity may be calculated by using several curves along the length of a vessel (Fig. 6–3). Dilution curves are used to provide the time delay between the arrival of dye at two points. By measuring the distance between those points and knowing the time it takes blood to pass between them, one can calculate the velocity of the dye.[80]

Dilution Analysis of ICG Angiography

The Glaucoma Research and Diagnostic Center (GRDC) has applied video dye-dilution technology to ICG angiograms. This is known as *area dilution analysis* (ADA)[76]. The brightness of six areas of the choroid is quantified. Brightness of fluorescence is proportional to the concentration of ICG in the choroidal vasculature. By graphing brightness over time, dye concentration is graphed, creating a dye-dilution curve.

Unlike the femoral artery, which was used to study dilution curves in the 1920's, the choroid contains a complex layer of overlapping arteries. It is

Concentration

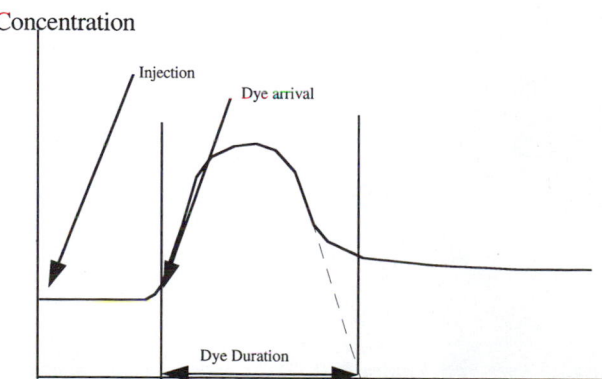

Figure 6–2. The dye-dilution curve displays the concentration of an injected indicator. Concentration is monitored at an arterial location and graphed over time.

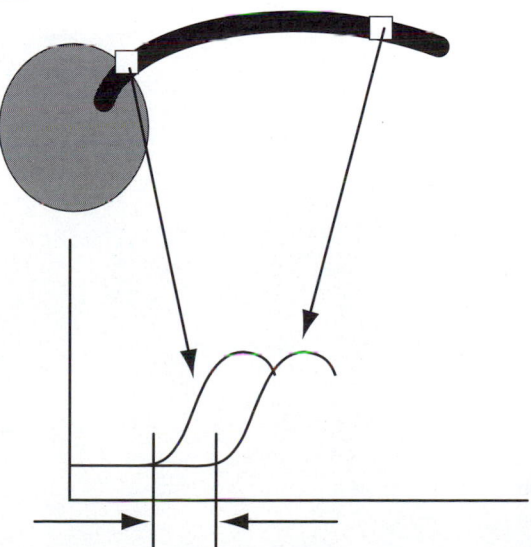

Figure 6–3. Mean dye velocity within a single artery can be calculated from dye-dilution curves from two points on an artery. Arrows indicate time between dye travel to two points of an artery.

impractical to attempt to create dilution curves for each one. Given this, one may attempt to choose some subset of vessels and create dilution curves for them. Unfortunately, the attempt to choose some small number of vessels for dye-dilution analysis would create an unacceptable bias. The new ADA method creates curves from regions of the vascular bed. The number of vessels within that region is not of direct concern to the technique.

The GRDC has developed a technique in which the entire 40° ICG angiogram is divided into a number of small regions, and dilution curves are created for each region. Although it is difficult to use fluorescence to measure the exact concentration of ICG within the choroid, simultaneous acquisition of dye-dilution curves from different locations within the choroid in a single angiographic exam allows comparison of relative concentrations between different locations. Six locations on the image were identified for analysis (Fig. 6–4). The size and position of these sample areas were chosen to coincide with the perimacular and temporal perimacular measurement areas of automated visual fields (approximately 6° of the visual field). The average brightness of the area contained in each box was computed for each frame of the angiogram. Area brightness was graphed with time on the X-axis and brightness on the Y-axis. ADA identifies three parameters from the brightness maps: slope, 10% arrival time, and dye duration. The slope represents the speed of blood as it enters the choroid. The slopes of the six curves are analyzed individually, as a mean of the six areas, and as the regional

spread or maximum slope minus minimum slope. Similarly, the 10% arrival time is the amount of time required to reach a degree of brightness 10% above baseline, and this is analyzed for each individual area, the mean of the six areas, and the maximum minus the minimum. Finally, the dye-duration time as described above is analyzed for each individual area, as a mean of the six areas, and as the maximum minus the minimum.

In a pilot study, ICG angiograms were recorded from 7 NTG patients and 8 age-matched controls. There was no significant difference between normals and NTG patients in mean slope, 10% arrival time, or dye duration. Regional arrival spread time was significantly greater in NTGs than in normals (3.436 vs. 1.167 s., $p = 0.04$). The choroid of some glaucoma patients presents with areas of slow filling, which are not present in age-matched normals. NTGs also displayed a trend toward increased dye duration spread.

Dye-dilution techniques have been used in hemodynamic studies for more than 70 years. From direct blood samples to non-invasive measurement of an indicator in the blood-stream, the basic structure of the dilution curve remains the same. Applying dilution-curve analysis to ICG angiograms, ADA is able to quantify differences in choroidal hemodynamics between NTGs and age-matched controls. The data suggest that some glaucomatous eyes present with select regions of slow choroidal filling and sluggish movement of blood into and out of the choroid.

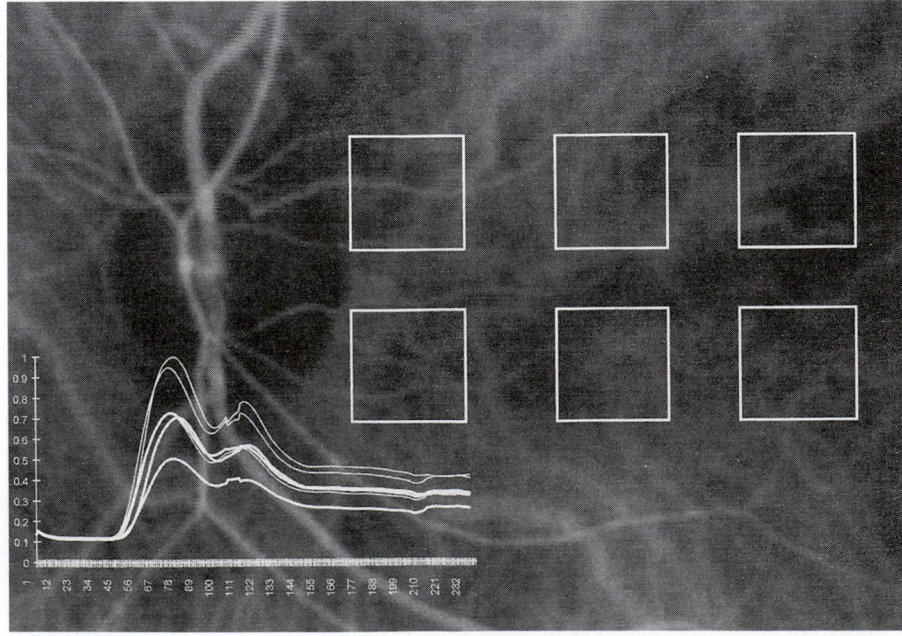

Figure 6–4. Using indocyanine green angiography, multiple dye-dilution curves have been used to compare hemodynamic characteristics from multiple areas of the choroid.

HEIDELBERG RETINAL FLOWMETRY

The Heidelberg Retinal Flowmeter (HRF, Heidelberg Engineering, Germany) is a non-invasive confocal scanning laser imaging device marketed for the mapping of flow magnitudes in the human fundus.[81] It has several unique characteristics.[82,83] Quantification of retinal blood flow is accomplished through a series of point measurements, each with a measurement resolution of approximately 10×10 μm on the retinal plane and a field depth of 400 μm. An average clinical measurement takes about 5 min, including post-processing. Users of this technology have published various studies measuring the effects of disease and medications on blood flow in the fundus;[84–86] however, many questions on the validity of HRF still remain. One concerns the arbitrary unit (a.u.) in the HRF report. Despite previous experiments,[29,87] physical units have not been successfully correlated to the arbitrary units. Furthermore, the functional range for these units, as well as the normal values, are yet to be determined. Can the HRF reliably differentiate glaucomatous disease processes from healthy ones based on these values? Are these values dependent on flow or other optical factors such as pallor? The GRCD has used HRF to measure changes in blood flow induced by hypercapnia and hyperoxia. Were these changes representative of true changes in volumetric retinal blood flow? Because the technology is plagued with these questions, a recent study is presented that was designed with two specific aims: (1) to determine the range of linear response, or functional range, of the HRF in a highly controlled environment and (2) to identify the effect of altered background brightness on HRF readings.

A flow model was constructed using a horizontal heparinized glass pipette. Bovine blood preserved and diluted with 3.2% sodium citrate solution (volume ratio approximately 1 in 10) was fed by gravity from a large surface reservoir. A constant hydraulic head was maintained during each experimental trial. Flow was determined by weighing the mass of blood collected after each timed trial. Flow velocity varied from zero to 30 mm/s. Images of the flow were taken by HRF without optical magnification. (Fig. 6–5) The experiment was conducted in two series. In the first, a velocity range from 0.3 to 2.67 mm/s was obtained, and a background of white paper was used to create a bright background. The second series of trials ran with mean velocities from 2.71 to 30 mm/s. Replacing the white paper with less reflective white gauze altered the background. The change in background simulates conditions where background and/or total image brightness is changed. Pixel brightness, labeled M (DC) in

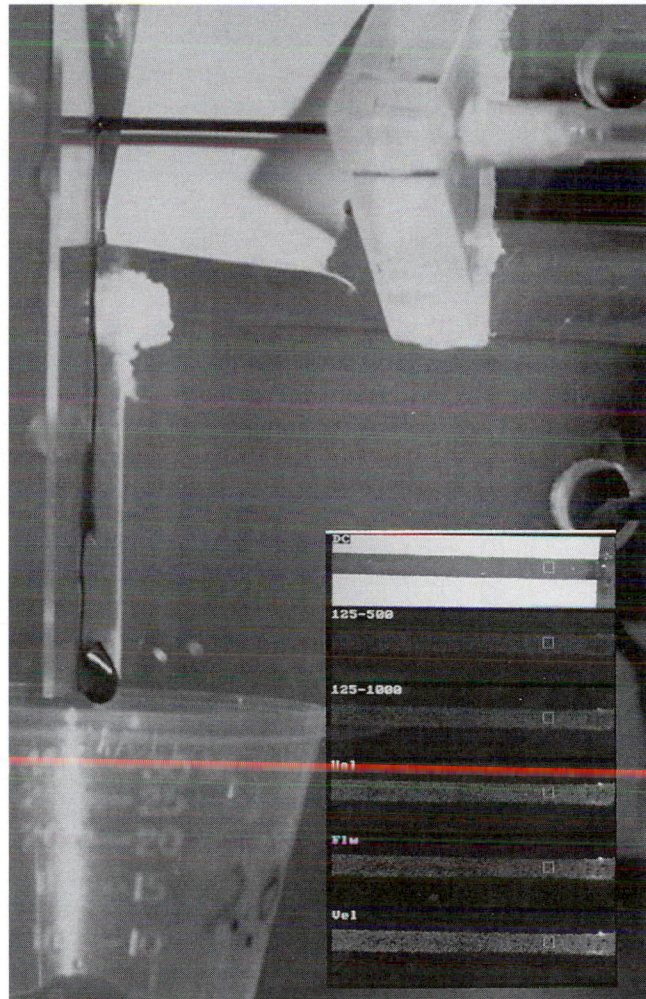

Figure 6–5. Bovine blood flowed through a heparinized capillary tube, and down a glass slide (to control surface tension). Images of the flow were taken by HRF without optical magnification.

HRF reports, is then tallied for each series to complete the analysis.

In both series of trials, HRF measurements were linearly correlated to the true velocity of blood within the tube. The upper limit of linearity occurred when blood in the tube was moving at 8.83 mm/s on average. The change of background scatter material between the two series induced a large change in the HRF velocity readings. The HRF velocity measurement is plotted against measured mean velocity in Fig. 6–6. It can be seen that the data were continuous within each operating condition, but both the slope and offset were altered by the change in background conditions.

The HRF noise estimation and correction algorithm, as conveyed in correspondences with Heidelberg Engineering, is based on the assumption that brighter images have proportionally more noise than darker images. In addition, it is dependent on the upper frequency band (1500–2000 Hz) of the power spectra. This algorithm has not been published or peer verified for flow-measurement applications. It would produce higher flow readings for darker areas, since only a small correction would be subtracted from the raw scan spectrum. Since these corrections are derived globally and subtracted locally, the reported values are distorted between regions of the same image and among different images. This has four clinical consequences. First, in performing repeated examinations of a single normal eye, it is imperative to align the image perfectly from one examination to the next. Misalignment would change image content and illumination, both of which affect global brightness. Second, the illumination must be consistently set to the same level between images, by control of the sensitivity setting and camera-to-eye distance. Variations will also induce changes in perceived noise. Third, different individuals would be expected to have different levels of fundus pigmentation and geometry. As a result, their noise corrections would be different. We believe that a simple intensity adjustment cannot compensate for the complex consequences of these noise corrections. Finally, and most damaging, the progressive disc pallor characteristic of glaucoma will result in progressively darker images in longitudinal measurements, even under strict control. A flow change reported in these circumstances is likely to be confounded by the optical properties of the fundus.

Our data are consistent with previous studies on the HRF.[29,87] Others found a linear relationship only between 0.1 and 1.0 mm/s.[29] Our experiment's resolution does not afford analysis below 0.1 mm/s, where our only data points have zero flow velocity, but it agrees with previous assessments of linear relationship. Other ophthalmic laser Doppler devices display the same characteristic linear range, ending at a plateau velocity, though at a level one order of magnitude higher than that of the HRF.[88]

Based on a regression gradient of 0.7 a.u. per mm/s, and an 8.8-mm/s velocity range, it can be deduced that the HRF can meaningfully report velocities in an arbitrary unit range of about 6. Arbitrary units of velocities in the teens may be aberrations of the noise correction in addition to effects of Doppler shifts. A similar argument would predict a range of about 2000 for the arbitrary unit of flow.

The plateau velocity of 8.8 mm/s cannot be applied universally as a clinical maximum. The sampling rate of 4000 Hz for the HRF would have predicted a plateau velocity of 0.78 mm/s, compared to the 8.8 mm/s here and 5 mm/s or so in others.[87] The apparent extension of capability observed in our experiment likely depends on two factors:

1. The penetration depth of the infrared laser in blood
2. The angle of incidence and scatter

Based on the physical properties of transmission of light[89] and the incidence angle, the data from this experiment would produce a calculated velocity limit of 0.54 mm/s, or ~70% of what was expected due to sampling rate limitations.

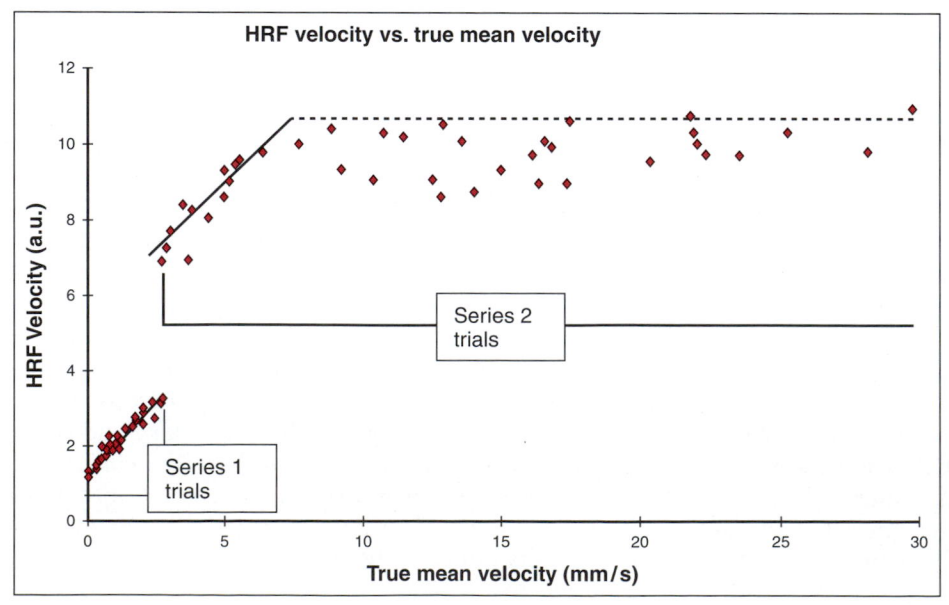

Figure 6–6. HRF measurements of velocity are drastically altered by changes in background brightness. In this series of experiments, changing the background material from paper to gauze induced a large shift in velocity measurements.

It is important to note that the above logic does not necessarily apply to the fundus or optic nerve head, where vessels are approximately 100 μm in diameter, where scatter from perfused tissue alters illumination directions, and where blood flow is no longer Newtonian. For comparison, the attenuation coefficient of perfused human dermal tissue in vivo is closer to 1.28, or one-fourth of that of whole blood. Thus the true absorption characteristics of retinal tissue will vary depending on the density of the vasculature. The random and competing effects of media scattering, in addition to angle of incidence, may explain the rest of the discrepancies. The effects of these variables were not measured in this study.

Due to its sensitivity to moving blood flow, the HRF is very successful in producing dramatic images of vasculature without intra-vessel contrast. However, it produces this flow-weighted vascular map while misrepresenting the numerical values it is supposed to report. The ideal flow-mapping system should discern and quantify velocity changes apart from brightness changes for three reasons. Velocity changes alone may be the early sign of a pre-symptomatic disease process. Second, physiologic changes or drugs may alter perfusion with local anatomic changes and hence brightness changes, (e.g., vasodilatation); but they can also produce pure velocity changes, (e.g., upstream pressure regulation). Finally, and most importantly, brightness is dependent on the image acquisition process, which introduces additional variations.

HRF measurements can be drastically altered by the brightness of an image. These results suggest that the HRF noise-reduction algorithm may account for much of the variations and false flow measurements produced by the instrument. These findings present a new dilemma for comparative studies using HRF:

1. Intersubject comparison may be unreliable with this software version, as eye image brightness depends on individual anatomy.
2. To track a single eye over time, great care must be taken to minimize variability of disc location within the image.
3. HRF sensitivity should be held constant between images during longitudinal follow up of individual eyes.
4. Changes in the scattering and reflective properties of the fundus, such as edema or disc pallor, may introduce significant changes in flow values as a result of noise correction.
5. Because of the optical characteristics of blood and human tissue, the HRF arbitrary units may relate to actual flow velocities by a com-

plex relationship involving angle of incidence, blood cell density, and vessel diameter.

The linearity and plateau of the HRF response curve are consistent with previous experiences of the technology. It is clear that the HRF is velocity-sensitive and that a linear response can be obtained with strict control over factors affecting the noise correction. In its present form, the HRF is not a reliable flow-measurement device. A long-term solution to enhance the usability of the HRF should begin with a re-examination of the noise-estimation and correction algorithm.

CONCLUSIONS

Each of these devices provides valuable hemodynamic data from the human eye; however, great caution must be used in interpreting the data they produce. None of these techniques have reached a "point-and-shoot" level of simplicity. A thorough understanding of the limitations discussed in this chapter is required to accurately interpret the data they produce. With such an educated approach, meaningful work in the area of ocular hemodynamics may be performed.

The literature contains numerous examples of altered blood flow in ophthalmic disease measured by these techniques. What do the differences between normals and various glaucoma groups mean? Current technologies cannot be used to determine whether altered blood flow is primary or secondary to nerve damage. Longitudinal studies may provide better insight into the role that deficits in ocular blood flow play in disease progression, but at a great cost in time and materials. As technology improves, more direct measurements may provide the answers to some basic questions:

- How great a blood flow deficit is necessary to cause glaucomatous damage?
- What is the threshold of perfusion deficit before nerve cell damage occurs?
- How can we identify this threshold?

Measurement of metabolism may provide the answer. Several types of measurements would be of interest, including retinal oximetry, quantification of metabolites, reduction/oxidation potentials, or perhaps ATP/NADH+ levels. Using spectral analysis of reflected light, work is underway in the development of retinal oximetry, but a system suitable for clinical use is still years the future. These measurements will allow us to fine-tune glaucoma medications as we gain a better understanding of how various drugs affect the environment in which neurons must survive.

REFERENCES

1. Davies EG, Sullivan PM, Fitzpatrick M, Kohner EM: Validations and reproducibility of laser Doppler velocimetry for the measurement of retinal blood flow. *Curr Eye Res.* 1992;11:633–640.

2. Mansberger S, Harris A, Caldemeyer K, et al: Acute effect of topical apraclonidine on perimacular and orbital hemodynamics: ARVO Abstract. *Invest Ophthalmol Vis Sci.* 1994;35(suppl):2176.

3. Lieberman MF, Maumenee AE, Green WR. Histologic studies of the vasculature of the anterior optic nerve. *Am J Ophthalmol* 1976;82:405.

4. Friedlander S, DeMaio R, Sinclair S, Werner E: The acute effects of betaxolol on human macular hemodynamics in normals. ARVO Abstract. *Invest Ophthalmol Vis Sci.* 1992;33(suppl):810.

5. Friedman E. A hemodynamic model of the pathogenesis of age-related macular degeneration. *Am J Ophthalmol.* 1997;124:677–681.

6. Harris A, Shoemaker JA, Burgoyne J, et al: The acute effect of topical beta-adrenergic antagonists on normal perimacular hemodynamics. *J Glaucoma.* 1995;4:36–40.

7. Hayreh SS. The central artery of the retina—its role in the blood supply of the optic nerve. *Br J Ophthalmol.* 1963;47:651.

8. Netland PA, Grosskreutz CL, Feke GT, Hart LJ, Color Doppler ultrasound analysis of ocular circulation after topical calcium channel blocker. *Am J Ophthalmol.* 1995; 119(6):694–700.

9. Niesel P, Gassman HB: Direkte fluorometrische Untersuchung am Augenhintergrund. *Ophthalmologica.* 1972; 165:297–302.

10. Langham ME, Tomey KF. A clinical procedure for the measurement of ocular pulse-pressure relationship and the ophthalmic arterial pressure. *Exp Eye Res.* 1978;27: 17–25.

11. Anderson DR, Hoyt WF: Ultrastructure of the intraorbital portion of human and monkey optic nerve. *Arch Ophthalmol.* 1969;82:506.

12. Christ TH, Stodtmeister R, Pillunat L. Okulo-Oszillo-Dynamographie nach Ulrich: Erste Ergebnisse bei Carotisstenosen. *Klin Mbl Augenheilk.* 1985;187:256–261.

13. Araki M. Anatomical study of the vascularization of optic nerve. *Acta Soc Ophthalmol Jpn.* 1975;79:101

14. Eisenlohr JE, Langham ME, Maumenee AE: Manometric studies of the pressure-volume relationship in living and enucleated eyes of individual human subjects. *Br J Ophthalmol.* 1962;46:536–548.

15. Hayreh SS. Inter-individual variation in the blood supply of the optic nerve head: Its importance in various ischemic disorders of the nerve head, and glaucoma, low-tension glaucoma, and allied disorders. *Doc Ophthalmol.* 1985;59:217.

16. Silver DM, Farrell RA, Langham ME, et al. Estimation of pulsatile ocular blood flow from intraocular pressure. *Acta Ophthalmologica Suppl.* 1989;191:25–29.

17. Sieker HO, Hickman JB, Gibson JF. The relationship between impaired retinal vasculature reactivity and renal function in patients with degenerative vascular disease. *Circulation.* 1955;12:64–8.

18. Arend O, Wolf S, Remky A, et al. Perifoveal microcirculation with non-insulin dependent diabetes mellitus. *Graefe's Arch Clin Exp Ophthalmol.* 232:225–231.

19. Arend O, Wolf S. Segmentation of fluorescence in the retinal microcirculation. Is it a valid indicator of blood cell flow? (reply). *Br J Ophthalmol.* 1992;76:510–511.

20. Arnold JV, Gates HW, Taylor KM. Possible errors in the measurement of retinal lesions. *Invest Ophthalmol Vis Sci.* 1993;34(8):2576–80.

21. Baxter GM, Williamson TH. Color Doppler flow imaging in central retinal vein occlusion: A new diagnostic technique? *Radiology.* 1993;187:847–850.

22. Portellos M, Riva CE, Cranstoun SD. Petrig BL. Brucker AJ : Effects of adenosine on ocular blood flow *Invest Ophthalmol Vis Sci.* 1995;36(9):1904–1909.

23. Baxter GM, Williamson TH. Color Doppler imaging of the eye: Normal ranges, reproducibility, and observer variation. *J Ultrasound Med.* 1995;14(2):91–96.

24. Baxter GM, Williamson TH, McKillop G, Dutton GN. Color Doppler ultrasound of orbital and optic nerve blood flow: Effects of posture and timolol 0.5%. *Invest Ophthalmol Vis Sci.* 1992;33:604–610.

25. Behrendt T. Scanning densitometer for photographic fundus measurements. *Am J Ophthalmol.* 1966;62:689–693.

26. Ben-Nun J, Constable JJ: Segmentation of fluorescence in the retinal microcirculation. Is it a valid indicator of blood cell flow? (letter). *Br J Ophthalmol.* 1992;76:510.

27. Bennet AG, Rudnicka AR, Edgar DF. Improvements on Littmann's method of determining the size of retinal features by fundus photography. *Graefe's Arch Clin Exp Ophthalmol.* 232:361–367.

28. Berges O. Colour Doppler flow imaging of the orbital veins. *Acta Ophthalmologica Suppl.* 1992;204:55–58.

29. Chauhan BC, Smith FM. Confocal Scanning Laser Doppler Flowmetry: Experiments in a model flow system. *J Glaucoma.* 1997;6:237–245.

30. Bertram B, Wolf S, Fiehöfer S, Schulte K, Arend O, Reim M. Retinal circulation times in diabetes mellitus type 1. *Br J Ophthalmol.* 1991;75:462–465.

31. Bignell J. Investigations into the blood supply of the optic nerve with special reference to the lamina cribrosa region. *Trans Ophthalmol Soc Aust.* 1952;12:105.

32. Cranstoun SD, Petrig BL, Riva CE, Baine J. Optic nerve head blood flow in the human eye by laser Doppler flowmetry (LDF). ARVO Abstracts. *Invest Ophthalmol Vis Sci.* 1994;35:1658.

33. Anderson DR. Ultrastructure of human and monkey lamina cribrosa and optic nerve head. *Arch Ophthalmol.* 1969;82:800.

34. Pichot O, Gonzalvez B, Franco A, Mouillon M. Color Doppler ultrasonography in the study of orbital and ocular vascular diseases. *J Fr Ophthalmol.* 1996;19(1):19–31.

35. Wolf S, Jung F, Keisewetter H, Körber N, Reim M. Video fluorescein angiography: Method and clinical application. *Graefe's Arch Clin Exp Ophthalmol*. 1989;227: 145–151.

36. Riva CE, Petrig BO, Grunwald JE. Retinal blood flow. In: Shepherd AP, Öberg PÅ, eds. *Laser-Doppler Flowmetry*. Boston: Kluwer Academic Publishers: 1989;349–383.

37. Harino S, Riva CE, Petrig BL: Intravenous nicardipine in cats increases optic nerve head but not retinal blood flow. *Invest Ophthalmol Vis Sci*. 1992;33:2885–2890.

38. Nasemann JE, Müller M: Scanning laser angiography. In: Nasemann JE. Burk ROW, eds. *Scanning Laser Ophthalmoscopy and Tomography*. Munich: Quintessenz, 1990: 63–80.

39. Langham ME, Farrel R, Krakau T, Silver D. Ocular pulsatile blood flow, hypotensive drugs, and differential light sensitivity in glaucoma. In: Krieglstein GK, ed. *Glaucoma Update IV*. Berlin: Springer-Verlag, 1991;162–172.

40. Feman SS, Schaffer C, van Heuven WAJ. Advances in TV-fluoroangiography. *Doc Ophthalmol*. 1976;9:19–23.

41. Harris A, Arend O, Kopecky K, et al. Physiological perturbation of ocular and cerebral blood flow as measured by scanning laser ophthalmoscopy and color Doppler imaging. *Surv Ophthalmol*. 1994;38 (suppl):S81–6.

42. Sergott RC, Flaharty PM, Lieb WE, et al. Color Doppler imaging identifies four syndromes of the retrobulbar circulation in patients with amaurosis fugax and central retinal artery occlusions. *Tran Am Ophthalmol Soc*. 1992; 90.383–402.

43. Anderson DR. Vascular supply to the optic nerve of primates. *Am J Ophthalmol*. 1970;70:341.

44. Sieker HO, Hickam JB. Normal and impaired retinal vascular reactivity. *Circulation*. 1995;7:79–83.

45. Petrig BL, Riva CE. Retinal laser Doppler velocimetry: Towards its computer-assisted use. *Appl Optics*. 1988; 27:1126–1134.

46. Am A. Ocular circulation. *Adler's Physiol Eye*. 1992;6:198.

47. Tamaki Y, Nagahara M, Yamashita H, Kikuchi M. Analysis of blood flow velocity in the ophthalmic artery by color Doppler imaging: 2. Studies on diabetic eyes. *J Jpn Ophthalmol Soc*. 1993;97:961–966.

48. Shimizu K: Sectorial order of fluorescein filling in the disc area. In Shimizu K. ed. *Fluorescein Angiography. Tokyo International Symposium, 1972*. Tokyo: Igakua Shoin, 1974;349.

49. Taylor KJW and Holland S. Doppler US part I: Basic principles, instrumentation, and pitfalls. *Radiology*. 1990; 174:297–307.

50. Bioeffects Report Sub-Committee of the AIUM Bioeffects Committee: Bioeffects considerations for the safety of diagnostic ultrasound. *J Ultrasound Med*. 1988;7:S1–S38.

51. Pourcelot L. Indications de l'ultrasonographie Doppler dans l'étude des vaisseaux périphériques. *Rev Prat*. 1975;25:4671–4680.

52. Onda E, Cioffi GA, Bacon DB, Van Buskirk EM: Microvasculature of the anterior human optic nerve. *Am J Ophthalmol*. 1995;120(1):92–102.

53. Williamson TH, Harris A, Martin BJ. Reproducibility of color Doppler imaging assessment of blood flow velocity in orbital vessels. *J Glaucoma*. 1995;4:281–286.

54. Dennis KJ, Dixon RD, Winsberg F, Ernest JT, Goldstick TK. Variability in measurement of central retinal artery velocity using color Doppler imaging. *J Ultrasound Med*. 1995;14(6):463–466.

55. Lieb WE, Flaharty PM, Sergott RC, Medlock RD, et al. Color Doppler imaging provides accurate assessment of orbital blood flow in occlusive carotid artery disease. *Ophthalmology*. 1991;98(4):548–52.

56. Beach KW, Hatsukami T, Detmer PR. Carotid artery intraplaque hemorrhage and stenotic velocity. *Stroke*. 1993 24(2): 314–319.

57. Johnston KW, Baker WH, Burnham SH, Hayes AC, Kupper CA, Poole MA. Quantitative analysis of continuous-wave Doppler spectral broadening for the diagnosis of carotid disease: results of a multicenter study. *J Vascular Surg*. 1986;4(5):493–504.

58. Flaharty PM, Sergott RC, Lieb W *et al.*: Optic nerve sheath decompression may improve blood flow in anterior ischemic optic neuropathy. *Ophthalmol*. 1993;100:297–305.

59. Hayreh SS, Beach DW, Discussion of: Optic nerve sheath decompression may improve blood flow in anterior ischemic optic neuropathy. *Ophthalmol*. 1993;100:303–305.

60. Evans DH, Barrie WW, Asher MJ, Bentley S, Bell PR. The relationship between ultrasonic pulsatility index and proximal arterial stenosis in a canine model. *Circ Res*. 1980;46(4):470–475.

61. Legarth J, Nolsoe C. Doppler blood velocity waveforms and the relation to peripheral resistance in the brachial artery. *J Ultrasound Med*. 1990;9(8):449–453.

62. Norris CS, Pfeiffer JS, Rittgers SE, Barnes RW. Noninvasive evaluation of renal artery stenosis and renovascular resistance. Experimental clinical studies. *J Vascular Surg*. 1984;1(1):192–201.

63. Eberli B, Riva CE, Feke GT: Mean circulation time of fluorescein in retinal vascular segments. *Arch Ophthalmol*. 1979;97:145–148.

64. Hoskins PR, Haddad NJ, Johnstone FD, Chambers SE, McDicken WN: The choice of index for umbilical artery Doppler waveforms. *Ultrasound Med Biol*. 1989;15(2): 107–111.

65. Spencer JA, Giussani DA, Moore PJ, Hanson MA. *In vitro* validation of Doppler indices using blood and water. *J Ultrasound Med*. 1991;10(6):305–308.

66. Pope JC, Hernanz-Schulman M, Showalter PR, Cole TC *et al.*: The value of Doppler resistive index and peak systolic velocity in the evaluation of porcine renal obstruction. *J Urol*. 1996;156(2 pt.2):730–733.

67. Yura T, Yuasa S, Fukunaga M, Badr KE, Matsuo H. Role for Doppler ultrasound in the assessment of renal circulation: Effects of dopamine and dobutamine on renal hemodynamics in humans. *Nephron*, 1995;71(2): 168–175.

68. Harris A, Sergott RC, Spaeth GL, et al. Color Doppler analysis of ocular vessel blood velocity in normal tension glaucoma. *Am J Ophthalmol*. 1994;118:642–649.

69. Marion J, Hornyak W. *Physics for Science and Engineering, Part 1*. Philadelphia, CBS College Publishing 1982;743.

70. Curry TS, Dowdey J, Murry R: *Christensen's Introduction to the Physics of Diagnostic Radiology*, 4th ed. Malvern, PA: Lea & Feviger 1990.

71. Flower RW, Hochheimer BF. Clinical infrared absorption angiography of the choroid (letter). *Am J Ophthalmol.* 1972;73:458–459.

72. Hochheimer BF. Angiography of the retina with indocyanine green. *Arch Ophthalmol.* 1971;86:564–565.

73. Kogure K, Choromokos E. Infrared absorption angiography. *J Appl Physiol.* 1969;26:154.

74. Cherrick GR, Stein SW, Leevy CM, et al: Indocyanine green: Observations on its physical properties, plasma decay, and hepatic extraction. *J Clin Invest.* 1960;39:592.

75. O'Brart DP, de Souza Lima M, Bartsch DU, Freeman W, Weinreb RN. Indocyanine Green angiography of the peripapillary choroid in glaucoma using a confocal scanning laser ophthalmoscope. *Am J Ophthalmol.* 1997; 123:657–66.

76. Kagemann L, Harris A, Cantor LB, Chung HS, Kristinsson, JK. A new method for evaluating choroidal blood flow in glaucoma: Area dilution analysis. *Invest Ophthalmol Vis Sci.* 1997;38(suppl):1049.

77. Zieler K, Symposium on Indicator-Dilution Techniques. *Cir Res.* 1962;10:377–407.

78. Kinsman M, Moore JW, Hamilton WF, Studies of the Circulation. I. Injection Method: Physical and Mathematical Considerations. *Am J Physio.* 1929;89:323–339

79. Symposium on diagnostic applications of indicator-dilution techniques. *Proceedings of the staff meeting of the Mayo Clinic.* 1957;32:463–508

80. Wolf S, Toonen H, Koyama T, Meyer-Ebrecht D, Reim M. Scanning laser ophthalmoscopy for the quantification of retinal blood-flow parameters: a new imaging technique. In: Nasemann JE and Burk ROW eds. *Scanning Laser Ophthalmoscopy and Tomography.* Munich, Quintessenz, 1990;91–96.

81. Michelson G, Schmauss B. Two-dimensional mapping of the perfusion of the retina and optical nerve head. *Br J Ophthalmol.* 1995;79:1126–1132.

82. Riva CE, Cransoun SE, Grunwald JE, Petrig BL. Choroidal blood flow in the foveal region of the human ocular fundus. *Inves Ophthal Vis Sci.* 1994;35(13):4273–4281.

83. Riva CE, Petrig BL, Grunwald JE. Near infrared retinal laser Doppler flowmetry. *Lasers in Ophthal.* 1987;1(4): 211–215.

84. Kagemann, L., Harris, A., Chung, H. S., Evans, D., Buck, S., Martin, B. Heidelberg retinal flowmetry: Factors affecting blood flow measurement. *Br J Ophthalmol.* 1998; 82:131–136.

85. Ness T, Muller-Velten R, Funk J. No changes in ocular blood flow of the retina after topically applied Timolol: Heidelberg Retina Flowmeter parameters in healthy volunteers. ARVO abstracts. *Invest Ophthalmol Vis Sci.* 1997;34(4):S777.

86. Park K-H, Choi SY, Park KH, Lee J. Evaluation of parafoveal blood flow in branch retinal vein occlusion (BRVO) patients using Heidelberg Retina Flowmeter (HRF). ARVO Abstracts. *Invest Ophthalmol Vis Sci.* 1997; 34(4):S774.

87. Van Heuven Waj, Kiel JW, Elliot WR, Harrison JM, Sponsel WE. Evaluation of the Heidelberg Retina Flowmeter. *Inv Ophthalmol Vis Sci.* 1996;37(3):S967.

88. Obeid AN, Barnett NJ, Dougherty G, Ward G. A critical review of laser Doppler flowmetry. *J Med Engrg Tech.* 1990;14(5):178–181.

89. Cui WJ, Ostrander LE, Lee BY. In vivo reflectance of blood and tissue as a function of light wavelength. *IEEE Trans Biomed Engrg.* 1990;37(6):632–639.

Chapter 7

BLOOD FLOW IN GLAUCOMA

David Evans

Ocular vascular insufficiency is now well documented in glaucoma. As clinical management of the disease moves away from complete reliance on reduction of intraocular pressure (IOP), it is important to recognize the prevalence of ocular circulatory irregularities and to understand how these are affected by various glaucoma treatments. This chapter reviews recent research describing blood flow abnormalities that occur in four different ocular vascular beds of glaucoma patients. The hemodynamic outcome of surgical and medical ocular hypotensive and vasorelaxant therapies for glaucoma is discussed.

EVALUATION OF THE INTRAOCULAR PRESSURE PULSE WAVE AS AN ESTIMATE OF OCULAR BLOOD FLOW

Chapter 6 thoroughly reviewed the testing methodologies that can be used to specifically measure movement of blood through ocular vessels and tissues. In addition to these techniques, there are several indirect methods that may be used to estimate ocular perfusion. One technique that is gaining wider clinical acceptance is the measurement of ocular pulsatility through evaluation of the continuous IOP pulse wave. A brief description of the technique is provided here.

Ocular pulsatility results from the influx of blood to the eye during cardiac systole and accordingly fluctuates with the cardiac cycle; the greater the pulse amplitude, the greater the bolus of blood entering the eye.[1,2] The ocular pulse can be measured using a pneumotonometer, which rests on the corneal surface and senses the variation in intraocular pressure associated with changing globe volume during the cardiac cycle. This pressure variation is then used to estimate pulsatile ocular blood flow using two assumptions: (1) that Langham's pressure/volume relationship is similar for all eyes[3,4] and (2) that the venous outflow is constant and not pulsatile.[4-6] Since choroidal blood flow accounts for nearly 90% of ocular perfusion, it has been suggested that the measurement of ocular pulsatility provides an indirect assessment of choroidal blood flow. This suggestion is supported by several studies that noted reduced ocular pulsatility in conditions associated with reduced choroidal volume, such as retinitis pigmentosa and choroidal atrophy.[7] The results of this technique are more fully discussed below, under "Choroidal Circulation."

VASCULAR DEFICITS IN GLAUCOMA

Circulation of the Optic Nerve Head

The optic nerve head is the exit point from the eye for over 1 million nerve fibers. These fibers are unmyelinated until after they traverse the lamina cribrosa. Unmyelinated fibers require considerable nourishment, and there is a dense vasculature at the confluence of nerve fibers at the optic nerve head. It is well known that glaucoma is a disease characterized by excavation of the optic nerve head. This excavation is caused by loss of both optic nerve fibers and nerve head vasculature.[8] The first in vivo study of optic nerve head circulation in glaucoma patients was made possible by the advent of the fluorescein angiographic technique. Standard photographs of the optic disc area are taken following a 5-mL intravenous injection of 10% sodium fluorescein solution. Over 30 years ago, Hayreh and Walker used this technique to study glaucoma and reported an overall reduction in the fluorescence of the optic disc.[9] Since that time, a number of investigators have identified specific absolute defects of the optic nerve head vasculature in which some areas show no filling at any point during the cardiac cycle.[10] These defects are larger and more numerous in glaucomatous eyes than in those of normal subjects or patients with ocular hypertension.[11] In many cases there is a topographical correlation between the fluorescein defect and the location of a visual field defect. Frequently, patients who display fluorescein deficits without field loss subsequently develop visual field defects in the areas corresponding to the vascular defects.[12] Similar relationships have been observed between the location of optic nerve vascular defects and drop-out of the adjacent nerve fiber layer.[13]

Technical advances using video fluorescein angiography and laser Doppler flowmetry have made it possible to study the movement of blood through the tiny vessels that supply the area of the optic nerve head. During angiography, the speed of flow of the fluorescein dye, or transit velocity, is lower in eyes with glaucoma.[14] Laser Doppler flowmetry has also identified reduced blood flow and velocity in the rim of the optic nerve head[5,15,16] and in the peripapillary area.[16-18] It has been suggested that such vascular insufficiencies precede visual defects in glaucoma and are etiologic to the disease process.[19]

Retinal Circulation

Although glaucoma is not typically classified as a retinal disease, numerous studies have shown abnormalities of the retinal circulation in glaucoma patients. Video angiography has shown reduced transit velocities in the retinal arteries in glaucoma.[20] The arteriovenous passage time (the time for the dye to travel from a retinal entry point on an artery to a retinal exit point on the corresponding vein) is also increased.[21,22] These differences have been shown to be unrelated to blood viscosity.

Defects are also widely found in the retinal veins of glaucoma patients.[23] A close association between central vein occlusions and glaucoma is well documented.[24] Morphological studies describe extensive endothelial proliferations in the vessels of glaucoma patients.[24] Krakau noted that venous abnormalities occur long before the classic clinical indications of glaucoma and suggests that these may be very common signs of glaucoma.[23]

Choroidal Circulation

Hayreh was the first to implicate choroidal vascular insufficiency as a factor for the pathogenesis of glaucoma. He proposed the existence of watershed zones in the choroid—zones between choroidal areas supplied by different branches of the short posterior ciliary arteries.[9] These areas appear to have a lower vascular supply than other areas of the choroid and are presumably at higher risk for ischemia during elevated IOP. Recent data have directly demonstrated choroidal vascular defects in glaucoma. Jung et al. provided preliminary findings of reduced choroidal filling in glaucoma patients as determined by fluorescein filling times.[25,26] More recently, fluorescein refreshment rates in the disc margin have been used to show that choroidal filling is much slower in glaucoma patients than in normal subjects.[21] A computerized technique for indocyanine green analysis allows visualization of vessel beds deeper than the retinal pigment epithelium. Through the use of this method, the choroidal vasculature in glaucoma patients has been shown to have slower filling times in the macular region. These patients are also those who have reduced central vision as measured by contrast sensitivity.[14]

Ocular pulsatility measurements provide a global estimate of choroidal blood flow. It is widely recognized that pulsatile ocular blood flow and ocular pulse amplitudes are lower in open-angle glaucoma patients than in normal subjects.[1,2] Although vasospasm has been suggested as a cause of reduced ocular blood flow, ocular pulse amplitude is similarly reduced in patients with normal-tension glaucoma (NTG) even in the absence of peripheral vasospasm.[27] Further, untreated patients with primary open-angle glaucoma (POAG) have less ocular pulsatility than those with ocular hypertension who have been matched for IOP, suggesting that the vascular defect may be independent of IOP.[5] The largest blood flow study performed to date comprised 1500 subjects at six different centers in the United Kingdom. The data showed that NTG patients with unilateral field loss display lower ocular pulsatility in the eye with field loss than the contralateral eye and, perhaps more importantly, that glaucomatous eyes without field loss have significantly lower pulsatility than those of normal subjects.[28] These findings suggest that hemodynamic deficits precede the development of glaucoma.

Blood Flow into the Orbit and Retrobulbar Circulation

Retrobulbar circulation is studied with the use of color Doppler imaging. By this method it has been shown that glaucoma patients exhibit lower end-diastolic velocity and a higher resistance index in the central retinal artery[29-33] and short posterior ciliary arteries.[29,31,33] The reductions in ocular blood flow are more pronounced in the vessels of patients who exhibit uncontrolled intraocular pressure[34] or progressing visual field damage.[32,34,35] For the ophthalmic artery, it has been shown that NTG patients display lower end-diastolic velocity and a higher resistance index than age-matched subjects.[36] In patients with POAG, data on the ophthalmic artery are contradictory. Butt and colleagues showed that POAG patients have higher peak systolic velocity than normal subjects,[29] while other data show that POAG patients display lower peak systolic velocity than normals.[34] This apparent contradiction may highlight the limitation of examining data that investigate velocity rather than flow, but both studies confirm vascular abnormalities that extend to the vessels feeding the orbit, even as far posterior as the ophthalmic artery.

Hemodynamic abnormalities have been identified in the different ocular vascular beds in patients with glaucoma. These vascular irregularities appear to be present not only in glaucomatous eyes with field loss but also in the contralateral eyes of patients with asymmetric glaucoma and in eyes of patients suspected to have glaucoma. These data strongly suggest that deficits in blood flow play an important role in the pathogenesis of the disease.

BLOOD FLOW RESPONSE TO TREATMENT

A myriad of studies have been done to evaluate the impact of glaucoma medications on ocular blood flow. The vast majority of these studies investigated the effect of acute doses of medications in normal eyes or in eyes with stable disease. As glaucoma is a long-term, slowly developing disease, acute response studies provide limited information from a clinical management perspective. Further, it is difficult to directly assess the visual function consequences of these types of studies, as visual function is unlikely to change following an acute dose in normal subjects or in patients

with stable disease. Interestingly, a number of studies have recently demonstrated a clinically reliable recovery of central contrast sensitivity in patients with untreated or uncontrolled glaucoma after these patients had been placed on treatment. These authors have noted no correlation between the degree of IOP reduction and change in visual function, but they have demonstrated a link between the changes in ocular circulation and changes in central vision.[37-39]

Surgical Reduction of Intraocular Pressure

The change in ocular blood flow following surgical reduction of IOP by trabeculectomy has been widely evaluated. Trible and colleagues tested blood flow velocity in the retrobulbar vessels using color Doppler imaging in glaucoma patients before and then 2, 5, and 14 weeks following surgery.[40] They found a sustained increase in retrobulbar blood flow velocity at all periods following surgery. James demonstrated that pulsatile ocular blood flow increased by an average of 29% in glaucoma patients following trabeculectomy.[41] He also noted that the increase in blood flow was unrelated to the level of IOP reduction, such that a few patients with very large reductions in IOP showed no change in measures of ocular perfusion. In a related study, Gandolfi and associates evaluated central contrast sensitivity in patients with normal visual fields but with asymmetrically high IOP, 31 versus 16 mmHg, both before and then 6 months after trabeculectomy.[42] They found that before treatment, the eye with the elevated pressure had significantly lower contrast sensitivity at all spatial frequencies and that, 6 months following surgery, this deficit in vision had recovered to levels indistinguishable from those of the fellow (untreated) normotensive eye. He also observed that the improvement in contrast sensitivity was uncorrelated to IOP reduction for most spatial frequencies. These results, taken together, suggest that surgical reduction of IOP has, on average, a beneficial effect on both ocular blood flow and central visual function, but the improvement may be unrelated to the level of IOP reduction in some patients.

Medical Reduction of Intraocular Pressure

Medical therapy for IOP reduction remains the cornerstone of the treatment of glaucoma. The circulatory response to medical hypotensive treatment is very important when one is considering the management of patients and the potential impact on abnormal ocular blood flow in glaucoma. Evans et al. evaluated the retrobulbar flow velocity of age-matched normal subjects and compared these results to POAG patients evaluated after a 4-week drug washout and then again following 6 months of treatment with timolol in

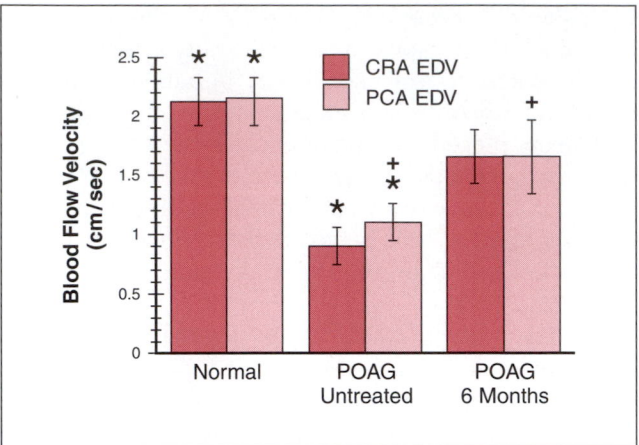

Figure 7–1. The end-diastolic blood flow velocity in the central retinal artery (CRA) and in the short posterior ciliary arteries (PCA) for normal subjects, untreated POAG patients, and these same patients following 6 months of treatment with timolol in Gelrite. The asterisk (*) represents a significant difference compared to normal subjects, while the plus sign (+) indicates a significant change from the untreated baseline. Note that after treatment, the POAG patients no longer have significantly lower blood flow velocity than normal subjects (Source: Evans DW, Harris A, Chung HS, Cantor L, Garzozi H. The effect of chronic hypotensive therapy on ocular hemodynamics in primary open-angle glaucoma: Non-selective beta blocker. *J Glaucoma.* 1999;8:12–17.)

Gelrite.[30] Figure 7–1 shows the end-diastolic velocities for the central retinal artery (CRA) and the posterior ciliary arteries (PCA). While untreated, glaucoma patients displayed a significant reduction in blood flow velocity; following 6 months of treatment, these measures improved to levels indistinguishable from those of normal subjects. The change in blood flow velocity was not correlated to the reduction in IOP. Significant improvements in contrast sensitivity have also been observed following chronic treatment with timolol in Gelrite in newly diagnosed and previously untreated patients.[43] These improvements also show no correlation in the level of IOP reduction. As with surgical reduction of IOP, these results suggest that, in general, medical ocular hypotensive therapy has a beneficial effect on ocular blood flow and visual function, but this level of recovery may be independent of IOP reduction in some patients.

Calcium Channel Blockade for the Treatment of Glaucoma

Several authors have suggested that vasodilator therapy may provide some benefit in glaucoma patients by dilating the ocular vessels and helping to preserve visual function.[44,45] The contractile status of vascular smooth muscle is dependent on the level of calcium

influx into the muscle tissue. Blockade of membrane-bound calcium channels does induce vascular dilation in susceptible subjects.[46] A number of studies have evaluated the effect of calcium channel blocker therapy on both central and peripheral visual function in NTG patients. These studies have demonstrated either better retention of or an improvement in visual field sensitivity and/or central contrast sensitivity following treatment.[47–50] These visual function results were attributed to recovery of ocular circulation, but ocular blood flow was not directly assessed. Harris and colleagues tested NTG patients for retrobulbar blood flow, visual field sensitivity, and contrast sensitivity after 4 weeks drug washout and then again after 6 months of treatment with a nifedipine sustained-release formulation (30 mg/day).[38] As a group, the patients showed no change in blood flow, visual field sensitivity, or IOP. Interestingly, however, a very tight correlation was found (Fig. 7–2) between the change in blood flow measures and the change in contrast sensitivity.

The subset of patients who demonstrated a significant improvement in contrast sensitivity displayed, on average, a 25% increase in blood flow velocity. However, those patients who showed no change in central visual function displayed a reduction in retrobulbar blood flow measures. One patient's blood flow velocity fell by as much as 90% in the ophthalmic artery. This dramatic change was coupled with an 8-dB reduction in visual field sensitivity and a log unit reduction of 0.6 in contrast sensitivity. After

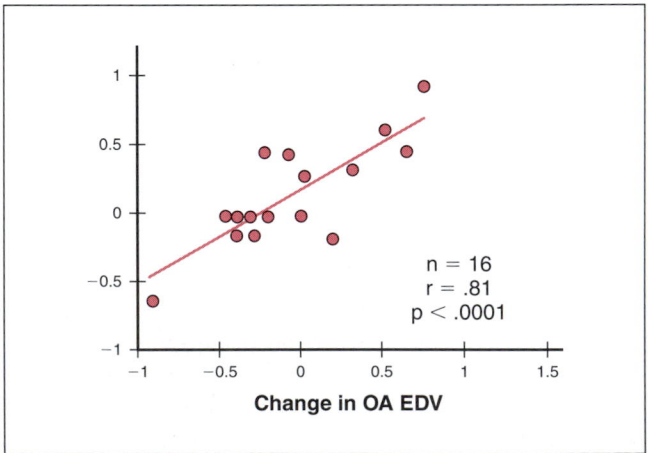

Figure 7–2. The tight coupling between change in ophthalmic artery end-diastolic velocity and in contrast sensitivity following 6 months of treatment with sustained-release nifedipine (30 mg/day). [Source: Evans DW, Harris A, Cantor L, Wilson M, Martin B. Changes in retrobulbar hemodynamics and visual function in low tension glaucoma patients after six months of treatment with nifedipine. *Invest Ophthalmol Vis Sci.* 1996;37(suppl):1253.]

cessation of treatment, these measures returned to baseline levels in this patient. These data suggest that vasodilatory therapy is beneficial for some NTG patients. These "responder" patients demonstrate a recovery of both blood flow and visual function, but this treatment is not a panacea for NTG. In some patients, calcium channel blocker therapy causes a reduction in both blood flow measures and visual function and as such would be contraindicated.

Combined Ocular Hypotensive and Vasodilatory Therapy

The recent focus on the circulatory status of glaucoma patients has heightened interest in pharmacological agents that may possess both ocular hypotensive and vasodilator capability. Carbonic anhydrase inhibition (CAI) has been used for many years in a dual role— by neurologists as a cerebral vasodilator to assess cerebral circulatory status[51] and in glaucoma therapy to reduce IOP.[52] As such, topical CAIs may possess this dual capability. Also, results from animal[53,54] and human studies[55] suggest that the beta$_2$-selective antagonist betaxolol has dual capability.

A recent crossover study by Harris et al. evaluated patients at washout, after 4 weeks of treatment with placebo, and after 4 weeks of treatment with the CAI dorzolamide.[56] Video fluorescein angiography data showed a significant hastening of arteriovenous passage time following treatment with dorzolamide but not with placebo. This increase in ocular blood flow was accompanied by a significant reduction in intraocular pressure and a significant improvement in contrast sensitivity (Fig. 7–3).

Dorzolamide treatment in these patients appears to provide the benefits of increased ocular circulation and improved visual function. It is unknown whether the improvement in visual function is due to IOP reduction, increased ocular circulation, or some other IOP-independent factor.

Evans et al. conducted a similar crossover study in which they compared a group of POAG patients, who tested positive for ocular vasospasm, for 4 weeks of timolol versus betaxolol treatment.[57] In this group of POAG patients, for whom the untreated level of IOP was relatively low (21.5 mmHg), timolol provided a significant reduction in IOP, but betaxalol did not. However, betaxalol did result in a significant change in retrobulbar hemodynamics and a significant improvement in contrast sensitivity. Interestingly, the change in color Doppler measures was significantly correlated to change in contrast sensitivity ($r = 0.70$; $p = 0.015$). For these patients, it appears that the change in ocular hemodynamics and visual function occurred independently of IOP reduction. Signif-

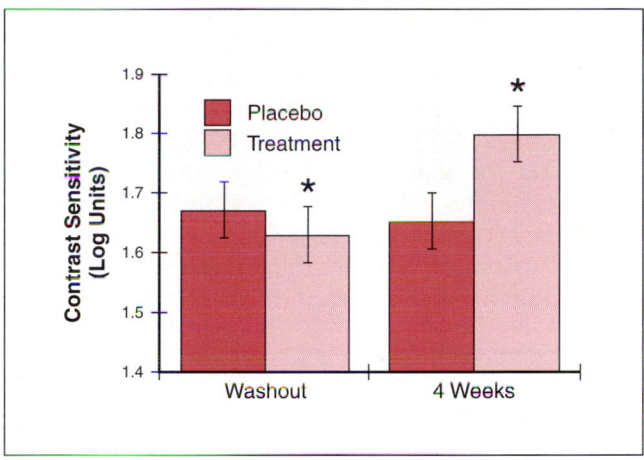

Figure 7–3. The central contrast sensitivity in NTG patients at washout and then following 4 weeks of treatment with either placebo or dorzolamide. The asterisk (∗) denotes a significant difference at $p < 0.05$. (Source: Harris A, Arend O, Kagemann L, Garrett M, Chung HS, Martin B. Dorzolamide, visual function, and ocular hemodynamics in normal-tension glaucoma. *J Ocul Pharm Ther.* 1999;15:189–197.

icant IOP reduction alone provided limited benefit for ocular circulation.

SUMMARY

A multitude of studies have demonstrated that glaucoma patients exhibit reduced ocular circulation and that this altered blood flow may be an important factor in the pathogenesis of the disease process. Contemporary treatments for glaucoma by reduction of IOP appear to have a beneficial effect on ocular blood flow and visual function. The specific level of recovery in some patients may be unrelated to the degree of IOP reduction. Vasodilator therapy, via systemic calcium channel blockade, provides concomitant improvements in ocular blood flow and contrast sensitivity in selected NTG patients. However, this treatment is contraindicated in some patients, as it may cause a loss of visual function and reduction in blood flow in some cases. Patients treated with calcium channel blocker therapy should be closely monitored after treatment for short-term changes in visual function in order to ascertain the potential benefit (or possible detriment) of this therapy. Drugs that possess both vasodilator and hypotensive characteristics have been found to be effective in providing circulatory and visual function benefits in both NTG and POAG patients with relatively low IOP. The effectiveness of these treatments in patients with higher IOP remains untested.

In conclusion, it seems that reduction of IOP, while providing obvious mechanical benefits, may also improve ocular circulation. It therefore remains central to the appropriate management of glaucoma. Vasodilator therapy is a potential adjunct to hypotensive therapy in glaucoma or as a "stand-alone" treatment in patients with NTG. Importantly, in some patients, the benefit in circulatory and visual function of IOP reduction and/or vasodilator therapy cannot be assessed by the measurement of IOP alone.

REFERENCES

1. Trew, DR, Smith, SE. Postural studies in pulsatile ocular blood flow. I. Ocular Hypertension and Normotension. *Br J Ophthalmol.* 1991;75:66–70.

2. Trew, DR, Smith, SE. Postural studies in pulsatile ocular blood flow. II. Chronic open-angle glaucoma. *Br J Ophthalmol.* 1991;75:71–75.

3. Eisenlohr JE, Langham ME, Maunemee AE. Manometric studies of the pressure/volume relationship in living and enucleated eyes of individual human subjects. *Br J Ophthalmol.* 1962;46:536–548.

4. Langham, ME, Farrell, RA, O'Brien, C. Estimation of pulsatile ocular blood flow from intraocular pressure. *Acta Ophthalmol.* 1989;191 (Suppl):9–13.

5. Kerr J, Nelson P, O'Brien C. A comparison of ocular blood flow in untreated primary open-angle glaucoma and ocular hypertension. *Am J Ophthalmol.* 1998;126: 42–51.

6. Silver DM, Farrell RA, Lanham ME, O'Brien V, Schilder P. Estimation of pulsatile ocular blood flow from intraocular pressure. *Acta Ophthalmol.* 1991;67:25–29.

7. Langham ME, Kramer T. Decreased choroidal blood flow associated with retinitis pigmentosa. *Eye* 1990;4:374–381.

8. Duke-Elder, S, Smith, J.H. Foundations of ophthalmology: clinical methods of examination, In: Duke-Elder S, ed. *System of Ophthalmology.* St Louis: CV Mosby; 1962;7:445.

9. Hayreh, SS, Walker, W.M. Fluorescent fundus photography in glaucoma. *Am J Ophthalmol.* 1967;63:982–989.

10. Schwartz B. Circulatory defects of the optic disk and retina in ocular hypertension and high pressure open-angle glaucoma. *Surv Ophthalmol.* 1994;38 (suppl):S23–S33.

11. Schwartz, B, Rieser, JC, Fishbein SL. Fluorescein angiographic defects of the optic disc in glaucoma. *Arch Ophthalmol.* 1977;95:1961–1974.

12. Fishbein SL, Schwartz B. Optic disc in glaucoma:topography and extent of fluorescein filling defects. *Arch Ophthalmol.* 1977;95:1975–1979.

13. Nanba K, Schwartz B. Nerve fiber layer and optic disc fluorescein defects in glaucoma and ocular hypertension. *Ophthalmology.* 1988;95:1227–1233.

14. Harris A, Chung HS, Kagemann L, Evans D, Martin B. The comprehensive ocular hemodynamic assessment in glaucoma. *Invest Opthalmol Vis Sci.* 1998;39(4 suppl):1011.

15. Grunwald JE, Piltz J, Hariprasad SM, DuPont J. Optic nerve and choroidal circulation in glaucoma. *Invest Ophthalmol Vis Sci.* 1998;39(12):2329–2336.

16. Nicolela MT, Hnik P, Drance S. Scanning laser doppler flowmeter study of retinal and optic disc blood flow in glaucomatous eyes. *Am J Ophthalmol.* 1996;122:775–783.

17. Chung HS, Harris A, Kagemann L, Martin B. Peripapillary retinal blood flow in normal tension glaucoma. *Br J Ophthalmol.* 1999;83:466–469.

18. Michelson G, Langhans MJ, Groh MJ. Perfusion of the juxtapapillary retina and neuroretinal rim area in primary open-angle glaucoma. *J Glaucoma.* 1996;5:91–98.

19. Piltz J, Grunwald JE, DuPont J, Harisprasad SM. Decreased optic nerve head blood flow precedes field defects in glaucoma suspect eyes. *Invest Ophthalmol Vis Sci.* 1999;15(suppl):2026.

20. Schwartz B, Kern J. Age, increased ocular and blood pressures, and retinal and disc fluorescein angiogram. *Arch Ophthalmol.* 1998;1980:1980–1986.

21. Duijm F, Van Den Berg JTP, Greve E. A comparison of retinal and choroidal hemodynamics in patients with primary open-angle glaucoma and normal-pressure glaucoma. *Am J Ophthalmol.* 1997;123:644–656.

22. Wolf, S., Arend O., Sponsel, E., Schulte, K., Cantor, L. Retinal hemodynamics using scanning laser ophthalmoscopy and hemorheology in chronic open-angle glaucoma. *Ophthalmol.* 1993;100:1561–1566.

23. Krakau CET. Disk Hemorrhages and Retinal Vein Occlusions in Glaucoma. *Surv Ophthalmol.* 1994;38:S18–S22.

24. Dryden, RM. Central retinal vein occlusion and chronic simple glaucoma. *Arch Ophthalmol.* 1965;73:659–663.

25. Jung, F., Kiesewetter, H., Korber, N. Quantification of characteristic blood-flow parameters in the vessels of the retina with a picture analysis system for video-fluoresccence angiograms:initial findings. *Graefes Arch Clin Exp Ophthalmol.* 1983;220:294–297.

26. Jung, F., Kiesewetter, H., Korbel, N., Wolf, S., Reim, M., Muller, G. Quantification of choroidal hemodynamics in glaucoma characteristic blood-flow parameters in the vessels of the retina with a picture analysis system for video-fluorescense angiograms: initial findings. *Graefes Arch Clin Exp Ophthalmol.* 1983;221:133–136.

27. Schmidt KG, Von Ruckman A, Mittag TW, Hessemer V, Piilunat LE. Reduced ocular pulse amplitude in low tension glaucoma is independent of vasospasm. *Eye.* 1997;11:485–488.

28. Fontana L, Poinoosawmy D, Bunce CV, O'Brien C, Hitchings RA. Pulsatile ocular blood flow investigation in asymmetric normal tension glaucoma and normal subjects. *Br J Ophthalmol.* 1998;82:731–736.

29. Butt Z, O'Brien C, McKillop G, Aspinall P, Allan P. Color Doppler imaging in untreated high- and normal-pressure open-angle glaucoma. *Invest Ophthalmol Vis Sci.* 1997;38(3):690–696.

30. Evans DW, Harris A, Chung HS, Cantor L, Garzozi H. The effect of chronic hypotensive therapy on ocular hemodynamics in primary open angle glaucoma: Nonselective beta blocker. *J Glaucoma.* 1999;8:12–17.

31. Kaiser H, Schoetzau A, Stumpfig D, Flammer J. Blood-flow velocities of the extraocular vessels in patients with

high-tension and normal-tension primary open-angle glaucoma. *Am J Ophthalmol.* 1997;123:320–327.

32. Nicolela M, Drance S, Rankin S, Buckley A, Walman B. Color Doppler imaging in patients with asymmetric glaucoma and unilateral visual field loss. *Am J Ophthalmol.* 1996;121:502–510.

33. Rankin SJA, Walman BE, Buckley AR, Drance SM. Color Doppler imaging and spectral analysis of the optic nerve vasculature in glaucoma. *Am J Ophthalmol.* 1995; 119:685–693.

34. Galassi F, Nuzzaci G, Sodi A, Casi P, Cappelli S, Vielmo, A. Possible correlations of ocular blood flow parameters with intraocular pressure and visual field alterations in glaucoma:A study by means of color doppler imaging. *Ophthalmologica.* 1994;208:304–308.

35. Yamazaki Y, Drance S. The relationship between progression of visual field defects and retrobulbar circulation in patients with glaucoma. *Am J Ophthalmol.* 1997; 124:287–295.

36. Harris A, Sergott RC, Spaeth GL, Katz JL, Shoemaker JA Martin BJ. Color Doppler analysis of ocular vessel blood velocity in normal-tension glaucoma. *Am J Ophthalmol.* 1994;118:642–649.

37. Evans DW, Harris A, Cantor L, Wilson M, Martin B. Changes in retrobulbar hemodynamics and visual function in low tension glaucoma patients after six months of treatment with nifedipine. *Invest Ophthalmol Vis Sci.* 1996;37(suppl):1253.

38. Harris A, Evans D, Cantor L, Edwards J, Martin B. Hemodynamic and visual function effects in normal tension glaucoma after treatment with oral nifedipine. *Am J Ophthalmol.* 1997;124(3):296–302.

39. Sponsel WE, DePaul K, Kaufman PL. Correlation of visual function and retinal leukocyte velocity in glaucoma. *Am J Ophthalmol.* 1990;109:49–54.

40. Trible JR, Sergott RC, Spaeth GL, et al. Trabeculectomy is associated with retrobulbar hemodynamic changes. *Ophthalmology.* 1994;101:340–351.

41. James CB. Effect of trabeculectomy on pulsatile ocular blood flow. *Br J Ophthalmol.* 1994;78:818–822.

42. Gandolfi S, Cimino L, Vecchi M. Improvement in spatial contrast sensitivity threshold after surgical reduction of intraocular pressure in unilateral glaucoma. *Acta Ophthalmol.* 1997;244(suppl):48.

43. Gandolfi S, Evans DW, Harris A. Comparison of ocular hypotensive and central visual function effects of levobunolol versus timolol gel formation in POAG. *Invest Ophthalmol Vis Sci.* 1997;38(4):abstr. No. 2588.

44. Flammer J, Gasser P, Prunte Ch, Yao K. The probable involvement of factors other than intraocular pressure in the pathogenesis of glaucoma. In: Drance SM, Van Buskirk EM, Neufeld A, eds. *Pharmacology of Glaucoma.* Baltimore:Williams & Wilkins;1992;273–283.

45. Gasser P. Ocular vasospasm:A risk factor in the pathogenesis of low-tension glaucoma. *Int Ophthalmol.* 1989; 13:281–290.

46. Swamy VC, Triggle DJ. The Calcium Channel Blockers, In: Craig CR, Stitzel RE, eds. in *Modern Pharmacology.* Boston: Little, Brown and Co, 1990:299–306.

47. Bose S, Piltz J, Breton M. Nimodipine, a centrally active calcium antagonist, exerts a beneficial effect on contrast sensitivity in patients with normal-tension glaucoma and in control subjects. *Ophthalmology.* 1995;102: 1236–1241.

48. Kitazawa Y, Shirai H, Go F. The effect of Ca^{2+}-antagonist on visual field in low-tension glaucoma. *Graefes Arch Clin Exp Ophthalmol.* 1989;227:408–412.

49. Netland PA, Chaturvedi N, Dreyer E. Calcium channel blockers in the management of low-tension and open-angle glaucoma. *Am J Ophthalmol.* 1993;115:608–613.

50. Sawada A, Kitazawa Y, Yamamoto T, Okabe I, Ichien K. Prevention of visual field defect progression with brovincamine in eyes with normal-tension glaucoma. *Ophthalmology.* 1996;103:283–288.

51. Ringelstein BE, Van Eyck S, Mertens I. Evaluation of cerebral vasomotor reactivity by various vasodilating stimuli:Comparison of CO_2 to acetazolamide. *J Cereb Blood Flow Metab.* 1992;12:162–168.

52. Becker B. Decrease in intraocular pressure in man by carbonic anhydrase inhibitor—Diamox: A preliminary report. *Am J Ophthalmol.* 1954;37:13–15.

53. Bessho H, Suzuki J, Tobe A. Vascular effects of betaxolol, a cardioselective beta-andrenoreceptor antagonist, in isolated rat arteries. *Jpn J Pharmacol.* 1991;55:351–358.

54. Hoste AM, Sys SU. The relaxant action of betaxolol on isolated bovine retinal microarteries. *Curr Eye Res.* 1994;13:483–487.

55. Harris A, Spaeth GL, Sergott RC, Katz LJ, Cantor LB, Martin BJ. Retrobulbar arterial hemodynamic effects of betaxolol and timolol in normal-tension glaucoma. *Am J Ophthalmol.* 1995;120:168–175.

56. Harris A, Arend O, Kagemann L, Garrett M, Chung HS, Martin B. Dorzolamide, visual function and ocular hemodynamics in normal-tension glaucoma. *J Ocul Pharm Ther.* 1999;15:189–197.

57. Evans DW, Harris A, Chung HS, Cantor L. Primary open angle glaucoma patients characterized by ocular vasospasm demonstrate a different ocular vascular response to timolol versus betaxolol. *J Ocul Pharm Ther.* 1999;15(6):479–487.

Chapter 8

NEUROPROTECTION

Evan Benjamin Dreyer

All currently recognized therapies for the treatment of glaucoma are based on the theory that the lowering of intraocular pressure (IOP) may retard or stop the progression of damage in glaucoma. The direct mechanical theory of glaucomatous optic nerve damage states that increased IOP leads to backward bowing of the lamina cribrosa sheets. This may, in turn, cause compression of the nerves, which then may decrease retrograde transport. This theory is based on early findings by Müller that high IOP leads to compression and death of optic nerve neurons.[1] Experiments have shown that axonal damage is diffuse rather than focal. This could be expected in a nerve with a localized kinking defect due to mechanical factors.

Another theory to explain the cause of damage from glaucoma suggests that vascular factors may be the principal causes of damage.[2] Studies using fluorescein angiography have shown that there are regions of transient hypoperfusion corresponding to areas of visual field loss in glaucomatous eyes.

In 1968, a new theory arose among investigators, proposing that glaucoma might interfere with axoplasmic flow, perhaps at the level of lamina cribrosa.[3] Interference with axoplasmic flow could impede normal transport of necessary trophic factors to the ganglion cell body, ultimately resulting in cell death. Ganglion cell death appears to be caused at least in part by loss of trophic factor influence following blockage of retrograde axonal transport. Impeded retrograde transport may cause cells to initiate a suicide response consistent with apoptosis. Although this response is found at normal IOP levels, it is increased with raised IOP. More recently, Quigley et al. have shown that the ganglion cell death seen in glaucoma is apoptotic in nature, which is consistent with the type of cell loss seen with trophic factor deprivation. In addition, these cells also have other features characteristic of apoptosis, such as chromatin condensation.[4,5] These insights suggest two possible therapies to lessen glaucomatous injury: (1) delivery of trophic factors and (2) manipulation of genetic expression in ganglion cell control over programmed cell death.

Nitric oxide has also been suggested as an important mediator in the death of retinal ganglion cells. In patients with primary open-angle glaucoma, investigators have found that the optic nerve head shows increased levels of one isoform of nitric oxide synthase, NOS-2. This finding may indicate that nitric oxide has a neurodestructive effect on the optic nerve head. Inhibitors of NOS-2 may potentially be useful in the treatment of glaucomatous nerve disorders.[6]

In our laboratory, we have established that the excitatory amino acid glutamate is elevated in the vitreous of glaucoma patients.[7] During the last three decades, studies in the central nervous system have found that excessive levels of glutamate and other excitatory amino acids can mediate both traumatic and ischemic neuronal injury. Both ischemic and traumatic insults have been implicated in optic nerve damage from glaucoma. Glutamate-mediated excitotoxicity has been demonstrated in a wide array of central nervous system disorders such as epilepsy, stroke, trauma, Huntington's disease, AIDS dementia, and amyotrophic lateral sclerosis. Since the retina is part of the central nervous system, excitatory amino acids may play a role in the ganglion cell loss seen in glaucoma.

Increased vitreal glutamate may be caused directly by glaucomatous elevated IOP levels or other pathological steps might be involved. However, if the glutamate level in the rat eye is chronically doubled by serial injections, 50% of the retinal ganglion cells are killed within 3 months.[8] Therefore, even if glutamate elevation is only an epiphenomenon of glaucoma, it still may significantly contribute to ganglion cell loss in humans. The discovery of an intervention that retards the toxic effects of glutamate might be able to slow visual loss in glaucoma.

The toxic effect of glutamate in the mammalian retinal ganglion cell layer has been well established. In 1957, Lucas and Newhouse reported the effects of glutamate on the mammalian eye.[9] While investigating another disorder, they serendipitously found that subcutaneous injection of glutamate in mice leads to massive destruction of the inner retinal layers, with most damage occurring to the ganglion cell layer. Olney demonstrated similar glutamate-induced retinal toxicity in neonatal mice and coined the term *excitotoxic* to refer to the process of neuronal damage resulting from excess stimulation by an excitatory amino acid.[10] Glutamate injections into the vitreous of adult rats were performed by Sisk and coworkers, who reported consequent degeneration of the ganglion cell layer. In addition to ganglion cell death, distinct cupping of the optic nerve has been shown in response to elevated intraocular glutamate by Azuma and coworkers. The retinal changes throughout these studies are markedly similar to those seen in glaucoma.

In our work, we have shown that in the vitreous of glaucoma patients, glutamate is present at toxic levels. We found a glutamate concentration of 28.3 ± 5.2 μM, compared to 10.3 ± 2.4 μM in control eyes. Although there is a clear disparity in glutamate in the two groups of eyes, no other amino acids differed between the two eyes. Ambati et al. have confirmed that glutamate is elevated in the vitreous of glaucoma patients.[11]

Similar results are found in a form of rabbit glaucoma. First described a century ago, buphthalmia in the rabbit is associated with markedly elevated IOP and deep excavation of the optic nerve as well as enlarged corneas, abnormalities in the structure of the iridocorneal angle, and ciliary process atrophy.

We investigated whether an elevation in vitreal glutamate was present in the buphthalmic rabbit eye. The mean glutamate level in the buphthalmic rabbit eye was 135 ± 13 mM/L, compared to a mean of 23 ± 13 mM/L in control eyes ($p < 0.001$). These results indicate a sixfold elevation over normal in vitreous glutamate concentration in the buphthalmic rabbit eye.[12]

In collaboration with Dr. Dennis Brooks (University of Florida), we have further found that glutamate levels are elevated in the vitreous of dogs with glaucoma.[13]

As mentioned above, in recent groundbreaking work, Quigley and coworkers have shown that ganglion cell death in glaucoma proceeds through an apoptotic mechanism as opposed to a necrotic demise.[4]

Although there are several classes of glutamate receptors, excitotoxic loss of retinal ganglion cells is mainly due to glutamate binding to the N-methyl-D-aspartate (NMDA) subtype. NMDA toxicity to retinal ganglion cells is found in vivo, as in the glutamate findings. A single intravitreal injection of only 20 nmol of NMDA can kill 70% of the retinal ganglion cells in the adult rat retina, sparing the other retinal layers.

Excitotoxicity to retinal ganglion cells is mediated by overstimulation of the NMDA subtype of glutamate receptor, which, in turn, leads to excessive levels of intracellular calcium. Eventual cell death correlates with the excessive levels of calcium. This association of cellular toxicity with excessive calcium levels suggests that a causal relationship exists, perhaps mediated through calcium-dependent enzymes. These enzymes include those translational and transcriptional enzymes that have been implicated in apoptotic death.

We therefore considered whether agents that can interfere with translation or transcription are also effective at preventing NMDA excitotoxicity.[14] In the presence of NMDA, cycloheximide or actinomycin D could prevent NMDA-mediated cell loss. Blockade of either translation or transcription effectively prevented retinal ganglion cell death resulting from exposure to low concentrations of NMDA. Either of these agents could be added 2 hours after the initial NMDA insult and still protect against excitotoxicity. The addition of 25 mM NMDA to retinal ganglion cells initiates a cascade of cellular events, including both translational and transcription events leading to cell death. Interruption of this schema with either actinomycin D or cycloheximide is sufficient to prevent cellular toxicity.

The low dose of glutamate that we have postulated may play a role in glaucomatous loss appears to trigger an apoptotic death, the mechanism of cell death in glaucoma.

As reviewed above, although a bolus of glutamate is acutely toxic to mammalian retinal ganglion cells and other central neurons, less is known about chronic perturbations of glutamate levels (as might be seen in glaucoma). We therefore explored the toxicity of a two-to-threefold increase in intravitreal glutamate as well as the ability of the NMDA antagonist memantine to protect against any such toxicity.[8] The glutamate level in the rat eye was elevated to ~30 mM by serial injections and ganglion cell survival was assessed. After 3 months of glutamate injection, there was a significant loss of ganglion cells. However, when animals were treated with the NMDA antagonist memantine concurrently with chronic glutamate administration, significantly more ganglion cells survived after 3 months. Memantine is therefore protective in this paradigm. It appears that a relatively minor but chronic elevation of glutamate over normal vitreous levels (similar to what we have observed in the human eye with glaucoma) can be toxic to retinal ganglion cells.

One unusual aspect to glaucomatous optic neuropathy is that larger retinal ganglion cells are preferentially damaged. In the mammalian retina, researchers have extensively studied the distribution of retinal ganglion cell size and size implications for cell function, but little is known about whether cell size affects sensitivity to glutamate. Previously, it had been demonstrated that larger retinal ganglion cells show greater susceptibility to glutamate-induced cell stress. We therefore chose to explore whether larger retinal ganglion cells were more sensitive to glutamate-mediated neuronal cell death both in vitro and in vivo.[15]

Most surprisingly, smaller retinal ganglion cells were not sensitive to the addition of exogenous glutamate. In vitro, exogenous glutamate administration only killed larger retinal ganglion cells. In the whole animal eye, the results were consistent with the in vitro results outlined above. NMDA was injected into rodent eyes and the animals were sacrificed. As was the case in vitro, NMDA had little effect on smaller retinal ganglion cells. Larger retinal ganglion cells were killed by intraocular NMDA; they are more sensitive to NMDA receptor–mediated neurotoxicity than smaller ganglion cells both in vivo and in vitro. If glutamate does indeed play a role in retinal ganglion cell loss secondary to glaucoma, this may explain why larger retinal ganglion cells are lost first.

One of the surprising aspects of glutamate toxicity in the retina is its selectivity for ganglion cells. Retinal ganglion cells are unique in the retina because they have extremely long processes. This raises the possibility that long neurites predispose retinal ganglion cells to excitotoxic damage. However, the precise role played by various subclasses and locales of glutamate receptors remains obscure. Therefore, we explored whether NMDA receptors located on neurites contribute to excitotoxicity. Our findings indicate that retinal ganglion cells without processes were far less susceptible to NMDA-mediated excitotoxicity than retinal ganglion cells with neurites. Furthermore, susceptibility to NMDA toxicity correlated positively with process length.[16]

We have suggested that cell loss in glaucoma may be mediated by glutamate excitotoxicity. Glutamate toxicity is predominantly mediated through activation of the NMDA subtype of glutamate receptor. If glutamate is indeed part of the pathophysiology of the neuronal loss in glaucoma, then agents that perturb the NMDA receptor might affect the course of the disease.[17]

The activity of the NMDA receptor–channel complex can be modulated at several sites on the receptor. The redox modulatory site consists of multiple sulfhydryl groups, forming one or more disulfide bonds on the receptor. This site is of particular interest since it acts as a "gain" control for current flux through NMDA receptor–operated channels and can affect the degree of neurotoxicity produced by excessive NMDA receptor activation. Activity of the NMDA receptor is enhanced by reducing agents such as dithiothreitol, which break disulfide bonds. Contrariwise, NMDA receptor activity is diminished (as well as related neurotoxicity) by administration of oxidizing agents such as 5,5-dithio-bis-2-nitrobenzoic acid, which form disulfide bonds from vicinal or paired free thiol groups.

Nitroglycerin and other drugs that generate nitric oxide can downregulate NMDA receptor function, in part by oxidizing this redox modulatory site via their generation of NO. Nitric oxide can thereby limit activation of the NMDA receptor. Nitroglycerin and other common nitrovasodilator drugs could, under certain circumstances, limit NMDA receptor–mediated neurotoxicity.

For more than 100 years, nitrates have been a major part of the internist's arsenal for the treatment of angina. In 1915, Wessely first reported that the administration of amyl nitrite led to a rise in IOP. Since Wessely's report, the effects of nitroglycerin in humans with glaucoma have received much attention, with inconclusive results.

Given that we have suggested that glutamate may play a role in the visual loss seen in glaucoma, nitroglycerin is an excellent candidate drug for limiting such glutamate-mediated damage in the retina precisely because of its ability to modulate the NMDA receptor. We therefore explored whether nitroglycerin preparations, taken for nonophthalmic reasons, had an effect on the rate of glaucomatous damage. We retrospectively compared two groups of patients with documented glaucoma. Glaucoma patients taking nitrates for cardiac reasons were matched to the group of glaucoma patients not taking nitrates. We compared optic nerve and visual field deterioration between the two groups.

In comparison to the control group, optic nerve deterioration and visual field deterioration was significantly lower in the patient population taking nitrate preparations. The difference between the two groups was backed up by statistical analysis. By controlling for IOP statistically, the risk was found to be about 20 times lower for optic nerve deterioration and 4 times lower for visual field deterioration in the nitroglycerin population than the control group.

These results support the surprising conclusion that the concurrent administration of nitrates for nonglaucomatous reasons was beneficial in terms of retarding both visual field loss and glaucomatous optic neuropathy. However, several flaws are inherent in this study, which must be examined. Most importantly, the cardiac health of the nitrate-taking population was not adequately controlled for. Presumably, patients in the nitrate group were in poorer cardiac health. A related confounding variable is the issue of compliance. Patients who are reliably taking nitrate preparations to avoid anginal symptoms may be more compliant with all medications. Prospective administration of nitrates to a glaucoma population without cardiac compromise would be necessary to conduct a study of this nature that does not have the above confounding variables.

Nevertheless, there are several explanations to account for the potential beneficial effects of nitrates on the glaucomatous eye. Systemic nitrates may have an effect on the IOP. Although our analysis does not support this hypothesis, our sample size may not have been large enough. Although we found no significant difference in overall IOP, nitrates may induce a lower pressure in the diurnal cycle that is not detectable by routine clinical tonometry. Alternatively, there may have been a beneficial effect on the optic nerve vasculature from chronic use of nitrates.

Nonetheless, we have hypothesized that chronic glutamate-mediated ganglion cell excitotoxic damage plays a role in glaucoma. Animals maintained on chronic nitroglycerin preparations are resistant to such an excitotoxic challenge. Consequently, nitrate preparations may be directly neuroprotective, causing retinal ganglion cells to be more resistant to the toxic effects of the glaucomatous process. Chronic nitrate

therapy, through its ability to downregulate sensitivity to glutamate, may protect ganglion cells against glaucoma-associated excitotoxicity. It is intriguing that agents known to perturb the NMDA receptor also retard glaucomatous damage.

CONCLUSION

The research reviewed above suggest that glutamate is elevated in the vitreous of glaucomatous eyes (in humans, dogs, and rabbits). This elevation rises to a level that might be toxic to retinal ganglion cells. Ganglion cells with longer processes and those with larger cell bodies are more susceptible to glutamate toxicity. The low doses of glutamate that we propose to be implicated in glaucoma have been demonstrated to cause apoptotic cell death, as has been described in glaucoma. However, this is not sufficient evidence to conclude that the blocking of glutamate toxicity can prevent blindness in glaucoma. Over 600 papers have been written on the pathophysiology of glaucoma to date. Future investigation may identify the source of the elevated glutamate in patients with glaucoma and establish whether agents that block excitotoxicity can be useful in the management of glaucoma. Presently, the pathophysiology underlying glaucomatous optic neuropathy remains something of an enigma. Hopefully, the next 600 papers will shed light on the precise etiology of the ganglion cell loss and blindness that accompany glaucoma.

REFERENCES

1. Müller H. Anatomische Beitrage zur Ophthalmologie: Ueber Nervean-Veranderungen an der Eintrittsstelle des Schnerven. *Arch Ophthalmolol*. 1858;4:1.
2. von Jaeger E. Ueber Glaucom und seine Heilung durch Iridectomie. *Z Ges Aertze Wien*. 1858;14:484.
3. Lampert PW, Vogel MH, Zimmerman LE. Pathology of the optic nerve in experimental acute glaucoma: Electron microscopic studies. *Invest Ophthalmol*. 1968;7:199–213.
4. Quigley HA, Nickells RW, Pease ME, et al. Retinal ganglion cell death in experimental monkey glaucoma and axotomy occurs by apoptosis. *Invest Ophthalmol Vis Sci*. 1995;36:774–786.
5. Kerrigan LA, Zack DJ, Quigley HA, Smith SD, Pease ME. TUNEL-positive ganglion cells in human primary open-angle glaucoma. *Arch Ophthalmol*. 1997;115:1031–1035.
6. Neufeld AH, Hernandez MR, Gonzalez M. Nitric oxide synthase in the human glaucomatous optic nerve head. *Arch Ophthalmol*. 1997;115:497.
7. Dreyer EB, Zurakowski D, Schumer RA, Podos SM, Lipton SA. Elevated glutamate in the vitreous body of hu-

mans and monkeys with glaucoma. *Arch Ophthalmol.* 1996;114:299–305.

8. Vorwerk CK, Lipton SA, Hyman BT, Sobel BA, Dreyer EB. Chronic low dose glutamate is toxic to retinal ganglion cells; toxicity blocked by memantine. *Invest Ophthalmol Vis Sci.* 1996;37:1618–1624.

9. Lucas DR, Newhouse JP. The toxic effect of sodium L-glutamate on the inner layers of the retina. *Am Med Assoc Arch Ophthalmol.* 1957;58:193–201.

10. Olney JW. Glutamate-induced retinal degeneration in neonatal mice: Electron microscopy of the acutely evolving lesion. *J Neuropathol Exp Neurol.* 1969;28:455–474.

11. Ambati J, Chalam KV, Chawla DK, et al. Elevated gamma-aminobutyric acid, glutamate, and vascular endothelial growth factor levels in the vitreous of patients with proliferative diabetic retinopathy. *Arch Ophthalmol.* 1997;115:1161–1166.

12. Dreyer EB. Amino acid abnormalities in the vitreous of the buphthalmic rabbit. *Vet Comp Ophthalmol.* 1997; 7:192–195.

13. Brooks DE, Garcia GA, Dreyer EB, Zurakowski D, Franco-Bourland RE. Vitreous body glutamate concentrations in dogs with glaucoma. *Am Jo Vet Res* 1997;58: 864–867.

14. Dreyer EB, Zhang D, Lipton SA. Transcriptional or translational inhibition blocks low dose NMDA-mediated cell death. *Neuroreport.* 1995;6:942–944.

15. Dreyer EB, Pan ZH, Storm S, Lipton SA. Greater sensitivity of larger retinal ganglion cells to NMDA-mediated cell death. *Neuroreport.* 1994;5:629–631.

16. Heng JE, Moscaritolo K, Dreyer EB. NMDA sensitivity is neurite enhanced. *Neuroreport.* 1995;6:1890–1892.

17. Zurakowski D, Chaturvedi N, Nichols DP, Lipton SA, Dreyer EB. Nitrates slow progression of glaucomatous optic neuropathy. *Invest Ophthalmol Vis Sci.* 1995;36:999.

Chapter 9

GENETICS AND GLAUCOMA

Lori R. Reminick

Diseases that are not infectious in origin are probably due to the genetic makeup of the individual. The genetic composition may be varied because of a mutation in a gene that leads to abnormal functioning or because a gene that regulates other genes may not be working properly. For many years there was awareness that genetic expression may play a role in the pathogenesis of some forms of glaucoma.[1-3] Recently documentation has occurred that several glaucomas are hereditary in origin; in some situations, the responsible gene has been sequenced. New methods to treat glaucoma may develop based upon genetics, allowing for either an earlier diagnosis or gene replacement therapy. For example, genes involved in the rate of fluid secretion or aqueous drainage from the eye may be manipulated. For the optic nerve, genes involved in the mechanisms that lead to cell death may be deactivated, while those that promote nerve cell regeneration may be emphasized. Although these approaches are new, they have the potential for becoming significant methods for managing glaucoma in the future, as the Human Genome Project progresses.

Although the exact mode of heredity remains unknown, indirect evidence suggests a polygenetic or multifactorial inheritance.[4] The term *polygenetic* refers to determination by many genes, with small additive effects.[5,6] Multifactorial inheritance is determined by multiple genetic and nongenetic (environmental) factors, each making a small contribution to the phenotype.[5,6] In polygenetic and multifactorial inheritance, there is a higher risk of the disorder among relatives of the affected person as compared with the general population.[6] Usually, the risk is approximately 3 to 5% for first-degree relatives (siblings and children) and approximately half that for second-degree relatives (uncles, aunts, nephews, and nieces).[6] A well-recognized risk factor in the development of primary open-angle glaucoma is the presence of a family member with the disease.[7,8] Studies have shown 13 to 25% of patients with glaucoma have a family history of the disease.[1,3] Additionally, many of the ocular components evaluated in the diagnosis of glaucoma—such as intraocular pressure (IOP), cup-to-disc ratio, steroid-responsiveness, ocular dimensions, and outflow facility—have a genetic component.[9]

Breakthroughs in the discipline of molecular genetics over the past decade have led to an improved understanding of many diseases, including glaucoma.[7] The positions of genes responsible for certain kinds of glaucoma have been localized to specific regions on individual chromosomes.[7] To date, six primary open-angle glaucoma and two congenital glaucoma genes have been mapped.[10] The Human Genome Organization/Genome Database designates "GLC" as the general symbol for glaucoma genes, with numbers 1, 2, and 3 representing open-angle, angle-closure, and congenital glaucoma, respectively. The letters A, B, and C indicate the first, second, and third genes mapped in each subgroup (Table 9–1).[10] Recent advances include the identification of the TIGR (trabecular meshwork inducible glucocorticoid response)/myocilin gene for the adult as well as the juvenile glaucoma GLC1A gene, a P450 gene for GLC3A congenital glaucoma, and a bicoid-homeobox transcription factor gene REIG for developmental glaucoma.[11]

The condition of glaucoma is classified according to age of onset (congenital versus juvenile versus adult), anatomy of the anterior chamber angle (open versus narrow), and etiology (primary versus secondary).[12] This chapter reviews the heritable factors contributory to the development of glaucoma, forms of glaucoma that have been shown to have a heritable component, and advances in our current understanding of the genetics of glaucoma.

INTRAOCULAR PRESSURE

Studies have shown that IOP is genetically determined and the mode of inheritance is polygenetic and multifactorial in nature.[13] IOP is higher in individuals with a family history of glaucoma,[8,14] and the prevalence of elevated IOP in patients with a positive family history was found to be three times greater than in the general population.[8] Approximately 9% of these patients will go on to develop glaucoma,[8] approximately 10 times greater than the prevalence of glaucoma in the general population.[8] Finally, with aging, individuals with a positive family history have an increasing chance of developing an IOP greater than 21 mmHg.[8]

TABLE 9–1. MAP OF GLAUCOMA GENES

Type of Glaucoma	Location	Locus	Mutation
Primary Congenital Glaucoma			
Buphthalmos	2p21	GLC3A	P-450
	1p36	GLC3B	
Secondary Congenital Glaucoma			
Aniridia type 1	2	AN1	
Aniridia type 2	11p13	AN2	
Rieger syndrome	4q25	Rieg 1	REIG
	13q14	Rieg 2	
Associated Congenital Glaucoma			
Lowe's syndrome	Xq24–q26		
Primary Open-Angle Glaucoma			
Juvenile-onset (JOAG)	1q23–q25	GLC1A	TIGR
	1q21–q31	GLC1A	
Adult-onset (COAG)	2cen–q13	GLC1B	
	3q21–q24	GLC1C	
	8q23	GLC1D	
Normal tension	10p15–p14	GLC1E	
Pigment dispersion	7q35–q36	GLC1F	

CUP-TO-DISC RATIO

The cup-to-disc ratio has been seen to be genetically determined and controlled by multifactorial inheritance.[15] Among the reported factors that determine susceptibility to glaucomatous damage are racial origin and size of the optic nerve head.[16] Normotensive blacks have a larger cup-to-disc ratio and disc area than age-matched whites, which may increase their susceptibility to pressure-induced axonal damage.[16] Additionally, IOP has been reported to be higher in individuals with a large cup-to-disc ratio.[17]

STEROID RESPONSE

A rise in IOP with topical corticosteroid therapy has been well documented.[18–20] Armaly[18] and Becker[19] found the rise in IOP in response to dexamethasone 0.1% tid is greater in the glaucomatous eye. Furthermore, this effect is of equal magnitude in normal-tension and primary open-angle glaucoma, indicating similarity of the two disease categories.[18] Patients with primary open-angle glaucoma also have been seen to respond to topical betamethasone with IOP elevation in spite of continued antiglaucoma medication.[21] Armaly hypothesized a polygenetic inheritance for chronic open-angle glaucoma, with the gene for the topical corticosteroid response being one of the genes involved.[22] Becker's hypothesis postulated the dominant transmission of the steroid-responsive trait and a recessive inheritance of glaucoma.[19] The intraocular response to steroids has shown three degrees of responsiveness where nn relates to the homozygous poor responder, ng to the heterozygous responder, and gg to the homozygous greater responder.[21]

OCULAR DIMENSIONS

Ocular dimensions of patients with angle-closure glaucoma compared with those of normal control subjects show smaller corneal heights and diameters, shallower anterior chambers, thicker and more anteriorly positioned lenses, and smaller axial lengths.[23] Ocular dimensions of siblings and offspring of patients with angle-closure glaucoma show similar anatomic variants as compared to the normal population.[23] Previous population studies have demonstrated a shallow anterior chamber as an inherited characteristic of Eskimos, explaining their high prevalence of primary angle-closure glaucoma.[24]

OUTFLOW FACILITY

Aqueous outflow facility is determined by multifactorial inheritance.[25] Outflow facility is correlated among siblings, regardless of whether a family history of glaucoma exists.[25] A decrease in outflow facility has been observed in close relatives of patients with glaucoma.[1]

HERITABLE GLAUCOMAS

Although it is believed that congenital glaucoma has a genetic basis, reports vary as to the precise mode of inheritance.[26] Congenital glaucoma may be primary, secondary, or associated.[27] Over two dozen disorders with a mendelian inheritance pattern are associated with glaucoma (Table 9–2). This chapter focuses on the more common disorders.

CONGENITAL (INFANTILE) GLAUCOMA

Primary congenital glaucoma (PCG), also known as buphthalmos, is characterized by persistence of embryonic mesodermal tissue at the iridocorneal angle accompanied by increased ocular size and pressure.[28] It is believed to be transmitted as an autosomal recessive, sex-controlled trait with variable penetrance.[27] A gene is said to be dominant if the phenotype of the heterozygote is the same as that of the homozygote for that gene.[5] A recessive trait is expressed only in individuals homozygous for the gene concerned.[5] The frequency of consanguinity of the parents in PCG exceeds 8%.[27] Some authors accept multifactorial heredity, where intrauterine or postnatal factors can play an unfavorable role in the development of the disease.[27] PCG has been mapped to mutations in the P450 gene CYP1B1 (the short arm of chromosome 2 at the 2p21 region) and named locus GLC3A, as well as the 1p36 region and named locus GLC3B.[29–31] Secondary congenital glaucoma is usually associated with other ocular anomalies or malformations such as aniridia and iridocorneal dysgenesis.[27]

ANIRIDIA

Aniridia is a rare congenital abnormality in which the iris is partially or totally absent.[32] Patients with aniridia may develop glaucoma early in life, but they usually do so in the preadolescent or adult years.[33] In approximately 85% of patients, aniridia is inherited as an autosomal dominant trait, with complete penetrance and variable expressivity.[6] Two autosomal

dominant genes for aniridia have been identified: aniridia type I, called AN1 and linked to a locus on chromosome 2, and aniridia type II, called AN2 and located on chromosome 11.[32] A single break at 11p13 is associated with isolated aniridia, while deletion of 11p13 results in aniridia combined with Wilms' tumor, genitourinary abnormalities, and mental retardation.[32] This is called the WAGR complex.[32]

AXENFELD-RIEGER SYNDROME

Axenfeld's anomaly consists of a white line in the posterior aspect of the cornea, near the limbus (posterior

TABLE 9–2. DISORDERS ASSOCIATED WITH GLAUCOMA AND HAVING A MENDELIAN INHERITANCE PATTERN

Disorder	Inheritance Pattern
Aniridia	Autosomal dominant*
Neurofibromatosis	Autosomal dominant
von Hippel–Lindau syndrome	Autosomal dominant
Axenfeld-Rieger syndrome	Autosomal dominant†
Familial hypoplasia of the iris	Autosomal dominant
Oculodentodigital dysplasia	Autosomal dominant
Familial microcoria	Autosomal dominant
Posterior polymorphous dystrophy	Autosomal dominant
Microcornea and absence of frontal sinuses	Autosomal dominant
Familial histiocytic dermatoarthritis	Autosomal dominant
Osteogenesis imperfecta	Autosomal dominant†
Stickler's syndrome	Autosomal dominant
Neovascular inflammatory vitreoretinopathy	Autosomal dominant
Juvenile glaucoma	Autosomal dominant†
Ectopia lentis	
Simple ectopia lentis	Autosomal dominant
Marfan's syndrome	Autosomal dominant
Weill-Marchesani syndrome	Autosomal recessive‡
Homocystinuria	Autosomal recessive
Ectopia lentis et pupillae	Autosomal recessive
Zellweger's syndrome	Autosomal recessive
Morquio's syndrome	Autosomal recessive
Hurler's syndrome	Autosomal recessive
Nanophthalmos with retinal degeneration	Autosomal recessive‡
Walker-Warburg syndrome	Autosomal recessive
Cystinosis	Autosomal recessive
Hunter's syndrome	X-linked recessive
Lowe's syndrome	X-linked recessive

*Aniridia may also be associated with a deletion on chromosome 11 or an autosomal recessive inheritance pattern.
†Some cases are sporadic.
‡Autosomal dominant inheritance has also been described.
Source: Reproduced with permission from Netland et al. *Int Ophthalmol Clin.* 1993;33(2):101–120.

embryotoxon); tissue strands extend from the peripheral iris to this prominent line.[34] Rieger's anomaly has additional iris involvement including corectopia, atrophy, and hole formation.[34] Rieger's syndrome includes ocular anomalies plus developmental defects of the teeth and facial bones.[34] All patients with the Axenfeld-Rieger syndrome share the same general features, consisting of bilaterality, frequent family history of the disorder with an autosomal dominant inheritance, and a high incidence of associated glaucoma.[34] Cytogenic analysis has revealed a deletion at chromosome 4q23–q27.[35] Recently, the REIG gene has been cloned; it encodes a novel bicoid-related homeobox transcription factor responsible for Rieger's syndrome. It maps to the 4q25–q27 region.[36]

Peters' anomaly includes buphthalmos, bilateral central corneal opacities, and adhesions to the iris.[34] The condition is usually present at birth and is bilateral.[34] There are reports of autosomal recessive inheritance and, less commonly, autosomal dominant inheritance; however, most cases are sporadic.[37,38] It has been reported both with and without systemic abnormalities.[38] Because of the varied genetic and nongenetic patterns, it is more likely to be a morphological finding than a distinct entity.[39]

ASSOCIATED CONGENITAL GLAUCOMA

Congenital glaucoma can be associated with numerous systemic conditions.[34] Lowe's (oculocerebrorenal) syndrome is a sex-linked disorder characterized by mental retardation, renal rickets, aminoaciduria, hypotonia, acidemia, and irritability.[34] It is commonly associated with bilateral cataracts, and—approximately two-thirds of the time—glaucoma.[34] Localization to breaks in chromosome Xq25 or the Xq24–q26 region has been detected.[40,41]

JUVENILE GLAUCOMA

Juvenile open-angle glaucoma (JOAG) is a form of open-angle glaucoma usually diagnosed during childhood or early adulthood and often having a strong family history.[42] JOAG has been defined as the subgroup of primary congenital glaucoma that occurs between 3 years of age and early adulthood[43] and is frequently reported as an autosomal dominant disease.[42–46] In a study by Johnson et al. of a multigenerational family with autosomal dominant JOAG, the average age at diagnosis was 18, and the IOPs were commonly more than 50 mmHg when the patients were first examined.[42] Topical medications were

initially effective in controlling IOP, but surgery was usually required for long-term pressure control. JOAG has been reported to have a higher incidence among African-American patients.[47] In 1993 the disease was first mapped to the 1q21–q31 chromosome; it was subsequently bracketed to a 3-cM region associated with 1q23–25.[43–45] The locus was named GLC1A.[43–45] The first set of mutations was mapped to a novel myosin-like protein, the TIGR (trabecular meshwork inducible glucocorticoid response) protein gene, also known as myocilin.[48] The TIGR gene was originally identified and isolated by induction of primary cultured cells of trabecular meshwork (TM) tissue with glucocorticoids.[48] The responding protein was named TIGR and was shown to be present in the TM and the ciliary body.[48] Recently, researchers in the field of molecular cloning have described a novel myosin-like protein that was named myocilin because it has homology to myosin and is expressed predominantly in the photoreceptor cells of the retina; it is localized particularly in the rootlet and basal body of the connecting cilium.[48,49] The nucleotide sequence of the human myocilin cDNA, designated MYOC, is identical to the TIGR gene with the exception of an additional GA at position 107–108, which shifted the initiation codon of ATG to position 109.[48]

The TIGR gene initiation codon is located at position 65 of the MYOC gene, and it has recently been confirmed that these two genes are identical.[48] Mutations in the GLC1A gene, which produces a protein that is induced in trabecular meshwork cells by treatment with dexamethasone (TIGR or myocilin), have been identified as responsible for GLC1A.[50] Wiggs et al. found that only 8% of JOAG pedigrees had identifiable mutations in the TIGR/myocilin gene. The small number of pedigrees with mutations suggests that additional genes are likely to be responsible for this disease.[51]

PRIMARY OPEN-ANGLE GLAUCOMA

Primary open-angle glaucoma (POAG) is believed to have a genetic basis.[4] The late-onset form of this condition rarely starts before the ages of 35 to 40 and is the most prevalent form of all glaucomas.[9,48,52] The majority of sufferers exhibit the disease after the age of 50 or 60, by which time their parents are usually deceased, making it difficult to identify families with multiple living generations that can be studied genetically.[53] Even when they are identified, family members are sometimes unable to cooperate with testing because of their advanced age.[53] As a consequence, it has been difficult to determine the exact mode of inheritance.

Although the role of heredity is well established, autosomal dominant, autosomal recessive, and multifactorial modes of heredity have all been reported.[9] The pedigree structure of the majority of families used in genetic linkage analysis suggests autosomal dominance with reduced penetrance.[48]

A family history of POAG puts a person at higher risk for developing the disease.[8] The disorder is present in 1 to 2% of those over the age of 40, and the prevalence increases with age.[8,52–54] The incidence of open-angle glaucoma in first-degree relatives with the disease has been reported up to be five times greater than that in the general population.[55] There is concordance in monozygotic twins[55] and no sex predominance, with women being affected as often as men.[55]

Five loci for adult-onset POAG have been discovered. Genetic studies have mapped this condition to the 2cen–q13, 3q21–q24, 8q23, 10p15–p14, and 7q35–q36 regions.[56–58] These locations have been named GLC1B, GLC1C, GLC1D, GlC1E, and GLC1F, respectively.[56–58] In addition to most juvenile-onset glaucoma families, 3% of individuals with adult-onset POAG also have mutations in the TIGR gene.[50] The precise relationship between the TIGR gene, corticosteroid-response glaucoma, and POAG is still uncertain.[10]

NORMAL-TENSION GLAUCOMA

The prevalence of POAG is greater in families of patients with normal-tension glaucoma (NTG) than in the general population.[59] The genetic association between POAG and NTG suggests some common causal factors.[59] Autosomal dominant transmission as well as NTG in identical twins have been reported.[60,61] Mutations in the GLC1B gene are found in a large number of individuals with normal-tension glaucoma, which may render the optic nerve abnormally sensitive to IOP or produce damage independent of IOP.[10] Localization of the fourth locus to the 10p15–p14 region (GLC1E) was discovered in a family with NTG.[56]

ANGLE-CLOSURE GLAUCOMA

Closed-angle glaucoma has reportedly been transmitted through multifactorial heredity.[54] The risk that first-degree relatives will develop angle-closure glaucoma is 2 to 5%.[54] Siblings and offspring of patients with angle-closure glaucoma share the same ocular parameters of smaller corneal heights and diameters, shallower anterior chamber depths, and increases in lens thickness.[23] These are the typical ocular dimensions of hypermetropia. Angle-closure glaucoma occurs most frequently but not exclusively in eyes that are hypermetropic.[23] Racial differences in the incidence of angle-closure glaucoma may indicate a genetic predisposition. It is more frequent among Eskimos, Asians, the aborigines of Australia, and the Maori of New Zealand.[54] Additionally, acute angle-closure glaucoma is a rare occurrence in African Americans.[62] The topical corticosteroid response does not appear to be related to the development of angle closure[9] and angle-closure glaucoma genes have not yet been identified.[9,10]

PIGMENTARY GLAUCOMA

Numerous studies suggest a hereditary basis for pigmentary glaucoma.[9] Pigment dispersion syndrome may be inherited in an autosomal dominant or autosomal recessive fashion.[63] Less than 50% of the cases of pigment dispersion develop into pigmentary glaucoma.[64] Shafer proposed a close genetic correlation between pigmentary glaucoma and open-angle glaucoma because the former patients exhibit the same increase in pressure response to corticosteroids as do those with POAG.[65] Investigators have found significant linkage between the disease phenotype and genetic markers located on the long arm of chromosome 7 (7q35–q36), named GLC1F.[10,66]

EXFOLIATIVE GLAUCOMA

Heredity may play an important role in pseudoexfoliation.[67] There is evidence that it could be associated with a gene influencing three characteristics—namely, an abnormality of the drainage mechanism, production of the pseudoexfoliation material, and degeneration of the pigment epithelium of the iris.[67] Pohjanpelta and Hurskainen[68] found exfoliation in 8% of relatives of patients with exfoliation syndrome with or without glaucoma. The response to corticosteroids more closely resembles that of normal individuals than that of patients with chronic open-angle glaucoma, suggesting a condition genetically distinct from chronic open-angle glaucoma.[69]

MOLECULAR GENETIC APPROACHES TO GLAUCOMA

Research is under way in the area of molecular genetics to identify additional genes responsible for the various forms of glaucoma. The search for diseased genes continues, utilizing several molecular techniques, and it appears to involve multiple genetic loci. The study of chromosomal abnormalities can help pinpoint a potential region in which a disease-causing gene might lie.[7] The candidate-gene approach can be of value if a disease is thought to be caused by one or more of a limited number of known genes.[7] In glaucoma, however, selecting proteins at random in attempts to explore tissues for candidate genes may not be as fruitful a method as positional cloning, which seeks to find the location of the gene as the basis for cloning.[70] Linkage analysis has been the most valuable tool in attempts to unfold the genetics of POAG.[7] It relies on the fact that genes that lie close to one another on a chromosome are less likely to be separated by the process of recombination during meiosis than those lying far apart.[7] Linkage to a chromosome implies that the gene is on the chromosome, but it does not mean that the gene has yet been identified, or cloned.[70]

Genetic markers are used to define regions of human chromosomes. Showing that a particular trait, such as glaucoma, is inherited with a particular genetic marker means that the gene responsible for the trait is located near the marker. Once the chromosomal location of the gene is known, the gene can be isolated using a variety of molecular techniques. Once the gene has been cloned, the DNA sequence can be used to predict the amino acid sequence of the protein encoded by the gene.[70] Ultimately, the protein's function can be determined, providing critical information as to how mutations in the gene cause defective protein and may thereby lead to the disease under investigation.[70]

If a limited number of genes are found to be responsible for glaucoma, genetic testing could be one method for diagnosing glaucoma at an earlier stage of disease. Additionally, progress in molecular genetics holds promise for the future therapy of glaucoma, as the discovery of the first six POAG and two congenital glaucoma genes may lead to the treatment of patients based on their genetic profiles. The genes discovered to date, however, may represent only a small fraction of the total glaucoma population, thus indicating the diversity of glaucoma genetics. It is likely that many more glaucoma genes exist, since there are many families with glaucoma whose genes do not localize to the already discovered regions.[10]

Genetic mapping and isolation of mutations will enable the development of DNA tests that can be used for earlier diagnosis. This flood of new information will have benefits for patient care as well as raising ethical issues regarding informed consent for DNA testing.[71] Continuous advances in the genetics of glaucoma will help to strengthen the role of genetic counseling for glaucoma patients. This includes providing information about the risks of glaucoma in children and other close relatives.[6] In glaucomas associated with polygenic or multifactorial inheritance, the role of genetic counseling is less obvious than in glaucomas associated with disorders exhibiting mendelian inheritance.[6] However, the need exists to educate patients about the higher risk in relatives of patients affected with glaucoma. There may eventually be testing with noninvasive methods, such as buccal scrapings, to identify POAG.[10] Earlier detection through genetic testing could therefore enable us to provide preventive treatment for this disease.

REFERENCES

1. Becker B, Kolker A, Roth D. Glaucoma family study. *Am J Ophthalmol.* 1960;50:557–567.
2. Biro I. Notes on the heredity of glaucoma. *Ophthalmologica.* 1939;98:43–50.
3. Biro I. Notes upon the question of hereditary glaucoma. *Ophthalmologica.* 1951;122:228–238.
4. Shields BM. *Textbook of Glaucoma,* 4th ed. Baltimore: Williams & Wilkins; 1998:153–176.
5. Nora JJ, Fraser FC, Bear J, et al. *Medical Genetics: Principles and Practice,* 4th ed. Philadelphia: Lea & Febiger; 1994:418–436.
6. Netland PA, Wiggs JL, Dreyer EB. Inheritance of glaucoma and genetic counseling of glaucoma patients. *Int Ophthalmol Clin.* 1993;33:101–120.
7. Booth A, Curchill A, Anwar R, et al. The genetics of primary open angle glaucoma. *Br J Ophthalmol.* 1997;81:409–414.
8. Rosenthal R, Perkins E. Family studies in glaucoma. *Br J Ophthalmol.* 1985;69:664–667.
9. Johnson AT, Alward W, Sheffield VC, et al. Genetics and glaucoma. In: Ritch R, Shields BM, Krupin T, eds. *The Glaucomas II.* St. Louis: Mosby; 1996:39–54.
10. Wirtz MK, Acott TS, Samples JR, et al. Prospects for genetic intervention in primary open-angle glaucoma. *Drugs Aging.* 1998;13(5):333–340.
11. Polansky JR, Nguyen TD. The TIGR gene, pathogenic mechanisms, and other recent advances in glaucoma genetics. *Curr Opin Ophthalmol.* 1998;9:15–23.
12. Shields MB, Ritch R, Krupin T. Classification of the glaucomas. In: Ritch R, Shields BM, Krupin T, eds. *The Glaucomas II.* St. Louis: Mosby; 1996:717–725.
13. Armaly MF. The genetic determination of ocular pressure in the normal eye. *Arch Ophthalmol.* 1967;78:187.
14. Armaly MF. On the distribution of applanation pressure. *Arch Ophthalmol.* 1965;73:11.
15. Armaly MF. Genetic determination of cup/disc ratio of the optic nerve. *Arch Ophthalmol.* 1967;78:35–43.
16. Chi T, Ritch R, Stickler D, et al. Racial differences in optic nerve head parameters. *Arch Ophthalmol.* 1989;107:836–814.

17. David R, Zangwill L, Stone D, et al. Epidemiology of intraocular pressure in a population screened for glaucoma. *Br J Ophthalmol.* 71(10):1987;71:766–771.

18. Armaly MF. Effect of corticosteroids on intraocular pressure fluid dynamics. *Arch Ophthalmol.* 1963;70:492

19. Becker B, Chevrette L. Topical corticosteroid testing in glaucoma siblings. *Arch Ophthalmol.* 1966;76:484.

20. Shields BM. *Textbook of Glaucoma*, 4th ed. Baltimore: Williams & Wilkins; 1998:323–328.

21. Becker B. Intraocular pressure response to topical corticosteroids. *Invest Ophthalmol.* 1965;4(2):198–205.

22. Armaly MF. Inheritance of dexamethasone hypertension and glaucoma. *Arch Ophthalmol.* 1967;77:747–751.

23. Tomlinson A, Leighton DA. Ocular dimensions in the heredity of angle-closure glaucoma. *Br J Ophthalmol.* 1973;57:18.

24. Alsbirk PH. Anterior chamber depth, genes and environment. *Acta Ophthalmol.* 1982;60:223–234.

25. Armaly MF, Monstavicius BF, Sayegh RE. Ocular pressure and aqueous outflow facility in siblings. *Arch Ophthalmol.* 1968;80:355–360.

26. Shields BM. *Textbook of Glaucoma,* 4th ed. Baltimore: Williams & Wilkins; 1998:195–197.

27. Francois J. Congenital glaucoma and its inheritance. *Ophthalmologica.* 1980;181:61–73.

28. Demenais F, Bonaiti C, Briard M, et al. Congenital glaucoma: Genetic models. *Hum Genet.* 1979;46:305.

29. Sarfarazi M, Akarou AN, Hossain A, etal. Assignment of a locus (GLC3A) for primary congenital glaucoma (buphthalmos) to 2p21 and evidence for genetic heterogeneity. *Genomics.* 1995;30:171–177.

30. Bejjani BA, Lewis RA, Tomey KF, et al. Mutations in CYP1B1, the gene for cytochrome P4501B1, are the predominant cause of primary congenital glaucoma in Saudi Arabia. *Am J Hum Genet.* 1998;62:325–333.

31. Akarsu AN, Turacki ME, Aktan SG, et al. A second locus (GLC3B) for PCG (buphthalmos) maps to the 1p36 region. *Hum Mol Genet.* 1996;5:1199–1203.

32. Moore JW, Hyman S, Atonarakis SE, et al. Familial isolated aniridia with a translocation involving chromosomes 11 and 22[t(11;22)(p13;q12.2)]. *Hum Genet.* 1986;72:297.

33. Grant WM, Walton DS. Progressive changes in the angle in congenital aniridia, with development of glaucoma. *Am J Ophthalmol.* 1974;78:842–847.

34. Shields BM. *Textbook of Glaucoma,* 4th ed. Baltimore: Williams & Wilkins; 1998:207–225.

35. Litguitic I, Brecevic L, Petovic I, et al. Interstitial deletion 4q and Rieger syndrome. *Clin Genet.* 1981;20:323.

36. Semina EV. Cloning a novel bicoid-related homeobox transcription factor gene. *Nature Genet.* 1996;14:392–399.

37. DeRespinis PA, Wagner RS. Peters' anomaly in a father and son. *Am J Ophthalmol.* 1987;104(5):545–546.

38. Holmstrom GE, Reardon WP, Baraitser M, et al. Heterogeneity in dominant anterior segment malformation. *Br J Ophthalmol.* 1991;75:591–597.

39. Kivlin JD, Fineman RM, Crandall AS, et al. Peters' anomaly as a consequence of genetic and nongenetic syndromes. *Arch Ophthalmol.* 1986;104:61–64.

40. Hodgson SV, Heckmatt JZ, Hughes JA, et al. A balanced de novo X/autosome translocation in a girl with manifestations of Lowe syndrome. *Am J Med Genet.* 1986;23:837–847.

41. Mueller OT, Hartsfield JK, Gallardo LA, et al. Lowe oculocerebrorenal syndrome in a female with a balanced X;20 translocation: Mapping of the X chromosome breakpoint. *Am J Hum Genet.* 1991;49:804–810.

42. Johnson AT, Drack AV, Kwitek BS, et al. Clinical features and linkage analysis of a family with autosomal dominant juvenile glaucoma. *Ophthalmology:* 1993;100(4):524–529.

43. Angius A, De Gioia E, Loi A, et al. A novel mutation in the GLC1A gene causes juvenile open-angle glaucoma in 4 families from the Italian region of Puglia. *Arch Ophthalmol.* 1998;116:793–797.

44. Sheffield VC, Stone EM, Wallace LM, et al. Genetic linkage of familial open angle glaucoma to chromosome 1q21–q31. *Nature Genet.* 1993;4:47–50.

45. Richards JE, Lichter PR, Boehnke M, et al. Mapping of a gene for autosomal dominant juvenile-onset open-angle glaucoma to chromosome 1q. *Am J Hum Genet.* 1994;54:62–70.

46. Fleck BW, Cullen JF. Autosomal dominant juvenile onset glaucoma affecting six generations in an Edinburgh family. *Br J Ophthalmol.* 1986;70:715.

47. Lotufo D, Ritch R, Szmyd L, et al. Juvenile glaucoma, race, and refraction. *JAMA.* 1989;261(2):249–252.

48. Sarfarazi M. Recent advances in molecular genetics of glaucomas. *Hum Mol Genet.* 1997;6(10):1667–1677.

49. Kubota R, Noda S, Wang Y. A novel myosin-like protein (myocilin) expressed in the connecting cilium of the photoreceptor: Molecular cloning, tissue expression, and chromosomal mapping. *Genomics.* 1997;41:360–369.

50. Stone EM, Fingert JH. Identification of a gene that causes primary open angle glaucoma. *Science.* 1997;275:668–670.

51. Wiggs JL, Allingham RR, Vollrath D, et al. Prevalence of mutations in TIGR/myocilin in patients with adult and juvenile primary open-angle glaucoma. *Am J Hum Genet.* 1998;63:1549–1552.

52. Alward WLM, Fingert J, Coote MA, et al. Clinical features associated with mutations in the chromosome 1 open-angle glaucoma gene (GLC1A). *N Engl J Med.* 1998;338:1022–1027.

53. Quigley HA. The search for glaucoma genes—Implications for pathogenesis and disease detection. *N Engl J Med.* 1998;338:1063–1064.

54. Francois J. Genetic predisposition to glaucoma. *Dev Ophthalmol.* 1981;3:1–45.

55. Miller SJH. Genetics of glaucoma and family studies. *Trans Ophthalmol Soc UK.* 1978;98:290–292.

56. Sarfarazi M, Child A, Stoilova D, et al. Localization of the fourth locus (GLC1E) for adult-onset primary open-angle glaucoma to the 10p15-p14 region. *Am J Hum Genet.* 1998;62:641–652.

57. Trifan OC, Traboulsi EI, Stoilova D, et al. A third locus (GLC1D) for adult-onset primary open-angle glaucoma maps to the 8q23 region. *Am J Ophthalmol.* 1998;126(1):17–28.

58. Wirtz MK, Samples JR, Rust K, et al. GLC1F, a new primary open-angle glaucoma locus, maps to 7q35-q36. *Arch Ophthalmol*. 1999;117:237–241.

59. Levene RZ. Low tension glaucoma: A critical review and new material. *Surv Ophthalmol*. 1980;24(6):621–664.

60. Bennett SR, Wallace LM, Alward MD, et al. An autosomal dominant form of low-tension glaucoma. *Am J Ophthalmol*. 1989;108:238–244.

61. Ofner S, Samples JR. Low-tension glaucoma in identical twins. *Am J Ophthalmol*. 1992;114(6):764–765.

62. Alper MG, Laubach JL. Primary angle-closure glaucoma in the American Negro. *Arch Ophthalmol*. 1968;79:663–668.

63. Mandelkorn RM et al. Inheritance and the pigment dispersion syndrome. *Ophthalm Paediatr Genet*. 1985;6:85.

64. Scheie HG, Fleischhauer HW. Idiopathic atrophy of the epithelial layers of the iris and ciliary body. *Arch Ophthalmol*. 1958;59:216–228.

65. Shafer RN. Pigment and glaucoma. In: *Symposium on Glaucoma: Transactions of the New Orleans Academy of Ophthalmology*. St. Louis: Mosby; 1975:238.

66. Scerra C. Genetic studies continue to yield new information on glaucoma. *Ophthalmol Times*. 1998;23(22):1.

67. Tarkkanen A. Pseudoexfoliation of the lens capsule. *Acta Ophthalmol*. 1962;(suppl)/71:1–98.

68. Pohjanpelta P, Hurskainen L. Studies on relatives of patients with glaucoma simplex and patients with pseudoexfoliation of the lens capsule. *Acta Ophthalmol*. 1972;50:225–261.

69. Gillies WE. Corticosteroid-induced ocular hypertension in pseudoexfoliation of lens capsule. *Am J Ophthalmol*. 1970;70:90–95.

70. Lichter PR. Genetic clues to glaucoma's secrets: The L Edward Jackson memorial lecture, part 2. *Am J Ophthalmol*. 1994;117:706–727.

71. Della NG. The revolution in molecular genetics and its impact on ophthalmology. *Aust N Z J Ophthalmol*. 1996;24(2):86–95.

Part II

DIAGNOSIS

individuals. The distribution of IOP data is not symmetrical around the means, and non-Gaussian analysis must be employed. Leydecker published normative data using the Schiotz tonometer,[15] while Armaly established the range of normal for the Goldmann instrument.[16] The average value was found to be 16 mmHg for both instruments. The standard deviation for the Goldmann tonometer was ± 2.5 mmHg, indicating that, assuming IOP was distributed in a Gaussian fashion, 95% of the population would have an IOP equal to or less than 21 mmHg, and 98% would have an IOP of 24 mmHg or less. It is important to again emphasize that these upper limits of "normal" IOP are derived statistically, not clinically. Although an IOP of 22 mmHg may represent only 1 mmHg higher than 95% of "normal" individuals and is within the tolerance of accuracy for all tonometers, many patients have been labeled as "suspect" or started on a lifetime of treatment for glaucoma because of a misinterpretation of the actual clinical significance of this level of pressure (Fig. 10–1).

The causal relationship between IOP and glaucoma was further confused by a misinterpretation of IOP levels and the corresponding number of patients with glaucoma. If a group of individuals whose IOPs are elevated outside the statistically normal range are examined, the prevalence of glaucoma among them is much higher than it is in the general population.[9,10,17] This was felt to support the role of elevated IOP as the cause of damage. However, although there is a higher prevalence of glaucoma in patients with elevated IOP, the total number of individuals with glaucoma without elevated IOP has been estimated to be equal to the total number with elevated IOP at the

time of initial diagnosis.[11,18,19] It is easier to find people with glaucoma by concentrating on the smaller number of patients with elevated IOP, thus the higher yield and the reinforcement of the misconception. Because a vast majority of the population do not have elevated IOP, finding the glaucoma patients who have statistically normal IOP is akin to finding a needle in a haystack. Further, examination of these data shows that a majority of patients with elevated IOP never develop field loss, thus undermining the concept of causality.[11,20–22]

AGE AND RACE

Inspection of the data from Leydecker,[15] Armaly,[16] and others shows that the distribution of IOP is not symmetrical around the mean but includes a greater proportion of patients with IOP above than below normal limits. This skewing of data toward a greater proportion of higher IOP made the determination of limits of normal by the usual Gaussian model inaccurate. Examination of the population of patients in this higher-IOP tail of the distribution showed that most were above the age of 40. The higher values of IOP were associated with increased age. While the 95% limit is 21 mmHg in a general population, it ranges to 28 mmHg in a subgroup of individuals aged 75 to 84.[23]

More recently, the concept of increased IOP with age has been challenged.[24,25] The mean IOP, which increases with age, is greatly influenced by values that lie well above the average. A few very high pressures will increase the mean IOP while the median IOP will remain the same. Also, when blood pressure, which rises with age, is factored in, the real level of IOP does not increase with age.[14]

The relationship between IOP and race is somewhat confusing. Early studies were flawed by lack of racial diversity within the study populations.[15,16] The Baltimore Eye Survey, which examined an inner-city, racially diverse population, found no difference in IOP between blacks and whites, although the prevalence of glaucoma was four times higher in blacks.[25] However, a later study done in Barbados, which separated the population into blacks, whites, and mixed races, found a higher mean IOP in blacks than in whites, with the mixed-race group in between.[26] The prevalence of glaucoma was found to be consistent with that of the Baltimore Eye Study. There may be genetic differences within the individual study's defined "black" populations to explain these conflicting data. The Japanese literature shows a lower IOP in Japan than in the West[27,28] and a decrease in IOP with age.[19] This has been attributed to lower rates of obe-

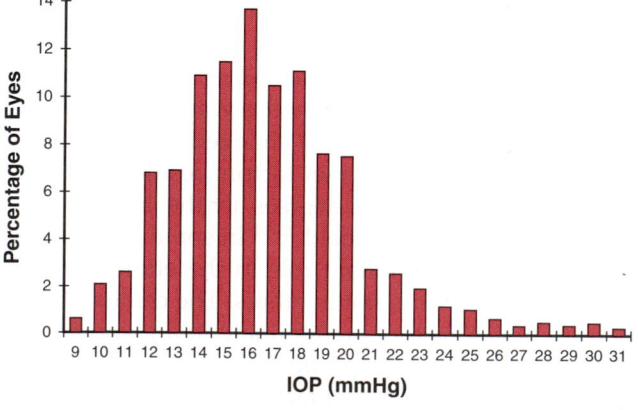

Figure 10–1. IOP versus frequency. Distribution of IOPs from 5220 eyes in the Framingham Eye Study. Distribution is unimodal but not Gaussian, with a skew to the higher pressures. (Redrawn with permission from Colton T, Ederer F. The distribution of intraocular pressures in the general population. *Surv Ophthalmol.* 1980;25: 123–129.)

sity and high blood pressure in the Japanese population than in Western populations.[29]

FACTORS AFFECTING THE MEASUREMENT OF INTRAOCULAR PRESSURE

Physiological Factors

Diurnal Variation

The level of IOP fluctuates in most individuals during each day (24-hour period).[30,31] Therefore, repeated tonometry measurements at various times of the day are necessary to plot the diurnal curve. It is not possible to predict the time of day at which an individual's IOP will reach its highest or lowest levels.[32] Intraocular pressure is usually but not always highest in the morning and lowest in the evening.[30,31] At least 50% of individuals will have a peak IOP outside normal office hours.[33]

The average diurnal variation in IOP is normally 4 mmHg or less.[30] Fluctuation in IOP within a day is directly proportional to the IOP level; the higher the initial IOP, the greater the diurnal fluctuation.[34] Glaucoma suspects are frequently found to have a diurnal variation greater than 6 mmHg.[30,35,36] Patients with normal-tension glaucoma exhibit a diurnal variation identical to that of normals.[37]

Intraocular pressure can vary from hour to hour, day to day, and season to season (Fig. 10–2).[38] The shape and peak of the diurnal plot of IOP was found to change for most individuals with glaucoma and ocular hypertension from month to month.[32] In this same study, about one-third of glaucoma patients showed different diurnal curves between eyes. This difference complicates evaluation of the therapeutic effect of a uniocular medical trial, requiring several readings on different days to confirm the true effect. Initiation of therapy may also alter the diurnal peak, with one study showing that the highest IOP while patients were on timolol occurred in the late afternoon.[39]

Arterial (Ocular) Pulse

The expansion of intraocular arterioles during systole may cause a momentary rise in IOP. The IOP will fluctuate 1 to 2 mmHg in most patients between systole and diastole and can rise to as much as 4 mmHg in others.[38]

Position of Measurement

A 2- to 3-mmHg increase occurs when the IOP is measured with the patient lying down rather than sitting up. This can be even higher if the head is below the level of the heart. The increase is believed to be secondary to a rise in episcleral venous pressure, with a resulting increase in resistance to aqueous outflow.[40]

Blood Flow

A decrease in blood flow in the carotid arteries can decrease perfusion to the ciliary body with less aqueous being produced, resulting in a lower IOP.[38] When

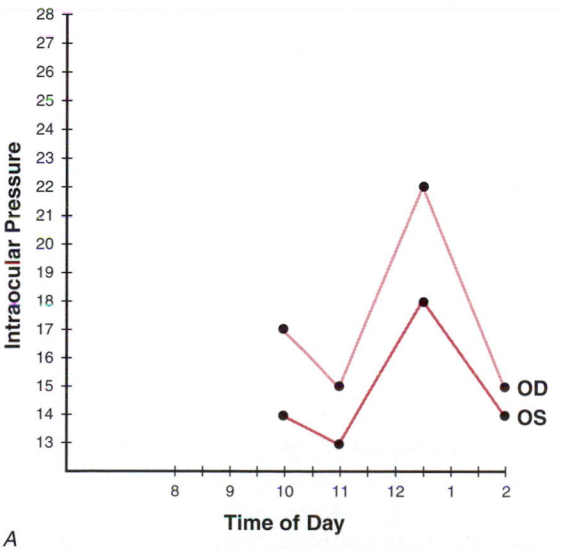

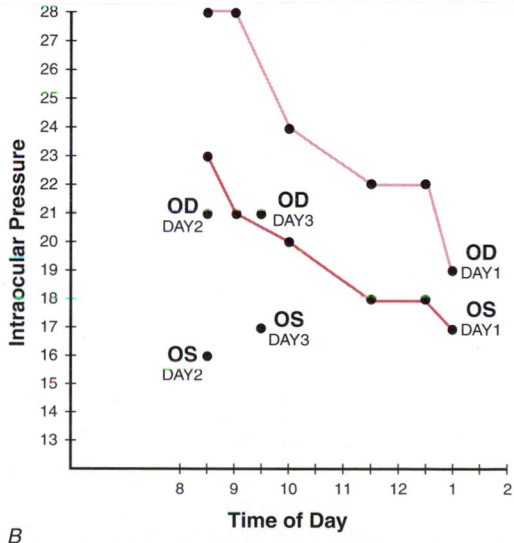

Figure 10–2. Diurnal curves. *A.* An IOP spike, occurring over 2 hours, is seen. *B.* On day 1, the IOP was elevated in the morning, decreasing to normal by 1 P.M. However, on days 2 and 3, the IOP was not elevated in the morning. While IOP can fluctuate during the day, it may also fluctuate for the same time from day to day.

the IOP differs by more than 4 mmHg between eyes, the clinician is confronted with a dilemma: is there a unilateral elevation (e.g., glaucoma) or a contralateral depression of IOP due to a decreased perfusion of blood? If the finding is repeatable on different days and the optic nerve and nerve fiber layer appear normal, then both etiologies should be pursued.

When venous drainage from the head-neck region is compromised, the outflow of aqueous is decreased, with a subsequent increase in the IOP. Venous pressure can be increased by restrictive clothing, such as a tight collar and tie.[41] Increased venous pressure can also be induced by a Valsalva maneuver when the patient holds his or her breath during tonometry.[42,43] The change in IOP is variable, with most normal patients showing an increase of about 4 to 5 mmHg.[41]

Exercise

A 20% decrease in IOP can be obtained in some patients undergoing aerobic training.[44] The reduction will be sustained as long as the individual continues with the exercise regimen, but it reverts to the pre-training IOP level within 3 weeks of cessation of training.[44] The effect of IOP reduction by exercise is additive to both selective and nonselective beta blockade.[45]

Accommodation

Accommodation increases the facility of aqueous outflow, thereby lowering IOP. Young patients can reduce their IOP by as much as 4 mmHg after 4 min of accommodation.[46] The effect is less in older patients, with a 2-mmHg decrease. Therefore, the patient's fixation should be directed to infinity before and during tonometry.

Corneal Thickness

In Goldmann's original calculations for applanation tonometry, he assumed a central corneal thickness of 0.520 mm, with minimal normal variation from this value.[47] Corneas thinner than this would result in underestimation of IOP, and thicker corneas would lead to overestimation. Subsequent studies have established that the average central thickness is not 0.520 mm and that the range of central corneal thickness can vary by as much as 0.080 mm above and below the mean.[48,49] A study of cadaver eyes found that a thin cornea may cause the IOP to be underestimated by as much as 5 mmHg and thicker corneas may cause it to be overestimated by as much as 7 mmHg.[50] The effect of variation in corneal thickness on IOP measurement depends on the correction factor used to adjust the reading. This has been estimated to be as little as 0.19 mmHg for every 10-μm increase in thickness to as much as 0.71 mmHg for every 5 μm.[49,51]

Attention has recently been drawn to how the artifact induced by central corneal thickness in IOP measurement might lead to an erroneous diagnosis.[52] In one study, Herndon et al. found that individuals with ocular hypertension tend to have thicker-than-average corneas. Sixty-five percent of those who were originally classified as having ocular hypertension were shown to have normal IOP when their readings were adjusted for corneal thickness.[49] Further, other studies have shown corneas to be thinner in patients with normal-tension glaucoma.[53,54] All of these studies imply that some patients may be overmanaged or misclassified on the basis of the artifact induced by central corneal thickness. However, as Brubaker[55] has pointed out, the true impact of corneal thickness may be minimal, depending upon which correction factor is used to modify the reading.

Corneas that are physiologically thicker should be differentiated from those that are thickened pathologically from edema. Edematous corneas will have applanation pressures that may be 9 to 10 mmHg *lower* than the true IOP, which is the opposite of the case with normally thick corneas.[56]

With the advent of photorefractive surgery, the effect of corneal thickness on IOP measurement has been rediscovered. Patients who have undergone photorefractive procedures that result in a thinner cornea will subsequently have an underestimation of their IOP. In general, the greater the degree of myopia treated, the greater the effect.[57] The exact amount of underestimation differs from predicted values and seems to be dependent on the type of tonometer, the amount of myopia corrected, and the type of procedure performed. For the majority of patients with less than 5 diopters spherical equivalent of myopic correction, there is no more than 1- to 2-mmHg underestimation of IOP with Goldmann tonometry.[58] For patients whose IOP was measured with the Nidek noncontact tonometer, a greater effect was found.[56]

Clinical Factors

Medications

Common systemic medications given to control blood pressure, such as clonidine and oral beta blockers, can cause a significant lowering of the IOP. Eighty milligrams of propranolol (common dose) has the same IOP-reducing effect as Timoptic (timolol) 0.5%.[59] Despite obvious cupping and field loss, the IOP may be "normal" because the systemic antihypertensive medications are also lowering the IOP.

Steroids, both oral and especially topical ophthalmic drops, are well known to cause an increase in

IOP in susceptible individuals. Finally, both marijuana and alcohol can lower the IOP.[60-62]

Trauma and Inflammation

Depending on its severity, inflammation may cause either a decrease or an increase in IOP. An inflammatory reaction may clog the trabecular meshwork with debris, leading to a subsequent increase in the resistance to aqueous outflow and a resulting rise in the IOP. Even with inflammatory debris present in the trabecular meshwork, there may be a decrease in aqueous production secondary to inflammation of the ciliary body, resulting in a decrease in IOP.[63]

Artifacts

Intra- and Interobserver Variability

Repeated tonometric measurements of the same eye with the same instrument will give varying results.[64-66] Measurements repeated by the same observer will be within 1 to 2 mmHg for 92% of patients. When two different observers measure the same patients, 25 to 50% of the readings will differ by 2 mmHg or more and 20 to 30% will differ by 3 mmHg or more.[65,66]

External Pressure on the Globe

IOP increases normally as the eye blinks. Involuntary, forceful closure of lids (blepharospasm) can cause a large increase in IOP as the lid muscles compress the globe.[38,67] Therefore, practitioners should try to control the lids during tonometry. Care must be exercised, since even light digital pressure on the globe can cause an increase in the IOP ranging from 5 to 20 mmHg. Enlargement of the extraocular muscles or other space-occupying lesions in the orbit can also cause an increase in IOP when they compress the globe. Patients with Graves' orbitopathy can show an increase in IOP especially if the enlarged muscle contracts at the time of IOP measurement.[68]

Children

IOP has been thought to be lower in children under age 10. This may be an artifact, since estimates have varied depending on the instrument used, with some investigators finding no difference.[69-71] Eisenberg has shown that the accuracy of tonometers varies significantly with patients under the age of 10.[72] Applanation tonometry underestimates the IOP to an amount based on the following formula: Ta = 0.71 age (years) +10. The Tono-Pen is not accurate enough and only the pneumatonometer accurately determined the IOP in newborn and small children.[71] Once a child reaches the age of 10, applanation tonometry is accurate and useful for clinical practice.

Contact Lenses

Studies of tonometry performed with the Goldmann tonometer, Tono-Pen, and Pneumotonometer over contact lenses have produced variable results.[73-75] In general, the IOP is minimally influenced by thin, plano power bandage lenses. Depending on the instrument used and type of cosmetic contact lens, the IOP can be 3 to 4 mmHg higher with nonbandage soft contact lenses (even thin, −1.00-diopter lenses). Still, in situations requiring a bandage contact lens, it is probably better to leave the lens in place when doing tonometry. The slight inaccuracy of 1 to 2 mmHg is inconsequential, and accurate readings may not even be possible on a diseased cornea once the lens is removed. However, all patients with cosmetic lenses should remove their lenses prior to tonometry.

Tonometry

The introduction of the Maklokoff and Schiotz tonometers at the turn of the century made the measurement of IOP a simple in-office procedure.[76] Further improvements in design and accuracy occurred in the late 1950s with the introduction of the Goldmann tonometer.[47] The dawn of the "electronic age" in the 1960s introduced the MacKay-Marg tonometer,[77] quickly followed by the American Optical noncontact tonometer (AONCT) in the early 1970s.[67] The 1980s, with new microchip technology, allowed a reduction in the size of the electronic tonometers and improvement in their ease of operation.[78,79] Yet all these different instruments are based on one of two principles: indentation or applanation.

Indentation

Indentation tonometry is similar in concept to pushing your thumb into a basketball to check the pressure; the more air in the ball, the greater the effort required to indent its surface. Indentation tonometry involves measuring the resisting force of the IOP while pushing on the cornea with a known weight or force until it bows backward. The amount of indentation will vary inversely to the IOP. The results of indentation tonometry are influenced by the rigidity of the cornea and sclera to indentation. This rigidity varies from eye to eye and introduces a potential measurement error.[38] During indentation tonometry, there is a simultaneous and significant increase in the outflow of aqueous,[80] causing repeated tonometry readings to decrease.[81]

Applanation

Applanation tonometry is based on the Imbert-Fick formula, which states that pressure (IOP) equals force/area. IOP is determined by measuring either force or area while holding the other variables constant. For instance, Goldmann tonometry takes a given area of the cornea and measures the force required to flatten it to a plano surface. Therefore IOP is directly related to the force needed to flatten (not indent) the cornea.

The area of the cornea that is flattened (applanated) is always the same for every patient. However, the amount of force necessary to push against the cornea to flatten it to a known size will vary by the amount of IOP that is pushing back from inside the eye. Unlike indentation tonometry, the artifact of ocular rigidity is rendered minimal by the forces of capillary attraction between the tonometer tip and the precorneal tear film. Goldmann determined empirically that when the area of the cornea that was applanated was approximately 3 mm in diameter, the artifact of rigidity was essentially neutralized.[82]

Other types of applanation tonometers apply a known force (weight) and measure how large an area of the cornea is flattened to determine IOP (Table 10–1). Because true applanation instruments displace very little aqueous, repeated IOP measurements remain accurate.

Instruments and Their Techniques

Goldmann Tonometer

Since its introduction, the Goldmann applanation tonometer has been the standard to which all other tonometers are compared. It has earned this reputation based on its accuracy, reliability, and ease of operation. Goldmann tonometric readings have been shown to be within 3% of the true IOP[38] as determined with cadaver eyes that are cannulated and attached to a column of mercury and within 1 to 2 mmHg for repeated readings.[83] It is used most commonly in conjunction with a slit lamp (Fig. 10–3), but hand-held models are available (Fig. 10–4).

The edge of the area of the cornea being flattened is discernible by a fluorescent tear meniscus located between the cornea and the tip of the probe. The greater the force against the cornea, the larger the diameter of the circular area being flattened. The tip

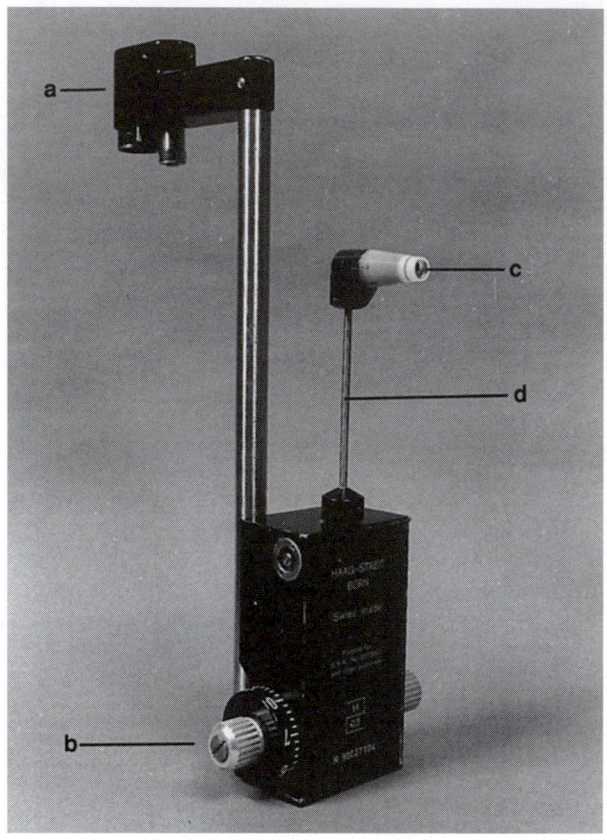

Figure 10–3. Goldmann applanation tonometer. The components of the slit-lamp mounted version: mounting arm (a); measuring drum (b); probe tip (c); probe arm (d). (Reproduced with permission from Casser L, Fingeret M, Woodcome HT. *Atlas of Primary Eyecare Procedures*, 2nd ed. Stamford, CT: Appleton & Lange; 1997.)

of the tonometer probe is 7 mm in diameter; therefore, to determine when a circle of exactly 3.06 mm in diameter is obtained, doubling prisms of proper power are located in the probe. The image of the circle is split in half horizontally and referred to as mires. Increases in the force of applanation on the cornea bring the circles closer together, while decreases in the force move them further apart. The prisms are optically set so that the circles interlock when the desired diameter is flattened. When the area applanated is 3.06 mm in diameter, the force of the applanation measured in grams is related to the level of the IOP in mmHg by a 10:1 ratio. Thus, 1 g of force on the measuring drum will equal 10 mmHg of IOP.

Some practitioners anesthetize the cornea with proparacaine and use a sterile fluorescein strip to prepare the cornea. This can be done before slit-lamp examination, allowing time for the anesthesia to take effect and saving the practitioner the extra step of having to get up to instill the drops later. If insuffi-

TABLE 10–1. TYPES OF TONOMETERS

Applanation	Indentation	Features of Both
Goldmann	Schiotz	MacKay-Marg
Noncontact		Tono-Pen
		Pneumatonometer

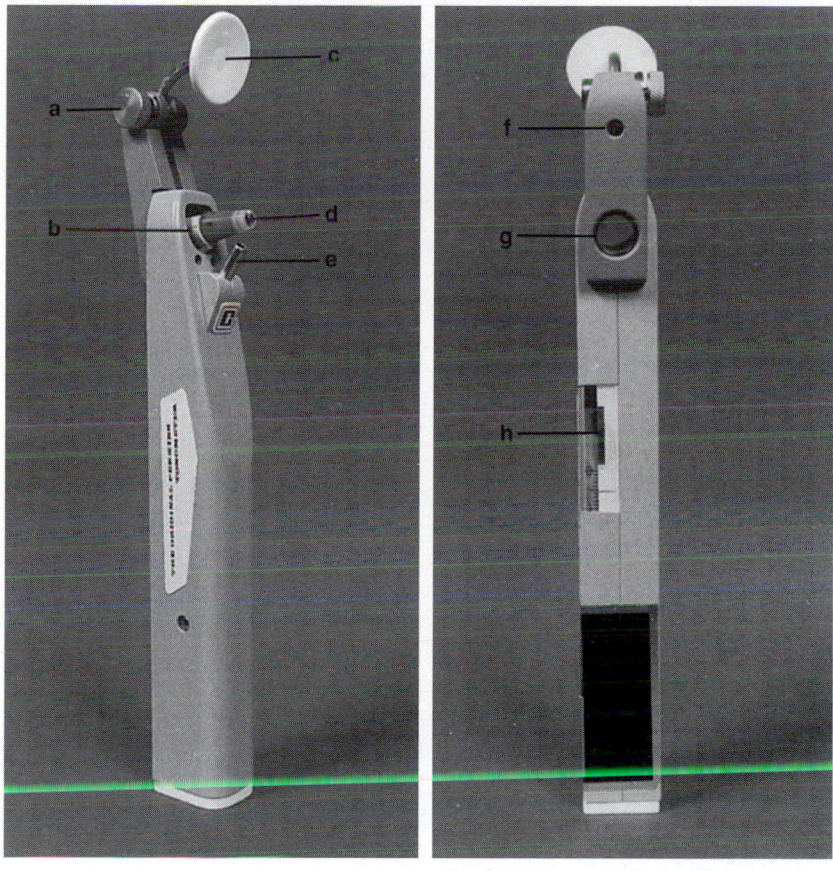

Figure 10–4. Perkins hand-held Goldmann tonometer. The components of the tonometer are as follows *A.* Forehead rest set screw (a); applanating probe holder (b); patient forehead rest (c); probe (d); illumination source (e). *B.* Examiner forehead rest mount (f); eyepiece (g); measuring knob (h). (Reproduced with permission from Casser L, Fingeret M, Woodcome HT. *Atlas of Primary Eyecare Procedures*, 2nd ed. Stamford, CT: Appleton & Lange; 1997.)

A   *B*

cient fluorescein is instilled, the true IOP may be underestimated by as much as 9 mmHg.[84]

Other practitioners prefer a combination drop with an anesthetic and fluorescein. Care should be exercised with some brands because to improve contact time they are made excessively viscous. This can lead to mires that are too thick, resulting in too much force being applied to align the mires and in an overestimation of IOP. Also, viscous drops complicate tonometer cleaning and require that the eye be copiously irrigated before soft contact lenses can be reinserted.

The commonly taught technique for the measurement of IOP with the Goldmann tonometer and a slit lamp is to set the magnification at 10× and swing the tonometer arm into click stop. The right eye is usually measured first, so the illumination column of the slit lamp is positioned to the doctor's left at an angle of 45 degrees or less with the oculars. The slit illumination is opened fully for maximum brightness. The measuring drum is set at approximately 10 mmHg and the tip is slowly and gently brought in contact with the cornea.

At first it is best for the examiner to view the actual placement of the tip on the cornea with his or her head out from behind the oculars of the slit lamp. With experience, most practitioners will approach the cornea until the probe is close to the cornea and then view the patient with one eye while the other views the placement on the cornea through an ocular.

The tonometer tip is visible through only one ocular; for most slit lamps, it is on the left. Therefore it is pointless to position both of the examiner's eyes behind the slit lamp during a reading. Rather, one may keep the right eye in front of the left ocular, allowing the left eye to view the patient. When contact is achieved, the examiner will notice the tip of the tonometer move backward and simultaneously observe mires in the ocular. The probe's position on the cornea is adjusted until the mires are of equal size and shape and are well centered in the view (Fig. 10–5). The measuring drum is adjusted until the inside edges of both mires just touch. When a strong ocular pulse is present, it is difficult to determine the endpoint because the mires are pulsating. An "average"

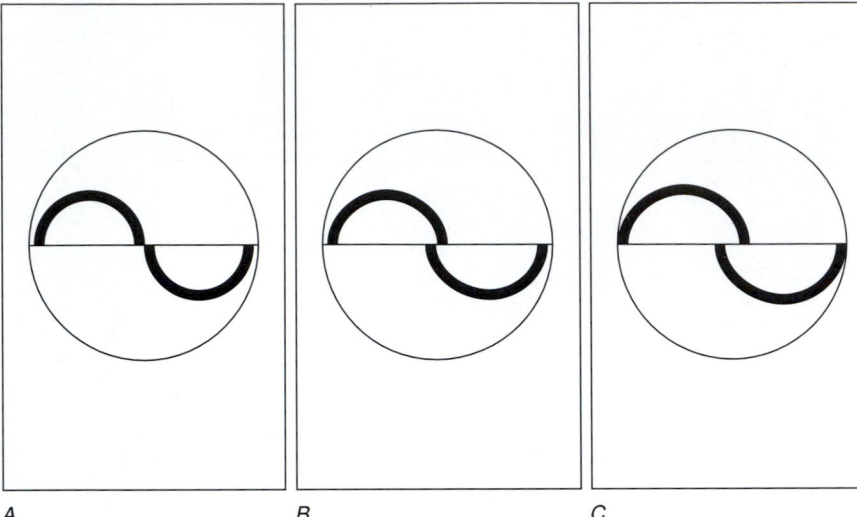

A   B   C

Figure 10–5. Goldmann tonometer mires pattern. *A.* Not enough pressure, turn measuring drum clockwise. *B.* Correct endpoint, read measuring drum. *C.* Too much pressure, turn measuring drum counterclockwise. (Reproduced with permission from Casser L, Fingeret M, Woodcome HT. *Atlas of Primary Eyecare Procedures,* 2nd ed. Stamford, CT: Appleton & Lange; 1997.)

value is obtained by setting the mires such that the gap between them during systole is equal to the amount they overlap during diastole.

Corneas with more than three diopters of cylinder will give an elliptical shape to the mires, which may affect the accuracy of the IOP measurement. To remedy this situation, the probe tip should be rotated so that its markings are 45 degrees away from the minus cylinder axis. An alternative approach is to take the first reading as usual, then repeat the measurement with the prism rotated 90 degrees. The average of these two readings should be used.[85] If the cornea is irregular or edematous, there will be a poor image of the mires, preventing an accurate measurement. This is one disadvantage of all applanation tonometers (Table 10–2).

The illumination column does not have to be swung around to the opposite side when the other eye is tested. As long as the slit beam is open wide, the probe tip should be adequately illuminated from almost any angle. When an angle of approximately 45 degrees or greater is used, the illumination column will not be in the way when the slit lamp is moved to measure the other eye.

A question that is often asked is whether the lids should be controlled during tonometry. If the patient blinks and touches the tonometer, a blepharospasm may occur, complicating the IOP measurement. If the lids are properly held against the orbital rim, there should be no artifact elevating the IOP (Fig. 10–6). Once a reading has been obtained, the practitioner slowly releases control of the lids. If the mires begin to move together, the practitioner can assume that an artifact was induced. The reading was probably

too high and must be retaken with less control of the lids.

Some uncooperative patients will not allow an accurate reading to be obtained, either because their eyes go into blepharospasm or because they fixate poorly. This response can usually be anticipated when the patient "fights" the instillation of anesthetic drops. In these situations, a screening technique is recommended. The practitioner sets the measuring drum to

TABLE 10–2. ADVANTAGES AND DISADVANTAGES OF GOLDMANN TONOMETRY

Advantages

Reference standard for accuracy
Calibration easily checked, rarely goes out of calibration
Displaces little aqueous, allowing repeatable readings
Extremely quick with a cooperative patient
Minimal disruption of corneal epithelium
Relatively inexpensive to buy and operate
Compact, mounts easily on any slit lamp
Hand-held models available for restricted patients
May be delegated, but needs a very competent technician
Mechanical device, no electronics, very reliable with little maintenance

Disadvantages

Requires topical anesthesia
Poor or invalid results with edematous cornea
Adjustment of calibration must be done by factory
Usually mounted on slit lamp, some patients cannot be positioned at slit lamp
Doctor's task; hard to delegate
Easily influenced by external pressure (fingers, lids)
No permanent record
Not accurate for children under 10
Not as accurate with thick or thin corneas

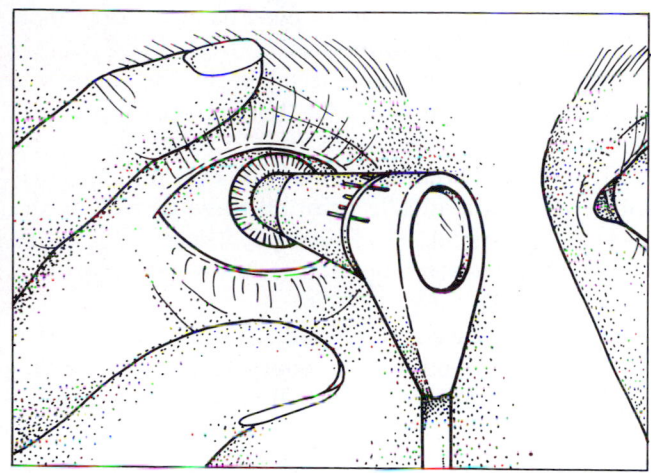

Figure 10-6. Controlling the lids. Gently retract the upper and lower lids. Artifact is avoided if the lids are held against the orbital rim. (Reproduced with permission from Casser L, Fingeret M, Woodcome HT. *Atlas of Primary Eyecare Procedures*, 2nd ed. Stamford, CT: Appleton & Lange; 1997.)

22 mmHg before approaching the cornea. He or she attempts to control the lids and, just as the cornea is touched, observes the mires. If they overlap, the IOP is 21 mmHg or less. If the mires do not overlap, one may try to release control of the lids slowly. The mires may then be seen to approach and overlap each other as external pressure on the globe is released. While not providing a precise measurement, this technique will allow you to determine whether the IOP is elevated above 22 mmHg.

When a patient cannot be positioned at the slit lamp for standard Goldmann tonometry, a hand-held model can be employed (Fig. 10-4). For very obese patients who have difficulty positioning themselves, the slit-lamp tonometer may overestimate IOP by an average of 4 to 5 mmHg, while the hand-held tonometer is accurate for both normal and obese patients.[86,87]

Although routine Goldmann tonometry is a rather simple procedure, poor technique will result in erroneous readings. When one is learning, it is best to compare the reading obtained to to that of an experienced practitioner to make sure that the technique has been properly mastered.

The risk of infection with adenovirus and human immunodeficiency virus (HIV) is present with contact tonometry; therefore the tip must be properly sterilized after use. Swabbing the tonometer tip thoroughly with an alcohol prep pad and allowing it to air-dry for approximately 10 min has been shown to be quite effective for HIV[88] and has been recommended by the American Academy of Ophthalmology.[89] However, the Centers for Disease Control

recommend first wiping the tonometer tip and then soaking it in one of three solutions: alcohol, 3% hydrogen peroxide, or a 1:10 dilution of household bleach.[90,91] Wiping the tip with alcohol is effective against all organisms except hepatitis B and C and *Acanthamoeba*.[92-94] A 10-min soak in hydrogen peroxide 3% will eliminate all organisms except *Acanthamoeba*, which requires a 2-h soaking.[92,93] Unfortunately, soaking (not swabbing) the tips in alcohol will damage the internal prisms, while bleach will remove the external markings.[95] Therefore, if one chooses to soak the tips, hydrogen peroxide should be used. Since hydrogen peroxide is toxic to the corneal epithelium, extreme care should be taken to rinse the tip thoroughly before use. If soaking is used, several tips can be kept in the examination room, with some soaking and others drying.

Thorough calibration of the tonometer should be performed quarterly, with more frequent checks recommended for older instruments or those with heavy use. A daily check is possible without using the calibration counterweight. The measuring drum is rotated counterclockwise until the scale reads just below zero. The tip will then be in the upright position. Next, the drum is rotated very slowly clockwise while the probe tip is watched. The drum's rotation is stopped the instant the tip drops forward; the scale is then read. It should read within 1 mmHg of zero if the tonometer is in calibration. The quarterly check should include verification of accuracy at 20 and 60 mmHg with the counterweight supplied with the tonometer (Fig. 10-7).

Noncontact Tonometer

The introduction by American Optical of the noncontact tonometer (NCT) in 1972 was a milestone in the history of optometric practice.[66] Without the use of topical anesthetics, accurate measurement of the IOP was not available to most optometrists. The NCT changed that by making accurate, reliable, and repeatable IOP measurements possible without the use of anesthesia, since the cornea was "touched" only by a pulse of air.[96] The fact that the instrument is still in wide use today is a credit to its other attributes.

The third-generation NCT instrument (Reichert XPERT) was redesigned, taking advantage of microchip technology to improve ease of operation (Fig. 10-8). This version employs a new alignment system that includes a video monitor of the eye being applanated, requiring the proper positioning of cross hairs to initiate automatic applanation (Fig. 10-9). Owing to the instrument's vague similarity to a video game, its operation is more readily mastered by office personnel than that of its predecessors. The instru-

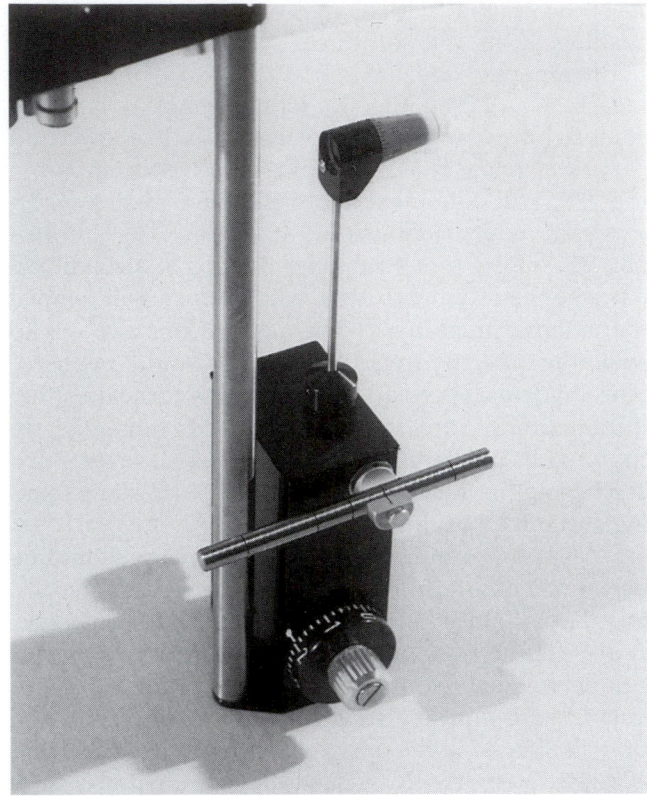

Figure 10–7. Goldmann calibration. The counterweight is in position and set to check the calibration at 20 mmHg. The first marking from the middle is used with the larger part of the counterweight toward the examiner. With the measuring drum set to less than 20, it is rotated clockwise until the probe tip drops forward. Calibration is similarly checked at zero (the center mark) and at 60 mmHg (the outermost mark).

ment now provides a printed copy of the tonometry results to serve as a permanent record in the chart. There is also an RS-232 port for connections to computerized office systems.

The design of the NCT employs the same principle as the Goldmann tonometer, measuring the amount of force required to applanate a fixed area. However, the NCT is more complex in its mechanical, optical, and electronic components. The apex of the cornea is progressively flattened over a period of 2 to 8 milliseconds by a puff of air that increases its force in a linear fashion. A beam of light is aimed at the cornea, which, when flattened to an exact area, acts like a plano mirror. This causes most of the light to be reflected to a sensor. At the instant of applanation, the piston generating the puff of air is electromechanically braked and the instrument computes the IOP based on the amount of air pressure at the time of applanation. In previous designs, the piston did not stop and a forceful puff was delivered to every eye. Since the piston now stops at the instant of applanation, the

puff of air delivered to most eyes has less force than was the case with prior models.

Because the instrument takes an instantaneous reading, it will measure the IOP at various points along the ocular pulse. With the XPERT version of the NCT, three readings are taken per eye, and the machine will automatically print all three as well as the average. In large-scale screenings, it is not necessary to take all three readings if at least one measurement is less than 20 mmHg.

As in the case of the Goldmann tonometer, poor results are obtained with an edematous cornea. However, IOP can be determined through a soft contact lens.[97,98] With an irregular or edematous cornea, a thin, soft contact lens can be placed on the eye, creating a smooth surface; IOP is then measured by either the Goldmann or the NCT. The only contraindication is the inability of the cornea to tolerate a contact lens (Table 10–3).

Electronic verification is used to check calibration in the office; however, the result must still be validated against another instrument. For this, the patient is checked with the NCT and the result is immediately compared with that obtained with a Goldmann tonometer. Studies have shown that two Goldmann tonometers will agree within 1 to 3 mmHg of each other. Therefore, the averaged NCT reading should be within 2 to 3 mmHg of the Goldmann reading. It is recommended that this check be performed quarterly, and more often if the

TABLE 10–3. ADVANTAGES AND DISADVANTAGES OF THE NONCONTACT TONOMETER

Advantages
 Accurate when compared with a Goldmann tonometer, varies slightly when IOP is >30 mmHg
 Requires no anesthetic
 Displaces virtually no aqueous, allowing repeatable readings
 Can be delegated to technician with little training
 No damage to corneal epithelium
 Takes little time with a cooperative patient
 Can measure edematous cornea through soft lens
 Portable model (Keeler) can be used for restricted patients

Disadvantages
 Some patients are apprehensive of the "puff" and refuse measurement
 Expensive
 Bulky, heavy, requires separate table
 Cannot be used on restricted patients (Reichert version)
 Cannot be calibrated or fixed by user
 Uncooperative patients can be time-consuming
 Repeat readings required, since single reading may be measuring height of ocular pulse
 Edematous corneas cannot be measured without soft contact lens

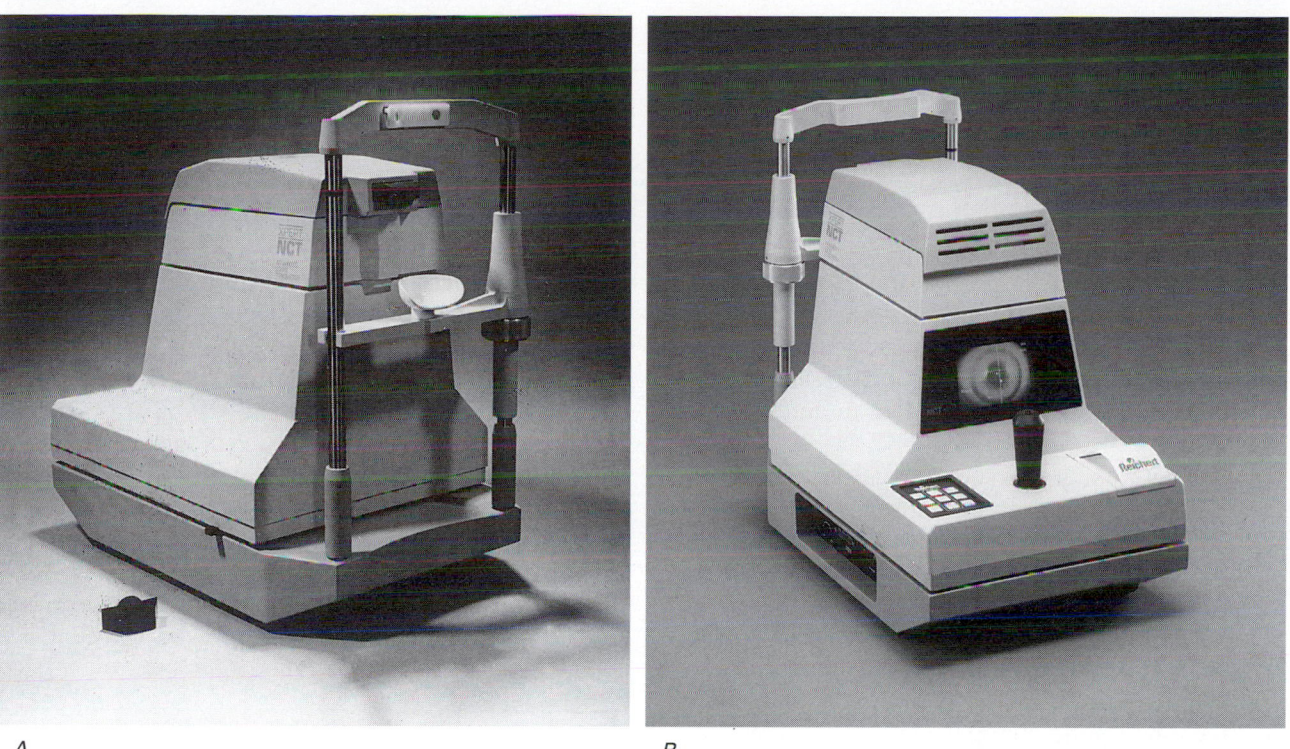

A   *B*

Figure 10–8. XPERT NCT. *A.* Patient's view of instrument. *B.* Operator's view. (Reproduced with permission from Myers K, Lalle P, Litwak T, et al. XPERT NCT: A clinical evaluation. *J Am Optom Assoc.* 1990;61:863–869.)

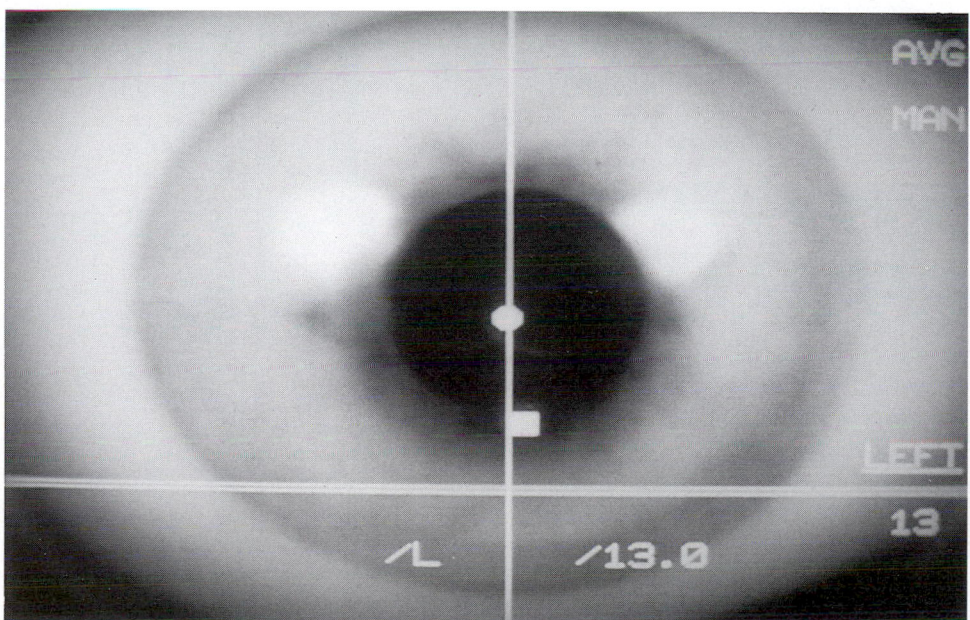

Figure 10–9. XPERT NCT. Operator's view of alignment video display. In this example, the alignment is too low and too far from the left eye. (Reproduced with permission from Myers K, Lalle P, Litwak T, et al. XPERT NCT: A clinical evaluation. *J Am Optom Assoc.* 1990;61:863–869.)

instrument has recently been transported (e.g., to a screening).

Only the chin and forehead rest need to be wiped with alcohol after every use; there is nothing to sterilize. Occasionally, the video lens should be cleaned, since it can become soiled by lashes and tears.

Pneumatonometer

This instrument, also developed in the 1970s, can measure IOP with the patient in any position.[40] Its main use has been in hospitals and clinics, where patients frequently present in wheelchairs and stretchers. It is also valuable for measuring the IOP of infants. A tired, hungry baby is given first anesthetic drops and then its bottle. Most infants will soon fall asleep. The sleeping baby can be held over a parent's shoulder, the lids held open, and a reading taken. It is also used in the immediate postoperative period on patients whose corneas are irregular or edematous, since it is more accurate than the Goldmann tonometer in these situations. Recently, it has been shown to provide more accurate IOP readings than the Goldmann in patients who have undergone myopic excimer keratectomy and have reduced corneal thickness.[99]

The instrument consists of a source of pressurized gas, a handpiece, and a console (Fig. 10–10). A piston with a hollow core is driven out of the handpiece by the gas pressure. (The gas can be supplied by either a pressurized can or a small compressor that uses room air.) Gas flows down the inside of the piston into a small, flexible tube before entering a tiny pancake-shaped chamber. The ocular-surface side of this chamber is a flexible membrane, 5 mm in diameter; the other side is a round disc with holes through

which the gas escapes. As the membrane is pushed against the convex cornea, it bows back into the chamber until it covers the escape holes. This creates a back pressure in the hollow core of the piston that is electromechanically measured in the console. The pressure inside the piston increases until it pushes the front of the membrane and the cornea back, reopening the escape holes and restoring the flow of gas (Fig. 10–11). The IOP is determined at this point, reflecting the amount of pressure needed to maintain a flow of gas when the probe is against the cornea. The IOP can be displayed as a printed waveform or a digital readout at the console. The waveform provides a continuous, ongoing reading, while the digital display provides an ongoing average.

The technique requires the eye to be anesthetized with proparacaine. Viscous combination drops are to be avoided, as they can clog the membrane's escape holes. The piston in the handpiece will jump forward when it is pressurized; therefore it should be directed away

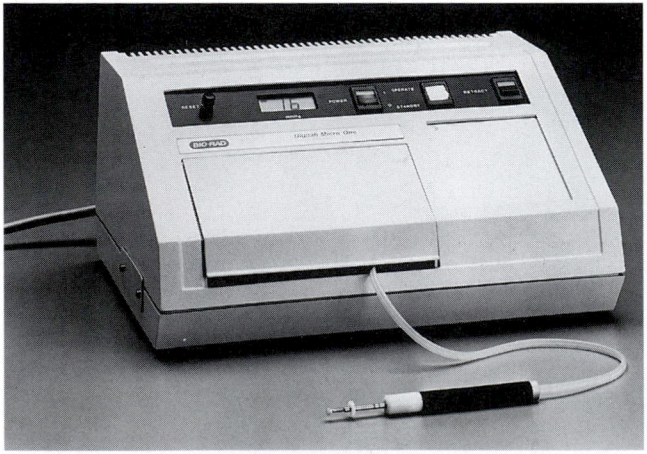

Figure 10–10. Digilab pneumatonometer. Console with a digital readout. Probe is in the foreground. (Courtesy of BIO-RAD, Cambridge, MA.)

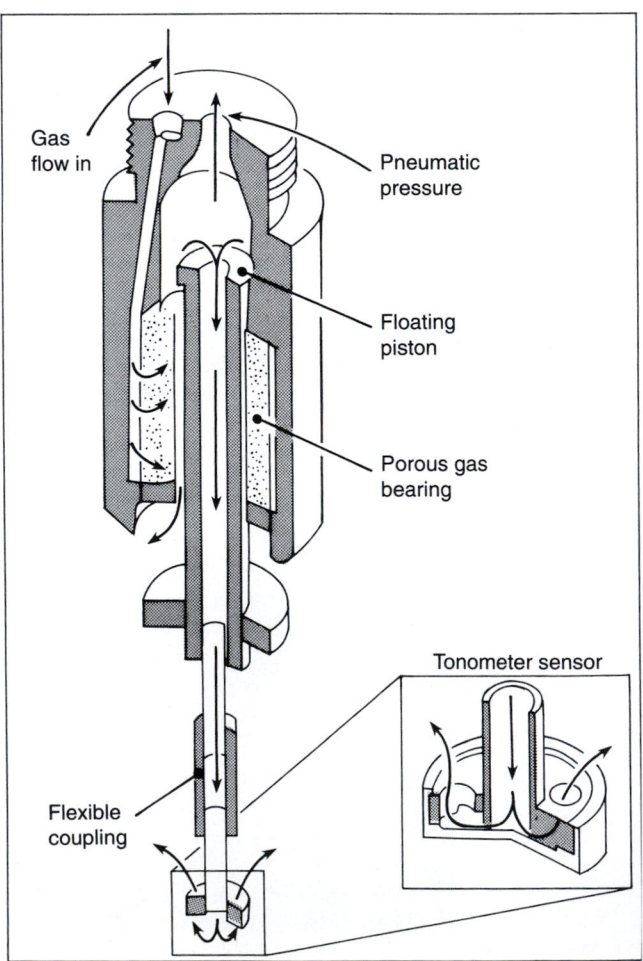

Figure 10–11. Digilab pneumatonometer. Cross section of pneumatonometer probe tip.

from the patient when the gas is turned on. The lids are controlled, if necessary, and the probe tip is pressed lightly against the apex of the cornea. The probe tip must be held against the cornea for a minimum of 5 s but no more than 10 s. The reading is initially higher in the first 1 to 2 s. On average, the pneumatonometer will slightly overestimate the IOP as compared to Goldmann tonometry. Although considered an applanation tonometer, this instrument will displace a significant amount of aqueous with each reading. Repeated readings, therefore, will be lower than the initial one and care should be taken for patients with shallow or flat anterior chambers (Table 10–4).[100]

For calibration, the instrument is provided with a pressurized membrane connected to a pressure gauge. The probe tip is positioned against the pressurized membrane and the instrument's reading is compared to that of the pressure gauge. However, there is wide variability between instruments, and it is strongly recommended that frequent comparisons be made with another tonometer to verify calibration.

For disinfection, the tip should be liberally swabbed with alcohol. It is not practical to remove the tip for cleaning after each use.

MacKay-Marg Tonometer and Tono-Pen

The MacKay-Marg tonometer was first introduced for the purpose of taking IOP readings through the sclera without the need for anesthesia. These readings were not accurate, and only those taken through an anesthetized cornea proved valid.[101] The original instrument's readings were in the form of a printed waveform that was difficult to obtain and interpret. A lot of skill was required to master the instrument, and many users became discouraged.

With the advent of microchip technology, allowing internal refinements and miniaturization, the principles of the MacKay-Marg tonometer have been incorporated into a newer instrument, the Tono-Pen.[78] The entire instrument is contained within a large, tubular handpiece that has a small foot plate at the end (Fig. 10–12). Within the foot plate is a protruding plunger connected to a sensitive electrical position transducer. As the instrument is pushed against the cornea, both the corneal rigidity and the IOP resist indentation, and the plunger is forced back into the foot plate. When the cornea is flattened by the foot plate, corneal rigidity is largely negated and an equilibrium exists between the plunger's force and the IOP. Therefore, the IOP is determined when the tip of the plunger is in the same plane as the foot plate.

Four valid readings are taken per eye, with internal circuits determining whether a reading is valid. The measurements are displayed as a digital readout, eliminating the waveform printout. The digital display also shows a percent indication regarding the range of the readings. The Tono-Pen tends to overestimate low IOPs and to underestimate high IOPs.[102,103]

The Tono-Pen's greatest asset is that it is the most accurate tonometer when used on a scarred or edematous cornea, especially with postoperative patients. It can also be used on patients in any position.[71] This, combined with its portability, also makes it very convenient for use in hospitals or nursing homes (Table 10–5). However, its accuracy compared to that of the Goldmann tonometer is only fair at best, and it is not recommended for routine office use, especially in children below 10 years of age.[72,105]

Each instrument is internally calibrated by the

TABLE 10–4. ADVANTAGES AND DISADVANTAGES OF PNEUMATONOMETER

Advantages

More accurate than Goldmann with irregular corneas (not as accurate as MacKay-Marg)
Very quick with a cooperative patient
Can be used in any position, especially with restricted patients. Used extensively in infants and patients in wheelchairs and stretchers
Compact, lightweight, portable
Can be delegated, easy to use
Minimal, if any, epithelial damage
Permanent copy of readings available
Accurate with children under 10
Accurate on corneas after radial keratotomy

Disadvantages

Not as accurate as Goldmann or noncontact tonometer (in adults)
Anesthesia required
Moderately expensive instrument
Expensive supplies (gas and membranes)
Displaces a significant amount of aqueous, inaccurate for repeat readings
Calibration is tedious; if out of calibration, must go back to factory
Patient must be able to hold eye still for at least 5 s

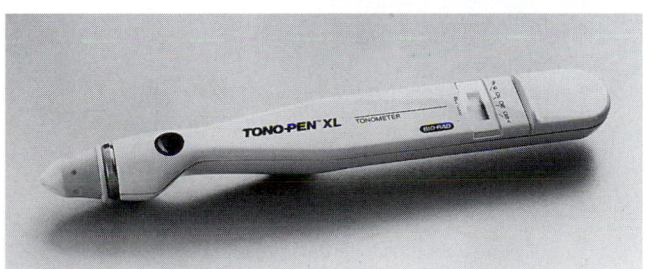

Figure 10–12. Oculab Tono-Pen. Disposable probe covering in place. (Courtesy of BIO-RAD, Cambridge, MA.)

TABLE 10–5. ADVANTAGES AND DISADVANTAGES OF THE TONO-PEN

Advantages
Most accurate tonometer with a scarred or edematous cornea
Fairly quick with a cooperative patient
Minimal disruption to corneal epithelium
Can be used in restricted patients
Portable, compact, lightweight, ideal for hospital and nursing home rounds

Disadvantages
Accuracy not reliable enough for routine office use
Since the instrument interprets the waveform, there is no way to verify the accuracy of a reading
Calibration of the handpiece is factory set, must be checked frequently by comparison to instrument
No user serviceable parts, expensive to repair
Requires anesthesia to obtain reliable results
Expensive instrument, requires supplies (tonotips)
Displaces significant amount of aqueous, may affect repeatability
Influenced by external pressure of fingers or lids

factory but should be checked periodically against another tonometer. Like the original instrument, the probe tip is covered with a single-use, disposable sleeve to ensure a sterile tip for each use.

The Schiotz Tonometer

From the early 1900s through the late 1960s, Schiotz tonometry was the accepted standard for measuring IOP. However, the need for anesthesia kept it out of optometrists' offices. By the time diagnostic drugs became available to optometrists, the Goldmann tonometer had replaced it as the standard. Because of this, most optometrists are not familiar with the instrument. Its simple, highly portable, and inexpensive

TABLE 10–6. ADVANTAGES AND DISADVANTAGES OF SCHIOTZ TONOMETRY

Advantages
Reliable, mechanically simple, no electronic component
Very inexpensive to buy and maintain
Can be used on restricted patients
Calibration simple to check

Disadvantages
Patients very apprehensive with procedure
Patient positioning is cumbersome and time consuming
Anesthesia required
Good patient cooperation is required
Corneal abrasion a distinct possibility with uncooperative patients
Readily influenced by external pressure or poor technique
Must be disassembled after each use to clean and disinfect
Must be performed by doctor, rarely delegated
Displaces significant amount of aqueous, affecting repeat measurements

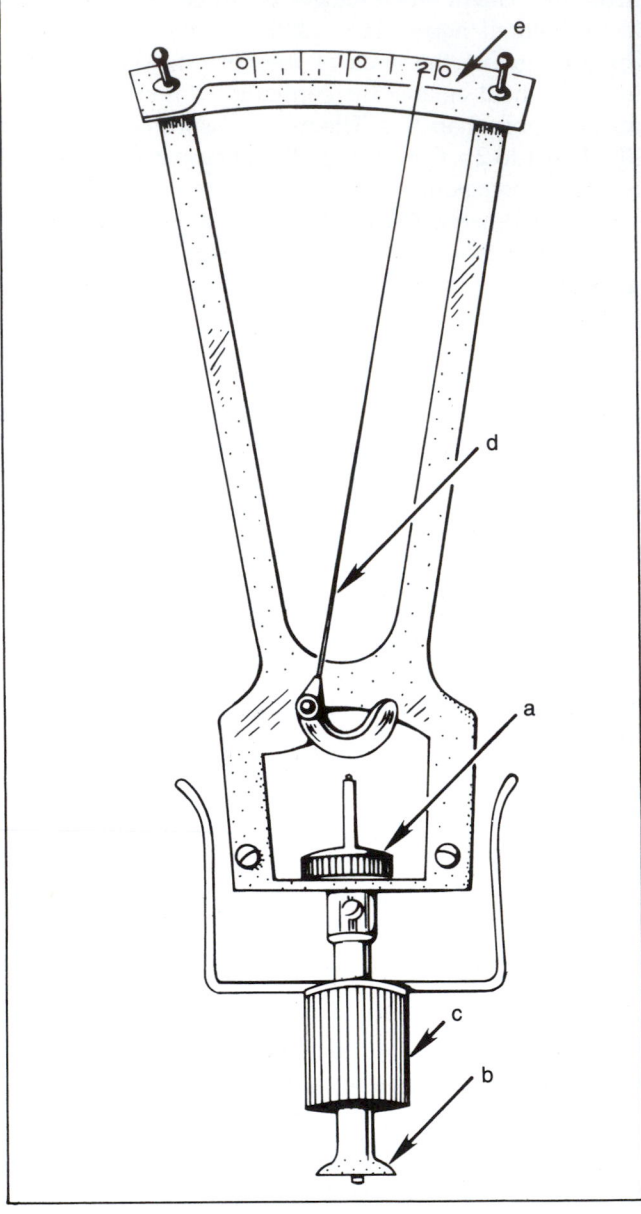

Figure 10–13. Schiotz tonometer: a, weighted plunger; b, footplate; c, outer sleeve; d, pointer; e, scale.

design makes it an ideal backup tonometer for the modern office (Table 10–6).

A weighted plunger inside a foot plate, surrounded by an outer sleeve, is brought in contact with the cornea and then indents it (Fig. 10–13). The amount of indentation is directly related to the weight of the plunger and inversely related to IOP and ocular rigidity. The amount of indentation is measured by a lever resting on top of the plunger, with a pointer connected to the lever. For each 0.05 mm that the plunger indents the cornea, the pointer moves up one marking on the scale. With an IOP of 16 mmHg, the scale reading is 5.5, which represents only 0.275 mm of indentation. Eyes with elevated IOPs will have lower scale readings. The measuring scale is logarithmic, with the lower scale values representing a disproportionate range of IOP values. Therefore, eyes with increased IOP need more weight on the plunger to further indent the cornea and get a higher, more accurate scale reading.

The tonometer is assembled with the 5.5-g weight attached to the plunger. If additional weights are needed, they are added on top of the 5.5-g weight. The eye is anesthetized with proparacaine, since viscous combination drops can affect accuracy by gumming up the cylinder in which the plunger travels. The patient is asked to recline so that the eyes are able to look straight up. The examiner stands either behind the patient or to one side. The patient holds up his or her hand and looks at his or her thumb for fixation. Make sure the measuring scale is visible before placing the tonometer on the eye. Gently place the foot plate on the cornea and continue to bring the tonometer handle a few millimeters further down so that the outer sleeve of the tonometer is floating freely. Note the scale reading and gently remove the tonometer. The needle may be seen to pulsate in some patients (ocular pulse). The midpoint between the highest and lowest reading should be used.

A table is supplied to convert the scale reading to pressure in millimeters of mercury. Any scale reading below 3 needs to be repeated with a heavier weight. Place the 7.5-g weight on top of the initial 5.5-g weight. The weight marked "7.5" is actually a 2-g weight that equals 7.5 g when added on top of the 5.5. The weight marked "10" is likewise added on top of "5.5" to equal 10 g. Additional weight is added until a scale reading of at least 3 is obtained.

Since it is an indentation tonometer, the Schiotz tonometer is significantly influenced by ocular rigidity, requiring that measurements on highly myopic or highly hyperopic eyes be confirmed with an applanation instrument.

Before each use, calibration should be checked by placing the tonometer on the metal block provided. Its front curvature exactly matches the curvature of the foot plate and prevents the plunger from protruding. The scale reading should be zero, and no error is tolerated. The instrument should be sent out for service if it is found to be out of calibration.

The tonometer should be completely disassembled after use and the tip soaked in alcohol. A pipe cleaner dipped in alcohol is used to ream out the cylinder. Dried tears or anesthetic will cause the plunger to bind up and give erroneous readings if the cylinder is not cleaned properly. The tonometer should be stored disassembled to indicate to the next user that it was carefully cleaned before storage.

FINAL CONSIDERATIONS

The choice of instruments for tonometry is an individual preference, because all will perform reasonably well if they are used within their limitations. From a theoretical standpoint, that which displaces the least amount of aqueous and is least affected by ocular rigidity should be the most accurate—i.e., the Goldmann or NCT. Also, it is important for every office to have at least one backup instrument so that, if one tonometer is broken, another will be available. The backup tonometer can also be used to double check suspicious findings. Ideally, the primary instrument should be accurate and easy to use. The backup instrument does not have to be as accurate and should be relatively inexpensive, since it will rarely be used.

Accurate and legible tonometry readings must be placed in the patient's chart. The numerical measurements are recorded in millimeters of mercury. The use of "wnl" or "normal" is not acceptable and leaves the practitioner vulnerable to malpractice claims. If different types of tonometers are used in the office, the type of tonometer should be recorded next to the reading. The time at which tonometry is performed is also recorded, since this provides useful information regarding diurnal fluctuations in IOP.

The age at which tonometry should be performed on a patient is open to debate. Waiting until a patient is age 40 to perform tonometry is no longer acceptable.[106] Since tonometry has minimal complications, the best advice is to measure the IOP of every patient regardless of age. The exception would be infants and small children who do not display any signs of congenital glaucoma.

If a patient refuses tonometry, the chart should well document that the risk of not doing tonometry was explained and that the patient understands and accepts the risk. Some doctors even make the patient sign a waiver. Likewise, whenever it is not possible to obtain a reliable reading (e.g., in case of edematous cornea or blepharospasm), the circumstances should be documented in the patient's record. Therefore it is incumbent on each practitioner to perform tonometry on every patient capable of being tested regardless of age or physical limitations. Tonometry, even with its limitations, remains a key test in the diagnosis and treatment of glaucoma.

REFERENCES

1. Mackenzie W. *Glaucoma: A Practical Treatise of the Diseases of the Eye*. London: Longman, Rees, Orme, Braun and Green; 1830:580.

2. Pederson JE, Anderson DR. The mode of progressive disc cupping in ocular hypertension and glaucoma. *Arch Ophthalmol.* 1980;98:490–495.

3. Eddy DM, Billing J. The Quality of Medical Evidence and Medical Practice: Report prepared for the National Leadership Commission on Health Care, 1988.

4. Olson RJ. How exposed are we? Is there a better way? *Arch Ophthalmol.* 1989;107:1131.

5. Lichter PR. A wolf in sheep's clothing. *Ophthalmology.* 1988;95:149–150.

6. Rossetti L, Marchetti I, Orszlesi N, et al. Randomized clinical trials on medical treatment of glaucoma: Are they appropriate to guide clinical practice? *Arch Ophthalmol.* 1993;111:96–103.

7. Keltner JL, Johnson CA, Spurr JO, Kass MA, et al. Classification of visual field abnormalities in the Ocular Hypertension Treatment Study. *Invest Ophthalmol Vis Sci.* 1999;40S:S69.

8. Heijl A, Leske MC, Bengtsson B, Hyman L, and the EMGT Group. The Early Manifest Glaucoma Trial: Study aims and design. *Invest Ophthalmol Vis Sci.* 1999;40S:S567.

9. Davanger M, Ringvold A, Blika S. The probability of glaucoma at different IOP levels. *Acta Ophthalmol (Copenh).* 1991;69:565–568.

10. Armaly MF, Krueger DE, Maunder L, et al. Biostatistical analysis of the Collaborative Glaucoma Study: I. Summary report of the risk factors for glaucomatous visual-field defects. *Arch Ophthalmol.* 1980;98: 2163–2171.

11. Hollows FC, Graham PA. Intraocular pressure, glaucoma and suspects in a defined population. *Br J Ophthalmol.* 1966;50:570–586.

12. Rojanapongpun P, Drance SM. The response of blood flow velocity in the ophthalmic artery and blood flow of the finger to warm and cold stimuli in glaucomatous patients. *Graefes Arch Clin Exp Ophthalmol.* 1993;231: 375–377.

13. Rankin SJ, Walman BE, Buckley AR, et al. Color Doppler imaging and spectral analysis of the optic nerve vasculature in glaucoma. *Am J Ophthalmol.* 1995; 119:685–693.

14. Tielsch JM, Katz J, Sommer A, et al. Hypertension, perfusion pressure and primary open-angle glaucoma: A population-based assessment. *Arch Ophthalmol.* 1994; 113:216–221.

15. Leydecker W. Zur Verbeitung des Glaucoma simplex in der scheinbar gesunden, augensichtlich nicht behandelten Bevolkerung. *Doc Ophthalomol.* 1959;13: 359–380.

16. Armaly MF. On the distribution of applanation pressure. *Arch Ophthalmol.* 1965;73:11–18.

17. David R, Livingston DG, Luntz MH. Ocular hypertension. A long term following of treated and untreated patients. *Br J Ophthalmol.* 1977;61:668.

18. Bengtsson B. The prevalence of glaucoma. *Br J Ophthalmol.* 1981;65:46–49.

19. Sommer A. Intraocular pressure and glaucoma. *Am J Ophthalmol.* 1989;107:186–188.

20. Armaly MF. Lessons to be learned from the Collaborative Glaucoma Study. *Surv Ophthalmol.* 1980;25:139–144.

21. Bengtsson B. The prevalence of glaucoma. *Br J Ophthalmol.* 1981;65:46–49.

22. Bankes JL, Perkins ES, Tsolakis S, et al. Bedford glaucoma survey. *BMJ.* 1968;1:791–796.

23. Colton T, Ederer F. The distribution of intraocular pressure in the general population. *Surv Ophthalmol.* 1980; 25:123–129.

24. Shiose Y. The aging effect on intraocular pressure in an apparently normal population. *Arch Ophthalmol.* 1984;102:883–887.

25. Tielsch JM, Katz J, Royall RM, et al. Racial variations in the prevalence of primary open-angle glaucoma. *JAMA.* 1991;266:369–374.

26. Leske MC, Connell AM, Wu SY, et al. Distribution of intraocular pressure: The Barbados Eye Study. *Arch Ophthalmol.* 1997;115:1051–1057.

27. Shiose Y, Kitazawa Y, Tsukahara S, et al. Epidemiology of glaucoma in Japan—A nationwide glaucoma survey. *Jpn J Ophthalmol.* 1991;35:133–155.

28. Quigley HA. The number of persons with glaucoma worldwide. *Br J Ophthalmol.* 1996;80:389–393.

29. Shiose Y. Intraocular pressure: New perspectives. *Surv Ophthalmol.* 1990;34:413–435.

30. Drance SM. The significance of the diurnal tension variations in normal and glaucomatous eyes. *Arch Ophthalmol.* 1960;64:494–501.

31. Armaly MF. Ocular pressure and visual fields. A ten-year follow-up study. *Arch Ophthalmol.* 1969;81: 25–40.

32. Wilensky JT, Gieser DK, Dietsche ML, et al. Individual variability in the diurnal intraocular pressure curve. *Ophthalmology.* 1993;100:940–944.

33. Zeimer RC: Circadian variations in intraocular pressure. In: Ritch R, Shields MB, Krupin T, eds. *The Glaucomas.* St. Louis: CV Mosby; 1989:319–335

34. Sacca SC, Rolando M, Marletta A, et al. Fluctuations of intraocular pressure during the day in open-angle glaucoma, normal-tension glaucoma and normal subjects. *Ophthalmologica.* 1998;212:115–119.

35. Leydhecker W. The intraocular pressure: Clinical aspects. *Ann Ophthalmol.* 1976;8:389–399.

36. Kitazawa Y, Horie T, Aoki S, et al. Untreated ocular hypertension. A long-term prospective study. *Arch Ophthalmol.* 1977;95:1180–1184.

37. De Vivero C, O'Brien C, Lanigan L, et al. Diurnal intraocular pressure variation in low-tension glaucoma. *Eye.* 1994;8(pt 5):521–523.

38. Stamper RL. Intraocular pressure: Measurement, regulation, and flow relationships. In: Duane TD, Jaeger EA, eds. *Biomedical Foundations of Ophthalmology II.* Philadelphia: Harper & Row; 1987:1–30.

39. Rota-Bartelink AM, Pitt A, Story I. Influence of diurnal variation on the intraocular pressure measurement of treated primary open-angle glaucoma during office hours. *J Glaucoma.* 1996;5:410–415.

40. Buchanan RA, Williams TD. Intraocular pressure, ocular pulse pressure, and body position. *Am J Optom Phys Optom.* 1985;62:59–62.

41. Bain WE, Maurice DM. Physiological variations in the

intraocular pressure. *Trans Ophthalmol Soc UK*. 1959;79: 249–260.

42. Rosen DA, Johnston VC. Ocular pressure patterns in the Valsalva maneuver. *Arch Ophthalmol.* 1959;62:810–815.

43. Maurice DM. A recording tonometer. *Br J Ophthalmol.* 1958;42:321–335.

44. Passo MS, Goldberg L. Exercise training reduces intraocular pressure among subjects suspected of having glaucoma. *Arch Ophthalmol.* 1991;109:1096–1098.

45. Harris A, Malinovsky V, Martin B. Correlates of acute exercise-induced ocular hypotension. *Invest Ophthalmol Vis Sci.* 1994;35:3853–3857.

46. Armaly MF, Rubin ML. Accommodation and applanation. *Arch Ophthalmol.* 1961;65:415–423.

47. Goldmann H, Schmidt T. Uber Applanationstonometrie. *Ophthalmologica.* 1957;134:221–242.

48. Wolfs RC, Klaver CC, Vingerling JR, et al. Distribution of central corneal thickness and its association with intraocular pressure: The Rotterdam Study. *Am J Ophthalmol.* 1997;123:767–772.

49. Herndon LW, Choudri SA, Cox T. Central corneal thickness in normal, glaucomatous, and ocular hypertensive eyes. *Arch Ophthalmol.* 1997;115: 1137–1141.

50. Whitacre MM, Stein, RA, Hassanein K. The effect of corneal thickness on applanation tonometry. *Am J Ophthalmol.* 1993;115:592–596.

51. Ehlers N, Bramsen T, Sperling S. Applanation tonometry and central corneal thickness. *Acta Ophthalmol.* 1975;53:34–43.

52. Argus W. Ocular hypertension and central corneal thickness. *Ophthalmology.* 1995;102:1810–1812.

53. Morad Y, Sharon E, Hefetz L, et al. Corneal thickness and curvature in normal-tension glaucoma. *Am J Ophthalmol.* 1998;125:164–168.

54. Copt R, Thomas R, Mermoud A. Corneal thickness in ocular hypertension, primary open angle glaucoma, and normal tension glaucoma. *Arch Ophthalmol.* 1999; 117:14–16.

55. Brubaker RB. Tonometry and corneal thickness. *Arch Ophthalmol.* 1999;117:104–105.

56. Simon G, Small RH, Ren Q, et al. Effect of corneal hydration on Goldmann applanation tonometry and corneal topography. *J Refract Corneal Surg.* 1993;9:110–117.

57. Chatterjee A, Shah S, Bessant DA, et al. Reduction in intraocular pressure after excimer laser photorefractive keratectomy: Correlation with pretreatment myopia. *Ophthalmology.* 1997;104:335–359.

58. Mardelli PG, Piebenga LW, Whitacre MM, et al. The effect of excimer laser photorefractive keratectomy on IOP measurements using the Goldmann applanation tonometer. *Ophthalmology.* 1997;104:945–949.

59. Ohrstrom A, Kattstrom O, Palland W, et al. Oral and topical beta-receptor blockers in glaucoma treatment: A multi-center study. *Acta Ophthalmol (Copenh).* 1984; 62:681–695.

60. Hepler RS, Frank IR. Marijuana smoking and intraocular pressure. *JAMA.* 1971;217:1392–1398.

61. Green K. Marijuana smoking vs cannaboids for glaucoma therapy. *Arch Ophthalmol.* 1998;116:1433–1437.

62. Fraunfelder FT, Meyer SM. Agents affecting the central nervous system. In: Fraunfelder FT, Meyer SM, eds. *Drug-Induced Ocular Side Effects and Drug Interactions.* Phildelphia: Lea & Febiger; 1989:135–139.

63. Epstein DL. Glaucoma due to intraocular inflammation. In: Epstein DL, ed. *Chandler and Grant's Glaucoma.* Philadelphia: Lea & Febiger; 1986:353–354.

64. Thorburn W. The accuracy of clinical applanation tonometry. *Acta Ophthalmol (Copenh).* 1978;56:1–5.

65. Sudesh S, Moseley MJ, Thompson JR. Accuracy of Goldmann tonometry in clinical practice. *Acta Ophthalmol (Copenh).* 1993;71(2):185–188.

66. Phelps CD, Phelps GK. Measurement of intraocular pressure: A study of its reproducibility. *Graefes Arch Clin Exp Ophthalmol.* 1976;198:39–43.

67. Forbes M, Pico G, Grolman B. A noncontact applanation tonometer. *Arch Ophthalmol.* 1974;91:134–140.

68. Zappia RJ, Winkelman JZ, Gay AJ. Intraocular pressure changes in normal subjects and the adhesive muscle syndrome. *Am J Ophthalmol.* 1971;71:611–618.

69. Jaafar MS, Kazi GA. Normal intraocular pressure in children: A comparative study of the Perkins applanation tonometer and the pneumatonometer. *J Pediatr Ophthalmol Strabismus.* 1993;30:284–287.

70. Radtke ND, Cohan BE. Intraocular pressure measurement in the newborn. *Am J Ophthalmol.* 1974; 78: 501–504.

71. Bordon AF, Katsumi O, Hirose T. Tonometry in pediatric patients: A comparative study among Tono-Pen, Perkins, and Schiotz tonometers. *J Pediatr Ophthalmol Strabismus.* 1995;32:373–377.

72. Eisenberg DL, Sherman BG, McKeown CA, et al. Tonometry in adults and children. *Ophthalmology.* 1998; 105:1173–1181.

73. Lim L, Ng TP, Tan DT. Accurate intraocular pressure measurement in contact lens wearers with normal pressures. *CLAO J.* 1997;23:130–133.

74. Scibilia GD, Ehlers WH, Donshik PC. The effects of therapeutic contact lenses on intraocular pressure measurement. *CLAO J.* 1996;22:262–265.

75. Panek WC, Boothe WA, Lee DA, et al. Intraocular pressure measurement with the Tono-Pen through soft contact lenses. *Am J Ophthalmol.* 1990;109:62–65.

76. Duke-Elder S. *System of Ophthalmology VI: The Physiology of the Eye and of Vision.* St. Louis: CV Mosby; 1968.

77. Mackay RS, Marg E. Fast automatic electronic tonometers based on an exact theory. *Acta Ophthalmol (Copenh).* 1959;37:495–501.

78. Meyers K, Lalle P, Litwak A, et al. XPERT NCT: A clinical evaluation. *J Am Optom Assoc.* 1990;61: 863–869.

79. Boothe WA, Lee DA, Panek WC, et al. The Tono-Pen: A manometric and clinical study. *Arch Ophthalmol.* 1988;106:1214–1217.

80. Freidenwald JS: Calibration of tonometers, in Standardization of Tonometers Decennial Report, by the Committee on Standardization of Tonometers. *Acad Ophthalmol Otolaryngol.* 1954;129.

81. Stocker FW. On changes in the intraocular pressure after application of the tonometer. In the same eye and in the other eye. *Am J Ophthalmol.* 1958;45:192–196.

82. Goldmann H. Applanation tonometry. In Newell FW, ed. *Glaucoma. Transactions of the Second Conference.* New York: *Josiah Macy, Jr., Foundation;* 1957:167–220.

83. Dielemans I, Vingerling JR, Hofman A, Grobbe DE, de Jong PT. Reliability of intraocular pressure measurements with the Goldmann applanation tonometer in epidemiological studies. *Graefes Arch Clin Exp Ophthalmol.* 1994;232:141–144.

84. Moses RA. Fluorescein in applanation tonometry. *Am J Ophthalmol.* 1960;49:1149–1155.

85. Holladay JT, Allison ME, Prager TC. Goldmann applanation tonometry in patients with regular corneal astigmatism. *Am J Ophthalmol.* 1983;96:90–93.

86. Baskett JS, Goen TM, Terry JE. A comparison of Perkins and Goldmann applanation tonometry. *J Am Optom Assoc.* 1987;57:832–834.

87. Gonzaga dos Santos M, Makk S, Berghold A, et al. Intraocular pressure difference in Goldmann applanation tonometry versus Perkins hand-held applanation tonometry in overweight patients. *Ophthalmology.* 1998;105:2260–2263.

88. Pepose J, Linette G, Lee S, et al. Disinfection of Goldmann tonometers against human immunodeficiency virus type I. *Arch Ophthalmol.* 1989;107:983–985.

89. Lichter P. Controlling risks of the possible transmission of human immunodeficiency virus. *Ophthalmology.* 1989;96:1.

90. Centers for Disease Control. Recommendations for preventing transmission of human T-lymphotropic virus type III/lymphadenopathy-associated virus from tears. *MMWR.* 1987;34:533–534.

91. Centers for Disease Control. Recommendations for prevention of HIV transmission in health care setting. *MMWR.* 1987;36:35–185.

92. Ventura L, Dix R. Viability of herpes simplex type 1 on the applanation tonometer. *Am J Ophthalmol.* 1986;103:48–52.

93. Bond W, Favero M, Petersen N, et al. Inactivation of hepatitis B virus by intermediate-to-high-level disinfectant chemicals. *J Clin Microbiol.* 1983;18:535–538.

94. Silvany R, Dougherty J, McCulley J, et al. The effect of currently available contact lens disinfection systems on *Acanthamoeba castellanii* and *Acanthamoeba polyphaga. Ophthalmology.* 1989;97:286–290.

95. Lingel N, Coffey B. Effects of disinfecting solutions recommended by the Centers for Disease Control on Goldmann tonometer biprisms. *J Am Optom Assoc.* 1992;63:43–48.

96. Meyers K, Lalle P, Litwak A, et al. XPERT NCT: A clinical evaluation. *J Am Optom Assoc.* 1990;61:863–869.

97. Rubenstein JR, Deutsch TA. Pneumotonometry through bandage contact lenses. *Arch Ophthalmol.* 1985;103:1660–1661.

98. Khan JA, LaGreca BA. Tono-Pen estimation of intraocular pressure through bandage contact lenses. *Am J Ophthalmol.* 1989;108:422–425.

99. Abbasoglu OE, Bowman RW, Cavanagh HD, et al. Reliability of intraocular pressure measurements after myopic excimer photorefractive keratectomy *Ophthalmology.* 1998;105:2193–2196.

100. Quigley HA, Langham ME. Comparative intraocular pressure measurements with the pneumotonograph and Goldmann tonometer. *Am J Ophthalmol.* 1975;80:266–273.

101. Moses RA, Marg E, Oeschli R. Evaluation of the basic validity and clinical usefulness of the MacKay-Marg tonometer. *Trans Am Acad Ophthalmol Otolaryngol.* 1962;66:88–95.

102. Armstrong TA. Evaluation of the Tono-Pen and the pulsair tonometers. *Am J Ophthalmol.* 1990;109: 716–720.

103. Kooner KS, Cooksey JC, Barron JB, et al. Tonometer comparison: Goldmann vs Tono-Pen. *Ann Ophthalmol.* 1992;24:29–36.

104. Kao SF, Lichter PR, Bergstrom TJ, et al. Clinical comparison of the Oculab Tono-Pen to the Goldmann applanation tonometer. *Ophthalmology.* 1987;94(12):1541–1544.

105. American Optometric Association. Care process. In: Scheiman MM, Amos CS, Ciner EB, et al, eds. *Optometric Clinical Practice Guideline: Pediatric Eye and Vision Examination.* St. Louis: AOA; 1994:7–26.

Chapter 11

GONIOSCOPY

G. Richard Bennett

Gonioscopy is a procedure used in the examination of the anterior chamber angle and its related structures. The technique requires competency with the instrumentation as well as knowledge of both normal and pathologic anterior chamber findings associated with glaucoma. Gonioscopy is a critical component of the diagnostic regimen for glaucoma since it allows the establishment of the type of glaucoma and may be the sole indicator of the specific mechanism for the disease. Gonioscopy must be performed on all individuals with glaucoma as well as glaucoma suspects. Periodically during the course of therapy for glaucoma, gonioscopy must be repeated to rule out the development of new mechanisms.

In 1907 Trantas visualized the anterior chamber angle of an eye with keratoglobus by indenting at the limbus; he used the term *gonioscopy* to describe this technique. Salzmann introduced a goniolens in 1914, which was refined by Koeppe. This 50-diopter concave lens served as the prototype for direct gonioscopy. Troncoso developed a monocular gonioscope in 1921 and continued to modify and improve the contact lenses of Salzmann and Koeppe. Goldmann established indirect gonioscopy by the development of a gonioprism in 1938. Barkan is credited with establishing the role of gonioscopy in the management of glaucoma. The reader is referred to Gorin's text on slit-lamp gonioscopy for a detailed history of the technique.[1]

METHODS AND TECHNIQUE OF GONIOSCOPY

The critical angle is the angle of incidence of light passing from an optically dense to a less dense (lower index of refraction) medium at which the angle of refraction will be 90 degrees. Light rays that approach the cornea-air interface at an angle exceeding the critical angle will be internally reflected. Thus, to view the internal angle of the eye optically, one must neutralize the difference in the index of refraction at the cornea-air interface. This is accomplished by placing a goniolens on the corneal surface and either directly (direct gonioscopy) or indirectly through internal mirrors in a gonioprism (indirect gonioscopy) viewing the structures of the eye (Table 11–1).

DIRECT GONIOSCOPY—THE KOEPPE GONIOLENS

The Koeppe goniolens is a 50-diopter concave lens with a convex, bubble-shaped outer surface and a diameter of 17.0 to 22.5 mm.[2] The lens is placed on the eye with the patient in the supine position. Topical

TABLE 11–1. GONIOSCOPY LENSES

Goniolens	Type of Lens	Goniogel Required*	Pressure Gonioscopy	Comments
Koeppe	Direct	Yes	No	Requires external light source
Goldmann 1-mirror	Indirect	Yes	No	Smaller size is easier to rotate
Goldmann 3-mirror	Indirect	Yes	No	Additional mirrors for peripheral fundus exam
Zeiss 4-mirror	Indirect	No	Yes	No rotation required; difficult in uncooperative patients
Posner 4-mirror	Indirect	No	Yes	Lighter than Zeiss; mounted handle angled steeper than Zeiss
Sussman 4-mirror	Indirect	No	Yes	Hand-held version of Zeiss

*Less viscous solutions, such as contact lens wetting solution or unpreserved artificial tears, can be substituted for goniogel to reduce corneal impairment following the procedure. Newer forms of goniolenses are available that do not require a coupling solution.

anesthesia and gonioscopic gel or saline are required. A hand-held gonioscope or slit lamp is used with a broad beam of light to obtain a high-quality, panoramic view of the angle structures. The technique is considered superior to the indirect methods of gonioscopy as it allows a more natural view with fewer induced artifacts. Unfortunately, Koeppe gonioscopy is cumbersome and time-consuming; it also requires a high degree of skill to perform. In addition, there are limited magnification options and the hand-held gonioscope cannot produce an optic section. Fewer than 2% of ophthalmic practitioners use direct gonioscopy, but the technique should be appreciated from a historical perspective.[3]

INDIRECT GONIOSCOPY

Indirect gonioscopy utilizes mirrors mounted within the gonioprism. These reflect light from a slit-lamp lighting source, making it possible to view a section of the angle that is 180 degrees from the position of the mirror. The image of the angle is inverted but not reversed laterally. Thus to view a structure in the angle at 12 o'clock, the mirror should be located at 6 o'clock. The gonioprism may be tilted to view over a steep iris insertion into the angle and rotated to view different sections of the chamber angle. A slit lamp is used with the goniolens to provide illumination and obtain a binocular view of the angle. An optic section may be produced, allowing identification of iris structures and determination of the iris insertion. The optic section also allows identification of the anterior termination of the angle at Schwalbe's line by locating the junction of the posterior (endothelium) and anterior (epithelium) corneal focal lines.

Major disadvantages of indirect gonioscopy include artifacts produced by tilting the gonioprism or applying excessive pressure, leading to distortion of the normal angle anatomy and degradation of the view due to folds in Descemet's membrane.

The technique of dynamic or compression gonioscopy is performed with a four-mirror goniolens and involves the intentional application of pressure to differentiate appositional from synechial closure.[4] Pressure from the gonioprism will cause aqueous to be pushed into the angle recess, opening an angle closed by apposition. Compression gonioscopy will not open the angle when synechial closure is present.

LENSES FOR INDIRECT GONIOSCOPY

Goldmann Lenses

The Goldmann-style indirect lenses are the ones most commonly used for gonioscopy. They are available in several sizes and variations, including a three-mirror "universal" lens. With the three-mirror lens, one mirror is angled for gonioscopy (59 degrees), one for the midperipheral retina (73 degrees), and one for the far peripheral retina (67 degrees). The three-mirror lens is supplied with a central fundus lens. Smaller versions of the Goldmann lens include the one-mirror lens with a single 62-degree mirror for gonioscopy and a central fundus lens; and a two-mirror version with a central lens and two mirrors angled at 62 degrees oriented 180 degrees apart. Most of these lenses require the use of a viscous coupling solution or less viscous artificial tears. Recently several manufacturers have introduced lenses that do not require coupling solutions.

The Goldmann lens must be rotated to view all quadrants with artifacts introduced by the suction created by the tight adherence of the goniolens. The smaller Goldmann-style lenses are easier to insert because of their small size and reduced tendency to adhere to the cornea. The small one- and two-mirror

Goldmann lenses tend to give a reduced view with a higher vantage point due to the mirror orientation. The large three-mirror Goldmann lens provides a stable and clear view of the angle. Although it is more difficult to insert because of its large size, the view through the three-mirror lens is easier to achieve for the beginning gonioscopist.

Goldmann Lens Technique

The patient should be comfortably positioned at the slit lamp with the chin and forehead firmly in place. Careful attention should be paid to fixation and the patient instructed to keep both eyes open while attending to the fixation target. If tonometry has been performed immediately prior to gonioscopy, no addi-

tional anesthetic is required. Otherwise one drop of a topical anesthetic, such as proparacaine, may be instilled in each eye. The coupling solution should be carefully instilled onto the concave surface, trying to avoid creating bubbles, which would interfere with the view of the angle structures. Either a commercial goniogel solution or a tear agent such as Celluvisc may be used (Fig. 11–1), filling the cavity of the lens about two-thirds full. After educating the patient concerning gonioscopy, instruct him or her to look up as the lower portion of the lens is rocked into the inferior cul-de-sac. The patient then looks straight ahead as the upper portion of the lens is placed onto the eye (Fig. 11–2). The lens is then maintained in position with gentle pressure.

The superior lid must be controlled until the lens is secured in position. If bubbles are present, it is sometimes possible to remove them by tilting the lens, allowing them to escape under the upper edge. Otherwise the lens must be removed and reinserted. If excess suction makes removal difficult, ask the patient to look up while applying gentle pressure next to the lens through the lower lid. The examiner's elbow should rest on the instrument table or arm rest to avoid placing excessive pressure on the lens. An elbow rest may be used for support if necessary. The suction achieved with proper lens insertion should be sufficient to maintain position using only the index finger, as the thumb and middle finger are used to rotate the Goldmann lens.

With one-mirror lens designs, it is more convenient to place the mirror initially at the 12 o'clock position to view the inferior angle, normally the deepest and easiest to view. The lamp tower should initially be in alignment with a narrow parallelepiped placed perpendicular to the flat surface of the mirror. A continuous focus should be maintained with the joystick, since gonioscopy is a dynamic technique. The lens can be tilted or the patient asked to rotate the eye toward the mirror so that previously obscured angle structures may be viewed. In this way, structures in a narrow angle may be visualized (Fig. 11–3). The goniolens must be rotated to view all four quadrants of the angle. The examiner should mentally record the appearance of the iris surface, the iris contour and angle of insertion, the location of iris insertion, and any abnormalities such as pigment, neovascularization, exfoliative material, synechiae, inflammatory material, or significant anatomic variations. These findings should be clearly documented in the record after gonioscopy is performed. If a viscous goniogel has been used, the eyes should be irrigated once the lens has been removed.

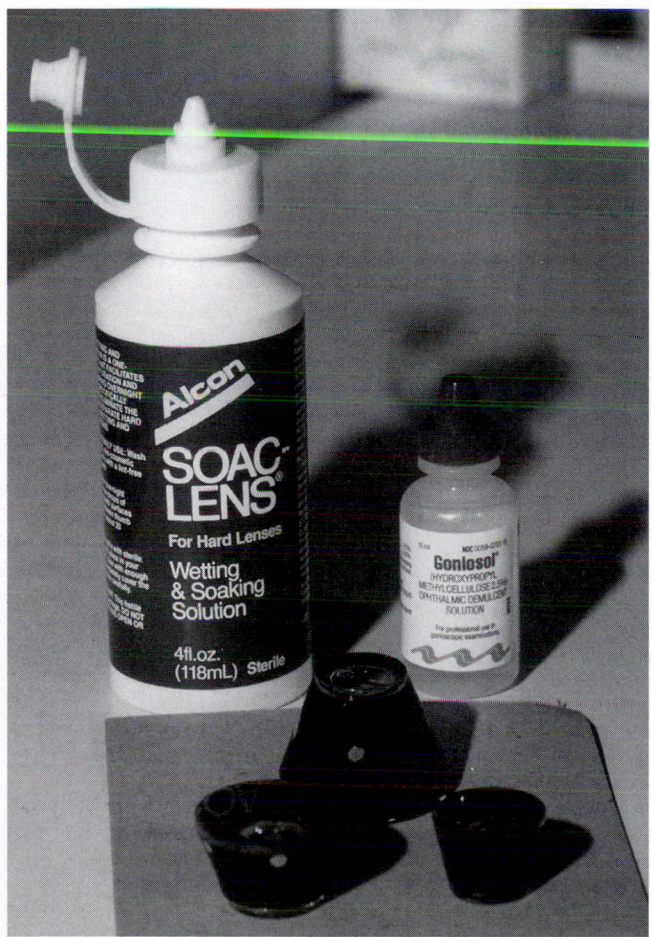

Figure 11–1. Less viscous solutions such as Soaclens or Celluvisc can be substituted for the more copious gels such as Goniosol. These solutions maintain corneal clarity for fundus examination and photography.

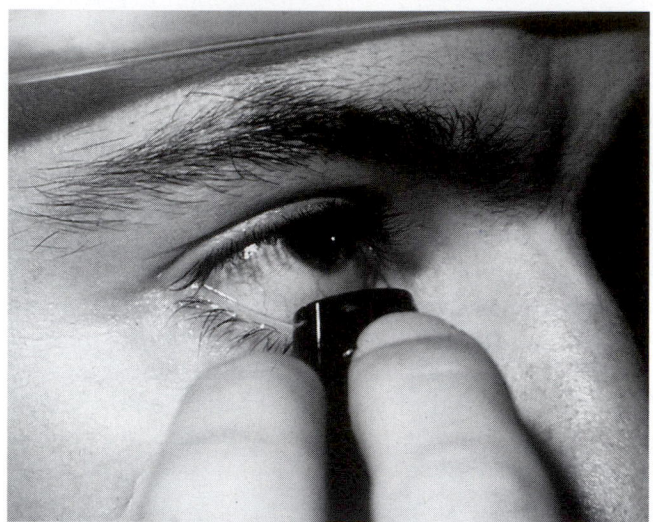

A

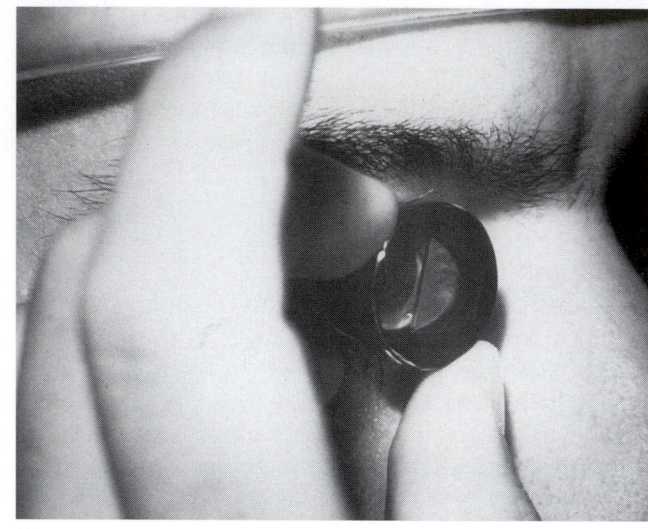

B

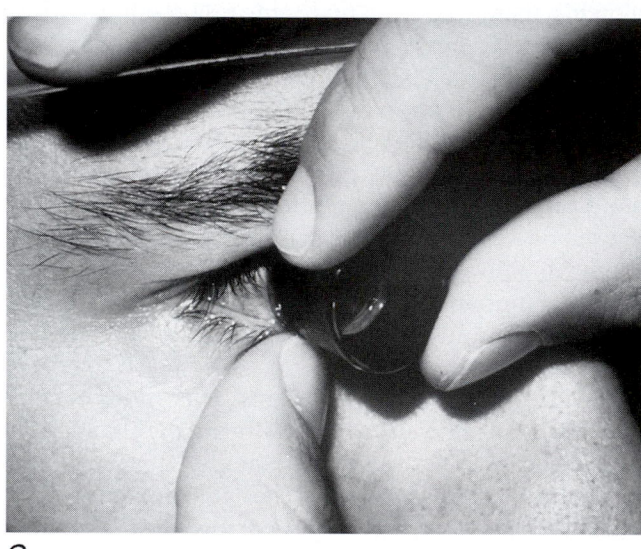

C

Figure 11–2. Technique for one- or three-mirror Goldmann gonioscopy. *A.* The goniolens is inserted quickly and gently onto the eye with the patient looking up and the lower lid held down with the goniolens. *B.* The goniolens is rotated 360 degrees with the slit beam following the mirror, so the entire angle can be examined. *C.* The lens is removed by gently pressing beneath the goniolens on the lower lid to break the lens suction on the eye.

Four-Mirror Lens Technique

The four-mirror lens has several advantages over its Goldmann-style counterparts. No coupling solution is required, which makes the technique quicker, more comfortable for the patient, and less likely to compromise the cornea; the last of these precludes a clear view of the fundus after gonioscopy. No rotation is necessary because of the lens has four mirrors. Four-mirror lenses are ideal for compression (dynamic) gonioscopy because of their flat base-curve, small-diameter design (Figs. 11–4 and 11–5). Unfortunately, some skill and experience is required before one becomes comfortable with their use. Even with experience, an uncooperative patient with poor fixation may be difficult or impossible to examine with a four-mirror goniolens. The lens is less stable on the eye than the Goldmann, leading to an unstable view. The lens is used only to view the angle and not to examine the peripheral retina.

The Zeiss four-mirror lens, the Posner lens, and the Sussman lens are examples of the four-mirror design (Fig. 11–6). The Zeiss four-mirror lens has four 64-degree-angled mirrors with a central fundus lens and an Unger grooved holding fork used to secure the lens. The Posner lens is a lighter version of the Zeiss, with the aluminum handle embedded in the lens. The Sussman lens and a recent Zeiss four-mirror design eliminate the handle; they are used in a hand-held manner, like a small Goldmann lens.

The procedure of four-mirror gonioscopy is similar to Goldmann lens gonioscopy. The patient is in-

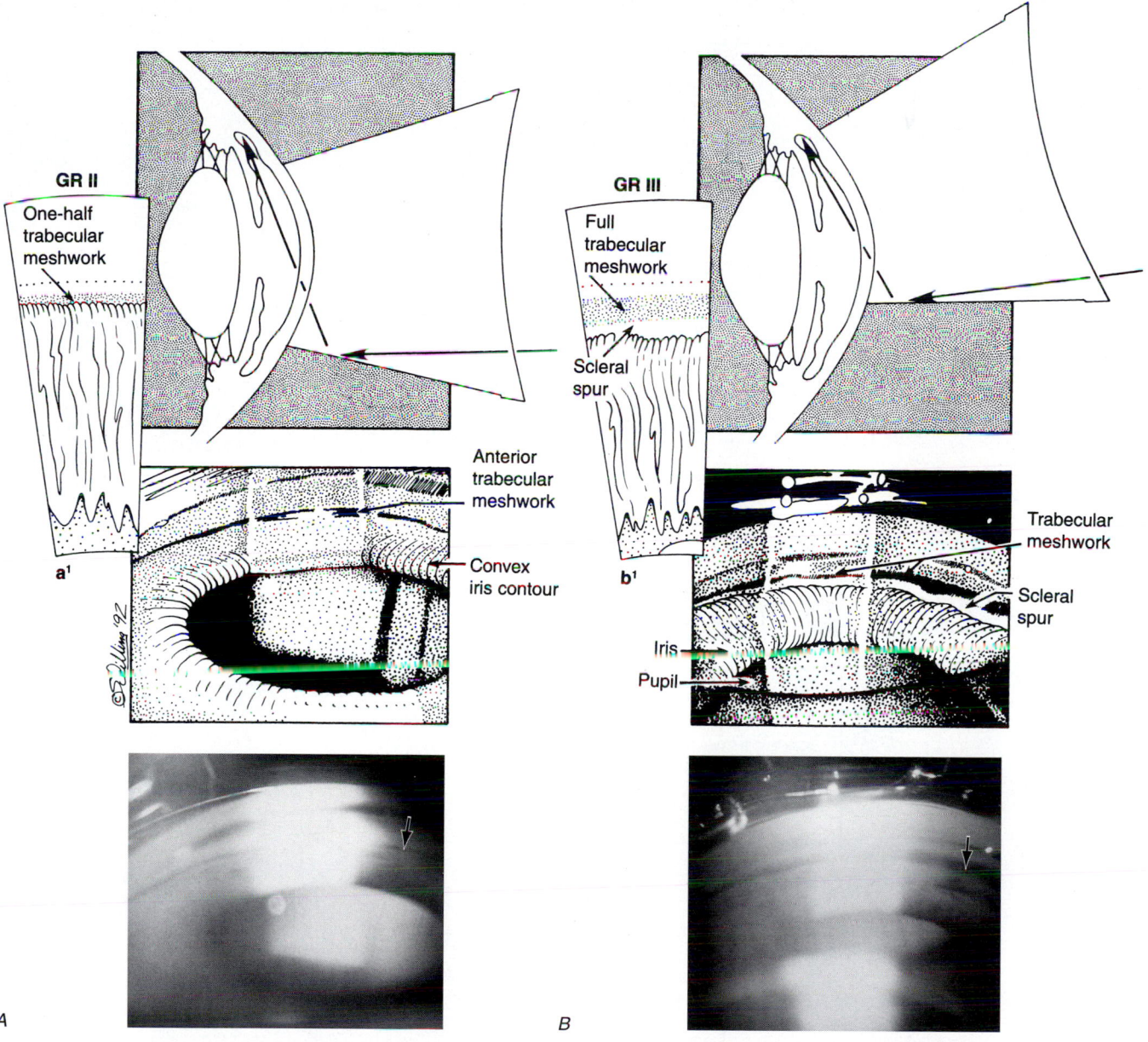

Figure 11–3. Lens tilting to view deeper into the angle. *A.* Angle view in the primary gaze position. Note convex iris contour with only anterior trabecular meshwork visible. *B.* Angle view tilting the goniolens away from the mirror or having the patient look slightly into the mirror. Note deeper view into the angle with full trabecular meshwork and scleral spur visible. (Courtesy of Tony Litwak, O.D.)

structed to maintain fixation and the procedure is described. The corneas are anesthetized with topical proparacaine and the gonioprism is placed directly against the cornea without goniogel (Fig. 11–7). A drop of contact lens wetting solution or artificial tears may be used but is generally unnecessary. All four quadrants are examined by moving the slit beam vertically and laterally onto the appropriate mirror.

The focal line technique may be used to identify the anatomic angle landmarks. An optic section is placed on a mirror of the gonioprism and the lamp tower is tilted. This produces a "V" along the angle wall, with one line representing the anterior cornea and the other the posterior cornea. Schwalbe's line (the end of Descemet's membrane) is located at the point of the "V." If the beam of light running along the iris intersects the point of the "V" above the tra-

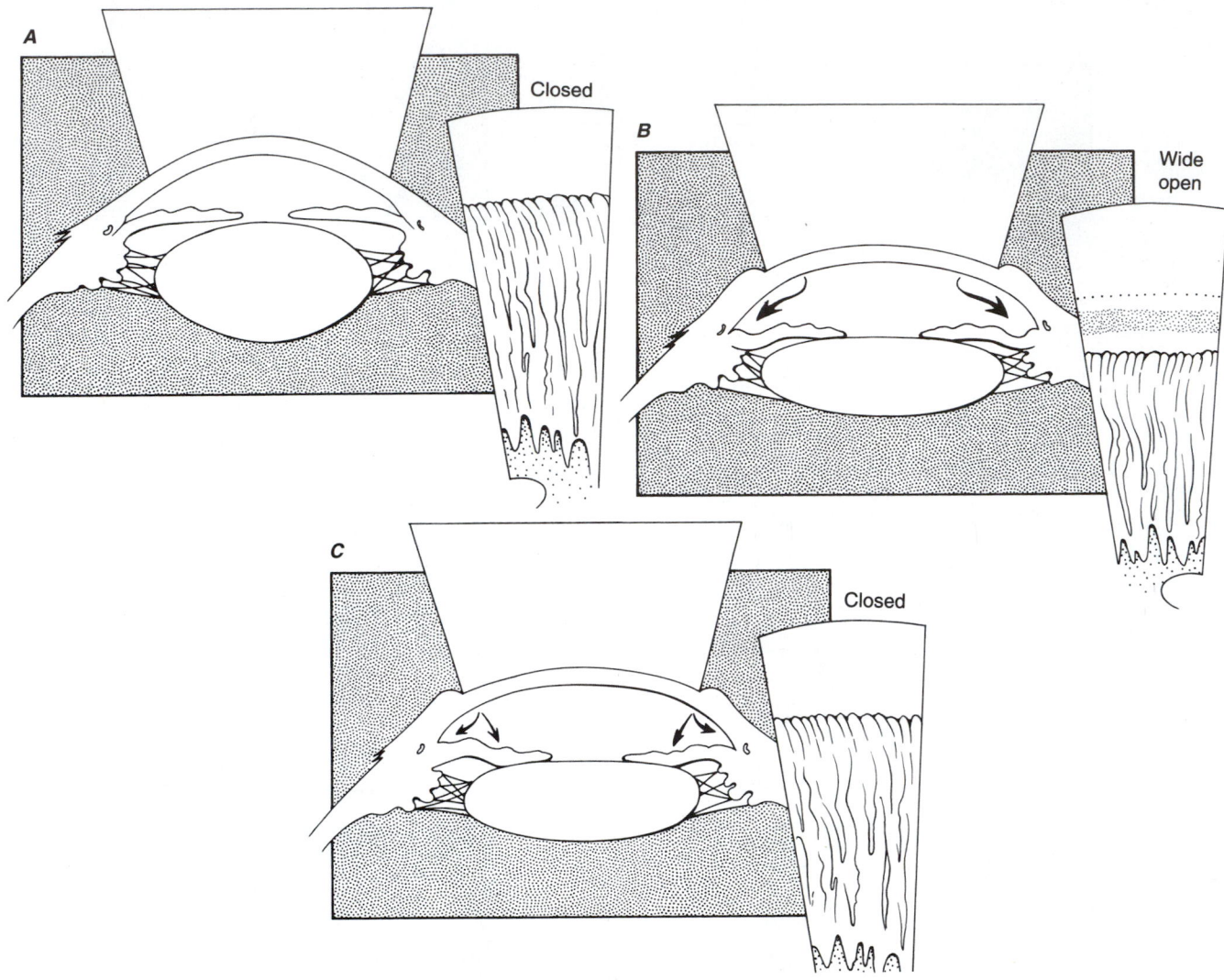

Figure 11–4. *A.* Pressure gonioscopy in a narrow-angle patient. *B.* With pressure directed on the goniolens perpendicular to the cornea, the peripheral iris is pushed back and the angle deepens. Pressure gonioscopy can help differentiate appositional angle closure from peripheral anterior synechia (PAS). *C.* When PAS has formed, the peripheral iris will not fall back with pressure gonioscopy.

becular meshwork, the angle is closed at that point. If the iris beam does not meet the point of the "V," there is parallax and the angle is wider than it appears.

Goniolens Disinfection

It is important to clean and disinfect the goniolens after use. Isopropyl alcohol is commonly used but is not considered to be a high-level disinfection agent. The lens may be disinfected by soaking in glutaraldehyde for 20 min or sterilized by oxide gas. A practical method of disinfection is to clean the lens carefully with tap water and disinfect it with sodium hypochlorite (household bleach mixed one part bleach to four

parts water). The lens should be rinsed with sterile saline and stored dry in the case.

ANTERIOR CHAMBER ANGLE ANATOMY

The anterior chamber angle is the recess bordered anteriorly by the cornea and posteriorly by the iris root. The anterior chamber angle is actually a recess and forms a true angle only in synechial closure. It is important to recognize the gonioscopic landmarks and how they relate to the anatomy of the angle (Figs. 11–8 and 11–9). The principal structures visible

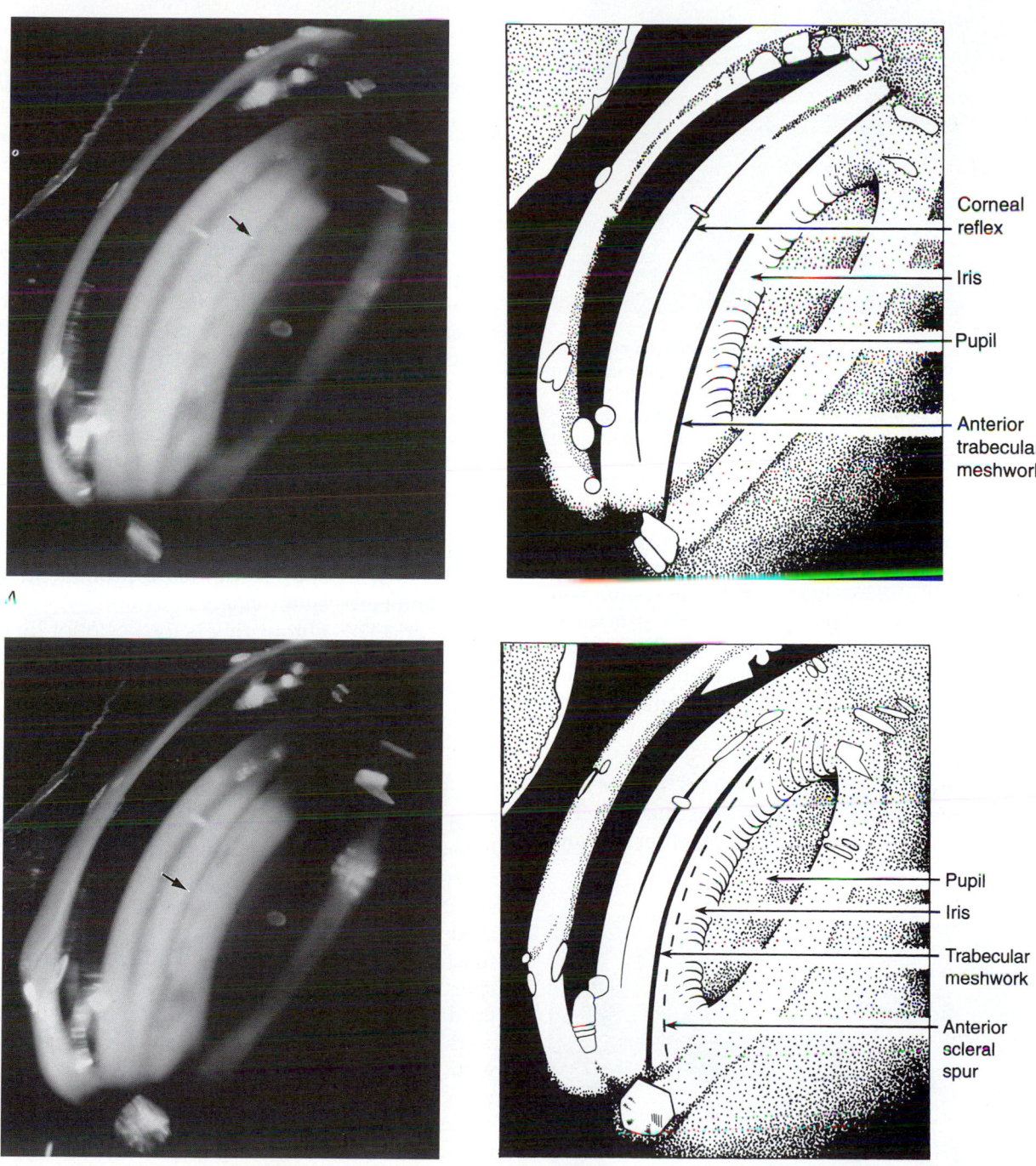

Figure 11–5. Pressure gonioscopy with the four-mirror goniolens. *A*. Narrow angle with only anterior trabecular meshwork visible. *B*. With pressure, the trabecular meshwork and scleral spur become visible with no evidence of PAS. (Courtesy of Tony Litwak, O.D.)

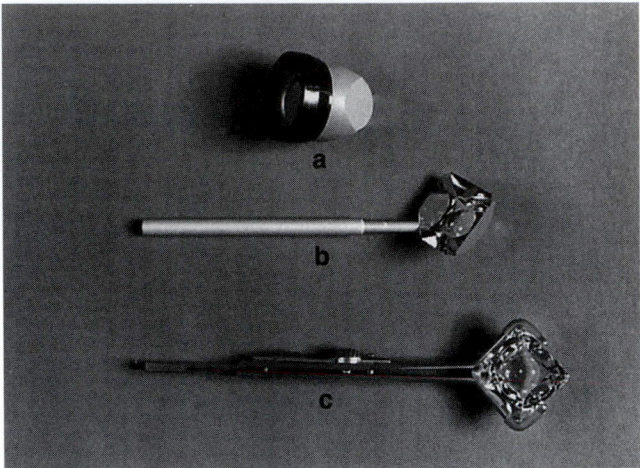

Figure 11–6. Four-mirror goniolens (a). Sussman hand-held four-mirror lens. (b). Posner four-mirror with a permanently mounted handle. Zeiss four-mirror with an Unger holding fork (c). (Reproduced with permission from Casser L, Fingeret M, Woodcome HT. *Atlas of Primary Eyecare Procedures*, 2nd ed. Stamford, CT: Appleton & Lange, 1997.)

through a goniolens, viewing anterior to posterior, are Schwalbe's line (the internal limit of Descemet's membrane), the trabecular meshwork, the scleral spur, and the ciliary body. In addition to the angle structures, the iris is visible in an open angle as it inserts onto the inner wall of the anterior chamber angle. A more detailed description of the anterior chamber angle may be found in Chap. 3.

The examiner should begin the gonioscopic examination by viewing the iris-pupil border and moving peripherally toward the angle structures. The contour of the iris plane should be observed and

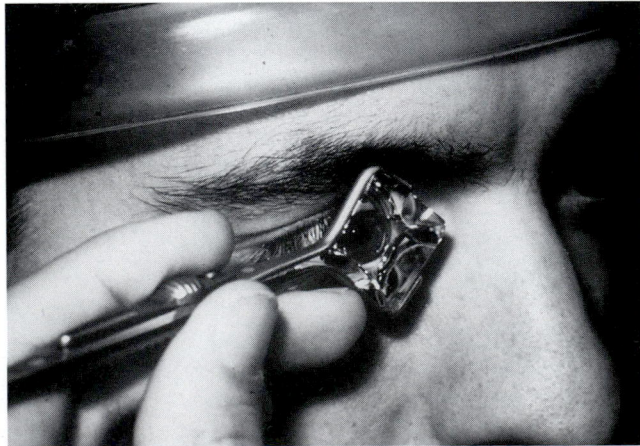

Figure 11–7. Four-mirror gonioscopy using the Zeiss goniolens. The slit beam is moved into the four mirrors to view the four angle quadrants.

described as flat, convex, or concave, with any abnormalities noted. The angle between the peripheral iris and the angle wall should be estimated; it is wider in angles with a posterior iris insertion.

The ciliary body is the most posterior structure of the angle; it is located anterior to the iris root and posterior to the scleral spur. The color of the ciliary body ranges from a chocolate brown to a gray-white in lighter eyes, with many variations. The width of the ciliary body band depends upon the contour and location of the insertion of the iris root. Iris processes, colored light to dark brown, are fine pigmented strands crossing the scleral spur from the iris root to the functional trabecular meshwork (Fig. 11–10). Iris processes tend to be open and lacy in appearance, in contrast to more solid and uniform peripheral anterior synechiae, which are full-thickness attachments of the anterior iris face to the angle wall (Figs. 11–11 and 11–12). Prominent iris processes may make the view of the ciliary body difficult. Iris processes inserting above the trabecular meshwork are observed in anterior cleavage anomalies such as Axenfeld's syndrome and should be considered abnormal.

The scleral spur is seen as a prominent white-gray band between the ciliary body and the trabecular meshwork. This fibrous ring is the posterior lip of the scleral sulcus; Schlemm's canal lies just anterior to its border. The scleral spur represents an important gonioscopic landmark, since its visibility means that functioning trabecular meshwork is not obstructed in that quadrant.

The trabecular meshwork is seen as a pigmented band extending from the scleral spur to Schwalbe's line. It has been described as having a characteristic grayish, finely granular texture or a band of pigment granules slightly translucent in appearance.[5] The trabecular meshwork is generally darker in appearance over the functional trabecular meshwork adjacent to the scleral spur and less pigmented in the nonfunctional anterior third adjacent to Schwalbe's line. The trabecular meshwork is relatively nonpigmented in early childhood, with pigmentation increasing after puberty. The meshwork is a sieve-like structure composed of fibrocellular sheets that acts as a filter for the aqueous draining from the anterior chamber into the Schlemm's canal. The degree of pigmentation and the color of the trabecular meshwork is quite variable and ranges from almost white to dark brown. Schlemm's canal lies directly beneath the middle functional trabecular meshwork and cannot be seen gonioscopically unless it is filled with blood. If excessive force is used with the gonioscopic lens, blood will regurgitate into Schlemm's canal, where it appears as a pink or red band.

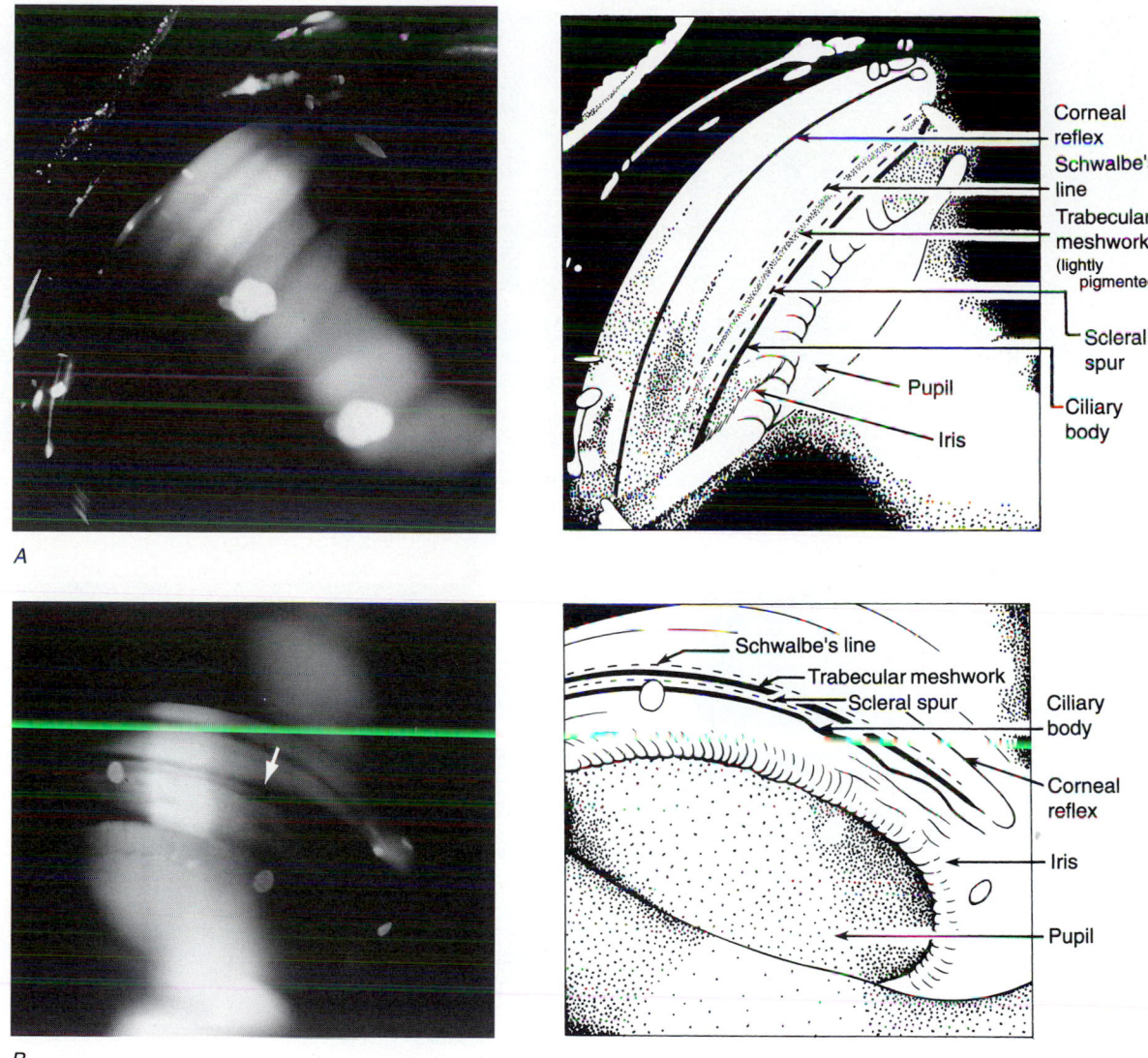

Figure 11–8. Normal angle anatomy. Note ciliary body, scleral spur, trabecular meshwork, and Schwalbe's line. The patient in *A* has very little pigmentation in the trabecular meshwork. The patient in *B* has a heavily pigmented trabecular meshwork. There may be considerable variation in the clinical appearance of the normal angle. (Courtesy of Tony Litwak, O.D.) (*See also Color Plate 4.*)

The anterior demarcation of the anterior chamber angle is Schwalbe's line, a ring of connective tissue fibers supported by collagen material and elastic fibers. Schwalbe's line represents the end of Descemet's membrane and the beginning of the trabecular meshwork; it may appear as a glistening white opaque line or be rather indistinct. Pigmentation may be found adjacent to Schwalbe's line (called Sampaolesi's line) and confused with the pigmented trabecular meshwork. The use of the focal line technique will aid the clinician in identifying this landmark. Schwalbe's line may be anteriorly displaced, allowing identification during routine slit-lamp examination as a posterior embryotoxin.

ANGLE GRADING SYSTEMS

It is important to record the gonioscopic appearance of the anterior chamber angle, including the angle configuration, the most posterior landmark observed, the degree of pigmentation, and abnormal structures or material present. There is no shortage of classification systems, but unfortunately they tend

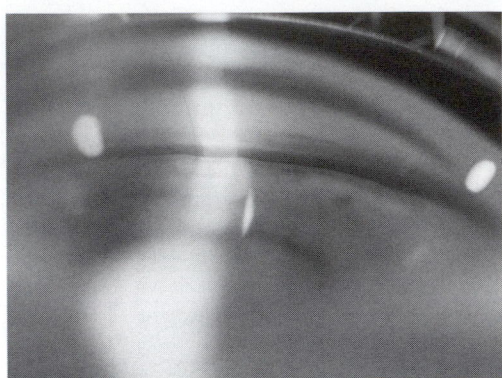

Figure 11–9. An image of the normal angle anatomy. All structures are visible. (Courtesy of Kelly Dignam, O.D.) (*See also Color Plate 5.*)

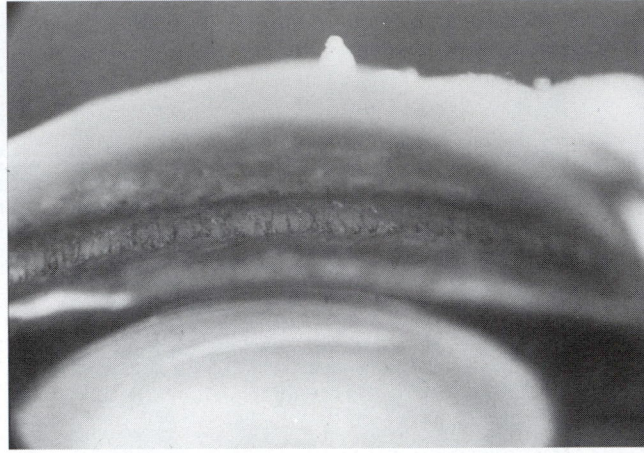

Figure 11–10. Iris processes are visible, obscuring some detail of other anterior angle structures. (Courtesy of Kelly Dignam, O.D.) (*See also Color Plate 6.*)

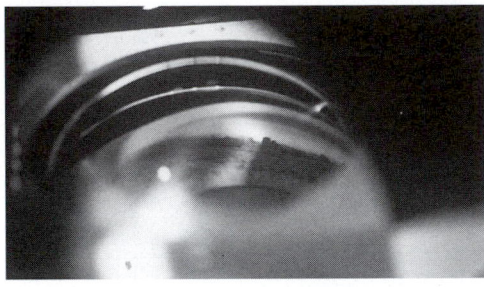

Figure 11–11. A peripheral anterior synechia. (Courtesy of Kelly Dignam, O.D.)

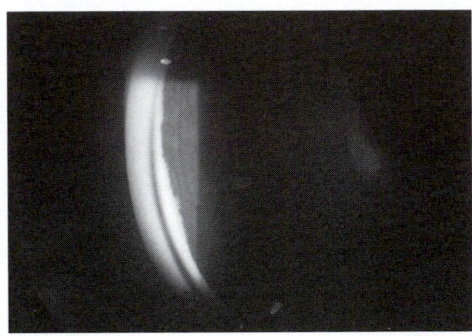

Figure 11–12. A low-lying peripheral anterior synechia. (Courtesy of Kelly Dignam, O.D.)

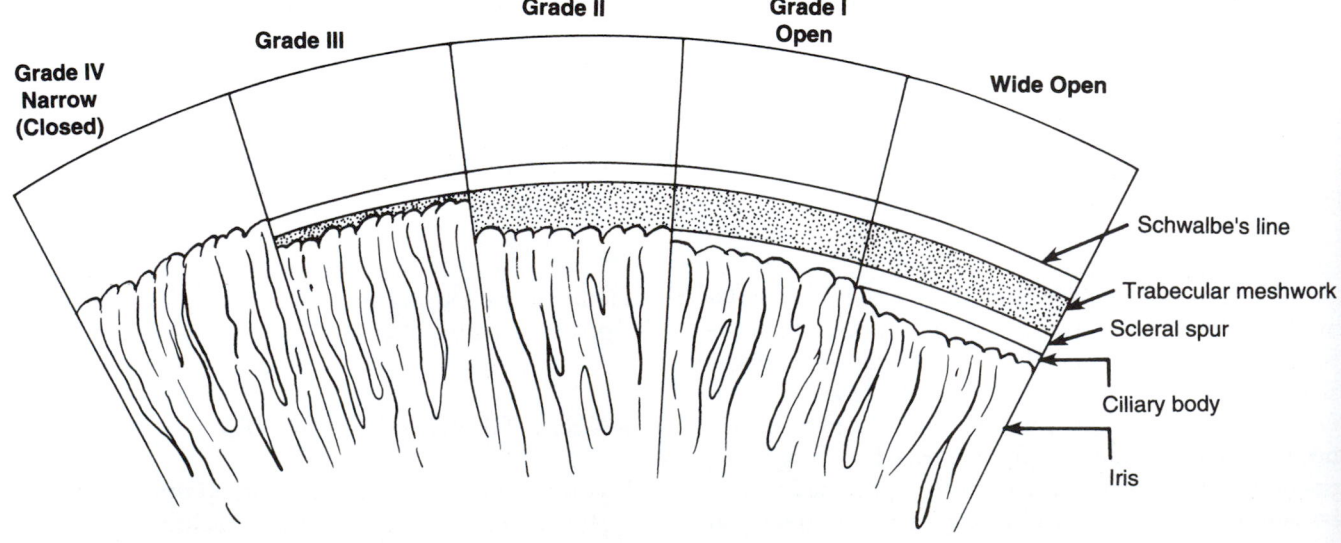

Figure 11–13. Scheie's angle classification; the grading system is based on the anatomical landmarks seen. This system is rarely used, as it is opposite to the more commonly used grading methods. (Modified with permission from Shields MB. *Textbook of Glaucoma*, 4th ed. Baltimore: Williams & Wilkins; 1998:183.)

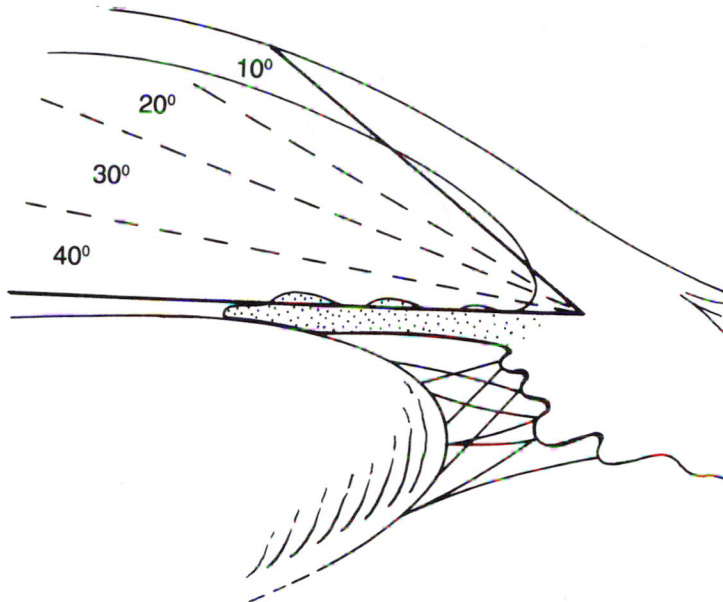

Figure 11–14. Schaefer angle classification. The grading system is based on the angular width between the posterior corneal surface and the anterior surface of the iris. The system also predicts the risk of angle closure. (Modified with permission from Shields MB. *Textbook of Glaucoma*, 4th ed. Baltimore: Williams & Wilkins; 1998:183.)

to be confusing and contradictory (i.e., a grading of zero may mean closed in one system and wide open in another). This can lead to confusion among clinicians and lack of uniformity. A written description of the angle with an accompanying diagram is often the most useful clinically. Some clinicians prefer to use a goniogram to document their gonioscopic observations, as this is an excellent method to record normal and abnormal findings.

Several different systems are used to grade the anterior chamber angle. The Scheie system grades the angle based upon the most posterior angle structure visualized from no structures seen (grade IV narrow, closed) to all structures seen (grade O, wide open).[6] Figure 11–13 shows the major grades of this classification system, which is interesting from a historic perspective but inadequately describes the configuration of the angle, and the numbering system (IV closed) is the opposite of other systems.

Figure 11–14 shows Shaffer's gonioscopic classification, which is based upon the angular width of the angle recess.[7] Shaffer's system grades a closed angle as zero, a moderately narrow angle of 20 degrees as grade 2, and a wide open angle of 45 degrees as grade 4. Shaffer's system attempts to predict the risk of closure, but there is no standard location for the iris frame of reference. Also, this system does not describe the depth of configuration of the angle recess.

Spaeth has developed a system using the evaluation of three variables, including angular width of the angle recess, configuration of the peripheral iris, and insertion of the iris root (Fig. 11–15).[8] Spaeth defines the location of the iris reference point in determining the angular width as the angle created by a line drawn tangentially to the inner surface of the trabecular meshwork and a line drawn tangentially to the iris surface one-third of the distance from the most peripheral portion of the iris. The iris insertion is graded from "A" to "E," where "A" is insertion onto the cornea and "E" is deep ciliary body. The angle width is recorded in degrees from 10 to 40 degrees. The contour of the most peripheral iris is recorded as "r" for regular (flat), "q" for queer (concave), and "s" for steep (convex). Pigment is graded 0 to 4+ and iris processes are described. Table 11–2 and Fig. 11–15 summarize Spaeth's angle grading system.

GONIOSCOPIC FINDINGS

A variety of normal variations and pathological findings may be observed during gonioscopy. Pigment should be evaluated in the angle and graded from 0 to 4+, with 0 representing no pigmentation and 4+ designating extensive pigmentation. If extensive pigmentation is noted in the angle, one should check

TABLE 11–2. SPAETH'S ANGLE GRADING SYSTEM

Grade	Description of Iris Insertion
A	Iris insertion on cornea
B	Insertion at trabecular meshwork
C	Insertion at scleral spur
D	Insertion at ciliary body
E	Deep ciliary body

Angle Width in Degrees	Peripheral Iris Contour
40	R: Regular, flat appearance
30	Q: Queer, concave iris
20	S: Steep, convex iris, narrow approach
10	

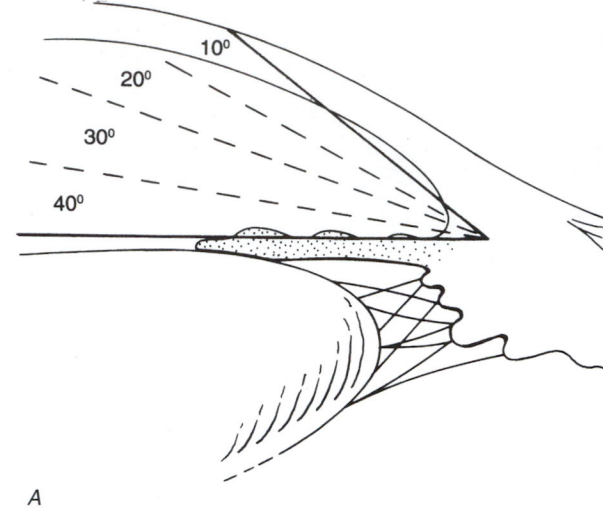

A

carefully for iris transillumination defects and a deposit of pigment located in a vertical pattern on the corneal endothelium (Krukenberg spindles), suggesting pigment dispersion syndrome (Fig. 11–16).

The angle should be evaluated for the presence of inflammatory material, blood, or ghost cells. Peripheral anterior synechiae (PAS) are broad-based adhesions that result from appositional angle closure, inflammation, trauma, or congenital conditions (Fig. 11–17). Table 11–3 lists some of the causes of PAS. Dynamic (compression) gonioscopy helps differentiate appositional closure without PAS from actual synechiae. It is important to do a gonioscopic examination at least yearly of a patient with narrow angles or previously diagnosed angle closure. The use of topical miotics may exacerbate a critically narrow angle. With extensive PAS, surgical intervention is often necessary to control intraocular pressure adequately.

Neovascularization of the angle may result from hypoxic conditions of the retina, such as proliferative diabetic retinopathy or central retinal vein occlusion (Figs. 11–18 and 11–19). The retinal hypoxia produces a vasoproliferative substance that induces neovascularization of the iris (usually beginning as fragile, feathery vessels at the pupillary margin) and independently in the angle. If prompt panretinal

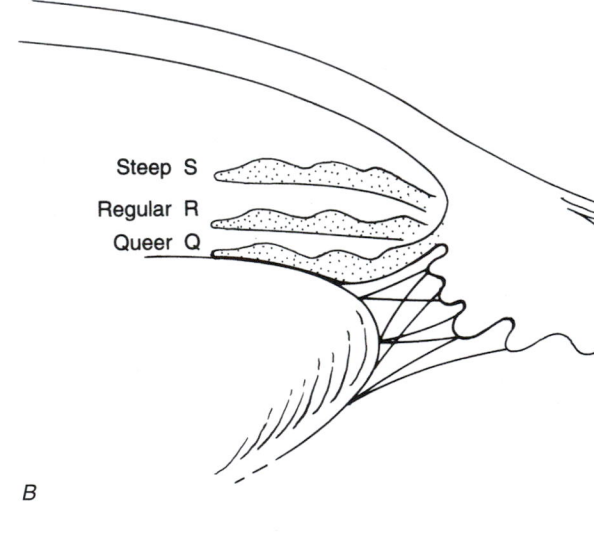

B

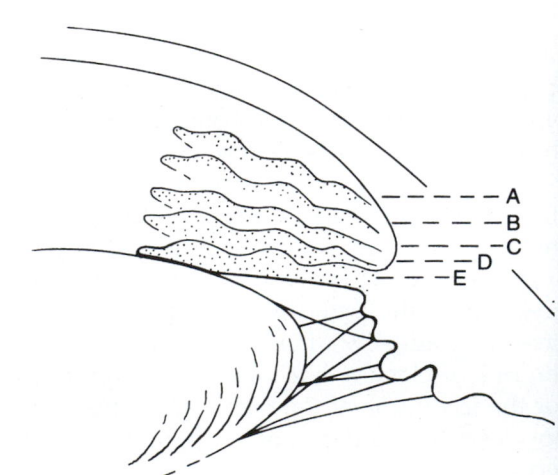

C

Figure 11–15. Spaeth's angle classification. The Spaeth system is ▶ a modification of the Schaefer classification. In addition to estimation of the angular width (*A*), the classification adds the configuration of the iris contour (*B*) and the insertion of the iris root into the angle (*C*). (Modified with permission from Shields MB. *Textbook of Glaucoma*, 4th ed. Baltimore: Williams & Wilkins; 1998:184.)

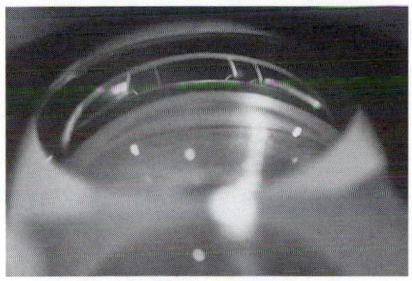

Figure 11–16. Fine, dense pigment is seen in the trabecular meshwork of this individual with pigment dispersion syndrome. (Courtesy of Kelly Dignam, O.D.)

TABLE 11–3. ETIOLOGY OF PERIPHERAL ANTERIOR SYNECHIAE (PAS)

Chronic iritis or uveitis
Chronic apposition angle closure
Angle neovascularization
Blunt trauma
Hyphema
Iridocorneal endothelia (ICE) syndromes[1]
Congenital anomalies
Complicated intraocular surgery
Flat anterior chamber after filtering surgery
Penetrating trauma

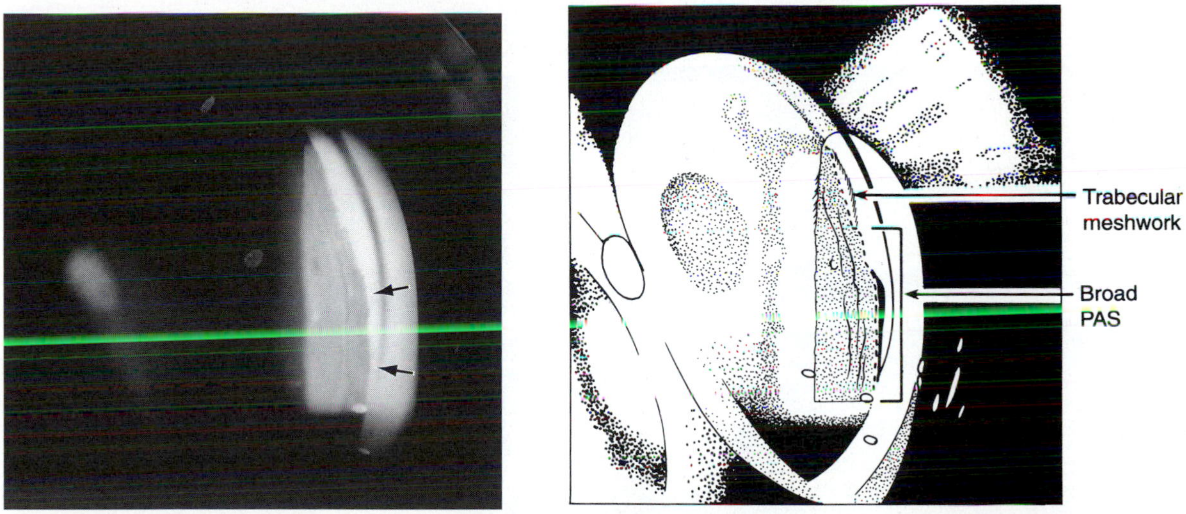

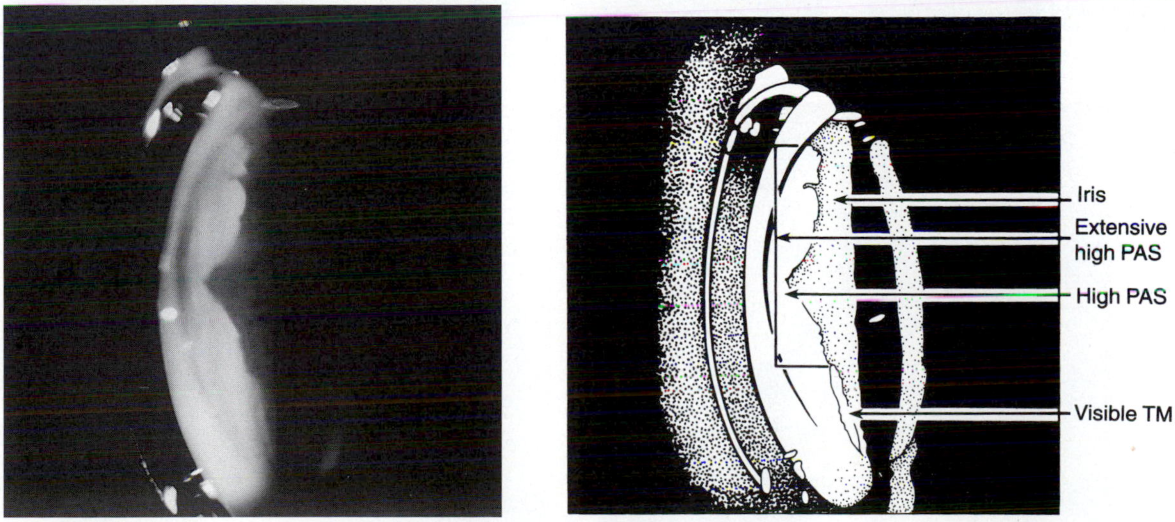

A

Trabecular meshwork

Broad PAS

B

Iris

Extensive high PAS

High PAS

Visible TM

Figure 11–17. Peripheral anterior synechiae (PAS) in a patient with chronic uveitis; PAS are broad adhesions of the peripheral iris into the trabecular meshwork. *B.* High PAS in a patient with a previously flat anterior chamber after glaucoma filtering surgery. The PAS extend well above Schwalbe's line. (Courtesy of Tony Litwak, O.D.)

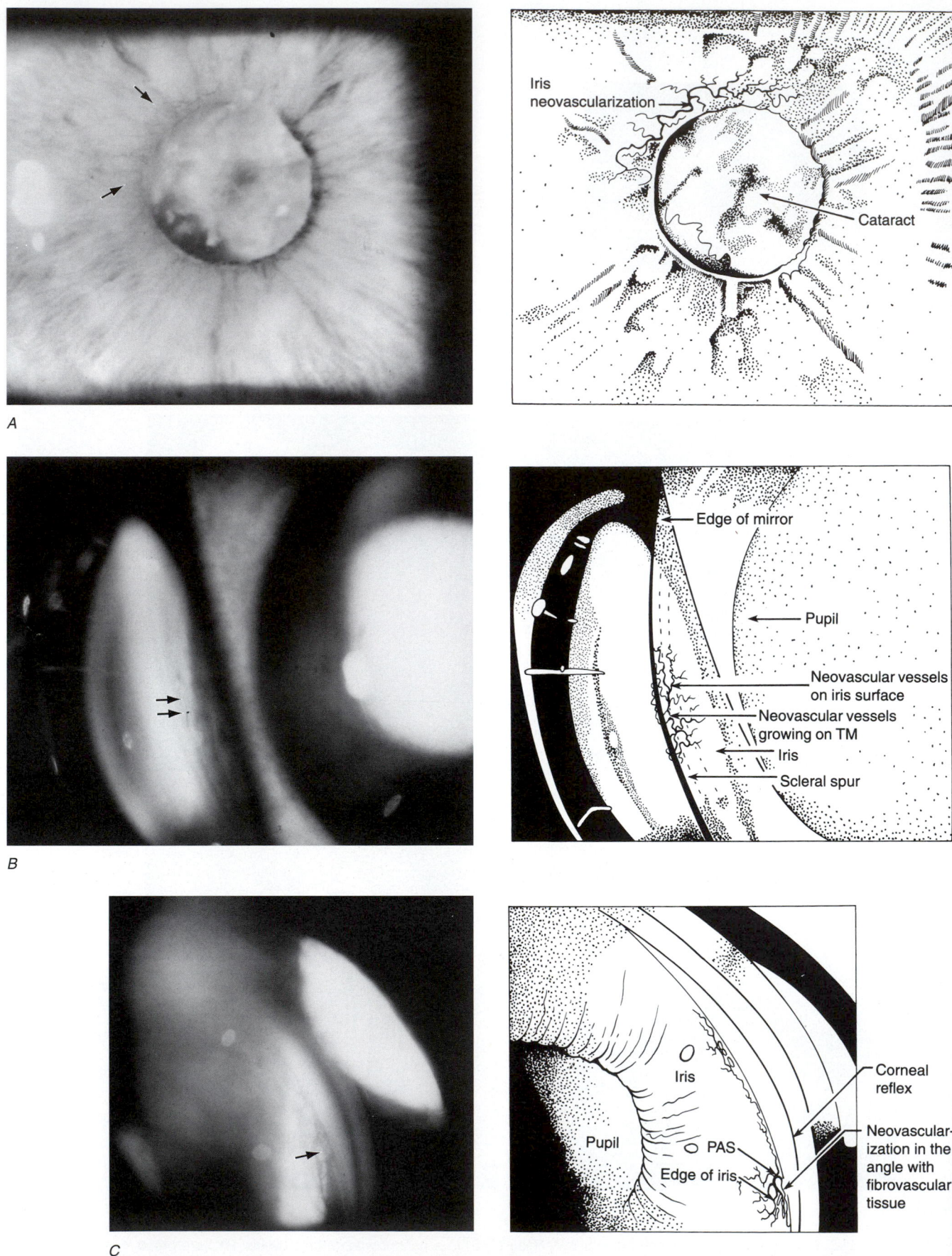

Figure 11–18. Iris neovascularization. Neovascular vessels typically occur at the pupillary margin of the iris (*A*) after an ischemic event to the retina. These vessels may grow into the angle (*B*) along with fibrovascular tissue forming PAS (*C*) and neovascular glaucoma. (Courtesy of Tony Litwak, O.D.). (*See also Color Plate 7.*)

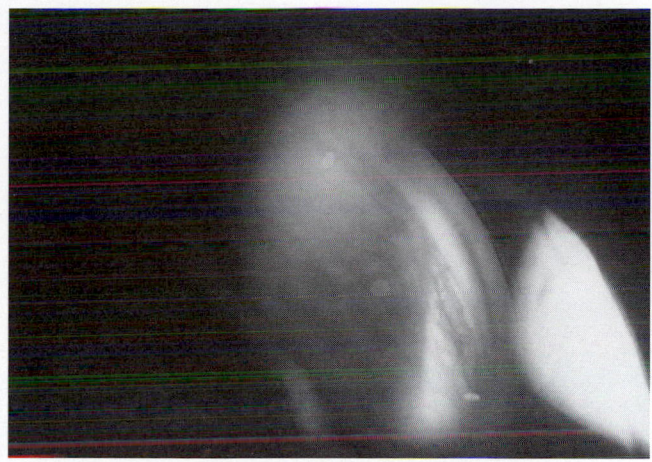

Figure 11–19. Neovascularization is visible in the anterior chamber angle. (Courtesy of Kelly Dignam, O.D.)

photocoagulation of the retina is not performed, the neovascularization will proceed across the iris onto the trabecular meshwork. Significant tractional forces from the fibrovascular tissue may contract, effectively closing the angle with elevation of the intraocular pressure.

Blunt trauma may cause a tear, known as angle recession, between the longitudinal and circular muscles of the ciliary body (Figs. 11–20 and 11–21). Gonioscopy will reveal an abnormally wide band of ciliary body in the quadrant with associated PAS. Angle recession may involve only one quadrant or be present in all 360 degrees. The eye should be carefully examined and followed, as traumatic glaucoma may develop years later (see Chap. 28). Blunt trauma may also cause hyphema from bleeding of the small branches of the major arterial circle of the iris.[9]

Regurgitation of blood into Schlemm's canal by excessive gonioscopic pressure has been described

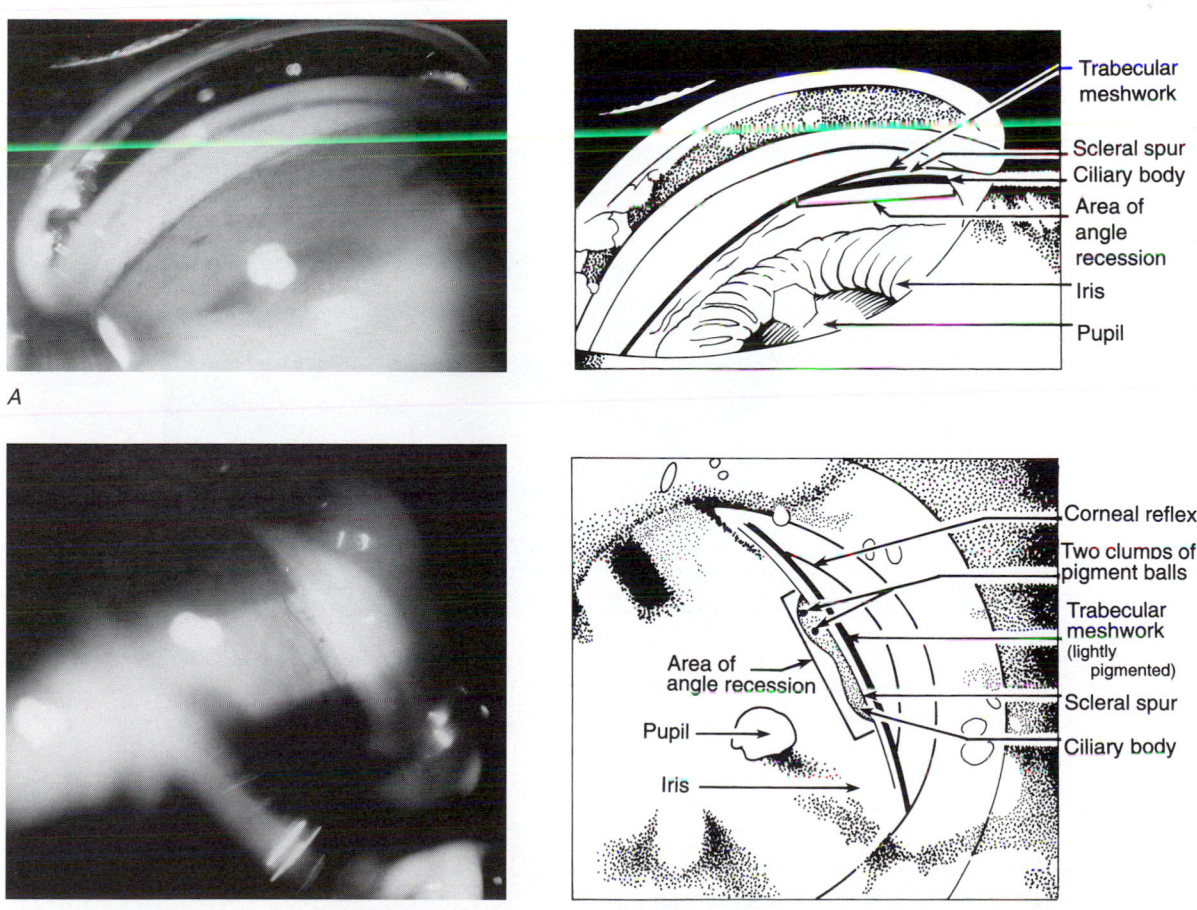

Figure 11–20. Angle recession after blunt trauma. *A.* Note visibility of scleral spur and ciliary body in area of angle recess. *B.* Angle recession or clumps of pigment in the angle are indicators of possible damage to the trabecular meshwork and development of traumatic glaucoma. (Courtesy of Tony Litwak, O.D.) (*See also Color Plate 8.*)

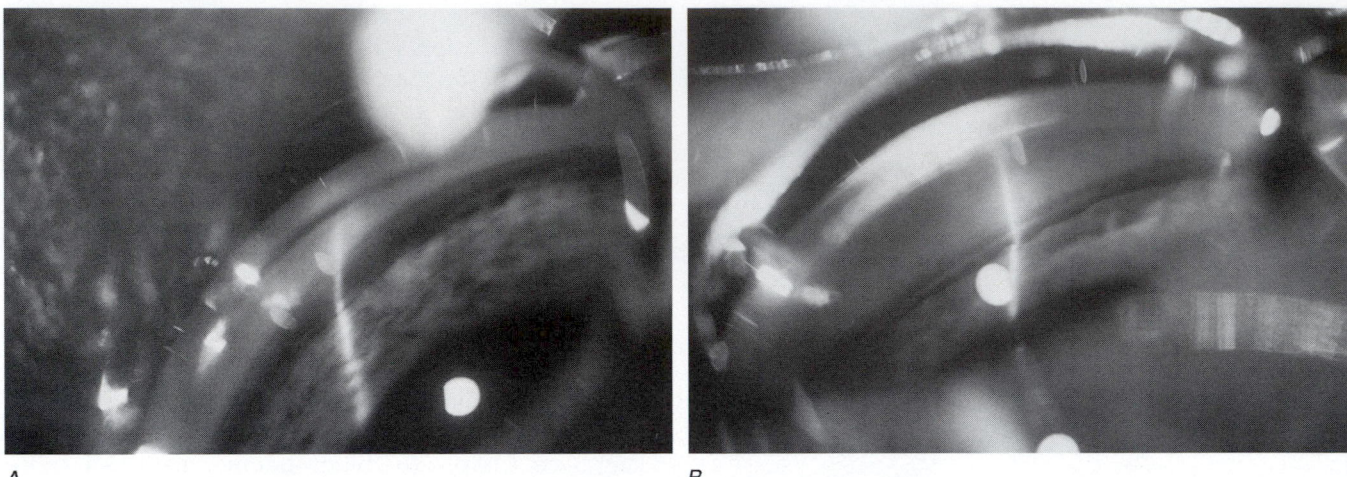

A   B

Figure 11–21. *A.* An angle recession is seen in the superior view of this patient, who suffered trauma. Note the extent to which the ciliary body is visible, especially in comparison to the fellow eye. *B.* The fellow eye of this patient. Note the normal-appearing angle with a visible ciliary body. (Courtesy of Kelly Dignam, O.D.) (*See also Color Plate 9.*)

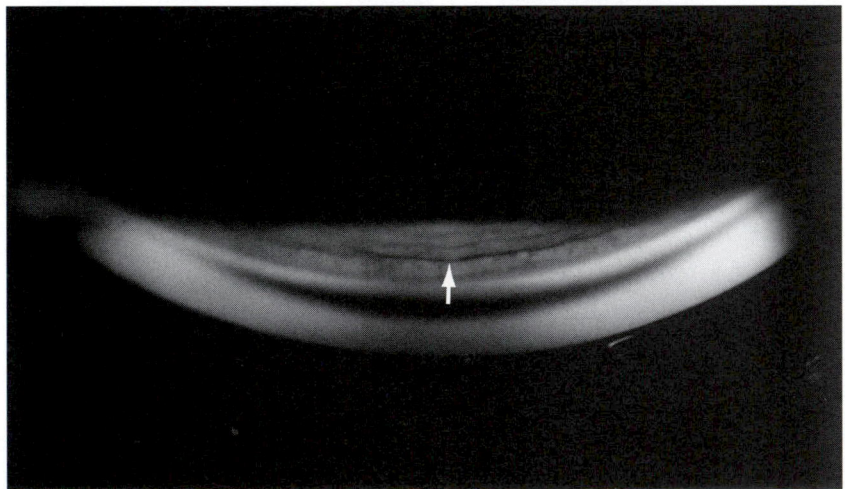

Figure 11–22. Blood in Schlemm's canal, a sign of elevated episcleral venous pressure. Schlemm's canal lies directly behind the trabecular meshwork and is not normally visible unless blood is present. (Courtesy of Tony Litwak, O.D.)

(Fig. 11–22). Spontaneous blood reflux into Schlemm's canal may be caused by elevated episcleral venous pressure, and one must rule out thyroid eye disease, superior vena cava syndrome, retrobulbar tumor, Sturge-Weber syndrome, arteriovenous fistulas, and orbital varices.

CONCLUSION

Gonioscopy is a critical technique in the diagnosis and management of glaucoma and should be performed on all glaucoma patients, glaucoma suspects, and individuals with anatomic narrow angles. Careful

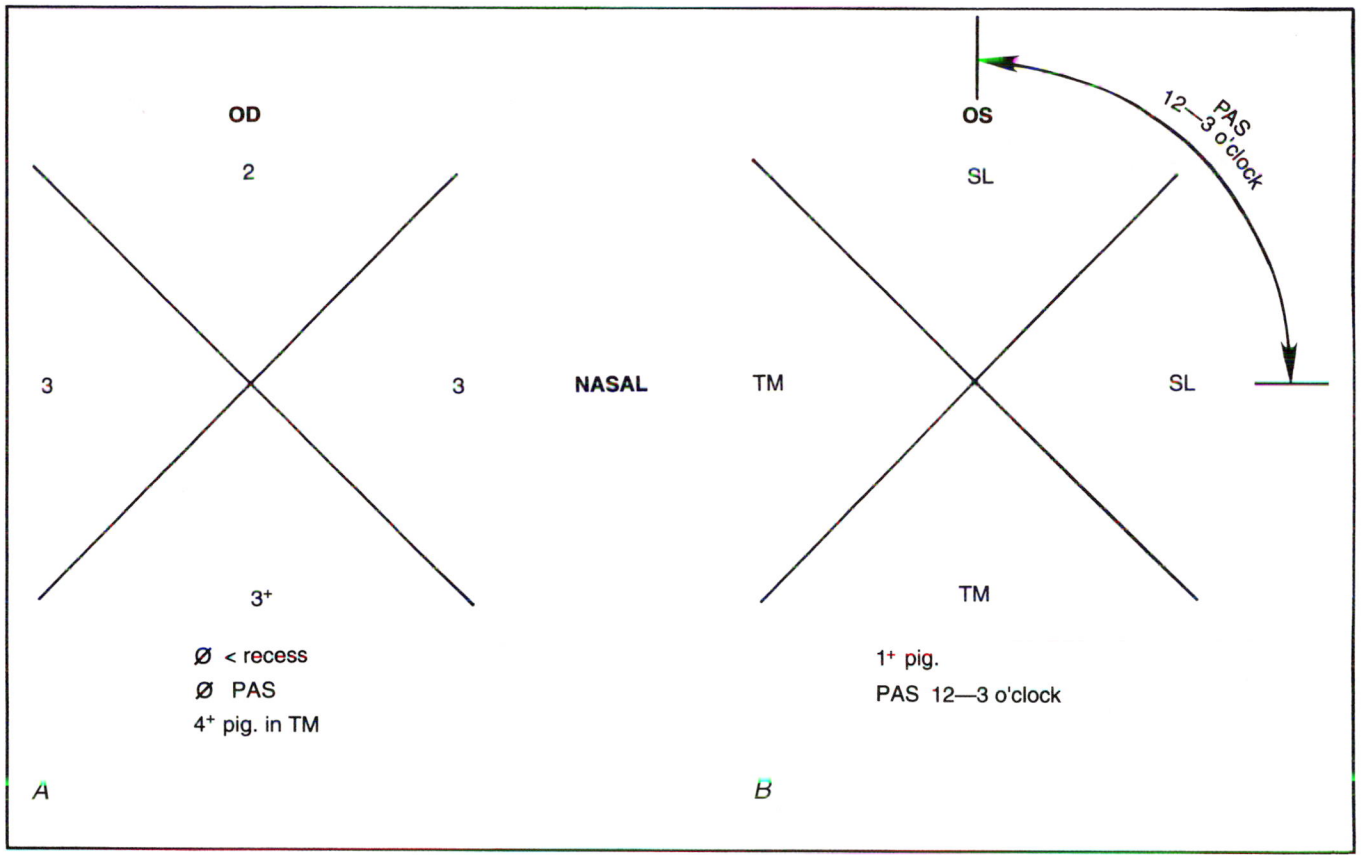

Figure 11–23. Documentation of gonioscopy findings. *A.* Crossed lines can be used for entering numerical grading classifications corresponding to the superior, temporal, inferior, and nasal quadrants. *B.* The most posterior angle structure seen can be recorded in a similar manner. Abnormal angle findings (such as pigmentation in the trabecular meshwork, PAS, angle neovascularization, angle recess) should be recorded. When these are not present, negative documentation is important.

documentation of the gonioscopic observations should be made in the patient's chart, using a uniform grading system (Fig. 11–23).

REFERENCES

1. Gorin G, Posner A. *Slit-Lamp Gonioscopy*, 3rd ed. Baltimore: Williams & Wilkins; 1967.
2. Casser L, Fingeret M, Woodcome HT. *Atlas of Primary Eyecare Procedures*. Norwalk, CT: Appleton & Lange; 1998.
3. Palmberg P. Gonioscopy. In: Ritch R, Shields, MB, Krupin T, eds. *The Glaucomas, I: Basic Sciences*, 2nd ed. St. Louis: Mosby; 1996.
4. Forbes M. Indentation gonioscopy and efficacy of iridectomy in angle closure glaucoma. *Trans Am Ophthalmol Soc.* 1974;74:488–515.
5. Grant WM, Schuman JS. The angle of the anterior chamber. In: Epstein DL et al, eds. *Chandler and Grant's Glaucoma*, 4th ed. Baltimore: Williams & Wilkins; 1997.
6. Scheie HG. Width and pigmentation of the angle of the anterior chamber. A system of grading by gonioscopy. *Am J Ophthalmol.* 1957;58:510.
7. Shaffer RN. Symposium: Primary glaucomas: III. Gonioscopy, ophthalmoscopy, and perimetry. *Trans Am Acad Ophthalmol Otol.* 1960;62:112.
8. Spaeth GL. The normal development of the human anterior chamber angle: A new system of descriptive grading. *Trans Ophthalmol Soc UK.* 1971;91:709.
9. Shields MB. *Textbook of Glaucoma*, 4th ed. Baltimore: Williams & Wilkins; 1998:329.

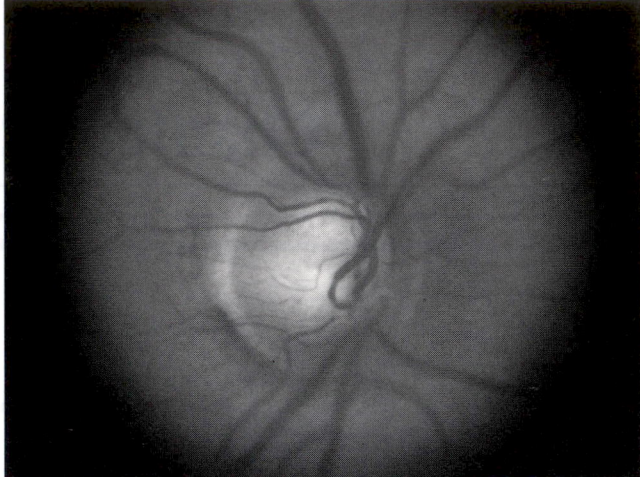

A

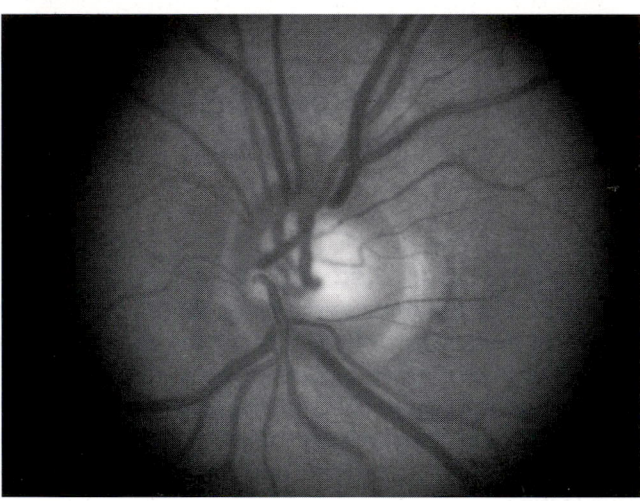

B

Figure 12–1. *A.* Optic nerve head asymmetry is present as well as a slightly enlarged optic disc area: OD>OS. Extensive cupping is judged to be 0.70/0.75 OD, with inferior overpass cupping and superior baring of the circumlinear vessel. *(See also Color Plate 10.)* *B.* Cupping OS is judged to be 0.65/0.60, with a slight temporal slope. Peripapillary atrophy is also present, with zone β approximately 5% of the disc area OD; zone α 5%; and zone β 5% of the disc area OS. No defects in the nerve fiber layer, hemorrhages, or areas of vasoconstriction are seen OD or OS. *(See also Color Plate 11.)*

TABLE 12–1. SYSTEMATIC APPROACH TO ASSESSMENT OF THE OPTIC NERVE HEAD

Optic disc size and shape
Physiological cuppimg

Generalized Signs of Optic Nerve Damage
   Generalized enlargement of the cup-to-disc ratio
   Increased depth of cupping
   Saucerization
   Vertical elongation of the cup-to-disc ratio
   Cup-to-disc asymmetry
   Loss of the neuroretinal rim
   Parapapillary atrophy
   Laminar dot sign
   Pallor

Localized Signs of Optic Nerve Damage
   Focal notching
   Acquired pit of the optic nerve

Abnormalities of the Retinal Vasculature
   Hemorrhage of the nerve fiber layer
   Focal narrowing
   Vascular attenuation
   Baring of the circumlinear vessels
   Overpass cupping
   Nasalization of the retinal vasculature
   Bayonet sign
   Optic disc shunt vessels

to be of similar size to those in patients with open-angle glaucoma (OAG).[13] Another study suggested that the optic discs in patients with pseudoexfoliation syndrome and pseudoexfoliation glaucoma were significantly smaller in size than those in patients with OAG, but in all other aspects similar.[12] Comparisons between glaucomatous eyes showed that the disc area was generally largest in eyes with normal-tension glaucoma.[13,14] Investigators have suggested that the lamina cribrosa of a larger disc may be more suscepti-

ble to poor perfusion and may therefore have a lower threshold for damage due to intraocular pressure (IOP). Another report was unable to confirm this finding.[15]

Evaluation of the size of the optic nerve head in severe myopia showed that the disc area varied with the degree of myopia for refractive errors greater than −8D. Disc area was found to increase with the degree of myopia for individuals with severe myopia but was independent of refractive error for those with mild to moderate myopia.[16,17]

Clinically, differences in the size and area of the optic disc are important. Interocular differences can help to explain corresponding cup-to-disc asymmetry and variations in neuroretinal rim area. Practitioners can roughly estimate the size of the optic disc and specify its shape using a technique described by Gross and Drance.[18] These investigators determined that the smallest aperture of a two aperture or middle sized aperture of a three aperture Welch Allyn ophthalmoscope. When the 5-degree aperture is positioned at the anterior focal point of the eye (17 mm in front of the cornea), a circular spot of light approximately 1.5 mm in diameter and 1.8 mm² in area is projected onto the retina. This circular image is independent of the refractive error or axial length of the eye. A disc that has an area substantially larger than this spot of light can be interpreted to be unusually large. Careful comparison between the two eyes can reveal an asymmetry in optic disc area that accounts for differences in other qualitative and quantitative characteristics (Fig. 12–2A and B).

Physiological Cupping

Physiological cupping corresponds to the congenital depression in the center of the optic nerve head created by the absence of neural tissue and glial elements. The mean cup-to-disc ratio in a normal population was previously described as 0.40 with a Gaussian distribution[19] (0.39 ± 0.28 in the horizontal meridian and 0.34 ± 0.25 in the vertical meridian[4]).

The size of the physiological cup is determined in part by heredity, in both a multifactorial and a poly-

genic fashion.[20,22] Physiological cupping is also strongly correlated with the size of the optic disc[4,21] and is generally symmetrical.[19,22,23]

Studies have shown significant differences between physiological cupping in various races. Patients of African descent were found to have a larger optic disc area and corresponding cup-to-disc ratio than Caucasian patients.[24–26] One study[26] found the differences in the vertical cup-to-disc ratio to be clinically significant, while another found both the horizontal and vertical cup-to-disc ratios to be different in these two populations.[24,25]

The effect of age on physiological cupping is unclear. Some studies have suggested that cupping changes with age,[4,19,27–29] while other investigations have found insignificant changes in cup-to-disc ratio with age.[24] Schwartz et al. documented a small but significant increase in cup-to-disc ratio with age. These investigators emphasized that individual variation can account for considerable changes in the cup-to-disc ratio over time, and that this progression could be diagnosed as a pathological finding in some eyes.[19]

Clinicians must differentiate between congenital and acquired changes of the optic nerve head. In physiological cupping, the neuroretinal rim is generally uniformly thick and full, with a distinct border. Other intrapapillary and parapapillary characteristics can help to distinguish physiological cupping from progressive optic neuropathy and are discussed below.

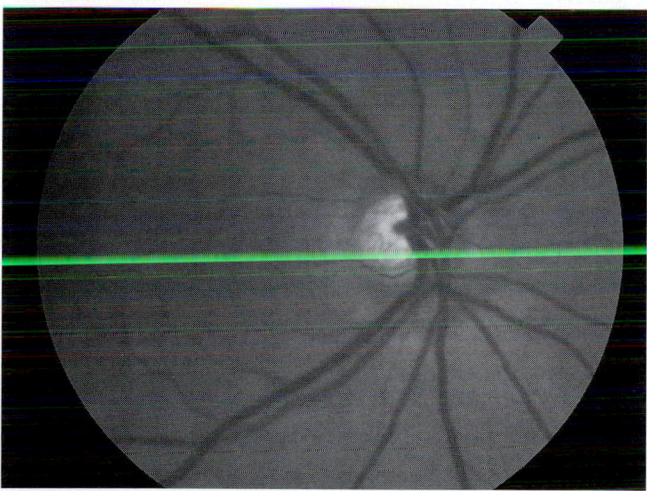

A

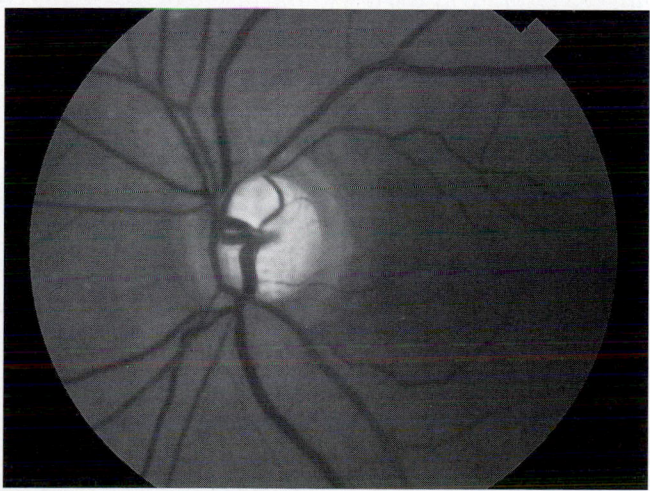

B

Figure 12–2. Cup-to-disc asymmetry is present, but it is related to the significant asymmetry in optic disc size. The left optic nerve (*B*) is twice the size of the right optic nerve (*A*). *(See also Color Plate 12.)*

GENERALIZED SIGNS OF GLAUCOMATOUS NERVE DAMAGE

General Enlargement of the Cup-to-Disc Ratio

Acquired optic nerve cupping may be superimposed upon preexisting physiological cupping, so that generalized enlargement of the cup-to-disc ratio may be the initial sign of glaucomatous damage (Fig. 12–3). Initially, the temporal region of the disc demonstrates loss of neuroretinal rim tissue with expansion toward superior and inferior regions of the optic disc.[30] This pattern of optic disc damage occurs more frequently in younger patients with glaucoma and also in patients with higher pretreatment pressures.[31]

Pederson and Anderson have reported that concentric enlargement of the cup was the most common type of change in progressive glaucoma, occurring in 79% of patients. This disc change was found to precede visual field loss by several years. These investigators concluded that treatment was indicated for eyes with progressive nerve damage in the presence

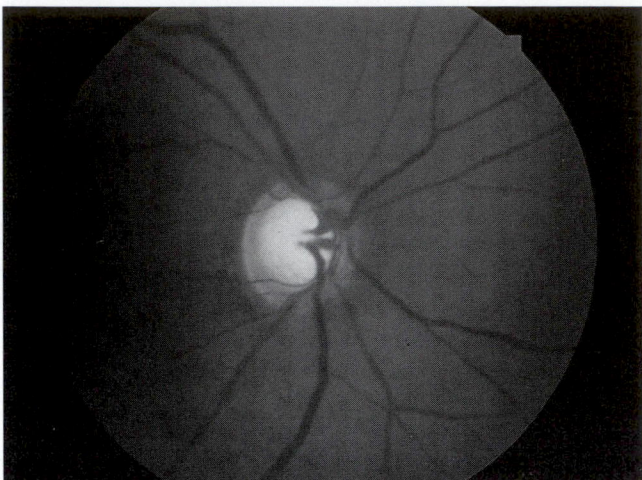

Figure 12–3. Moderate concentric enlargement of the optic cup. The width of the neuroretinal rim is relatively uniform around the nerve circumference.

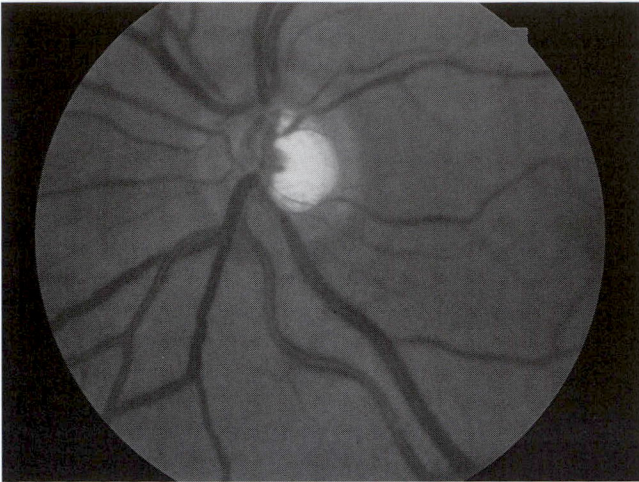

Figure 12–4. Concentric cupping with increased depth of cupping. Although this is more easily evaluated stereoscopically, vessel deviation and cup contour can provide valuable clues.

of normal fields.[32] Generalized enlargement of the cup-to-disc ratio was more commonly observed in normal-tension glaucoma[15] as well as in primary open-angle glaucoma.[33] Planimetric analysis of the neuroretinal rim area confirmed diffuse loss as the most frequent pattern of neuroretinal rim loss in early glaucoma.[34] In ocular hypertension, eyes that progressed to visual field loss over time were shown to develop significant generalized enlargement of the cup-to-disc ratio more frequently than those eyes that did not develop visual field defects.[35]

Concentric enlargement of the cup-to-disc ratio has been associated with other optic nerve conditions in addition to glaucoma. Acquired cupping of the optic nerve head has been attributed to optic nerve infarction, hereditary optic neuropathies, optic neuritis, trauma, and compressive disease. Compressive lesions can simulate glaucoma by causing acquired visual field defects as well as increased cupping.[36]

Increased Depth of Disc Cupping

Increased depth of cupping is not a specific finding for glaucoma, (Fig. 12–4). Depth of cupping can be affected by factors including disc area, ethnicity, refractive error, and severity of glaucoma. A previous study has shown that depth of disc cupping was independent of cup size,[2] while another observed that greater disc area was associated with increased cup volume and depth.[26] African Americans were found to have a greater cup depth relative to Hispanics, Asians, and Caucasians.[24] A study of severe myopia and glaucoma determined that cup depth was shallower for high myopes than for low to moderate myopes.[17] An experimental monkey study showed that cup depth was significantly associated with loss of nerve fiber

layer in an investigation comparing glaucomatous and nonglaucomatous eyes.[37]

In the advanced stages of glaucoma, the optic nerve may demonstrate "beanpot cupping."[38,39] The floor of the cup appears to be bowed posteriorly and the wall of the cup appears to be excavated (Fig. 12–5).

Saucerization

Saucerization of the optic nerve head is observed as a diffuse, shallow cupping that extends to the disc margin (Fig. 12–6). It becomes more difficult to quantify the degree of optic nerve cupping in these eyes. An investigation will show a difference in height between

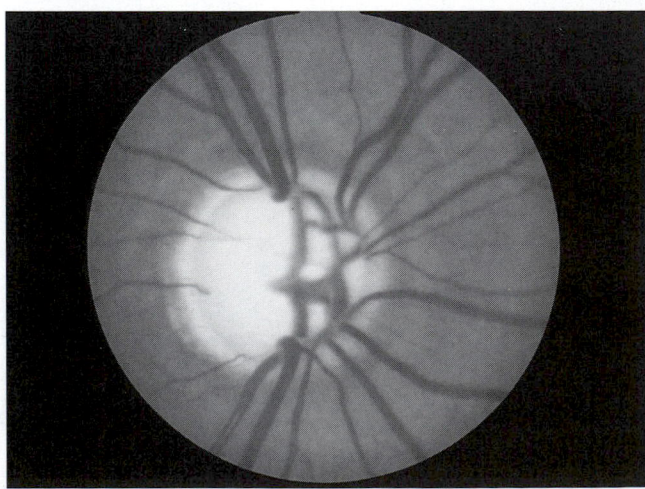

Figure 12–5. Absolute optic nerve cupping, demonstrating a beanpot appearance. Blood vessels angulate over the edge of the disc rim and follow the wall of the cup, disappearing from view before progressing along the floor of the cup.

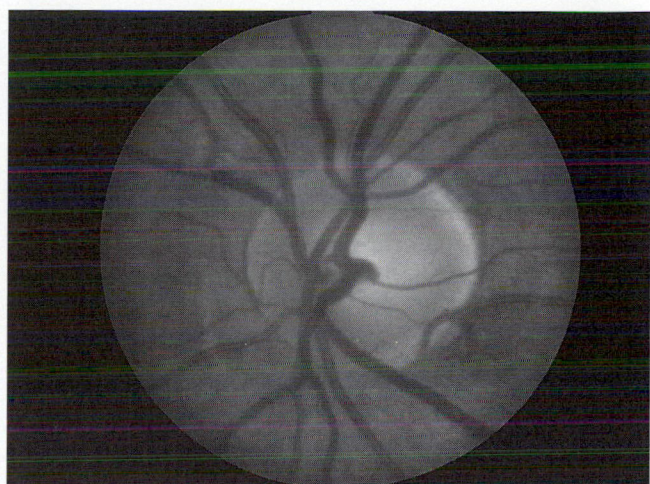

Figure 12–6. Saucerization makes estimation of the cup-to-disc ratio difficult because of the shallow erosion of the neuroretinal rim.

the midpoint of the neuroretinal rim and a point on the retina just outside the edge of the disc, which will be less in glaucomatous eyes than in control eyes. Relative to the optic disc edge, the neuroretinal rim was thinned from the superior nasal sector to the inferior position in glaucomatous eyes. Saucerization has been suggested as an early sign of glaucoma.[40]

Vertical Elongation

Vertical elongation develops secondarily to the loss of the neuroretinal rim at the superior and inferior poles.[10,41,45] Vertical elongation greater than 0.2 has been suggested as an acquired change that is infrequent in patients without field loss. Glaucomatous eyes with visual field defects have demonstrated vertical elongation of cupping more often than normal eyes.[42] This pattern of glaucomatous nerve damage occurred less frequently than generalized enlargement of the cup in early glaucoma, but it is clinically significant, because this change can precede the development of visual field defects by several years.[32] A significant number of eyes that did not initially demonstrate this finding might develop vertical elongation with progression of the disease, even though the first changes were observed as generalized enlargement, focal notching, or both.[43]

Normally, the horizontal cup-to-disc ratio is greater than the vertical cup-to-disc ratio. Therefore, optic nerves with vertical elongation should be considered suspect for glaucoma.[4,27,30] In a population with ocular hypertension, a change in the vertical cup-to-disc ratio of at least 0.10 was found to be a significant predictor for the development of visual field loss, progressive optic nerve damage, or both.[44] Reports evaluating vertical elongation with age present conflicting results: One study found a mild associa-

tion between increasing vertical elongation and age,[11] but this was not observed in another study.[24]

Clinically, vertical elongation is a significant acquired change that can be associated with progressive nerve head damage. Other causes for apparent vertical elongation should be ruled out, including an oblong nerve head or the presence of significant astigmatic refractive error.

Cup-to-Disc Asymmetry

Unusual cup-to-disc asymmetry may occur if the cup area in one eye is exceptionally large or the cup area in the fellow eye is exceptionally small. A cup-to-disc asymmetry of 0.2 or less has been observed in 96% of eyes.[4] Further, a cup-to-disc difference of more than 0.2 between fellow eyes occurs in only 1% of a normal population, and a difference of greater than 0.1 between fellow eyes occurs in only 8%.[22] Cup-to-disc asymmetry is generally considered clinically significant when it is greater than 0.20.

Cup-to-disc asymmetry occurs commonly in glaucomatous eyes[23] but may be attributed to other congenital or acquired conditions. Asymmetry of the optic disc area or significant anisometropia can help to explain differences in cupping.

Congenital conditions may cause an apparent asymmetry in cup-to-disc ratio. An optic nerve with prominent optic disc drusen may appear to be less cupped than the fellow eye, while a colobomatous disc or a disc with "morning-glory syndrome" may exhibit significantly greater cupping than the fellow eye. Compressive lesions of the optic chiasm and optic nerves (e.g., pituitary adenoma, meningioma, craniopharyngioma, or aneurysm) may cause significant asymmetry in cup-to-disc area as well as visual compromise.[36]

Loss of Neuroretinal Rim

Loss of the neuroretinal rim in glaucoma can precede visible changes in the optic nerve head. An animal model demonstrated that the neuroretinal rim area was correlated with loss of nerve fiber layer.[37] If loss of nerve fiber layer and neuroretinal rim occurs in a generalized fashion, concentric enlargement of the cup will result. Localized loss may manifest as vertical elongation or focal notching of the neuroretinal rim (Fig. 12–7).

The neuroretinal rim area in normal eyes can vary up to sixfold,[4] with the average area reported as 2.26 ± 0.58 mm^2. Morphological studies have shown that the neuroretinal rim is generally wider inferiorly than superiorly or nasally, with the width of the temporal rim smallest.[4,10,45] When glaucomatous loss of the neuroretinal rim occurred, the inferotemporal region was affected early in the course of the disease. This

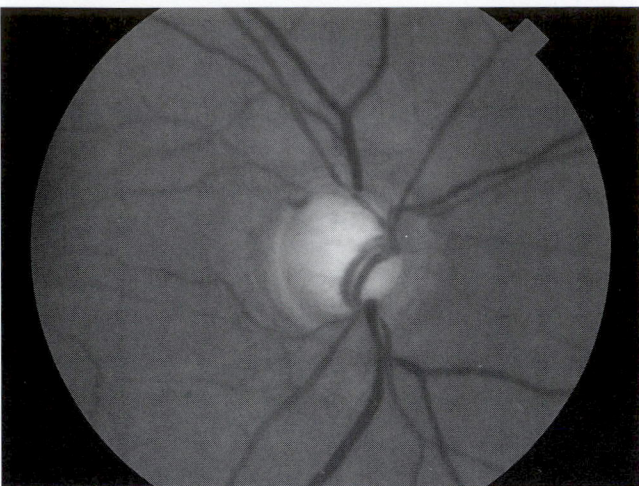

Figure 12–7. Advanced loss of the neuroretinal rim is observed by the loss in temporal rim tissue, with associated changes in vessel contour. The superior temporal rim is significantly damaged: There is also a hemorrhage of the nerve fiber layer.

neuroretinal rim loss was followed by changes to the superotemporal, temporal, inferonasal, and superonasal sectors. This alteration in the configuration of the neuroretinal rim corresponded to morphological changes in the lamina cribrosa.[45] A planimetric study of patterns of neuroretinal rim area loss in early glaucoma showed that diffuse loss occurred most frequently. Other less common patterns of neuroretinal rim loss included multisectorial and selective inferotemporal defects.[34] In glaucomatous eyes, the inferotemporal rim was observed to be thinner than the superotemporal rim.[57] Progressive loss of the neuroretinal rim has also been observed in patients with ocular hypertension. This change has been useful in predicting the conversion of these patients to glaucomatous discs, or visual field changes.[44]

The neuroretinal rim area can be affected by disc size[26,46] and age. Race is not a factor.[26] A significant normal age-related loss of rim area was observed in a study comparing young and elderly populations.[46] Investigators have suggested that studies evaluating rim-to-disc ratio instead of neuro-rim area are more sensitive in differentiating age-related changes from disease-related changes over time.[47]

Even when normal age-related loss of the neuroretinal rim area was considered, there was more rapid loss of rim tissue in glaucomatous eyes and eyes of glaucoma suspects.[48] A planimetric study of neuroretinal rim loss in glaucomatous eyes with and without initial visual field defect showed that the rate of loss was similar for both groups. Progression of optic nerve damage occurred more frequently than changes in the visual field for patients without initial

visual field defects. In early glaucoma, careful examination of the optic nerve was especially important due to the high ratio of disc change to field change.[49]

Pressure-dependent loss of the neuroretinal rim was also found to be significant in cases of normal-tension glaucoma (NTG). After correction for optic disc size, the neuroretinal rim area decreased with increasing intraocular pressure (IOP) even when IOP was less than 21 mmHg. This study suggested that intraocular pressure plays a role in nerve damage even though the optic nerve damage in NTG has been suggested to be vascular in origin. Based on these findings, these investigators concluded that IOP should be lowered in NTG to prevent further progression of optic neuropathy.[50]

Clinically, assessment of the neuroretinal rim can be affected by the presence of a temporal crescent or by zones of parapapillary atrophy. Evaluation can be further complicated by an anomalous insertion of the optic nerve, including the oblique insertion observed in myopic eyes. Disc size plays an important role in the configuration of the neuroretinal rim and should be carefully assessed. A description of contour and profile of the neuroretinal rim can help in monitoring progressive nerve head changes.

Parapapillary Atrophy

Parapapillary atrophy is a nonspecific nerve head sign[56] corresponding to areas of irregular pigmentation adjacent to the optic disc in normal and glaucomatous eyes.[51] Areas of parapapillary atrophy have been classified as zone alpha and zone beta.[52] Zone alpha occurs outside of zone beta and appears as irregular parapapillary pigmentation (Fig. 12–8). Zone alpha may represent a precursor to zone beta in glaucomatous eyes and should be noted as a significant finding.[56]

Zone beta represents the chorioscleral crescent that occurs in conjunction with retraction of retinal pigment epithelium. There is increased visibility of the choroidal vessels or exposure of sclera. Irregular pigmentation may also be present. Zone beta rarely occurs without an adjacent area of zone alpha and has been suggested to be found in some normal eyes.[53,54] This area was found to correspond histologically to an area with loss of the retinal pigment epithelium and overlying photoreceptors.[54]

Parapapillary atrophy occurs more frequently in glaucomatous eyes[55,56,58] and has been shown to correspond to diffuse loss of nerve fiber layer and shallow cupping of the optic disc.[58] Parapapillary atrophy was not related to refractive error when high myopes were excluded from the evaluation.[57] But caution should be observed in patients with severe myopia (refractive error greater than −8D), since a larger area for zone

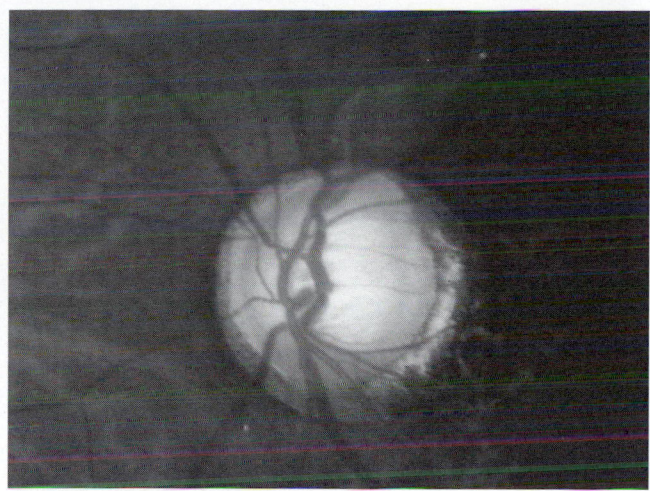

Figure 12–8. The darker area distal to the scleral crescent is zone alpha (α). Irregular parapapillary pigmentation is present.

beta would be an expected finding in these patients with[17] or without glaucoma.[16]

Parapapillary atrophy had good predictive value in distinguishing between normal and glaucomatous eyes.[57] In normal eyes, zone alpha was generally larger than zone beta. Both zones were widest in the temporal sector and narrowest in the nasal sector in normal eyes.[52,58] Zone beta was found to occur more frequently in glaucomatous eyes, and both zones were larger when glaucomatous eyes were compared with normal eyes (Fig. 12–9). Parapapillary atrophy occurred to a greater extent temporally in glaucomatous eyes; however, the nasal sector was the most clinically significant in differentiating between normal and glaucomatous eyes. Further, the extent and frequency of parapapillary

atrophy was found to increase with the severity of glaucoma.[52,58]

Parapapillary atrophy was observed more frequently in NTG than in either primary open-angle glaucoma (POAG) or ocular hypertension.[59,60] Ischemia may be a factor in the development of parapapillary atrophy in these patients. This finding was more often associated with advanced optic nerve damage and progressive glaucoma than with stable glaucoma or ocular hypertension.[51] When eyes were matched for the severity of neuroretinal rim loss, there was no significant difference between the extent and area of parapapillary atrophy in eyes with NTG and POAG.[60]

When eyes with ocular hypertension were evaluated, the area of parapapillary atrophy was larger than in normal eyes.[61] A recent study showed that both an increased parapapillary-to-disc area and increased zone beta-to-disc area were associated with conversion of ocular hypertension to glaucoma.[44,62] Further, these factors seemed to correlate positively with the development of glaucomatous optic nerve changes, visual field loss, or both. The zone alpha-to-disc area parameter was less significant as a predictive factor.[44] This progression of parapapillary atrophy was more frequent in patients with a positive family history of glaucoma and also a larger initial area and extent of zone beta.[62]

The presence of zone beta or a large zone alpha should suggest glaucomatous optic neuropathy. When compared to nonglaucomatous optic neuropathies, it was found that parapapillary atrophy was less frequent in nonglaucomatous optic neuropathies and was observed with a smaller zone beta.

Patients with a diagnosis of glaucoma or risk factors for glaucoma should be evaluated for the presence and extent of parapapillary atrophy. This finding can help practitioners to distinguish between eyes at risk for conversion to glaucoma and those with glaucoma, as well as between stable and progressive disease.

Laminar Dot Sign

The laminar dot sign was described as the exposure of the laminar structure due to loss of neural tissue.[30] These laminar pores became more obvious in eyes with significant glaucomatous nerve damage (Fig. 12–10). Although nonspecific for glaucoma, the laminar dot sign has frequently been observed in glaucomatous eyes.[35,57] This change in structural support may be related to shearing and compressive forces applied to the lamina cribrosa.[63]

In advanced stages, the laminar pores appear slit-like rather than round (Fig. 12–11).[64,65] An in vivo study using scanning laser ophthalmoscopy found almost

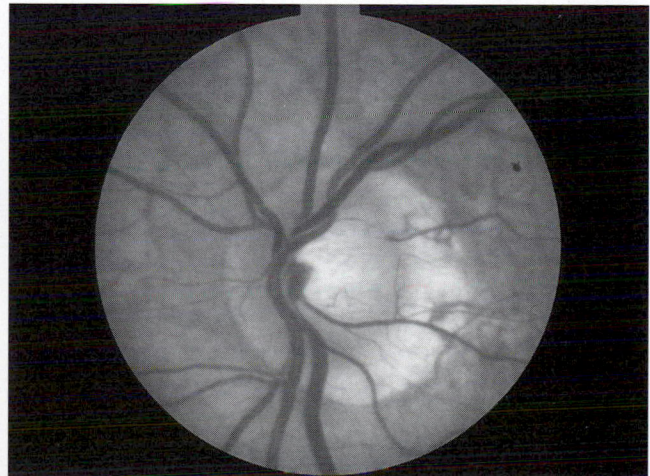

Figure 12–9. Extensive temporal parapapillary atrophy is present. The extent of zone beta (β) is greatest temporally and minimal nasally.

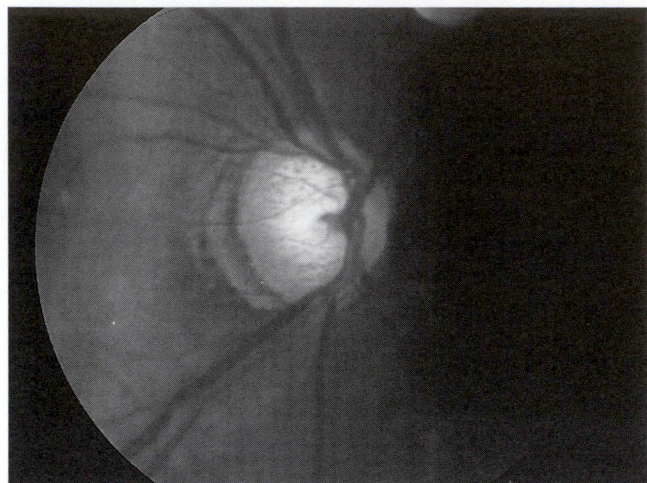

Figure 12–10. The laminar pores appear darker than the underlying scleral meshwork. These pores become more obvious as cupping progresses.

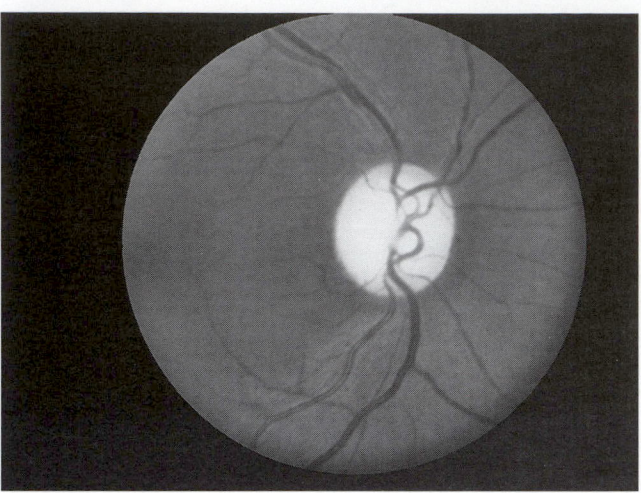

Figure 12–12. Pallor of the optic nerve due to pituitary adenoma. Pallor is greater than the extent of cupping. *(See also Color Plate 13.)*

round laminar pores in normal eyes and elongated laminar pores in glaucomatous eyes. The lengthening of the pores was positively correlated with the severity of visual field loss.[63]

Pallor

Pallor of the optic disc is not caused by loss of capillaries but by the increased visibility of supporting structures.[66] Optic disc pallor and cupping are not equivalent, since estimation of the cup-to-disc ratio is a study of contour rather than color. In glaucoma, cupping is most often greater than pallor[57,67,68]; while in optic atrophy, the area of pallor is greater than the degree of cupping (Fig. 12–12).[68,69]

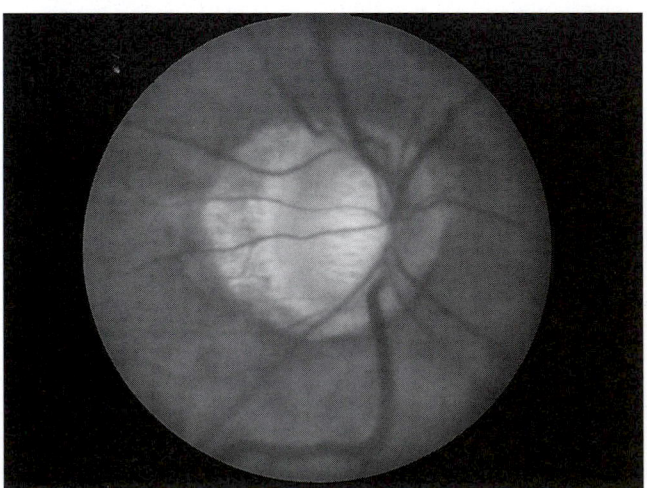

Figure 12–11. Advanced optic nerve cupping is associated with posterior bowing of the lamina cribrosa. Laminar pores appear elongated—the "laminar slit sign."

The degree of pallor is greatest in glaucomatous eyes, followed by ocular hypertensive and then normal eyes.[29,70] The inferior and nasal regions of the disc were most helpful in differentiating between normal and glaucomatous eyes. A three-dimensional analysis showed that pallor of the optic disc was initially observed at the bottom of the cup and ascended the cup wall as it progressed.[70]

The mismatch between the extent of cupping and area of pallor has high specificity in distinguishing between glaucomatous and normal eyes.[57] The clinician must evaluate the deviation of the retinal vessels when judging cup-to-disc ratio rather than the area of maximal color contrast. Estimation of the area of disc pallor is made more difficult by yellowing of the crystalline lens, which may give the disc a falsely "rosy" glow.

LOCALIZED SIGNS OF GLAUCOMATOUS NERVE DAMAGE

Focal Notching

Focal notching represents an area of localized damage to the neuroretinal rim (Fig. 12–13). Notching has been described in association with a pattern of glaucomatous optic neuropathy termed *focal ischemia*. This type of nerve damage was found to demonstrate corresponding localized visual field defects, with a greater number of these defects posing a threat to fixation.[31]

Focal notching may be preceded by hemorrhage of the nerve fiber layer (Fig. 12–14).[74] Most frequently located at the inferotemporal or superotemporal aspect of the disc, focal notching may lead to an acquired vertical elongation of the cup-to-disc ratio.[30,38,39,43,45] An ini-

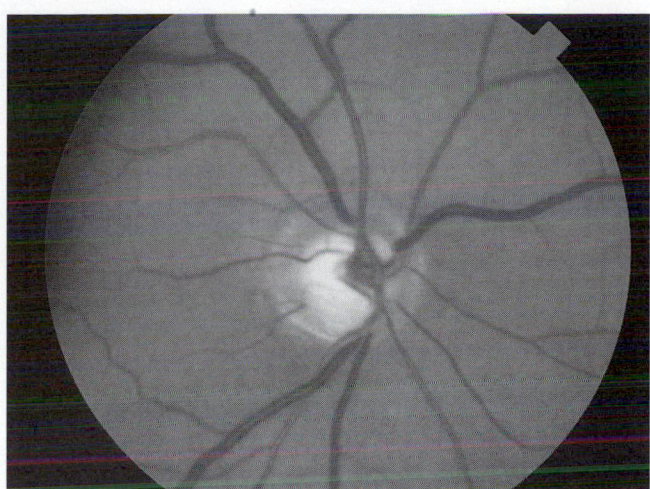

Figure 12–13. A focal notch is present at 7 o'clock. This notch is associated with a wedge defect of the nerve fiber layer. *(See also Color Plate 14.)*

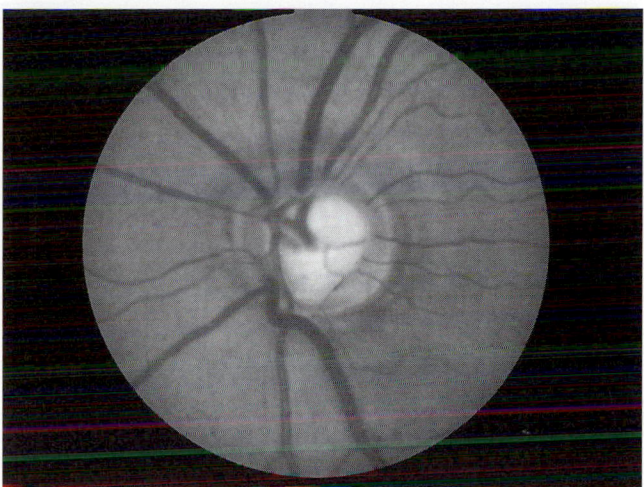

Figure 12–14. This focal notch at 5 o'clock is accompanied by a resolving hemorrhage of the nerve fiber layer and a wedge defect of the nerve fiber layer. *(See also Color Plate 15.)*

tially small defect can deepen over time to develop a "sharpened polar nasal edge" or a deviation of the retinal vasculature over the sharpened edge called "bayonetting of the retinal vessels."[30]

Focal notching is a localized sign of optic nerve damage that may be more common in smaller optic discs. Focal notching with or without a defect of the nerve fiber layer has been correlated clinically to loss of visual field using short-wavelength perimetry in a small population.[71] This optic disc finding is clinically significant, since focal notching of the neuroretinal rim with or without diffuse enlargement of the cup was found to be as common as diffuse enlargement of the cup in early stages of optic nerve progression.[42]

Acquired Pit of the Optic Nerve

An optic disc pit appears as a hole in the nerve tissue due to a localized absence of tissue. There is a deep localized depression within the neuroretinal rim and loss of the normal architecture of the lamina cribrosa. Optic disc pits have been described as an acquired change of the optic nerve head (Fig. 12–15).

Acquired pit of the optic nerve (APON) is suggested to represent focal glaucomatous damage and has also been called *focal glaucoma* or *focal ischemic glaucoma*. This abnormality is usually unilateral and located inferiorly or inferotemporally at the disc margin (Fig. 12–16).[72,73] APONs were found more commonly in a population with NTG and occurred up to 16 times more frequently than in OAG.[72] This disc finding may represent an area of increased vulnerability to nerve damage. Disc hemorrhages were also observed more often in patients with APON, and re-

current disc hemorrhages were found only in patients with APON. Interestingly, patients who developed APON during the course of this study had a history of disc hemorrhage in the same location.[73]

The loss of visual field associated with APON was most frequently located centrally or paracentrally. A dense scotoma was found to involve fixation in some patients. However, this study reported that visual field loss in NTG patients with APON was not substantially different for age-matched NTG patients without APON.[72] Ugurlu et al. determined that APON was associated with more frequent progression of optic disc damage or visual field loss.[73]

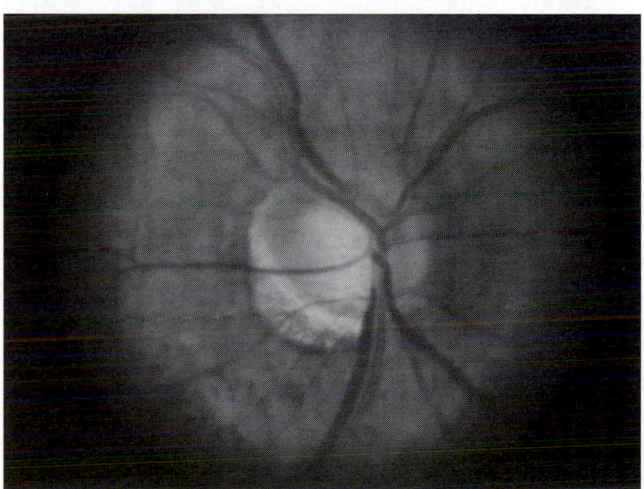

Figure 12–15. An acquired pit of the optic nerve (APON) is present at 6 o'clock. APON appears as a focal gray defect at the disc margin. This defect is associated with a dense arcuate scotoma with threat to fixation. *(See also Color Plate 16.)*

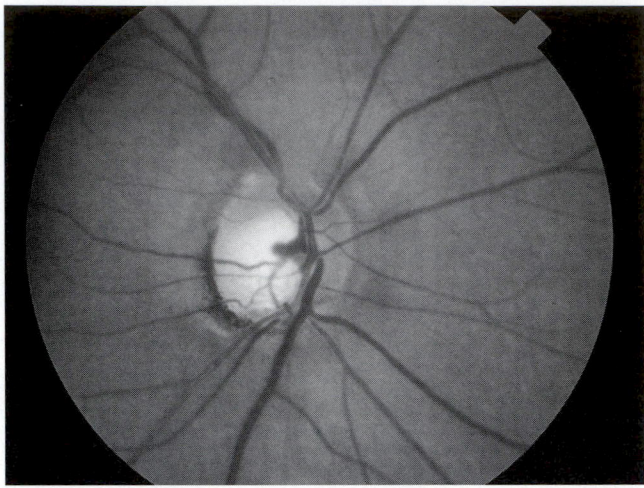

Figure 12–16. APON can appear as an enlarged laminar pore, although it is usually more extensive in size. The defect is present at 7 o'clock. *(See also Color Plate 17.)*

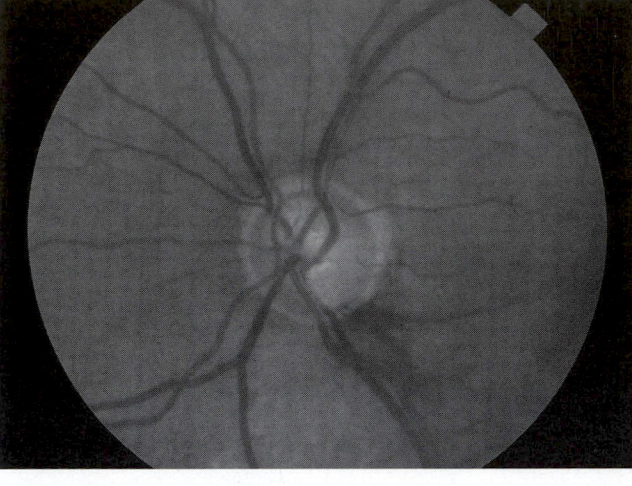

Figure 12–17. An extensive hemorrhage of the nerve fiber layer is present at 5 o'clock. This flame-shaped hemorrhage is associated with severe loss of the neuroretinal rim. *(See also Color Plate 18.)*

These investigators concluded that APON represented a distinct type of focal glaucomatous nerve damage and was a significant risk for the progression of glaucoma.

RETINAL VASCULATURE

Hemorrhage of the Nerve Fiber Layer

Hemorrhages of the nerve fiber layer are flame-shaped and extend from the optic disc into the nerve fiber layer (Fig. 12–17). Those that originate from deeper vessels have a blot appearance. Disc hemorrhages occur most frequently at the temporal aspect of the disc,[79,80] more often inferotemporally,[74,80,82,86] although they may be seen at any position around the disc margin. The location of the disc hemorrhage is most often superotemporal in NTG and inferotemporal in primary OAG.[80]

Disc hemorrhages have been shown to be highly specific for glaucoma,[75] although they may occur in association with systemic conditions such as anemia or systemic hypertension. In glaucomatous eyes, patients with systemic conditions such as hypertension[76,79] and diabetes[77,78] demonstrated more frequent disc hemorrhages. One study found an increased frequency of disc hemorrhages in patients with a history of migraine headaches. These investigators suggested that vasospastic activity of the retinal vasculature could lead to disc hemorrhage.[79] In a nonglaucomatous eye, disc hemorrhages may occur with ischemic optic neuropathy, diabetic retinopathy, optic disc drusen, or posterior vitreous detachment. Other risk factors for the development of disc hemorrhage in nonglaucoma-

tous eyes include the presence of pseudoexfoliation and vertical elongation of the cup-to-disc ratio.[79,80]

Disc hemorrhages occur more frequently in glaucomatous eyes and are more prevalent in eyes with NTG.[60,79–81] Studies have estimated the prevalence of disc hemorrhages in nonglaucomatous eyes varies from 0.02 to 0.4%[75,82] and up to 1.4% in an older general population.[79] Comparatively, the prevalence of disc hemorrhages in normal-tension glaucoma varies from 20.5 to 35.3% and from 4.2 to 10.3% for OAG.[79,81] Kitazawa et al. suggested that there is a subgroup of patients diagnosed with NTG that is susceptible to disc hemorrhages and another group that is not.[75]

Hemorrhages of the retinal nerve fiber layer can remain visible from 2 to 35 weeks[75] and may be followed by focal arteriolar narrowing or notching of the neuroretinal rim (Fig. 12–18).[74] Disc hemorrhages tend to recur more frequently in NTG (67% in one study[80]) than in POAG (12 to 29%[81,83]). These hemorrhages have been associated with inadequate IOP control or progressive nerve damage. The role of localized ischemia has been discussed.[81]

Disc hemorrhages may precede a visual field defect,[83–86] change in the nerve head,[86] or defect in the nerve fiber layer.[87] In one study, the average interval following the observation of disc hemorrhage to progression of visual field defects was 17 months, and that of optic nerve changes was 24 months.[86] There is a significant risk for visual field deterioration in patients with NTG or POAG with a history of disc hemorrhage.[85]

The presence of a hemorrhage of the nerve fiber layer or disc should prompt the clinician to evaluate

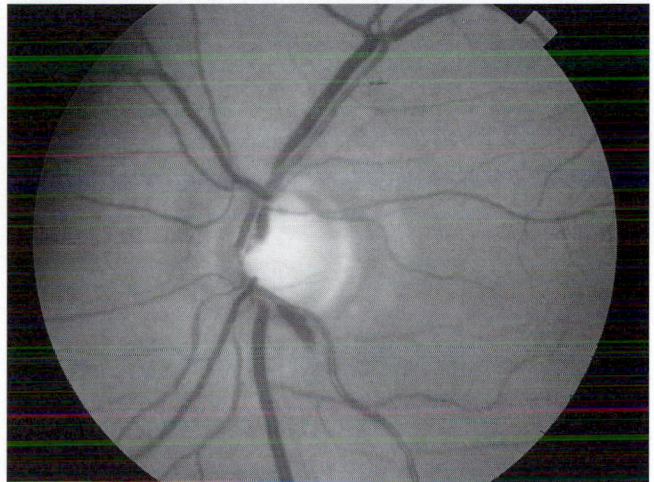

Figure 12–18. A hemorrhage of the nerve fiber layer can recur or develop in other sectors of the optic nerve. This finding can be followed by a change in the visual field, nerve fiber layer, or vascular caliber. *(See also Color Plate 19.)*

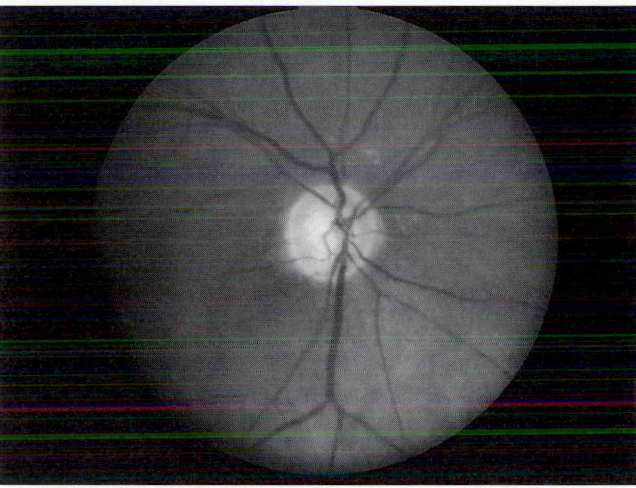

Figure 12–19. Focal arteriolar narrowing at 4 and 6 o'clock is observed as an irregularity in vessel diameter at the margin of the optic disc. *(See also Color Plate 20.)*

the efficacy of therapy and to rule out other possible causes of disc hemorrhage. In glaucoma patients, disc hemorrhages are ominous signs, since they can portend future optic disc or visual field defects.

Focal Narrowing

Focal narrowing has also been called proximal constriction and refers to constriction of the retinal arterioles at or just beyond the disc margin (Fig. 12–19). This finding has been described in association with glaucomatous eyes as well as eyes with other forms of optic neuropathy. The degree of focal narrowing also increases with age.[88]

A retrospective review of fundus photographs in patients with glaucoma and other forms of nonglaucomatous optic neuropathy determined that 42% of patients with glaucoma had proximal constriction, as compared with 5% of normal patients. Most of the constricted vessels were observed to occur in areas where cupping of the optic disc was most significant (90%) and adjacent to areas with the most prominent parapapillary atrophy (Fig. 12–20). Focal narrowing was found to be more common in patients with a history of nonarteritic anterior ischemic optic neuropathy (NAION), glaucoma, NTG, descending optic atrophy, or nonischemic optic neuritis. These investigators have suggested that focal narrowing was caused by decreased metabolic demand in local areas.[89]

Other investigators suggested that the focal narrowing was due to local vasospasm caused by the release of vasoconstrictive factors or by autoregulation in response to reduced metabolic demand following ganglion cell loss.[88] Again, focal narrowing occurred

more frequently in association with NAION than with POAG; however, analysis of glaucoma subgroups determined that focal narrowing was present as frequently in patients with NTG as in those with NAION. Therefore, the degree of local arteriolar narrowing was similar for patients with NAION and NTG but greater than in patients with either POAG or pseudoexfoliation glaucoma (PXG).

Comparisons between patients with glaucoma and ocular hypertension showed that focal narrowing was also more common in glaucoma (66%) than in ocular hypertension (5%)[90] and specifically more

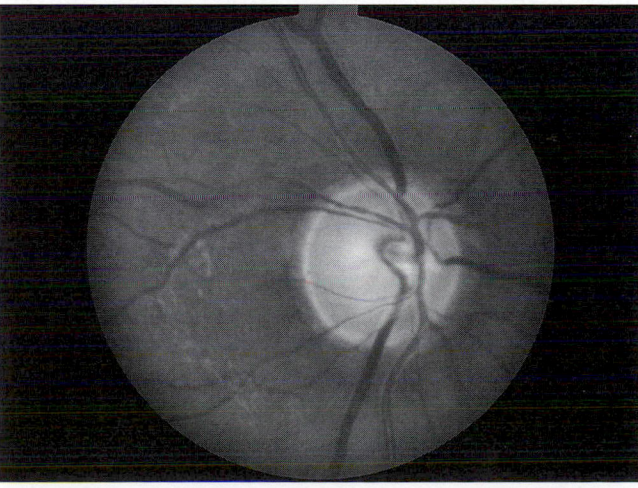

Figure 12–20. Vascular sheathing can occur in association with focal arteriolar narrowing. Focal vasoconstriction may be obvious (10 o'clock) or more subtle (11 o'clock). *(See also Color Plate 21.)*

frequent in NTG than in OAG or ocular hypertension.[60]

Although focal narrowing is a nonspecific sign for glaucoma, it may indicate that the optic nerve is suffering from a localized form of vascular insufficiency or may highlight areas in which severe axonal loss has previously occurred. Corresponding visual field defects have been found more frequently in eyes that demonstrate focal narrowing than in those without focal narrowing.[90] The presence of focal narrowing should alert the clinician to the progression of glaucoma.

Vascular Attenuation

Vascular attenuation has been observed in optic nerve disease. When glaucomatous eyes and eyes affected by other optic neuropathies were compared with normal eyes, there was a significant decrease in the caliber of the vessels on the optic nerve.[56,89] This finding was believed to develop following retinal ganglion cell loss in response to the decreased metabolic demand.

In normal eyes, the caliber of the retinal vessels has been found to be larger in areas where the nerve fiber layer has increased visibility. Retinal arterioles were widest at the inferotemporal aspect of the optic disc, followed by the superotemporal, superonasal, and inferonasal regions.[91] The diameters of these vessels were significantly narrower in glaucomatous eyes than in normal eyes even after correcting for age.[92,93] The difference was most pronounced for the inferotemporal and superotemporal arteries.[92]

Vascular attenuation worsened with increasing severity of glaucoma and was observed in the same sector of the optic nerve where loss of the neuroretinal rim and nerve fiber layer was most severe.[93] Decreased vessel caliber was also associated with an overall loss of sensitivity on visual field testing. The effects of vascular diseases such as diabetes, arterial hypertension, and vasoactive medications on these results was not evaluated.

The degree of generalized arteriolar narrowing has been shown to correspond with the degree of optic nerve damage independent of its etiology. Greater amounts of generalized vascular constriction have been observed in severe optic nerve disease[89] and more frequently in glaucomatous eyes than in nonglaucomatous eyes.[92,93] In the clinical setting, practitioners should recognize generalized arteriolar narrowing as a nonspecific sign of optic neuropathy (Fig. 12–21).

Baring of Circumlinear Vessels

Circumlinear vessels are small branches of the retinal vasculature that follow the margin of the cup. These vessels originate from the main vessels of the optic

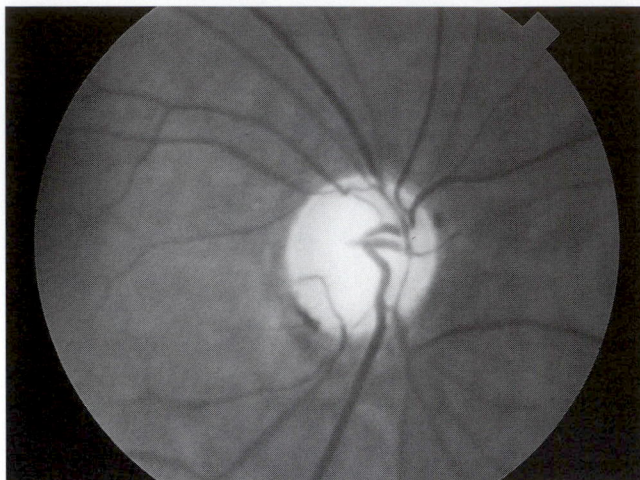

Figure 12–21. Severe vascular attenuation can occur in association with glaucoma and other optic neuropathies. *(See also Color Plate 22.)*

nerve and extend to the temporal aspect of the disc. Baring of the circumlinear vessels occurs when the cupping of the optic disc extends beyond the circumlinear vessel (Fig. 12–22). An area of pallor between the circumlinear vessel and the cup margin may be present.[94]

Baring of the circumlinear vessel is not specific for glaucoma[95,96] and has been observed in other optic nerve conditions including optic atrophy.[32] This sign has more frequently been seen in eyes with glaucoma[57,94] or ocular hypertension.[96,97] Baring of the circumlinear vessel can represent acquired enlargement of cupping but is sometimes present in normal eyes. This change in the retinal vasculature

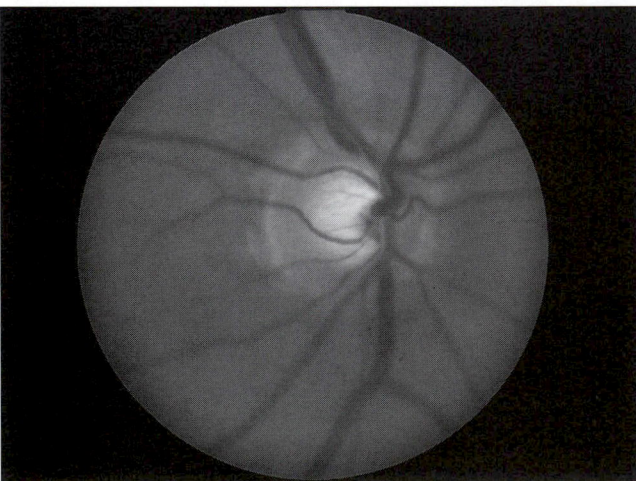

Figure 12–22. Baring of the circumlinear vessels occurs when cupping progresses. *(See also Color Plate 23.)*

may help to distinguish glaucoma suspects from converters, especially early in the disease process. Baring of the circumlinear vessel may represent an early sign of nerve loss in eyes with ocular hypertension and occurs more frequently in eyes with significant cup-to-disc asymmetry.[97]

Overpass Cupping

Overpass cupping may occur due to secondary shifting of vessels following loss of the neuroretinal rim. In overpass cupping, the circumlinear vessels that course over the optic cup appear to be unsupported by neural tissue. Overpass cupping occurs due to loss of tissue underneath nerve head vessels and collapse of vessels to the bottom of the deepened cup.[30] This disc finding may be more easily seen when visualized with stereoscopic viewing.[39]

Nasalization of Retinal Vasculature

Nasal displacement of the retinal vasculature has been described with enlargement of the cup-to-disc ratio[41] and also with physiological cupping.[98] Because this sign is nonspecific for glaucoma,[99] nasalization of the retinal vasculature is a less significant finding than other vessel changes.

Bayonet Sign

Areas of the neuroretinal rim that are affected by focal notching may also develop a sharpening of the nasal border of the notch. This localized atrophy may allow the retinal vasculature to deviate from its normal course, demonstrating what is called the "bayonet sign" (Fig. 12–23). These vessels have a "z" appear-

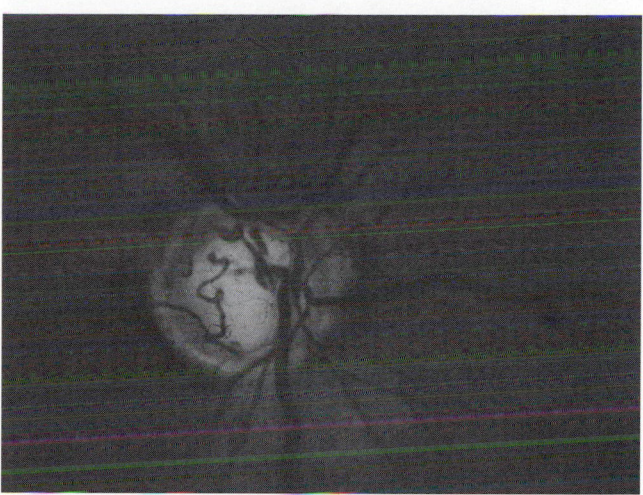

Figure 12–24. Disc collateral vessels in a patient with advanced open-angle glaucoma and no history of retinal vascular occlusion. *(See also Color Plate 25.)*

ance as they travel along the bottom of the cup, emerging at a sharp angle over the lip of the cup to pass over the disc margin.[30] This finding rarely occurs in nonglaucomatous eyes[100] and serves as a localized sign of advanced optic nerve damage.

Optic Disc Shunt Vessels

Optic disc shunt vessels are collateral vessels that develop between the central retinal vein and peripapillary veins or between two retinal veins (Fig. 12–24). This vascular anomaly was found to occur in 3% of patients with a history of glaucoma and no previous history of vein occlusion or venous stasis retinopathy. Investigators have proposed that these optic disc shunt vessels result from small venous occlusions at the optic disc.[101] Patients with these abnormal vessels are asymptomatic, but should be evaluated for other vascular conditions such as arterial disease.[102]

REVERSAL OF CUPPING

Reports have shown that the cupping of the optic disc can vary with intraocular pressure, suggesting that mechanical deformation of the glial tissue plays a role. Schwartz et al. documented four cases in which changes in optic disc cupping and visual field were noted after reduction of intraocular pressure by medical and surgical means, although corresponding changes in optic disc pallor were inconsistent.[103] Postsurgical improvement in optic disc cupping was also observed by Greenidge et al.; however, regression and increased optic nerve pallor in individual cases were documented.[104] Pederson and Herschler demon-

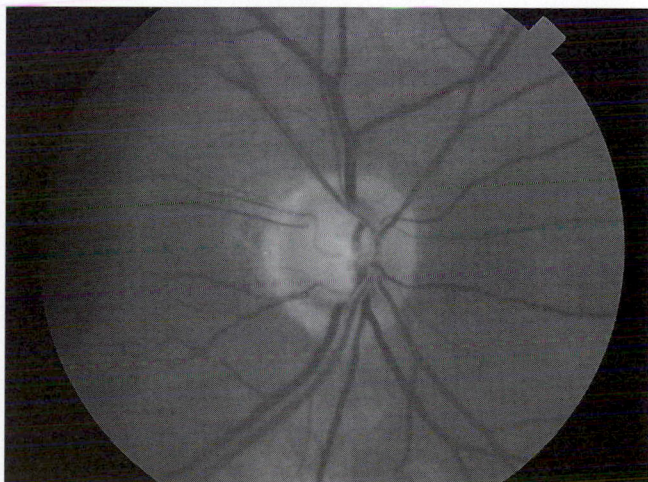

Figure 12–23. Bayonetting of retinal vessels is present at 6 o'clock. The vein overlying the disc margin turns back beneath the rim and then turns again to lie along the floor of the cup, forming a "Z" pattern. *(See also Color Plate 24.)*

strated similar findings, with significant pressure reduction following trabeculectomy in five patients and also after resolution of a glaucomatocyclitic crisis in another patient.[105] These investigators suggested that the decrease in optic disc cupping might be partially attributed to a reduction in the posterior bowing of the lamina cribrosa. Their findings are supported by the work of Parrow et al., who showed that even short-term changes in intraocular pressure affect the cup-to-disc ratio and rim area and that these changes are reversible.[106]

It appears that the degree of IOP reduction may affect the reversibility of optic disc cupping. A study comparing two groups of patients with varying degrees of IOP reduction showed the frequency of optic disc and visual field improvement was more significant when intraocular pressure was decreased by at least 30% from baseline. Reversibility in optic disc cupping was not observed when IOP reduction was less than 20% of baseline.[107]

The reversibility of optic disc cupping may occur because of a number of factors, including the elasticity of the lamina cribrosa, acute or prolonged disc edema, restoration of normal axoplasmic flow, and increased size and/or number of supportive glial elements.[104]

DIFFERENTIAL DIAGNOSIS OF GLAUCOMATOUS OPTIC NERVE HEADS

Ischemic Optic Neuropathy

Ischemic optic neuropathy (ION) is a disease that presents with classic signs and symptoms. This condition can be classified as arteritic (caused by giant-cell arteritis) or nonarteritic (caused by other diseases). Nonarteritic forms of ischemic optic neuropathy have frequently been associated with conditions such as arterial hypertension, diabetes mellitus, ischemic heart disease, thyroid disease, chronic obstructive pulmonary disease, and cerebrovascular disease.[108]

Initially, patients experience a sudden painless loss of vision. Visual field testing may reveal an inferior nasal sectoral defect, altitudinal hemianopia, or central scotoma. Pupillary testing demonstrates a relative afferent defect, and color vision may be affected. The optic disc generally shows marked localized edema with or without associated hemorrhages of the nerve fiber layer.

Later, resolution of the ischemic event is followed by the attenuation of the retinal vasculature, loss of nerve fiber tissue, and atrophy and pallor of the optic disc. In many cases of optic atrophy following ar-

teritic ION, the color of the disc has been described as "chalky white." Sectoral cupping occurs later and may be difficult to distinguish from glaucomatous cupping. The erosion of disc tissue occurs secondarily to the interruption of blood flow through the posterior ciliary arteries to the optic nerve. Clinically, the extent of disc pallor is key, since the degree of pallor is generally larger than the cupping of the nerve. The neuroretinal rim should be evaluated carefully for maximal color contrast, since this tissue appears pale following resolution of ION.[109]

Optic Disc Drusen

Asymmetry of optic disc cupping may be caused by the presence of optic disc drusen. Disc drusen may be buried or superficial and appear as globular deposits anterior to the lamina cribrosa (Fig. 12–25). These hyaline deposits have been associated with progressive optic atrophy and compromise of the nerve fiber layer.

Optic disc drusen may occur in an autosomal dominant fashion with variable penetrance. In the general population, this phenomenon is estimated to occur in approximately 0.34%. A recent survey[110] found optic disc drusen present in 9.2% of patients with retinitis pigmentosa.

If optic disc drusen are suspected as a cause of elevated nerve heads, specialized testing should include β-scan ultrasound. Ultrasonography can demonstrate the presence of optic disc drusen without requiring costly imaging studies such as magnetic resonance imaging or computed tomography.[111] Tests to assess optic nerve integrity are important in these

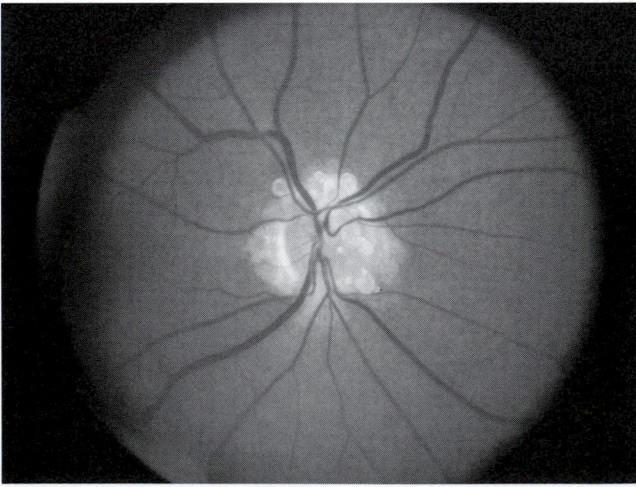

Figure 12–25. Optic disc drusen appear as refractile globular deposits on the surface or within the disc substance. Defects or hemorrhages of the nerve fiber layer can occasionally be associated. *(See also Color Plate 26.)*

patients, since the presence of disc drusen may make evaluation of the nerve head difficult. A recent study demonstrated the benefit of optical coherence tomography in two patients with drusen of the optic nerve head and glaucoma. These patients showed a loss of nerve fiber layer that was not consistent with the appearance of the optic nerve.[112]

Other retinal findings may include vascular anomalies such as venous stasis retinopathy.[113] There is potential for mechanical compression of the retinal vasculature by disc drusen, resulting in vasoocclusive events.[114] Retrospective case analysis has shown disc hemorrhages to be present in approximately 70% of patients and vascular shunts in almost 7% of patients with disc drusen.[115]

Patients with optic disc drusen and elevated intraocular pressures are at risk for progressive nerve damage due to mechanical factors. Further, patients with significant asymmetry in cupping should be evaluated for possible buried disc drusen.

Optic Disc Pit

Although optic disc pits have been described as acquired changes of the nerve head, there are similar findings that have been suggested to represent a congenital anomaly.[122] These findings are not generally associated with systemic syndromes. Histologically, congenital optic disc pits are found to be localized areas of abnormal retinal tissue that protrude posteriorly through a defect in the lamina cribrosa.[122]

Congenital disc pits are more frequently observed in the temporal aspect of the nerve head (Fig. 12–26),[116] in contrast to acquired pits of the optic nerve, which are more often seen in the inferior or inferotemporal sectors. Associated retinal findings may include a defect of the nerve fiber layer with a corresponding visual field defect or serous maculopathy. Optical coherence imaging of optic disc pits has shown that an inner layer separation of the retina is connected to the optic disc pit and that schisis formation may precede the serous macular detachment.[117–119] Visual symptoms are related to the detachment of the outer layer of the retina that may overlie the fovea. Gas tamponade has been used to resolve such detachment, with associated improvement in visual acuity.[120] Other surgical treatments for serous maculopathy associated with optic disc pits include vitrectomy with autologous platelet application.[121]

"Morning Glory Syndrome"

Morning glory syndrome has been described as a funnel-shaped staphyloma of the nerve head, which appears large in size, with a pink color and central depression within which Bergmeister's papilla may be

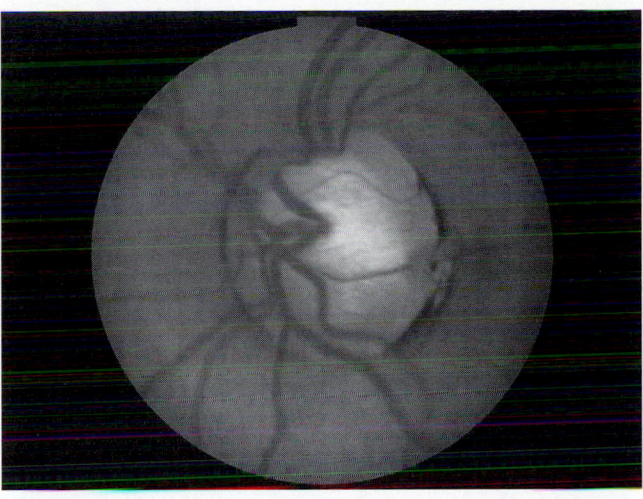

Figure 12–26. A congenital pit in the optic disc is generally observed temporally on the disc margin as a localized depression. This is in contrast to acquired optic disc pits, which are more common superiorly or inferiorly. *(See also Color Plate 27.)*

present. A grayish ring corresponding to an area of chorioretinal pigment disruption generally surrounds the nerve head. The retinal vasculature is also abnormal and appears to originate from the peripheral region of the disc. These vessels appear more numerous and attenuated in caliber. The retinal vessels radiate outward over the disc margin. An initial report by Kindler differentiated this optic nerve appearance from optic disc coloboma by the pinkish color of the optic disc.[122] The pale or white color associated with the appearance of a disc coloboma was related to the presence of only scleral and retinal tissue.

Visual acuity is generally reduced in eyes with morning glory syndrome; however, 20/20 vision has been reported in some cases. An association between morning glory syndrome and the transphenoidal form of basal encephalocele has been documented, with risk for multisystem abnormalities including respiratory, endocrine, and neurological dysfunction. Morning glory syndrome does not appear to be an inherited condition and is rarely bilateral. Ocular associations include an increased risk of retinal detachment.[122]

Optic Disc Coloboma

If the embryonic fissure of the eye fails to close during the eighth week of development, an optic nerve coloboma may result. Other ocular structures may be involved, including the retina, choroid, or iris. Optic nerve coloboma appears as a well-demarcated, deeply excavated depression in an enlarged optic canal. The color of the coloboma is white, with minimal chorioretinal pigmentation, such as is seen in morning glory syndrome. The inferior aspect of the excavated disc is deeper than the superior portion owing to the incomplete closure of the embryonic fissure (Fig. 12–27). Other characteristics that differentiate optic nerve coloboma from morning glory syndrome include the absence of a central glial tuft and the presence of normal retinal vasculature.[123]

Chorioretinal colobomata are diagnosed by funduscopic evaluation; other imaging techniques can be used to evaluate them. If radiological studies are undertaken, computed tomography should be recommended over ultrasonography or magnetic resonance imaging.[124] Patients with this condition may have other congenital syndromes or disorders, including trisomy 13, acro-renal-ocular syndrome, or Aicardi syndrome. Visual acuity may be unaffected or decreased due to direct involvement of the macula, retinal detachment, or subretinal neovascularization.[125]

Optic nerve coloboma has been associated with serious retinal complications, including serous macular detachment. Retinal detachment is also a concern but occurs more frequently in retinochoroidal coloboma rather than optic nerve coloboma.[123] Various combinations of vitrectomy, laser photocoagulation, and gas tamponade can successfully treat retinal detachment in such eyes.[126] Other treatments include relaxing retinotomy and retinopexy with cyanoacrylate to resolve retinal detachment associated with choroidal coloboma.[127] Eyes with abnormally large cupping and optic nerve size should be carefully evaluated for congenital optic nerve abnormalities including optic nerve coloboma.

Tilted Discs

The tilted-disc syndrome is easily recognized as a bilateral congenital condition in which the superotem-

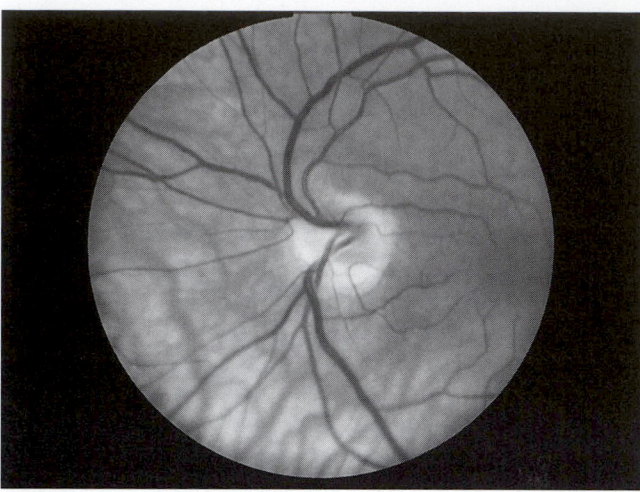

Figure 12–28. Tilted optic disc demonstrates relative crowding of the superior nerve fibers and inferior scleral crescent. *(See also Color Plate 29.)*

poral portion of the optic nerve is elevated and the inferonasal portion of the optic nerve is posteriorly displaced. This appearance occurs because of crowding of axons in the superior portion of the disc with relative absence toward the inferior aspect (Fig. 12–28). A characteristic inferotemporal chorioretinal hypoplasia can be observed bilaterally.[128] This inferior crescent can be associated with a "pseudo–bitemporal hemianopia." These visual field defects differ from those observed in neurological conditions, since they do not respect the vertical midline. Imaging studies should be completed for patients with congenital tilted-disc syndrome who demonstrate visual field defects that respect the vertical midline, since reports have documented suprasellar tumors in several cases.[129]

TECHNIQUES OF EVALUATION

Various examination techniques can be employed in evaluation of the optic nerve head. Caprioli et al. suggested that qualitative methods of analyzing the optic disc and nerve fiber layer may detect focal changes, whereas quantitative methods of analyzing the height or thickness of the nerve fiber layer may detect subtle, diffuse changes.[140]

Detection of progressive nerve damage can be further complicated by variations in examination technique and by observer bias. For example, evaluation of the optic nerve using a stereoscopic technique such as indirect biomicroscopy generally produces a larger cup-to-disc ratio than a monoscopic technique such as direct ophthalmoscopy.[130–132] The variation in estimation by expert observers was found to be significant as

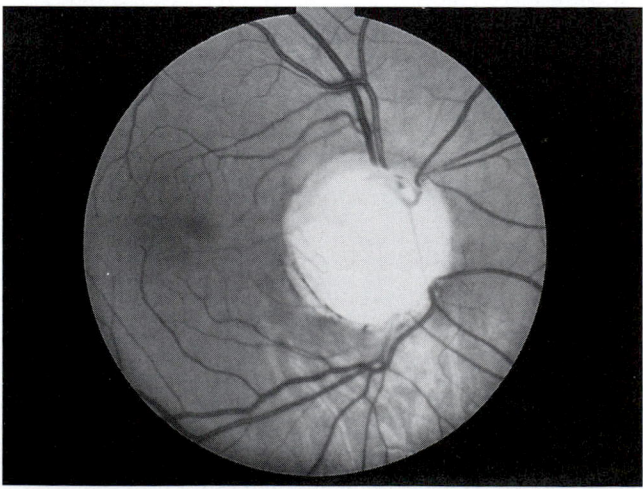

Figure 12–27. An optic nerve coloboma may occur with incomplete closure of the embryonic fissure. *(See also Color Plate 28.)*

well: cup-to-disc estimates differed by at least 0.2 ratio units in as many as 50% of subjects studied.[132] In this study, the intraobserver agreement was high compared to interobserver estimation. This suggests that a clinician will use similar criteria for evaluating the optic nerve (good intraobserver agreement), although these criteria may differ between practitioners (poor interobserver agreement). Drawings of the optic nerve were found to be similar to serial stereoscopic disc photographs in the ability to detect progression of optic nerve damage, even with significant interobserver variation.[133] There is a need for standardized methods of interobserver evaluation. Regular stereophotographs (e.g., annually) should be considered for patients being monitored by multiple clinicians so as to reduce the possibility of over- or undertreatment.

Direct ophthalmoscopy has the advantages of ease and familiarity of use for most clinicians. The relatively high magnification of the image (15×)[134] allows the observer to carefully evaluate the parapapillary tissue for hemorrhages in the nerve fiber layer as well as other vessel changes. Unfortunately, this technique provides a relatively small field of view and produces a monoscopic image. Contour is generally appreciated by movement of the light spot across the surface of the optic disc, while depth is inferred from other monocular cues. The use of polarizing filters in direct ophthalmoscopy is not recommended because of the reduction in maximal color contrast.

The Hruby lens is a slit lamp–mounted −55D lens that can be used in evaluating the optic nerve head; however, this lens is less frequently used due to the poor quality of the image and reduced stereopsis as compared with other fundus lenses. The Hruby lens provides a slight exaggeration in the depth of cupping, and its image provides a limited field of view. Good patient fixation is generally required for this technique.

A variety of fundus lenses are available for indirect biomicroscopy. This technique produces an inverted, real image with a larger field of view than that obtained with direct methods of nerve assessment. Magnification of the image and working distance from the eye decrease with higher dioptric powers, while field of view increases. These condensing lenses tend to underestimate the apparent cup depth.[135] Clear lenses are generally preferred for examination of disc pallor. Use of a binocular indirect ophthalmoscope is not recommended for optic nerve assessment due to the relatively low magnification of the image (3×).[134]

Several fundus contact lenses provide the truest image of the optic disc, although there is a slight apparent decrease in the cup depth.[135] A Goldmann one-, two-, or three-mirror lens can be used as a fundus contact lens. Other gonioscopic lenses that can be used as fundus contact lenses include Zeiss, Posner, and Sussman goniolenses. Improvements in the profile of the contact lens surface allow these lenses to be used with or without a coupling solution. Caution should be exercised when using coupling agents for patients who will require fundus photography, since corneal defects and edema may reduce the quality of the photographic image.

Stereodisc photography provides a means by which the appearance of the disc can be objectively documented. (Image analyzers are discussed elsewhere.) True stereoscopic photos are taken by simultaneous imaging of the optic disc, while "pseudostereoscopic" photos are taken by slightly varying the position of the image. Evaluation of optic cup depth may vary depending upon the method of analysis. Images taken using a Nidek 3-Dx split-frame technique (true stereoscopic image) showed better interobserver reliability than those obtained with a Zeiss full-frame technique (pseudostereoscopic).[136] Serial photographs can be viewed and assessed for subtle changes in rim contour and positional shifts in the retinal vasculature.

In eyes with opaque media, A-scan ultrasound has been suggested as an alternative technique to evaluate the optic nerve because of the high cost of other imaging techniques, such as magnetic resonance imaging. A-scan ultrasound can be used to measure optic nerve diameter indirectly. A comparison between normal and glaucomatous eyes showed that the diameter of the optic nerve in glaucomatous eyes was smaller. In a pilot study, the optic nerve diameter significantly correlated with neuroretinal rim area, narrowing of retinal arterioles, decreased retinal nerve fiber layer, increasing mean defect of visual field, and zones of parapapillary atrophy.[137] These results support previous histological data suggesting that optic nerve diameter decreases with loss of nerve fiber tissue.[138] Unfortunately, this technique is unable to distinguish between glaucomatous and nonglaucomatous causes of optic nerve damage and is further complicated by the significant overlap between normal and glaucomatous eyes. Even so, this method can be of benefit in assessing patients with hazy media in whom other methods of assessing the nerve head are not possible.

CONCLUSION

The optic nerve head should be systematically assessed for findings consistent with a diagnosis of glaucoma and other optic neuropathies. The optic disc should be evaluated for size and asymmetry of size. The cup-to-disc ratio should be specified in the horizontal and vertical meridians, with careful examination for generalized concentric enlargement, vertical elongation of the cup-to-disc ratio, and asymmetry in cupping. Irregularities in the profile and contour of the neuroretinal rim suggest diffuse loss, saucerization, or localized loss, including focal notching of the neuroretinal rim and acquired pit of the optic nerve. The area and extent of parapapillary atrophy should be measured. Pallor of the neuroretinal rim can help to differentiate between glaucomatous and nonglaucomatous optic neuropathy.

Careful examination of the retinal vasculature is also important. The presence or absence of hemorrhages in the nerve fiber layer should be noted. Vessel changes that occur with optic nerve damage include focal narrowing or generalized vascular attenuation. Nonspecific signs, such as baring of the circumlinear vessels, overpass cupping, nasalization of the retinal vasculature, the bayonet sign, and optic disc shunt vessels should be noted if present.

Investigators have shown that qualitative disc evaluation has better diagnostic precision than qualitative assessment of the nerve fiber layer, quantitative measurement of the optic nerve, height of the nerve fiber layer, or planimetric measurement of rim area in detecting patients with early glaucomatous loss of visual field.[139, 140] Careful examination of the optic nerve head, retinal vasculature, and parapapillary tissue can help to identify those patients with glaucoma as well as those with risk for development of glaucoma or with progressive disease.

REFERENCES

1. Jonas J. Letter to the editor. *J Glaucoma.* 1997;6:436.
2. Kee C, Koo H, Ji Y, Kim S. Effect of optic disc size or age on evaluation of optic disc variables. *Br J Ophthalmol.* 1997;81:1046–1049.
3. Jonas JB, Gusek GC, Guggenmoos-Holzmann I, Naumann GOH. Variability of the real dimensions of normal human optic discs. *Graefes Arch Clin Exp Ophthalmol.* 1988;226:332–336.
4. Jonas JB, Gusek GC, Naumann GO. Optic disc, cup and neuroretinal rim size, configuration and correlation in normal eyes. *Invest Ophthalmol Vis Sci.* 1988; 29(7):1151–1158. [Published errata in 32(6):1893, 1991 and 32(2):474–475, 1992.]
5. Jonas JB, Fernandez MC, Naumann GOH. Glaucomatous optic nerve atrophy in small discs with low cup-to-disc ratios. *Ophthalmology.* 1990;97:1211–1215.
6. Heijl A, Mölder H. Optic disc diameter influences the ability to detect glaucomatous damage. *Acta Ophthalmol.* 1993;71:122–129.
7. Jonas JB, Zach FM, Gusek GC, Naumann GO. Pseudoglaucomatous physiologic large cups. *Am J Ophthalmol.* 1989;107:137–144.
8. Quigley HA, Katz J, Derick RJ, Gilbert D, Sommer A. An evaluation of optic disc and nerve fiber layer examinations in monitoring progression of early glaucoma damage. *Ophthalmology.* 1992;99:19–28.
9. Iester M, Broadway DC, Mikelberg FS, Drance SM. A comparison of healthy, ocular hypertensive, and glaucomatous optic disc topographic parameters. *J Glaucoma.* 1997;6:363–370.
10. Jonas JB, Gusek GC, Naumann GOH. Optic disc morphometry in chronic primary open-angle glaucoma. *Graefes Arch Clin Exp Ophthalmol.* 1988;226:522–530.
11. Garway-Heath DF, Wollstein G, Hitchings RA. Aging changes of the optic nerve head in relation to open angle glaucoma. *Br J Ophthalmol.* 1997;81:840–845.
12. Tuulonen A, Airaksinen PJ. Optic disc size in exfoliative, primary open angle, and low-tension glaucoma. *Arch Ophthalmol.* 1992;110:211–213.
13. Jonas JB, Papastathopoulos KI. Optic disk appearance in pseudoexfoliation syndrome. *Am J Ophthalmol.* 1997; 123:174–180.
14. Burk ROW, Rohorschneider K, Noack H, Volcker HE. Are large optic nerve heads susceptible to glaucomatous damage at normal intraocular pressure? A three-dimensional study by laser scanning tomography. *Graefes Arch Ophthalmol.* 1992;230:552–560.
15. Eid TE, Spaeth GL, Moster MR, Augsburger JJ. Quantitative differences between the optic nerve head and peripapillary retina in low-tension and high-tension primary open-angle glaucoma. *Am J Ophthalmol.* 1997; 124:805–814.
16. Jonas JB, Gusek GC, Naumann GOH. Optic disc morphometry in high myopia. *Graefes Arch Clin Exp Ophthalmol.* 1988;226:587–590.
17. Jonas JB, Dichtl A. Optic disc morphology in myopic primary open-angle glaucoma. *Graefes Arch Clin Exp Ophthalmol.* 1997;235:627–633.
18. Gross PG, Drance SM. Comparison of a simple ophthalmoscope and planimetric measurement of glaucomatous neuroretinal rim areas. *J Glaucoma.* 1995;4:314–316.
19. Schwartz JT, Reuling GH, Garrison RJ. Acquired cupping of the optic nerve head in normotensive eyes. *Br J Ophthalmol.* 1975;59:216–222.
20. Teikari JM, Airaksinen JP. Twin study on cup-disc ratio of the optic nerve head. *Br J Ophthalmol.* 1992;76: 218–220.
21. Britton RJ, Drance SM, Schulzer M, Douglas GR, Mawson OK. The area of the neuroretinal rim of the optic nerve in normal eyes. *Am J Ophthalmol.* 1987;103: 497–504.
22. Armaly M. Genetic determination of cup/disc ratio of the optic nerve. *Arch Ophthalmol.* 1975;78:35–43.
23. Fishman RS. Optic disc asymmetry: A sign of ocular hypertension. *Arch Ophthalmol.* 1970;84:590–594.
24. Varma R, Tielsch JM, Quigley HA, et al. Race-, age-, gender-, and refractive error–related differences in the normal optic disc. *Arch Ophthalmol.* 1994;112:1068–1076.
25. Beck RW, Messner DK, Musch DC et al. Is there a racial difference in physiologic cup size? *Ophthalmology.* 1985; 92:873–876.

26. Tsai CS, Zangwill L, Gonzalez C et al. Ethnic differences in optic nerve head topography. *J Glaucoma.* 1995;4: 248–257.

27. Carpel EF, Engstrom PF. The normal cup-disc ratio. *Am J Ophthalmol.* 1981;91:588–597.

28. Bengtsson B. The alteration and asymmetry of cup and disc diameters. *Acta Ophthalmol.* 1980;58:726–732.

29. Schwartz B. Optic disc changes in ocular hypertension. *Surv Ophthalmol* 1980;25:148–154.

30. Read RM, Spaeth GL. The practical clinical appraisal of the optic disc in glaucoma: The natural history of cup progression and some specific disc-field correlations. *Trans Am Acad Ophthalmol Otolaryngol.* 1974;89:255–274.

31. Nicolela MT, Drance SM. Various glaucomatous optic nerve appearances: Clinical correlations. *Ophthalmology.* 1996;103:640–649.

32. Pederson JE, Anderson DR. The mode of progressive disc cupping in ocular hypertension and glaucoma. *Arch Ophthalmol.* 1980;98:490–495.

33. Caprioli J, Spaeth GL. Comparison of the optic nerve head in high- and low-tension glaucoma. *Arch Ophthalmol.* 1985;103:1145–1149.

34. Garway-Heath DF, Hitchings RA. Quantitative evaluation of the optic nerve head in early glaucoma. *Br J Ophthalmol.* 1998;82:352–361.

35. Motolko M, Drance SM. Features of the optic disc in preglaucomatous eyes. *Arch Ophthalmol* 1981;99: 1992–1994.

36. Bianchi-Marzoli S, Rizzo JF, Brancato R, Lessel S. Quantitative analysis of optic disc cupping in compressive optic neuropathy. *Ophthalmology.* 1995;102:436–440.

37. Yucel YH, Bupta N, Kalichman MW, et al. Relationship of optic disc topography to optic nerve fiber number in glaucoma. *Arch Ophthalmol.* 1998;116:493–497.

38. Spaeth GL, Hitchings RA, Sivalingam E. The optic disc in glaucoma: Pathogenetic correlation of five patterns of cupping in chronic open-angle glaucoma. *Trans Am Acad Ophthalmol Otolaryngol.* 1976;81:217–223.

39. Hitchings RA, Spaeth GL. The optic disc in glaucoma: I. Classification. *Br J Ophthalmol.* 1976;60:778–785.

40. Phillips CI, Tsukahara S, Makino F, et al. Saucerisation (recession) of neuro-retinal rim is characteristic of glaucoma. *Jpn J Ophthalmol.* 1993;37:171–177.

41. Kirsch RE, Anderson DR. Clinical recognition of glaucomatous cupping. *Am J Ophthalmol.* 1973;75:442–454.

42. Weisman RL, Asseff CF, Phelps CD, et al. Vertical elongation of the optic cup in glaucoma. *Trans Am Acad Ophthalmol Otolaryngol.* 1973;77:157–161.

43. Tuulonen A, Airaksinen PJ. Initial glaucomatous optic disk and retinal nerve fiber layer abnormalities and their progression *Am J Ophthalmol.* 1991;11:485–490.

44. Tezel G, Kolker AE, Kass MA, et al. Parapapillary chorioretinal atrophy in patients with ocular hypertension. I. An evaluation as a predictive factor for the development of glaucomatous damage. *Arch Ophthalmol.* 1997;115:1503–1508.

45. Jonas JB, Fernandez MC, Sturmer J. Pattern of glaucomatous neuroretinal rim loss. *Ophthalmology.* 1993; 100(1):63–68.

46. Caprioli JM, Miller J. Optic disc rim area is related to disc size in normal subjects. *Arch Ophthalmol.* 1987;105: 1683–1685.

47. Tsai CS, Ritch R, Shin DH, et al. Age-related decline of disc rim area in visually normal subjects. *Ophthalmology.* 1992;99:29–35.

48. Airaksinen PJ, Tuulonen A, Alanko HI. Rate and pattern of neuroretinal rim area decrease in ocular hypertension and glaucoma. *Arch Ophthalmol.* 1992;110: 206–210.

49. Zeyen TG, Caprioli J. Progression of disc and field damage in early glaucoma. *Arch Ophthalmol.* 1993;111: 62–65.

50. Jonas JB, Grundler AE, Gonzales-Cortes J. Pressure-dependent neuroretinal rim loss in normal-pressure glaucoma. *Am J Ophthalmol.* 1998;125:137–144.

51. Rockwood EJ, Anderson DR. Acquired peripapillary changes and progression in glaucoma. *Graefes Arch Clin Exp Ophthalmol.* 1988;226:510–515.

52. Jonas JB, Nguyen NX, Gusek GC, Naumann GOH. Parapapillary chorioretinal atrophy in normal and glaucoma eyes: I. Morphometric data. *Invest Ophthalmol Vis Sci.* 1989;30:908–918.

53. Fantes F, Anderson DR. Clinical histologic correlation of human peripapillary atrophy. *Ophthalmology.* 1989, 96:20–25.

54. Kubota T, Jonas JB, Naumann GOH. Direct clinico-histological correlation of parapapillary chorioretinal atrophy. *Br J Ophthalmol.* 1993;77:103–106.

55. Jonas JB, Naumann GOH. Parapapillary chorioretinal atrophy in normal and glaucoma eyes: II. Correlations. *Invest Ophthalmol Vis Sci.* 1989;30:919–926.

56. Jonas JB, Fernandez MC, Naumann GOH. Parapapillary atrophy and retinal vessel diameter in non-glaucomatous optic nerve damage. *Invest Ophthalmol Vis Sci.* 1991;32:2942–2947.

57. Jonas JB, Nguyen NX, Naumann GOH. Non-quantitative morphologic features in normal and glaucomatous optic discs. *Acta Ophthalmol.* 1989;67:361–366.

58. Jonas JB, Fernandez MC, Naumann GOH. Glaucomatous parapapillary atrophy: Occurrence and correlations. *Arch Ophthalmol.* 1992;110:214–222.

59. Buus DR, Anderson DR. Peripapillary crescents and haloes in normal tension glaucoma and ocular hypertension. *Ophthalmology.* 1989;96:16–19.

60. Tezel G, Kass MA, Kolker AE, Wax MB. Comparative optic disc analysis in normal pressure glaucoma, primary open-angle glaucoma, and ocular hypertension. *Ophthalmology.* 1996;103:2105–2113.

61. Jonas JB, Konigsreuther KA. Optic disk appearance in ocular hypertensive eyes. *Am J Ophthalmol.* 1994;117(6): 732–740.

62. Tezel G, Kolker AE, Wax MB, et al. Parapapillary chorioretinal atrophy in patients with ocular hypertension: II. An evaluation of progressive changes. *Arch Ophthalmol.* 1997;115:1509–1514.

63. Fontana L, Bhandara A, Fitzke FW, Hitchings RA. In vivo morphometry of the lamina cribrosa and its relation to visual field loss in glaucoma. *Curr Eye Res.* 1998; 17:363–369.

64. Susanna R Jr. The lamina cribrosa and visual field defects in open angle glaucoma. *Can J Ophthalmol.* 1984; 18:124–126.

65. Miller KM, Quigley HA. The clinical appearance of the lamina cribrosa as a function of the extent of glaucomatous nerve damage. *Ophthalmology.* 1988;95: 135–138.

66. Quigley HA, Hohman RM, Addicks EM. Quantitative study of optic nerve head capillaries in experimental optic disc pallor. *Am J Ophthalmol.* 1982;93:689–699.

67. Jonas JB, Zach FM, Gusek GC, Naumann GO. Pseudoglaucomatous physiologic large cups. *Am J Ophthalmol.* 1989;107(2):137–144.

68. Schwartz B. Cupping and pallor of the optic disc. *Arch Ophthalmol.* 1973;89:272–277.

69. Jonas JB, Nguyen NX, Naumann GOH. Optic disc morphometry in simple optic nerve atrophy. *Acta Ophthalmol.* 1989;67:199–203.

70. Sagaties MJ, Schwartz B. Three-dimensional evaluation of optic disc pallor in open angle glaucoma. *Acta Ophthalmol.* 1993;71:308–314.

71. Yamagishi N, Anton A, Sample PA, et al. Mapping structural damage of the optic disk to visual field defect in glaucoma. *Am J Ophthalmol.* 1997;123:667–676.

72. Javitt JC, Spaeth GL, Katz LJ, et al. Acquired pits of the optic nerve: Increased prevalence in patients with low-tension glaucoma. *Ophthalmology.* 1990;97: 1038–1044.

73. Ugurlu S, Weitzman M, Nduaguba C, Caprioli J. Acquired pit of the optic nerve: A risk factor for progression of glaucoma. *Am J Ophthalmol.* 1998;125:457–464.

74. Airaksinen PJ, Mustonen E, Alanko HI. Optic disc hemorrhages: Analysis of stereophotographs and clinical data of 112 patients. *Arch Ophthalmol.* 1981;99: 1795–1801.

75. Kitazawa Y, Shirato S, Yamamoto T. Optic disc hemorrhage in low-tension glaucoma. *Ophthalmology.* 1986; 93:853–857.

76. Kottler MS, Drance SM. Studies of hemorrhage on the optic disc. *Can J Ophthalmol.* 1976;11:102–105.

77. Poinoosawmy D, Gloster J, Nagasubramanian S, Hitchings RA. Association between optic disc hemorrhages in glaucoma and abnormal glucose tolerance. *Br J Ophthalmol.* 1986;70:599–602.

78. Tuulonen A, Takamoto T, Wu DC, Schwartz B. Optic disc cupping and pallor measurements of patients with disc hemorrhages. *Am J Ophthalmol.* 1987;103:505–511.

79. Healey PR, Mitchell P, Smith W, Wang JJ. Optic disc hemorrhages in a population with and without signs of glaucoma. *Ophthalmology.* 1998;105:216–223.

80. Hendrickx KH, van den Enden A, Rasker MT, Hoyng PFJ. Cumulative incidence of patients with disc hemorrhages in glaucoma and the effect of therapy. *Ophthalmology.* 1994;101:1165–1172.

81. Drance SM. Disc hemorrhages in the glaucomas. *Surv Ophthalmol.* 1989;33:331–337.

82. Diehl DL, Quigley HA, Miller NR, et al. Prevalence and significance of optic disc hemorrhage in a longitudinal study of glaucoma. *Arch Ophthalmol.* 1990;108: 545–550.

83. Shihab ZM, Lee PF, Hay P. The significance of disc hemorrhage in open-angle glaucoma. *Ophthalmology.* 1982;89:211–213.

84. Bengtsson B. Optic disc hemorrhages preceding manifest glaucoma. *Acta Ophthalmol.* 1990;68:450–454.

85. Rasker MT, van den Enden A, Bakker D, Hoyng PF. Deterioration of visual fields in patients with glaucoma with and without optic disc hemorrhages. *Arch Ophthalmol.* 1997;115:1257–1262.

86. Seigner SW, Netland PA. Optic disc hemorrhages and progression of glaucoma. *Ophthalmology.* 1996;103: 1014–1023.

87. Airaksinen PJ, Mustonen E, Alanko HI. Optic disc hemorrhages precede retinal nerve fiber layer defects in ocular hypertension. *Acta Ophthalmol (Copenh).* 1981; 59: 627–641.

88. Papastathopoulos KI, Jonas JB. Focal narrowing of retinal arterioles in optic nerve atrophy. *Ophthalmology.* 1995;102:1706–1711.

89. Rader J, Feuer WJ, Anderson DR. Peripapillary vasoconstriction in the glaucomas and the anterior ischemic optic neuropathies. *Am J Ophthalmol.* 1994; 117:72–80.

90. Rankin SJA, Drance SM. Peripapillary focal retinal arteriolar narrowing in open angle glaucoma. *J Glaucoma.* 1996;5:22–28.

91. Jonas JB, Schiro D. Visibility of the normal retinal nerve fiber layer correlated with rim width and vessel caliber. *Graefes Arch Clin Exp Ophthalmol.* 1993;231: 207–211.

92. Jonas JB, Nguyen NX, Naumann GOH. Parapapillary retinal vessel diameter in normal and glaucomatous eyes. I. Morphometric data. *Invest Ophthalmol Vis Sci.* 1989;30:1599–1603.

93. Jonas JB, Naumann GOH. Parapapillary retinal vessel diameter in normal and glaucomatous eyes. II. Correlations. *Invest Ophthalmol Vis Sci.* 1989;30:1604–1611.

94. Balazi G, Werner EB. Relationship between baring of circumlinear vessels of the optic disc and glaucomatous visual field loss. *Can J Ophthalmol.* 1983;18:333–336.

95. Osher RH, Herschler J. The significance of baring of the circumlinear vessel: A prospective study. *Arch Ophthalmol.* 1981;99:817–818.

96. Sutton GE, Motolko MA, Phelps CD. Baring of a circumlinear vessel in glaucoma. *Arch Ophthalmol.* 1983; 101:739–744.

97. Herschler J, Osher RH. Baring of the circumlinear vessel: An early sign of optic nerve damage. *Arch Ophthalmol.* 1980;98:865–869.

98. Varma R, Spaeth GL, Hanai C, Steinmann WC, Feldmann RM, et al. Positional changes in the vasculature of the optic disk in glaucoma. *Am J Ophthalmol.* 1987; 104:457–464.

99. Armaly MF. The optic cup in the normal eye. I. Cup width, depth, vessel displacement, ocular tension, and outflow facility. *Am J Ophthalmol.* 1969;69:401–407.

100. Boeglin RJ, Caprioli J. Contemporary clinical evaluation of the optic nerve in glaucoma. *Ophthalmol Clin North Am* 1991;4:711–731.

101. Tuulonen A. Asymptomatic miniocclusions of the optic disc veins in glaucoma. *Arch Ophthalmol.* 1989;107:1475–1480.

102. Anderson DP, Khalil M, Lorenzetti DW, Saheb NE. Abnormal blood vessels on the optic disc. *Can J Ophthalmol.* 1983;18:108–114.

103. Schwartz B, Takamoto T, Nagin P. Measurements of reversibility of optic disc cupping and pallor in ocular hypertension and glaucoma. *Ophthalmology.* 1985;92:1396–1407.

104. Greenidge KC, Spaeth GL, Traverso CE. Change in appearance of the optic disc associated with lowering of intraocular pressure. *Ophthalmology.* 1985;92:897–903.

105. Pederson JE, Herschler J. Reversal of glaucomatous cupping in adults. *Arch Ophthalmol.* 1982;100, 426–431.

106. Parrow KA, Shin DH, Tsai CS, et al. Intraocular pressure-dependent dynamic changes in optic disc cupping in adult glaucoma patients. *Ophthalmology.* 1992;99:36–40.

107. Katz LJ, Spaeth GL, Cantor LB, et al. Reversible optic disk cupping and visual field improvement in adults with glaucoma. *Am J Ophthalmol.* 1989;104:485–492.

108. Hayreh SS, Joos KM, Podhajsky PA, Long CR. Systemic diseases associated with nonarteritic anterior ischemic optic neuropathy. *Am J Ophthalmol.* 1994;118:766–780.

109. Hayreh SS. Anterior ischemic optic neuropathy. *Clin Neurosci.* 1997;4:251–263.

110. Grover S, Fishman GA, Brown J. Frequency of optic disc or parapapillary nerve fiber layer drusen in retinitis pigmentosa. *Ophthalmology.* 1997;104:295–298.

111. Kheterpal S, Good PA, Beale DJ, Kritzinger EE. Imaging of optic disc drusen: A comparative study. *Eye.* 1995;9:67–69.

112. Roh S, Noecker RJ, Schuman JS. Evaluation of coexisting optic nerve head drusen and glaucoma with optical coherence tomography. *Ophthalmology.* 1997;104:1138–1144.

113. Austin JK. Optic disc drusen and associated venous stasis retinopathy. *J Am Optom Assoc.* 1995;66:91–95.

114. Boldt HC, Byrne SF, DiBernardo C. Echographic evaluation of optic disc drusen. *J Clin Neurophthalmol.* 1991;11:85–91.

115. Borruat FX, Sanders MD. Vascular anomalies and complications of optic disc drusen. *Klin Monatsbl Augenheilkd.* 1996;208:294–296.

116. Brown GC, Shields JA, Goldberg RE. Congenital pits of the optic nerve head. II. Clinical studies in humans. *Ophthalmology.* 1980;87:51–65.

117. Rutledge BK, Puliafito CA, Duker JS, Hee MR, Cox MS. Optical coherence tomography of macular lesions associated with optic nerve head pits. *Ophthalmology.* 1996;103:1047–1053.

118. Krivoy D, Gentile R, Liebmann JM, et al. Imaging congenital optic disc pits and associated maculopathy using optic coherence tomography. *Arch Ophthalmol.* 1996; 114:165–170.

119. Rutledge BK, Puliafito CA, Duker JS, Hee MR, Cox MS. Optical coherence tomography of macular lesions associated with optic nerve head pits. *Ophthalmology.* 1996;103:1047–1053.

120. Lincoff H, Krelssig I. Optical coherence tomography of pneumatic displacement of optic disc pit maculopathy. *Br J Ophthalmol.* 1998;82:367–372.

121. Rosenthal G, Bartz-Schmidt KU, Walter P, Heimann K. Autologous platelet treatment for optic disc pit associated with persistent macular detachment. *Graefes Arch Clin Exp Ophthalmol.* 1998;236:151–153.

122. Kindler P. Morning glory syndrome: Unusual congenital optic disk anomaly. *Am J Ophthalmol.* 1970;69:376–384.

123. Brodsky MC. Congenital optic disk anomalies. *Surv Ophthalmol.* 1994;39:89–112.

124. Murphy BL, Griffin JF. Optic nerve coloboma (morning glory syndrome): CT findings. *Radiology.* 1994;191:59–161.

125. Steahly LP. Retinochoroidal coloboma: Varieties of clinical presentations. *Ann Ophthalmol.* 1990;22:9–14.

126. McDonald HR, Lewis H, Brown G, Sipperley JO. Vitreous surgery for retinal detachment associated with choroidal coloboma. *Arch Ophthalmol.* 1991;109:1399–1402.

127. Hotta K, Hirakata A, Shinoda K, Miki D, Hida T. Characteristics of retinal detachment in eyes with choroidal colobomas. *Nippon-Ganka-Gakkai-Zasshi.* 1998;102:207–214.

128. Brazitikos PD, Safran AB, Simona F, Zulauf M. Threshold perimetry in tilted disc syndrome. *Arch Ophthalmol.* 1990;108:1698–1700.

129. Keane JR. Suprasellar tumors and incidental optic disc anomalies: Diagnostic problems in two patients with hemianopic temporal scotomas. *Arch Ophthalmol.* 1977;95:2180–2183.

130. Lichter PR. Variability of expert observers in evaluating the optic disc. *Trans Am Ophthalmol Soc.* 1976;74:532–572.

131. Houston GL, Shipp MD. Reliability of assessing the cup/disc ratio using a 90-D lens photograph. *Optom Vis Sci.* 1989;66:78–81.

132. Varma R, Steinmann WC, Scott IU. Expert agreement in evaluating the optic disc for glaucoma. *Ophthalmology.* 1992;99:215–221.

133. Coleman AL, Sommer A, Enger C, et al. Inter-observer and intra-observer variability in the detection of glaucomatous progression of the optic disc. *J Glaucoma.* 1996;5:384–389.

134. Jupiter DG. The introduction of new condensing lenses for fundus examination. *J Am Optom Assoc.* 1995;66:42–46.

135. Repka MX, Uozato H, Guyton DL. Depth distortion during slit-lamp biomicroscopy of the fundus. *Ophthalmology.* 1986;93(S):47–51.

136. Boes DA, Spaeth GL, Mills RP, et al. Relative optic cup depth assessments using three stereo photograph viewing methods. *J Glaucoma.* 1996;5:9–14.

137. Dichtl A, Jonas JB. Echographic measurement of optic nerve thickness correlated with neuroretinal rim area and visual field defect in glaucoma. *Am J Ophthalmol.* 1996;122:514–519.

138. Jonas JB, Schmidt A, Muller-Bergh JA, Naumann GOH. Optic nerve fiber count and diameter of the retrobulbar optic nerve in normal and glaucomatous eyes. *Graefes Arch Clin Exp Ophthalmol.* 1995;223:421–424.

139. O'Connor DJ, Zeyen T, Caprioli J. Comparisons of methods to detect glaucomatous optic nerve damage. *Ophthalmology.* 1993;100:1498–1503.

140. Caprioli J, Prum B, Zeyen T. Comparison of methods to evaluate the optic nerve head and nerve fiber layer for glaucomatous change. *Am J Ophthalmol.* 1996;121:659–667.

Chapter 13

EVALUATION OF THE RETINAL NERVE FIBER LAYER

Pait Teesalu
P. Juhani Airaksinen

Glaucoma is a disease of multifactorial etiology that causes damage to the ganglion cell axons in the fundus of the eye. The loss of nerve fibers gives a typical glaucomatous configuration to the optic nerve head. In the retina, the loss of nerve fibers is associated with decreased visibility of the retinal nerve fiber layer (RNFL). Hoyt et al.[1] first described glaucomatous abnormalities in the visible RNFL. The first observable changes he found were thin, slit-like defects or grooves in the arcuate area of the RNFL. In more advanced cases, wedge-shaped localized defects developed. Two distinct patterns of neural tissue loss are recognized: localized and diffuse (called also widespread or generalized). In an individual patient, one or the other pattern may predominate, or both patterns may occur (Fig. 13–1).[2,3] It has been found that diffuse or generalized loss of axons is the most common pattern in early glaucoma, but that a mixed pattern of diffuse and localized loss is more common as a later finding.[4]

NORMAL ANATOMY

The RNFL is the innermost layer of the fundus and is separated from the vitreous by an internal limiting membrane. Healthy RNFL appears as regularly oriented striations, which are formed by the retinal ganglion cell axon bundles and compartmentalized in tunnels formed by Mueller's cell processes. These striations are seen because the light is reflected back from the nerve bundles and the separating glial septa. The organization of the nerve fibers in the retina is probably such that the more peripherally originated fibers are situated closer to the pigment epithelium; the fibers originating from more proximal ganglion cells pierce them and proceed closer to the vitreous. In the optic nerve head, the superficial nerve fiber bundles are located centrally, whereas the more peripherally originating fibers are located closer to the edge of the chorioscleral canal (Fig. 13–2).

Papillomacular bundles have an almost straight horizontal course, while the upper and lower temporal fibers form an arch around the macula. This pattern determines the typical appearance of glaucomatous arcuate defects in the visual field. The superior and inferior temporal bundles are bounded by the temporal raphe, which extends from the foveola to the temporal periphery of the retina. Nasal nerve fiber bundles proceed radially to the optic disc (Fig. 13–3). The axons come together at the disc, bend backwards, and form the neuroretinal rim of the optic disc. The width on the neuroretinal rim and the size of optic disc cupping are dependent on the size of the optic disc and the number of nerve fibers passing through the scleral canal.

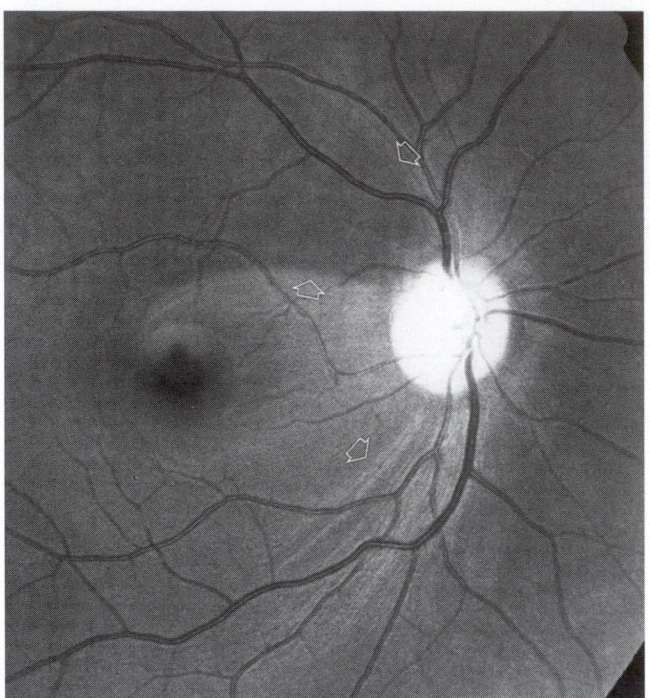

Figure 13–1. Generalized loss of axons with a narrow, localized defect inferotemporally *(arrow)* and an even deeper and wider localized sector-shaped dropout of axon bundles superotemporally *(arrows). (See Color Plate 30.)*

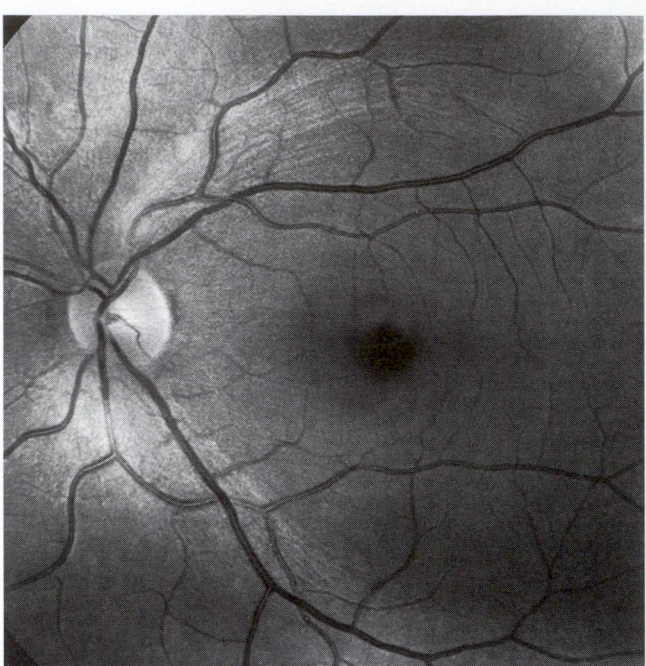

Figure 13–3. Normal nerve fiber layer showing typical pattern of the arcuate, papillomacular, and nasal bundles. *(See Color Plate 31.)*

EXAMINATION TECHNIQUES

The RNFL can be assessed ophthalmoscopically or with wide-angle red-free photography. In the white light of an ophthalmoscope, the healthy nerve fiber bundles appear slightly opaque, with radially oriented striations covering the vessels. They are most easily detected in the peripapillary region and in the area of arcuate fibers above and below the optic disc, where the RNFL is thickest. In the upper and lower temporal arcuate regions, the RNFL is up to 300 μm thick and the number of nerve bundles is substan-

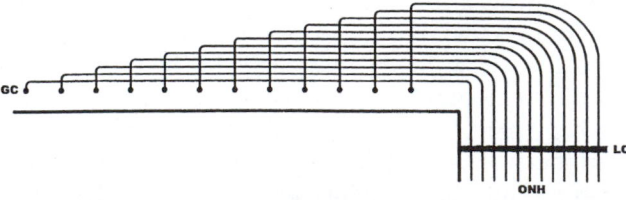

Figure 13–2. Arrangement of the axon bundles in the nerve fiber layer. The peripherally originating axons are located closer to the pigment epithelium while the more proximally originating fibers are located more superficially, closer to the vitreous. In the optic disc, the fibers originating peripherally are closer to the disc edge and the fibers originating proximally are closer to the center of the nerve.

tially greater than the number of light striations.[5] The nerve fiber layer is more difficult to visualize in the thin nasal and papillomacular areas, where the thickness of the nerve fiber layer is only one-fifth of that in the upper and lower temporal regions. In these areas there is one nerve bundle which is seen for each light striation.[5]

In the white light, atrophy of the RNFL appears as a darker red area in which visibility of the normal striation pattern is reduced or absent. A much better visibility of the nerve fiber layer and its defects can be achieved with a green or blue light. The advantage of red-free ophthalmoscopy was probably first noted by Vogt in 1917.[6] The reason is that the short-wavelength light does not penetrate beyond the RNFL but is reflected from the superficial layers of the retina back to the camera except in areas where the nerve fiber layer is destroyed and the light is absorbed by the underlying pigment epithelium. The dark pigment epithelium provides the contrast between the normal and degenerated areas. Defective areas appear darker and with less detail than the healthy areas (Fig. 13–1).

One can follow the striped pattern of the RNFL with a simple ophthalmoscope, but use of the fundus lens or a contact lens with the slit lamp will provide a binocular overview. The 78-diopter lens provides more magnification and detail, but the 90-diopter lens has a wider field of view and can often be used in the presence of a smaller pupil. Both fundus lenses convert the slit lamp into an indirect ophthalmoscope. In order to achieve the best image, the pupils should be maximally dilated and the room lighting dimmed.

By taking a wide-angle red-free photograph, one can evaluate the RNFL more easily while also obtaining a permanent record. Any defect visible by clinical examination can generally be demonstrated in photographs. Although many localized sector-shaped RNFL defects can be detected easily with funduscopy, some will be visible only in good photographs. Diffuse nerve fiber loss is difficult to detect by slit-lamp examination and usually requires photographs.

A monochromatic light was introduced into ophthalmic photography by Behrendt and Wilson.[7] Using interference filters and black-and-white film, they noticed that the RNFL was invisible for red light, that its visibility increased in green-blue and blue light from 549 to 477 nm, and that it began to disappear at 431 nm. Airaksinen[8] and later Peli et al.[9] reported easier detection of defects in the nerve fiber layer with a wide-angle fundus camera, using high-resolution, fine-grain, black-and-white film with a blue narrow-band interference filter of 495 nm wavelength. This technique was used in the RNFL photographs of this chapter. Other wavelengths and films have also been used successfully.[3,7,10,11] In another method, the nerve fiber layer is first photographed on color film using white light; then the color transparency is reproduced on black-and-white film through a green filter to eliminate the disturbing image of the deeper retina and choroid.[12] Delori et al.,[10] however, reported that with monochromatic light, nerve fibers can be observed two to three times further away from the optic disc than with white light. In part this may be explained by the higher resolving power of low-sensitivity black-and-white films as opposed to color films.[12,13]

The RNFL itself is very difficult to see through the camera. To achieve good results, the photographer should focus on the blood vessels about half a disc diameter away from where they emerge from the disc. The RNFL will be out of focus if the photographer focuses on the disc, because the disc is deeper than the RNFL. Pupillary dilation is not essential when photographs are taken with a nonmydriatic fundus camera.[14] Otherwise, patients should be instructed to discontinue miotic therapy for 2 days to allow the pupils to dilate maximally. It is important that intraocular pressure not be measured with fluorescein before photography because of the fluorescein exciter filter used. This would lead to a gray and poor contrast image.

Lens opacities and lens yellowing have an effect on RNFL visibility, and in some patients the RNFL cannot be adequately visualized. The quality of photographs of the RNFL also depends on how well the blue light is absorbed by the retinal pigment epithelium. A darkly pigmented epithelium as a background greatly enhances visibility of the axon bundles; but in eyes with anomalies of fundus pigmentation, the RNFL cannot be well evaluated (e.g., in lightly pigmented myopic eyes).

CLINICAL EVALUATION OF RETINAL NERVE FIBER LAYER DEFECTS

In half of the eyes that develop glaucoma, the first detectable RNFL abnormality is diffuse loss of axons—in other words, generalized thinning of the RNFL.[4] Diffuse loss of the RNFL is visible as generalized reduction of the RNFL pattern and is usually considerably more difficult to detect than localized RNFL defects. A typical sign of diffuse RNFL damage is a mottled appearance of the retina (Fig. 13–4). When there is total or subtotal atrophy of the fibers, the fundus looks dark because no light is reflected back.

Where diffuse damage is suspected, it is particularly helpful to evaluate the visibility of blood vessels and capillaries. In healthy eyes, blood vessels are embedded in the RNFL; therefore small vessels

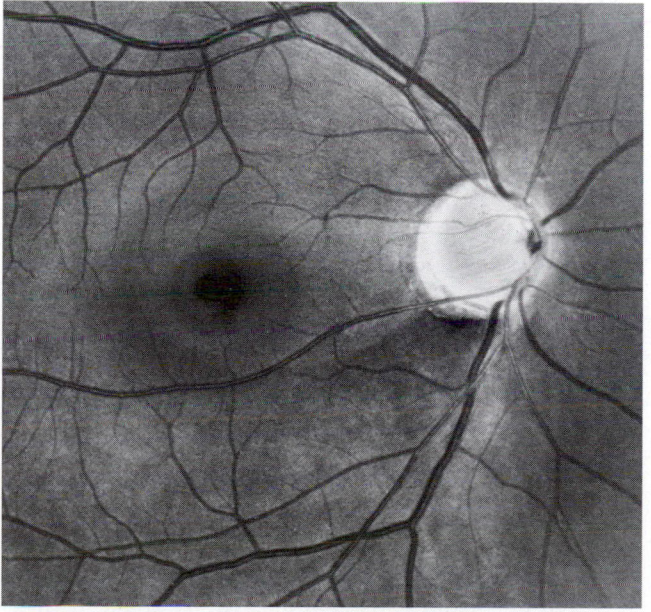

Figure 13–4. Diffuse or generalized loss of nerve fibers inferiorly. Note the mottled appearance of the pigment epithelium and sharp wall images of the small retinal vessels. *(See Color Plate 32.)*

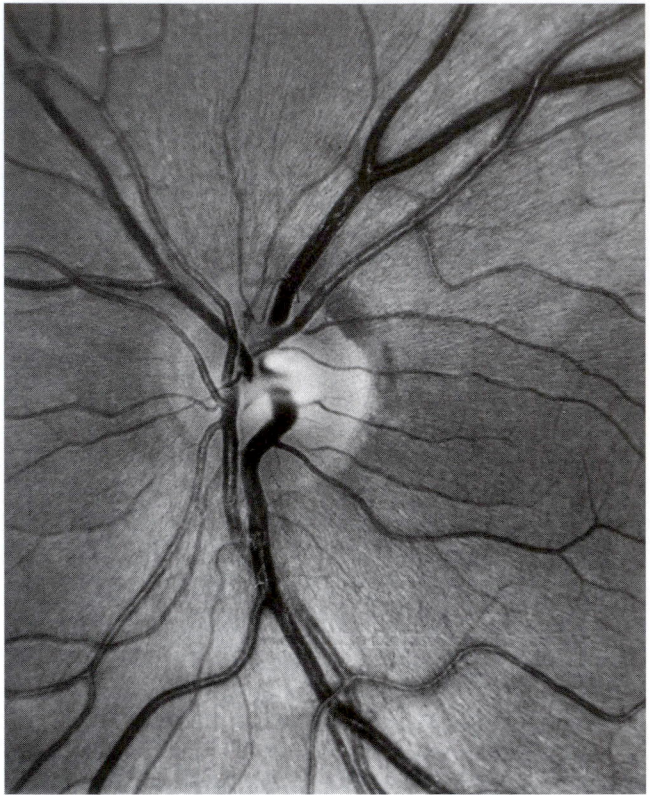

Figure 13–5. Normal retinal nerve fiber layer. The margins of the small vessels appear blurred and cross-hatched, as they are within the healthy nerve fiber layer. *(See Color Plate 33.)*

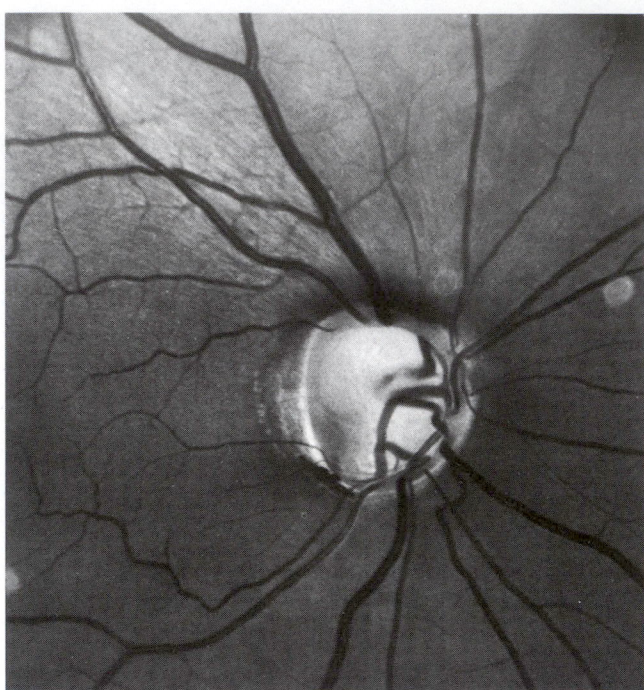

Figure 13–6. Severe diffuse or generalized loss of nerve fibers in the inferior half of the right fundus. The vessels are not covered by the pattern of the retinal nerve fiber layer and can be visualized very clearly. Also, the fundus appears darker inferiorly than superiorly, as only a little light is reflected back to the camera from the defective area.

appear blurred and cross-hatched (Fig. 13–5). In defective areas, the retinal vessels are covered only by the inner limiting membrane and the vessel walls stand out sharply. In mild or moderate RNFL atrophy, the first-order branches of vessels are bare (sharp wall images). If the pattern of RNFL is absent and even second-order vessels are clearly not covered by the pattern, severe diffuse atrophy is present (Fig. 13–6).

In cases where the RNFL cannot be visualized, the following possible reasons should be considered:

1. The patient may suffer from advanced loss of nerve fibers.
2. Media opacities may be hampering the visibility of the nerve fibers. In this case, the photographs look gray and fuzzy rather than dark. In addition, it is useful to compare the visibility of the superior and inferior fibers within the same eye. Comparison of up to down is the best way to see whether a somewhat attenuated RNFL pattern is due to media haze or mild atrophy, as cataracts rarely make it difficult to see at least half of the RNFL (Fig. 13–6).
3. The fundus may be very lightly pigmented.
4. The photographs may be out of focus.

Slit-like or wedge-shaped RNFL defects can be more easily detected because defective areas appear dark and are outlined sharply against the more silvery hue of intact RNFL. The narrowest tip of the wedge is found at the optic disc margin or peripapillary area close to the disc supero- (Fig. 13–7) or inferotemporally. The frequency of localized RNFL defects in glaucomatous eyes increases significantly from early- to moderate-stage glaucoma and decreases again in advanced glaucoma.[15] In the advanced stage, the defects are usually no longer detectable because of the pronounced loss of nerve fibers in the entire fundus (Fig. 13–8A through G). The localized defects of the RNFL should not be confused with RNFL slits, which appear in 10% of normal individuals and are often spindle-shaped, rarely wider than a retinal vessel, and often do not extend to the border of the optic disc.

Retinal Nerve Fiber Layer, Optic Disc, and Visual Field in Glaucoma

Visual field defects and changes in the optic nerve head (ONH) and RNFL are widely regarded as important and definite signs of glaucoma. As a clinician should

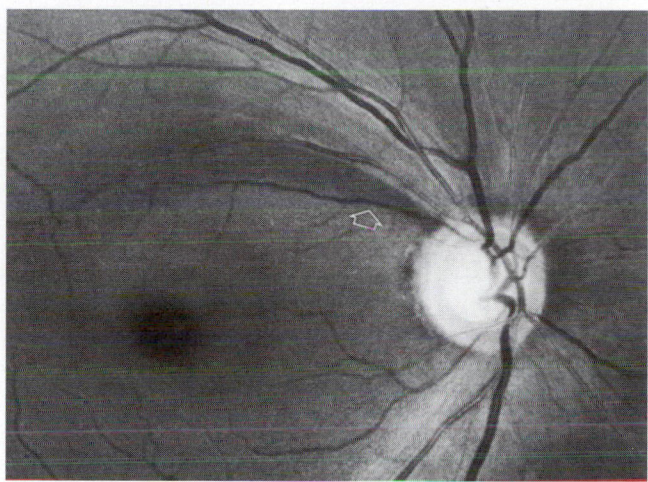

Figure 13–7. A wedge-shaped defect in the upper arcuate fibers *(arrow)* that developed after an optic disc hemorrhage (not shown). The narrowest tip of the wedge is located at the 11-o'clock position of the optic disc.

always use all clinical information available, it is helpful to compare the RNFL findings with the appearance of the optic disc and the visual field. One could first assess the optic nerve or the visual field and then see whether the appearance of the RNFL confirms these findings. On the other hand, localized abnormalities in the RNFL may call attention to a specific location on the optic disc or visual field, thus helping the examiner to detect very early disc changes.

It has long been recognized that glaucoma is associated with an increase in the absolute size of the optic cup as well as in the cup-to-disc ratio. Neither by itself is very helpful in distinguishing the normal from the glaucomatous disc, since both are functions of the size of the disc, which varies tremendously in the normal population. The normal optic cup does, however, display characteristic features related to its shape and configuration, which may be more helpful than the size alone. The normal optic cup is rarely vertically oval. Since early localized loss of nerve fibers and rim tissue tends to occur mainly at the superior and inferior poles of the disc, the cup is most likely to enlarge more vertically than horizontally. The upper and lower temporal areas of the optic disc are affected first, probably because of weaker architecture of the lamina cribrosa in these areas.[16] Usually the affected fibers originate from ganglion cells located about 15 to 20 degrees from the fovea, close to the temporal raphe. Atrophy of the ganglion cells cannot be visualized clinically, but the loss of respective axons appears as a wedge-shaped RNFL defect and a small notch at the optic disc margin (Figs. 13–7 and 13–8C). Corresponding to this localized decline in

ganglion cells is an isolated scotoma in the mirror-image hemifield close to the horizontal meridian.

It is also useful to look at the peripapillary RNFL stereoscopically in the stereo–photographs of the optic disc. The observer can then assess both the optic disc and the adjacent RNFL in detail simultaneously. One should, however, keep in mind that in the early stages of development, the visibility of an RNFL defect near the optic disc is poor because undamaged, more proximally originating axons cover the defect. When the proximally originating axons are also degenerated, the RNFL defect can be visualized all the way to the optic disc. The notch of the neuroretinal rim reaches the optic disc margin at the same time as the arcuate visual field defect connects to the blind spot. Further progression of the glaucomatous damage can be seen as widening of the RNFL defect (Fig. 13–8C, E, and G) and visual field defect. When the papillomacular bundles are affected, the visual field defect comes closer to fixation. In the far advanced stage, there is a total or subtotal atrophy of nerve fibers as well as a totally cupped optic disc, and the patient has advanced visual field defects.

In glaucoma, the anatomic loss of neural tissue goes along with deterioration of function. Several studies have investigated the association of the RNFL abnormalities with various functional and structural variables indicating the degree of glaucomatous optic nerve damage.

Scoring the Retinal Nerve Fiber Layer

Because the information obtained from RNFL photographs is qualitative in nature, grading systems that attempt to quantify the RNFL abnormalities have been developed.[2,17,18] We have used a semiquantitative scoring system where the optic disc is divided into 10 sectors: two sectors for the papillomacular bundles, both extending 20 degrees above and below the horizontal; two sectors for the nasal area, both extending 60 degrees to either side of the horizontal; and three sectors each for the superior and inferior arcuate areas, each extending 30 degrees to the nasal side of the vertical meridian.[2,19] Each sector is scored from 0 to 3 separately for localized and diffuse loss of nerve fibers (with 0 = no damage; 1 = mild atrophy; 2 = moderate atrophy; and 3 = severe atrophy). The localized and diffuse scores are added together to provide an overall score. Quigley and associates[17] have proposed a four-level grading system with three features assessed: the brightness of the reflexes, the RNFL's texture, and the degree to which the RNFL obscures the view of retinal blood vessels. Readings were performed by comparing the areas above and below the optic disc to that directed toward the fovea. On the basis of these three features, diffuse atrophy was divided into mild, moderate, and

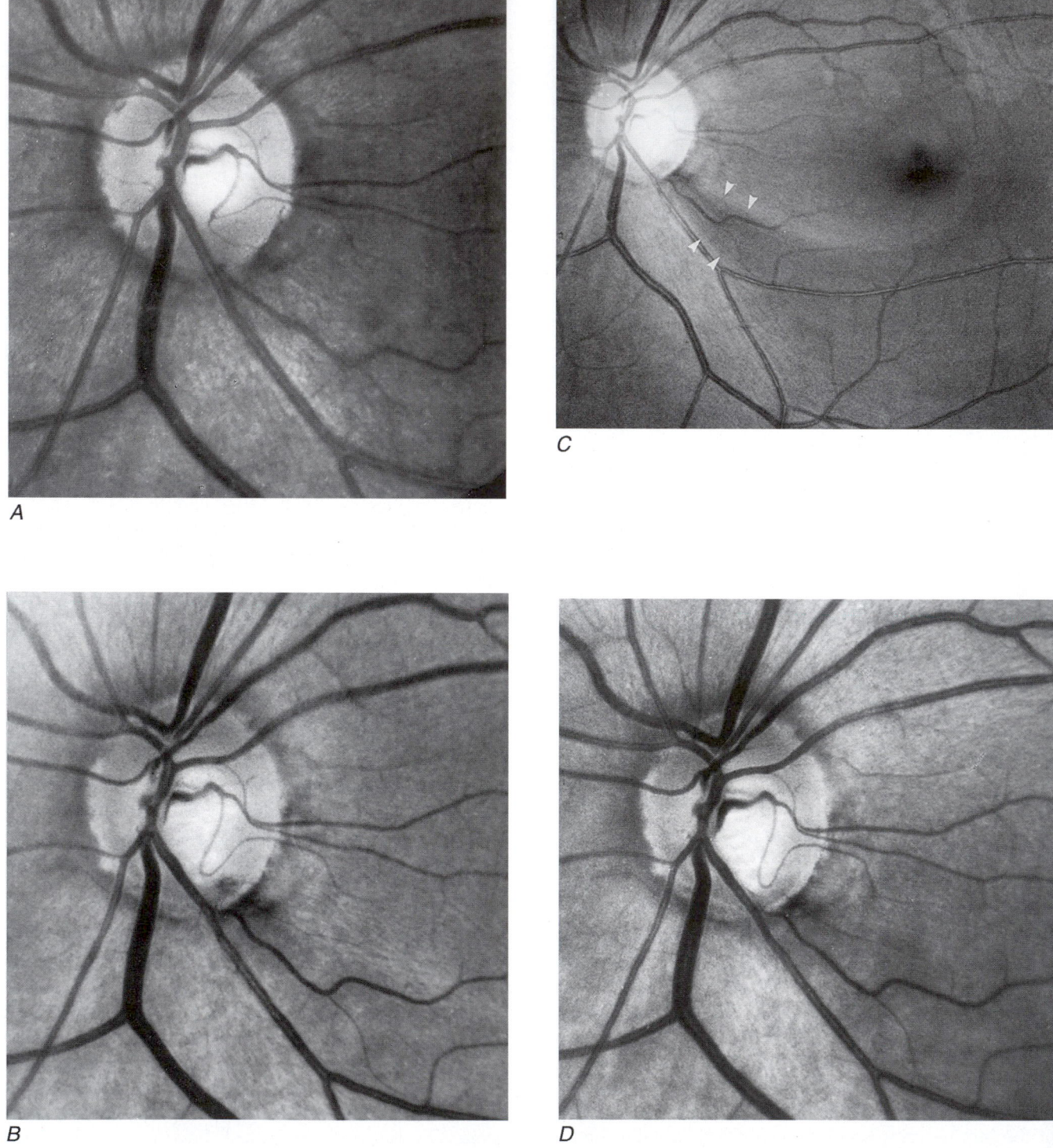

Figure 13–8. *A.* Optic disc with normal and healthy appearance of the optic disc neural tissue as well as normal peripapillary retinal nerve fiber layer (RNFL) in 1973. *B.* In a photograph taken 16 years later, in 1989, notching of the neural rim has developed in association with repeated optic disc hemorrhages at the 5 o'clock position. Note also how the optic disc vessels at 5 o'clock have changed in position owing to loss of underlying neural tissue. *C.* In this RNFL photograph taken with a wide-angle camera on the same day as the one in Fig. 13-8*B,* an associated wedge-shaped defect of the RNFL can be seen *(arrows). D.* By 1991, the disc notch has become wider and deeper. *(Continued on page 183)*

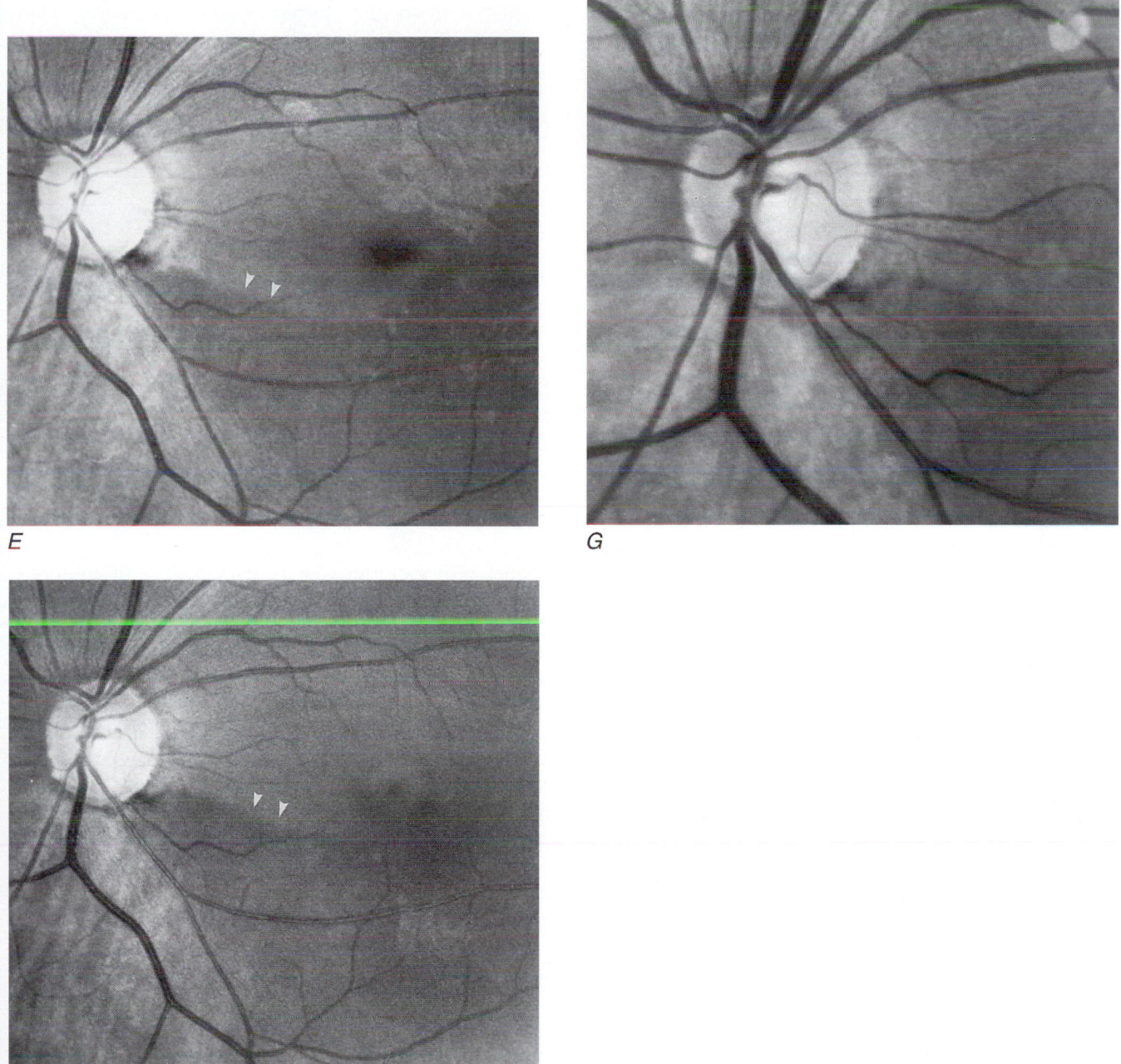

Figure 13–8. *(Continued).   E.* The RNFL defect is touching the papillomacular nerve fiber bundles. *F.* Some 4 years later, in 1995, further progression of the optic disc damage and *(G)* widening of the RNFL defect are seen. The inferior margin of the defect can no longer be visualized because the local defect is progressing and developing into a widespread or more generalized loss of axons.

severe grades, and localized (wedge) atrophy was graded in two levels. For a final score, diffuse and wedge types of atrophy were combined into a single score. Milder wedge defects were included with mild diffuse atrophy and more severe wedge defects with moderate diffuse atrophy. Niessen et al.[18] used a visu-ally supported grading system where the patient's photograph was compared with a set of 25 reference photographs, numbered from 25 (broad, clearly striated nerve fiber bundles) to 1 (no nerve fibers visible). Their classification system was based on grading diffuse atrophy separately for upper and lower halves.

The Retinal Nerve Fiber Layer and Perimetry

The correlations between RNFL semiquantitative scores and measures of visual function have been evaluated in several studies.[19–25] Lachenmayr et al.[23] found that RNFL scores were highly correlated with mean flicker frequency of flicker perimetry. A statistically highly significant correlation was also found between the results of high-pass resolution perimetry and semiquantitative RNFL scoring in a patient population including normals and patients with ocular hypertension or glaucoma.[24] Examination of the color vision of early glaucoma patients with an anomaloscope showed that the yellow-blue and green-blue matching ranges correlated significantly with diffuse loss of nerve fibers.[25]

A variety of clinical correlations reflect the fact that the RNFL may be damaged both diffusely and locally. Airaksinen and associates[20] found that semiquantitative RNFL scores were highly correlated with "Octopus" visual-field indices, although more with the mean defect index (expressing generalized reduction of light sensitivity) than with the corrected loss variance index (expressing localized visual field abnormalities). In our recent study,[19] the mean deviation (MD) values obtained using short-wavelength automated perimetry (SWAP) and conventional white-on-white (W-W) perimetry (Humphrey 24-2) were both statistically highly significantly related to the total score for diffuse and overall loss of RNFL, but no correlation was found between MD values and total localized score of the RNFL loss.

The detectable abnormalities in the RNFL and optic disc usually precede criteria referred to, in achromatic perimetry, as *typical glaucomatous field loss.*[26–28] Sommer et al.[27] retrospectively examined photographs taken sequentially in patients with increased intraocular pressure and found that RNFL abnormalities were the first observable changes in patients with glaucoma and preceded visual field damage by as much as 6 years. They found RNFL defects in both hemispheres of over 80% of eyes when visual field loss was first documented. In contrast, visual field loss (by kinetic and suprathreshold static perimetry) involved both hemifields in only 14% of eyes.

In evaluating the seemingly unaffected hemifields of glaucoma patients, we[29] found that regression analysis using SWAP hemifield data classified 38% of normal W-W hemifields as abnormal; 52% were classified as abnormal when optic nerve head parameters were measured by Heidelberg retinal tomography (HRT). In another study,[19] we showed that there was an abnormal RNFL in 84% of hemispheres respective to the seemingly healthy W/W hemifields in early glaucoma patients. A high association was found between RNFL assessment and SWAP in patients with ocular hypertension and early glaucoma;[19,30] this also suggests that in the progression of glaucoma, the results of SWAP and RNFL assessment follow each other more closely than do results of the conventional perimetry.

On the other hand, the function of the ganglion cells may be impaired even if the RNFL appears clinically normal. In an experimental study, Quigley and Addicks[5] found that localized RNFL defects can be detected clinically if more than 50% of the thickness of the RNFL is lost. In our study,[19] the analysis of variance showed a statistically significant difference between the SWAP visual field results in normal subjects and in those with ocular hypertension (with zero RNFL loss score) but no statistically significant difference between ocular hypertensive patients and the early glaucoma group.

CONCLUSION

Damage of the optic disc is associated with an abnormal appearance of the RNFL. Airaksinen and Drance[31] found that the neuroretinal rim area was statistically highly significantly correlated with the scores rating nerve fiber loss. Jonas and associates[32] demonstrated that the locations of RNFL defects were correlated with neuroretinal rim notching as well as with peripapillary chorioretinal atrophy. More recently, Eid et al.[33] found that RNFL height measured with HRT was correlated strongly with topographic optic disc parameters such as rim volume, rim area, and cup-to-disc ratio.

The splinter hemorrhages on the optic disc (Figs. 13–7 and 13–8B) seem to precede both the development and progression of glaucoma damage and to predict its location. Airaksinen et al.[34] reported that most of the time the RNFL defect appeared at locations where disc hemorrhages had been seen 6 to 8 weeks earlier. In a study of eyes with increased intraocular pressure, Airaksinen and Heijl[21] found changes of the RNFL to be the only abnormal feature present in 46% of eyes with disc hemorrhages and in 26% of eyes without disc hemorrhages.

The axons are gathered together in the optic nerve head but spread out in a thin layer in the retina. Therefore, examination of the RNFL may, in fact, provide information on the minor losses of axons that cannot be detected by evaluating the neuroretinal rim of the optic nerve head. There are several studies suggesting that RNFL examination is, in fact, more sensitive than evaluation of the optic disc in detecting early progressive glaucoma damage. Caprioli[35] found, in a cross-sectional study, that RNFL height was the best of the structural parameters used to discriminate between normal and glaucomatous eyes. In a 5-year follow-up study, Quigley et al.[36] compared the value of serial optic disc and RNFL examinations in detecting progressive changes of converters—that is, patients with ocular hypertension in whom glaucoma was developing. They found that the RNFL examination was more sensitive than optic disc evaluation in detecting early progressive glaucoma damage. The higher sensitivity of RNFL evaluation was also confirmed in our recent study.[37]

The diagnosis is always a summary of all the clinical information available. Although analysis of the RNFL takes some time to learn, it is a worthy adjunct to evaluation of the optic disc and visual field. The assessment of RNFL is subjective and qualitative, and today's high-technology systems for analyzing the optic disc and RNFL are probably superior in the follow-up of disease and in patients with small pupils and opacities of the optic media. However, RNFL evaluation as a readily available method should be part of every routine ophthalmoscopy.

REFERENCES

1. Hoyt WF, Frisèn LL, Newman NM. Funduscopy of nerve fiber layer defects in glaucoma. *Invest Ophthalmol.* 1973;12:814–829.
2. Airaksinen PJ, Drance SM, Douglas GR, Mawson DK, Nieminen H. Diffuse and localized nerve fiber loss in glaucoma. *Am J Ophthalmol.* 1984;98:566–571.
3. Iwata K, Nanba K, Abe H. Typical slit-like retinal nerve fiber layer defect and corresponding scotoma. *Acta Soc Ophthalmol Jpn.* 1981;85:1791–1803.
4. Tuulonen A, Airaksinen PJ. Initial glaucomatous optic disk and retinal nerve fiber layer abnormalities and their progression. *Am J Ophthalmol.* 1991;111:485–490.
5. Quigley HA, Addicks EM. Quantitative studies of the retinal nerve fiber layer defects. *Arch Ophthalmol.* 1982;100:807–814.
6. Vogt A. Die Nervenfaserstreifung der menschlichen Netzhaut mit besonderer Berücksichtigung der Differentialdiagnose gegenüber pathologischen streifenförmigen Reflexen (präretinalen Fältelungen). *Klin Monatsbl Augenheilkd.* 1917;58:399–411.
7. Behrendt T, Wilson LA. Spectral reflectance photography of the retina. *Am J Ophthalmol.* 1965;59:1079–1088.
8. Airaksinen PJ, Nieminen H, Mustonen E. Retinal nerve fiber layer photography with a wide angle fundus camera. *Acta Ophthalmol (Copenh).* 1982;60:362–368.
9. Peli E, Hedges TR, McInnes T, Hamlin J, Schwartz B. Nerve fiber layer photography: A comparative study. *Acta Ophthalmol (Copenh).* 1987;65:71–80.
10. Delori FC, Gragoudas ES, Francisco R, Pruett RC. Monochromatic ophthalmoscopy and fundus photography: The normal fundus. *Arch Ophthalmol.* 1977;95:861–868.

11. Manor RS, Schleinn N, Yassur Y, Svetliza E, Ben-Sira I. Narrow-band (540 nm) green-light stereoscopic photography of the surface details of the peripapillary retina. *Am J Ophthalmol.* 1981;91:774–780.
12. Frisen L. Photography of the retinal nerve fiber layer: An optimised procedure. *Br J Ophthalmol.* 1980;64:641–650.
13. Ducrey NM, Delori FC, Gragoudas ES. Monochromatic ophthalmoscopy and fundus photography: II. The pathological fundus. *Arch Ophthalmol.* 1979;97:288–293.
14. Tuulonen A, Airaksinen PJ, Montagna A, Nieminen H. Screening for glaucoma with a non-mydriatic fundus camera. *Acta Ophthalmol (Copenh).* 1990;68:445–449.
15. Jonas JB, Schiro D. Localized wedge shaped defects of the retinal nerve fiber layer in glaucoma. *Br J Ophthalmol.* 1994;78:285–290.
16. Quigley HA, Addicks EM. Regional differences in the structure of the lamina cribrosa and their relation to glaucomatous optic nerve damage. *Arch Ophthalmol.* 1981;99:137–143.
17. Quigley HA, Reacher M, Katz J, Strahlman E, Gilbert D, Scott R. Quantitative grading of the nerve fiber layer photographs. *Ophthalmology.* 1993;100:1800–1807.
18. Niessen AGJE, Van den Berg TJTP, Langerhorst CT, Bossuyt PM. Grading of retinal nerve fiber layer with a photographic reference set. *Am J Ophthalmol.* 1995;120: 577–586.
19. Teesalu P, Airaksinen PJ, Tuulonen A. Blue-on-yellow visual field and retinal nerve fiber layer in ocular hypertension and glaucoma. *Ophthalmology.* 1998;105:2077–2081.
20. Airaksinen PJ, Drance SM, Douglas GR, Schulzer M, Wijsman K. Visual field and retinal nerve fiber layer comparisons in glaucoma. *Arch Ophthalmol.* 1985;103:205–207.
21. Airaksinen PJ, Heijl A. Visual field and retinal nerve fiber layer in early glaucoma after optic disc haemorrhage. *Acta Ophthalmol (Copenh).* 1983;61:186–194.
22. Drance SM, Airaksinen PJ, Prince M, Schulzer M, Douglas GR, Tansley BW. The correlation of functional and structural measurements in glaucoma patients and normal subjects. *Am J Ophthalmol.* 1986;102:612–616.
23. Lachenmayr BJ, Airaksinen PJ, Drance SM, Wijsman K. Correlation of retinal nerve-fiber-layer loss, changes at the optic nerve head and various psychophysical criteria in glaucoma. *Graefes Arch Clin Exp Ophthalmol.* 1991; 229:133–138.
24. Airaksinen PJ, Tuulonen A, Välimäki J, Alanko HI. Retinal nerve fiber layer abnormalities and high-pass resolution perimetry. *Acta Ophthalmol (Copenh).* 1990;68: 687–689.
25. Airaksinen PJ, Lakowski R, Drance SM, Price M. Color vision and retinal nerve fiber layer in early glaucoma. *Am J Ophthalmol.* 1986;101:208–213.
26. Hitchings RA, Poinoosawmy D, Poplar N, et al. Retinal nerve fiber layer photography in glaucomatous patients. *Eye.* 1987;1:621–625.
27. Sommer A, Katz J, Quigley HA, et al. Clinically detectable nerve fiber atrophy precedes the onset of glaucomatous field loss. *Arch Ophthalmol.* 1991;109:77–83.
28. Tuulonen A, Lehtola J, Airaksinen PJ. Nerve fiber layer defects with normal visual fields: Do normal optic disc

and normal visual field indicate absence of glaucomatous abnormality? *Ophthalmology.* 1993;100:587–598.

29. Teesalu P, Vihanninjoki K, Airaksinen PJ, Tuulonen A. Hemifield association between blue-on-yellow visual field and optic nerve head topographic measurements. *Graefes Arch Clin Exp Ophthalmol.* 1998;236:339–345.

30. Polo V, Abecia E, Pablo LE, Pinilla I, Larrosa JM, Honrubia FM. Short-wavelength automated perimetry and retinal nerve fiber layer evaluation in suspected cases of glaucoma. *Arch Ophthalmol.* 1998;116:1295–1298.

31. Airaksinen PJ, Drance SM. Neuroretinal rim area and retinal nerve fiber layer in glaucoma. *Arch Ophthalmol.* 1985;103:203–204.

32. Jonas JB, Nguyen NX, Naumann GOH. Die retinale Nervenfaserschicht in Normal- und Glaukomaugen: II. Korrelationen. *Klin Monatsbl Augenheilkd.* 1989;195: 308–314.

33. Eid TM, Spaeth GL, Katz LJ, Azuara-Blanco A, Agusburger J, Nicholl J. Quantitative estimation of retinal nerve fiber layer height in glaucoma and the relationship with optic nerve head topography and visual field. *J Glaucoma.* 1997;6:221–230.

34. Airaksinen PJ, Mustonen E, Alanko HI. Optic disc hemorrhages precede retinal nerve fiber layer defects in ocular hypertension. *Acta Ophthalmol (Copenh).* 1981;59: 627–641.

35. Caprioli J. Discrimination between normal and glaucomatous eyes. *Invest Ophthalmol Vis Sci.* 1992;33:153–159.

36. Quigley HA, Katz J, Derick RJ, Gilbert D, Sommer A. An evaluation of optic disc and nerve fiber layer examination in monitoring progression for early glaucoma damage. *Ophthalmology.* 1992;99:19–28.

37. Vihanninjoki K, Teesalu P, Burk ROW, Läärä E, Tuulonen A, Airaksinen PJ. Determination of an optimal combination of structural and functional parameters for the diagnosis of glaucoma. Multivariate analysis of confocal scanning laser tomographer, blue-on-yellow visual field and retinal nerve fiber layer: ARVO abstracts. *Invest Ophthalmol Vis Sci.* 1998;39:S701.

Chapter 14

IMAGING OF THE OPTIC NERVE AND NERVE FIBER LAYER IN GLAUCOMA

John G. Flanagan

Evaluation of the optic nerve head and nerve fiber layer is critical in the diagnosis and management of glaucoma. The last decade has seen a revolution in our ability to objectively document and quantify these ocular structures. Advances in digital imaging technology have enabled the three-dimensional reconstruction of the optic nerve and retina, making possible the noninvasive, objective assessment of morphological change in glaucoma. The three approaches explained in detail are scanning laser tomography, (a technology based upon confocal scanning laser microscopy and analogous to CT scanning), optical coherence tomography, and scanning laser polarimetry. The former technology is based on the optical principles of low-coherence interferometry, analogous to B-scan ultrasound imaging. The latter uses the optical phenomenon of birefringence to distinguish the nerve fiber layer.

Most research into these new techniques has concentrated on the clinical classification of the glaucomatous optic nerve and nerve fiber layer in strictly cross-sectional studies. Although this is a necessary period in the development of these new technologies, the potential strength of topographic imaging is its ability to detect and monitor change in the optic nerve. Because of the large physiological variation within the normal population,[1,2] even an ideal imaging system, whether concentrating on the optic nerve or nerve fiber layer, would face frustration in attempting to identify early glaucoma accurately in a single session. Similarly, it is unlikely that comparison with normative data will enable the techniques to realize their full potential in the accurate identification of glaucomatous damage. Studies are now beginning to appear that investigate the instruments' ability to detect structural change over time for both the initial diagnosis and later management of progressive disease.[3,4] The implications of their findings, combined with the rapidly decreasing costs associated with the technologies involved, are about to dramatically change the standard of practice for the early detection and management of the glaucomas.

CONFOCAL SCANNING LASER TOMOGRAPHY

Scanning laser tomographers are amongst the most common of the new imaging systems for the optic nerve. They are based upon the optical principles of confocal scanning laser ophthalmoscopy, which, in turn, are based upon confocal microscopy. The confocal imaging system uses a light source focused to a single point at the object. The light reflected from each point of the object is focused through a confocal pinhole to a detector that is conjugate to the focal plane, as shown in Fig. 14–1. The purpose of the pinhole is to exclude light reflected or scattered from adjacent structures, in both the axial and lateral planes, ensuring that only light reflected from structures at the focal plane is registered by the detector. In scanning laser systems, the laser light acts as the point source and is deflected periodically in two dimensions (the x and y planes) by scanning mirrors. A scan of a series of point sources within a specified (x,y) dimension is performed and used to construct a two-dimensional view of the ocular tissue. Single two-dimensional sectional images are displayed in a digital format and can be viewed in real time.

Scanning laser ophthalmoscopes (SLOs) use these imaging principles to record images of the ocular fundus. Scanning laser tomographs (SLTs) record a series of images along the axial axis of the eye, thus enabling three-dimensional reconstruction of the surface of the retina and/or the optic nerve head. They were first introduced in the late 1980s[5–8] and have been marketed principally for use in glaucoma, although they have also proven to be useful in the monitoring of retinal disease.[6,9–12] There are presently three commercially available instruments: the Topographic Scanning System (TopSS) (Laser Diagnostic Technologies Inc., San Diego, CA), the Heidelberg Retina. Tomograph (HRT) (Heidelberg Engineering GmbH., Heidelberg, Germany), and, from the same company, the HRT II, launched in May 1999. All of these systems are based on similar optical and analytical principles, but most of the published information concerns the HRT. Consequently the following sections focus mainly on the HRT (for review, see Refs. 5 and 13 to 17).

The Heidelberg Retina Tomograph

The HRT was designed for the three-dimensional imaging and measurement of the in vivo optic nerve and retina. The system is computer-controlled via proprietary software and consists of a scanning laser camera, stand, and an image-acquisition control panel. The diode laser source used by the HRT camera operates at a wavelength of 670 nm (780 nm for the TopSS) and has a maximum laser output intensity of 180 μW. This results in a maximum radiance of approximately 15 mW/cm^2/sr, considerably less than the maximum radiance of a typical fundus camera (650 mW/cm^2/sr). The HRT scans 32 optical sections, approximately equally spaced, perpendicular to the optic axis during a single image acquisition (Fig. 14–2). The acquisition time is 1.6 s (0.9 s for the TopSS), and each image section has a pixel resolution of 256×256. Each pixel corresponds to a single point source image in the x,y plane prior to deflection. The location of the focal plane can be adjusted in 0.25-DS increments, from -12.00 DS to $+12.00$ DS, and usually corresponds to the 11th image plane in the series of 32. The total scan depth can be adjusted from 0.5 to 4 mm in 0.5-mm steps and the field of view can be selected as 10, 15, or 20 degrees. Theoretically, the optimal lateral resolution is therefore approximately 11 μm. The axial resolution (full width at half maximum) is approximately 300 μm and is limited principally by ocular aberrations. Theoretically, the optimal accuracy of the obtained height value is 16 μm. This represents the ability of the instrument to distinguish peaks in the reflectance intensity across the 32 image planes and is sometimes referred to as the *axial resolution*.

Following acquisition, each of the 32 section images can be viewed in rapid sequence ("cartoon" mode) in order to qualitatively assess the magnitude of any eye movements. If the sections are considered acceptable, the image series is registered so that the sequential sections can be aligned. This allows the effect of inherent, subtle eye movements to be corrected when the 32 sections are stacked to construct the three-dimensional image. A topographic surface, or height image, is generated by determining the position of maximum reflectance intensity along the optical axis for each pixel. This is assumed to correspond to the position of greatest change in refractive index—i.e., the vitreous/internal limiting membrane interface. This topography image provides the three-dimensional information for the analysis of the retina and optic nerve. The height values are color-coded along a yellow to red axis, such that the light yellow color depicts depression and the dark red color depicts elevation. In addition, the reflectivity at each image plane can be plotted for each pixel location. This plot of reflectance intensity per unit depth is termed the z-profile (Fig. 14–2). A reflectivity image is generated by summating the reflectivity measurements along the z-axis for each aligned pixel.

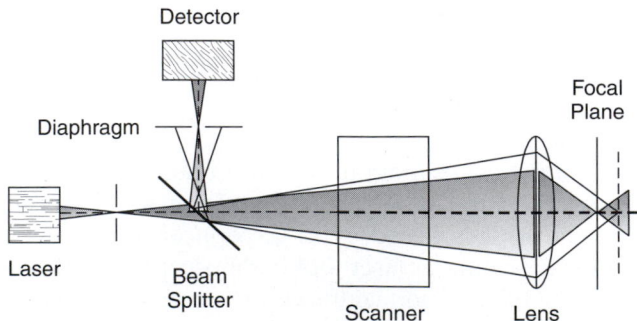

Figure 14–1. Schematic illustration of the optical components of the Heidelberg Retina Tomograph. A confocal pinhole aperture is conjugate with the focal plane and reduces the effect of scattered light. (Reproduced with permission from Heidelberg Engineering.)

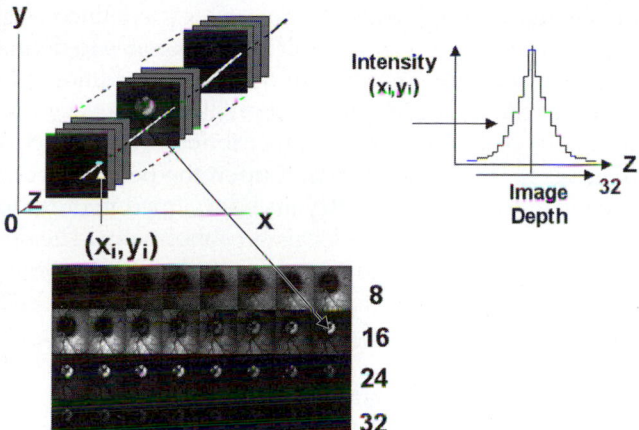

Figure 14–2. Schematic illustration of the registration of the 32 image scans and the construction of the z profile, a plot of reflectance intensity versus scan depth. The peak reflectance of the z profile determines the height value allocated to the x, y pixel coordinate of the topography image. (Reproduced with permission from Heidelberg Engineering.)

Knowledge of the topographical surface allows for the correction of rotation, height offset, and tilt between images. The absolute mean height and the tilt of the retinal surface are determined by establishing a reference ring along the margins of the topography image (Fig. 14–3). The reference ring is circular and centered on the topography image; its outer diameter is 94% of the image size and the width of the ring margin is 3% of the image size. The mean height of the reference ring is set as zero, and all height values are measured relative to this zero position. The tilt of the reference ring with respect to the optical axis is used to define a plane parallel to the retinal surface. Correction of retinal orientation or of problems caused by misalignment of the laser during image acquisition is made relative to this plane.

The proprietary software permits interactive measurement of height profiles and detailed image analysis within a defined area of interest—e.g., the optic nerve. For this to happen, it is necessary to define a contour line that encompasses the region of interest. The contour line may be a user-defined circle, or it may be free-drawn to precisely define the optic nerve head. The height along the contour line is displayed as a line plot (Fig. 14–4), with the temporal aspect defined as zero degrees. A normal height variation will have a "double hump" appearance, where the peaks correspond to the thicker nerve fiber layer at the superior and inferior aspects of the optic nerve head. The contour line coordinates can be exported to subsequent images to enable analysis of change in the same region. It has been reported that contour lines drawn by trained observers give measurements with a high level of concordance.[18]

Topographical information within the contour line is measured with respect to a reference plane. The standard reference (as used in software versions 1.11 and above) is located 50 μm below the mean contour line height in the papillomacular bundle (Fig. 14–5) and is determined for a wedge between -10 and -4 degrees.

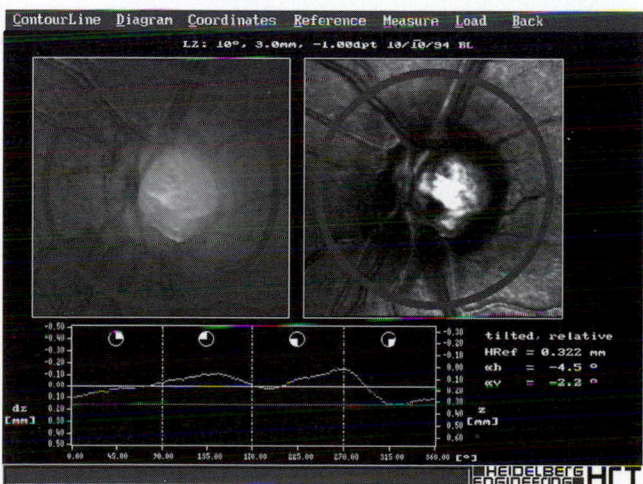

Figure 14–3. The reference ring is illustrated in blue on this HRT printout of a glaucomatous patient. The absolute mean height and the tilt of the retinal surface are determined relative to the reference ring. The mean height of the reference ring is set to zero and all height values are measured relative to this zero position. (Courtesy of Dr. S. Hosking.) (*See Color Plate 34.*)

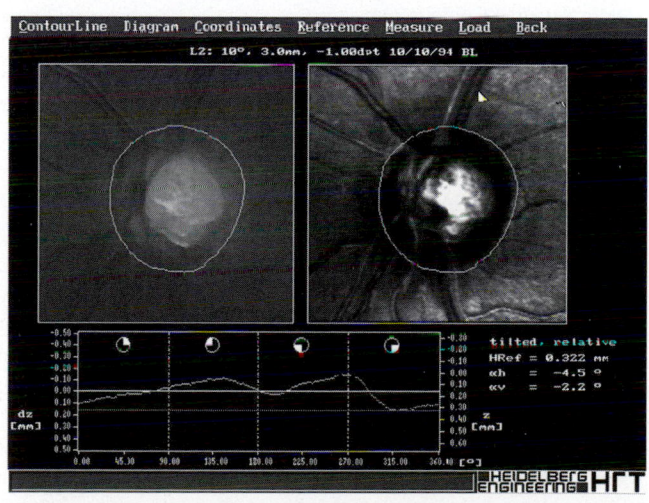

Figure 14–4. HRT printout showing a contour line drawn around the optic nerve head and identifying an area of interest for subsequent analysis. On the bottom of the printout is a plot of the height values along this contour line. (Courtesy of Dr. S. Hosking.) (*See Color Plate 35.*)

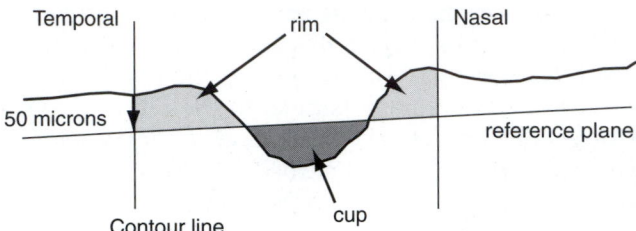

Figure 14–5. Schematic illustration showing the reference plane, corrected for tilt relative to the retinal surface. (Reproduced with permission from Heidelberg Engineering.)

It is assumed that this region is least affected by glaucomatous damage and therefore helps establish a relatively stable reference plane for serial analysis of the optic nerve head.[16] Alternatively, the stereometric parameters can be calculated relative to a curved surface plane defined by the contour line (see Table 14–1).

The parameters generated for assessment of the optic nerve head are defined in Table 14–1 and illustrated in Fig. 14–6. They can be calculated globally (Fig. 14–6) or divided into segments. There are six predefined segments, as shown in Fig. 14–7. It is also possible to define a custom segment, specified in degrees. In addition, parameters can be illustrated as cumulative frequency distributions or ranked segment distribution (RSD) curves (Fig. 14–8).[19,20] These are based upon the Bebie curves[21] used in automated perimetry and developed in order to visualize both diffuse and localized abnormality. The optic nerve is divided into thirty-six 10-degree segments, with each segment compared to the group mean and 95% confidence limits of normality.

Accuracy, Validity, and Reproducibility

The accuracy of depth measurements obtained with the HRT has been assessed using a model eye.[22] The relative error ranged from approximately 11% for cup-volume parameters to 4% for retinal elevations. The two-dimensional accuracy was explored in the human eye by comparing HRT measurements with direct ocular measurements during vitrectomy[23] and was found to vary with the degree of ametropia. All current software versions have accordingly incorpo-

TABLE 14–1. SUMMARY OF THE STEREOMETRIC PARAMETERS GENERATED BY THE HEIDELBERG RETINA TOMOGRAPH FOR THE STRUCTURE OF THE OPTIC NERVE HEAD

Disk Area (area), mm²	Total area within contour line
Effective Area, mm²	Area within contour line and below curved surface
Cup Area (area below reference), mm²	Area within contour line and below reference plane
Cup/Disk Area Ratio	Cup area/disk area.
Rim Area, mm²	Area above reference plane
Mean Radius, mm	Mean radius of contour line
Mean Height of Contour, mm	Mean height (z position) of retinal surface along contour line
Height Variation Contour, mm	Height variation of retinal surface along contour line, representing the difference between most elevated and most depressed point of contour line
Cup Volume (volume below reference), mm³	Volume within contour line and below reference plane
Rim Volume (volume above reference), mm³	Volume within contour line and above reference plane
Volume below Surface, mm³	Volume within contour line and below curved surface
Volume above Surface, mm³	Volume within contour line and above curved surface
Mean Depth in Contour, mm	Mean depth within contour line
Mean Cup Depth (effective mean depth), mm	Mean depth inside contour line and below curved surface
Maximum Cup Depth, mm	Maximum depth inside contour (relative to curved surface)
Cup Shape Measure (third moment)*	Third central moment of frequency distribution of depth values within contour line and below curved surface
Mean RNFL† Thickness, mm	Mean distance between retinal surface along contour line and reference plane
RNFL Cross-Sectional Area, mm²	Mean distance between retinal surface along contour line and reference plane, multiplied by length of contour line
Classification	Classification of examined optic nerve head as "normal" or "glaucoma"[44]
Mean Variability	Mean standard deviation of height measurements (only for mean topography images)
Center $x/y/z$, mm	x, y, z coordinates of center of gravity of surface within contour line

*Normal nerve heads may exhibit negative values of this parameter because the cup is relatively flat and small depth values are most frequent. Glaucomatous optic nerve heads will have positive values because the slope at the boundary of the cup is steep and the cup is often deep.

†RNFL, retinal nerve fiber layer.

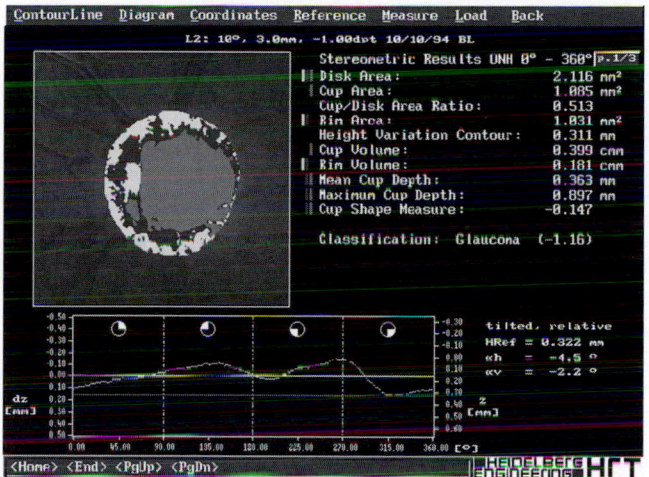

Figure 14–6. HRT printout of a glaucomatous patient showing the global analysis of the optic nerve head as defined by the contour line. The "cup" is illustrated in red and defined as the height values distal to the reference plane. The "rim" is illustrated in green and blue and defined by the height values proximal to the reference plane. The stereometric parameters generated for assessment of the optic nerve head are defined in Table 14-1. (Courtesy of Dr. S. Hosking.) (*See Color Plate 36.*)

rated correction factors for ametropia. Several studies have found the HRT to overestimate the neuroretinal rim and underestimate the cup-to-disc ratio.[24,25] It is believed that the inclusion of retinal vessels as part of the rim is primarily responsible.

It has been suggested that an advantage of the HRT is that there is a decreased need for pupil dilation and clear media.[26–28] But although it is often possible to obtain acceptable image quality without dilation,

ContourLine Diagram Coordinates Reference Measure Load Back
L2: 10°, 3.0mm, -1.00dpt 10/10/94 BL

Parameter [dim]	global	temporl	tmp/sup	tmp/inf	nasal	nsl/sup	nsl/inf
Area [mm²]:	2.116	0.515	0.274	0.280	0.514	0.260	0.274
Effect. Area [mm²]:	1.649	0.491	0.210	0.216	0.345	0.175	0.210
Area bel Refr [mm²]:	1.085	0.423	0.136	0.152	0.159	0.098	0.117
Height in Cont [mm]:	0.425						
MeanHeight Cont[mm]:	0.155	0.261	0.166	0.149	0.126	0.094	0.055
PeakHeight Cont[mm]:	0.010	0.192	0.133	0.010	0.053	0.055	0.012
Height Var Cont[mm]:	0.311						
Vol bel Surfce[cmm]:	0.599	0.189	0.078	0.091	0.107	0.058	0.075
Vol abv Surfce[cmm]:	0.025	0.001	0.004	0.002	0.011	0.005	0.002
Vol bel Refrnc[cmm]:	0.399	0.143	0.052	0.066	0.064	0.033	0.040
Vol abv Refrnc[cmm]:	0.181	0.006	0.021	0.023	0.065	0.035	0.032
Maximum Depth [mm]:	0.897	0.818	0.810	0.914	0.951	0.821	1.027
Third moment []:	-0.147	-0.040	-0.087	-0.115	-0.255	-0.152	-0.188
Mean radius [mm]:	0.821						

Figure 14–7. HRT printout of a glaucomatous patient showing the six predefined segments for the stereometric analysis of the optic nerve head. The parameters generated are defined in Table 14-1. (Courtesy of Dr. S. Hosking.)

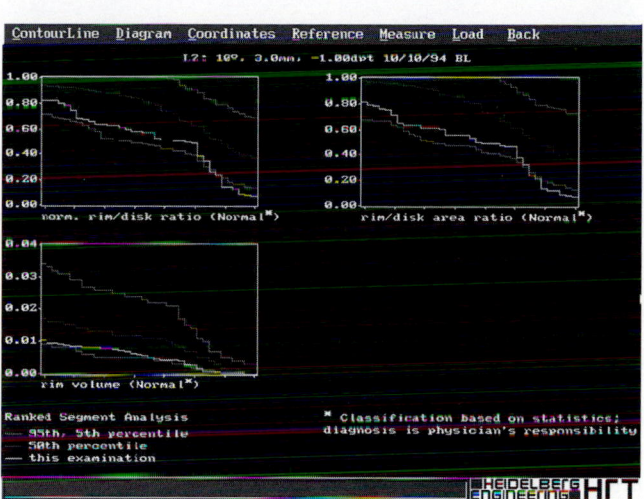

Figure 14–8. HRT printout showing the parameters illustrated as cumulative frequency distributions or ranked segment distribution (RSD) curves. The display was developed in order to visualize both diffuse and localized abnormality. The optic nerve is divided into thirty-six 10-degree segments, with each segment compared to the group mean and 95% confidence limits of normality. (Courtesy of Dr. S. Hosking.)

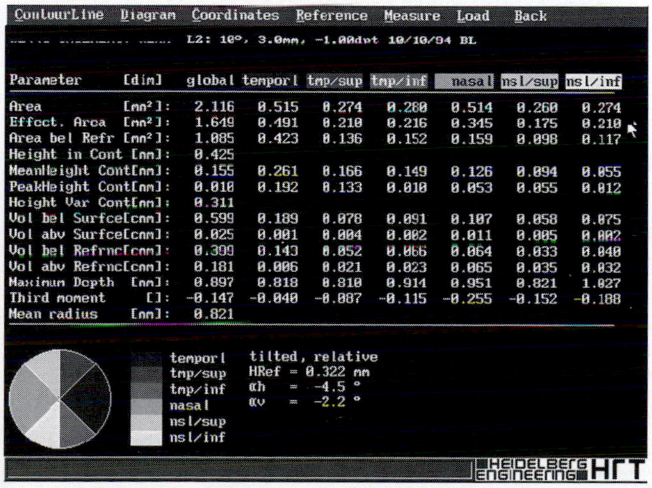

there are many instances when miotic pupils, particularly when accompanied by cataract, require dilation.[16,29] In addition, in a recent study of the reproducibility of HRT measurements at the macula, it was found that height measurements were better in dilated eyes than with the natural pupil.[9] Chauhan et al.[30] reported a significant increase in variability with advancing age in glaucomatous eyes, which was significantly larger than that observed in healthy eyes.

In spite of these differences, it is the reproducibility of the instrument's results that will dictate its ability to detect change. This factor alone will ultimately determine the clinical usefulness of the technique. Several studies have provided encouraging evidence to suggest a level of reproducibility that will permit the detection of glaucomatous progression.[26,30–35] The coefficient of variation of the stereometric parameters for the optic nerve head is generally less than 5%, with single-pixel variability of less than 30 μm.

Clinical Application

The clinical application of scanning laser tomography in the detection and management of glaucoma has been hypothesized since the technique's inception.[8] Recent cross-sectional studies have shown that the parameters generated by the HRT are capable of discriminating between normal optic nerve heads and those of patients with ocular hypertension[36] and early glaucoma.[36–40] Similarly, this discriminative ability has been demonstrated between the optic nerve heads of

these patients[38,41] and even between glaucomatous optic nerve heads with and without loss of visual field.[41]

The stereometric parameters best able to separate normal from glaucomatous optic nerve heads include cup shape, cup area, cup/disc area ratio, rim area, cup volume, and rim volume.[37,40,42,43] Of particular interest is the recent work of Wollstein et al.,[40] who have reported exceptional sensitivity (96.3%) and specificity (84.3%) in using the 99% prediction interval from the linear regression of the optic disc area against the log rim area.

The parameters that were best able to differentiate between ocular hypertension and glaucoma before and after functional loss were rim volume, cup shape, and mean height of contour.[41] Across all the studies, cup shape appears to be the parameter that is most consistently useful in differentiating subject groups with and without glaucoma, irrespective of study design or recruitment criterion.

Relationship of Parameters and Visual Fields

The HRT parameters for the optic nerve head have been compared to the extent of glaucomatous visual field damage.[33,43–49] Parameters including cup shape, cup area, cup/disc area ratio, rim area, cup volume, rim volume, maximum depth, and height variation exhibit a cross-sectional correlation with visual field indices and/or the location and depth of visual field abnormality. Of these, cup shape was the parameter that most consistently exhibited a correlation with functional loss.

Mikelberg et al.[44] investigated the ability of the HRT to differentiate between subjects with early glaucomatous visual field defects and normal eyes without visual-field loss. Forward selection discriminant function analysis was used to determine which characteristics of the optic nerve head were best able to differentiate between the two groups. Using software version 1.11, the sensitivity was 89% and the specificity 84%. It is from this research that the classification that defines the probability of an optic nerve being normal is derived; it is included on the standard HRT analysis (see Table 14-1).

Longitudinal Studies

The greatest potential for scanning laser tomography is in the detection of change in the topography of the optic nerve head over time. The first longitudinal studies are starting to appear in the literature. Kamal et al.[3] outlined a study whereby the HRT was used to follow nearly 300 mid- to high-risk ocular hypertensive subjects, of whom 13 developed glaucomatous visual field loss during the follow-up period. When this group of

13 patients was compared to a normal control group, it was found that there was a significant group difference in both the global and the segmental HRT parameters. Cup area, cup volume, and cup/disc area ratio increased, while rim area and rim volume decreased. Interestingly, cup shape was not found to be of value. Farra et al.[4] designed a prospective cohort study from which a sample of 39 patients was recruited. Of the 39 patients, 13 had progressive glaucomatous visual field loss established over a 5-year period; they formed the experimental group. Thirteen age- and visual field–matched subjects with stable visual fields over time and 13 age-matched ocular hypertensive subjects with pretreatment elevated intraocular pressure (IOP) and no visual field loss were recruited as control groups. The HRT was able to detect structural change in the optic nerve heads of patients with progressing visual fields. The parameters most effective at identifying this change were peak height of contour, maximum cup depth, and cup volume. Other preliminary studies[50,51] support the parameters found by Farra et al.[4] Again, cup shape was not found to be of significance in these studies, in contrast to the findings of the cross-sectional studies.

Other studies of interest in establishing the ability of the HRT to detect subtle changes in the optic nerve head include the monitoring of optic nerve head topography following trabeculectomy,[52,53] whereby it was possible to show a significant association between decrease in IOP and parameters corresponding to a reduction in cup size and enlargement of rim size. Yan et al.[54] demonstrated the ability of the HRT to detect both global and regional deformation in the optic nerve head of a human eye model in which IOP was manipulated. Hosking and Flanagan have shown that scaling errors are incurred for subjects in whom the refractive error setting[55] or keratometry reading[56] is altered between visits. These studies indicate that care must be taken in any longitudinal study to make sure that the focus setting and keratometry values remain constant, compensating with supplementary refractive correction if necessary.

New Developments

The Glaucoma Panel of the Committee on Ophthalmic Procedures Assessment of the American Academy of Ophthalmology has recently evaluated several new optic nerve head imaging technologies including the HRT.[28] They list advantages to include the ability to obtain images without dilation, the use of low light intensity, real-time imaging for immediate evaluation, and the HRT's axial resolution as compared with previous technologies. The major disadvantage was considered to be the dependence of measurements on a reference plane. In spite of the encouraging clinical results discussed earlier in this chapter, it would indeed be desirable to find measurement techniques that were independent of a reference plane, which is assumed to remain stable across both images and time.

Reference Plane–Independent Analysis

Yan et al.[54] have suggested a new method of analysis that computes the location of the point of maximum slope within a 10-degree sector of the optic nerve head as well as the magnitude of this slope. The technique, termed *inflection-point analysis* (IPA), was designed to be robust to the potential artifacts of image translation, reference plane location, and the subjective determination of a contour line. Using a human eye model in which the IOP could be controlled, IPA showed several advantages over standard HRT parameters. It was insensitive to artifacts due to tilt, was able to objectively delineate the boundary between the optic cup and neuroretinal rim, and could sensitively track changes in the location of this margin. The technique needs to be further tested in longitudinal studies of progressive glaucoma. Chauhan[57] introduced probability-map analysis for the reference plane–independent detection of localized change in topography images. In the event of a height change, the pooled variability of baseline and follow-up examinations will be greater than the within-variability of the baseline or follow-up examinations. The analysis requires a minimum of three baseline and three follow-up images and divides each image into 4×4 superpixels in order to quantify the variability within each 16-pixel cell. Change is then quantified for each superpixel between images, and this results in a two-dimensional map of F-test error probabilities.

HRT II

The new HRT II (Fig. 14–9) operates on the same principles as the original HRT but with a few notable refinements aimed at improving the standardization of the technique. The field of view is restricted to 15×15 degrees, while the two-dimensional resolution has been increased to 384×384 pixels (i.e., the digital resolution is the same as with the previous 10×10 degree field of view with a 256×256 pixel resolution). Following a similar philosophy, the scan depth is adjustable in 0.5-mm steps between 1.0 and 4.0 mm, but the axial resolution is kept constant, with the number of scan images varying as a function of scan depth. Sixteen scans are used per millimeter of scan depth. A 2-mm scan depth with 32 image scans has a quicker 1-s acquisition time (24 ms per scan), down from 1.6 s, although the 4-mm scan depth will take 2 s. The light source

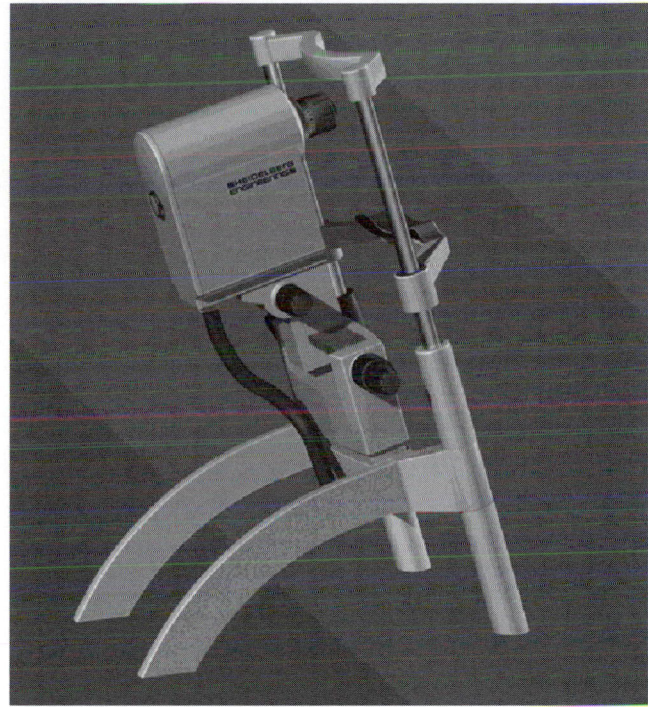

Figure 14–9. Illustration of the HRT II. (Reproduced with permission from Heidelberg Engineering.)

remains a 670-nm diode laser and the focus range remains spherical between -12 and $+12$ diopters.

OPTICAL COHERENCE TOMOGRAPHY

The optical coherence tomograph (OCT) (Humphrey Systems Inc., San Leandro, CA) uses low-coherence interferometry to enable noncontact, high-resolution, cross-sectional imaging of the retina (for review, see Refs. 58 to 63) (Fig. 14–10). A superluminescent diode provides a near-infrared (830-nm), low-coherence source, which, before each light path goes back to a detector, is divided between a reference device and the eye. The reference beam is then compared with the measurement beam, scattered, and reflected from the ocular tissue of interest. Axial resolution in air has been reported to be between 14[63] and 17 μm[64] for the 830-nm light source available on the commercial instrument (Humphrey Systems Inc., San Leandro, CA), with a penetrance of several millimeters. Retinal resolution is somewhat reduced from these levels. Recent advances have seen the development of an instrument with a claimed 4-μm axial resolution using a source of 1,300 nm.[65] Lateral resolution is theoretically 25 μm, diffraction limited by the eye.[64] A practical resolution limit is dictated by the instrument design, in which 100

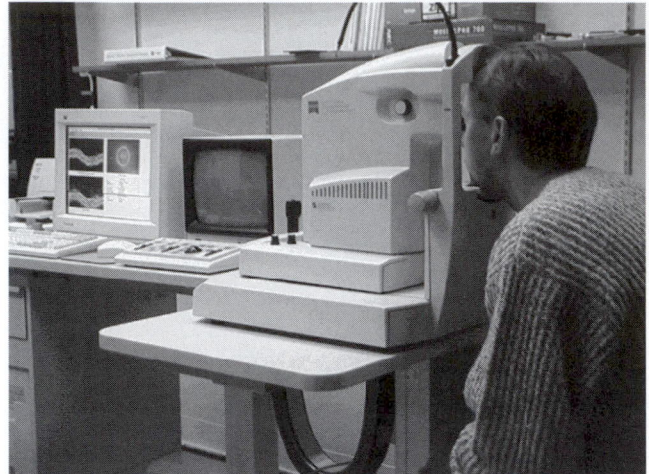

Figure 14–10. The optical coherence tomograph (OCT) showing a patient seated at the camera, with the OCT scan on the far monitor and a monitor for direct observation of the subject's fundus and OCT scan location. (Courtesy of Dr. T. Simpson).

individual axial scans are combined to give a scan series, irrespective of the field size selected. The scan series is corrected for axial eye-movement artifacts and the image is color-coded for reflectivity (Fig. 14–11). The reflectivity value recorded is a combination of actual reflectivity and the scattering and absorption properties of the ocular media.[66] A typical section image, or OCT tomogram, depicts a four-banded retina. The brightest inner band has been related to the nerve fiber layer; the outermost bright band to the retinal pigment epithelium/choriocapillaris; in between are the plexiform and the photoreceptor layers.[66,68] However, recent findings have challenged the ability to identify anatomically meaningful retinal structure.[64]

OCT has been used to image a wide variety of retinal and optic nerve head conditions.[69–79] Applications to glaucoma include the measurement of the thickness of the nerve fiber layer, peripapillary circular tomograms that map the retinal thickness around the optic nerve head, and radial tomograms to assess the cross-sectional profile of the optic nerve.[71,78,80,81]

Accuracy, Validity, and Reproducibility

Two studies have attempted to correlate OCT images with retinal histology. Toth et al.[67] concluded that there was a high correlation between the two. Chauhan and Marshall[64] have recently disagreed with these findings, stating that the OCT images could not be considered tissue-specific. They reported that the highly reflective outer band was made up of both nerve fiber ganglion cell layers and, outside of the macular region, also the inner plexiform layer. This gave results that were between three and eight times

greater than expected by light microscopy. However, this does not preclude the usefulness of following change in the thickness of the nerve fiber layer or, more accurately, the reflective inner band over time.

The reproducibility of measurements of the nerve fiber layer was considered good, but the variability was found to be better within a visit than between visits.[82] It has been proposed that this is due to the adjustable polarization setting, an operator-defined variable, which is therefore easier to maintain at a constant level within a session than between sessions.[64] In a recent critical appraisal of the OCT, it was considered that measures of total retinal thickness were precise and accurate but that intraretinal layers could not be assessed with certainty.[64]

Clinical Application of the Optical Coherence Tomograph

In a study of 33 glaucoma patients, Schuman et al.[71] found that the OCT's assessment of the nerve fiber layer correlated well with the visual field results and better than optic nerve head cupping or neuroretinal rim area. The nerve fiber layer was found to thin with age, and there was a significant difference between normal and glaucomatous subjects.[71] OCT measurements of the nerve fiber layer were found to correlate well with the clinical assessment of focal defects in patients with glaucoma.[78]

New Developments

The Glaucoma Panel of the Committee on Ophthalmic Procedures Assessment of the American Academy of

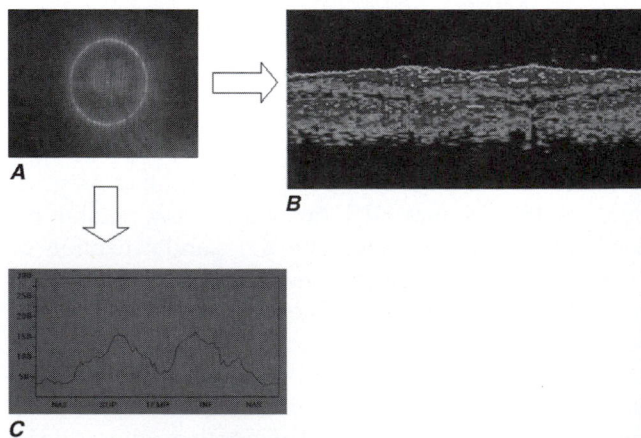

Figure 14–11. OCT tomogram sampled from a peripapillary circle (A), showing the retinal thickness around the optic nerve head. The retina is illustrated as a typically four-banded retina (B). The brightest inner band has been related to the nerve fiber layer and the outermost bright band to the retinal pigment epithelium/choriocapillaris. The in-between layers are considered as the plexiform layer and the photoreceptor layer. The thickness of the nerve fiber layer is illustrated as a line graph (C). (Courtesy of Dr. T. Simpson.) (See Color Plate 37.)

Ophthalmology[28] considered the advantages of OCT to include its independence from the refractive status of the eye and from a reference plane in quantifying the thickness of the nerve fiber layer. Disadvantages were listed as problems in imaging through subcapsular and cortical cataracts and the need for pupil dilation. The panel also recommended that assumptions linking the band of high reflectivity labeled with the nerve fiber layer be carefully validated.

Optical coherence tomography offers a remarkable technology for imaging the optic nerve and retina. With the promise of quicker acquisition times (currently 2.4 s), higher resolution, and reduced costs, the technique has the potential to contribute significantly to the future management of glaucoma.

SCANNING LASER POLARIMETRY

Scanning laser polarimetry combines scanning laser ophthalmoscopy with polarimetry to measure the retardation of polarized laser light due to the birefringent properties of the nerve fiber layer (for review, see Refs. 83 through 91). The commercially available instrument is called the GDx/Nerve Fiber Analyzer (Laser Diagnostic Technologies, San Diego, CA) (Fig. 14–12). It uses a 780-nm diode laser source in which the state of polarization is modulated. A polarization

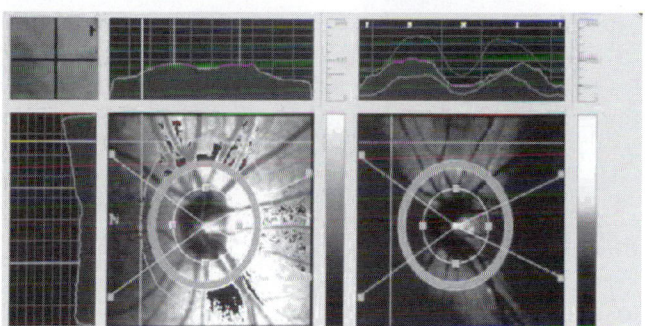

Figure 14–13. Retardation map of a normal subject produced by the GDx/Nerve Fiber Analyzer. The line plot in the top right of the image shows a thickness of the nerve fiber layer that falls within the confidence intervals for normality. (Reproduced with permission from Laser Diagnostics Technologies, Inc.) (*See Color Plate 38.*)

detector can measure the interaction of the polarized light with birefringent ocular tissue. The influence of the anterior segment is reduced through the use of proprietary techniques. A retardation map with 256×256 pixel resolution is produced with the assumption that the highest measured retardation corresponds to the thickest areas of the nerve fiber layer (Figs. 14–13 and 14–14). Image acquisition takes 0.7 s and the scan field is 15 degrees. Results are compared to an age- and race-matched normative database and a neural network is used to define the likelihood that a map is normal or from a glaucoma patient.

Accuracy, Validity, and Reproducibility

In vitro studies have shown that the retardation values are linearly related to the thickness of the nerve fiber layer and well correlated with histological measurements.[83] The resolution was estimated at 13 μm. Retardation values are highest at the superior and

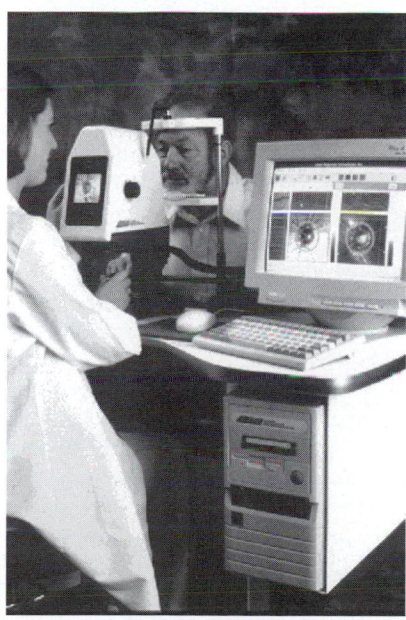

Figure 14–12. The GDx/Nerve Fiber Analyzer showing a patient seated at the camera and a typical retardation map on the monitor. (Reproduced with permission from Laser Diagnostics Technologies, Inc.)

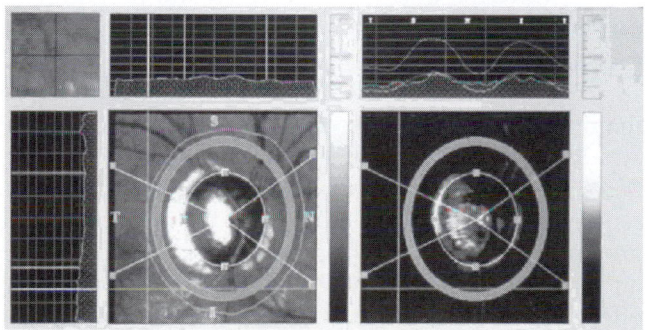

Figure 14–14. Retardation map of a patient with glaucoma as produced by the GDx/Nerve Fiber Analyzer. The line plot in the top right of the image shows a thickness of the nerve fiber layer that falls outside the confidence intervals for normality. (Reproduced with permission from Laser Diagnostics Technologies, Inc.) (*See Color Plate 39.*)

inferior aspects of the optic nerve and low in the foveal region and over blood vessels.[87] Separate studies of reproducibility have stated a coefficient of variation of 4.5% or less for normal subjects and between 6 and 10% for glaucoma patients.[87,88,92–96]

Clinical Application of the Nerve Fiber Analyzer

Retardation values decrease with age, corresponding to an estimated thinning of the nerve fiber layer of 0.2 μm per year.[92] Normal values have shown considerable interindividual variability, corresponding to the range of values reported in histological studies.[87,92,97,98] This undoubtedly limits the ability to detect glaucoma on a cross-sectional basis—i.e., at a single diagnostic session[99]—but it does not necessarily limit the ability to detect change. However, there are reported studies that have found differences between normal subjects and ocular hypertensives[98,100] and normal subjects and patients with glaucoma. Significant correlation has also been claimed between retardation and glaucomatous loss of visual field.[91,101] Tjon-Fo Sang and Lemji[97] have reported extraordinarily high levels of sensitivity and specificity, although the results of other studies would suggest considerable overlap between normal and glaucoma groups. The differences in retardation recorded between the temporal quadrant and the superior and inferior quadrants appear to be exaggerated.[99,102] Concern is expressed as to the original calibration of the technique using histological studies of previously imaged monkey eyes[83] as well as to the influence of the polarization compensator used to correct for the birefringent properties of the anterior segment.[87]

Hudson[99] considered all these issues in a recent editorial, summarizing that "the obvious and exciting potential of scanning laser polarimetry should not overshadow the uncertainties which still remain concerning the underlying principles and assumptions of the technique."

The Glaucoma Panel of the Committee on Ophthalmic Procedures Assessment of the American Academy of Ophthalmology[28] lists among the advantages of scanning laser polarimetry its speed, that it requires no pupil dilation, and that the measurements are independent of reference plane, magnification, and ocular resolution. Disadvantages include the effect of other birefringent tissues in the eye and the increased retardation caused by peripapillary atrophy and chorioretinal scars.

The Glaucoma Panel[28] also referred to a study by Nakla and coworkers,[103] which compared the ability of all three techniques outlined in this chapter to detect glaucomatous damage to the optic nerve head.

The best performance was for the HRT, with a receiver operator curve area (representing a summary of sensitivity and specificity) of 91%; followed by the OCT, with 85%; and the GDx/Nerve Fiber Analyzer, with 78%. However, this study does not address the issue of detection of change, the key to the future of imaging techniques in the detection and management of the glaucomas.

CONCLUSION

The three technologies outlined in this chapter represent the dawning of a new era in clinical imaging of the optic nerve and nerve fiber layer. We need to be mindful of their limitations and embrace their potential. The relative costs will be reduced substantially over time and protocols for their optimal application will be developed. What is certain is that they will have a major impact on our future attitudes and the clinical standard for the primary care of the glaucomas.

ACKNOWLEDGMENTS

I would like to thank all students and colleagues past and present for their continual inspiration. Specifically with relation to this chapter I thank Wendy Hatch, Taline Farra, Graham Trope, Mustafa Rawji, Natalie Hutchings, Chris Hudson, and Sarah Hosking. Sarah's images are used with kind permission.

REFERENCES

1. Jonas JB, Gusek GC, Guggenmoos-Holzman I, Naumann GOH. Variability of the real dimensions of normal human optic discs. *Graefes Arch Clin Exp Ophthalmol.* 1988;226:332–336.
2. Jonas JB, Muller-Bergh JA, Schlitzer-Schrehardt UM, Naumann GOH. Histomorphometry of the human optic nerve. *Invest Ophthalmol Vis Sci.* 1990;31:736–744.
3. Kamal DS, Viswanathan AC, Garway-Heath DF, et al. Detection of optic disc change with the Heidelberg retina tomograph before confirmed visual field change in ocular hypertensives converting to early glaucoma. *Br J Ophthalmol.* 1999;83:290–294.
4. Farra T, Flanagan JG, Trope GE. The detection of glaucomatous progression using scanning laser tomography. *Invest Ophthalmol Vis Sci.* 1999;39(suppl):389.
5. Zinser G, Wijnaendts-van-Resandt RW, Dreher AW, Weinreb RN, Harbarth U, Schröder H, Burk ROW. Confocal laser tomographic scanning of the eye. *SPIE Proc.* 1989;1161:337–344.
6. Bartsch DU, Intaglietta M, Billie JF, et al. Confocal laser tomographic analysis of the retina in eyes with macular

hole formation and other focal macular diseases. *Am J Ophthalmol.* 1989;108:277–287.

7. Kruse FE, Burk ROW, Volcker HE, Zinser G, Harbrath U. Reproducibility of topographic measurements of the optic nerve head with laser tomographic scanning. *Ophthalmology.* 1989;96:1320–1324.

8. Weinreb RN, Dreher AW, Bille J. Quantitative assessment of the optic nerve head with the laser tomographic scanner. *Int J Ophthalmol.* 1989;13:25–29.

9. Menezes AV, Giunta M, Chisholm L, Harvey PT, Tuli R, Devenyi RG. Reproducibility of topographic measurements of the macula with a scanning laser ophthalmoscope. *Ophthalmology.* 1995;102:2;230–235.

10. Hudson C, Shah S, Flanagan JG, Brahma AK, Ansons A. Scanning laser tomography as an objective measure of the efficacy of the treatment of benign intracranial hypertension. *Lancet.* 1996;346:1435.

11. Hudson C, Charles SJ, Flanagan JG, Brahma AK, Turner GS, McLeod D. The objective morphological assessment of macular hole surgery by scanning laser tomography. *Br J Ophthalmol.* 1997;81(2):107–116.

12. Hudson C, Flanagan JG, McLeod D, Turner GS. Scanning laser tomography z-profile signal width as an objective index of macular retinal thickening. *Br J Ophthalmol.* 1998;82:121–130.

13. Weinreb RN, Lusky M, Bartsch DU, Morsman D. Effect of repetitive imaging on topographic measurements of the optic nerve head. *Arch Ophthalmol.* 1993; 111:636–638.

14. Burk ROW, Rohrschneider K, Volcker HE, Takamotot T, Schwartz B. Laser scanning tomography and stereophotogrammetry in three-dimensional optic disc analysis. *Graefes Arch Clin Exp Ophthalmol.* 1993;231:193–198.

15. Zinser G. Topographic measurements at the fundus with the Heidelberg Retina Tomograph. In: Elsner AE, ed. *Scanning Laser Ophthalmoscopy, Tomography and Microscopy.* New York: Plenum Press; 1994.

16. Chauhan BC. Confocal scanning laser tomography. *Can J Ophthalmol.* 1996;31:152–156.

17. Malinovsky VE. An overview of the Heidelberg Retina Tomograph. *J Am Optom Assoc.* 1996;67:457–467.

18. Hatch W, Flanagan JG, Trope GE, Williams-Lyn D, Buys Y, Farra T. Interobserver agreement of Heidelberg Retina Tomograph parameters. *J Glaucoma.* 1999;8:232–237.

19. Aaswaphureekorn S, Zangwill L, Weinreb RN. The ranked-segment distribution curve for interpretation of optic nerve topography. *J Glaucoma.* 1996;5:79–90.

20. Bartz-Schmidt KU, Sengersdorf A, Esser P, et al. The cumulative normalised rim/disc area ratio curve. *Graefes Arch Clin Exp Ophthalmol.* 1996;234:227–231.

21. Bebie H, Flammer J, Bebie T. The cumulative defect curve: Separation of local and diffuse components of visual field damage. *Graefes Arch Clin Exp Ophthalmol.* 1989;227:9–12.

22. Janknecht P, Funk J. Optic nerve head analyser and Heidelberg Retina Tomograph: Accuracy and reproducibility of topographic measurements in a model eye and in volunteers. *Br J Ophthalmol.* 1994;78:760–768.

23. Bartz-Schmidt KU, Weber J, Heiman K. Validity of two-dimensional data obtained with the Heidelberg Retina Tomograph as verified by direct measurements in normal optic nerve heads. *German J Ophthalmol.* 1994;3:400–405.

24. Dichtl A, Jonas JB, Mardin CY. Comparison between tomographic scanning evaluation of photographic measurement of the neuroretinal rim. *Am J Ophthalmol.* 1996;121:494–501.

25. Zangwill L, Shakiba S, Caprioli J, Weinreb RN. Agreement between clinicians and a confocal scanning laser ophthalmoscope in estimating cup:disc ratios. *Am J Ophthalmol.* 1995;119:415–421.

26. Lusky M, Bosem ME, Weinreb RN. Reproducibility of optic nerve head topography measurements in eyes with undilated pupils. *J Glaucoma.* 1993;2:104–109.

27. Zangwill L, Irak I, Berry CC, Garden V, Lima MD, Weinreb RN. Effect of cataract and pupil size on image quality with confocal scanning laser ophthalmoscopy. *Arch Ophthalmol.* 1997;115:983–990.

28. Lee DA (Chair, Committee on Ophthalmic Procedures Assessment, Glaucoma Panel). Optic nerve head and retinal nerve fiber layer analysis. *Ophthalmology.* 1999; 106:1414–1424.

29. Tomita G, Honbe K, Kitazawa Y. Reproducibility of measurements by laser scanning tomography in eyes before and after pilocarpine treatment. *Graefes Arch Clin Exp Ophthalmol.* 1994;232:406–408.

30. Chauhan BC, LeBlanc RP, McCormick TA, Rohers JB. Test-retest variability of topographic measurements with confocal scanning laser tomography in patients with glaucoma and control subjects. *Am J Ophthalmol.* 1994;118:9–15.

31. Mikelberg FS, Wijsman K, Schulzer M. Reproducibility of topographic parameters obtained with the Heidelberg retina tomograph. *J Glaucoma.* 1993;2:101–103.

32. Rohrschneider K, Burk RO, Kruse FE, Volcker HE. Reproducibility of the optic nerve head topography with a new laser tomographic scanning device. *Ophthalmology.* 1994;101:1044–1049.

33. Brigatti L, Caprioli J. Correlation of visual field with scanning confocal laser optic disc measurements in glaucoma. *Arch Ophthalmol.* 1995;113:1191–1194.

34. Orgül S, Cioffi GA, Bacon DR, Van Buskirk EM. Sources of variability of topometric data with a scanning laser ophthalmoscope. *Arch Ophthalmol.* 1996;114: 161–164.

35. Geyer O, Michaeli-Cohen A, Silver DM, et al. Reproducibility of topographic measures of the glaucomatous optic nerve head. *Br J Ophthalmol.* 1998;82:14–17.

36. Zangwill LM, VanHorn S, Lima MD, Sample PA, Weinreb RN. Optic nerve head topography in ocular hypertensive eyes using confocal scanning laser ophthalmoscopy. *Am J Ophthalmol.* 1996;122:520–525.

37. Uchida H, Brigatti L, Caprioli J. Detection of structural damage from glaucoma with confocal laser image analysis. *Invest Ophthalmol Vis Sci.* 1996;37:2393–2401.

38. Iester M, Broadway DC, Mikelberg FS, Drance SM. A comparison of healthy, ocular hypertensive, and glaucomatous optic disc topographic parameters. *J Glaucoma.* 1997;6:363–370.

39. Bathija R, Zangwill L, Berry CC, et al. Detection of early glaucomatous structural damage with confocal scanning laser tomography. *J Glaucoma*. 1998;7:121–127.

40. Wollstein G, Garway-Heath DF, Hitchings RA. Identification of early glaucoma cases with the scanning laser ophthalmoscope. *Ophthalmology*. 1998;105:1557–1563.

41. Hatch WV, Flanagan JG, Etchells EE, Williams-Lyn DE, Trope GE. Laser scanning tomography of the optic nerve head in ocular hypertension and glaucoma. *Br J Ophthalmol*. 1997;81:871–876.

42. Iester M, Mikelberg FS, Swindale NV, Drance SM. ROC analysis of Heidelberg Retina Tomograph optic disc shape measures in glaucoma. *Can J Ophthalmol*. 1997; 32:382–388.

43. Gramer E, Maier H, Messner EM. A measure for the thickness of the nerve fibre layer and the configuration of the optic disc excavation in glaucoma patients: A clinical study using the laser tomographic scanner. In: Mills RP, ed. *Perimetry Update. Proceedings of the Xth International Perimetric Society Meeting*. Amsterdam/New York: Kugler; 1993:207–213.

44. Mikelberg FS, Parfitt CM, Swindale NV, Graham SL, Drance SM, Gosine R. Ability of the Heidelberg Retina Tomograph to detect early glaucomatous visual field loss. *J Glaucoma*. 1995;4:242–247.

45. Tsai CS, Zangwill L, Sample PA, Garden V, Bartsch DU, Weinreb RN. Correlation of peripapillary retinal height and visual field in glaucoma and normal subjects. *J Glaucoma*. 1995;4:110–116.

46. Yamagishi N, Anton A, Sample PA, Zangwill L, Lopez A, Weinreb RN. Mapping structural change of the optic disc to visual field defect in glaucoma. *Am J Ophthalmol*. 1997;123:667–676.

47. Iester M, Mikelberg FS, Courtright P, Drance SM. Correlation between the visual field indices and Heidelberg Retina Tomograph parameters. *J Glaucoma*. 1997;6: 78–82.

48. Iester M, Swindale NV, Mikelberg F. Sector-based analysis of optic nerve head shape parameters and visual field indices in healthy and glaucomatous eyes. *J Glaucoma*. 1997;6:371–376.

49. Teesalu P, Vihanninjoki K, Airaksinen PJ, Tuulonen A. Correlation of blue-on-yellow visual fields with scanning confocal laser optic disc measurements. *Invest Ophthalmol Vis Sci*. 1997;38:2452–2459.

50. Flanagan JG, Hatch W, Williams-Lyn D, Trope GE. Change in HRT optic nerve head parameters in progressive glaucoma. *Invest Ophthalmol Vis Sci*. 1996;37:S664.

51. Hosking SL, Flanagan JG, O'Donoghue EP. Scanning laser tomography detects disease progression in glaucomatous optic neuropathy. *Invest Ophthalmol Vis Sci*. 1997;38:S828.

52. Irak I, Zangwill L, Garden V, Shakiba S, Weinreb RN. Change in optic disc topography after trabeculectomy. *Am J Ophthalmol*. 1996;122:690–695.

53. Flanagan JG, O'Donoghue EP. Topographic change in the optic nerve head following acute reduction of IOP in glaucoma. In: Mills R, Walls M, eds. *Perimetry Update 1994/95*. Kugler, 357.

54. Yan DG, Flanagan JG, Farra T, Trope GE, Ethier CR. Study of regional deformation of the optic nerve head using scanning laser tomography. *Curr Eye Res*. 1998; 17:903–916.

55. Hosking SL, Flanagan JG. Prospective study design for the Heidelberg Retina Tomograph: The effect of change in focus setting. *Graefes Arch Clin Exp Ophthalmol*. 1996; 234:306–310.

56. Hosking SL, Flanagan JG. Scanning laser tomography: Effect of change in keratometry values on retinal distance measures. *Ophthalmol Physiol Optom*. 1998;18(3): 182–185.

57. Chauhan BC. Analysis of changes in the optic nerve head. In: Anderson DR, Drance SM, eds. *Encounters in Glaucoma Research: 3. How to Ascertain Progression and Outcome*. Amsterdam: Kugler, 1996:195–208.

58. Huang D, Swanson EA, Lin CP, et al. Optical coherence tomography. *Science*. 1991;254:1178.

59. Izatt JA, Hee MR, Huang D, et al. Ophthalmic diagnostics using optical coherence tomography. In: Ren Q, Pavel JM, chairs/eds. *Proceedings of Ophthalmic Technologies III*. Los Angeles, January 16–18, 1992. Bellingham, WA: SPIE; 1993:136–144. (Progress in biomedical optics. *Proc SPIE*;v.1877.)

60. Izatt JA, Hee MR, Swanson EA, et al. Micrometer-scale resolution imaging of the anterio eye in vivo with optical coherence tomography. *Arch Ophthalmol*. 1994;112: 1584–1589.

61. Hee MR, Izatt JA, Swanson EA, et al. Optical coherence tomography of the human retina. *Arch Ophthalmol*. 1995;113:325–332.

62. Hee MR, Izat JA, Swanson EA, et al. Optical coherence tomography for micron-resolution ophthalmic imaging. *IEEE Eng Med Biol*. 1995;14(1):67–75.

63. Fujimoto J, Brezinski M, Tearney G, Boppart S, Bouma B, Hee M, Southern J, Swanson E. Optical biopsy and imaging using optical coherence tomography. *Nature Med*. 1995;1:970–972.

64. Chauhan DV, Marshall J. The interpretation of optical coherence tomography images of the retina. *Invest Ophthalmol Vis Sci*. 1999;40:2332–2342.

65. Brezinski M, Tearney G, Bouma B, Boppart S, Pitris C, Southern J, Fujimoto J. Optical biopsy with optical coherence tomography. *Ann NY Acad Sci* 1998;838:68–74.

66. Puliafito CA, Hee MR, Schuman JS, Fujimoto JG. *Optical Coherence Tomography of Ocular Diseases*. Thorofare, NJ: Slack;1996:17–34.

67. Toth CA, Narayan DG, Boppart SA, et al. A comparison of retinal morphology viewed by optical coherence tomography and by light microscopy. *Arch Ophthalmol*. 1997;115:1425–1428.

68. Hee MR, Puliafito AC, Wong C, Duker JS, Reichel E, Rutledge B, Schuman JS, Swanson EA, Fujimoto JG. Quantitative assessment of macular edema with optical coherence tomography. *Arch Ophthalmol*. 1995; 113:1019–1029.

69. Puliafito CA, Hee MR, Lin CP, Reichel E, Schuman JS, Duker JS, Izatt JA, Swanson EA, Fujimoto JG. Imaging of macular diseases with optical coherence tomography. *Ophthalmology*. 1995;102:217–229.

70. Hee MR, Puliafito CA, Wong C, Duker JS, Reichel E, Schuman JS, Swanson EA, Fujimoto JG. Optical coherence tomography of macular holes. *Ophthalmology*. 1995;102:748–756.

71. Schuman JS, Hee MR, Puliafito CA, Wong C, Pedut-Kloizman T, Lin CP, Hertzmark E, Izatt JA, Swanson EA, Fujimoto JG. Quantification of nerve fiber layer thickness in normal and glaucomatous eyes using optical coherence tomography. *Arch Ophthalmol*. 1995;113:586–596.

72. Wilkins JR, Puliafito CA, Hee MR, Duker JS, Reichel E, Coker JG, Schuman JS, Swanson EA, Fujimoto JG. Characterization of epiretinal membranes using optical coherence tomography. *Ophthalmology*. 1996; 103:142–151.

73. Hee MR, Baumal CR, Puliafito CA, Duker JS, Reichel E, Wilkins JR, Coker JG, Schuman JS, Swanson EA, Fujimoto JG. Optical coherence tomography of age-related macular degeneration and choroidal neovascularization. *Ophthalmology*. 1996;103:1260–1270.

74. Rutledge BK, Puliafito CA, Duker JS, Hee MR, Cox MS. Optical coherence tomography of macular lesions associated with optic nerve head pits. *Ophthalmology*. 1996;103:1047–1053.

75. Hee MR, Puliafito AC, Duker JS, Reichel E, Coker JG, Wilkins JR, Swanson EA, Fujimoto JG. Topography of diabetic macular edema with optical coherence tomography. *Ophthalmology*. 1998;105:369–370.

76. Sourdille P, Santiago PY. Optical coherence tomography of macular thickness after cataract surgery. *J Cataract Refract Surg*. 1999;25:256–261.

77. Ip M, Garza-Karren C, Duker JS, Reichel E, Swartz JC, Amirikia A, Puliafito CA. Differentiation of degenerative retinoschisis from retinal detachment using optical coherence tomography. *Ophthalmology*. 1999;106:600–605.

78. Pieroth L, Schuman JS, Hertzmark E, Hee MR, Wilins JR, Coker J, Mattox C, Pedut-Kloizman R, Puliafito CA, Fujimoto JG, Swanson E. Evaluation of focal defects of the nerve fiber layer using optical coherence tomography. *Ophthalmology*. 1999;106:570–579.

79. Trabucchi G, Brancato R, Pierro L, Introini U, Sannace C. Idiopathic juxtafoveolar retinal telangiectasis and pigment epithelial hyperplasia: An optical coherence tomographic study. *Arch Ophthalmol*. 1999;117:405–406.

80. Puliafito CA, Hee MR, Schuman JS, Fujimoto JG. *Optical Coherence Tomography of Ocular Diseases*. Thorofare, NJ: Slack; 1996:289–356.

81. Schuman JS. Optical coherence tomography for imaging and quantitation of nerve fiber layer thickness. In: Schuman JS, ed. *Imaging in Glaucoma*. Thorofare, NJ: Slack; 1997:95–130.

82. Schuman JS, Pedut-Kloizman T, Hertzmark E, et al. Reproducibility of nerve fiber layer thickness measurements using optical coherence tomography. *Ophthalmology*. 1996;103:1889–1898.

83. Weinreb RN, Dreher AW, Coleman A, Quigley H, Shaw B, Reiter K. Histopathologic validation of Fourier-ellipsometry measurements of retinal nerve fiber layer thickness. *Arch Ophthalmol*. 1990;108:557–560.

84. Dreher AW, Reiter K, Weinreb RN. Spatially resolved birefringence of the retinal nerve fiber layer of normal and glaucomatous eyes. *Am J Ophthalmol*. 1992;31: 3730–3735.

85. Dreher AW, Reiter K. Scanning laser polarimetry of the retina nerve fiber layer. *SPIE Proc*. 1992;1746:34–38.

86. Dreher AW, Reiter KR. Retinal laser ellipsometry: A new method for measuring the retinal nerve fiber layer thickness distribution. *Clin Vision Sci*. 1992;7:481–488.

87. Weinreb RN, Shakiba S, Zangwill L. Scanning laser polarimetry to measure the nerve fiber layer of normal and glaucomatous eyes. *Am J Ophthalmol*. 1995;119: 627–636.

88. Niessen AG, Van Den Berg TJ, Langerhorst CT, Greve EL. Retinal nerve fiber layer assessment by scanning laser polarimetry and standardized photography. *Am J Ophthalmol*. 1996;121:484–493.

89. de Souza Lima M, Zangwill L, Weinreb RN. Scanning laser polarimetry to assess the nerve fiber layer. In: Schuman JS, ed. *Imaging in Glaucoma*. Thorofare, NJ: Slack; 1997:83–92.

90. Zangwill LM, Williams JA, Weinreb RN. Quantitative methods for evaluating the retinal nerve fiber layer in glaucoma. *Ophthalmol Clin North Am*. 1998;11:1–9.

91. Weinreb RN, Zangwill L, Berry CC, Bathija R, Sample PA. Detection of glaucoma with scanning laser polarimetry. *Arch Ophthalmol*. 1998;116:1583–1589.

92. Chi Q, Tomita G, Inazumi K, Hayakawa T, Tadayoshi I, Kitazawa Y. Evaluation of the effect of aging on the retinal nerve fiber layer thickness using scanning laser polarimetry. *J Glaucoma*. 1995;4:406–413.

93. Tjon-Fo-Sang MJ, van Strik R, de Vries J, Lemji HG. Improved reproducibility of measurements with the nerve fiber analyzer. *J Glaucoma*. 1997;6:203–211.

94. Zangwill L, Berry CA, Garden VS, Weinreb RN. Reproducibility of retardation measurements with the nerve fiber Analyzer II. *J Glaucoma*. 1997;6:384–389.

95. Hoh ST, Ishikawa H, Greenfield DS, Liebmann JM, Chew SJ, Ritch R. Peripapillary nerve fiber layer thickness measurement reproducibility using scanning laser polarimetry. *J Glaucoma*. 1998;7:12–15.

96. Waldock A, Potts MJ, Sparrow JM, Karwatowski WS. Clinical evaluation of scanning laser polarimetry: I. Intraoperator reproducibility and design of a blood vessel removal algorithm. *Br J Ophthalmol*. 1998;82: 252–259.

97. Tjon-Fo Sang MJ, Lemji HG. The sensitivity and specificity of nerve fiber layer measurements in glaucomas determined with scanning laser polarimetry. *Am J Ophthalmol*. 1997;123:62–69.

98. Tjon-Fo-Sang MJ, de Vries J, Lemji HG. Measurement by nerve fiber analyzer of retinal nerve fiber layer thickness in normal subjects and patients with ocular hypertension. *Am J Ophthalmol*. 1996;122:220–227.

99. Hudson C. Nerve fibre layer thickness measurements derived by scanning laser polarimetry: The jury is out. *Br J Ophthalmol.* 1997;81:338–339.

100. Anton A, Zangwill L, Emdadi A, Weinreb RN. Nerve fiber layer measurements with scanning laser polarimetry in ocular hypertension. *Arch Ophthalmol.* 1997;115:331–334.

101. Weinreb RN, Shakiba S, Sample PA, et al. Association between quantitative nerve fiber layer measurement and visual field loss in glaucoma. *Am J Ophthalmol.* 1995;120:732–738.

102. Varma R, Skaf M, Barron F. Retinal nerve fiber layer thickness in normal human eyes. *Ophthalmology.* 1996; 103:2114–2119.

103. Nakla M, Nduaguba C, Rozier M, et al. Comparison of imaging techniques to detect glaucomatous optic nerve damage. *Invest Ophthalmol Vis Sci.* 1999;40 (suppl):397.

Chapter 15

THE VISUAL FIELD IN GLAUCOMA

Peter Åsman

Many new techniques for the diagnosis of glaucoma have recently been introduced. These include three-dimensional optic disc measurements, with raster and scanning laser tomography; retinal nerve fiber layer measurements with optical coherence tomography; and polarimetry. Despite these new technologies, clinical evaluation of automated visual field charts still remains the most widely accepted method to detect manifest glaucoma. The purpose of this chapter is to provide the reader with the structural foundations of glaucomatous visual field loss and to illustrate glaucomatous damage using several clinical examples.

SHORT HISTORICAL OVERVIEW

Glaucomatous visual field loss was first described by Albert von Graefe in 1869.[1] He presented campimetry results, obtained in a patient with advanced glaucoma, showing a central island and a peripheral temporal crest. Later, Landesberg[2] and Bjerrum[3] independently discovered an arcuate defect in the visual fields of patients with glaucoma. Landesberg described an isolated finding while Bjerrum presented a series of patients with this type of defect, which has often been called a *Bjerrum scotoma* and has been a hallmark of glaucomatous field loss ever since. The Bjerrum scotoma is one of the very few defect entities that has survived throughout the twentieth century as a

genuine sign of glaucoma. Although Landesberg presented an absolute defect, Bjerrum, with his refined campimetric technique, also detected relative defects of the arcuate shape.

In 1909, Rønne detected a nasal step in many patients.[4] The nasal step is another defect, along with the Bjerrum scotoma, that is definitely related to glaucoma. Rønne also presented the staging system for glaucomatous field loss.

There were two major breakthroughs in field testing during the twentieth century. The first was the standardization of manual perimetry made possible by the work of Hans Goldmann. The second was the advent of automated static threshold perimetry. With these new refined techniques, much controversy regarding glaucomatous field loss emerged. Several signs now known to be of no clinical relevance were strongly advocated as early signs of glaucoma. Enlargement of the blind spot and general constriction are probably the most widely known. During the last 10 years, much of this debate has settled and there is now little if any disagreement as to the nature of glaucomatous visual field loss.

THEORY

This section discusses the theoretical basis for interpretation of glaucomatous field loss in terms of diagnostics.

The aspects covered here are then applied in a number of clinical examples.

Anatomic Basis for Glaucomatous Visual Field Loss

The Arcuate Field Defect

Glaucomatous field defects occur as a result of damage to the retinal nerve fibers. The site of damage is not entirely understood, but is likely at the level of the optic disc. Nerve fibers project from the peripheral temporal retina to the optic disc in an arcuate pattern. Damage to nerve fibers at the optic disc will therefore result in diminished light sensitivity along these arcuate fibers (Fig. 15–1). The arcuate shape is most pro-

nounced in the parts corresponding to the superior and inferior retinal vascular arcades.

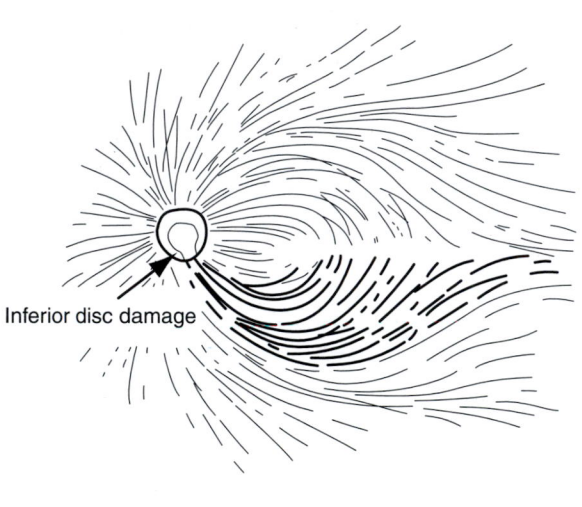

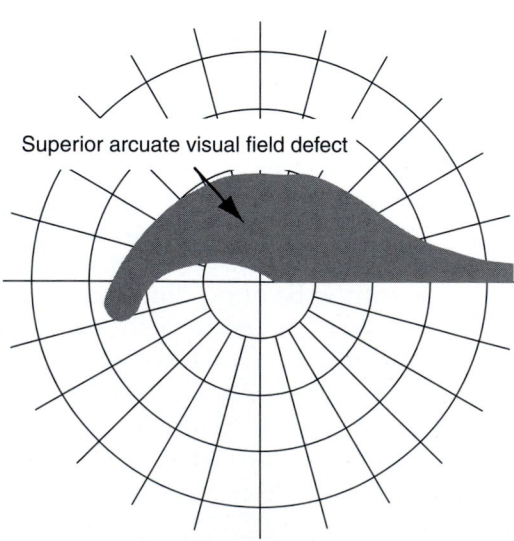

Figure 15–1. Arcuate visual field defect in superior hemifield (*bottom*) caused by notch at inferior disc pole (*top*). Nerve fibers project in an arcuate fashion from the peripheral retina to the optic disc; thus sensory impulses from those parts of the retina lying within the damaged nerve fiber layer will be diminished.

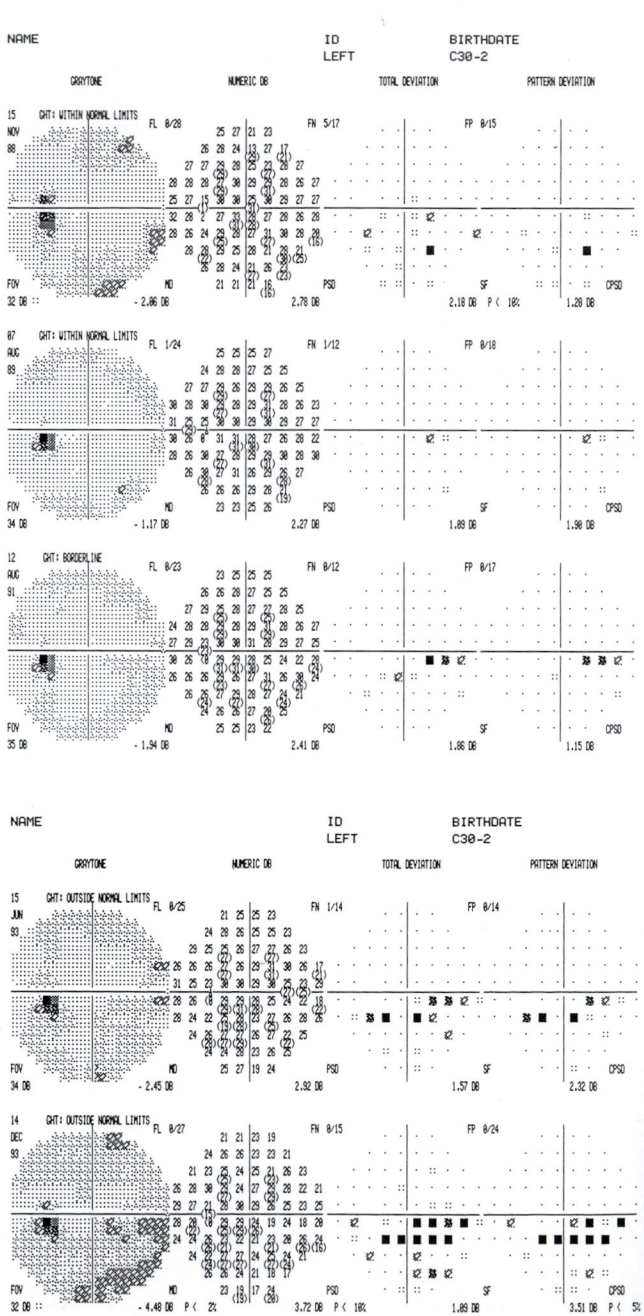

Figure 15–2. Development of a glaucomatous visual field defect. In the earliest phase (*top*), the gray-scale map is essentially normal. In the pattern-deviation map (*right column of maps*) increased scatter over time results in a nasal defect that comes and goes. The defect is not always in the same test point locations but usually in the same area. After this transitional time zone, a definite field defect appears (*bottom*) and is now also evident in the gray-scale printout. The Glaucoma Hemifield Test classification is "within normal limits" in the first two tests followed by "borderline" classification in the third test session. The final two tests had a classification "outside normal limits."

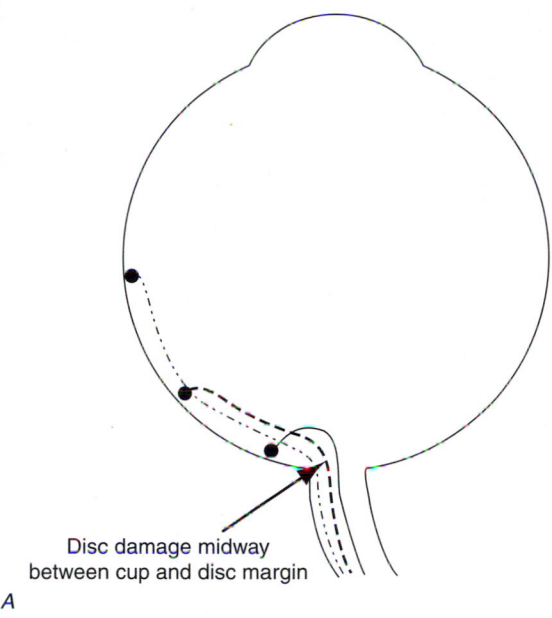

A

Disc damage midway
between cup and disc margin

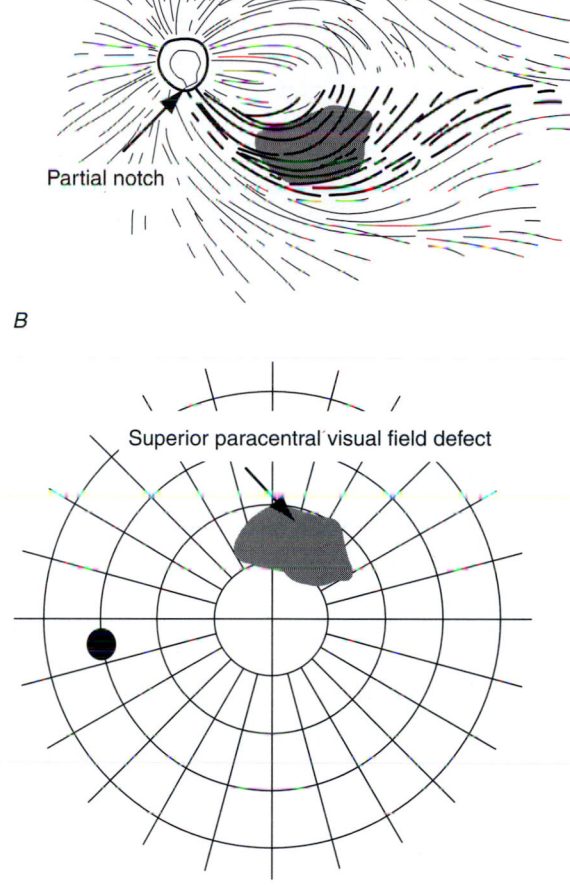

B

Partial notch

Superior paracentral visual field defect

C

Figure 15–3. Morphological basis for paracentral visual-field loss in glaucoma. *A.* Nerve fibers from the peripheral retina run close to the optic nerve sheath while fibers emanating from the peripapillary region run close to the central retinal artery within the nerve. Damage to nerve fibers midway between the cup and disc margin affects paracentral parts of the retina (*B*), resulting in a paracentral visual field defect (*C*).

The Nasal Step

Nerve fibers emanating from the superior retinal hemisphere reach the optic disc without crossing the horizontal midline. Temporal to the macula, nerve fibers project to enter the optic disc near the superior and inferior poles. Thus, damage at one of the optic disc poles will cause a defect that may be located in the nasal periphery of the visual field and reach the horizontal meridian. The other side of the meridian will, however, remain unchanged because fibers here reach the disc at the opposite pole (Fig. 15–2). Nasal steps will also frequently occur if there is damage at both the superior and inferior poles of the optic disc, since such disc damage is seldom entirely symmetrical.

The Paracentral Defect

Retinal nerve fibers entering the optic disc run through the optic disc at different eccentricities depending on their origin in the retina (Fig. 15–3*A*). Thus, fibers starting close to the disc margin run centrally in the optic nerve, close to the blood vessels. Fibers originating in the peripheral retina, on the other hand, run peripherally in the optic nerve close to the nerve sheath. Localized damage within the optic nerve midway from its center to its periphery will therefore result in field loss midway between the central and the peripheral field. If the damage occurs superiorly or inferiorly, which is the case in glaucoma, the defect will be paracentral (Fig. 15–3*B* and *C*).

Diffuse and Localized Field Loss

Visual field loss as so far discussed is focal or localized in nature. Diffuse loss of sensitivity has also been reported as an important sign of glaucomatous damage. Such loss is thought to be the result of loss of nerve fibers in all areas of the optic nerve head. In other words, no portion of the retinal nerve fiber layer is entirely spared from damage in early glaucoma. Diffuse and localized field loss has given rise to much controversy previously, and some authors have argued that diffuse loss is mandatory or at least a not unusual finding in early glaucoma,[5-7] while others have concluded that pure diffuse field loss is rare in early glaucoma.[8-10] In any event pure diffuse field loss should not be regarded as a finding specific for glaucoma but more likely as the result of cataract or miotic therapy. Therefore, in clinical practice, pure diffuse field loss is a sign with very little information with respect to glaucoma. On the other hand, combined diffuse and localized field loss seems to be quite a

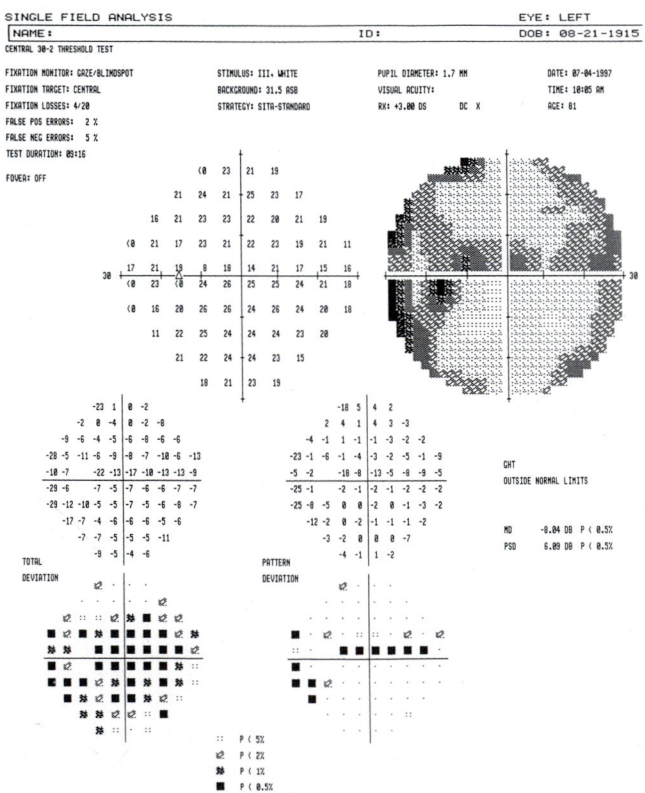

Figure 15–4. A thin, superior glaucomatous visual-field defect resulting in a row of highly significant test points above the horizontal meridian. A narrow notch at the 5 o'clock position explains the thinness of the defect. The total-deviation probability map is markedly darker due to coexisting cataract. Note that the total-deviation probability map is unable to reveal the glaucomatous scotoma. The Glaucoma Hemifield Test classification is "outside normal limits."

TABLE 15–1. STAGES OF GLAUCOMATOUS VISUAL FIELD LOSS*

Isolated pericentral scotomas or baring[†] in all its modalities

Bjerrum's scotoma or arcuate scotoma

Bjerrum's scotoma with a break through to the peripheral part of the field

Penultimate stage, with possible sparing of the central and temporal islands

Total blindness

*Classification suggested by Dubois-Poulsen based on the findings of Aulhorn and Harms in 1967.
[†]Reduced sensitivity adjacent to the blind spot.

common finding in glaucoma.[11] Such loss is best referred to as *widespread field loss* (Fig. 15–4).

Frequency Distribution of the Localization of the Earliest Defects

In Aulhorn and Harms' large study presented in 1967, the various stages of visual field loss throughout the course of glaucoma were nicely clarified (Table 15–1).[12] Later, careful studies have showed that the earliest defects in glaucoma occur in the paracentral visual field, predominantly superiorly.[13,14] Defects may also occur more peripherally,[15,16] but the increased physiological variability and abundance of peripheral test artifacts suggest that testing of the peripheral field with static threshold perimetry is of little or no clinical value. Before definite field loss occurs, the visual field often undergoes a long period of transient field defects.[15] These usually occur along the same retinal nerve fiber path but not necessarily with exactly the same eccentricity. The occurrence of such transient defects should raise suspicion of early but not manifest glaucoma in the presence of other signs of glaucoma, especially optic disc notches or disc hemorrhages.

There seems to be a preponderance of field defects in the superior hemifield. Disc changes in early glaucoma are also more frequent around the inferior pole. Unfortunately, common test artifacts are more common in the superior hemifield and may at times be misinterpreted as glaucomatous defects. It is therefore always wise to look for changes at the optic disc that can be related to a measured field abnormality.

Importance of Test Strategy

The topographical appearance of glaucomatous field loss is more or less independent of the technique used to measure the visual field. Thus, paracentral defects, arcuate scotomas, and nasal steps can all be demonstrated with Bjerrum's campimetric screen from 1889, the Goldmann manual kinetic perimeter, or the new third-generation automated static threshold measuring devices (SITA). However, the different testing methods detect these defects at entirely different stages of the disease. Shallow defects may be obvious and indisputable in probability maps from a SITA test and at the same time be totally missed with routine Goldmann perimetry. At the same time, one needs to bear in mind that the newer and faster thresholding algorithms result in decreased physiological threshold variability. Also, threshold values within glaucomatous field defects are often higher with SITA testing than with older tests. Therefore, field loss at the same stage may appear less evident in gray-scale printouts when SITA testing is performed. When the lower variability is taken into account by using probability maps, the defect becomes equally or often more evident than in the probability maps of older threshold-measuring techniques.[17]

Interpretation

Single visual fields can be judged either intuitively or with the help of computer-based analyses. Intuitive judgment is often quite sufficient to establish a diagnosis in the case of moderately advanced glaucoma. In early glaucoma, however, computer-assisted interpretation in the clinical routine becomes mandatory.

Intuitive Judgment

Intuitive judgment of visual fields in order to detect glaucomatous field loss relies on the recognition of localized depression or scotomas. These scotomas should have a shape that corresponds to the anatomy of the retinal nerve fiber layer. Deep nasal steps and arcuate scotomas not connected with the superior midperiphery are probably the easiest defects to recognize. In the absence of computer aids, peripheral defects of nonspecific shape should be judged with high suspicion of being test artifacts.

Computer-Assisted Interpretation

A large number of computer-assisted tools for visual field interpretation have been suggested and many have been used routinely in clinical settings. The simple ones are visual field indices.[18,19] These represent summary statistics for measured threshold values and should be avoided in the interpretation of the individual visual field. Graphical probability maps, on the other hand, are very useful because they indicate the likelihood that, pointwise, measured threshold values are within or outside the normal physiological variability.[20] Two such probability maps are available in the STATPAC programs of the Humphrey perimeter. The total deviation probability map (Fig. 15–5A) shows the significance of the raw measured threshold values after correction for age. Many diseases, including cataract, affect these threshold values either focally or homogeneously. Cataracts may therefore mask focal field loss due to glaucoma. In the pattern-deviation probability map (Fig. 15–5B) the deviations from age-corrected threshold values are adjusted homogeneously to compensate for any diffuse depressions in the visual field. In this way, only localized field loss is highlighted, which is the best method for revealing glaucomatous defects.

The Glaucoma Hemifield Test (GHT) (Fig. 15–5C) is a system based on the pattern deviation maps.[21] The GHT compares differences across the horizontal meridian in the pattern-deviation probability map with empirically determined normative limits. The results are then classified as within or outside the normal limits. Field results in the gray zone between normality and abnormality are classified as borderline. The GHT is the most widely accepted standard for computer-assisted interpretation and is used, for example, in the Early Manifest Glaucoma Trial in the definition of glaucomatous field loss.

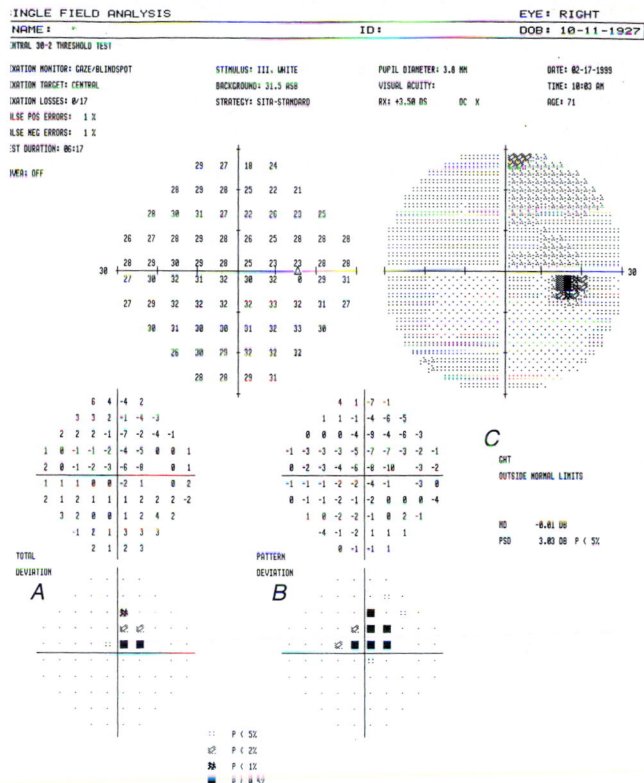

Figure 15–5. Early superior glaucomatous field defect. The gray scale is normal but total (*A*) and the pattern-deviation probability map (*B*) reveals a superior cluster of test points with significantly reduced sensitivity. The defect was due to glaucomatous narrowing of the neuroretinal rim at the inferior disc pole. The Glaucoma Hemifield Test classification (*C*) is "outside normal limits."

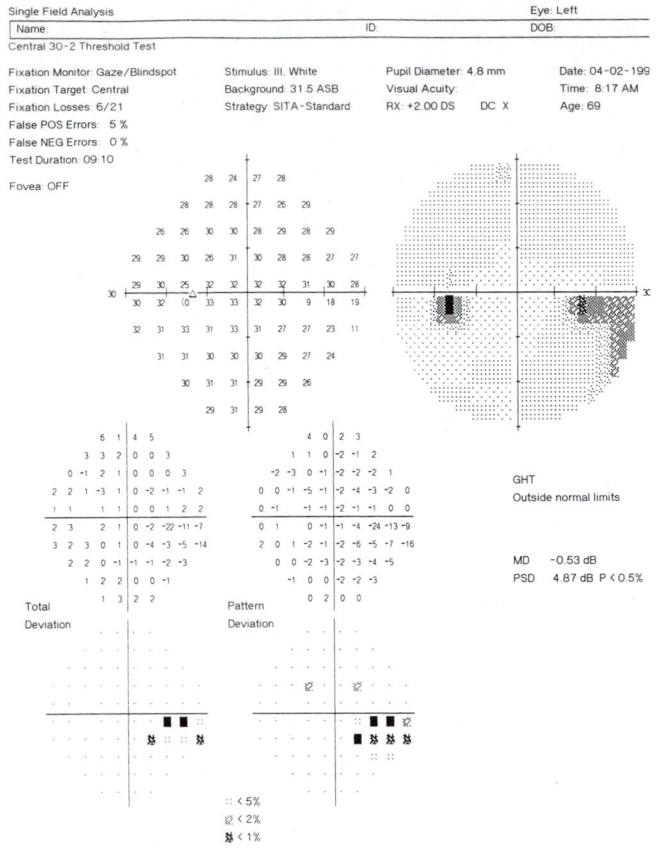

Figure 15–6. Early nasal step evident in gray-scale, total-deviation, and pattern-deviation probability maps. The defect was due to a partial superior glaucomatous notch in the optic disc. The Glaucoma Hemifield Test classification is "outside normal limits."

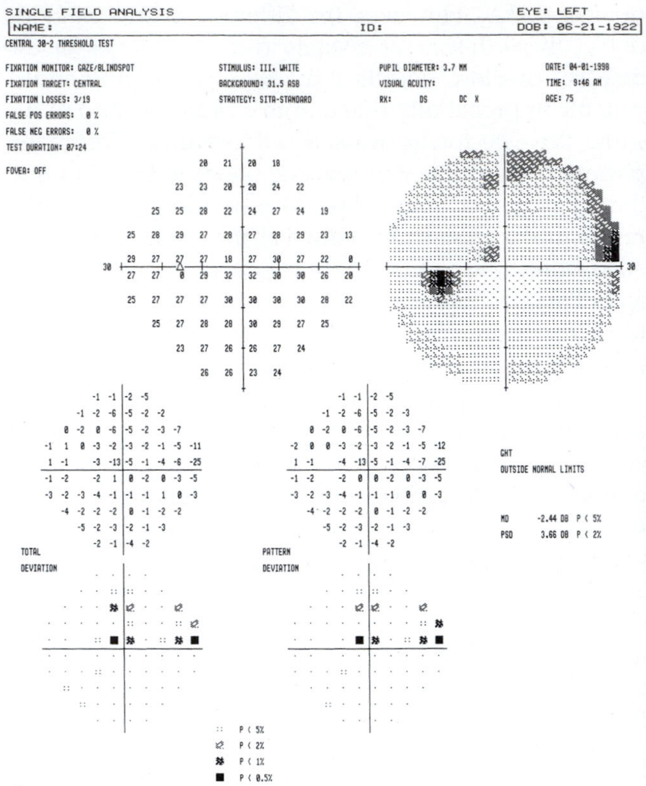

Figure 15–7. *A.* Early glaucomatous visual field damage in the superior hemifield. The defect has a central/paracentral part and a midperipheral part. An advanced but incomplete notch at the inferior disc pole corresponds with field damage. *B.* It can be seen that the defect's depth and shape change slightly over time, which is typical for glaucoma in earlier stages. The Glaucoma Hemifield Test classification is "outside normal limits." Tests were obtained 5 months apart.

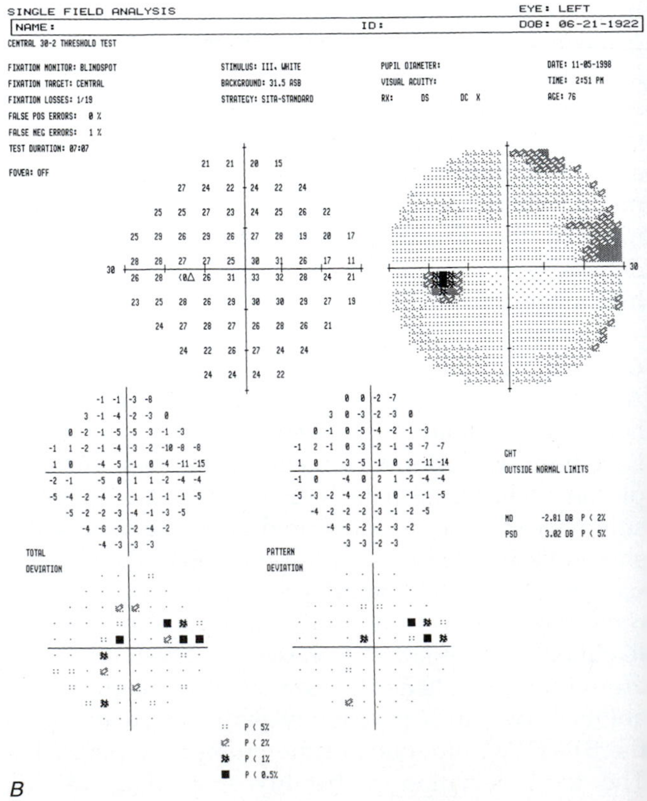

CLINICAL EXAMPLES

The following section is subdivided into two parts. The first illustrates true glaucomatous visual field defects. The second part shows some important differential diagnoses.

Glaucomatous Visual Field Defects

The various stages in the development of glaucomatous visual field loss are illustrated in Figs. 15–3 through 15–13. There is usually a good correspondence between optic disc findings and visual field appearance. Furthermore, the defects strongly correlate with the anatomy of the retinal nerve fiber layer.

Differential Diagnosis

Some important causes of visual field loss that can result in problems with differential diagnosis are shown in Figs. 15–14 through 15–17.

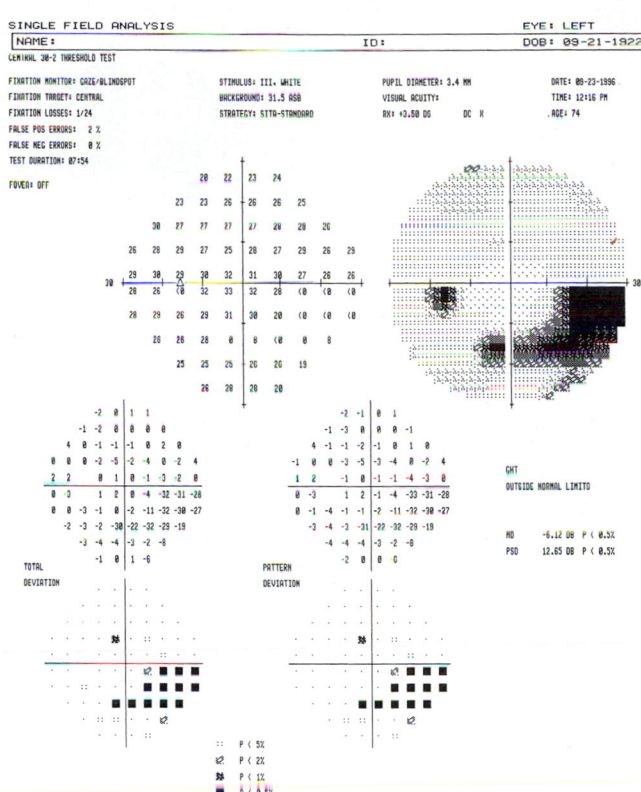

Figure 15–9. A deep arcuate scotoma in the inferior hemifield. Note the sharp edge at the horizontal meridian, which is typical for glaucomatous field loss. There is a zone of normal sensitivity between the defect and the blind spot. The optic disc has an incomplete glaucomatous notch at the superior pole. The Glaucoma Hemifield Test classification is "outside normal limits."

CONCLUSION

In evaluating a visual field chart for the detection of glaucoma, one should remember the following rules of thumb:

- Glaucomatous visual field loss is localized.
- The shape of glaucomatous field defects correlates well with the anatomy of the retinal nerve fiber layer.
- A field defect corresponding to an optic disc abnormality (notch or disc hemorrhage) strengthens the suspicion for glaucoma.
- A repeated visual field examination should be performed whenever there is doubt as to whether or not an apparent field defect represent abnormality or is just an expression of physiological variability or the learning curve.

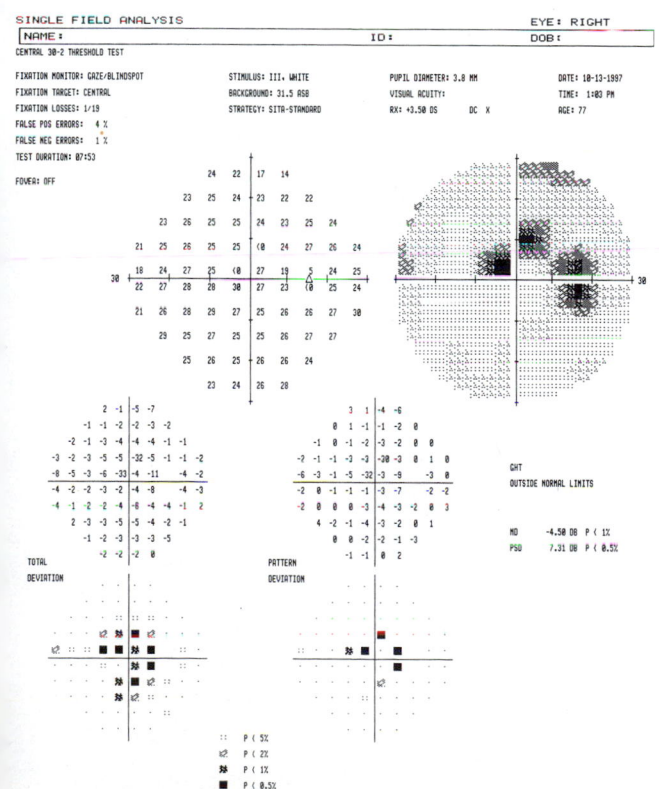

Figure 15–8. A deep absolute paracentral visual field defect. An incomplete glaucomatous notch at the inferior disc pole explains the defect, which has an arcuate shape. The Glaucoma Hemifield Test classification is "outside normal limits."

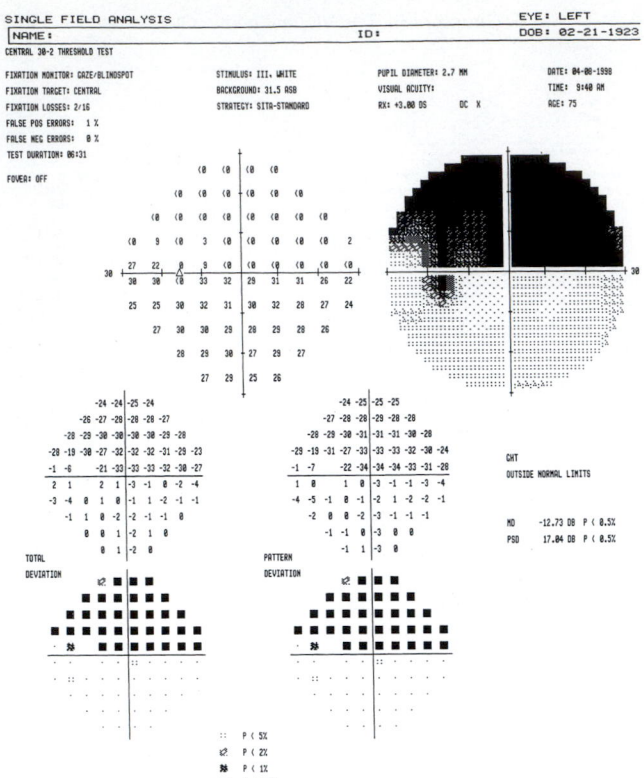

Figure 15–10. A complete superior glaucomatous altitudinal defect due to wide marginal disc cupping at the inferior pole. The Glaucoma Hemifield Test classification is "outside normal limits."

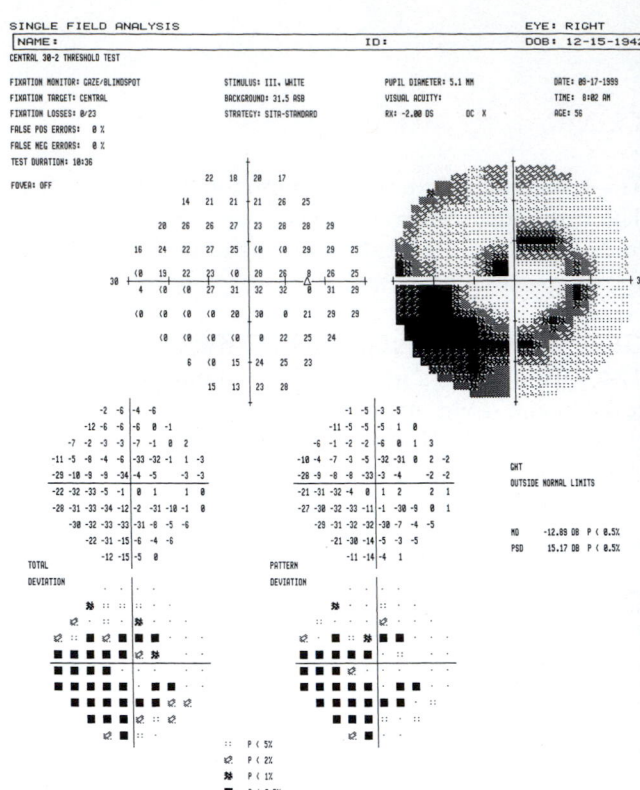

Figure 15–11. Advanced visual field loss involving both hemifields in a patient with primary open-angle glaucoma. There is a complete Bjerrum scotoma in the inferior hemifield connecting the blind spot with the midperiphery and a smaller but deep superior arcuate field defect. The Glaucoma Hemifield Test classification is "outside normal limits."

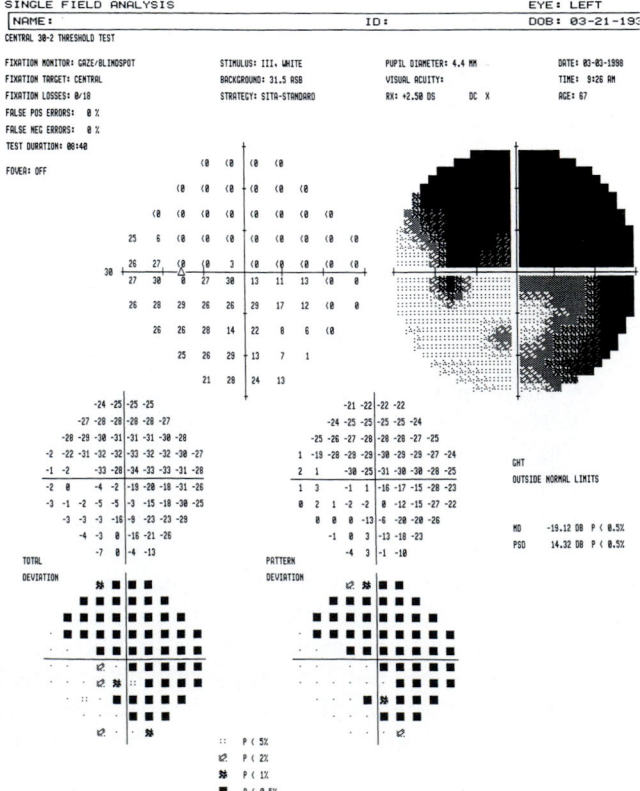

Figure 15–12. Advanced visual field loss in a patient with primary open-angle glaucoma. The entire superior hemifield is blind and there is a deep but incomplete arcuate defect in the inferior hemifield. The Glaucoma Hemifield Test classification is "outside normal limits."

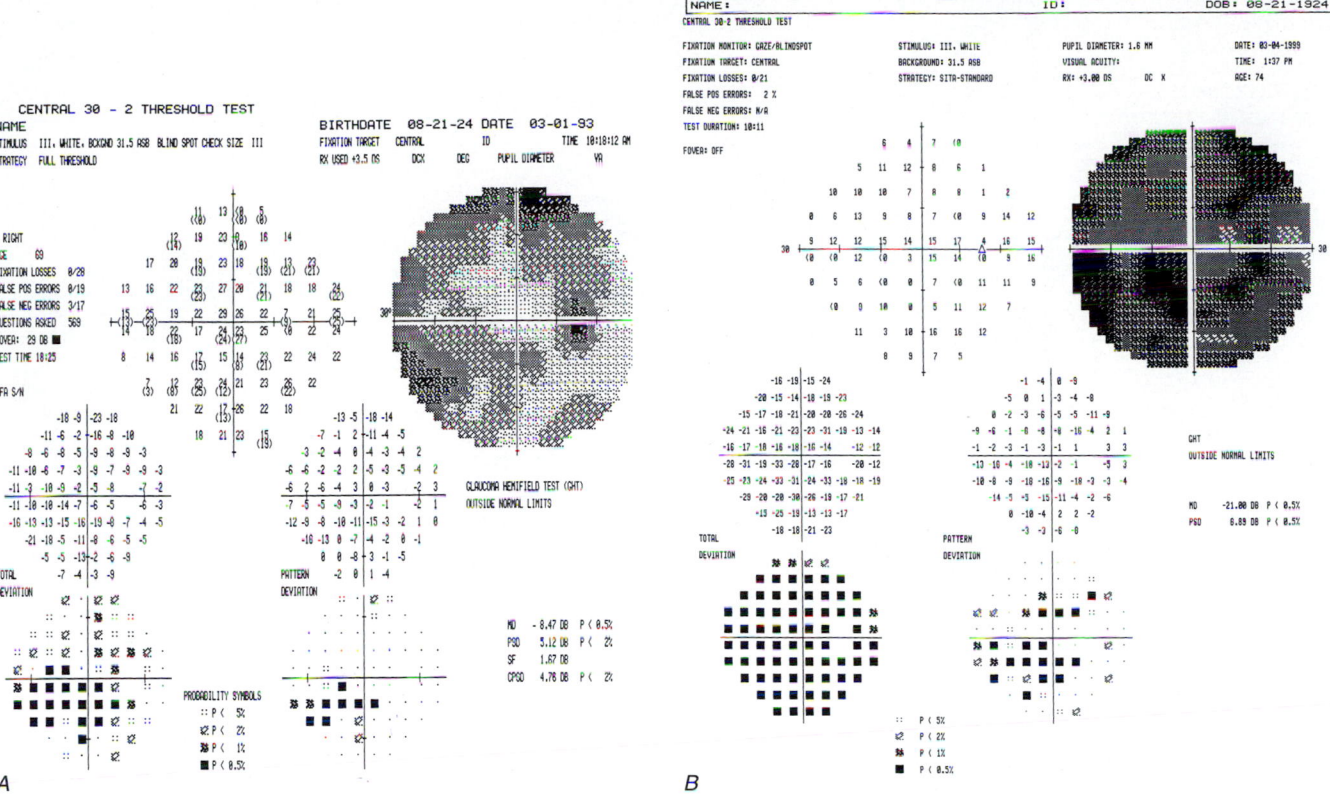

Figure 15-13. *A.* Effect of an increasing cataract on the glaucomatous visual field. An inferior defect of the arcuate visual field corresponds well with the disc findings. *B.* Six years later, the visual field is severely damaged by combined glaucoma and cataract (*right*). The gray scale is very dark and the entire visual field has highly significant sensitivity values. In the pattern-deviation probability map, the effect of cataract is filtered away, leaving only areas of significant localized field loss. The inferior glaucomatous visual field defect has increased only slightly and a smaller superior arcuate field defect has also appeared. The dramatic change in the appearance of this visual field was thus mainly due to increasing cataract. The Glaucoma Hemifield Test classification was "outside normal limits" on both occasions.

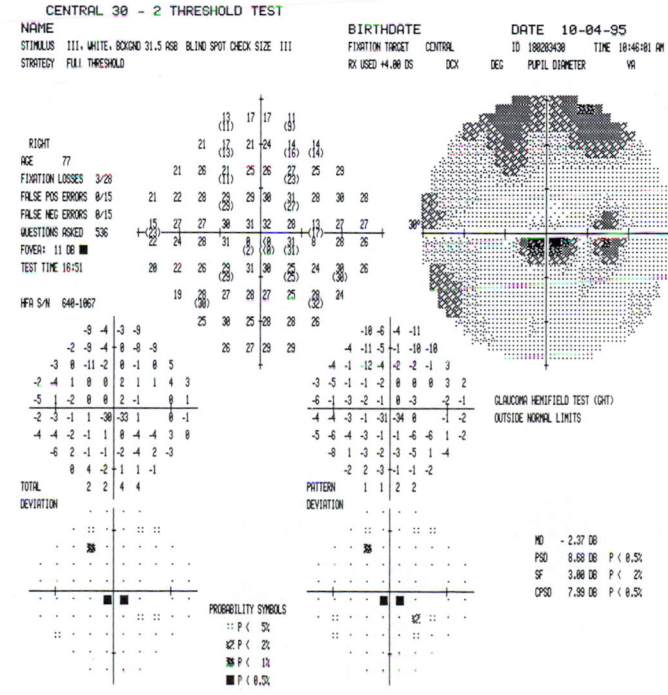

Figure 15-14. Central visual field defect due to age-related macular degeneration. Careful ophthalmoscopy reveals a normal optic disc and pigmented lesions in the macular region.

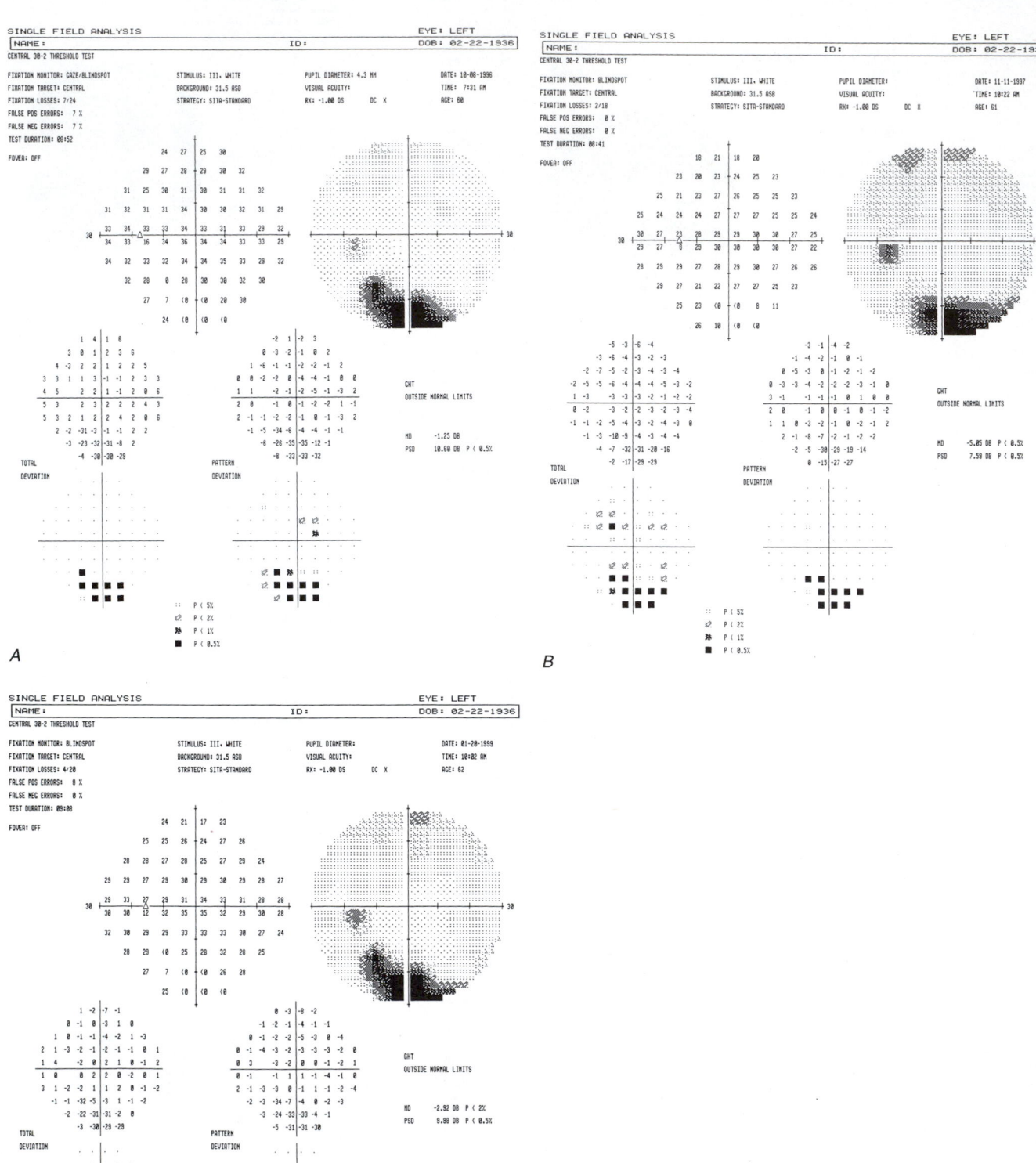

Figure 15–15. *A.* An inferior arcuate visual field defect caused by a retinochoroidal scar. The optic disc is completely normal. *B* and *C.* The defect has an identical appearance at repeated visual field testing, which is typical for retinal lesions. Glaucomatous defects usually have a much higher degree of fluctuation from one test to another.

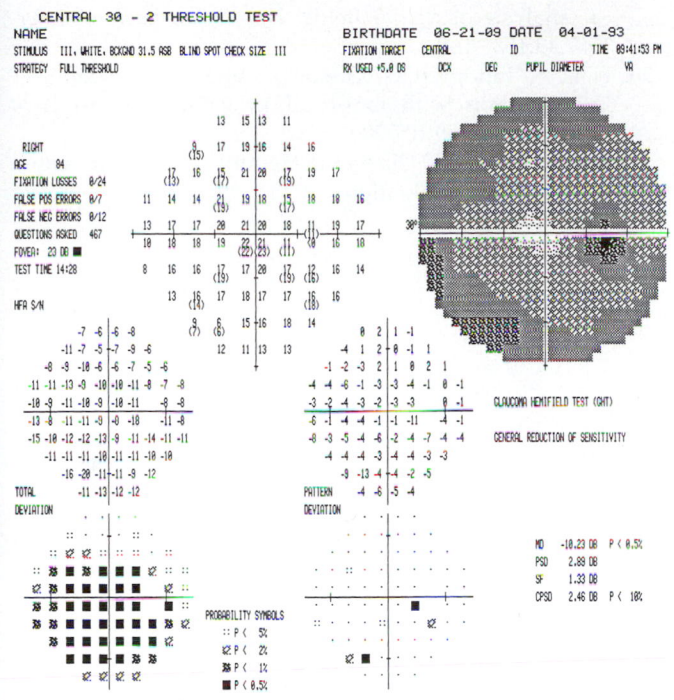

Figure 15–16. Homogeneously reduced visual field sensitivity in a patient with moderately advanced cataract. The total-deviation probability map is abnormal, with a majority of test points having significantly reduced sensitivity. The pattern-deviation probability map is normal, indicating that there is no localized field defect. The Glaucoma Hemifield Test classification is "general reduction of sensitivity." The optic disc was normal.

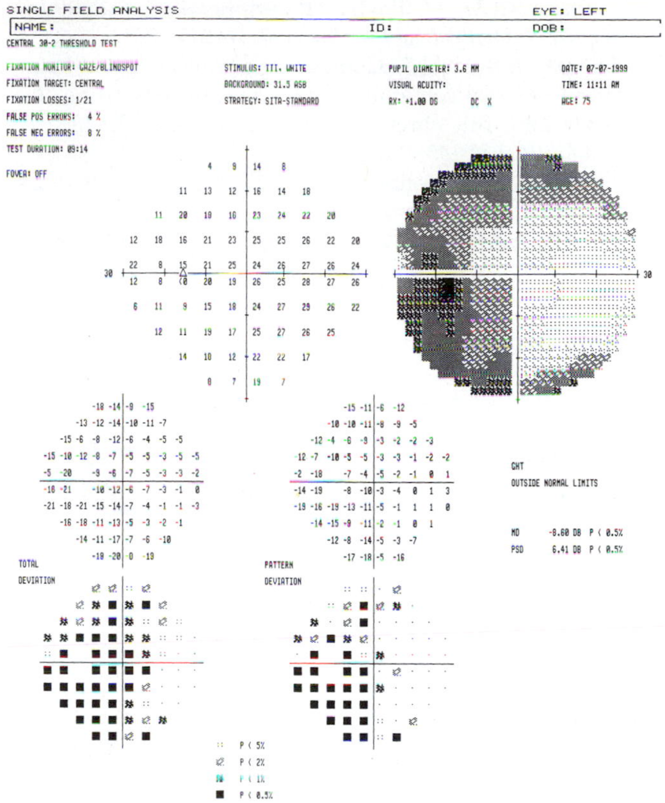

Figure 15–17. Neurological visual field defect due to pituitary tumor. A sharp vertical demarcation line between the nasal and temporal hemifields in the pattern-deviation probability map should always raise suspicion of damage at or posterior to the optic chiasm. Temporal disc pallor is typical for long-standing optic nerve compression. The other eye was blind.

REFERENCES

1. Von Graefe A. Beiträge zur Pathologie und Therapie des Glaucoms. *Arch Ophthalmol.* 1869;15:108–152.
2. Landesberg H. Ausbruch von Glaucom in Folge eines Streifschusses: Eigenthümliche Gesichtsfeldbeschränkung. *Arch Ophthalmol.* 1869;15:204–210.
3. Bjerrum J. Om en tilføjelse til den saedvanlige synsfeltundersögelse samt om synsfeltet ved glaukom. *Nordisk Ophthalmol Tidsskr.* 1889;2:141–185.
4. Rønne H. Ueber das Gesichtsfeld beim Glaukom. *Klin Monatsbl Augenheilkd.* 1909;47:12–33.
5. Anctil JL, Anderson DR. Early foveal involvement and generalized depression of the visual field in glaucoma. *Arch Ophthalmol.* 1984;102:363–370.
6. Glowazki A, Flammer J. Is there a difference between glaucoma patients with rather localized visual field damage and patients with more diffuse visual field damage? *Doc Ophthalmol Proc Ser.* 1987;49:317–320.
7. Drance SM. Diffuse visual field loss in open-angle glaucoma. *Ophthalmology.* 1991;98:1533–1538.
8. Werner EB, Saheb N, Patel S. Lack of generalized constriction of affected visual field in patients with visual field defects in one eye. *Can J Ophthalmol.* 1977;17: 53–55.
9. Heijl A. Lack of diffuse loss of differential light sensitivity in early glaucoma. *Acta Ophthalmol.* 1989;57: 353–360.
10. Langerhorst CT, van den Berg TJTP, Greve EL. Is there general reduction of sensitivity in glaucoma? *Int Ophthalmol.* 1989;13:31–35.
11. Weber J. *Topographie der funktionellen Schädigung beim chronischen Glaukom.* Heidelberg: Kaden Verlag; 1992.
12. Aulhorn E, Harms M. Early visual field defects in glaucoma. In: Leydhecker W, ed. *Glaucoma Tutzing Symposium.* Basel: Karger; 1967:151–186.
13. Aulhorn E, Karmeyer H. Frequency distribution in early glaucomatous visual field defects. *Doc Ophthalmol Proc Ser.* 1977;14:75–83.
14. Heijl A, Lundquist L. The frequency distribution of earliest glaucomatous visual field defects documented by automatic perimetry. *Acta Ophthalmol (Copenh).* 1984;62: 658–664.
15. Werner EB, Drance SM. Early visual field disturbances in glaucoma. *Arch Ophthalmol.* 1977;95:1173–1175.

16. LeBlanc RP, Lee A, Baxter M. Peripheral nasal field defects. *Doc Ophthalmol Proc Ser*. 1985;42:377–381.

17. Bengtsson B, Heijl A. Comparing significance and magnitude of glaucomatous visual field defects using the SITA and full threshold strategies. *Acta Ophthalmol Scand*. 1999;77:143–146.

18. Flammer J. The concept of visual field indices. *Graefes Arch Clin Exp Ophthalmol*. 1986;224:389–392.

19. Heijl A, Lindgren G, Olsson J. A package for the statistical analysis of visual fields. *Doc Ophthalmol Proc Ser*. 1987;49:153–168.

20. Heijl A, Lindgren G, Olsson J, Åsman P. Visual field interpretation with empirical probability maps. *Arch Ophthalmol*. 1989;107:204–208.

21. Åsman P, Heijl A. Glaucoma Hemifield Test: Automated visual field evaluation. *Arch Ophthalmol*. 1992;110:812–819.

Chapter 16

THE HUMPHREY VISUAL FIELD ANALYZER

Peter Lalle

HFA-1: HARDWARE

The original Humphrey visual field analyzer, the HFA-1, was introduced in 1984. Although not the first automated projection perimeter on the market, it has become the standard for automated perimetry in the United States. The HFA-1 consists of a rectangular box approximately 3 ft wide by $2^2/_3$ ft tall by 2 ft deep (Fig. 16–1). Contained within the box is a spherical cupula (bowl) with a radius of 33 cm.[1] The patient is positioned facing the inside of the cupula, with a forehead strap and a manually adjustable chin rest to provide alignment and proper positioning. Six motors control the projection of the stimulus onto the bowl. At startup, the accuracy of the positioning of the projector is checked by edge detectors. Likewise, the intensity of the bowl illumination and stimulus is checked and the perimetrist is alerted if the HFA-1 fails the calibration check.

There are three fixation targets inside the cupula. In the middle of the bowl is a round, 2-degree target that appears as an orange light to the patient and is the standard fixation target. Below the standard target are two additional diamond-shaped targets, one large and one small, each consisting of four light-emitting diodes. When these targets are used, the patient is

directed to keep fixation within the center of the illuminated diamond target.

The diamond pattern is employed either to measure foveal threshold or to compensate for a central scotoma. After foveal threshold has been determined, the patient is redirected to use the central fixation target for the remainder of the test. If a patient with a central scotoma cannot see the central fixation target without using eccentric fixation, he or she is instructed to gaze at the center of the diamond target. The patient is instructed to find the four points and maintain fixation in the center of the pattern. Depending on the size of the central scotoma, either the small or large target should be employed, preferably the small target. Steady fixation during the entire test is critical for accurate diagnosis and repeatable follow-up visual field tests. The test points of the visual field are shifted inferiorly to compensate for the inferior shift of fixation. Because fixation is directed inferiorly, parts of the inferior peripheral visual field cannot be tested when the diamond targets are employed. However, the entire central visual field can be tested with the diamond fixation targets. Many patients with reduced acuity secondary to a central scotoma can be tested readily with these targets. However, because fixation is steadier when the central fixation target is used, the

213

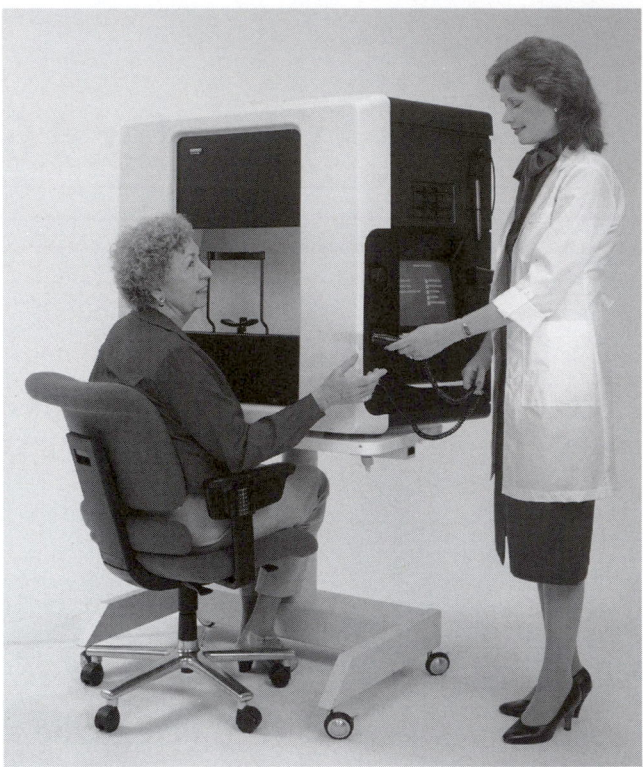

Figure 16–1. The Humphrey HFA-1 perimeter. (Reproduced with permission from Humphrey Systems, Inc.)

perimetrist should first attempt the test with the central target and switch to the diamond fixation targets only if needed.

Manual monitoring of the patient's fixation with the original HFA-1 was performed through a periscope with the central fixation spot in the cupula acting as the objective lens. Later versions replaced the periscope with a video camera, which displayed the image of the patient's eye as a small inset on the instrument's monitor. Exact, manual monitoring of fixation is not possible when the diamond targets are employed, although unsteady fixation can be detected by the blind spot check and attempts to correct fixation can be made by verbal instructions to the patient.

The central processing unit of the on-board computer is the older but dependable Intel 8088 microprocessor. A light pen is used in conjunction with the on-board monitor for data entry and command selections. As with other computers of this vintage, there is a problem with the recognition of the year 2000, and many of the early versions of the HFA-1 cannot be upgraded to recognize the correct year. The original versions of the HFA-1 used $5\frac{1}{4}$-in. double-sided, double-density floppy drives for storage of test data; these are now becoming harder to obtain. Later versions incorporated a hard drive as well a tape backup device.

Software for the operating system, test programs, and database interpretation programs are stored on erasable, programmable read-only memory chips (EPROMs) that were changed as upgrades became available. A serial port is available for data transmission to another HFA (either 1 or 2) or to a personal computer.

HFA-2: HARDWARE

The HFA-2 was introduced in 1994 as the next generation in perimeters. The more compact HFA-2 measures only 2 ft wide by 2 ft tall by $1\frac{1}{2}$ ft deep, with significant differences in the design of the bowl from the HFA-1 (Fig. 16–2). The central radius is shorter, 30 rather than 33 cm, and the bowl is now aspherical, with a "bullet" shape. Shortening of the peripheral radius alters the shape and size of a projected stimulus (and its apparent intensity) in the peripheral visual field compared to a spherical bowl. This alteration of the stimulus is predictable, and compensation has been incorporated into the intensity of the projected stimulus for the peripheral visual field. This compensation may introduce a minor error, but it is inconsequential given the high variability of threshold values

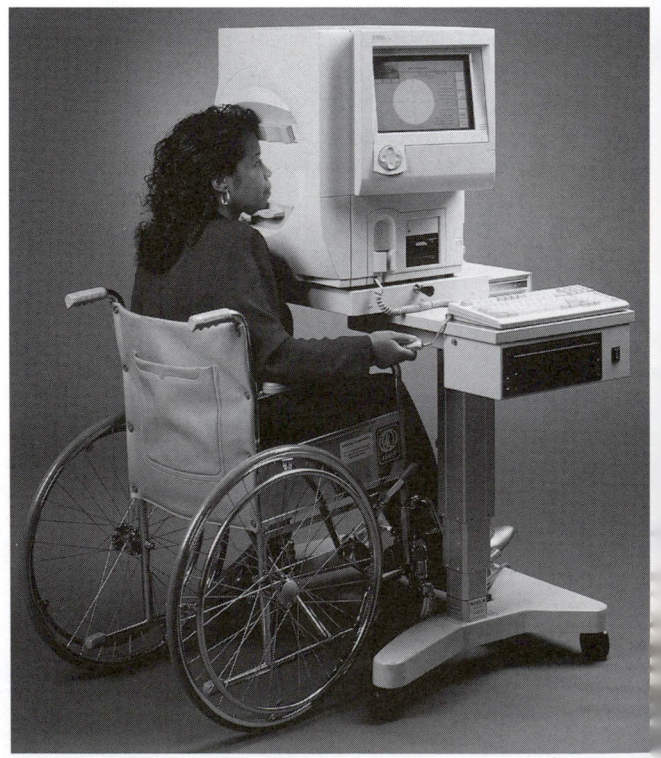

Figure 16–2. The Humphrey HFA-2 perimeter. (Reproduced with permission from Humphrey Systems, Inc.)

in the peripheral visual field. Precise measurement of the threshold value of the peripheral visual field is less important than knowing the clinical significance of the value obtained. A database of normal values for the peripheral visual field tested with the Swedish interactive thresholding algorithm (SITA) on the HFA-2 has been gathered and its release is anticipated shortly.

The alteration of the bowl has contributed to the compactness of the HFA-2. This compactness, along with an extendable tabletop, allows handicapped patients to be comfortably tested even while seated in a wheelchair. Chin-rest positioning is now controlled by electric motors and the forehead strap has been replaced by a contoured bar. Slight adjustments are made automatically during the examination as directed by the gaze-tracking unit to maintain alignment. The HFA-2 provides both a central fixation target and diamond targets, similar to the HFA-1.

Fixation is monitored by a gaze-tracking unit that can also detect when the patient's head moves backward (vertex monitoring). A corneal reflex generated by an infrared light-emitting diode (LED) adjacent to the fixation target serves as a stable reference point. The pupil is illuminated by infrared diodes on the back of the trial lens holder. When the trial lens holder is not in use, infrared LEDs at the bottom of the bowl are used. The center of the pupil is determined by real-time analysis of the video image of the pupil. By comparing the center of the pupil, which moves as the eye changes gaze, with the relatively stationary corneal reflex, the amount (and direction) of errant gaze can be determined.

Vertex monitoring compares the change in the spacing between other reflexes to determine if the eye is moving away from the instrument. The perimetrist is alerted whenever the vertex changes.

The HFA-2 employs a Motorola 68020 microprocessor with 4 megabytes of random access memory. Data and test selection are now entered by a touch screen and/or a keyboard. A software upgrade has made it possible to add a mouse for data entry and screen selection. All HFA-2s come with a $3\frac{1}{2}$-in. floppy drive and the option of a hard drive. A faster tape backup is available and its frequent use is strongly recommended. An optional external $5\frac{1}{4}$-in. floppy drive is available for those offices that need to continue to transfer data from an older HFA-1 to the HFA-2. Care must be taken that the hard drive and all its patient data are not corrupted. Likewise, data on the $5\frac{1}{4}$-in. floppy can become corrupted, and it is advised that a copy of the floppy be made before data transfer is attempted. Data transfer can also be accomplished via a cable utilizing the serial ports of both instruments. This method does not imperil the integrity of the contents of the hard drive. The hard drive stores the operating system and patient test data. Software is loaded and changed via the $3\frac{1}{2}$-in. floppy drive, a process familiar to most users of personal computers.

HFA-1 SOFTWARE

Software on the HFA-1 consists of three components: testing programs, reliability determination procedures, and statistical interpretation.

HFA-1 Testing Programs: Suprathreshold and Threshold

Suprathreshold

Suprathreshold testing is commonly referred to as a screening strategy. The purpose of a screening examination is *rapid detection*—that is, the visual field is tested for the purpose of determining the presence or absence of a defect in as little time as feasible. The qualities of the defect—its size, shape, and depth—are only estimated to save time. The algorithm used by the instrument to generate the "hill of vision" (HOV) for screening tests has a fixed shape that does not change with age,[1] only raising or lowering its height according to the central reference level. Although this rough estimate serves the purpose of a screening test adequately, it does not reflect the extent of the empirical data of STATPAC, which has shown that the hill of vision is not fixed and does change its shape with age.[2-4] The use of this fixed shape to the HOV across all age groups will cause some defects to be poorly defined.

Every screening examination begins with the determination of the overall height of the patient's HOV, which, in turn, raises or lowers the expected values. When the height is elevated, all points will be tested with dimmer stimuli than when the height is depressed, and careful determination of the height is critical for an accurate test. During a suprathreshold examination, each stimulus is presented four to six times brighter than what is expected to be necessary to be seen at each test location. The "expected" value of each stimulus is adjusted such that the peripheral portions of the visual field are tested with more intense stimuli than the more sensitive central visual field, based on the height of the HOV.

The height of the HOV can be determined either automatically or manually. The HFA can be allowed to determine the height automatically in one of two methods. The first method is "threshold related," which begins with a process referred to as *initialization*. Four points surrounding fixation undergo threshold testing. The second most sensitive point is used to estimate the height of the hill of vision. This method compensates for patients who may have an overall depression from cataracts, miosis, or normal aging. The height determined during initialization is referred to as the *central reference level* (CRL). Of the methods to estimate the height of the HOV, this is the most time-consuming, but it may be worth the investment in time because it obtains more meaningful results in older patients.

In the second method, the height of the HOV is determined by using the "age-related" method. The HFA-1 with software upgraded to STATPAC 2 allows the instrument to skip initialization and select the central reference level based upon stored, predicted values for different age groups derived from STATPAC, saving about 1 min of test time. One concern is that, in the original STATPAC database, there were no patients with significant cataract or miosis, both of which will cause an overall depression.[4-6] Older patients with an overall physiological depression, when tested using the age-related method for setting the height of the HOV, will be presented with stimuli that are too dim, resulting in a significant overestimation of visual field loss. Although all young and older patients with clear media and pupils of at least 3 mm can be reliably tested with the age-related estimate of the height of the HOV, threshold-related estimates should be employed when the media status is unknown.

Finally, the height of the HOV can be chosen manually by the perimetrist prior to the test. This would be useful when a screening test is being repeated and the perimetrist wants to make sure that the tests are comparable. However, it is not advisable to follow patients for change with suprathreshold tests. Once a patient has been screened, follow-up testing should be done with the more definitive threshold examinations.

The HFA-1 has four strategies to perform a screening test and attempt to define a defect: *single-intensity, threshold-related, three-zone,* and *quantify-defects.* The single-intensity strategy uses the same test stimulus for all test points. Although this strategy is useful for some disability examinations, it is not relevant for glaucoma testing. The quantify-defects strategy adds additional test time by thresholding missed points in an attempt to better define the defect, which defeats the purpose of a screening test. The information derived from the threshold procedure, defect depth, is meaningless without a database to interpret its significance. The interpretation of the results is left solely to the practitioner.

Clinically, only the threshold-related and three-zone strategies are of value as screening tests; the present discussion is limited to these. Confusing terminology is introduced at this point. In the HFA-1, *threshold-related* refers to both the method for determining the height of the HOV and the strategy for defining defects. In the HFA-2, the term *threshold-related* has been replaced by the more appropriate term *two-zone* in referring to the screening test strategy for defining defects. To eliminate confusion, the term *initialization* is used from here forward to refer to the method of determining the height of the HOV and *threshold-related (two-zone)* for the strategy of defining defects.

Threshold-Related (Two-Zone). After initialization, each point is tested with a stimulus 6 dB brighter than the test point's expected sensitivity as predicted by the HOV. If the age-related strategy is used to determine the height of the HOV, the stimulus will be 8 dB brighter at each test point. Central points will be tested with dimmer lights, although more peripheral points will be tested with brighter stimuli. This is known as eccentricity compensation. The printout will be a map of points seen and missed. Points seen will be assigned a zero. If a point is missed, it will be retested; if still missed, it will be marked with a black box on the printout. If a point is not seen, it is a scotoma of at least 6 dB in depth; this exceeds the Goldmann visual field standard of 5 dB for a scotoma to be considered significant.[7] The threshold-related (two-zone) strategy does not define defects well. It cannot discern whether a missed point is only a 7-dB defect versus an absolute defect (does not respond to the brightest light).

Three-Zone. This strategy is a modification of the threshold-related strategy (two-zone), retesting all missed points a third time with the light as bright as possible (10,000 asb). If a point is missed with the brightest stimulus, it is marked with a black box and considered an absolute defect. If missed only by the 6-dB suprathreshold stimulus but seen by the brightest light, it is marked with an X and considered a relative defect. Although not exactly quantifying the defect, it gives a little extra information to better define a defect and assurance that the point is not totally blind. In general, relative defects of 6 dB found within the central 20 degrees are usually considered significant. Outside 30 degrees, 6-dB defects are not significant unless they are arrayed in a pattern suggesting a nasal step or part of an arcuate defect.[2,3] More significance should be given to absolute defects in the periphery. In reviewing a screening examination, it is important to note whether the threshold-related (two-zone) or three-zone strategy was used, since the meaning of the black box is different. With abnormal visual fields, test time is lengthened by only a few minutes when using the three-zone rather than the threshold-related (two-zone) strategy.

Once the testing strategy is determined, the next step is the selection of the test point pattern. The HFA-1 has an extensive library of screening test point patterns to choose from, and many practitioners have individual preferences. However, to know the true value of any of these tests, one has to know its sensitivity and specificity. This can be determined only by way of a clinical trial, where known glaucoma patients and normal controls are tested with various patterns of points. Published clinical trials have been performed on only a few of the many screening tests available; therefore only a few can be recommended.

Central 76. This test uses the same point pattern as the central 30-2 threshold examination. Because this point pattern has been shown to be highly effective in the threshold examination, many practitioners elect to screen the patient first with the central 76, followed up by threshold examinations using the 30-2. Although this screening test has good sensitivity and specificity in patients with neuroocular disease, its value in glaucoma patients is unproved.[8] There is no accepted definition of what constitutes an abnormal visual field with this pattern. However, two or three contiguous defective points should warrant a follow-up threshold examination.

Armaly. This test employs the test pattern modeled after the visual field examination developed originally by Armaly and Drance for the Goldmann perimeter. A total of 52 points are distributed within the central 20 degrees, with an additional 12 points along the nasal step. The HFA version of this test was found to have a sensitivity of only 64% in one study, and the interpretation strategy used was not published.[9]

Full Visual Field 120 (F120). In all, 120 points—70 nasal and 50 temporal—are distributed throughout the central and peripheral visual fields. It will take approximately 6 min to examine a normal eye with this test, while a severely depressed visual field will take 9 to 10 min. Interpreting the test is rather simple. Kosoko and associates reported a remarkable sensitivity of 97% and a specificity of 88% for glaucoma by labeling all visual field tests with more than 17 missed points as abnormal.[10] However, it should be noted that the patients tested were experienced in perimetry prior to taking the F120. In clinical practice, the F120 is the first test a glaucoma suspect

takes, and points are often missed because of the patient's inexperience with the test. This would cause the F120 to falsely identify normal patients as having defective visual fields, thus reducing the published specificity. Further, the glaucoma patients in this study had well-established visual field defects as defined by kinetic perimetry. A defect that is readily detected with kinetic perimetry is found to be deeper and larger with static perimetry. [11-13] Overall, these patients usually have moderate to severe visual field loss in static perimetry. The reported sensitivity of the test may not be repeatable if patients with only mild defects are tested. Thus, the high sensitivity and specificity found in the clinical trial are often not duplicated in clinical practice. However, when the F120 is completely normal, the practitioner can assume that, at worst, only a mild defect may be missed. The age–reference level option was not employed in this clinical study.

Further interpretation of the F120 was provided by the Baltimore Eye Survey (BES), which used it in its initial screening of visual fields.[14] In addition to a total of 17 missed points as a criterion for abnormal, 8 missed points in any quadrant of the visual field was considered abnormal and follow-up testing was performed. It has been suggested that a difference of 10 missed points between the right and left eyes is suspicious of glaucoma, even if each eye missed less than 17 points.[15] Because this analysis makes no distinction as to whether the missed point represented a relative or an absolute defect, the threshold-related or three-zone screening strategies can be employed. However, the added information of the three-zone strategy may occasionally help to differentiate between artifact versus a true defect. Finally, even if Kosoko's or the BES's criteria are not met but a recognizable defect such as a nasal step or arcuate defect is present, the visual field should be considered abnormal. A positive finding with the F120 mandates a follow-up threshold visual field test to confirm the presence of a defect as well to define its size and depth. Because the F120 is the only HFA screening test that has undergone extensive clinical trials, it is the only one recommended for glaucoma suspects at this time (Fig. 16–3).

Threshold

Unlike screening tests that simply compare the patient's responses to an expected "normal" HOV, threshold tests determine the exact shape and contour of the patient's HOV and any defects that may be present. Although they are time-consuming, threshold tests provide the detailed information that allows a patient's visual field to be quantified and monitored closely for change. Since this is a cornerstone in the

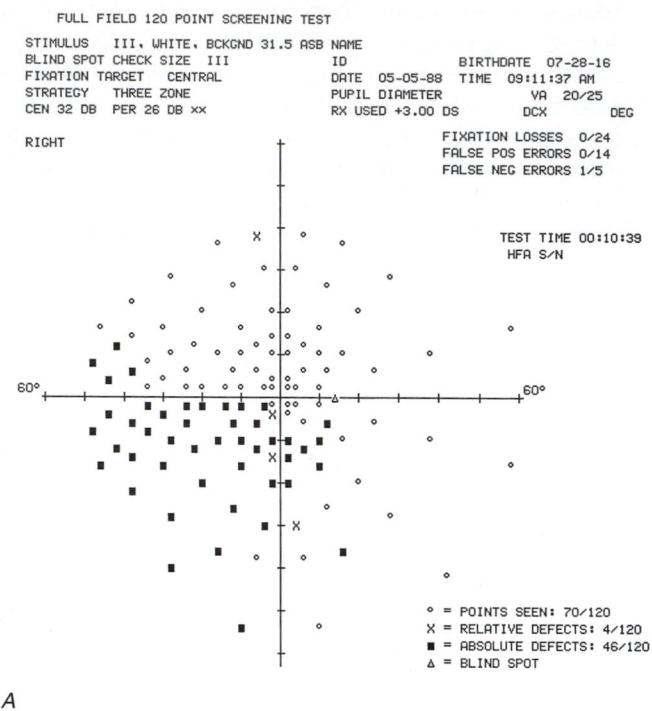

A

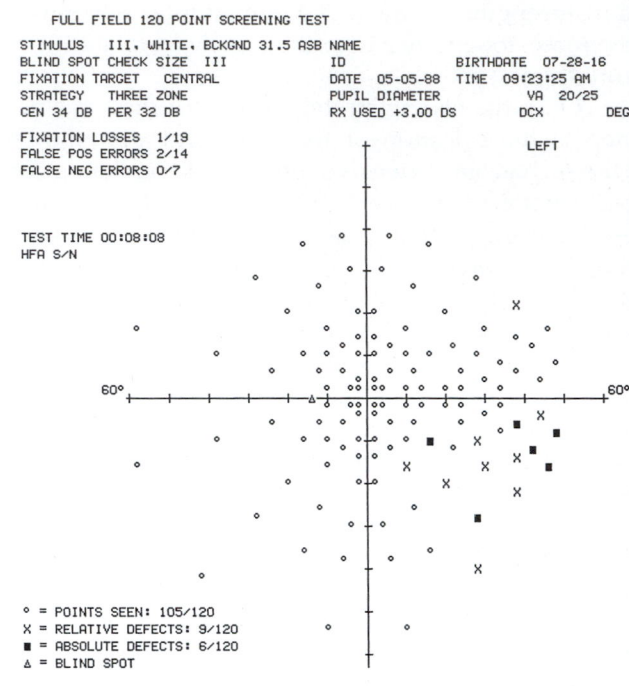

B

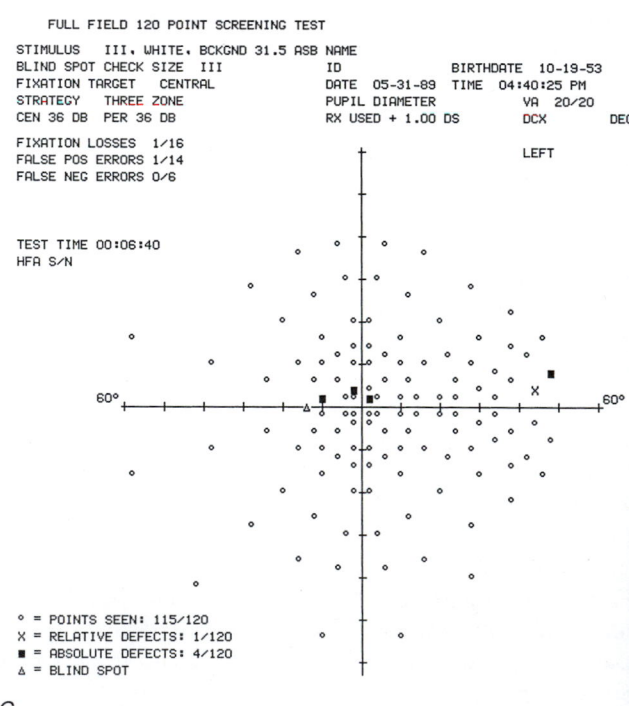

C

Figure 16–3. *A.* A large, broad, inferior arcuate scotoma with a nasal step below the horizontal raphe is seen with the Full Field 120 screening examination. Because a majority of the 50 missed points are absolute defects, the three-zone strategy indicates a very deep defect. A cup-to-disc ratio of 0.85 was noted in both eyes. *B.* This is the fellow eye showing an inferior nasal step of relative and absolute defects. Although the total number of missed points is below Kosoko's original criteria of 17 missed points,[10] the pattern clearly suggests a defect consistent with glaucoma. The Baltimore Eye Survey modified the criteria to include any field with eight or more points missed in any one quadrant.[14] Threshold testing with a 30-2 confirmed an early inferior nasal step with an uninvolved central field. *C.* A small arcuate scotoma is seen that does not meet either Kosoko's criteria or the modification by the Baltimore Eye Survey in this young patient with 0.9 cup-to-disc ratio. However, the missed points are consistent with an arcuate defect, which was later confirmed with threshold testing.

management of glaucoma, threshold testing is the only appropriate method for following glaucoma patients. The original HFA-1 in 1984 came with three thresholding strategies: *full, full from prior,* and *fast.* An optional upgrade added the FASTPAC threshold strategy in 1991.

By definition, the threshold value for any point is the intensity of a stimulus that will be seen 50% of the time it is presented. In discussing the fluctuation of threshold values, it is useful to remember the converse, that the stimulus is missed 50% of the time. Determining a threshold is more involved than screening a point. To begin a threshold procedure, a stimulus brighter than predicted from the estimated height of the HOV (determined during initialization) is presented. If the patient sees the stimulus, the stimulus is dimmed by 4 dB. If the patient still sees the stimulus, it is again dimmed by 4 dB. The process continues until the patient does not respond. The light is then brightened by 2 dB until the patient responds. Threshold is recorded as the value when the stimulus is seen again. If the patient does not see the initial stimulus, the process is reversed, with the stimulus brightness increased by 4-dB steps until seen. The stimulus is then dimmed by 2 dB until not seen. Threshold is recorded as the value of the last stimulus seen. This is the classic 4-2 double-cross staircase technique for determining the threshold value. The closer the initial presentation is to the actual threshold, the fewer the "steps" or test presentations the test must take. The testing procedure is randomized but, in general, central points are tested first and the periphery last.

Full-Threshold.

This is the established "gold standard" by which all other techniques are judged for accuracy.[7,16,17] The test begins with initialization of four central points, one in each quadrant. The values obtained at these points are used to estimate the starting points of the other test locations within the same quadrant. In general, central points are tested first and peripheral points last. As testing proceeds within a quadrant, the HFA "learns" from neighboring points. That is, if a point is unexpectedly found to be severely depressed, the HFA assumes that the surrounding points must be somewhat depressed as well and lowers the expected value for these untested points. Since this provides a better estimate of the probable threshold value, less time is spent thresholding the neighboring points.

Full from Prior.

This strategy utilizes a patient's previously stored threshold tests to determine the starting point for the staircase technique of the next visual field exam, thus skipping initialization and providing a better estimate of the expected threshold for each point. However, because the HFA-1 "learns" from adjacent points during a test, full-threshold from prior data decreases testing time minimally compared to the full-threshold and is generally not used. The printout is similar to the one for the threshold strategy.

Fast Threshold.

Perhaps misnamed, this strategy is more like the quantify-defect suprathreshold examination than a true threshold test. Using stored

results, the HFA presents stimuli 2 dB brighter than the threshold value found at a previous full-threshold test. If the stimulus is seen, it will be considered as stable and no thresholding will be done. If it is missed, the point will undergo thresholding. The printout will show stable points as a zero. For unstable points, the amount of change in decibels from the last visual field test is noted. Unlike the quantify-defect strategy, which adds time to a screening test, fast-threshold is quicker than a full-threshold test. More importantly, it uses the patient's own HOV for comparison, rather than one generated by the instrument. Because the amount of expected fluctuation within a defect of a stable glaucoma patient typically exceeds 2 dB, a large number of stable points will undergo thresholding, needlessly increasing test time. This threshold strategy is best used when the patient has a visual field with no more than mild defects.[18]

Because visual field tests using the "fast" strategy cannot be incorporated into certain printouts used to analyze change over time, this method should not be used for long-term follow-up. Rather, the fast-threshold test is indicated when a quick and immediate answer to the question of progression is needed in patients with minimal visual field loss.

FASTPAC.

In the 4-2 bracketing strategy, there are at least three stimulus presentations at each test point. Eliminating the last presentation, the double crossing of the threshold, would theoretically decrease test time by 33% but increase the uncertainty of the true threshold. FASTPAC takes 3-dB instead of 4-dB steps until threshold is crossed and then stops. Threshold is recorded as the last value seen. FASTPAC will typically decrease test time 25 to 30%, but visual fields with advanced visual field loss will have minimal time saving.[19] Accuracy of the threshold determination is sacrificed in the interest of time, and some subtle or shallow defects may be missed while others are not well defined.[19–21] Threshold tests done with this software cannot be analyzed with either the glaucoma hemifield test for abnormality or the glaucoma change probability analysis for progression. Therefore, FASTPAC may not be a desirable strategy for some glaucoma patients.

On the other hand, many patients fail to give interpretable visual field tests with the standard threshold strategy, as they become fatigued, progressively unresponsive, and unreliable during the test.[22,23] Switching to the faster test strategy of FASTPAC may allow the patient to finish the examination without tiring. A reliable FASTPAC examination is always preferable to an unreliable threshold test marred by fatigue artifact.[24] Further, fluctuation of threshold values between tests (long-term fluctuation) is considerable in glaucoma patients, with defects fluctuating in size and depth. FASTPAC does not increase long-term fluctuation compared to the standard threshold testing and may be appropriate to use in following some patients with serial visual fields.[25,26]

Threshold Test Patterns

Numerous studies have documented the excellent sensitivity of central threshold tests for glaucoma.[27,28] There are several test point patterns available on the HFA-1 to perform threshold tests, though in clinical practice only three point patterns are used for glaucoma patients: the central 30-2, the central 24-2, and the central 10-2.

Central 30-2. The 30-2 has been available since the HFA-1 was first introduced in 1984. Along with the full-threshold test strategy, it has been the gold standard for glaucoma testing. Seventy-six points are tested within 30 degrees, with the test points straddling the horizontal and the vertical midlines, spaced 6 degrees apart. For the first threshold visual field exam, both full-threshold and FASTPAC are available. On follow-up, "full from prior" or "fast" strategy can be employed, using the stored data from a previous full-threshold test. Using the full-threshold strategy, the average test time for most glaucoma patients is about 13 min per eye. A normal eye will take about 10 min, while a defective visual field may take up to 19 min.[29] FASTPAC results will be about 33% faster than the full-threshold strategy.[19]

While it remains the standard test for many studies, several factors limit the clinical usefulness of the 30-2. Compared to the 24-2, it takes several minutes longer. Because the peripheral points are tested last, they are frequently marred by fatigue artifact. Also, peripheral points vary more in their range of normal values as compared to central points, making it harder to judge whether depressions represent true disease or the lower end of a wide range of normal.[30] Thus, interpretation of the edge points in the 30-2 is challenging, even with statistical analysis. Therefore, many practitioners find the extra time spent testing the peripheral points in the 30-2 to be unproductive and have turned to the 24-2 instead. While time is saved with the 24-2, some knowledge of visual field is lost in the compromise between test time versus data gathering.

Central 24-2. The 24-2 test pattern was added as a software upgrade to the original HFA-1 in 1988. The test was designed to remove the superfluous edge points of the 30-2, thus shortening test time. The central 24-2 eliminates one-quarter of the 76 points from the 30-2 pattern, removing all edge points except for those above and below the nasal horizontal meridian. This leaves 54 points within 24 degrees, straddling the midlines and spaced 6 degrees apart. The 24-2 will save approximately 2 to 4 min per eye compared to a 30-2 using the same strategy. The same threshold strategies employed with the 30-2 are available to the 24-2.

The time saved by not testing the edge points comes at the expense of a wider view of the patient's visual field. In some instances, the extra data would allow the practitioner to decide whether a peripheral point missed with a 24-2 is truly a defect or perhaps a lens rim or lid artifact. It may be suggested that any patient who will be followed with 24-2 threshold visual fields have at least one suprathreshold evaluation of the peripheral visual field, with attention to the nasal periphery. One possible scenario would have the first visual field test be a F120 with all subsequent visual fields done as 24-2 threshold.

Central 10-2. The management of end-stage glaucoma presents a unique challenge. A 30-2 or 24-2 test on these patients will often show many severely depressed points and large areas of absolute defects, leaving only a small central isle inside 10 degrees and/or a temporal isle. It is a waste of time to continue to test the nonresponding points with the same stimulus. These nonresponding areas are not necessarily "blind," and if a larger target is used, a response may be elicited. When most of a 30-2 or 24-2 visual field appears as absolute defects, as in end-stage glaucoma, there are two options that can be explored, either simultaneously or separately.

The first option is to increase the size of the target to size V and retest the central visual field. This strategy will add about 10 dB to each point, with most of the prior absolute defects converting to single- or double-digit threshold values.[31] No STATPAC analysis is available for visual fields done with a size V target, but this is not necessary since it is already known that the visual field is highly abnormal. Visual field testing in end-stage glaucoma is done not to detect defects but rather to monitor for progression. Since these points were unresponsive to the size III target, there is no choice but to employ the size V. Changes in threshold values, not probability values, will be followed.

Although further loss of the central visual field can now be monitored, the critical area of fixation is still poorly defined because the test points are spaced 6 degrees apart. In clinical practice, the loss of fixation means loss of the acuity necessary to read, recognize faces, and carry out activities of daily living. Before fixation is totally extinguished, it is first "split."[32,33] When fixation is split, all sensitivity is lost either above or below the horizontal midline through fixation. The splitting of fixation is an ominous sign for the survival of central acuity and requires intensive therapeutic intervention. In a severely depressed visual field with only central vision remaining, the HOV is not circular but rather more depressed supranasally. This would suggest that the superior part of the remaining central island of vision is at greater risk for splitting fixation. However, even with size V targets, scotomas near fixation are usually poorly defined because test points will straddle fixation by 3 degrees on either side. Fixation cannot be followed with test point patterns spaced 6 degrees apart.

The second option is to test only the central 10 degrees of the visual field with greater resolution than the 24-2 or 30-2. The central 10-2 test uses a finer grid, placing 68 points inside the central 10 degrees, spaced 2 degrees apart and straddling the midlines. The closer spacing allows detection and definition of scotomas threatening fixation (Fig. 16-4A, B, and C).[34]

With severe, end-stage glaucoma, even the central 10-2 test may show a predominance of absolute defects. It may be necessary to use the size V target with the 10-2 visual field in order to follow the remaining visual function. Extreme caution must be exercised at this point, since STATPAC analysis is available only for 10-2 tests done with the size III target, not the size V. The interpretation of a size V, central 10-2 will be based solely on the clinician's experience, intuition, and interpretation of changes in the threshold values of patients with threatened fixation.

HFA-1 Reliability Catch Trials

With manual Goldmann perimetry, the perimetrist would write on the record if the patient maintained good fixation and good cooperation and gave consistent responses. This information would allow the doctor to judge if the test was reliable and valid. The HFA-1 has tried to supplement this subjective appraisal with objective measurements, the reliability catch trials (Table 16-1). Randomly interspersed between every 33 stimulus presentations will be one false-positive and one false-negative catch trial. In addition, fixation-loss catch trials are performed about every 20th presentation, with more presented earlier in the test to ensure that the patient is fixating properly, allowing the test to be stopped and the patient reinstructed if too many fixation losses occur. A score is given on each printout of how many times the patient responded improperly compared to the number of

times a catch trial was conducted. Those catch trials whose percentage of improper responses exceeds a predetermined limit will be flagged for the examiner's inspection. The limits were originally derived from a sample of patients by the manufacturer in order to guide the practitioner in determining whether a test is acceptable. A very wide range of values was found and the limits for false positives and false negatives were chosen because they were clearly abnormal.[35] The limit for fixation losses was stricter because it was assumed that practitioners would be more concerned about the effect of fixation loss than about false positives and false negatives. The manufacturer's recommendations were intended solely as a guide and were never meant to represent strict upper limits of normal. Unfortunately, in clinical practice, they have taken on that meaning, and many visual fields have been needlessly discarded.

Fixation Losses

To determine the patient's ability to maintain fixation, a stimulus is periodically presented in the blind spot. If the patient is not fixating properly, the stimulus will be seen as it falls on the retina and the response button will be pressed.[36] Approximately 5% of all presentations are devoted to blind-spot checking, although most of these occur toward the beginning of the test. The HFA-1 assumes an anatomically predicted location for the blind spot. If the patient misses the first or second fixation-loss catch trial, the HFA-1 will automatically stop testing, plot the blind spot, and then resume testing. Traditionally, if more than 20% fixation losses occurred during the test, the results would be considered unreliable and generally not used to make specific clinical decisions. Studies indicate that the most common cause for visual field tests to be

---

TABLE 16-1. ASSESSMENT OF RELIABILITY OF VISUAL FIELD

1. If FPs are flagged, discard field regardless of other indices. Reinstruct patient and repeat VF.
2. If FPs are not flagged but some are recorded, review threshold values and discard field if any values are over 37 dB.
3. If FLs are flagged, keep field if perimetrist vouches for good fixation based on perimetrist's observations during test.
4. If FNs are flagged and the patient is expected to have a field defect, keep field but view suspiciously.
5. If both FLs and FNs are flagged, discard field and use shorter test strategy.

Key: FP, false positive; FL, fixation loss; FN, false negative.
Note: Because the reliability indices require that the patient press the response button at an inappropriate time, a very unresponsive patient will appear falsely reliable. The absence of flagged indices does not guarantee reliability. The observations and assessment of the perimetrist remain the best gauge of reliability.

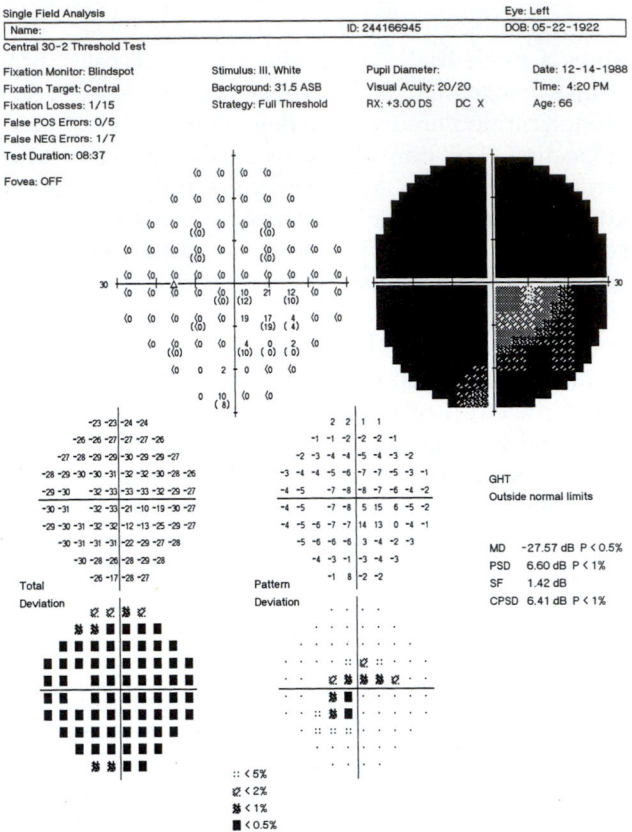 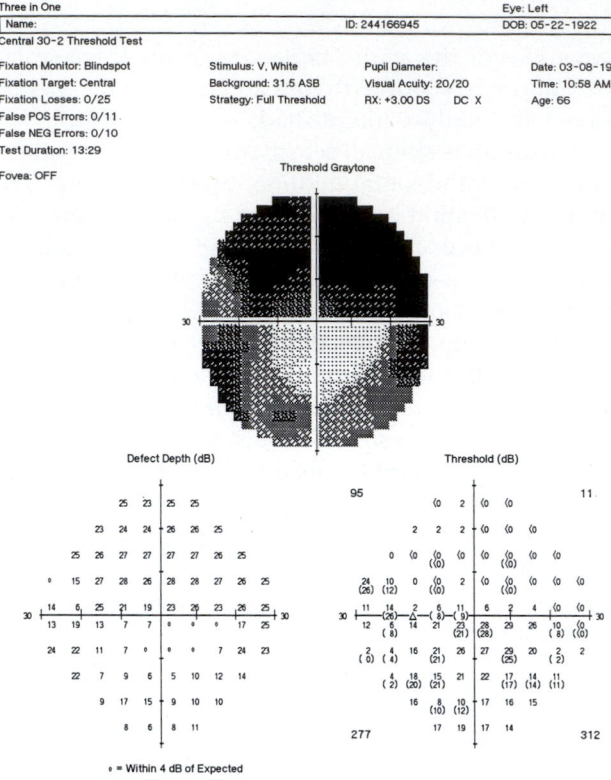

A

B

C

Figure 16–4. Patient with end-stage glaucoma with remaining small, central isle of vision. *A.* In the 30-2, only 10 out of 76 points responded to the standard size III target, with obvious splitting of fixation. *B.* When the patient was retested with the larger size V target, 43 points responded and the visual field inferior to fixation appeared intact. *C.* When the patient was tested with the 10-2 size III stimulus, the area below fixation was found to be involved and continued to progress despite optimal treatment. Because the 10-2 tests points 2 rather than 6 degrees apart, the defect that threatened fixation could be identified and defined with the improved resolution.

classified as unreliable is excessive fixation losses.[37-39] However, it has been shown that the majority of these visual fields are arbitrarily labeled as unreliable because of increased fixation losses that may instead be due to artifacts. Therefore 20% is probably too restrictive. In a few patients, the true position of the blind spot is not exactly where it is anatomically predicted, resulting in falsely reported fixation losses. More often the artifact occurs because the patient's head has tilted ever so slightly during testing, unnoticed by the perimetrist but enough to alter the position of the blind spot. If the perimetrist notices that two or more fixation losses have occurred during the first 10 trials, which is not enough to automatically stop the test, he or she should pause the test and ask the HFA-1 to plot the patient's true blind spot. If the HFA-1 still cannot find the blind spot, the fixation monitor should be turned off and fixation monitored manually.

In addition to poor fixation and an anomalous position for the blind spot, fixation losses can result from improper occlusion of the untested eye as well as from a visual field test that shows a high number of false-positive responses. The overall effect of a true increase in fixation losses is to make the visual field appear better than it really is, disguising or minimizing scotomas (Fig. 16–5).

False Negatives

To judge whether the patient's responses are consistent, a location that was previously tested is later retested with a stimulus 9 dB brighter than previously seen. If the patient fails to see this brighter stimulus, a false negative is recorded. False-negative responses occur in normal individuals if they become inattentive or fatigued or if they change their criteria for responding to the stimuli during the test. If more than 33% of these retested points are missed, false negatives are flagged, implying that the visual field is unreliable.

Although an increase in false negatives in normal patients should be considered as an unreliable test, this poses a diagnostic challenge because it is not known a priori that the patient is normal and that the visual field defect is an artifact of inconsistency. Even more perplexing is the fact that an increase in false negatives is expected in diseased eyes. Patients with real disease and visual field loss, including loss due to glaucoma, may give inconsistent responses because of their disease condition rather than because they are unreliable (Figs. 16-5 and 16-6). Both false negatives and the other measure of consistency, short-term fluctuation, are elevated when there is a loss of visual field. The doctor is faced with the dilemma of determining whether the patient is normal and gave unreliable responses or if this is true visual field loss with

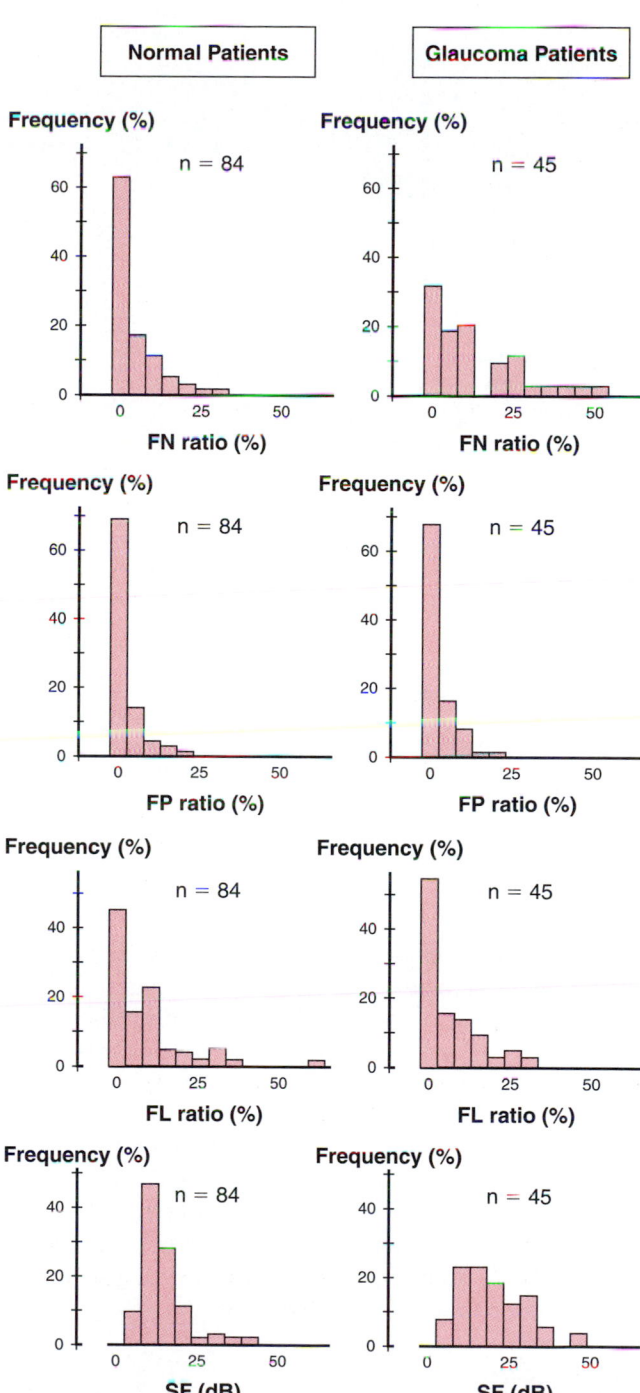

Figure 16–5. A comparison of the reliability indices for glaucoma patients versus normal controls is seen. Both groups displayed similar results for fixation losses and false positives. However, glaucoma patients showed a considerable increase in false negatives and short-term fluctuation. Both indices measure the amount of variability in a field, indicating that glaucoma patients have a large amount of intratest fluctuation. (Reproduced with permission from Heijl A, Lindgren G, Olson J. *Doc Ophthalmol Proc Ser.* 1987;49:593–600.)

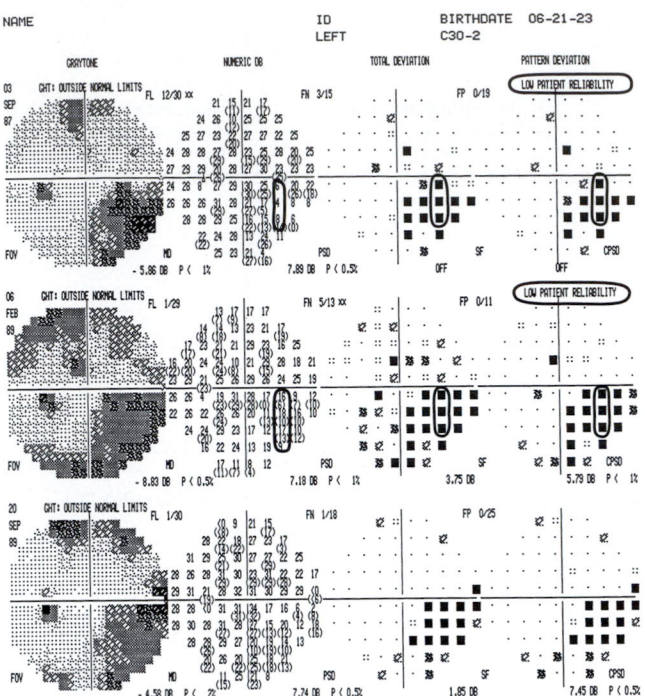

Figure 16–6. The patient's first field has an increase in fixation losses. While fixation losses improved on the second field, false negatives are now flagged and inspection of the "good" areas confirms excessive variability. By the third field, the reliability indicators are all normal. This improvement represents a learning effect. Note that between the first and second tests, three points greatly improved, yet remained plotted with a black box since they still deviated significantly from expected values.

the presence of expected false negatives. Because of these inconsistencies, one should be hesitant to consider discarding a visual field when only false negatives are flagged, especially where patients with known disease are concerned.

Even patients with known disease and established loss of visual field will occasionally have a "bad day," probably due to fatigue (Fig. 16–7). Visual fields taken on these "bad days" will further increase false-negative responses and cause an increase in the overall depression, with larger and deeper scotomas than before being documented.

False Positives

In the initial versions of the HFA-1, the motors that positioned the stimulus made a noise while moving between presentations. Overly anxious patients would key their responses to the sound of the motors and not to the visualization of the stimulus. To detect this behavior, the HFA-1 would intentionally pause and not make a stimulus presentation. A false-positive response was recorded if the patient responded. The newer HFA-1's have silent motors, but the HFA-1 will

still intentionally pause and allow the patient to respond when no presentation has been made. Thirty-three percent or more false-positive responses will be flagged by the HFA-1. Unlike fixation losses and false negatives, whose criteria for unreliability may be too restrictive, the criterion for false positives is too generous. One paper has shown that even a 10% false-positive rate will make the visual field appear better than it really is.

This pattern of behavior, responding when no stimulus is visible, may also affect responses when a stimulus is presented. The visual field may show areas of unusually high sensitivity as the patient responds to stimuli that are very dim and well below normal threshold ranges. The printout may show areas of white in the gray scale, representing false supersensitivity. These are sometimes termed "white scotomas" and, if they are randomly distributed throughout the area tested, can create the appearance of a "popcorn" pattern to the gray-scale printout. Because a stimulus was presented, it is not considered a false-positive catch trial and will not be counted as such in the total false positives reported

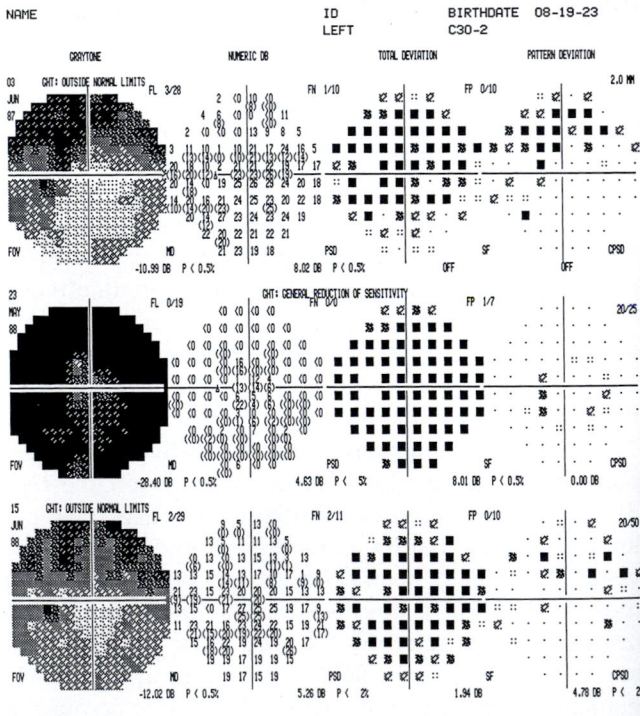

Figure 16–7. This uniocular patient with advanced glaucoma showed marked deterioration between the first and second field tests. The reliability indicators were normal. Since the patient was on maximum tolerated medical therapy, the field was repeated 1 month later to confirm a true progression before recommending filtering surgery. The third field showed improvement from the first rather than deterioration. A minimum of two fields is necessary to confirm true defects or progression.

by the HFA-1. Only careful inspection of the threshold values obtained or the box plots will reveal these "silent" false-positive responses. Because false positives will make the visual field appear better than it truly is, scotomas and the underlying disease may be missed.

Patients with elevated false positives frequently show elevated fixation loss catch trials despite good fixation. This is because a false-positive response is being made while the stimulus is on the blind spot. Also, some anxious patients may begin to search for the stimulus, increasing both false-positive responses and fixation losses (Fig. 16–8).

Properly instructing the patient at the beginning of the test that he or she is not expected to see all stimuli, probably no more than half, and to respond only when sure that a stimulus is seen will usually eliminate excessive false positives. The perimetrist should monitor during the test for any false positives or threshold values above 37 dB and pause the test immediately to reinstruct the patient if either occurs.

HFA-1: Assessing Reliability

Determining whether a visual field examination is reliable is a matter of examining the reliability indices as well as the perimetrist's comments and correlating the visual field with the clinical examination. One problem with the HFA-1's reliability catch trials is that they only "sample" the patient's response patterns—that is, a few trials are supposed to be representative of the entire test. Additionally, trials are designed for the patient to make "active" mistakes. Both fixation losses and false positives require the patient to press the response button at the wrong time. A poorly responsive or somnolent patient will generally not make these types of errors, because the overall response pattern of such patients is to respond infrequently. False negatives can be tested only at points where there has been a response and the stimulus can be made 9 dB brighter. In both end-stage glaucoma and very unresponsive patients, there may not be enough responding points to test false negatives. Hence, the least responsive patient will not have any catch trials flagged.

Assessing the overall reliability of an examination requires a systematic inspection. Beginning with increased fixation losses, the visual field may be reliable if the perimetrist's comments indicate that the patient was indeed fixating and that the HFA was in error. The perimetrist should always record his or her comments within the permanent patient record rather than the printout, as older printouts are discarded when follow-up visual fields are performed.

False positives should then be inspected. It is prudent, when any false positives are recorded, to examine the visual field carefully. The box plot of the visual field will quickly show whether there is at least one highly elevated point. Because threshold values should gradually decrease as one goes farther away from fixation, points that are more than 4 or 5 dB higher than surrounding normal points should be viewed skeptically. Because elevated false positives are more likely to hide true scotomas and lead to a false identification of the visual field as normal, it is recommended that the test be repeated and the patient carefully reinstructed. The perimetrist should also be instructed to redouble his or her efforts to identify false-positive responses when they occur and pause the test to reinstruct the patient.

False negatives should then be considered with the clinical examination as a reference. If the patient has an obviously glaucomatous optic nerve, visual field loss is expected. Because fluctuation is expected in patients with visual field loss, false negatives are not a measure of inconsistency in these patients and are of little value in the doctor's assessment of reliability. When false negatives are elevated in a patient with

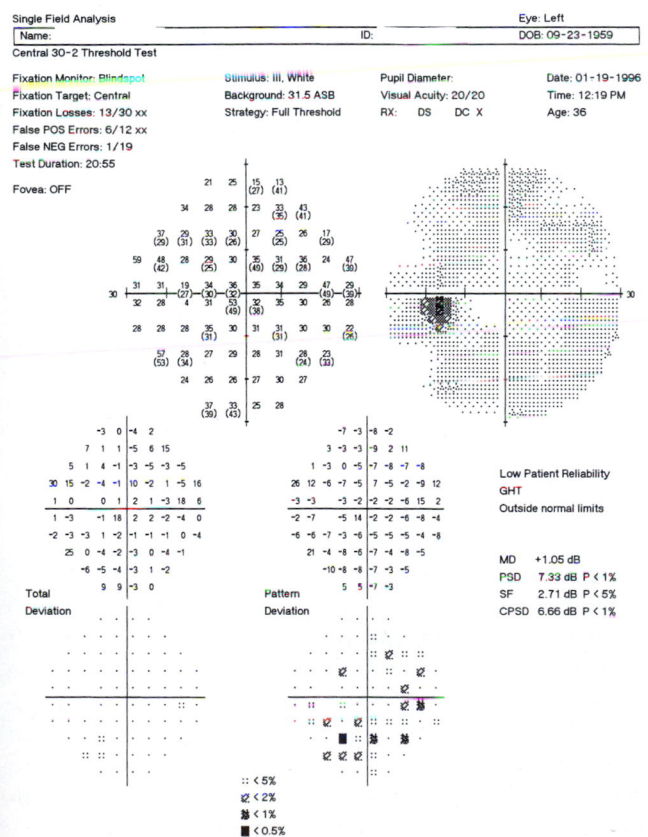

Figure 16–8. An example of a visual field marred by false positives (6/12). As expected, fixation losses are likewise elevated. The gray scale shows patchy white areas ("white scotoma") corresponding to threshold values in the 40 to 50dB range.

low risk factors and no visual field loss is anticipated, suspicion of inconsistency is justified. However, even when visual field loss is anticipated, patients may indeed be truly inconsistent and their elevated false negatives may reflect an accurate assessment. In these cases, both the perimetrist's assessment of the patient's attentiveness and the doctor's assessment of the consistency of the recorded visual field loss in relation to that anticipated is crucial for determining reliability.

In general, a visual field exam with elevated fixation losses may be kept if the perimetrist's comments testify to steady fixation. Likewise, elevated false negatives in a patient whose visual field loss was anticipated is not necessarily a cause for discarding the visual field. Correlation with the clinical examination and the perimetrist's assessment is critical. Finally, whenever there are elevated false positives, the patient should be reinstructed and the visual field test repeated with specific instructions to the perimetrist to increase his or her vigilance for identifying false positives during the test.

Despite the automation of the testing procedure and the objective scoring of the patient's reliability, nothing will replace the physical presence of a perimetrist in the room during the test. The technician should constantly monitor fixation as well as reposition the patients who start to lean. At the first recorded false positive, the test should be paused and the patient reinstructed to push the response button only when he or she is certain. The technician can continuously encourage and correct a hesitant or poorly motivated patient. The reliability of many visual field tests is improved markedly when the technician recognizes fatigue and pauses the test when needed. Typically, the test should be paused every 5 to 6 min to allow the patient to rest. Although the responsibility for determining how and where to test is now automatically determined, the technician still plays a vital role by determining when to override the software of the HFA-1.

Speeding up Threshold Examinations with the HFA-1

It became readily apparent, using the 30-2 with the full-threshold strategy in the original HFA-1, that test time was excessive for a significant number of patients, up to 19 to 20 min per eye. Although some patients were able to maintain attention and provide reliable responses, others would become fatigued, with poor responses, especially toward the end of the examination, when the peripheral points are tested. These visual fields typically showed a concentric, overall depression that could be extensive, masking true scotomas or falsely making the visual field look

abnormal.[40-43] To avoid fatigue artifacts and improve patient flow, there are three basic methods to speed up a threshold examination: test fewer points, decrease or eliminate catch trials, and shorten the actual threshold staircase. The 24-2 was the first step in decreasing test times. By eliminating about 25% of the point pattern, an immediate savings in time of roughly the same amount was realized. Although the 30-2 remains the preferred test in most clinical trials and academic centers, the demands of clinical practice have made the 24-2 the preferred alternative.

Catch trials can be partly eliminated in the HFA-1. Neither false positives nor false negatives can be turned off, but fixation losses can be, relying solely on the perimetrist's comments for an estimation of the patient's fixation. As discussed above, this may actually be preferable for many patients. Turning off fixation catch trials saves less than a minute.

While not technically a catch trial, short-term fluctuation serves as an indicator of consistency and therefore reliability, as 10 points undergo thresholding for a second time during the test. Of the 10 points, 4 are used in the initialization process and must always be retested, but the other 6 will not be retested if short-term fluctuation is turned off. In essence, short-term fluctuation "adds" 6 extra points to every test. As discussed below, short-term fluctuation adds little to the interpretation of the visual field and can be eliminated without detriment to interpretation.

The testing of the foveal threshold contributes little that cannot be inferred from the four points surrounding fixation and the visual acuity. While only one test point is involved, the overall delay in testing associated with redirecting fixation and giving special instructions to the patient is considerable but not reflected in the recorded test time.

All of the previously mentioned test modifications can be done either individually or together. They can be selected on a test-by-test basis, or the user-defined testing menu can be modified so that these changes become the default setting for all tests. Approximately 2 to 4 min is saved by using the 24-2 instead of the 30-2, and an additional 2 min (roughly) per eye of test time can be eliminated by turning off fixation catch trials and short-term fluctuation. None of the changes in either the test-point pattern or the reliability indices will have any detrimental effect on interpretation. Both the glaucoma hemifield test and the glaucoma change probability analysis are available for any of the tests suggested above.

The final choice for decreasing test time on the HFA-1 is to select the FASTPAC threshold strategy. With FASTPAC, fewer steps are taken in determining the stimulus threshold at the expense of accuracy.

Further detracting from the use of FASTPAC is the unavailability of either the glaucoma hemifield test or glaucoma change probability analysis for any test run under the FASTPAC strategy. Although the threshold values are less precise, a savings of up to 30% is obtained.[19]

In everyday clinical practice, using the 24-2 and modifying the reliability indices as suggested can make modest but significant savings in time without a loss in either accuracy or analysis techniques. The FASTPAC strategy should be used judiciously. If a patient has demonstrated a fatigue artifact even with the other time-shortening techniques, then the use of FASTPAC is justified. A visual field test that has a substantial fatigue artifact has no clinical usefulness, and the shortcomings of the FASTPAC strategy are quickly offset by obtaining a reliable visual field in a patient who did not tire. Using the 24-2, modifying the reliability indices, and employing FASTPAC results in about a 50% reduction in test time compared with a 30-2 done with the full-threshold strategy[44] (Fig. 16–9).

The overall effect of a faster test is the lessening or elimination of the fatigue artifact. In a normal patient, in addition to the peripheral depression, several points in the paracentral area may be missed because of the patient's fatigue, thus giving the false impression of both specific and nonspecific visual field loss. For these patients, a faster test will cause the visual field to revert to normal. For patients with real defects, the effect of fatigue will cause many of the defects to appear deeper and larger. Changing to a faster test will both eliminate the peripheral depression and lessen the depth and size of real defects. This improved visual field should be considered as the true visual field for the patient, and it is important to then revisit the original diagnosis and treatment plan. It may be possible to reduce the level of therapeutic intervention based on the improved visual field test.

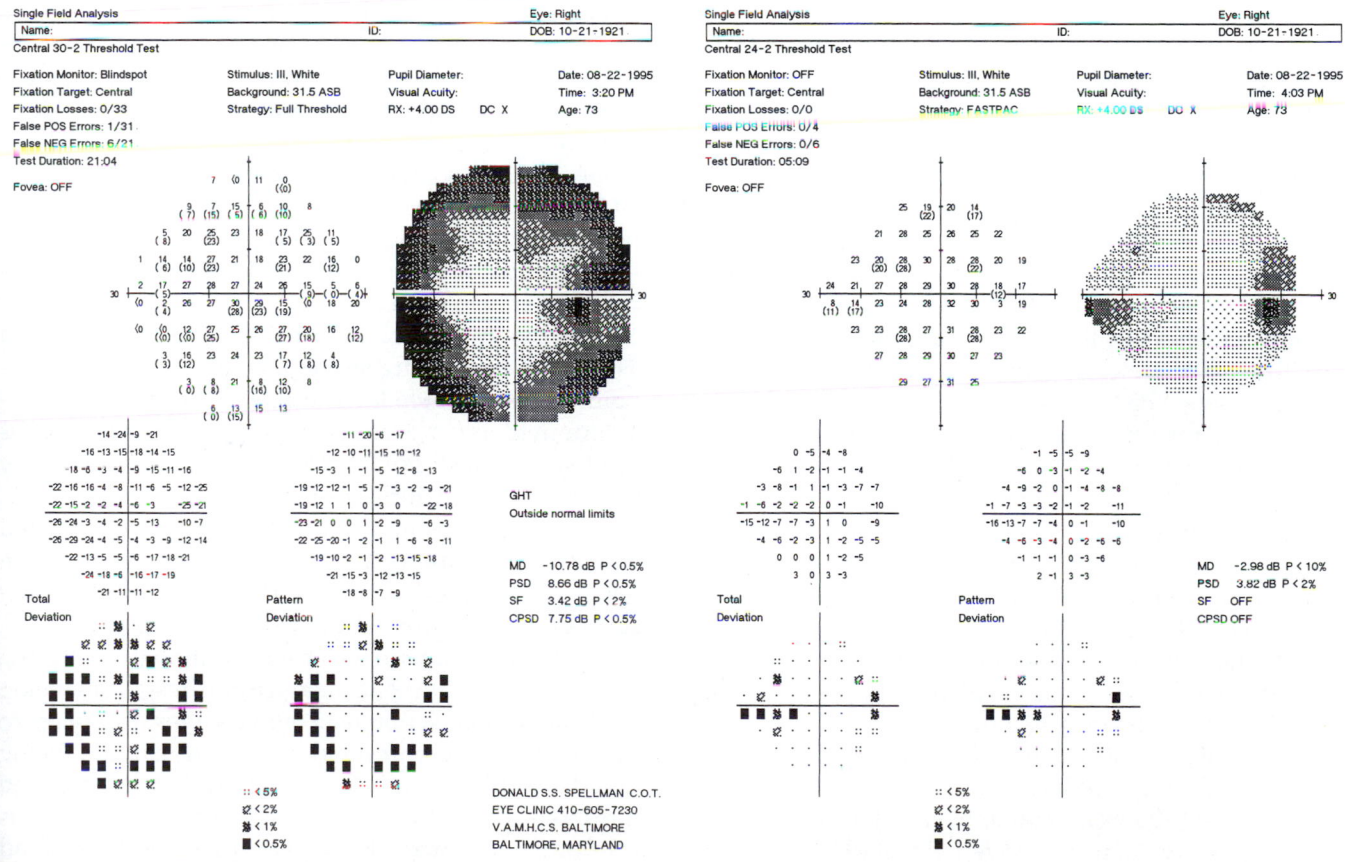

Figure 16–9. *A.* The full-threshold 30-2 test took 21:04 min and showed marked fatigue artifact. Visual fields did not correspond to the appearance of the patient's optic nerve. *B.* After the left eye was rested, patient underwent another visual field of the right eye on the same day but with the pattern changed to the 24-2, with SF and FL turned off and FASTPAC turned on. Total test time was 5:09 and the loss of visual field corresponded to the level of optic nerve damage.

HFA-2 SOFTWARE

Like the HFA-1, the HFA-2 has three software components: testing programs, reliability catch trials, and statistical interpretation. This section discusses the changes and additions to the testing programs and reliability catch trials of the HFA-2. Statistical interpretation for both units is discussed further on.

HFA-2 Testing Programs

Suprathreshold

The HFA-2 carries over most of the screening tests of the HFA-1, but the threshold-related screening strategy has been appropriately renamed the two-zone strategy. Both quantify-defect and single-intensity strategies are available, but their use is not recommended for clinical screening examinations. The same recommendations hold true for the HFA-2 as for the HFA-1: only the two-zone (threshold-related) and three-zone strategies are suggested for suprathreshold tests. As with the HFA-1, use of the age-related means for estimating the height of the HOV should be avoided in patients with small pupils or those in whom the status of the ocular media is uncertain.

Threshold

The HFA-2 deleted both the "fast" and "full from prior," leaving the "full" and FASTPAC threshold strategies. In 1997, two new threshold strategies became available via software upgrade: SITA standard (Swedish interactive thresholding algorithm) and SITA fast. The SITA strategies require greater computer processing power than is available on the HFA-1 as well as faster motors; thus they will not be available on the HFA-1 perimeters. The SITA strategies represent the culmination of 10 years of research and testing and constitute an entirely new approach to threshold tests.[45] The underlying approach to the development of SITA was to reduce test time without sacrificing accuracy. The SITA standard strategy matches the precision of the full-threshold strategy while reducing test time by half.[46,47] SITA fast matches the accuracy of FASTPAC but takes only half the time.[48]

Both SITA and SITA fast use four methods for reducing test time: reducing time between presentations, starting the examination of each location with a better estimate of the expected threshold, reducing the testing performed at each test point, and reducing the time spent in catch trials.

With full-threshold or FASTPAC strategies, the time it takes the patient to respond to the stimuli during the first 10 presentations is averaged and 0.85 s is added. This sum is then used by the HFA-1 or HFA-2

to either slow down or speed up the time between subsequent stimulus presentations. In general, the result is that the test is slowed down for many patients. For SITA tests in the HFA-2, response time by the patient is constantly monitored, and the time between presentations can again be adjusted either slower or faster. Unlike the HFA-1, the HFA-2 has motors that can reposition the projector faster, thus allowing for shorter time intervals between presentations. Considering that there are anywhere between 300 and 400 stimulus presentations, saving even 0.1 s per presentation can result in a half minute less per test. This time reduction is accomplished without sacrificing accuracy. More importantly, patient morale is improved by the faster pacing; and the test will speed up appreciably for those capable of the quicker presentations.

For full-threshold or FASTPAC strategies, the starting point for thresholding is determined by an extrapolation of the HOV based on the results obtained in that quadrant during initialization. Then, as the examination progresses, results are used to modify the estimate of the starting point for neighboring points. SITA further refines these concepts. First, it draws on its empirical databases for a more sophisticated knowledge of both the normal and glaucomatous HOV. Second, it integrates the results of more "neighboring points" into a sophisticated estimate of the patient's HOV and therefore a better estimate of the starting point for thresholding individual points. The closer the testing begins to the final threshold, the fewer the number of presentations required.

In the full-threshold or FASTPAC strategies, a "staircase" bracketing strategy is carried out on every point in the visual field. The size of the steps was predetermined by a frequency-of-seeing curve that is used for all test points. However, both eccentricity and disease will influence the shape of this curve. Thus, for some points, the endpoint may be reached quickly and with a large degree of certainty with fewer trials, while other points may need additional steps in the staircase to be sure of the endpoint.

SITA takes advantage of the additional computing power of the HFA-2 to analyze the responses being made at all points, not just completed test locations, to predict the final threshold value for a point being tested. As the examination progresses, the predicted threshold value for all points in the visual field is constantly updated. For every predicted threshold value, there is an estimate of its accuracy, or how certain SITA is of what the final value for that point will be. Once an estimate for the final threshold value reaches a predetermined level of certainty, that point is "closed" and further testing ceases at that point.[49] The major difference between SITA standard and SITA fast is how "certain" SITA must be before closing a point. Because SITA fast will accept a greater degree of uncertainty and therefore a less precise estimate of threshold in exchange for fewer stimulus presentations, it will result in a shorter examination. SITA standard will cross threshold at least once, whereas SITA fast is not always required to cross it. When there is a large degree of uncertainty because of variable responses from the patient, both SITA standard and SITA fast will end up double-crossing threshold, just like the standard full-threshold strategy.

Intuitively, the SITA approach to testing is appealing. For example, when the results of three contiguous test points are all normal and are at the predicted values, an untested point that is contiguous with the other three is very likely to be both normal and at the predicted value. As points around it are tested, the ability to predict the threshold value for this point continues to increase. It does not seem necessary, then, to proceed with the entire 4-2 staircase bracketing technique when it seems highly likely that the point is both normal and as predicted. Clinical testing of the algorithm has shown that its original goals have been reached. SITA standard will take about half as much time as the full-threshold strategy with no loss of accuracy, while SITA fast takes half the time of FASTPAC but has the same accuracy as FAST-PAC (Fig. 16–10A, B, and C).

It should be noted that when a patient is switched from the full-threshold to a SITA standard, there will be an increase in threshold values at all points but principally at the peripheral ones.[50,51] Since the threshold values will change, a comparison using the standard full-threshold will be different from one done with SITA. Therefore, direct comparison of these values is not recommended. At this point, the SITA test should be considered the new starting baseline test, and previous examinations should be placed in the back of the chart for reference only. In converting patients with established loss of visual field to SITA examinations, it may be necessary to repeat the standard full-threshold test one more time to rule out progression. Once the doctor is convinced that the visual field is stable, the patient can be switched to SITA. Patients with prior normal full-threshold visual fields can be converted directly to SITA.

The final technique for reducing test time is to eliminate and/or modify the catch trials. The HFA-2 has several new approaches for testing false positives and false negatives when using the SITA strategy.

Catch Trials

In addition to blind-spot monitoring, the HFA-2 has gaze-tracking capability that will monitor fixation during the examination. Either technique can be employed, or both can be used simultaneously. Unlike the HFA-1's blind-spot catch trials for fixation losses, which estimate fixation by random sampling, gaze tracking monitors fixation continuously throughout the entire test. Because no separate catch-trial presentation is required, time is saved *during* the test. However, before each eye is tested, the gaze tracker is calibrated by having the patient maintain fixation for 20 s without blinking. At each stimulus presentation, there is a simultaneous recording, in degrees, of the position of the patient's gaze in reference to the fixation target. It is displayed as a bar graph on the bottom of the screen and printout. If the patient is looking straight ahead, there is no deflection from the baseline. An upward deflection indicates that gaze was not on the fixation target, with the height of the deflection proportional to the extent of errant fixation. The maximum height corresponds to 10 degrees (or more) off fixation. There are six sizes of downward deflection. In general, the larger downward deflections are usually caused by a blink, while small deflections mean that the gaze tracker was unable to determine the direction of the patient's gaze. When a large number of downward deflections occur in a row, the test should be paused and gaze tracking reinitialized. Likewise, if a large number of tall, upward deflections occur in a row and the video monitor shows good fixation, the gaze tracker should be reinitialized.

As one examines the gaze-track display, fixation at any point during the test can be assessed. It is not uncommon to see fixation begin to wander toward the end of the test, with the onset of fatigue. This is often unnoticed by the blind-spot monitoring, which intentionally tests more often at the beginning of the test to correct the patient and fewer times toward the end. Occasionally there may be brief periods of fixation losses at any time during the test, which usually occur when the patient shifts his or her position in the instrument (Fig. 16–11).

Although blind-spot catch trials are subject to artifact, they do provide a quantifiable estimate of fixation with arbitrary criteria for reliability. Although gaze tracking provides a complete and accurate recording of fixation, it offers no guidelines for interpretation or criteria for reliability. It is suggested that as practitioners first begin working with the gaze track, they also employ standard blind-spot monitoring to serve as a reference as well as the perimetrist's comments. As clinical experience is accrued, the practitioner will become more comfortable with interpretation of the gaze-track display and eventually elect to turn off the blind-spot monitor, with a subsequent decrease in test time. One word of caution: In

the current sof
fixation losses c
those that exce
printout. There
of excessive los
have been an ov

False Negative

The underlying
label a patient
ally responsib
sponses. For fal
tests, time is s
stimulus than v
formation is al
actual threshol
separate catch
able responses
tained for a giv
any denial of s
nal threshold
tests ignore the
crossing of thre

When eith
HFA-2 examin
the testing of
when the stim
based on the fi
fluctuation in
tion with
consideration.5

stimulus faster than the preset criterion, the HFA-2 will consider it to be a false positive. Second, during the examination, the HFA-2 constantly monitors the patient's response time. It determines both an average response time and the range of response times in which most responses lie, and it formulates an "acceptance interval." Any response after the "acceptance interval" is usually considered a false response by the HFA-2. The HFA-2 knows when to reject a response as having occurred either too soon or too late after a stimulus presentation. False positives are reported as a percentage to indicate the estimated frequency of false-positive responses during the test. As with false negatives, there is no published criterion for when to reject a visual field based on false-positive responses.

Because no patient is perfect, the problem for the clinician is deciding what percent constitutes an unreliable visual field. Although, in theory, the new methods for determining false negatives and false positives are a marked improvement, at present there are no published criteria or research data to guide the clinician as to when a visual field is unreliable. When the HFA-1 was introduced, the company provided general guidelines for reliability. Later research and large-scale clinical use of the HFA-1 demonstrated that the criteria were, in many cases, too restrictive for fixation losses and false negatives and too forgiving for false positives. Clinicians have learned to modify the instrument's criteria based on their own experience and their perimetrists' subjective yet invaluable assessments of reliability. The company has plans to eventually provide some guidance based on the normative data collected in the gathering of the SITA databases. Unlike the data gathered in STAT-PAC, which excluded unreliable patients, the SITA database excluded only those patients whose fixation losses exceeded 20%. No patient was excluded on the basis of false negatives or false positives. Therefore a statistical analysis should be able to provide limits of normal for false negatives and false positives.

INTERPRETING THRESHOLD VISUAL FIELDS

The interpretation of visual fields, integral to the management of glaucoma, can be divided into two tasks: looking at a single visual field and deciding whether it is abnormal, and looking at a series of visual fields and determining whether the visual fields have become progressively worse. Typically, one decides to initiate therapy based on whether a visual field is abnormal, while the decision to intensify therapy is based on the presence of progressive visual field loss. Both the HFA-1 and HFA-2 employ similar methods of graphical data display as well as statistical analysis to aid practitioners in their evaluation of the visual fields. Because the techniques are almost identical for the two instruments, the following discussion combines information for the HFA-1 and HFA-2.

SINGLE VISUAL FIELD ANALYSIS

The purpose of single visual field analysis is to determine whether a glaucomatous defect is present. Implicit in any definition of "abnormal" is knowledge of what is normal. In psychophysical testing, there is no single value that defines "normal"; rather, there is a range of responses from normals. The first step in interpreting a visual field is to compare the values obtained against the known range of values from normals. Contained within the software of both the HFA-1 and HFA-2 are extensive empirical databases (STATPAC, STATPAC Plus, STATPAC for FASTPAC, STATPAC II, SWAPPAC, and the SITA STATPAC) gathered from hundreds of normal patients.

The STATPACs use empirically derived databases generated from the testing of normal patients, ranging in age from 20 to 80 years, from several different clinics. To be included in the original STATPAC database, a patient under the age of 65 had to have corrected 20/20 acuity and, if over age 65, an acuity no worse than 20/30. For all ages, no more than 20% fixation losses, 33% false negatives, and 33% false positives were allowed for a visual field to be included in the database. The SITA databases excluded patients with fixation losses greater than 20% but did not exclude those with elevated false positives or false negatives. The patients were tested three times and were free of ocular disease, cataracts, and miosis. Because the values obtained from first threshold visual field tests are much more variable than those from follow-up visual field tests, normalization of the data became too difficult and only the second and third visual field exams were used in the original STAPAC databases.[53,54]

Within the databases there is a continuous range of normal values with a gradual transition from common values to less common ones. Attention is paid to the ends of the spectrum—the values least likely to occur in a normal population. In patients with moderate to severe disease, values are likely to fall completely outside the range of normal values, while the values obtained from patients with early disease overlap the values obtained at the extreme ends of the range of normals. Thus, though the upper limits of normal will clearly identify those patients with frank disease, the real challenge is distinguishing patients with early disease from entirely normal patients with extreme values. Identification of the extreme values and how likely they are to occur in normals is the task of statistics.

In classic gaussian statistics, a bell-shaped curve is generated when values are plotted against frequency. The top of the curve represents both the median and the average values. By convention, the median value has become the "expected" value for a normal patient. However, there is a range of normal values that includes the "statistically abnormal" as well. Two standard deviations from the median represents the upper and lower values of the curve under which 95% of all normal values are contained. The values outside 2 SD occur in less than 5% of normals, and are "statistically significant." Again, note that even these extreme values were obtained from normals and do not constitute an "abnormal" finding. Rather, their "significance" is that they fall within the transition zone where normal values overlap those indicating early disease. The frequency with which these values are found among normal patients is indicated by a p value. However, the distribution of values from visual fields is not Gaussian; it has a greater proportion of lower sensitivity values. Values representing high sensitivity are ignored, since they are not part of the disease process. Probability values are assigned only to lower sensitivities.

In STATPAC, a "$p < 5\%$" means that the threshold value obtained from a patient for that specific point is expected to occur in less than 5% of normal patients of the same age. Similarly, a value with a $p < 1\%$ occurs in less than 1% of normal patients, while $p < 0.5\%$ occurs in less than 0.5% of all normals of the same age. Clinically, the p values of <1 and $<0.5\%$ are the most significant in helping to differentiate normal from abnormal findings.

A map of individual p values for each point in the visual field tested would present an awkward display of data. Schwartz first proposed using a modified gray scale to designate the clinical significance of the threshold value measured at a given point, and that idea has been incorporated in the probability plots for STATPAC.[55] An individual point is assigned a shading based on its significance. Unlike the standard gray-scale printout, there is no interpolation or extrapolation in the display. Therefore, the display will show individual points as either dots (normal) or small shaded boxes.

Although the probability plot display provides an easy, quick means of assessing the "normalcy" of each point, two caveats must be mentioned. First, while individual points are analyzed by STATPAC, it remains the clinician's task to analyze the entire visual field. Second, while a probability map will aid in the analysis of a single visual field test, it may hide progressive loss of visual field. Once a black box ($p < 0.5\%$) is assigned to a point, any further deterioration cannot be represented. Therefore, additional schemes must be employed other than using probability plots for following changes over time.

When the expected HOV is determined by empirical testing and statistical analysis is applied, several important facts must be kept in mind in interpreting the visual field. The range of normal responses in the HOV increases the further one tests away from fixation. Heijl found that points adjacent to fixation have 98% of their normal values within 5 dB of the average or expected value. At 15 degrees from fixation, the distribution of threshold values is non-Gaussian, with an asymmetrical distribution around the median. It was noted that at the 95th percentile, the value was 13 dB below the median, while at the 5th percentile it was 7 dB above. At a point 27 degrees directly above fixation, the curve was even more non-Gaussian, with some points being 20 dB less than the expected value yet still within the definition of normal.[54] Because of this increasing range of normal values with eccentricity, a 5-dB defect near fixation may be assigned a black box (most significant) while an 11-dB defect in the periphery may be represented by a dot (normal point) (Fig. 16–12).

Empirical testing showed not only that variability among normals increases with eccentricity but also that some quadrants are more variable than others, with the superior visual field showing the most variability. This means that not only will a point 15 degrees from fixation be more variable than a point 3 degrees from fixation but also a point 15 degrees superior to fixation will be more variable than one 15 degrees inferior to fixation. Finally, empirical data have shown that while each point decreases in sensitivity at a constant rate with age, different points will decrease at different rates. The superior visual field was found to steepen faster with age than the rest of the HOV.

Essentials of Single Visual Field Analysis

The output from a single visual field analysis with STATPAC consists of a printout that includes a numerical display of the actual threshold values, a graphical gray scale of the threshold values, total-deviation scores and corresponding probability plot, pattern-deviation scores with corresponding probability plots, global indices, and the results of the analysis of the glaucoma hemifield test (see Table 16–2). The printout also includes two separate sections listing the point pattern used, test strategy employed, size of the test target, patient's demographic data, date of test, length

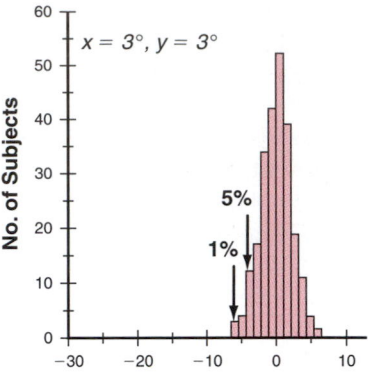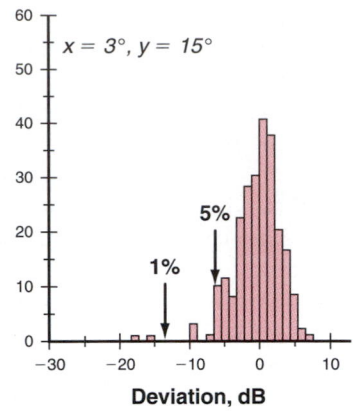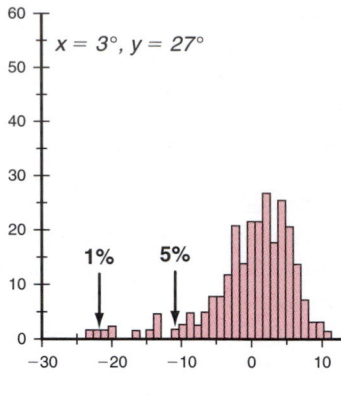

Figure 16–12. Three points in the superior quadrant at 3, 15, and 27 degrees from fixation were measured and the spread of normal values is displayed. Arrows indicate the 95th and 99th percentiles of normal. The further the point is from fixation, the greater the range of expected normal values, invalidating the simple rule that a 5-dB defect is significant. (Reproduced with permission from Heijl A, Lindgren G, Olsson J, Asman P. *Arch Ophthalmol.* 1989;107(2):204–208.)

of test, number of questions asked (number of times a stimulus was presented), refractive correction used, pupil size, and other items concerning the way in which the test was conducted. All data should be verified as correct, with special attention to the correction used and the patient's date of birth. Any analysis of the results begins with these two sections.

First, the practitioner should decide whether the proper test was performed. In clinical practice, either the 30-2 or 24-2 is acceptable for glaucoma. End-stage visual field loss requires a 10-2 to adequately monitor a threat to fixation. While the full-threshold test is the standard, faster threshold strategies are acceptable and encouraged for many patients. The length of the

---

TABLE 16–2. COMPONENTS OF SINGLE FIELD ANALYSIS

Gray scale: Used to identify defects but must be correlated with probability plots and threshold values. Easily influenced by artifacts to look abnormal.

Threshold values: Of limited value but can be used to recognize lid artifacts that cause straight rows of absolute defects.

Total-deviation probability plots: In the absence of media opacity or miosis, total deviation gives a true representation of focal and overall depression defects. These plots overcall defective points when media opacity or miosis is present.

Pattern-deviation probability plots: Remove overall depression from cataracts and miosis, revealing true focal defects. When overall depression is secondary to advanced disease, the pattern-deviation plot undercalls defects.

Global indices: Of limited value. Mean deviation can help assess severity of loss. CPSD and PSD can help identify abnormal fields. SF of little use.

Key: PSD, pattern standard deviation; CPSD, corrected pattern standard deviation; SF, short-term fluctuation.

test should be noted. When test time exceeds 10 min, many normal patients begin to experience fatigue, although some may tire even sooner. If analysis of the test determines the presence of a fatigue artifact, future tests should employ different test strategies to shorten test times.

The reliability indices should then be checked for any flagged index. Flagged indices require extra analysis to ensure the reliability of the visual field test. Judgment of reliability requires both a subjective assessment from the perimetrist and an a priori knowledge of expected visual field loss to interpret the indices properly. Inspection of the visual field then turns to the test results and their interpretation (Figs. 16–13, 16–14, and 16–15).

Threshold Values

The actual threshold value obtained for each point tested is printed in a display that presents both its value and its position in the visual field. With the HFA-1, the 10 test locations included in the determination of short-term fluctuation are tested twice, with both values displayed. Similarly, those points whose values fell 4 dB below the expected value are retested and both values are displayed. With the SITA strategies, only one threshold value per point is determined and printed. These raw data have not been subjected to statistical analysis and are usually of limited value. However, they are of value in four distinct circumstances. First, for non-SITA tests, the fluctuation in "good" areas of the visual field can be compared with the "bad" areas to see whether the visual field is reliable (see "Short-Term Fluctuation,"

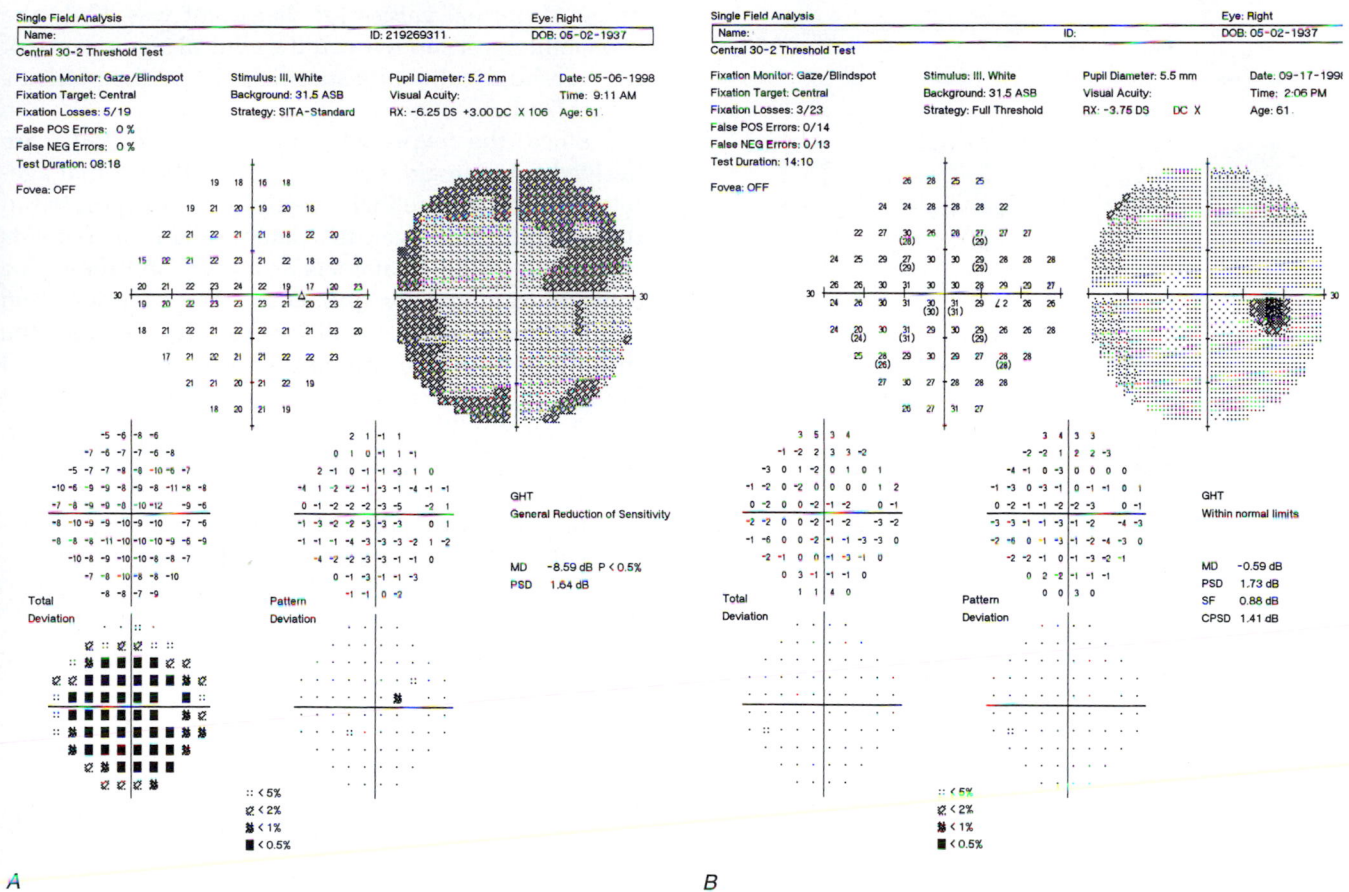

Figure 16–13. Three prior visual fields (not shown) were normal using −4.25 trial lens correction. *A.* By mistake a −6.25 +3.00×106 trial lens was used, and the resultant blur caused an overall depression seen on the 5-98 visual field. *B.* When retested in 9-98 with a −4.00 lens, the visual field was again normal.

below). Second, threshold values are useful in analyzing the visual field for progression. Third, certain artifacts such as those caused by trial lens rims and eyelids present with a distinctive pattern of absolute defects that can be recognized when the threshold values are inspected. Fourth, inspection of the threshold values for points above 37 dB can reveal hidden false positives.

Gray Scale
The graphical display of threshold values is performed by the gray scale, which was originally designed to replace the isopter plots that doctors had become accustomed to in interpreting Goldmann visual fields. Threshold values are grouped in 5-dB increments. Interpretation of the visual field on the basis of the gray scale is difficult owing to the large number of artifacts that influence its depiction. First, the difference between two shades of gray may be as little as 1 dB or as much as 9 dB. Second,

elderly patients normally have decreased retinal sensitivity and smaller pupils. Therefore, a normal 20-year-old's gray scale will always look "better" than a normal 70-year-old's gray scale. Third, cataracts will further depress the visual field and darken the gray scale but will not represent true disease. Fourth, shallow defects may be missed by the gray scale and apparent defects may be only artifacts due to the significant amount of fluctuation that can occur, especially in the periphery, in normal individuals. Finally, the data from the individual test points are both interpolated and extrapolated to construct the gray scale.

Despite these limitations, the gray scale can be of value in interpreting a visual field. Attention is quickly drawn to areas of low sensitivity, and the shape of the defect can readily be inspected to determine whether it is similar to defects known to occur in glaucoma. The depth of the defect is readily indicated by the shading. As discussed further on, the

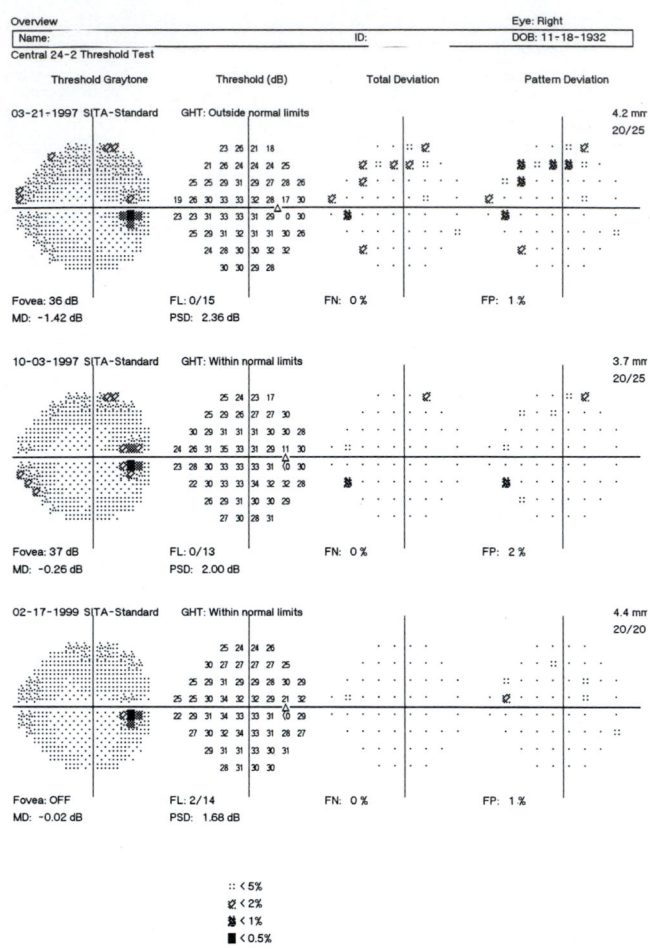

Figure 16-14. The first visual field showed superior field depression with an "outside normal limits" glaucoma hemifield test (GHT) message and a significant cluster of points. The next two visual fields showed a learning curve and turned out to be normal.

gray scale is invaluable in monitoring for progression. Also, the presence of unusually high sensitivity, called *white scotomas*, can readily be noted on the gray scale and the corresponding threshold value can be evaluated for false positives. Any threshold value over 37 dB should be considered suspect.

Total Deviation

The individual's threshold values are subtracted point by point from the expected values in STATPAC's age-matched database of normals and the difference is recorded. This is similar to the "defect-depth" table, which is part of older versions of the threshold printout, except that total deviation uses the empirically determined HOV from STATPAC. A probability plot is then generated from the total-deviation data and displayed next to the numerical display. The numerical display of deviation from expected is of little value unless the practitioner has knowledge of what the

range of normal values for that point was. Only the probability plot can tell you the clinical significance of the threshold value of a specific point in the patient's visual field.

Since the expected values in STATPAC are derived from an age-matched group, the normal age-related decline in retinal sensitivity is incorporated in the analysis. However, the database is from patients without significant cataracts or miosis, and these two artifacts can greatly influence the total-deviation display, causing an overall depression. Likewise, the first visual field of many patients is greatly depressed because of a learning effect. Although subsequent visual fields will improve if they were depressed due to "learning," those depressed secondary to cataracts, miosis, or glaucoma will not.

In patients free of these artifacts, the total deviation will identify those points that deviate significantly from the expected HOV. The Normal Tension Glaucoma Study employed an algorithm based on the total-deviation analysis to identify a cluster of defective

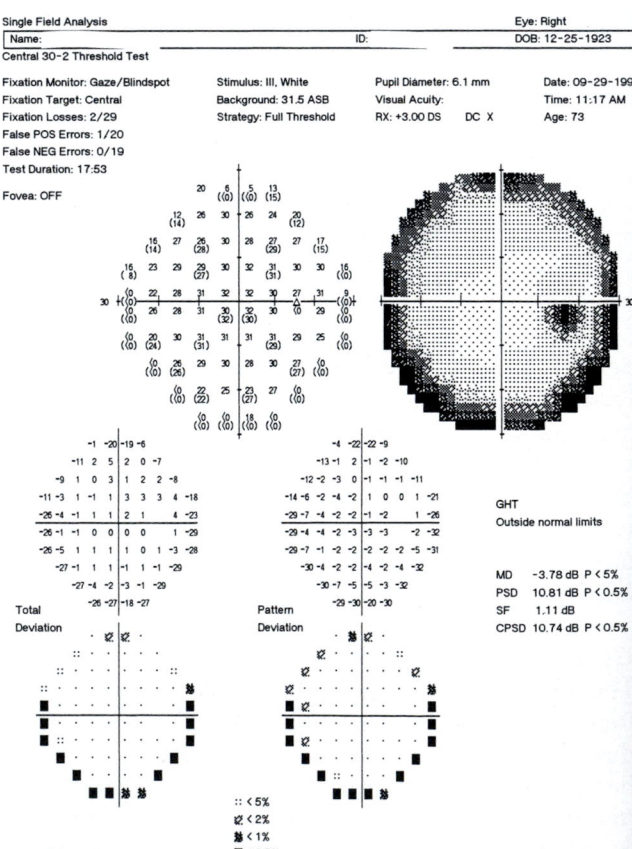

Figure 16-15. Rim artifact occurred with a +3.00 lens. Although a convex lens is more likely to cause a rim artifact, this usually occurs with powers greater than +4.00. In this patient, the technician positioned the lens too far from the eye.

points that constitute a visual field defect.[56] According to the algorithm, if three contiguous points on the same side of the horizontal meridian have a defect depth of at least 5 dB in two points and 10 dB in the third, the defect is considered significant. Other conditions of the algorithm attempt to minimize the effect of an overall depression. However, since cataracts and miosis are frequent findings in the elderly, an overlying generalized depression is almost always present, making it difficult to identify focal defects. Therefore, total deviation is good at identifying the overall visual field loss but of limited value in identifying focal defects if a general depression is present (Fig. 16–16).

Pattern Deviation

To compensate for overall or generalized depression, a statistically determined adjustment can be added to each individual threshold score. STATPAC ranks the total-deviation values from best to worst and then looks at the value of the point that represents the 85th percentile of non-edge points. Several points around the optic nerve are also excluded. This point is used to determine the "general height indicator." The difference between the obtained threshold value for the general height indicator and its expected value is then added to all points in the visual field. If the point used for the general height indicator is depressed, all threshold values in the visual field will be raised. By raising the values of the patient's actual threshold data before comparison with the expected HOV, the effects of cataracts or miosis can be minimized, thus allowing focal defects to become more apparent. This technique implies that cataracts and miosis will depress each point equally. Research indicates that different types of cataracts will not only lower the HOV but also change its shape.[57,58] More recently, however, one study has shown that pattern-deviation analysis is not clinically affected and remains reliable when a cataract is tested.[59]

A patient with a normal HOV but who has a significant cataract will have a markedly depressed visual field. The gray scale will be uniformly dark and the total-deviation probability plots will be made up almost entirely of black boxes. However, the pattern deviation will filter out the depression and the display of the pattern-deviation probability plot will be normal. If there is a significant cataract and localized visual field loss, the pattern-deviation display will show only the focal defects, having filtered out the depression from the cataract (Fig. 16–17).

There are two types of patients who will cause the general height indicator to lower all the threshold values. First, there are a small number of patients who are reliable and whose retinal sensitivity is higher than that of normals. The general height indicator will lower the HOV of these patients by a few decibels. This is useful because shallow scotomas would have been masked. Second, in unreliable patients with elevated false positives who have areas of false supersensitivity, the general height indicator may be falsely elevated, with a subsequent lowering of the HOV. This lowering may range from a few decibels to up to 15 dB or more.

The defect depth after adjustment, along with a probability plot, is displayed, assigning clinical significance to the recalculated deviation values. Since the effect of depression has been eliminated, the pattern-deviation probability plot display will now highlight focal defects in the HOV. Katz et al. recognized the inherent susceptibility of the normal-tension glaucoma (NTG) cluster criteria to false positives in the presence of a cataract and modified the criteria using the pattern-deviation probability plots.[60] To be considered a significant defect, there must be a cluster of three contiguous, non-edge, defective points that are part of the 24-2 pattern and are on the same side of the horizontal. Two points have to be significantly depressed at least to the $p < 5\%$ level, with the third point depressed to the $p < 1\%$ level. This modification, using

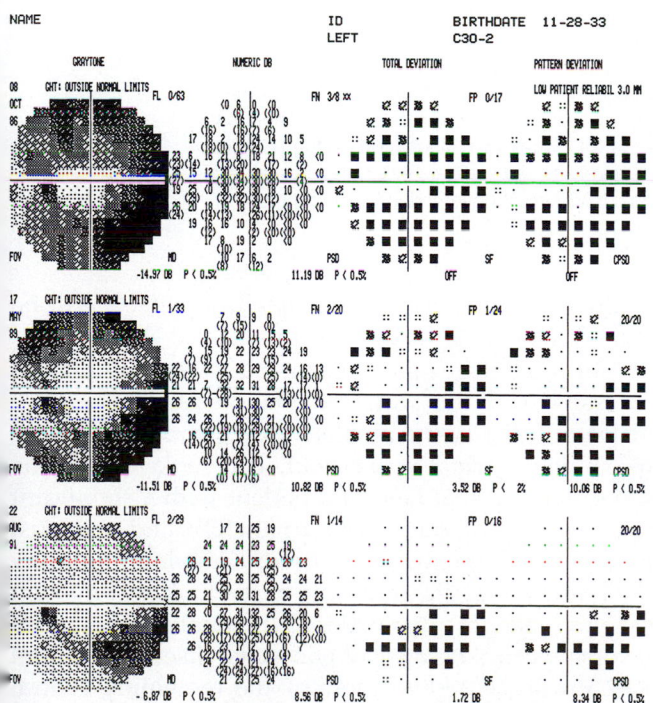

Figure 16–16. A patient with an inferior arcuate defect who showed a marked learning curve between his first, third, and fifth fields (second and fourth not shown). By the fifth field, the superior field looks normal and the inferior arcuate defect is clearly delineated.

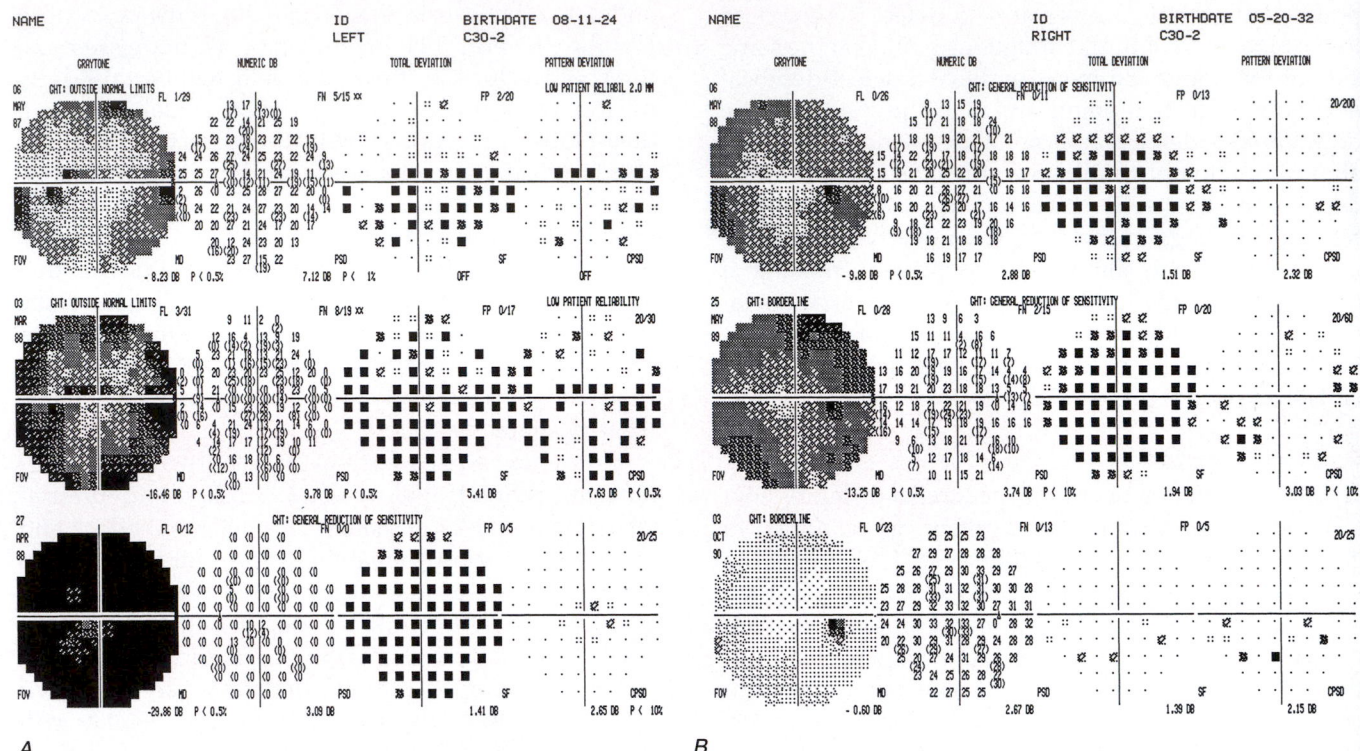

A *B*

Figure 16–17. *A.* This glaucoma patient experienced a dramatic loss of field between the second and third examinations. Note the worsening of both the gray scale and the total-deviation plot. However, the pattern-deviation plot "reverses" at the third field and appears normal. The pattern-deviation analysis is fooled by a severely depressed field, since there are no focal defects with end-stage disease. Although this patient is similar in appearance to the one in Fig. 16-17*B*, knowledge of the patient's media and cup-to-disc ratio will aid in the clinician's interpretation. *B.* This glaucoma suspect had a maturing cataract that was removed after the second field examination. Note the dramatic change in the gray scale. The total-deviation plot showed marked general depression, which reversed after cataract extraction and returned to normal. While the MD index was influenced by the cataract, the PSD index and the pattern deviation plots remained relatively stable. The GHT noted the general depression but remained "borderline" after the second field because of several depressed points.

pattern-deviation probability values, takes into account both cataracts and the eccentricity of the defects to avoid false positives. Cluster-analysis criteria along with the Glaucoma Hemifield Test have demonstrated exceptional sensitivity and specificity when Goldmann visual field loss is used as the gold standard.[60]

During the early stages of glaucoma, the pattern-deviation probability plot supplies very useful information for analyzing a visual field. With more advanced cases, in addition to focal defects, an overall depression begins to become apparent.[61] Both the gray-scale and total-deviation plots will show extensive loss, while the pattern deviation will remove the overall depression. Because the depression is caused by glaucoma rather than media opacification, the resultant pattern-deviation probability plot is misleading. All defects will be "corrected" by the general height indicator, which will then lessen the true depth

of the deepest defects, while shallow defects will be shown as normal points (Fig. 16–18).

In end-stage glaucoma, the overcorrection is excessive and the pattern-deviation plot "reverses"; instead of displaying all black boxes, the display may resemble a normal visual field. This looks almost the same as the visual field of a patient with a significant cataract and an otherwise normal HOV, and one must be able to differentiate the two. Knowledge of how the patient's media and optic nerve look will make it easy to make this distinction. When pattern-deviation reversal occurs because of end-stage disease, a central 10-2 threshold test to monitor the remaining central visual field is the proper examination.

Glaucoma Hemifield Test

Duggan et al.'s concept of mirror image analysis, comparing portions of the superior to the inferior half of

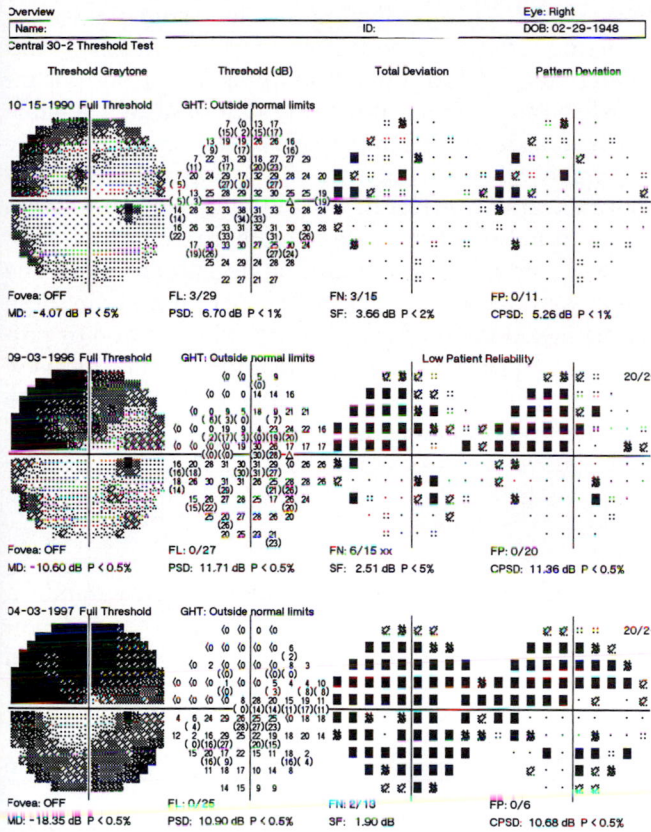

Figure 16-18. Between 1990 and 1996, the superior arcuate visual field defect both enlarged and deepened, as seen by the gray scale, total-deviation, and pattern-deviation probability plots. From 1996 to 1997, only the gray scale depicted further decline in the superior visual field. Note that the inferior visual field worsened significantly in the same time, as shown by both the gray scale and total-deviation plots. The pattern-deviation plot showed minimal change because it has been "corrected" for overall depression. However, in this 49-year-old patient, neither miosis nor media opacity is present and the overall depression is part of the disease process. If the patient is free of any cause for physiological depression, the total-deviation plot gives a more accurate assessment of the visual field.

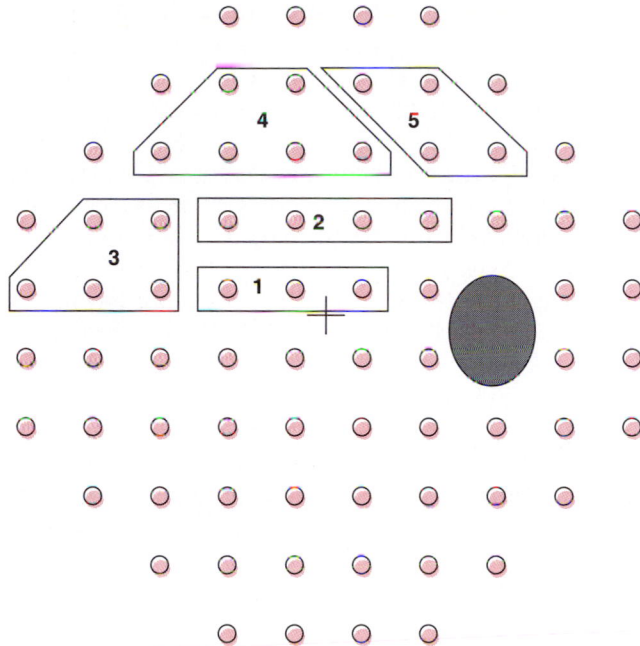

Figure 16-19. In the Glaucoma Hemifield Test (GHT), groups of points called zones are compared to their mirror image in the other half of the visual field. Statistical differences between matched zones are determined and compared to the likelihood of the same difference occurring with the STATPAC database of normals. (Reproduced with permission from Humphrey Systems, Inc.)

the visual field, is the basis for the Glaucoma Hemifield Test (GHT).[62-64] In the STATPAC version, probability values are used instead of raw threshold scores. Each of five zones in the superior half of the visual field is compared to its mirror-image zone in the inferior half (Fig. 16-19). Five possible interpretations or messages will appear on the printout:

1. *Outside Normal Limits*: This message will appear when one of two conditions occurs. First, a score is assigned to each member of the pair of matched zones on either side of the horizontal midline based on the percentile deviation from normal. The total score in one zone is compared to the total score in the matched zone. If the difference between the matched zones yields a sum that is found in less than 1% of normals, it is considered outside normal limits. This detects asymmetry across the midline, usually from focal defects. Second, if each zone in a matched pair yields a score that is outside the 0.5% level of probability, the message will also appear. Although there is no asymmetry, this finding reflects an overall depression that is affecting the superior and inferior visual hemifields equally. If the patient is reliable and has had previous experience with this type of testing, so that the learning effect is eliminated, this message correctly identifies most glaucoma patients with defects. A small number of patients with symmetrical focal defects will be undetected.

2. *Borderline:* The same matched zones will be analyzed, but the difference between zones yields a sum that is found in less than 3% of normals. There is no analysis for overall depression. When the GHT is borderline, careful scrutiny of other parts of the visual field printout may yield additional information that may contribute to the results being considered abnormal, e.g., the presence of significant cluster meeting Katz's criteria. With unreliable or

inexperienced patients, this is a frequent message, and a repetition of the visual field examination with close supervision and encouragement from the perimetrist is recommended.

3. *General Reduction of Sensitivity*: The GHT looks at the general height indicator determined for the pattern-deviation analysis. If the result is a positive value that occurs in less than 0.5% of normals in that age group, this message will appear. (If the condition for "borderline" is also met, this message will also appear.) It will identify patients with end-stage glaucoma and/or advanced cataracts who have significant depressions that are equal above and below the horizontal midline. The optic nerve should have severe glaucomatous damage to account for this level of general reduction in sensitivity; otherwise media opacity or fatigue artifact should be suspected.

4. *Abnormally High Sensitivity:* If the patient's general height indicator is higher than indicators occurring in less than 0.5% of individuals in that age group of the STATPAC's database, this message will be displayed. With "abnormally high sensitivity" appearing, all other GHT messages will be suppressed. This message occurs in unreliable patients with a high number of false positives, and the visual field should be discarded. The patient should be retested at a later date and reinstructed to respond only when he or she is sure that a stimulus is seen.

5. *Within Normal Limits*: This message appears when none of the above conditions are met and the visual field is considered normal. However, the GHT can miss subtle defects. Small, shallow paracentral defects may be present but not considered abnormal by the GHT. If these defects show up consistently on follow-up visual fields, the visual field should be viewed suspiciously even though the message indicates normalcy. Other indicators of abnormality, such as cluster defects and/or abnormal corrected pattern standard deviation (CPSD), should be compared with the clinical appearance of the optic nerve and nerve fiber layer even when the GHT is normal.

The GHT is automatically generated and displayed on the printout only for full-threshold, SITA standard, and SITA fast visual field examinations. Katz and coworkers found high sensitivity and specificity for both the GHT and the cluster criteria based on pattern-deviation plots, although no technique

was perfect.[60] In analyzing single visual fields, the practitioner should both note the GHT message and search the pattern-deviation plots for a significant cluster. When both criteria are abnormal in a reliable patient, a defect is almost certainly present. In early or equivocal cases, only one of the criteria may be abnormal, and the results of the clinical examination and evaluation of the patient's other risk factors must be weighed more heavily in the decision to treat. The GHT is not available when FASTPAC is used; in these cases the corrected pattern standard deviation or pattern standard-deviation global indices may be used and correlated to the appearance of the optic nerve and nerve fiber layer (Figs. 16–20, 16–21, and 16–22). The cluster criterion suggested by Katz can also be employed.[60]

Global Indices

The global indices (mean deviation, pattern standard deviation, short-term fluctuation, and corrected pattern standard deviation) summarize the information

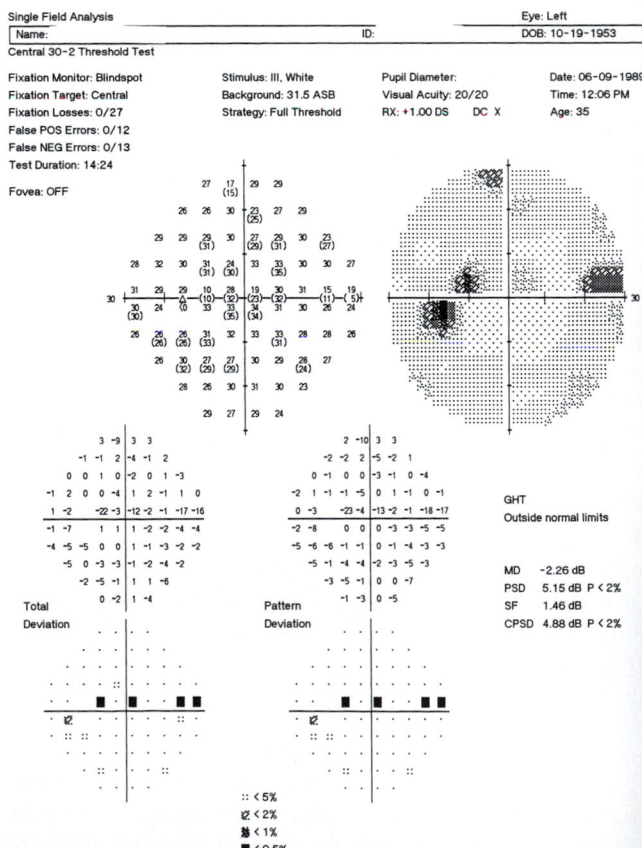

Figure 16–20. Superior arcuate visual field defect identified by the GHT message of "outside normal limits," but without a significant cluster of defective points meeting Katz's criteria. The defect is poorly seen by the gray scale.

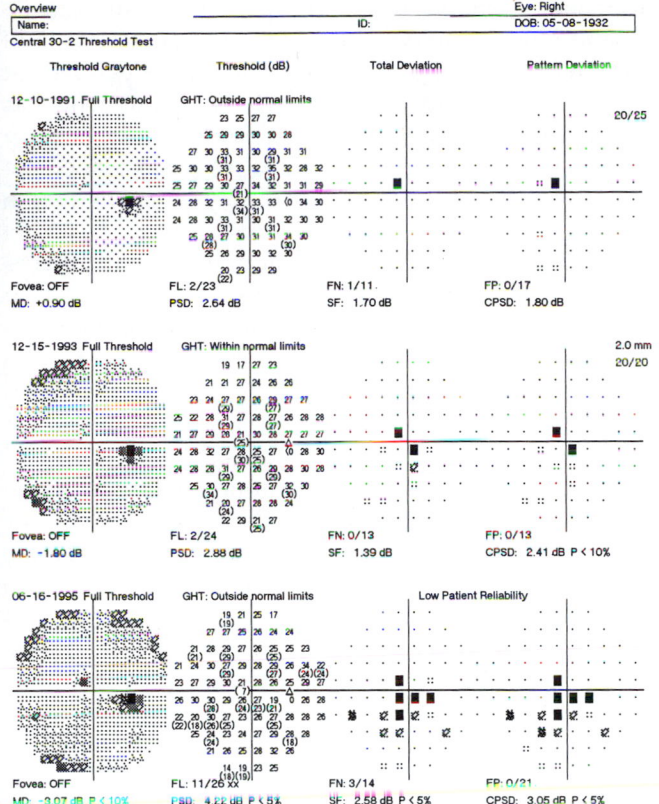

Figure 16–21. In 1991, two paracentral points generated a GHT message of "outside normal limits." In 1993, there was a paracentral visual field loss with a significant cluster of defective points seen in the pattern-deviation plot but normal GHT. The GHT message is normal because the defect within the zone is more or less symmetrical across the horizontal midline. In 1995 there was both a positive GHT message and a significant cluster.

provided in threshold values and the total- and pattern-deviation analysis. In a 30-2 test, these indices utilize information from all 76 points and reduce it to one number, much as an average test score is supposed to indicate how a whole class performed on a test. With the reduction of data, however, comes the inherent loss of spatial information. The index may indicate that a visual field is abnormal, but it does not tell you where the abnormality is located. Like the total- and pattern-deviation probability plots, the statistical significance of each global index is expressed as a *p* value to indicate whether the index is within the normal limits of the database. For single visual field analysis, these values play a limited role in determining if the results are abnormal.

Mean Deviation. The amount that each point in the visual field deviates from the expected STATPAC value is first weighted and then averaged. Points closer to fixation are weighted more heavily since

their deviation is clinically and statistically more significant. The mean deviation (MD) index is a summary of the "average" deviation of all points from the total-deviation analysis. If the visual field is uniformly affected, the MD index is a good indicator of general depression. An MD index of -3 to -4 dB represents a mild depression, while any visual field with an MD over -15 dB should be considered markedly depressed. Unfortunately, with this type of data reduction, spatial information is lost. For example, a stroke patient may show that the left half of his visual field is depressed by an average of -10 dB but that the right half is normal. The MD index will show only an average of a -5-dB deviation, suggesting a mild depression but losing the spatial information of a hemianopic defect.

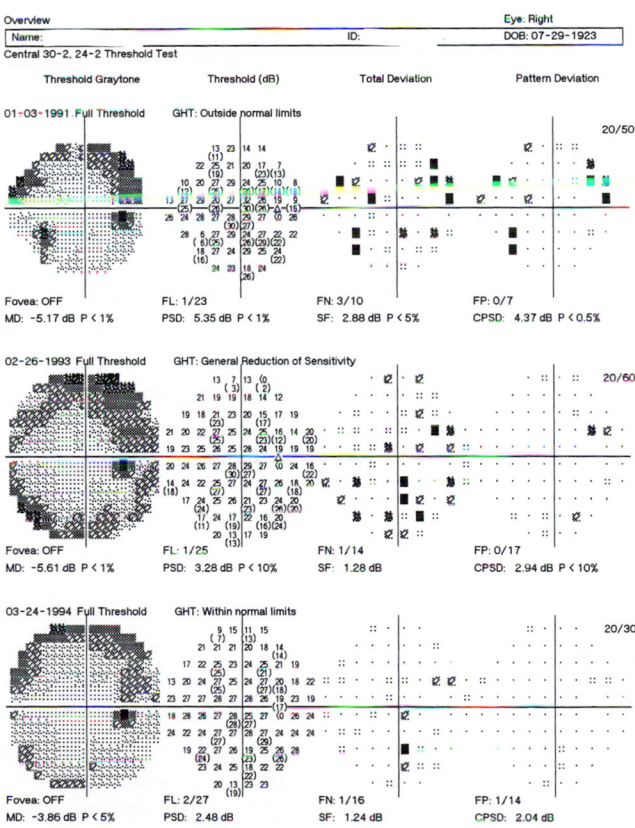

Figure 16–22. The initial visual field showed scattered defective points without an obvious glaucomatous defect, commonly referred to as *patchy loss*. Defects are significant on both total- and pattern-deviation plots. Although defects are nonspecific for glaucoma, focal asymmetry is present in certain zones and the GHT message displayed "outside normal limits." The second visual field showed an overall depression on the gray-scale and total-deviation plots, but no focal defects were noted in the pattern deviation. GHT indicated a "general reduction in sensitivity." By the third visual field, the patient's learning curve had flattened and the results were now "within normal limits."

It is better to look first at the total- and pattern-deviation probability plots to assess the nature of the visual field loss and then use the MD index to judge the overall severity. Since MD index is easily influenced by the same factors that affect total deviation, the probability values assigned to an individual MD index have not been shown to be useful for detecting glaucoma.[65] However, it has been suggested that if the media changes are symmetrical, a difference of 2 dB in MD index between a patient's eyes is significant and should be viewed suspiciously.[66]

Pattern Standard Deviation

The amount that each test location deviates from the expected STATPAC value after it has been adjusted for a general depression or supersensitivity is weighted and then averaged. The pattern standard deviation (PSD) index is the standard deviation around the mean of the total deviations. Conceptually, the PSD is supposed to indicate how evenly the visual field loss is spread across the visual field, being extremely valuable in identifying local or focal visual field defects. It is minimally influenced by a mild or moderate cataract. However, just like the pattern-deviation probability plot analysis, it cannot differentiate between a significant cataract and end-stage glaucoma. Therefore, the PSD index will appear normal when the pattern-deviation probability plot "reverses." In the absence of end-stage glaucoma, studies have shown that the PSD index is a relatively sensitive indicator and is somewhat useful clinically in identifying abnormal visual fields if the test is reliable and the PSD index has a p value of 5% or less. However, the GHT and Katz's cluster criteria usually outperform the PSD index.[60]

Short-Term Fluctuation

Patients usually show some variation in response when a point is tested a second time during the same test. The short-term fluctuation (SF) index is a measure of the consistency and implied reliability of the patient's responses. During the test, 10 points are retested and compared to the first threshold value. The SF index is calculated as the root mean square of the variation and usually ranges between 2.00 and 3.00 dB for normal patients.[67] This indicates that a point with a threshold value of 32 dB and a SF of 1.5 dB is expected to give you a value of between 30.50 and 33.5 dB when retested. A probability (p) value is assigned to the SF index values that are significantly different from the STATPAC normals.

When the SF index is abnormal, a corresponding increase in false negatives is expected. There are two reasons why the SF index may be abnormal. First,

unreliable patients will give unreliable visual fields. The unreliable patient is likely to have increased fixation losses as well. More importantly, the perimetrist who performed the test will offer the comment that the patient was not reliable. Second, patients with true glaucoma will give variable responses, since the defective area of the visual field may be unstable as a consequence of the disease process.

Both unreliable patients and those with visual field loss may have increased false negatives and an abnormal SF index. One can differentiate the two by looking at the threshold values for the retested points, which appear in parentheses below the first value. An unreliable patient will have increased fluctuation at most of the retested points. However, those with real disease will have large fluctuation in the defective areas but little fluctuation in the normal areas. Although it helps to explain the dynamics of perimetry, the SF index has not been shown to assist in separating normal from abnormal visual fields. It is not tested in the SITA strategies because of its limited value, and it is recommended that it be turned off in the interest of reducing test times with standard threshold and FASTPAC strategies.

Corrected Pattern Standard Deviation

In patients with an elevated SF index and visual field loss, some defects may be overemphasized; that is, a 6-dB defect may only be a 3-dB defect if retested. The corrected pattern standard deviation (CPSD) represents the PSD index adjusted for SF to help differentiate defects or depressions due to normal fluctuation from those due to disease. The values are weighted by location and the CPSD looks for focal defects. Therefore, with increased SF, it is possible to have an abnormal PSD index but a normal CPSD index. SF can be turned off in the user-defined menu of the HFA-1 and HFA-2; this is strongly encouraged to save test time. Although the CPSD will not be calculated, the PSD index is still calculated and the visual field is better analyzed by the GHT and cluster analysis.

The global indices are conveniently graphed in the change-analysis format to enable the practitioner to tell quickly whether a trend is evident. It remains the clinician's task to determine whether the trend is clinically significant (Tables 16–3 and 16–4).

FOLLOWING FOR CHANGE OVER TIME

Perhaps no task in perimetry is more vexing than judging progressive visual field loss. A number of confounding variables are encountered. First, many glaucoma patients are of the age when small pupils

TABLE 16–3. CRITERIA FOR ABNORMALITY WITH FULL THRESHOLD, FASTPAC, AND SITA FIELDS

1. GHT marked "outside normal limits" (not available with FASTPAC)
2. Cluster criteria
3. Abnormal CPSD global index (not available with any SITA fields, not available when SF is turned off)

Key: GHT, glaucoma hemifield test; CPSD, corrected pattern standard deviation; SITA, Swedish interactive thresholding algorithm; SF, short-term fluctuation.
Note: In patients with moderate to advanced disease, one or more of these criteria are expected to be met. In mild disease, only one may be met and close correlation with the rest of the clinical presentation is required.

TABLE 16–4. STEPS FOR SINGLE FIELD ANALYSIS

1. Verify that the correct test and strategy have been used.
2. Establish that the field is reliable.
3. Examine gray scale for any areas of concern, verify with threshold values and probability plots.
4. Apply criteria for abnormality (see Table 16–3):
   Look for significant cluster of abnormal points in pattern-deviation plots.
   Look at GHT message.
   Look at CPSD global index if available.

Key: GHT, glaucoma hemifield test; CPSD, corrected pattern standard deviation.
Note: Random defects occur in normal patients, especially in the first few fields. To be considered abnormal, a field defect should be repeatable over at least two fields.

and progressive cataract formation are prevalent, adding an overall depression that may mimic or mask true progression. Second, older patients are more susceptible to artifacts such as dermatochalasis or fatigue, which may increase as the patient ages (Fig. 16–23).[43] Third, the deeper the initial defect, the greater the random fluctuation in threshold values at the next test.[68,69] Long-term fluctuation, which increases as the visual field worsens, is the primary obstacle to detecting progression. It is against this background of artifact-generated noise that the practitioner must determine whether there is sight-threatening progression.

Two types of patients are followed for progression: those with normal visual fields and those with established defects.

In following patients with normal visual fields, the practitioner will apply the techniques for single visual field analysis to determine whether the visual field has progressed. The practitioner simply has to decide whether the visual field is now abnormal.

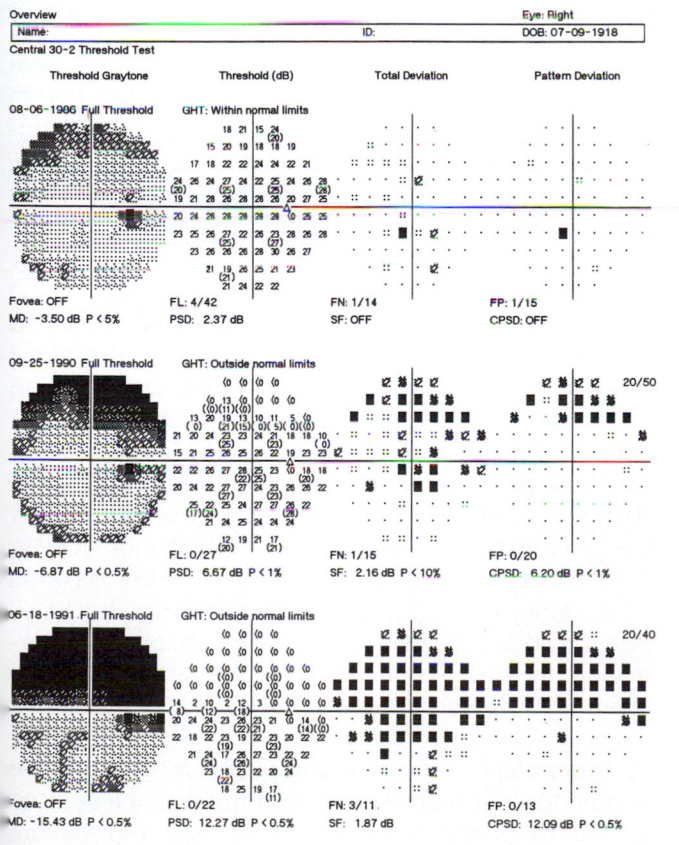
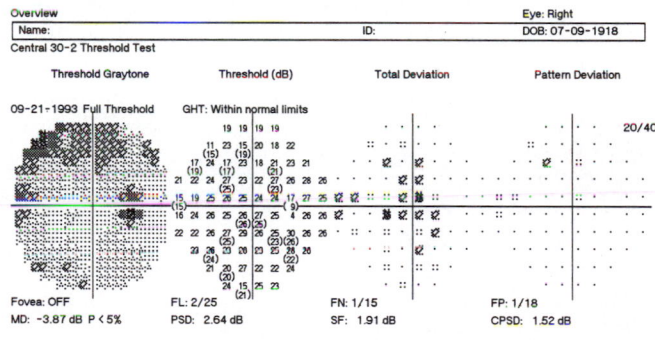

Figure 16–23. *A.* Monocular patient with apparent glaucomatous progression over 5 years. *B.* When the upper lid was taped to correct dermatochalasis, the visual field reverted to normal. Inspection of threshold values in suspected areas of progression showed straight rows of absolute defects superiorly corresponding to a ptotic upper lid. Temporally, there were absolute defects from the dermatochalasis.

When a visual field suddenly converts to abnormal in a patient with an unchanged clinical course, caution is urged. Numerous investigators have documented that reliable, normal patients will demonstrate apparent defects in their visual fields. In addition to random points, which can be depressed by as much as 11 dB, contiguous points, too, can appear depressed in some normal visual fields.[70,71] The main difference between these random fluctuations in a normal patient and true visual field defects due to disease is that true defects are repeatable. When the normal patient is retested, random defects due to normal physiological variation will be in other locations or absent.[72] True defects, though they may fluctuate in depth, will occur in the same point or region consistently, underscoring the importance of spatial information for accurate interpretation. Therefore, in order to be sure that the patient has a true defect, the visual field test must be repeated to demonstrate that the defect is reproducible.[73,74] In the case of very early, shallow defects, up to three visual fields may be needed to prove that an abnormality is present (Figs. 16–24, 16–25, and 16–26).

In a patient with an established visual field loss, follow-up visual fields are used to confirm that a defect is reproducible as well as to determine whether the visual field is stable or deteriorating. Since visual field defects are known to progress in glaucoma despite normalized

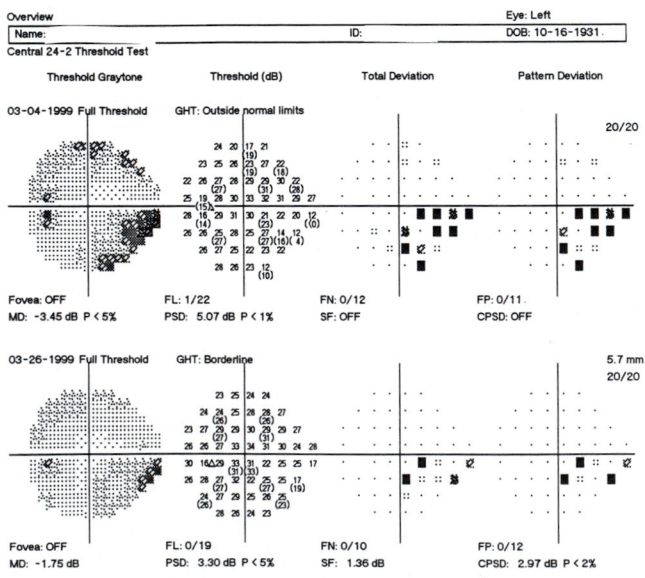

Figure 16–24. Inferior arcuate defect in the initial visual field with a significant cluster of defective points as well as a GHT message of "outside normal limits." Visual field testing was repeated less than 1 month later. The defect was smaller and shallower but repeatable (same area is defective in two consecutive visual field tests). The GHT message was now "borderline," but there was still a significant cluster of defective points.

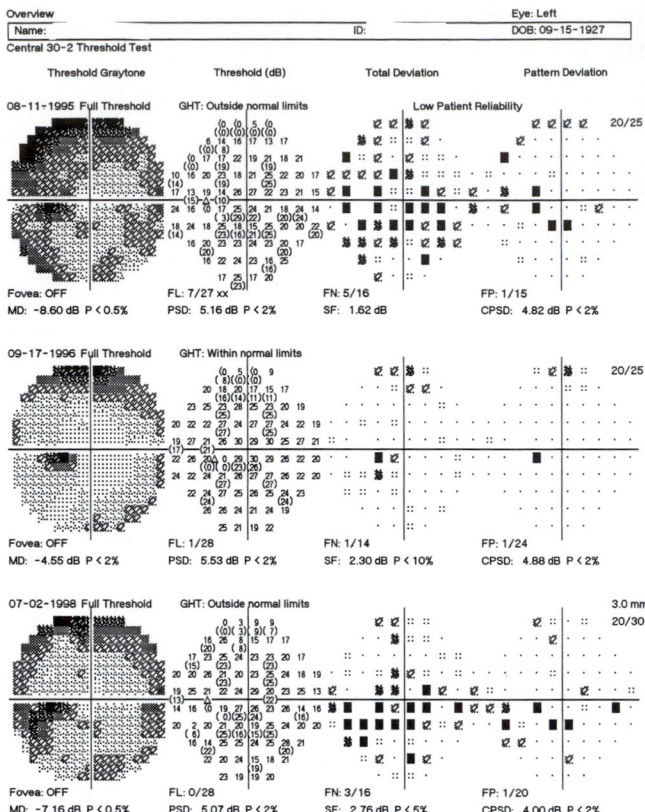

Figure 16–25. Initial visual field from 1996 showed an inferior arcuate visual field defect as revealed by the pattern-deviation plot and an overall depression seen in the gray scale and total-deviation plot. In 1996, neither the overall depression nor the inferior arcuate defect was present. In 1998, the inferior arcuate defect is again present, involving the same points. Small, shallow defects may frequently fluctuate between normal and abnormal. Although not present on consecutive visual field tests, the involved area should be considered a true defect if it is present on a majority of tests.

IOP, they play a key role in the management of the disease. Visual fields will typically progress in one of three ways: First, an existing defect may enlarge, involving previously normal contiguous points. Second, it may get deeper, with defective points losing additional sensitivity. Third, previously normal areas of the visual field not contiguous with established defects may become abnormal. Progression may occur in any combination of these three ways, though most commonly a defect becomes deeper (Fig. 16–27).[75] Although the analysis of a single visual field entails assimilating a large amount of information, the analysis of change over time demands the ability to assimilate the information from several visual fields simultaneously.

Any display of serial visual fields for the purpose of monitoring progression should involve one or more of the following components: spatial information, depth of defect information, trend of the visual field

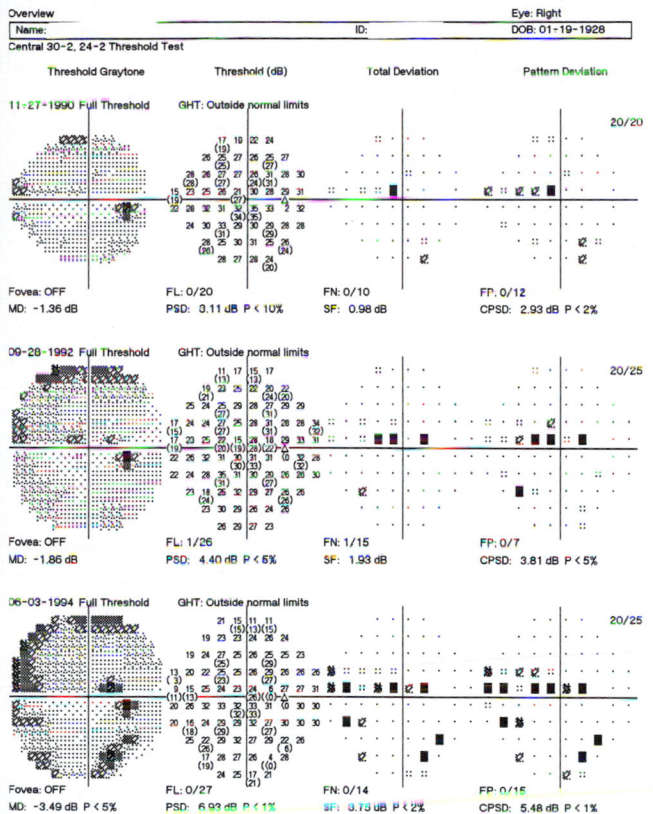

Figure 16–26. Progression in shallow superior arcuate visual field defect over 8 years (not all visual fields shown) Note that in 1990, the superior arcuate defect was clearly identifiable by the probability plots but was too shallow to be noted on the gray scale. As the defect continued to deepen and enlarge, the probability plots depicted this change fairly accurately. In mild loss of visual field, small, shallow defects are best followed with the probability plots.

status, and the significance of any change displayed. Spatial information will identify which points are changing, whether the size of the defects is increasing, the pattern of the defect, whether new defects are present, and if so, where they are. Depth information will show the deviation from normal and may also calculate the change from baseline. The trend of the visual field status is the overall view of the direction in which the visual field is headed. Trends may be displayed with or without statistical interpretation. Significance of change attempts to interpret the trend of the visual field. It employs statistical analysis such as linear regression of data, empirical databases, or intuitive algorithms to interpret the change and decide whether the change represents true progression.

The HFA-1 and HFA-2 use two techniques to aid in monitoring change over time. First, the presentation format is altered to allow easier viewing of several visual fields simultaneously. This is accomplished either by the overview or by the change-analysis printout.

The second technique employs both a format change and statistical analysis; the glaucoma change probability analysis serves to identify change and to determine whether it is statistically significant.

Overview

In this format the gray scale, threshold values, and the total and pattern-deviation probability plots are reduced in size and displayed across the page. Pupil size, visual acuity, fixation loss, false negatives, false positives, GHT messages, and the global indices are also displayed in a compact format. Up to 16 visual fields from one eye can be printed on a continuous sheet with the internal dot matrix printer on the HFA-1 or up to three visual fields to a page with an external laser printer.

The gray scales, which can show which areas are suspect and the pattern of the loss, should be scanned

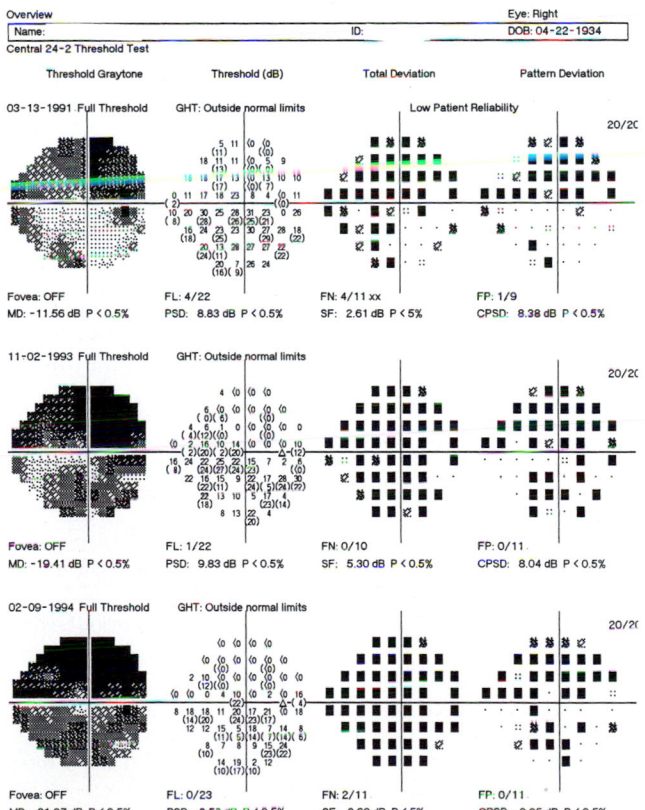

Figure 16–27. Progression in a deep superior arcuate defect in the visual field over 3 years (not all visual fields shown). In 1991, the superior visual field was severely depressed, with most points reaching a *p* value of <0.5%. Most threshold values were in the teens. By 1994, most of the points in the superior visual field were absolute defects. The probability plots remained unchanged while the gray scale readily depicted the decline. Once points are assigned a "black box" in the probability plots, further loss cannot be depicted. In visual fields with moderate to severe loss, more attention should be paid to the gray scale and threshold values.

for any apparent changes. Unlike the probability plots, the gray scale is capable of representing deepening of scotomas. By scanning the gray scales, an overall trend in the visual field is quickly ascertained. Gray scales are very susceptible to artifacts, and the other components of the printout must be used to confirm the significance of the gray-scale findings. By examining the magnitude of the change in the raw threshold values that was highlighted by the gray scale, some sense of significance is obtained. Any change of 10 dB merits attention. Still, serial examination of all 54 or 76 data points over multiple visual fields is tedious and not feasible. It is usually done with those points highlighted by the gray scale or probability plots.

In watching for progression, the pattern-deviation plot and threshold values are important displays in early to moderate disease. New defects and enlarging defects will be easily spotted by observing the pattern-deviation plots. However, it must be kept in mind that probability plots have a limited ability to recognize deepening of a defect. As a defect deepens, this change in threshold values is readily reflected in the change in the probability plots, but only up to a point. For most central points, less than 25% of the expected sensitivity has to be lost before it is represented by the highest level of significance, the black box representing $p < 0.5\%$. Once a black box is assigned to a point, no further reduction in sensitivity can be represented. The actual threshold values for all points with a $p < 0.5\%$ (black box) must be monitored

with extreme vigilance to determine whether the point has worsened on follow-up. This can be a daunting task when many points over several visual fields must be checked manually. Tables 16–5, 16–6, and 16–7 list guidelines for considering whether a change in threshold values is clinically significant and represents true progression of a defect (Figs. 16–28 and 16–29).

Change Analysis

The change-analysis printout graphs the global indices for each visual field performed on a patient, allowing the practitioner to look for trends. Still, global indices fail to account for spatial information—i.e., which part of the visual field is changing. For example, a decline in the MD index may represent a small decline at all points or a dramatic loss in a few. Therefore, although a graph of the indices may show a trend, it remains incumbent on the practitioner to determine whether it is significant. With regard to the MD index, one study has suggested that if the first visual field is mildly to moderately abnormal, a change in MD index of about 5 to 7 dB is required to represent a clinically significant change.[76] True progression of the visual field may occur with a smaller change in the MD, but since the visual fields of glaucoma patients are known to fluctuate markedly, only a large change can be considered true progression. If five threshold visual fields are available, STATPAC will perform a linear regression analysis to determine whether the change over time is different from that seen in normals. A probability value is assigned to indicate whether the rate of decline in the MD index is significant. Global indices are best used to highlight trends that should direct the examiner's attention to the other displays to determine whether true progression has occurred.

The change-analysis printout also includes a modified bar graph, called a box plot, of the threshold values. The amount that each value deviates above

TABLE 16–5. CRITERIA FOR PROGRESSION BASED ON THE NORMAL-TENSION GLAUCOMA STUDY[56]

1. Establish "baseline field" for comparison:
   Average two or three fields, select fields that are reliable and accurate.
   Note all values obtained for each point in the baseline fields.
2. For areas that were normal in the baseline, to progress to abnormal:
   Three contiguous points on the same side of horizontal must decrease.
   One point has to decrease by 10 dB as indicated on the total-deviation values.
   Two points must decrease by at least 5 dB as seen on the total-deviation values.
   New abnormal value must be greater than any value in baseline for that point.
3. For areas that were abnormal in the baseline:
   At least two contiguous points on the same side of horizontal must decrease by at least 10 dB or three times the average STF in the baseline, whichever is the higher value.
   New value for the point suspected of progressing must be lower than any value recorded in the baseline tests for that specific point.

TABLE 16–6. ANALYZING FOR PROGRESSION USING GLAUCOMA CHANGE PROBABILITY

1. Verify that the correct baseline fields have been selected.
2. Compare gray scale for enlarging or deepening defect (watch for artifact).
3. Compare total deviation probability plots.
4. Look at deviation from baseline decibel values. Identify any change of 10 dB.
5. Look at change probability plots for clusters of points that have progressed.
6. To be suspect for progression, change should involve at least two points and be repeatable over at least two other confirming fields.

TABLE 16-7. OVERALL APPROACH TO ASSESSING FOR PROGRESSION

1. Print out overview.
2. Assess gray scales and probability plots for areas of concern.
3. Correlate suspected areas with threshold values.
4. Review clinical course and select appropriate baseline fields.
5. Apply Normal-Tension Glaucoma Study criteria (see Table 16-5).
6. Select appropriate baseline and print out glaucoma change probability.
7. Assess gray scales and total-deviation plots.
8. Apply glaucoma change probability criteria (see Table 16-6).

Note: When in doubt, repeat field in 1 to 3 months.

(+) or below (−) the age-matched STATPAC database is rank-ordered from the best to worst points. The median value of these deviations is noted by a stripe in the box and 1 SD of good and bad points is noted by the ends of the box. The box represents 70% of the deviation values. Extending from the top of the box (better points) is a tail that will stop at the value of the best point. Extending from the bottom of the box (worse points) is a tail that will stop at the value of the

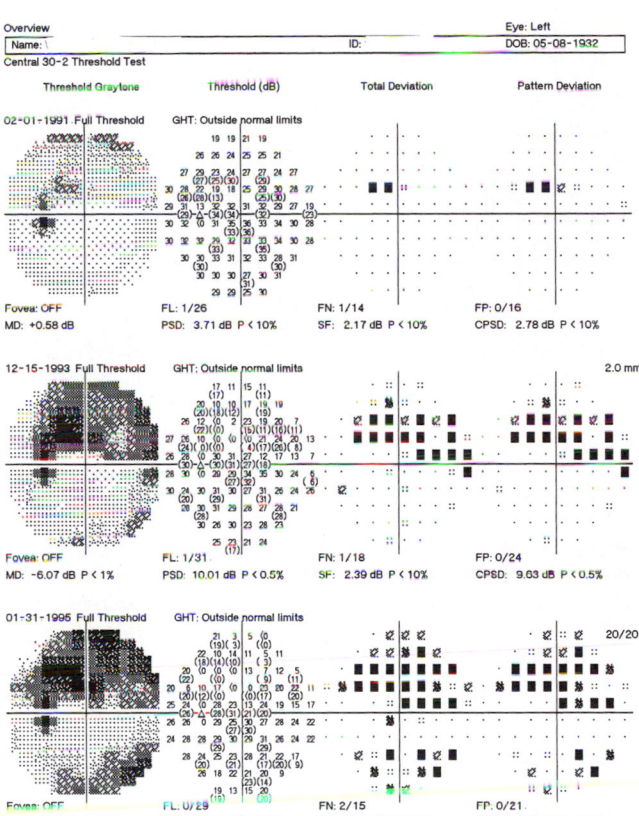

Figure 16–29. Rapid rate of progression in a superior arcuate defect over 5 years. The superior defect deepened and widened during this time. A new defect began in the inferior visual field in 1995.

worst point. At the left of the display is a box plot representing a normal patient for that age. By comparing the height and shape of the patient's box plot to that of the normal, valuable information can be quickly ascertained.

If the box plot looks identical to the normal, yet continues to be graphed lower on follow-up, it indicates that the HOV is not changing shape but is becoming depressed, probably secondary to a cataract. If the bottom of the box plot remains at about the same level and the tail begins to extend downward, it is an indication that a scotoma may be deepening. If the bottom of the box gets lower while the median remains the same, a scotoma may be enlarging. If the bottom of the box elongates and the top shrinks while the median is getting worse, then a scotoma is getting larger and/or new scotomas are appearing. Note that once the tail or bottom of the box reaches −22 dB, no further deepening can be represented on the graph (Fig. 16–30).

Glaucoma Change Probability

The Glaucoma Change Probability (GCP) is based on empirical data collected from a small group of stable

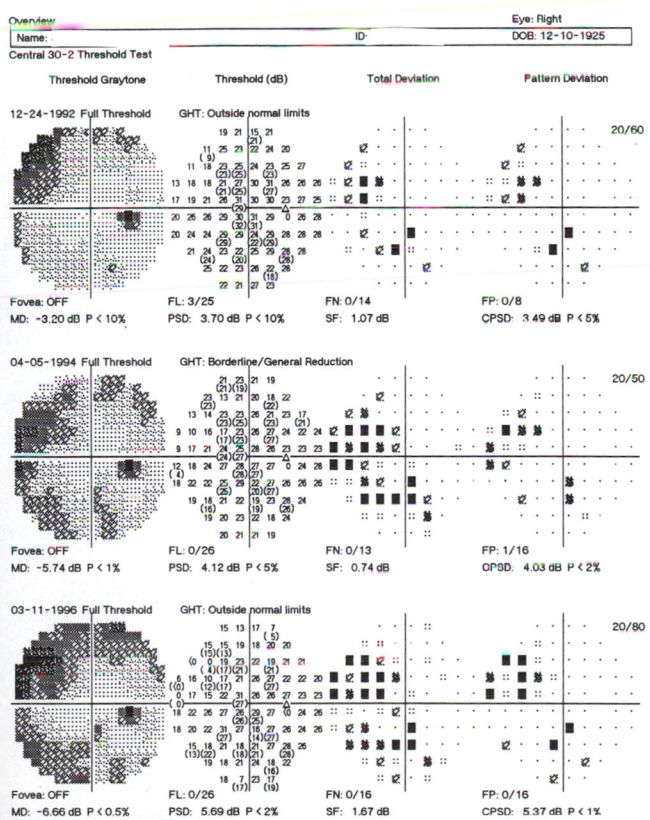

Figure 16–28. Medium rate of progression in a superior nasal step defect over 5 years. Most points lost approximately 10 dB. Both gray scale and probability plots indicate a worsening.

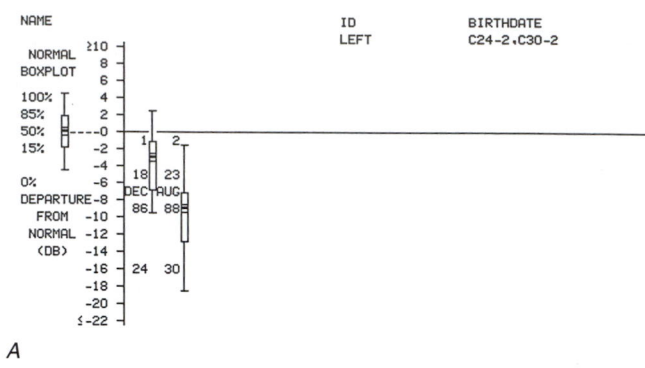

A

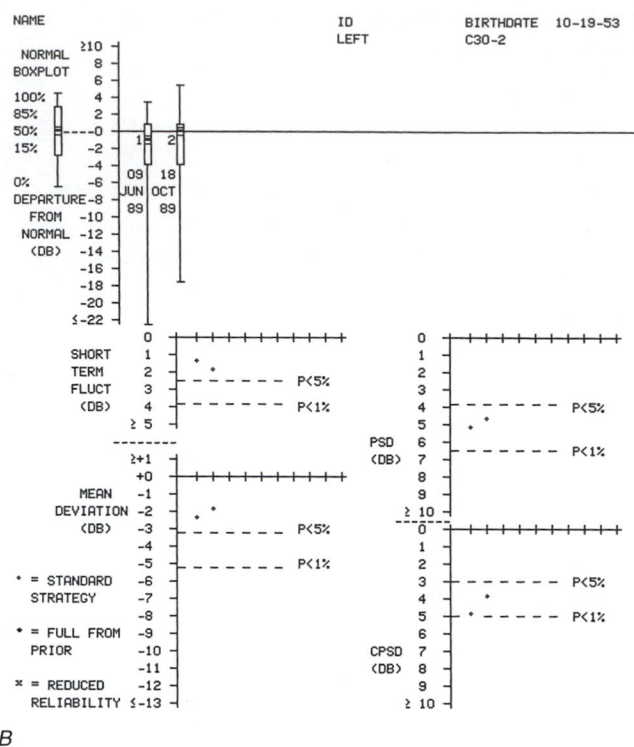

B

Figure 16–30. *A.* In this box plot display of two visual fields, the body of the box (70% of all points) did not elongate in the second test; rather, it shifted downward, indicating an increased overall depression. Both tails elongated, increasing the difference between the worst and best points. *B.* Note that the better half of the visual field (above the median) improved between tests, but the tail remained elongated because of several significantly depressed points. The MD index showed improvement (learning effect), while the PSD index remained abnormal (focal loss).

glaucoma patients. The data were derived by repeating the field every week for a month, measuring the fluctuation between tests of the individual points. An assumption was made that since the database was collected within a month while the IOP was controlled, no progression occurred. Any change in threshold values reflects long-term fluctuation rather than worsening of the disease. Both the initial depth of the defect and its eccentricity were found to influence the amount of long-term fluctuation, requiring these points to demonstrate a greater change to be considered clinically significant.

The GCP is available for all standard threshold visual fields on the HFA-2 and on those with the STATPAC II upgrade to the HFA-1. At present, no GCP is available for visual fields performed with the SITA strategy, but the database has been gathered and its release is anticipated.

A minimum of three visual fields are necessary for this analysis. The GCP will average the first two threshold visual fields and use them as the baseline. Each subsequent visual field is then compared to the baseline. The GCP will attempt to recognize a poor initial visual field and discard it if it is not similar to the second visual field. However, this determination by the GCP is often inaccurate, and it is incumbent on the practitioner to select the visual fields to be used for the baseline. Additionally, once a documented progression

has occurred, it is necessary to reset the baseline to the most recent visual fields and disregard earlier visual fields. This must be done by the perimetrist prior to printing the test as directed by the practitioner.

The glaucoma change probability format will print a gray scale and a total-deviation probability plot, similar to the overview printout. The GCP will also display the degree to which each point has changed, in decibels, as compared with the baseline. These values can rapidly be scanned for points that have progressed by 10 dB or more. A new probability plot is generated by the GCP. When a point has decreased from the baseline more than predicted from the database of controlled glaucoma patients, a black triangle appears. Statistically, the probability that this change occurred by chance rather than because of disease is < 5%. If the point has improved significantly, an open triangle appears. If there is no significant change, a dot is shown. Because of the statistics and the level of probability involved, a stable visual field can show a few improved points and a few progressing points each time the analysis is performed. Subsequent visual fields are needed to confirm any suspected worsening (Figs. 16–31 and 16–32).

The GCP analysis for detecting change over time in the visual fields of a glaucoma patient has several limitations. First, there is very little information in the database for very depressed points (a mean deviation

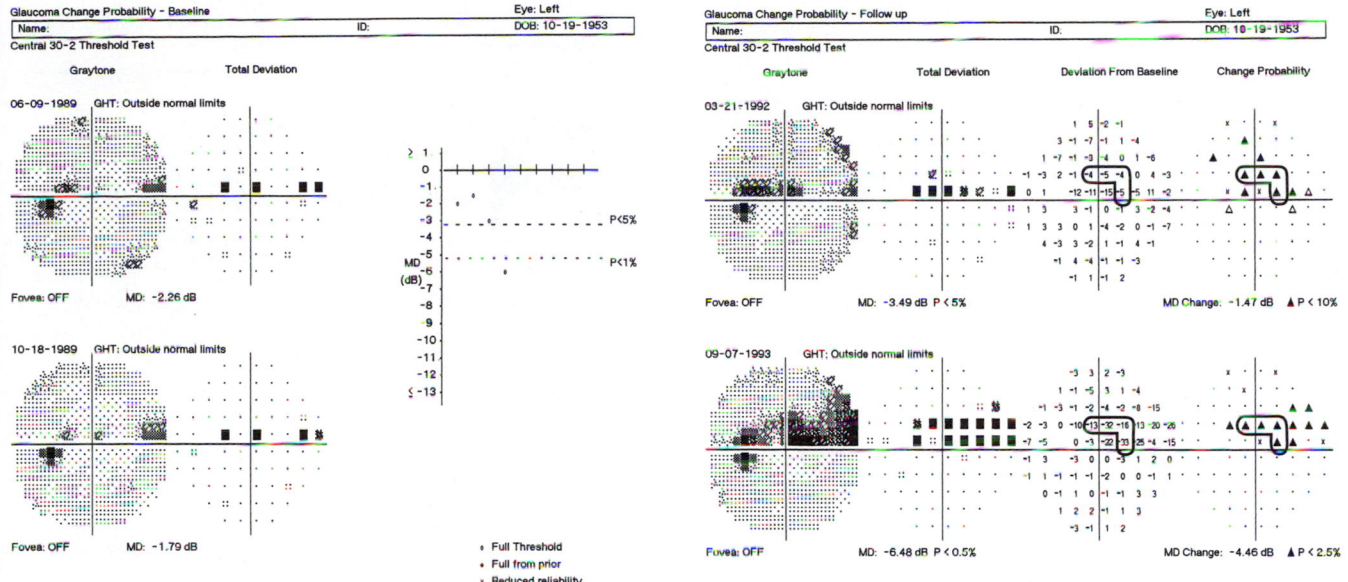

Figure 16–31. Aggressive progression is seen with glaucoma change probability (GCP). Baseline visual fields in 1989 showed a partial arcuate defect with paracentral points and nasal step. The paracentral point closest to the optic nerve averaged 13 dB in the baseline, while the point next to fixation averaged 20 dB. By 1992, these two points had decreased by 12 and 15 dB, respectively, as noted on the delta dB from baseline display. The point between these two had decreased by 11 dB as well. Three contiguous points decreasing by 10 dB meets a common rule of thumb for progression. All three have decreased significantly according to the empirically derived database and are marked by a black delta *(triangle)*. Also note the four adjacent points that are highlighted. In 1992 they had declined by only 4 to 5 dB, yet they were noted to have changed significantly when compared to the empirical database. By 1993, these four points had decreased by 13 to 33 decibels.

greater than –15 dB), and it will not be able to determine the significance of change over time in these points. These points are marked with an "x." This is unfortunate, since these areas are the ones closest to blindness. Similarly, there is little information on glaucoma patients with either normal visual fields or minimal visual field loss. Points from these visual fields that have improved or have minimal loss will also be marked with an "x," making the visual field difficult to interpret. The GCP should not be used with normal visual fields; rather, the patient should be followed with the overview display with attention to the GHT and looking out for new significant clusters of defects. Once a defect is established, the GCP will be appropriate for use in follow-up visual fields.

Second, the software used to select the baseline often exercises poor judgment. Thus, it may appear the patient is improving or remaining stable simply because subsequent visual fields are compared to an inappropriate baseline, contaminated by an artificially depressed initial visual field. Remember, too, that current tests are compared to a baseline that may be years old and are not compared to the most recent visual field examination.

Third, the practitioner must reset the baseline once a worsening in the visual field has been recognized. A patient may truly progress between his or her third and fourth tests and then stabilize. If the practitioner continues to compare subsequent visual fields to the old baseline, a false impression of continued progression will be made. The most recent visual fields after progression has been documented must be set as the baseline.

Fourth, the GCP display does not take into account any change in sensitivity from cataracts or miosis. Although the analysis does factor in a decrease in sensitivity with age as it judges change from baseline, overall depression from cataracts and miosis is indistinguishable from disease to the GCP, and points will be erroneously flagged as progressed. Subsequent versions of this software not yet released will try to correct for overall depression, perhaps with the general height indicator, before analyzing for progression.

Two final issues must be discussed concerning progression. First, *how many* visual field examinations are necessary to confirm progression? Long-term fluctuation remains the biggest confounding variable, causing large random changes in threshold values,

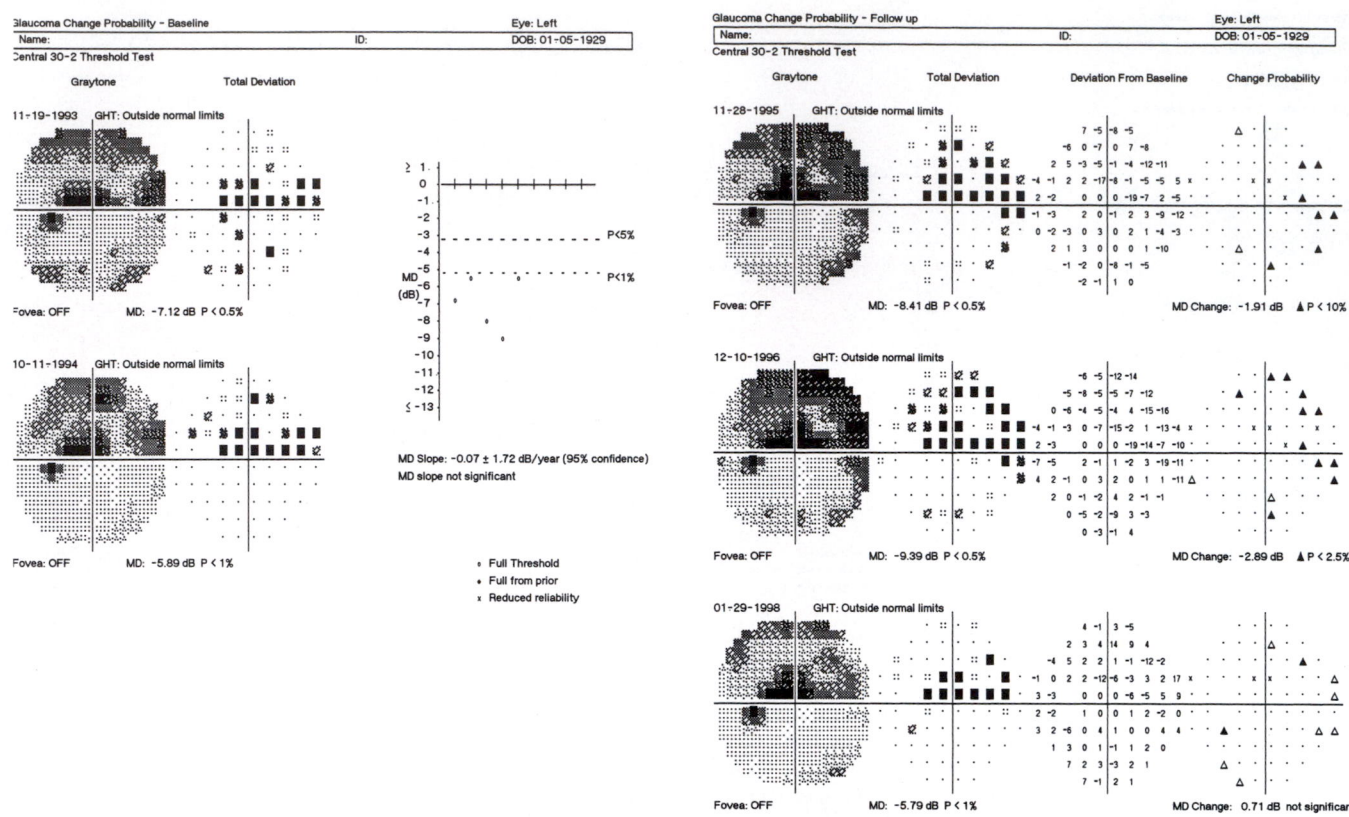

Figure 16–32. After baseline established in 1994, apparent progression occurred in the superior arcuate defect in 1995 and was "confirmed" in 1996. However, subsequent visual fields in 1998 reverted to approximately baseline status. Large fluctuations occurring in the same location consecutively can mimic progression. When the intraocular pressure has been well controlled and the optic nerve appears unchanged, it is essential to repeat the visual field test several times to confirm progression. Even in 1998, there still appear to be three points that have progressed in the superior visual field. The two points above fixation are marked with "x" because of the limited information in the GCP database. Inspection of the threshold values (not shown) for these points showed that the first two points had markedly decreased between the 1993 and 1994 baseline and had remained unchanged, but the value in subsequent visual fields was still significantly lower than the average value used in the baseline. Only the superior nasal point had declined since the baseline.

particularly those points that are most depressed. Conventional wisdom has dictated that a minimum of two or more visual fields are necessary to confirm progression. When the clinical course of the disease is poor, with failure to control IOP or suspected disc progression, perhaps only two visual fields are necessary to "confirm" progression. However, if the IOP has been at the target pressure during the interval under question and the optic nerves appear unchanged, three visual fields may be necessary to convince the skeptical practitioner that further therapeutic intervention is warranted. This skepticism is further justified when surgical intervention is contemplated.

Second, *how often* should visual field examinations be performed? When trying to detect change, two paths may be chosen, and the number of visual fields

depends on the path. If one is trying to determine the earliest change, with minimal progression, the small change in threshold values will be difficult to discern against long-term fluctuation. Only multiple visual fields, as employed by the NTG study with up to six visual fields in 6 months, may be able to reliably detect a subtle change against long-term fluctuation. The other path is to allow a greater change (loss) in threshold sensitivity to occur, requiring fewer visual fields to be certain that long-term fluctuation is not responsible. Clinically, the second path is typically chosen, as there is a limit to how many visual field examinations a patient is willing to undergo.

What is known clinically is that some patients progress rapidly, with marked visual field loss occurring within several years or less, while other patients will show minimal loss over 5 years or longer. More visual field examinations should be performed on those patients with the highest risk factors for progression: large cup-to-disc ratio, extensive loss of nerve fiber, defects approaching fixation, poorly controlled IOP, and so on. Perhaps those patients who have exhibited stable visual fields over several years with no change in their clinical course could have visual field examinations performed at 2-year intervals. Finally, the life expectancy of the patient should be weighed against the known aggressiveness of the disease. Clearly, the approach to an 80-year-old patient with minimal visual field loss is different from that to the 50-year-old with defects approaching fixation. The former might receive no more than an annual visual field examination, while the latter would need perhaps two to three visual field examinations per year to assure stability and preservation of acuity (Table 16–8).

CONCLUSION

Visual field examinations are critical to the diagnosis and management of glaucoma. The presence of a defect confirms the diagnosis of glaucoma even in the absence of a detectable elevation of IOP. Progressive visual field loss despite IOP "control" is also common; therefore, perimetry provides the best monitor for the disease. Today's state-of-the-art instruments allow automated static threshold perimetry to be performed in an accurate, reproducible fashion in any office. Automated perimetry represents the greatest advancement in glaucoma management in the past 30 years.

The deficiencies of the instrument must also be recognized. Although automated perimetry is a very sensitive test of visual function, up to 20% of the optic nerve may still be lost before a defect is detectable.[77] The absence of a visual field defect does not rule out the diagnosis of glaucoma in the presence of other compelling clinical findings.[78] Some patients give unreliable responses during testing some of the time, while others give unreliable answers most of the time. Multiple attempts with different test strategies may be necessary before the clinician is convinced that the patient is incapable of performing an automated visual field examination and that manual techniques will be needed. Automation of the testing procedure has not eliminated the need for a skilled and diligent technician to be present with the patient during the test. The greater the technician's skills, the more likely he or she will be to recognize an artifact or patient fatigue and intercede to modify the test. The skilled technician will eliminate the need to discard many "unreliable" visual fields.

Perhaps the greatest challenge confronting the clinician is mastering the interpretation of the results and the integration of these findings into the total clinical picture. The cornerstone of modern perimetry is the statistical database of visual field test results from normal patients, which aids in the decision-making process. Although these databases are invaluable, they do not remove responsibility from the practitioner in the decision-making process. It is incumbent on the clinician always to remember that statistics deal with numerical events, while the clinician deals with patients and their disease.

TABLE 16–8. VISUAL FIELD TESTING SCHEME

Glaucoma suspect, first field:
Start with full field 120
If normal, do threshold in 3 to 6 months
If abnormal, do threshold in 1 to 3 months
or
Start with FASTPAC 24-2 or 30-2
If normal, do full threshold in 3 to 6 months
If abnormal, do full threshold in 1 to 3 months
or
Start with SITA Standard 24-2 or 30-2
If normal, repeat as dictated by severity of disease
Known glaucoma patient:
Follow with full threshold or SITA standard
Repeat until no learning curve/artifact
Thereafter, twice a year for end-stage disease or suspicion for aggressive progression
Repeat once a year for well-controlled patients, consider every 2 years if patients are well controlled and there has been no documented change in at least 5 years of yearly field exams
If progression is suspected:
Repeat in 1 to 3 months

ACKNOWLEDGMENT

The author wishes to express his deepest gratitude and appreciation to Vincent Michael Patella, O.D., for his technical assistance, guidance, and unlimited patience in the preparation of this chapter.

REFERENCES

1. Haley MJ. The Field Analyzer Primer. San Leandro, CA: Humphrey Instruments, Inc; 1987.
2. Heijl A, Lindgren G. Normal variability of static threshold values across the central visual field. *Arch Ophthalmol.* 1987;105:1544–1549.
3. Katz J, Sommer A. Asymmetry and variation in the normal hill of vision. *Arch Ophthalmol.* 1986;104:65–68.

4. Heijl A, Lindgren G, Olsson J. A package for the statistical analysis of visual fields. *Doc Ophthalmol Proc Ser.* 1987;49:153–168.

5. Budenz DL, Fuer, WJ, Anderson, DR. The effect of simulated cataract on the glaucomatous visual field. *Ophthalmology.* 1993;100:511–517.

6. Lam BL, Alward WL, Kolder HE. Effect of cataract on automated perimetry. *Ophthalmology.* 1991;98:1066–1070.

7. Aulhorn E, Harms H. Early visual field defects in glaucoma. In: Leydecker W, ed. *Glaucoma: Tutzig Symposium.* Basel: Karger; 1967:151–186.

8. Siatowski RM, Lam BL, Anderson DR, et al. Automated suprathreshold static perimetry screening for detecting neuro-ophthalmologic disease. *Ophthalmology* 1996;103: 907–917.

9. Marraffa M, Marchini G, Albertini R, Bonomi L. Comparison of different screening methods for the detection of visual field defects in early glaucoma. *Int Ophthalmol.* 1989;13:43–45.

10. Kosoko O, Sommer A, Auer C. Screening with automated periphery using a threshold-related three level algorithm. *Ophthalmology.* 1986;93:882–886.

11. Katz J, Tielsch JM, Quigley HA, et al. Automated perimetry detects visual field loss prior to manual Goldmann perimetry. *Ophthalmology.* 1995;102:21–26.

12. Trope GE, Britton R. A comparison of Goldmann and Humphrey automated perimetry in patients with glaucoma. *Br J Ophthalmol.* 1987;71:489–493.

13. Beck RW, Bergstrom TJ, Lichter PR. A clinical comparison of visual field testing with a new automated perimeter, the Humphrey field analyzer and the Goldmann perimeter. *Ophthalmology.* 1985;92:77–82.

14. Tielsch JM, Sommer A, Katz J, et al. Racial variations in the prevalence of primary open-angle glaucoma. The Baltimore Eye Survey. *JAMA.* 1991;266:369–374.

15. Lalle PA, Fingeret M, Eiden SB. Automated perimetry in the management of glaucoma. *J Am Optom Assoc.* 1989; 60:900–911.

16. Heijl A. Automatic perimetry in glaucoma visual field screening: A clinical study. *Graefes Arch Clin Exp Ophthalmol.* 1976;200:21–27.

17. Heijl A, Lundqvist L. The location of earliest glaucomatous defects documented by automatic perimetry. *Doc Ophthalmol Proc Ser.* 1983;35:153–158.

18. Araujo ML, Feurer WJ, Anderson DR. Evaluation of baseline-related suprathreshold testing for quick determination of visual field progression. *Arch Ophthalmol.* 1993;11:365–369.

19. Flanagan JG, Wild JM, Trope GE. Evaluation of FASTPAC, a new strategy for threshold estimation with the Humphrey field analyzer, in a glaucomatous population. *Ophthalmology.* 1993;100:949–954.

20. O'Brien C, Poinoosawmy D, Hitchings R. Evaluation of the Humphrey FASTPAC threshold program in glaucoma. *Br J Ophthalmol* 1994;78:516–519.

21. Schaumberger M, Schafer B, Lachenmayr BJ. Glaucomatous visual fields: FASTPAC versus full threshold strategy of the Humphrey field analyzer. *Invest Ophthalmol Vis Sci.* 1995;7:1390–1397.

22. Searle AET, Wild JM, Shaw DE, et al. Time-related variation in normal automated static perimetry. *Ophthalmology.* 1991;98:701–707.

23. Heijl A, Drance SM. Changes in differential threshold in patients with glaucoma during prolonged perimetry. *Br J Ophthalmol.* 1983;67:512–516.

24. Jay JL. Computerised perimetry—the emperor's new clothes? *Br J Ophthalmol.* 1994;78:513–515.

25. Hatch W, Flanagan JG, Trope GE. Evaluation of repeatability of FASTPAC in glaucoma. In: Mills RP, Walls M, eds. *Perimetry Update 1994/1995: Proceedings of the XIth International Perimetric Society Meeting, Kyoto, 1994.* Amsterdam: Kugler; 1995: 239.

26. O'Donnel NP, Birch MK, Wishart PK. FASTPAC error is within the long-term fluctuation of Standard Humphrey threshold field testing. In: Mills RP, Walls M, eds. *Perimetry Update 1994/1995.* Amsterdam: Kugler; 1995:231.

27. Heijl A. Automatic perimetry in glaucoma visual field screening: A clinical study. *Graefes Arch Clin Exp Ophthalmol.* 1976;200:21–27.

28. Duggan C, Sommer A, Auer C, Burkhard K. Automated differential threshold perimetry for detecting glaucomatous visual field loss. *Am J Ophthalmol.* 1985;100:420–423.

29. Anderson DR, Patella VM. *Automated Static Perimetry.* St. Louis: Mosby; 1999:94.

30. Young WO, Stewart WC, Hunt H, et al. Static threshold variability in the peripheral visual field in normal subjects. *Graefes Arch Clin Exp Ophthalmol.* 1990;228:454–457.

31. Anderson DR, Patella VM. *Automated Static Perimetry.* St. Louis: Mosby; 1999;247.

32. Kolker AE. Visual prognosis in advanced glaucoma: A comparison of medical and surgical therapy for retention of vision. *Trans Am Ophthalmol Soc.* 1977;75:539–555.

33. Weber J, Schultze T, Ulrich H. The visual field in advanced glaucoma. *Int Ophthalmol.* 1989;13:47–50.

34. Zhang L, Drance DM, Douglas GR. Automated perimetry in detecting threats to fixation. *Ophthalmology.* 1997;104:1918–1920.

35. Heijl A, Lindgren G, Olsson J. Reliability parameters in computerized perimetry. *Doc Ophthalmol Proc Ser.* 1987; 49:593–600.

36. Heijl A, Krakau CET. An automatic static perimeter: Design and pilot study. *Acta Ophthalmol [Copenh].* 1975; 53:293–310.

37. Katz J, Sommer A. Reliability indices of automated perimetric tests. *Arch Ophthalmol.* 1988;106:1252–1254.

38. Katz J, Sommer A, Witt K. Reliability of visual field results over repeated testing. *Ophthalmology.* 1991;98:70–75.

39. Sanabria O, Feuer WJ, Anderson DR. Pseudo-fixation loss in automated perimetry. *Ophthalmology.* 1991; 98:76–78.

40. Hudson C, Wild JM, O'Neill EC. Fatigue effects during a single session of automated static threshold perimetry. *Invest Ophthalmol Vis Sci.* 1994;35:268–280.

41. Heijl A. Time changes of contrast thresholds during automated perimetry. *Acta Ophthalmol (KBH).* 1977;55: 696–708.

42. Heijl A, Drance SM. Changes in differential threshold in patients with glaucoma during prolonged perimetry. *Br J Ophthalmol.* 1983;67:512–516.

43. Fujimoto N, Adachi-Usami E. Fatigue effect within 10 degrees visual field in automated perimetry. *Ann Ophthalmol.* 1993;25:142–144.

44. Fingeret M. Clinical alternative for reducing the time needed to perform automated threshold perimetry. *J Am Optom Assoc.* 1995;66:699–705.

45. Bengtsson B, Olsson J, Heijl A, et al. A new generation of algorithms for computerized perimetry: SITA. *Acta Ophthalmol.* 1997; 75:368–375.

46. Bengtsson B, Olsson J, Heijl A. Evaluation of a new threshold visual field strategy, SITA, in normal subjects. *Acta Ophthalmol.* 1998;76:165–169.

47. Bengtsson B, Heijl A. Evaluation of a new perimetric threshold strategy, SITA, in patients with manifest and suspect glaucoma. *Acta Ophthalmol.* 1998;76:268–272.

48. Bengtsson B, Heijl A. SITA Fast, a new rapid perimetric threshold test: Description of methods and evaluation in patients with manifest and suspect glaucoma. *Acta Ophthalmol.* 1998;76:431–437.

49. Anderson DR, Patella VM. *Automated Static Perimetry.* St. Louis: Mosby; 1999:85–86.

50. Bengtsson B, Heijl A. Inter-subject variability and normal limits of the SITA standard, SITA fast, and the Humphrey full threshold computerized perimetry strategies, SITA STATPAC. *Acta Ophthalmol Scand.* 1999; 77:125–129.

51. Bengtsson B, Heijl A. Comparing significance and magnitude of glaucomatous visual field defects using the SITA and full threshold strategies. *Acta Ophthalmol Scand.* 1999;77:143–146.

52. Olsson J, Bengtsson B, Rootzen H. Improving estimation of false positive and false negative responses in computerized perimetry. In Mills RP, Wall M, eds: *Perimetry Update 1994/95.* Amsterdam: Kugler; 1995:265.

53. Heijl A, Lindgren G, Olsson J. The effect of perimetric experience in normal subjects. *Arch Ophthalmol.* 1989; 107:81–86.

54. Heijl A, Lindgren G, Olsson J, Asman P. Visual field interpretation with empiric probability maps. *Arch Ophthalmol.* 1989;107:204–208.

55. Schwartz B, Nagin P. Probability maps for evaluating automated visual fields. *Doc Ophthalmol Proc Ser.* 1985; 42:39–48.

56. Schulzer M. Normal-tension Glaucoma Study Group: Errors in the diagnosis of visual field progression in normal-tension glaucoma. *Ophthalmology.* 1994;101:1589–1595.

57. Guthauser U, Flammer J. Quantifying visual field damage caused by cataract. *Am J Ophthalmol.* 1988;106:480–484.

58. Wood JM, Wild JM, Smerdon DL, Crews SJ. Alterations in the shape of the automated perimetric profile arising from cataract. *Graefes Arch Clin Exp Ophthalmol.* 1989;227:157–161.

59. Lam BL, Alward WLM, Kolder HE. Effect of cataract on automated perimetry. *Ophthalmology.* 1991;98:1066–1070.

60. Katz J, Sommer A, Gaasterland D, Anderson DR. Comparison of analytic algorithms for detecting glaucomatous visual field loss. *Arch Ophthalmol.* 1991;109: 1684–1689.

61. Heijl A. Computerized perimetry in glaucoma management. *Acta Ophthalmol.* 1989;67:1–12.

62. Duggan C, Sommer A, Auer C, Burkhard K. Automated differential threshold perimetry for detecting glaucomatous visual field loss. *Am J Ophthalmol.* 1985;100:420–423.

63. Asman P, Heijl A. Glaucoma hemifield test: Automated visual field evaluation. *Arch Ophthalmol.* 1992;110: 812–819.

64. Asman P, Heijl A. Evaluation of methods for automated hemifield analysis in perimetry. *Arch Ophthalmol.* 1992; 110:820–826.

65. Enger C, Sommer A. Recognizing glaucomatous field loss with the Humphrey STATPAC. *Arch Ophthalmol.* 1987;106:1355–1357.

66. Feuer WJ, Anderson DR. Static threshold asymmetry in early glaucomatous visual field loss. *Ophthalmology.* 1989;96:1285–1297.

67. Fankhauser F, Bebie H. Threshold fluctuation, interpolations, and spacial resolution in perimetry. *Doc Ophthalmol.* 1979;19:296–306.

68. Heijl A, Lindgren A, Lindgren G. Test re-test variability in glaucomatous visual fields. *Am J Ophthalmol.* 1989; 108:130–135.

69. Werner EB, Petrig B, Krupin T, Bishop KI. Variability of automated visual fields in clinically stable glaucoma patients. *Invest Ophthalmol Vis Sci.* 1989;30:1083–1089.

70. Sommer A, Duggan C, Auer C, Abbey H. Analytic approaches to the interpretation of automated threshold perimetric data for the diagnosis of early glaucoma. *Trans Am Ophthalmol Soc.* 1985;83:250–267.

71. Heijl A, Asman P. A clinical study of perimetric probability maps. *Arch Ophthalmol.* 1989;107:199–203.

72. Wilensky JT, Joondeph BC. Variation in visual field measurements with an automated perimeter. *Am J Ophthalmol.* 1984;97:328–330.

73. Hoskins HD, Magee SD, Dreake MV, Kidd MN. Confidence intervals for change in automated visual fields. *Br J Ophthalmol.* 1988;72:591–597.

74. Katz J, Quigley HA, Sommer A. Repeatability of the Glaucoma Hemifield Test in automated perimetry. *Invest Ophthalmol Vis Sci.* 1995;36:1658–1664.

75. Mikelberg FS, Drance SM. The mode of progression of visual field defects in glaucoma. *Am J Ophthalmol.* 1984; 98:443–445.

76. Hoskins HD, Magee SD, Dreake MV, Kidd MN. Confidence intervals for change in automated visual fields. *Br J Ophthalmol.* 1988;72:591–597.

77. Quigley HA, Dunkelgerger BS, Green WR. Retinal ganglion cell atrophy correlated with automated perimetry in human eyes with glaucoma. *Am J Ophthalmol.* 1989; 107:453–464.

78. Sommer A, Katz J, Quigley HA, et al. Clinically detectable nerve fiber atrophy precedes the onset of glaucomatous field loss. *Arch Ophthalmol.* 1991;109:77–83.

Chapter 17

THE OCTOPUS PERIMETER

Michael A. Chaglasian

In 1976 Octopus introduced the first automated perimeter, the Octopus 201. Currently available instruments include the Octopus 1-2-3 and Octopus 101. The 1-2-3 unit utilizes the unique principle of direct retinal projection, while the 101 is a traditional bowl-projection unit. These instruments have a wide variety of clinical applications and their features, their operation, and the interpretation of their printouts are covered in this chapter.

OCTOPUS 1-2-3

Features

In 1989 Octopus introduced the 1-2-3 perimeter, which allows for the projection of a light stimulus directly onto the patient's retina (Fig. 17–1). Surrounding background light and a fixation target are also visualized by the patient with this system. One advantage that this instrument offers is its compact size. The base of the 1-2-3 measures 16×16 in., and the unit itself weighs only 55 lb. The projection unit rises above the base and has a small joystick to control its movement. Examinations do not have to be performed in a darkened room because stray light does not affect the background illumination. In addition, the optics of the instrument create a stimulus as if from an infinite point; thus a trial lens is used only for distance correction. A monitor screen contains both the menu selections and a video display of the

patient's eye. The keypad is located on the base, where the examiner enters patient data and makes selections from the menu items displayed on the monitor. Joystick movement of the projection head allows for patient alignment without any need to move the patient.[1]

The Octopus 1-2-3 uses a background illumination of 31.4 asb. This level is consistent with the Goldmann perimeter and other automated perimeters. This level also allows the patient to be examined under normal room illumination without concern for adaptation. For normal test programs, the stimulus size is set at Goldmann size III; for the low-vision program, a Goldmann size V stimulus is used. The duration of stimulus presentation is fixed at 100 ms. The optical projection system of the 1-2-3 limits the measurable visual field to the central 30 degrees from fixation. However, this is not usually a significant limitation, because approximately 90% of all glaucomatous and neurological field defects will initially present within this central 30-degree field. In addition, automated evaluation of the peripheral field (30 to 60 degrees) is often unreliable owing to artifact and variability.[2]

Another unique feature of the 1-2-3 is the fixation monitor, which will not allow a test stimulus to be presented unless the patient is attending to the fixation target. An infrared CCD camera system continuously monitors the patient's pupil in relation to a fixed centered cursor. If the patient moves his or her eye off of fixation or closes the eye during the examination, the

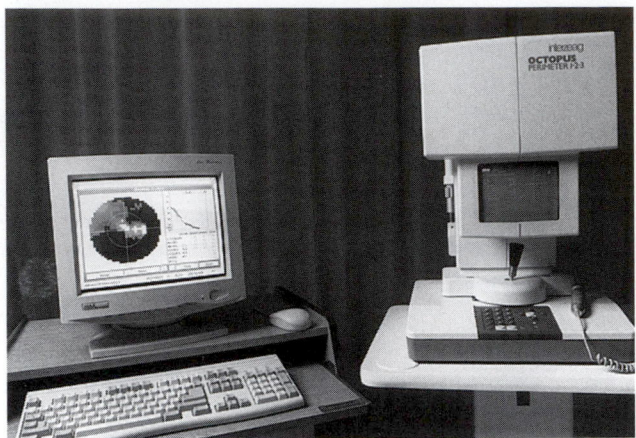

Figure 17–1. Setup of Octopus 1-2-3 perimeter with cable hook-up to a Windows personal computer running the PeriExe/PeriTrend data analysis program.

instrument will not present a test stimulus, thus preventing the patient from making an inappropriate response. If the patient blinks or moves his or her eye at the same time as a stimulus is presented, the unit will repeat the stimulus question. When a loss of fixation lasts longer than 3 s, an audible signal alerts the examiner to direct the patient to attend to the fixation target. Because of this system, the Octopus 1-2-3 does not need to utilize the traditional Heijl-Krakow method of blind-spot checks, which would add to the test time. Thus, a fixation quotient will not be found on the printout. This monitor helps to improve the validity and reliability of patient responses during the entire course of the test (Fig. 17–2).

Octopus perimeters offer a variety of testing programs to suit the needs of many different types of patients. Each program offers unique test patterns, stimulus locations, test strategies, and algorithms. The most commonly employed programs include (1) the G1X, a threshold program designed for glaucoma patients and other neurological conditions; (2) the

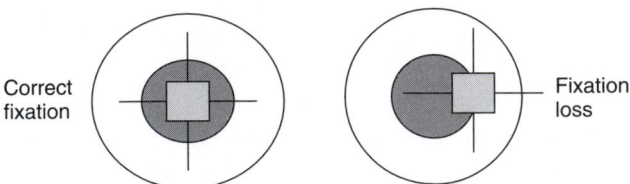

Correct fixation   Fixation loss

Figure 17–2. Fixation monitor. Fixation is constantly monitored during the exam. Fixation loss is reported when the pupil moves away from the cursor; the test is then suspended until the patient regains proper fixation. This prevents any invalid stimuli from being used. (Reproduced with permission from *Octopus Visual Field Digest*, 4th ed. Schlieren, Switzerland: Interzeag AG; 1998.)

STX, a screening test program; (3) the M2X, a central 10-degree macular test thresholding program; and (4) the LVC, a low-vision program for the central 30 degrees that utilizes a large (size V) test stimulus. These test programs work with the Octopus staging technology, which offers flexibility in controlling the length of any test exam.

Results from the Octopus 1-2-3 can be printed via an externally connected printer. Commonly an ink-jet printer is utilized; but laser printers can also be used. Because the Octopus 1-2-3 unit will store only the 11 most recently completed exams, some practitioners may wish to link the unit to a Windows-based personal computer. When used in conjunction with Octopus PeriExe/PeriTrend software, a personal computer (PC) can receive transmitted visual field exams from the 1-2-3 unit, allowing for long-term data storage. The PeriExe/PeriTrend program provides additional statistical analysis and printout options for a sequence of visual fields performed over time.

Instrument Setup

After the unit is turned on, a short calibration is performed. This procedure is initiated by pushing the green "OK" button on the keypad. The next menu screen on the monitor offers several choices for the examiner. In most cases, the CODE option is selected. This submenu holds all of the specific test program options that have been defined and entered by the examiner. Thus CODE 01 may begin the normal threshold test program, CODE 02 may begin the dynamic threshold strategy, CODE 03 may begin the TOP test strategy, CODE 04 the screening program, and so on.

The next menu screen asks for patient data. The patient's birth date is the minimal information that must be correctly entered for proper comparison with the normative database. Additional information (name, gender, acuity, pupil size, diagnosis, etc.) can be input via a keyboard or entered later if the exam is to be transmitted to the PeriExe/PeriTrend program on a linked personal computer. The next menu screen in sequence will initiate the test program once the patient has been properly positioned. This screen also displays the video eye monitor and other data that can be followed during the course of the visual field test (Fig. 17–3).

Patient Setup

The patient setup is similar to that of other automated perimeters. The nontested eye is patched and an appropriate trial lens is inserted into the holder, which is based on the patient's distance correction. A spherical equivalent is usually used for up to 2.00 D of cylinder.

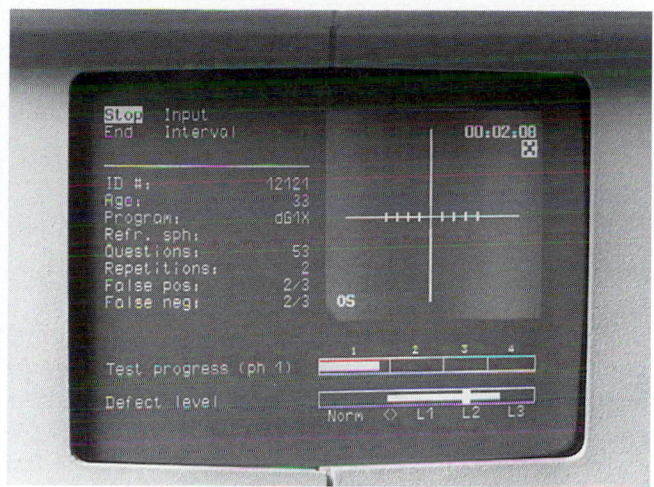

Figure 17–3. Closeup of the menu screen on the 1-2-3 perimeter as it would appear during a patient examination.

The table height is set at a comfortable position and the chin and forehead are placed on the rests. Right and left eye testing is automatically selected based on the positioning of the instrument in front of the patient. Using the joystick and following the video eye monitor, the patient's pupil is centered on the crosshairs and proper focusing is achieved. Patients are instructed to attend to the fixation light and to push the response button when they believe that they have seen a light stimulus. They are encouraged to relax and blink normally. Remind patients that for threshold tests, only half of the test stimuli will be visible. If necessary, the test can be paused and restarted if a short break is needed. Verbal feedback during the test also helps patients improve the accuracy of their responses. Proper setup and instructions are among the most important steps in achieving reliable results with an automated perimeter.

Tracking the Examination

The Octopus 1-2-3 has several features that help the examiner to monitor the patient and the test results during the examination. As described earlier, the fixation monitor assures that test stimuli are presented only when the patient is looking at the fixation light. The progress indicator, a horizontal bar graph near the bottom of the monitor screen, tracks the course of the exam through its completed stages. It is helpful to share this information with the patient. For example, when nearing the end of the exam, let the patient know how much time remains. Elapsed test time is also displayed within the video eye monitor. An additional bar graph at the bottom of the screen is the defect-level indicator. This is a combination of two scales based on the patient's responses during the test. The solid vertical bar indicates the mean defect and is read on the basis of its position within the window. A normal mean defect will be located to the far left, borderline will be in the middle, and depressed will be to the far right. The horizontal bar that is placed over the indicator bar tracks the variability of the patient's responses. The defect-level indicator can be used as a guide to shorten the test time for certain patients (Fig. 17–4). When the indicators are both showing very normal patient responses (far left and narrow), most exams can be safely terminated early; the staging feature of data collection allows this. When the defect-level indicator shows an abnormal field, the exam should continue to its proper completion.

OCTOPUS 101

The Octopus 101 is a traditional hemispheric bowl perimeter that allows for testing of the peripheral

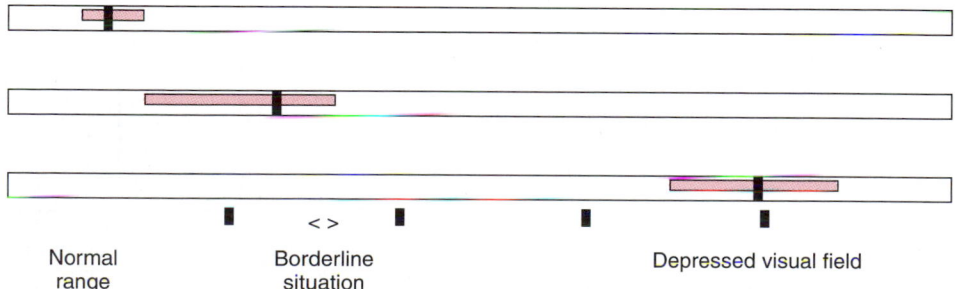

Normal range   < >   Borderline situation   Depressed visual field

Figure 17–4. Defect level indicator. This indicator, which is located on the bottom of the monitor screen, provides a real-time assessment on the current field. The vertical bar estimates the mean defect, and the horizontal bar shows test variability. The indicator is used as a guide for identifying normal tests that may be terminated early without loss of accuracy. (Reproduced with permission from *Octopus Visual Field Digest*, 4th ed. Schlieren, Switzerland: Interzeag AG; 1998.)

field out to 90 degrees. The perimeter is controlled by a separate personal computer running the Windows operating system. The 101 runs the same standard threshold and screening programs that are found on the 1-2-3, with numerous additional tests also available.

As compared with the Octopus 1-2-3 unit, other automated perimeters, and the Goldmann perimeter, the 101 uses a lower background illumination of 4 asb. This flattens the patient's hill of vision and provides a higher dynamic range.[1] Several studies have looked at the differences in results among automated perimeters. These comparisons are quite complex because of the different background illu-minations, range and decibel scale of target luminance, target presentation patterns, and duration of stimulus presentation used by various manufacturers. However, in comparing the values of the Octopus with Humphrey threshold values on earlier in-struments, a 2- to 3-dB difference (indicating less sensitivity) has been measured.[3–5] However, fundamental mechanical and operational procedures between the two units explain this difference as arti-fact and not a true difference in sensitivity.[6] A later comparison between the Humphrey 640 model and the Octopus 1-2-3 found a negligible difference in mean sensitivity values.[7] Formulas for converting data results between the two instruments have sub-sequently been derived.[8] Practically speaking, there are sufficient differences between all automated perimeters that threshold values cannot be directly compared to each other, and the formulas are too cumbersome for regular use in clinical practice.

The Octopus 101 is also capable of running a blue-yellow test program. Short-wavelength automated perimetry (SWAP) has been proven over the past decade to be able to identify glaucomatous defects 3 to 5 years before traditional white-on-white perimetry.[9,10] As an option on the 101, the blue-yellow configuration meets the recommended technical standards and can be an asset for practices examining a large number of glaucoma suspects. Blue-yellow perimetry can be a helpful additional test for glaucoma suspects and ocular hypertensives with normal white-on-white fields.

The Octopus 101 also has a kinetic perimetry option. This is a computer-assisted (semimanual) procedure that moves the test stimulus along meridians chosen by the examiner and operated via a PC mouse. Isopters are plotted automatically, and a combination of static and kinetic testing can be done during a single test.

EXAMINATION PROGRAMS

Octopus perimeters offer a variety of threshold and screening programs. These programs alter the specific test pattern as well as the testing strategy in order to best meet the needs of the patient.

Staging Technology and Exam Phases

Data collection during an Octopus test program is broken down into stages. Weighting and prioritizing all of the test locations has been performed, and this information is in the unit's database. With this information, the G1X test program is conducted in such an order that the essential questions are asked at the beginning of the exam. Each stage consists of a grouping of 13 to 16 test points from within the pattern. Thus, after approximately 50% of the test time, 80% of the information has been collected. Four exam stages make up phase one of a test program. At the completion of phase one, all of the test locations will have been evaluated once by the perimeter. The exam does not have to reach the end of phase one in order to print results. The ability of the unit to save and print this information prior to its completion, combined with the defect-level indicator as a real-time examination monitor, allows the examiner to interrupt and end the exam early for some patients. Although it is possible to conclude testing after one stage (16 test locations), it is recommended that at least two stages be completed to avoid an underestimation of visual field damage (Fig. 17–5).[11]

After a pause, the examination proceeds into phase two and two additional stages (5 and 6) are completed. In screening tests, this allows for the quantification of relative defects found in the first phase; in

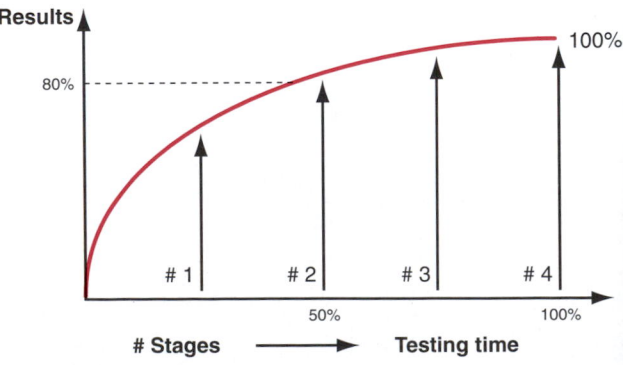

Figure 17–5. Staging concept. By dividing the test into four stages and prioritizing locations, the test program will have obtained approximately 80% of the information halfway through the test. The exam can then be terminated, saved, and printed. (Reproduced with permission from *Octopus Visual Field Digest*, 4th ed. Schlieren, Switzerland: Interzeag AG; 1998.)

threshold tests, it allows short-term fluctuation to be measured by repeat questions at all locations. The use of various stages and phases is under the control of the examiner and can be programmed into preselected CODE exams. In some cases a CODE exam can be programmed to end the exam after phase one (four stages), while another option for the same exam would be for it to continue on to phase two. For example, CODE 03 is programmed for an STX test that ends after phase one for every patient. For CODE 04, an STX test is programmed that continues on to phase two.

In summary, staging and phases break down lengthy test programs into components that permit the evaluation and interpretation of data in a more efficient manner. The ability to end exams early allows results to be obtained on patients who fatigue quickly and cannot continue the test.

Screening Programs

The STX screening program consists of 59 test locations in the central 30 degrees. The distribution of test points is modeled after the G1X threshold program. When programmed for phase one testing only, the examination is usually completed in 2 to 3 min. The screening algorithm proceeds in the standard fashion; suprathreshold test questions are asked based upon the normative database. As with all screening programs, it is designed to evaluate the visual field quickly and will not find subtle or shallow defects. Results are displayed on the printout in the following manner: a plus sign (+) indicates a response that was within 4 dB of normal, an open rectangle (□) indicates a relative defect, and a black square (■) indicates an absolute defect. A relative defect means that the patient did not respond to the initial presentation of a stimulus but did respond when a brighter one was presented at the same location. An absolute defect means that the patient did not respond after the second, brighter stimulus was presented. If the program is allowed to go on into phase two, decibel values will be displayed as the screening program quantifies the abnormal responses (Fig. 17–6).

Threshold Programs

Test Patterns

The G1X program is designed to meet the needs of most testing situations requiring a threshold strategy and is adapted for glaucoma. It represents an evolution of the original program 32, which is the classic grid of 76 test points distributed over the central 30 degrees, with 6 degrees of resolution. Program G1 was an earlier version on older Octopus perimeters that did not having the staging technology. The G1X

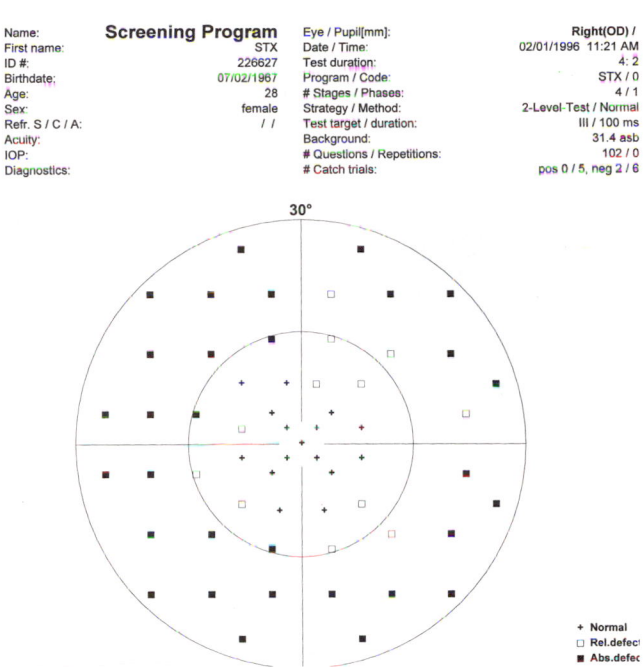

Figure 17–6. Example of an STX (screening) program. For this patient, testing was completed in four stages. Further quantification of abnormal responses can be obtained by extending the test to six stages. The test pattern is the same as that of the G1X program.

has its test locations in a nonsymmetrical distribution. They are arranged to follow the pattern of the retinal nerve fiber bundle, as this is the most frequent location of early glaucomatous defects. The locations are concentrated in the paracentral region with as little as 2.8 degrees of separation. Important nasal test locations are retained out to 30 degrees, while unnecessary edge and peripheral points are eliminated. There are only 59 total test points in the G1X program, which can provide a 30% saving of time over the standard program 32. Overall, the G1X allows for the identification of localized defects and generalized depression in an efficient and anatomically sound manner (Fig. 17–7).[12–14]

When the staging and phase features are applied, the most important test locations are completed after stage 2 (phase one). Although this is only halfway along, approximately 80% of the information will have been collected, and if the defect-level indicators are normal, the exam can be ended at this point. Practically speaking, however, it is customary to complete phase one for most patients. For additional data analysis and statistical information, stages 5 and 6 (phase two) can be completed on patients who are able to sit for slightly longer exams. Program 32 is retained as an option for patients who have used this program previously or for comparison with similar programs from

final measured value is calculated as the midpoint between the last two stimuli after a change in the patient's response. With these two modifications, dynamic strategy reduces test times by about 40%. Normal G1X programs are completed in about 6 to 7 min. Overall, the accuracy of dynamic strategy is comparable to that of the normal strategy.[15, 16]

There are some drawbacks with the dynamic strategy. In the normal and borderline regions of the visual field, sensitivity and accuracy are maintained. Still, there is greater fluctuation and somewhat less precision in the abnormal regions because of the larger steps taken. Also, an increase in the short-term fluctuation value may be noted as compared to normal strategy. For most patients the trade-off is in favor of the dynamic strategy because the test time being shorter improves reliability. One model is to utilize the dynamic strategy as the default program, holding the normal strategy in reserve for special situations where the subject is a good test taker who can sit through a lengthy exam or where a detailed evaluation of an abnormal area is required.

Tendency-Oriented Perimetry/TOP Strategy

TOP is a recent development in fast thresholding programs, with its algorithm a departure from the traditional bracketing technique. The decrease in testing time is dramatic, a reduction of 80% from older programs as all tests (normal and abnormal) are completed in less than 3 min. The TOP strategy is based on the principle that neighboring test points are likely to have a similar sensitivity and decibel value. During testing, a normal point will have a positive influence on surrounding points, while an abnormal point will have a negative influence. This proximal interdependence or "tendency" between the thresholds of adjacent zones allows for a significantly fewer number of questions to be asked during the exam. Indeed, only one test question is asked per location; however, the algorithm uses that single answer many times to influence the values at up to eight neighboring points.[17,18]

The details of the TOP strategy are briefly highlighted as follows. With TOP, all of the test locations in the pattern are divided into four matrices, which consist of intermingled grids (Fig. 17–11). The matrices are tested in sequence, with every location in the grid tested once in random order. Testing starts with a stimulus intensity equal to $\frac{1}{2}$ of the age-corrected normal value. Positive and negative responses are used as "vectors" that will affect test points in subsequent matrices. In the second matrix, a step size equal to $\frac{1}{4}$ of the age-corrected normal value will be added or subtracted to the start values for adjoining test locations.

		1	4	1	4				
	2	3	2	3	2	3			
1	4	1	4	1	4	1	4		
2	3	2	3	2	3	2	3	2	3
4	1	4	1	4	1	4	1	4	1
2	3	2	3	2	3	2	3	2	3
4	1	4	1	4	1	4	1	4	1
	3	2	3	2	3	2	3	2	
		4	1	4	1	4	1		
			3	2	3	2			

Figure 17–11. TOP matrices. This plot shows how the TOP program divides up the test pattern into four uniform groups with an equal number of test locations. Each group is tested in succession and values are added or subtracted to the start values for adjoining test locations. Each location is tested only once, allowing the test to be completed for all patients in under 3 min. (Reproduced with permission from *Octopus Visual Field Digest*, 4th ed. Schlieren, Switzerland: Interzeag AG, 1998.)

Thus all test locations are affected by as many as six neighboring points (top, bottom, sides, diagonal). Testing continues through the remaining grids, with all test data being used to update and influence the intermediate value of neighboring points, although each location is actually tested only once (Figs. 17–12 and 17–13).

Although all tests are completed in less than 3 min, two studies have shown excellent correlation between TOP and the normal strategy.[19,20] However, there are two differences that should be noted. In TOP, the mean sensitivity can be 1 dB higher and the mean defect 1 dB lower than with conventional examinations. This is probably because the shorter test does not produce a "retinal fatigue effect," where patients show a slight loss of sensitivity when maintaining steady fixation for a long period of time. Second, because the sharp and steep edges of deep hemianopic defects become smoothed or rounded by the algorithm, adjacent points across the vertical midline will appear to show an abnormality when in fact, neurologically (and anatomically), none is present. In evaluating patients with neurological disease, the TOP program has been able to clearly identify visual field abnormalities.[21]

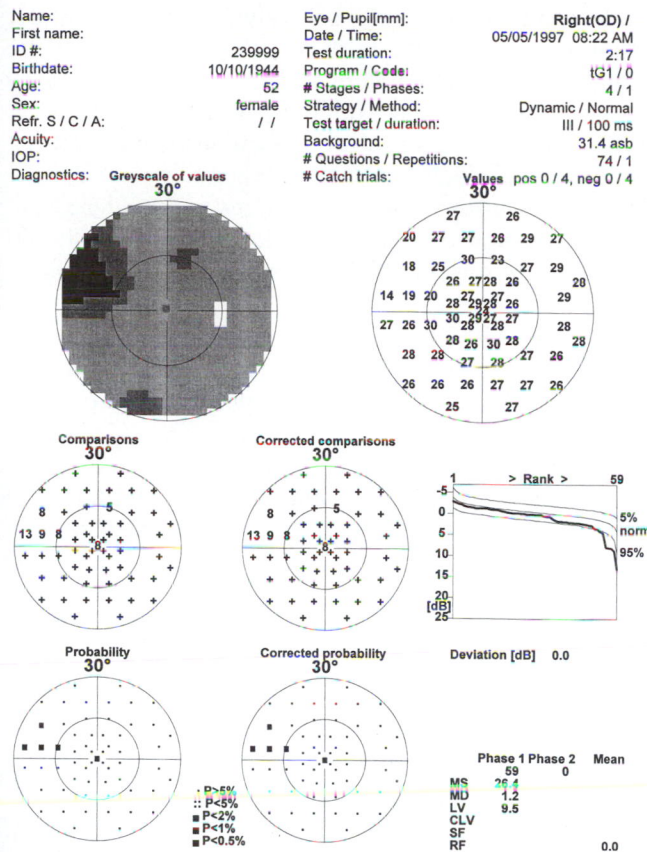

Figure 17–12. Example of TOP visual field for a patient with an early superior nasal step. Even with a test time of just over 2 min, the TOP program can identify early and shallow field defects.

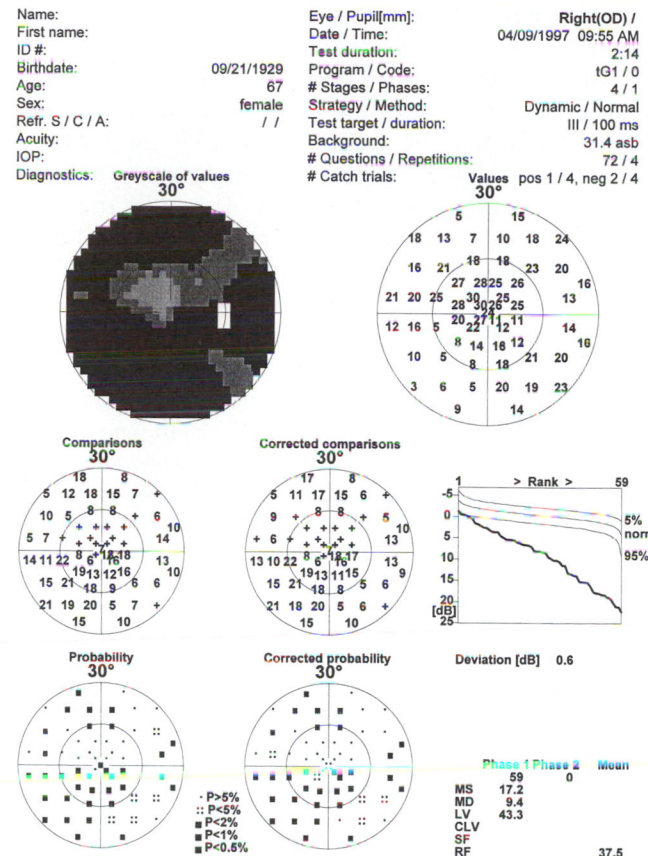

Figure 17–13. Example of TOP visual field for a patient with an advanced glaucomatous defect. This patient has a large, deep inferior altitudinal defect, yet the total test time is still just over 2 min.

The TOP program is a more recent testing algorithm, and continued experience will determine its role in perimetric practice. It offers the ability to perform threshold visual fields on patients who could not or would not sit for the longer programs. As compared with screening programs, it provides much greater quantitative information in about the same (or less) test time. Table 17–1 summarizes an overview of the indications for the various thresholding options.

INTERPRETING RESULTS: READING PRINTOUTS

Patient Data, General Information, and Reliability Indices

The complex-looking printout can be easily analyzed by taking a methodical and sequential approach to every visual field. It is generally best to begin at the top of the page and work down to the bottom.

The header contains basic information identifying the perimeter, software version, name of institution or office, and the printout format selected (e.g.,

seven-in-one). Just below that in the left-hand column is demographic information regarding the patient. The entering of names and some of the other data (refractive error, acuity, IOP, diagnosis) is optional and requires a separate keyboard or a connection to the PeriExe/PeriTrend program. A check to make sure

TABLE 17–1. COMPARISON OF OCTOPUS TEST STRATEGIES

Strategy	Approximate Test Time	Application
TOP Strategy	2–3 min	General threshold test for all conditions. Suited for elderly patients, children, or individuals who have a reduced attention span
Dynamic Strategy	6–8 min	Recommended exam for glaucoma suspects and patients
Normal Strategy	12–14 min	The most accurate exam, which is used in select situations

Source: Adapted with permission from Octopus: Visual Field Digest, 4th ed. Schlieren, Switzerland: Interzeag AG; 1998.

that the patient's age has been correctly entered is important to assure proper statistical analysis.

In the right-hand column, the tested eye is identified; testing date and time and test duration are also provided. Noting the duration can aid in the analysis; for example, longer exams are more likely to have artifacts and show patient fatigue. The program/code identifies the specific test that was run. The standard Octopus abbreviations will be listed: G1X, STX, M2X, etc. If the dynamic or TOP strategy was selected, a lowercase "d" or "t" will precede the test pattern listed. The next two lines identify the number of stages and phases completed and the test strategy used in the exam. This lets the clinician know how thorough the testing was and what type of statistical information will be provided. The technical specifications of stimulus size, stimulus duration, and background illumination are then provided on the following two lines. An increase in the stimulus size, as in the low-vision program, will be seen here.

The total number of stimulus questions presented is provided along with the test duration. Repetitions arise when the instrument has to present a second stimulus because the patient changed fixation or closed an eyelid. A high number indicates a patient who was not very cooperative during the testing procedure. The last line in the right-hand column contains important information regarding catch trials. Two types of catch trials are detected by the perimeter, false positives and false negatives. Both can provide critical information about the analysis and should be reviewed carefully.

False Positives

When a false positive is noted, it indicates that the patient responded to a stimulus that was not presented. The perimeter is designed to periodically pause to see if the patient is spontaneously pushing the response button or is responding to the sounds of the instrument. It identifies a patient who is anxious and "trigger happy." In these cases, the visual field may look better than it actually is because the patient might have been credited for seeing stimuli that were actually not seen. In looking at the comparisons versus corrected comparisons plots, one will note that the latter has more abnormal points than the former when false positives are high. A 15% or higher false-positive rate is considered unacceptable.

False Negatives

False negatives are recorded by the instrument when the patient fails to respond to a stimulus that should have been seen. For example, the perimeter will retest measured locations with a stimulus that is 9 dB brighter than that previously identified. Normally the

patient should respond positively. When the brighter stimulus is not seen, a false negative is recorded. False negatives are interpreted as occurring because the patient is tiring, losing attention, or even falling asleep. When the percentage of false negatives is high, the visual field will look worse than it actually is. A 25% or higher percentage of false negatives is considered unacceptable, and thus interpretation of the field should be done cautiously or the test repeated (Fig. 17–14).

Plots and Graphs

The middle section of the printout includes a number of plots and graphs used in the interpretation process.

Value Table

This plot of numbers displays the final values of retinal sensitivity for each test location as measured in decibels. These are the raw data upon which all of the other plots and graphs are based. Because it is rather cumbersome to analyze this array of numbers, we rely on other plots to tell us about their significance.

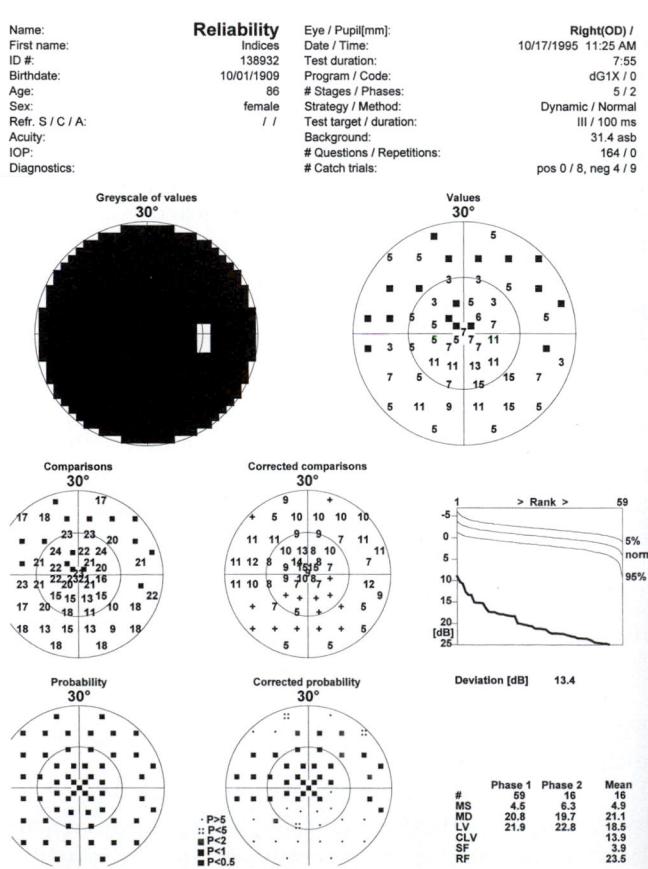

Figure 17–14. Reliability indices. This patient has a significant percentage of false-negative catch trials (4 of 9). The reliability factor (RF) at the bottom of the page is above 20%, indicative of an unreliable exam.

Numbers on the value table will be higher toward the middle (fixation point) on normal fields, as higher decibel values represent greater retinal sensitivity. Edge points will typically have lower values and show more fluctuation.

Gray Scale

The gray scale is used to identify the pattern, location, and general size and depth of field loss. It can quickly call attention to abnormal or depressed areas; however, it cannot be used for an accurate interpretation or diagnosis. On the Octopus, the normal gray scale is based on actual measured values. Darker areas indicate abnormal test points, while lighter-shaded areas are normal or close to normal. With the use of actual values, it is normal to see an increase in shading at the edge of the field. Octopus also provides a second gray scale, CO values, based on deviations from normal. With this scale, it is easier to identify only those areas that are abnormal. Overall, the gray scale is best used for patient education and is not considered to be a highly reliable source of information about the patient's visual field.

Defect Curve

The defect curve is also known as the *Bebie curve*. It is similar to the gray scale in that it is used to make quick, general characterizations and impressions about the field.[22] The plotted graph represents a ranking of the 59 test locations (G1X program) from most sensitive (upper left of the box) to least sensitive (lower right). Inside are two curves, one above and the other below, that represent the range of test points for 90% of all normal fields. The shape of the plotted curve relates to characteristics about the field. If the plotted curve falls within the normal band, the field is close to or within normal limits. Bebie curves can often be more accurate than the gray scale because they are not subject to similar artifacts. When the curve runs parallel to the normal curves but somewhat below, it indicates a generalized depression, with all points being reduced relative to normative values. When a majority of the curve is in the normal band but the right end of it drops off sharply, it indicates a localized scotoma. That is, most of the test points in the field were normal while a small cluster were significantly lower than normal. Although interpretation of the field cannot be made only on the basis of the defect curve, it does offers a good overview (Fig. 17–15).

The four plots in the lower 1/3 of the printout present most of the vital information used in reading any visual field. Through a comparison of the patient's threshold values to a normative database, these plots are designed to highlight a field defect, as opposed to the decibel plot or gray scale. The plots are designed to be read as a pair, starting on the left with the comparisons plot and then on to the corrected comparisons plot. Directly below each of these numerical plots are corresponding probability plots, which consist of shaded boxes. The final stop in analyzing the Octopus printout will be the table of visual field indices in the lower right corner.

Comparisons Plot

Statistical analysis of the visual field begins with the comparisons plot. This plot represents the difference (in decibels) between the patient's responses and the

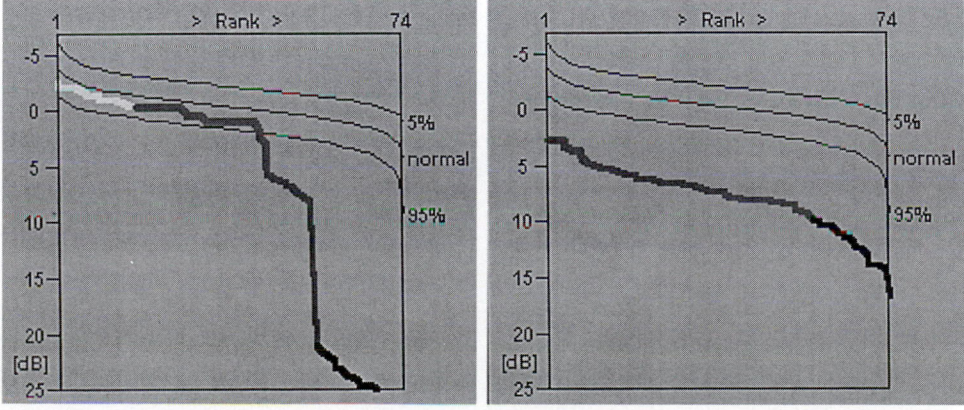

Figure 17–15. The defect curve. The defect curve ranks all 59 test locations from most to least sensitive, left to right along the curve. It allows for a quick assessment of the overall characteristics of the visual field. The curve on the left depicts a localized loss, with several points being significantly below normal. The curve on the right depicts a generalized depression.

age-corrected normal values as found in the perimeter's database. Any number in this plot is interpreted as a decrease in sensitivity from average/normal values for that location. For example, a value of 10 means that the stimulus had to be 10 dB brighter than average threshold in order for the patient to see it. Higher numbers indicate a more abnormal response and even lower sensitivity. Values that are within 4 dB of the age-corrected normal database are represented with a plus sign (+) and are considered to be within normal variation. The comparisons plot is used to identify all of the patient's responses that fall outside of normal limits; thus it shows both generalized and localized depressions to the visual field.

When there are a large number of abnormal locations on the comparisons plot, it can be challenging to review all of the information efficiently, including identifying the most abnormal from the less abnormal ones. The probability plots allow the examiner to do this.

Probability Plots

There are two probability plots, which are related to the numerical plots that lie directly above. This additional information gives the calculated probability that the location could be normal. In other words, it will identify the most statistically abnormal points. The shading of the boxes is based upon the scale displayed between the two plots. A probability value (*p*) of 0.5% is represented by a solid black box. A probability value is read as the chance that a normal person could have given the same response as the patient. A solid box at a single location is interpreted as meaning that "less than 0.5% of the normal population could have a sensitivity that low"—that is, this would be a highly abnormal response. More lightly shaded boxes are less abnormal. The range of probability values includes <0.5%, <1%, <2%, <5%, and >5%. The lower three (0.5 to 2%) values are the more significant and more important values to follow. The probability plot can be used to characterize the size, shape, and location of the patient's defect by looking at the particular distribution or grouping of the darkly shaded boxes (Fig. 17–16).

Corrected Comparisons Plot

The corrected comparisons plot is designed to highlight localized visual-field defects, separating them out from the information presented in the comparisons plot. Localized field defects are of great significance in many conditions as opposed to generalized depressions, which are frequently caused by media opacities and artifacts (small pupils, incorrect trial lens, and so on).

The corrected comparisons plot does this by performing an adjusted analysis of the patient's responses. By readjusting the hill of vision to "subtract out" the generalized component of the field loss, this plot will display the most significantly abnormal portions of the field (localized loss). Numerical decibel values are on the top plot, while the probability plot below will use the shaded boxes to highlight the responses with a lower *p* value (Fig. 17–17).

Visual Field Indices

Further statistical analysis for multiple visual fields is provided with the visual field indices. They are used both in the analysis of any single field and in a series of visual fields for the same person. Two important objectives are to identify any change or progression to the visual field as compared with baseline examinations and to quantify the amount of localized defect. The indices are located in a table in the lower right-hand margin.

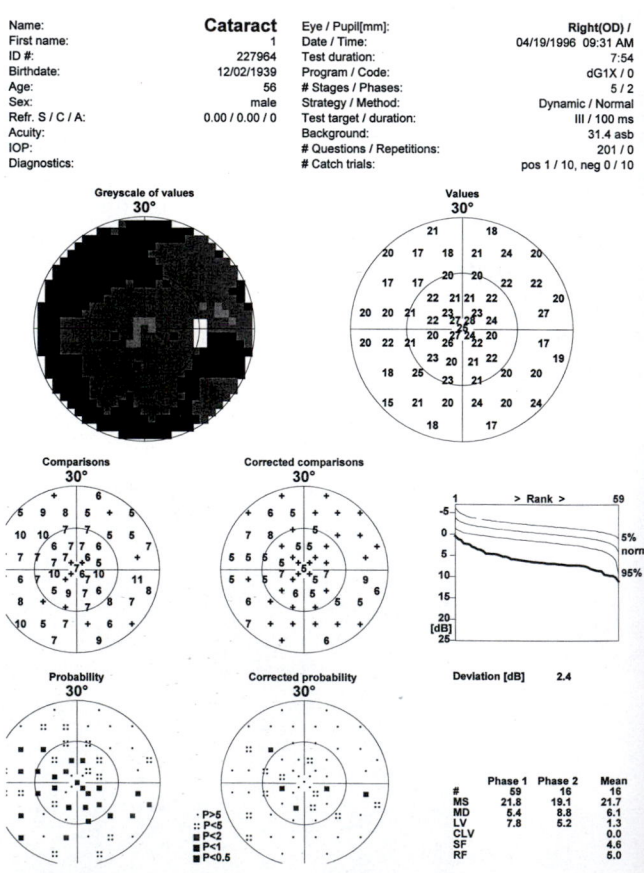

Figure 17–16. Example of a patient with a generalized depression from a cataract. There is a diffuse scattering of abnormal test locations and the mean deviation (MD) is high, while the loss variance value (LV) is low. The defect curve also shows a uniform reduction in sensitivity.

Mean Sensitivity

The mean sensitivity (MS) represents the arithmetic mean of all of the threshold values from the value (decibel) plot. High values indicate a more normal field. This index is not used regularly by itself.

Mean Defect

The mean defect (MD) is the average defect of all of the values from the comparisons plot. This index will identify an overall reduction in the visual field. Positive MD value represent a depression. If a negative value should appear, it would indicate a value that is more sensitive than normal. Clinicians should note that this is the opposite of the printout from the Humphrey field analyzer, where negative values represent depressed values. The normal range for MD values is between −2 and +2 dB.

Loss Variance

The loss variance (LV) value is designed to identify focal loss and irregularity in the hill of vision. While the MD reflects overall loss, the LV value will increase when there are significant focal alterations. This index is calculated from the individual deviations of all measured locations with the mean defect value. The LV is a measure of the degree to which the patient's hill of vision departs from its normal smooth shape. It specifically analyzes the shape, contour, and irregularity of the hill of vision and arrives at a numerical value (dB^2) that quantifies the amount of localized abnormality. Therefore it is a critical value to use when one is looking for early glaucomatous defects. It is also valuable for following a series of visual fields over time, where an increase in the LV could indicate a progression of the scotoma. On the Humphrey perimeter, LV is called pattern standard deviation.

One drawback with the LV value is that it includes any component of the patient's variability of responses during the test. The next two values will sort out the influence of that artifact on the field.

Short-Term Fluctuation

The short-term fluctuation (SF) value is a measurement of intratest variability. It is obtained by a second thresholding of all test locations during phase 2 of the examination. By statistically comparing the patient's first threshold response to the second one, done later in the exam, a measurement of the patient's reliability and consistency can be derived. Patients with high fluctuation may appear to have some localized defects that would be reflected in the loss variance value. It is desirable to eliminate the patient's fluctuation from these calculations. The SF value is then used to determine the corrected loss variance. Normal SF values range between 0 and 2 dB. High SF values are found when there are inconsistent responses. In the depressed area of the field, patients will show fluctuation in their threshold responses. Some of the earliest changes to the visual field in patients with glaucoma may appear as an increase in the short-term fluctuation value.

Corrected Loss Variance

The corrected loss variance (CLV) integrates the SF value with the LV value to give a more accurate measurement of localized field loss. The principle is that fluctuation during the test will have contributed to the calculated LV value. A high SF value will reduce the LV value, leaving a lower CLV. When the SF is low, the LV and CLV values will be approximately the same, as there is no significant variability from the patient that could influence the test results. Obtaining the SF value, and thus the CLV, requires additional test time in phase 2 (stages 5 and 6). Often

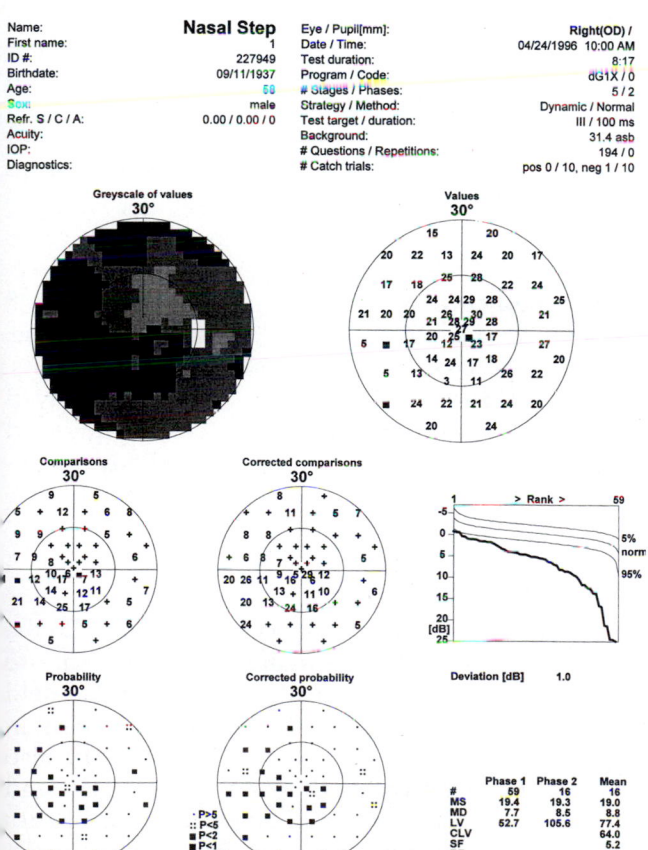

Figure 17–17. This patient has a large inferior nasal step. The MD is relatively low (8.8 dB), while the loss variance and corrected loss variance are very high (77.4 and 64.0 dB), correlating with this large localized scotoma.

this extra test time is very helpful in performing a more critical analysis of the visual field. However, for patients who have demonstrated normal responses through phase 1, this step may not be necessary. Like the LV, the CLV is best utilized to monitor the amount of localized defect for any progression over a series of visual field examinations.

Reliability Factor

The reliability factor (RF) is the final index listed in the chart. It is a percentage calculation based on the number of false positives, false negatives, and repeat questions identified during the test. It serves as a single quick check of the patient's overall performance and attention. A percentage greater than 15 to 20% is highly suggestive of poor reliability, which indicates that the test should be evaluated cautiously (Fig. 17–18).

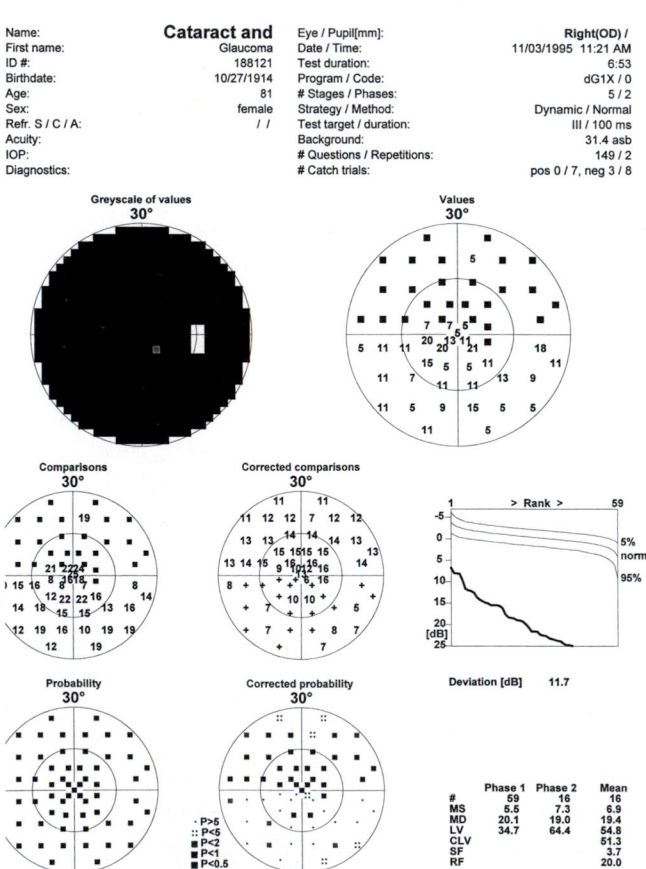

Figure 17–18. In this example, the patient has loss of visual field from both cataracts and glaucoma. This is best represented on the comparisons and corrected comparisons plots. The former shows all of the abnormal test points as a dense generalized depression. The corrected comparisons plot then reveals the superior altitudinal defect. The mean deviation and both the loss variance and corrected loss variance values are abnormal. In addition, the reliability factor (RF) at 20% is high, indicating patient fluctuation and inconsistency.

Printout Formats

Octopus perimeters offer a variety of different formats for printout. When the Octopus 1-2-3 has a direct connection to a printer, the pages will have a slightly different text font and appearance; however, all of the graphs and plots will be available. Additional options are available when the perimeter is linked to a PC and the PeriExe/PeriTrend software program is employed

Seven-in-One

This is the most commonly used printout, as it includes all of the vital information on a single page. All of the aforementioned plots, graphs, and numerical indices are presented in this format.

Large Graphics

This print option provides a single graph or plot (gray scale, comparisons, decibel, defect curve) on a single page. It can be useful in patient education or presentations.

PeriExe/PeriTrend Software Programs

The PeriExe/PeriTrend programs extend the versatility of an Octopus perimeter by allowing the long-term storage of data and the analysis of a series of visual fields for a given patient. The PeriExe program allows the transfer of fields from the perimeter to a Windows-based (3.1 or Windows95) computer. The PC can be a multiuse office computer in another room or a dedicated PC near the perimeter. The currently recommended PC configuration is a 90-MHz Pentium, 8 MB RAM, and a VGA monitor, keyboard, and mouse. A data transmission cable connects the two units. After the field is stored on the PC, it can be displayed and printed in a variety of formats. Viewing the field on a large color monitor has some obvious advantages over viewing it on the small monitor on the perimeter.

PeriTrend

The PeriTrend program is an optional addition to the PeriExe program. This component has the ability to display all the components of a single field (sequence function), as well as a series of fields in several presentations (series function). It can also perform a regression analysis of the series (trend function). For users who will be performing a series of visual fields on a patient over time—for example, on glaucoma patients—these features become extremely helpful in interpreting the results (Figs. 17–19 and 17–20).

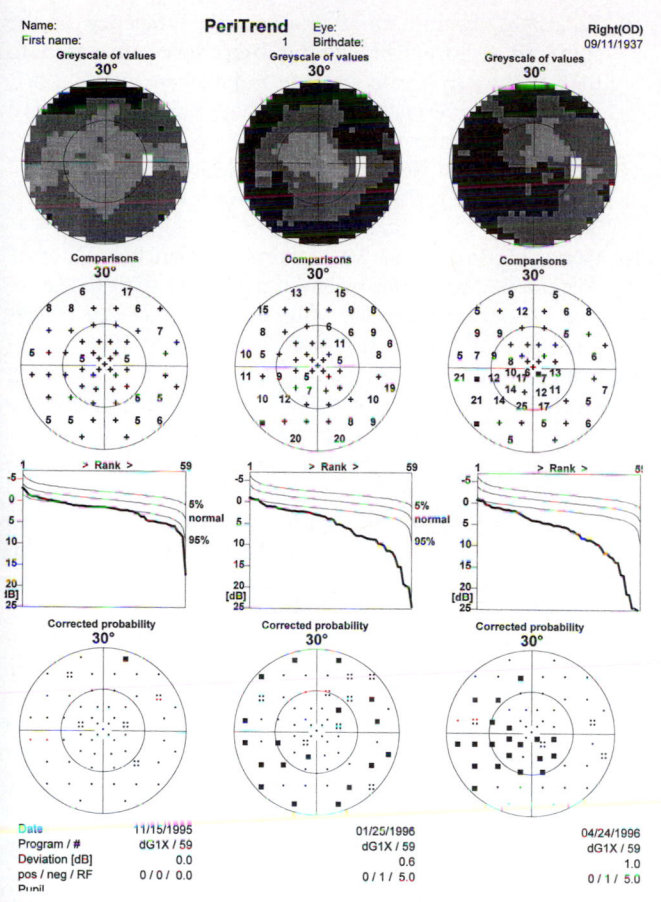

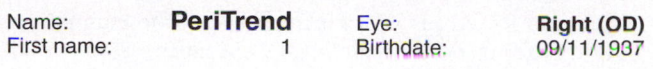

Figure 17-19. The PeriExe/PeriTrend software package is designed for advanced interpretation of a series of visual fields. In this example, rapid development of an inferior nasal step is seen in a patient with severe uncontrolled angle-recession glaucoma. The scotoma is also evident on the defect curve plots and the corrected probability plots.

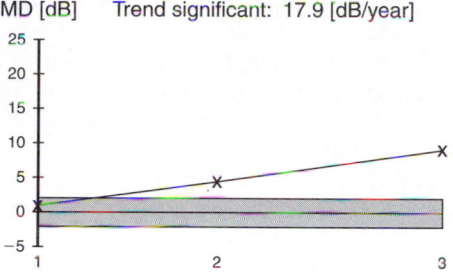

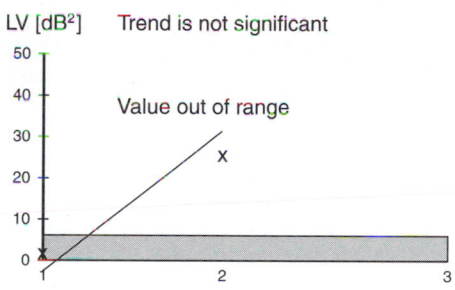

	1	2	3
Date	11/15/1995	01/25/1996	04/24/1996
Program	dG1X	dG1X	dG1X
# Testlocations	59/16	59/16	59/16
# Questions	183	196	194
MD	0.9	4.4	8.8
LV	0.8	24.5	77.4
SF	1.8	4.0	5.2
RF	0.0	5.0	5.0
Pupil			

Figure 17-20. The trend-analysis component of PeriExe/PeriTrend will graph the change in mean defect and loss variance value (LV) over the series of fields selected. This is the trend analysis for the patient in Fig. 17-19. For this example, the LV change is so dramatic that the values are out of range.

SUMMARY

The Octopus 1-2-3 perimeter offers a variety of features and testing options to evaluate patients for all types of visual field loss efficiently and accurately. The Octopus 101 has additional features, such as blue-yellow perimetry. Although automated perimeters are highly sophisticated instruments, it is the clinician's responsibility to choose the appropriate exam program and testing strategy in order to avoid artifact and attain the highest level of sensitivity. Interpretation of the printout is equally important. A thorough knowledge of the displayed plots and numerical indices is vital to assess the field accurately and then follow it for change over time. Octopus perimeters will continue to evolve, incorporating new technology as it becomes available. It is incumbent upon clinicians to stay abreast of the developments in automated perimetry and, when appropriate, offer them to their patients.

REFERENCES

1. *Octopus Visual Field Digest*, 4th ed. Schlieren, Switzerland: Interzeag AG; 1998.
2. Stewart W, Shields MB. The peripheral visual field in glaucoma: Reevaluation in the age of automated perimetry. *Surv Ophthalmol.* 1991;36:59–69.

3. Brenton RS, Argus WA. Fluctuations on the Humphrey and Octopus perimeters. *Invest Ophthalmol Vis Sci*. 1987; 28:767–771.

4. Anderson DR, Feuer WJ, Alward WLM, et al. Threshold equivalence between perimeters. *Am J Ophthalmol*. 1989; 107:493–505.

5. Heuer DK, Anderson DR, Feuer WJ, Gressel MG. The influence of decreased retinal illumination on automated perimetric threshold measurements. *Am J Ophthalmol*. 1989;108:643–650.

6. Fankhauser F, Bebie H, Flammer J. Fluctuations on the Humphrey and Octopus perimeters (letter). *Invest Ophthalmol Vis Sci*. 1988;29:1466.

7. Vivell PM, Lachenmayr BJ, Schaumberger MM, et al. Conversion of normal visual field data between the Humphrey Field Analyzer 640, the Rodenstock Perstat 433 and the Octopus 1-2-3. In: Mills RP, ed. *Perimetry Update 1992/93*. Amsterdam and New York: Kugler Publications, 1993.

8. Zeyen T, Roche M, Brigatti L. Formulas for conversion between Octopus and Humphrey threshold values and indices. *Graefes Arch Clin Exp Ophthalmol*. 1995;233:627–634.

9. Sample PA, Taylor JDN, Martinez G, et al. Short-wavelength color visual fields in glaucoma suspects at risk. *Am J Ophthalmol*. 1993;115:225–233.

10. Johnson CA, Adams AJ, Cassos EJ, et al. Blue-on-yellow can predict the development of glaucomatous visual field loss. *Arch Ophthalmol*. 1993;111:645–650.

11. Sugimoto K, Schtzau A, Bergamin O, Zulauf M. Optimizing distribution and number of test locations in perimetry. *Graefes Arch Clin Exp Ophthalmol*. 1998;236:103–108.

12. Flammer J, Jenni F, Bebie H, Keller B. The Octopus program G1. *Glaucoma*. 1987;9:67–72.

13. Messmer C, Flammer J. Octopus program G1X. *Ophthalmologica*. 1991;203:184–188.

14. Zeyen TG, Zulauf M, Caprioli J. Priority of test locations for automated perimetry in glaucoma. *Ophthalmology*. 1993;100:518–520.

15. Weber J, Klimaschka T. Test time and efficiency of the dynamic strategy in glaucoma perimetry. *German J Ophthalmol*. 1995;4:25–31.

16. Zulauf M, Fechlmann P, Flammer J. Efficiency of the standard Octopus bracketing procedure compared to that of the "dynamic strategy" of Weber. In: Mills RP, Wall M, eds. *Perimetry Update 1994/95*. Amsterdam and New York: Kugler Publications, 1995:263–264.

17. Gonzalez de la Rosa M, Bron A, Morales J, et al. TOP perimetry: A theoretical evaluation. *Vision Res*. 1996; 36:88–90.

18. Gonzalez de la Rosa M, Martinez A, Sanchez M, et al. Accuracy of tendency oriented perimetry with the Octopus 1-2-3 perimeter. In: Mills RP, ed. *Perimetry Update 1996/97*. Amsterdam and New York: Kugler, 1998.

19. Martinez A, Pareja A, Mantolan C, et al. Results of the tendency oriented perimetry in a normal population. *Vision Res*. 1996;36:153–156.

20. Gonzalez de la Rosa M, Morales J, Weijland A. A comparison of the tendency oriented perimetry method with normal threshold perimetry using a PC controlled Octopus 1-2-3 perimeter. Schlieren, Switzerland: Interzeag AG; 1998.

21. Morales J, Hoffman RS, Abdul-Rahim AS. TOP perimetry in patients with neurological abnormalities of the visual pathway. *Invest Ophthalmol Vis Sci*. 1997;38(suppl):26.

22. Bebie H, Flammer J, Bebie T. The cumulative defect curve: Separation of local and diffuse components of visual field damage. *Graefes Arch Clin Exp Ophthalmol*. 1989;227:9–12.

23. Flammer J. The concept of visual field indices. *Graefes Arch Clin Exp Ophthalmol*. 1986;224:389–392.

24. Flammer J, Drance SM, Augustiny A, et al. Quantification of glaucomatous visual field defects with automated perimetry. *Invest Ophthalmol Vis Sci*. 1985;26:176–181.

25. Chauhan BC, Drance SM, Douglas GR. The use of visual field indices in detecting changes in the visual field in glaucoma. *Invest Ophthalmol Vis Sci*. 1990;31:512–520.

26. Zulauf M, LeBlanc RP, Flammer J. Normal visual fields measured with the Octopus program G1: Global visual field indices. *Graefes Arch Clin Exp Ophthalmol*. 1994; 232:516–522.

Chapter 18

NEW DEVELOPMENTS IN PERIMETRY

Chris A. Johnson

Perimetry and visual field testing have been shown to be useful clinical tools for the detection of ocular and neurological pathology, differential diagnosis of eye disease, and monitoring of changes in visual status over time. Over the past 150 years, there have been many advances in perimetry and visual field testing, including improved instrumentation, better stimulus control and calibration, automation and standardization of procedures, statistical comparison of individual data to normal population characteristics, better methods of graphically presenting test results, and many other innovations.[1-4] However, the basic technique of detecting a small white target on a uniform background has remained essentially the same during that time.

Within the past 20 years, a large amount of information has been obtained concerning the properties of different types of ganglion cells.[5-8] Our current understanding indicates that there are several major groups of retinal ganglion cells that project to different portions of the lateral geniculate nucleus. One group of retinal ganglion cells projects to the parvocellular layers of the lateral geniculate (P cells); they tend to be concentrated in central vision, have slower conduction velocities and thinner axons, and are most responsive to high spatial frequencies (fine detail) and low temporal frequencies (steady stimulus presentations or slow changes).[5-8] P cells are believed to be primarily involved in the processing of color

information, spatial resolution, and form vision. Approximately 80% of all retinal ganglion cells are P cells. Recently, it has been reported that blue-sensitive retinal ganglion cells project to the koniocellular layers of the lateral geniculate nucleus (K cells).[9] These cells are believed to be involved in the processing of blue-yellow color opponent information and make up about 5% of the retinal ganglion cell population.

A third group of retinal ganglion cells projects to the magnocellular layers of the lateral geniculate (M cells); they tend to be distributed rather uniformly throughout the visual field, have fast conduction velocities and thicker axons, and are most responsive to low spatial frequencies (large objects or coarse patterns) and high temporal frequencies (rapid changes).[5-8] M cells are believed to be primarily involved in the processing of rapid flicker, motion, and related temporal visual functions. They make up about 15% of the total number of retinal ganglion cells. Thus, subsets of the M-, K-, and P-cell nerve fibers are believed to be primarily responsible for the organization and processing of specific types of visual functions.

This representation of the visual system is presented schematically in Fig. 18-1. Although this is a gross oversimplification,[10-13] it is a useful way of thinking about the primary functional properties of vision associated with particular groups of ganglion cells, particularly for clinical testing purposes. Our

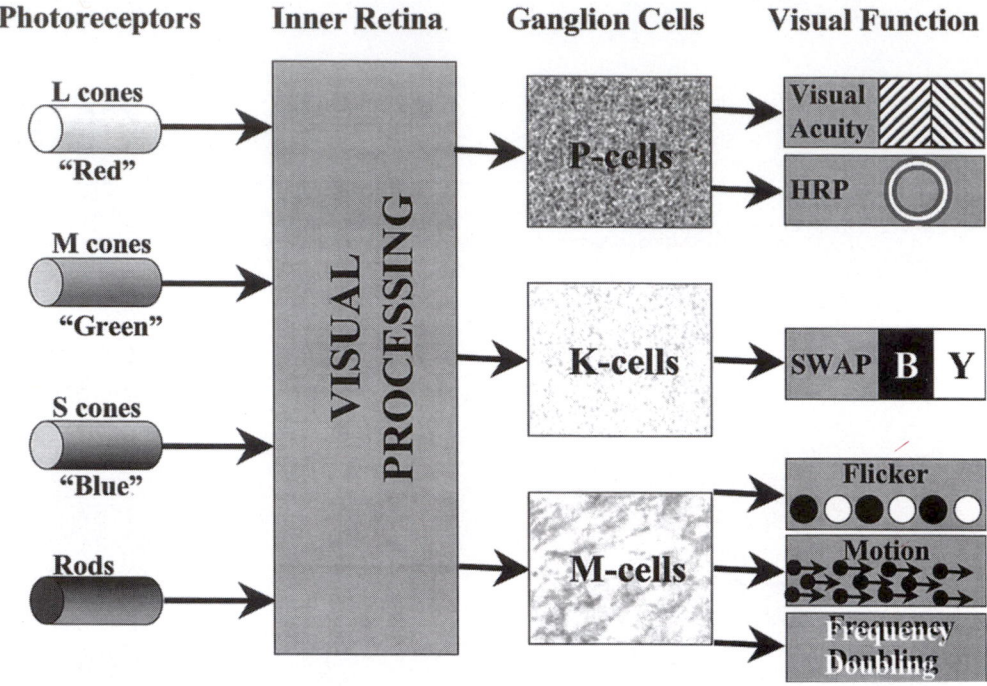

Figure 18–1. Schematic representation of the different populations of retinal ganglion cells and the various visual functions they subserve.

expanding knowledge in this area has recently prompted investigators to evaluate a number of psychophysical visual functions that are associated with specific types of retinal ganglion cells, especially in view of reports indicating that glaucoma may preferentially damage specific subgroups of ganglion cells.[14–20] As a consequence, we now have a number of techniques available for the perimetric evaluation of visual fields in glaucoma that are much more specific than the detection of a small white spot on a uniform background.

The ability to test different subsets of retinal ganglion cells underlying specific visual functions provides a more targeted means of examining glaucomatous damage. If there is a selective or preferential loss of particular types of ganglion cells, visual function tests that are predominantly determined by these cells can be evaluated to produce a more direct and sensitive measure of damage. Quigley and colleagues[14–16] have reported that there is a selective or preferential loss of large-diameter fibers in glaucoma. The examination of visual functions mediated by ganglion cells with larger-diameter axons could therefore provide a better assessment of glaucomatous loss. Similarly, a selective or preferential loss of M-cell pathways has also been reported in

glaucoma,[17,18] and tests mediated by M cells could therefore produce a more direct assessment of glaucomatous damage. Finally, it has been suggested that even if glaucomatous damage is not selective, subsets of retinal ganglion cells with sparse representation may be able to reveal early losses more readily because they have minimal redundancy.[19–21]

This chapter provides an overview of six of the new procedures for the detection and evaluation of visual function in glaucoma: short-wavelength automated perimetry (SWAP), frequency-doubling technology (FDT) perimetry, high-pass resolution perimetry (HRP), flicker perimetry, motion perimetry, and acuity (detection/resolution) perimetry. As indicated in Fig. 18-1, SWAP responses are probably mediated by K cells, while HRP and acuity (detection/resolution) perimetry functions are primarily determined by P cells. Similarly, FDT perimetry responses have been reported to be mediated by a subset of M cells, whereas motion and flicker perimetry responses are primarily determined by a larger group of M cells. Four of the new perimetric test procedures (SWAP, FDT, HRP, and flicker perimetry) are commercially available for the routine testing of patients; therefore particular emphasis is placed on the discussion of these techniques

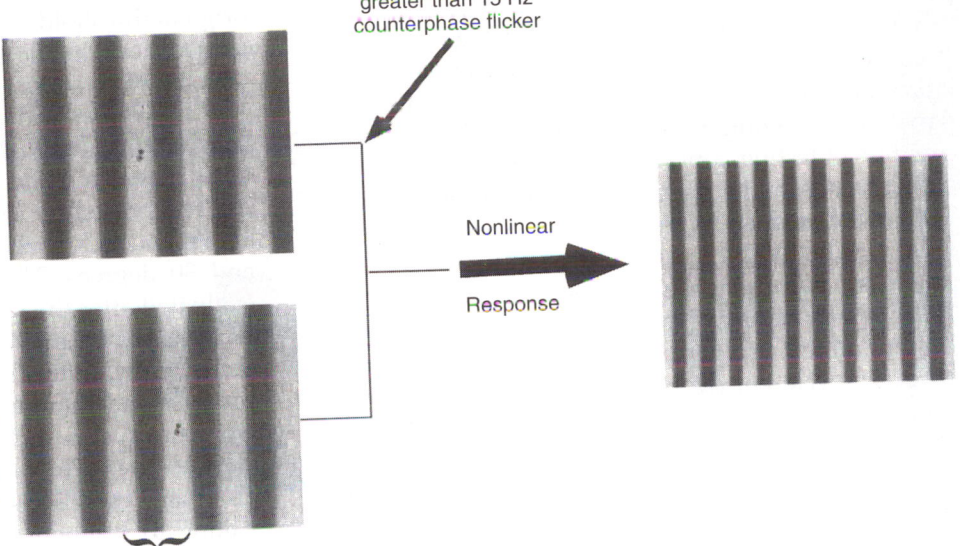

greater than 15 Hz
counterphase flicker

Nonlinear

Response

1 cycle/ degree or less

Figure 18–6. A schematic representation of the frequency doubling effect. (Reproduced with permission from Johnson CA, Samuels SJ. *Invest Ophthalmol Vis Sci.* 1997;38:413–425. Copyright ©1999 Association for Research in Vision and Ophthalmology.)

axons, frequency-doubling contrast-sensitivity measures should be well suited for demonstrating these deficits. Additionally, a selective loss to M-cell pathways would also be manifest by a contrast-sensitivity loss for frequency-doubled stimuli. Finally, because only a small percentage (3 to 4%) of all retinal ganglion cells are believed to be of the My type, this represents a very sparse system with minimal redundancy. Thus, early glaucomatous visual field losses should be more noticeable for this procedure than would be the case for other visual functions mediated by other ganglion cell populations with greater redundancy and overlap. No matter which of these hypotheses concerning the basis of early glaucomatous losses is correct, a perimetry test based on frequency-doubling stimuli should theoretically be very good for detecting early glaucomatous damage.

Maddess and Henry[72] initially reported that contrast sensitivity measures obtained for frequency-doubled stimuli presented to the central 20-degree visual field and the superior and inferior hemifields were able to distinguish glaucoma patients from normal subjects with reasonably good sensitivity and specificity. This test was subsequently extended by Johnson and Samuels[73] to utilize a greater number of smaller targets in order to enhance detection and to incorporate a more reliable threshold-testing strategy. These changes improved the sensitivity and specificity of the frequency-doubling test for detection of early glaucomatous visual field loss as well as substantially reducing test-retest variability. These modifications

formed the basis for the commercially available version of the frequency-doubling technology (FDT) perimeter jointly produced by Welch Allyn (Skaneateles, NY) and Humphrey Systems (Dublin, CA).

The current commercial version of FDT perimetry has been reported to be useful for the detection of glaucomatous visual field loss, both for the full-threshold test procedures[73–78] and for the rapid-screening procedures.[79,80] It has also been shown to be useful in the detection of visual field loss produced by a variety of neuroophthalmologic disorders.[81] FDT perimetry also has many other desirable attributes as a clinical diagnostic testing procedure. Test results are minimally affected by blur of up to 6 diopters, and changes in pupil size do not influence the findings as long as the pupillary diameter is above 2 mm.[82] Learning and practice effects are also minimal.[82] Unlike conventional automated perimetry, where test-retest reliability increases by a factor of more than 300% in areas of moderate to advanced visual field loss, FDT test-retest reliability increases by only about 30% when going from normal visual field regions to those with moderate to severe damage.[83] Thus, FDT threshold measures exhibit less variability in patients with glaucomatous visual field damage. Testing time is shorter than for conventional perimetry, with full-threshold procedures taking 4 to 5 min per eye and screening procedures taking between 45 and 90 s per eye. Because of this, most patients prefer the FDT test over conventional perimetry. Finally, the device requires minimal training to use, is relatively portable, and has an age-adjusted normative database[84] as well

SHORT-WAVELENGTH AUTOMATED PERIMETRY

Color perimetry as a clinical diagnostic technique has been investigated for many years, and its usefulness in evaluating early or subtle diseases of the retina and optic nerve has been well documented. Early investigations of color perimetry used chromatic targets that were superimposed on a uniform neutral background.[22,23] A more selective method of evaluating individual color-vision mechanisms can be achieved by using the two-color increment threshold technique developed by Stiles.[24] This procedure uses one color for the target, which is designed to optimally stimulate one color-vision mechanism, and another color for the background to adapt or reduce the sensitivity of other color-vision mechanisms. For example, short-wavelength-sensitive (blue) color-vision mechanisms can be isolated by using a bright yellow background to adapt the middle- (green) and long- (red) wavelength-sensitive mechanisms and a large blue target to stimulate the short-wavelength-sensitive mechanisms. This principle of selectively isolating the short-wavelength-sensitive pathways is the basis of blue-on-yellow or short-wavelength automated perimetry (SWAP), which is illustrated in Fig. 18–2.

Isolation of short-wavelength-sensitive color-vision mechanisms in a clinical ophthalmic setting was initially done by Marre,[25] King-Smith and colleagues,[26,27] Hart and colleagues,[28,29] and Kitahara.[30] These studies indicated that assessment of short-wavelength-sensitive mechanisms could provide useful information concerning early pathological changes in glaucoma and retinal disease. However, these procedures required careful calibration of stimuli and specialized custom equipment, and were able to test only a limited number of visual field locations. As a consequence, color perimetry did not truly become a viable clinical tool until two-color-increment threshold procedures were adapted for use in automated perimetry with the advent of SWAP in the late 1980s and early 1990s.[31–51]

As previously indicated, SWAP utilizes a bright yellow background and a large short-wavelength (blue) stimulus to isolate and measure the sensitivity of the short-wavelength-sensitive pathways. The bright yellow background suppresses the sensitivity of the middle- (green) and long- (red) wavelength mechanisms and permits the sensitivity of the short-wavelength-sensitive mechanisms to be evaluated. In an elegant set of experiments, it has been shown by Felius and colleagues that detection of the short-wavelength stimulus at threshold is mediated by the blue-yellow opponent chromatic mechanisms.[52] Moreover, their re-

Standard

Year 1

Year 2

Year 3

Year 4

Year 5

○ = Normal

Figure 18–4. An example [of visual] field loss on standard auto[mated perimetry] and inferior deficits are pre[sent on] automated perimetry result[s. The deficit] appears on standard auto[mated perimetry], then progresses through ye[ars with pro]-gressive loss for years 2 th[rough 5. Areas] within normal limits, gray ci[rcles are] normal 5% probability lev[el, black are] worse than the normal 1% p[robability level]...

patients with chiasma[l lesions] have normal visual fie[lds on standard] perimetry but have vi[sual field defects] ing that include vertica[l components]...

As with all perim[etry, there are] some disadvantages as[sociated with] factors that has compli[cated its] cal diagnostic proced[ures, including] yellowing of the lens...

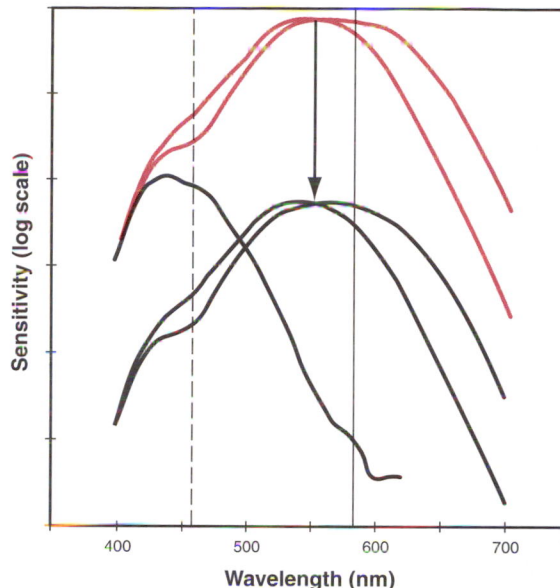

Figure 18–2. Sensitivity of short- (blue), middle- (green), and long- (red) wavelength color-vision mechanisms. Without a background luminance, the middle- and long-wavelength mechanisms (top curves in brown) are more sensitive to blue light than the short-wavelength mechanism (*solid curve, left*). When a bright yellow background is introduced, the sensitivity of the middle- and long-wavelength mechanisms is depressed, thereby permitting the blue stimulus to be detected by the short-wavelength mechanism. The dashed vertical line indicates the dominant wavelength of the blue stimulus used for SWAP, and the solid vertical line indicates the dominant wavelength of the yellow background.

sults and those of Demirel and Johnson[53] indicate that the blue-yellow opponent chromatic pathways are responsible for detecting the blue stimulus even in areas with extensive glaucomatous visual field loss. Using the optimum stimulus conditions for SWAP (implemented on the Humphrey Field Analyzer II–Model 750), approximately 17 dB of isolation can be achieved.[54] This means that the short-wavelength-sensitive (blue) mechanisms are 17 dB more sensitive for detecting the blue target than middle- (green) or long- (red) wavelength-sensitive mechanisms. At threshold, it is thus the short-wavelength-sensitive mechanisms that determine the response. The optimum stimulus conditions consist of a 100 cd/m^2 yellow background (Schott OG 530 filter), a size V stimulus, a 200-ms stimulus duration, and a narrow-band blue stimulus (Omega 440-nm filter, 27-nm bandwidth). These conditions provided the best isolation of short-wavelength-sensitive pathways, the greatest dynamic range, and the least amount of influence by age-related lens yellowing.

A substantial part of the initial development and validation of short-wavelength automated perimetry (SWAP) was conducted independently in the laboratory

the necessity of measuring lens transmission represented a major obstacle in the use of SWAP testing for routine clinical diagnostic evaluation. The use of a glaucoma hemifield test-analysis procedure to identify localized SWAP deficits without correcting for lens-transmission losses provides a viable means of introducing this procedure for large-scale clinical use.

A related problem is the influence of cataract on SWAP test results, since many patients with glaucoma and ocular hypertension are older and are therefore prone to develop cataracts. Moss and associates[68] evaluated a group of patients with cataract and age-matched normal control subjects with SWAP and conventional automated perimetry. The cataract group consisted of approximately equal numbers of patients with anterior cortical cataract ($n=7$), nuclear cataract ($n=7$), and posterior subcapsular cataract ($n=6$). Overall, the amount of sensitivity loss produced by cataract was approximately equal for standard automated perimetry and SWAP. Patients with anterior cortical cataract showed slightly greater amounts of sensitivity loss for standard automated perimetry than for SWAP; patients with posterior subcapsular cataract demonstrated greater losses for SWAP than for standard automated perimetry; and patients with nuclear cataract showed similar sensitivity reductions for both procedures. The authors account for their results on the basis of differences in stimulus size and background luminance for standard automated perimetry and SWAP. Standard automated perimetry uses a small (size III) target and a relatively low background luminance (10 cd/m²). At lower background luminances, pupil size becomes relatively larger, thereby permitting peripheral anterior cortical opacities to produce their maximal effect. This, combined with the fact that the contrast attenuation resulting from light scatter is greater for small stimuli, explains why standard automated perimetry is more affected than SWAP by anterior cortical cataract. Conversely, the higher-luminance background used by SWAP will cause the pupil to constrict about a centrally located opacity such as a posterior subcapsular cataract, thereby producing a greater attenuation of sensitivity for SWAP than for standard automated perimetry. Since the background luminance used by Humphrey Instruments for SWAP testing is considerably lower than that employed by Moss and colleagues, this effect is likely to be smaller for the commercial version of SWAP.

Another preretinal factor that can affect sensitivity to short-wavelength light is the density of macular pigment, because it also absorbs short-wavelength light.[69] Although macular pigment density must be taken into account for SWAP testing in macular degen-

eration and other retinal diseases affecting the foveal and macular regions, it is not particularly relevant for glaucoma, because visual field changes usually are not present within the central 3 to 4 degrees until very late in the disease process.

Finally, it has been reported that variability is somewhat greater for SWAP than for conventional automated perimetry.[70,71] The application of new, robust threshold-estimation procedures, such as maximum-likelihood procedures for SWAP, should be very helpful in reducing variability for SWAP. None of the difficulties mentioned above are problems that are critical to the efficacy of SWAP in glaucoma patients and glaucoma suspects. In spite of these factors, SWAP has clearly been shown to be a useful clinical diagnostic procedure for glaucoma, particularly in early stages of the disease.

FREQUENCY-DOUBLING TECHNOLOGY PERIMETRY

When a low spatial frequency sinusoidal grating (1 cycle per degree or less) undergoes high temporal frequency counterphase flicker (15 Hz or greater), the grating appears to have twice as many light and dark bars as are actually present, as shown schematically in Fig. 18–6. The frequency-doubling effect is produced by a nonlinearity that is present in the visual system's response to contrast. Most parvocellular (P-cell) and magnocellular (M-cell) mechanisms exhibit a linear response to contrast, although a small subset of M cells (approximately 25% of M cells) have been reported to have nonlinear response properties. These cells, sometimes referred to as My-type cells, have large-diameter axons and have been said by Maddess[72] and colleagues to be responsible for generating the frequency-doubling effect.

Because there is evidence suggesting that My-type cells might be damaged early in glaucoma, Maddess and Henry[72] have used the frequency-doubling effect as the basis of a test procedure for detecting glaucomatous loss of visual field. Contrast sensitivity for detection of a frequency-doubled stimulus is measured and compared with responses from normal observers. The rationale is that if there is damage to the My-type cells, more contrast will be required to detect the frequency-doubled stimulus—i.e., contrast sensitivity for detection of this stimulus will be reduced. Theoretically, this test procedures should be an excellent means of detecting glaucomatous loss of visual field. My-type cells are reported to have the largest-diameter axons; therefore, if glaucoma produces a selective or preferential loss of large-diameter

the location is classified as having a "severe" sensitivity loss.

Figure 18–11 presents an example of the printout for the C-20-1 screening procedure. The information at the top of the printout is similar to that presented for the full-threshold test procedures. Below this is a graphic representation of whether the sensitivity of the 17 visual field locations is within normal limits or whether the visual field loss is mild (worse than the 1% probability level), moderate (worse than the 0.5% probability level), or severe (unable to detect the 100% contrast stimulus) as designated by the various gray-scale levels.

The C-20-1 screening procedure uses a conservative test strategy to optimize specificity (i.e., minimizing the misclassification of persons with normal visual fields as being abnormal). Sensitivity for detecting early glaucomatous visual field loss is good, but because the strategy has been optimized to provide high specificity, some early glaucomatous visual field defects may not be detected. Because of its high specificity, this test strategy is most appropriate for mass screening and rapid evaluation of the population at large.

The second screening procedure is similar to the one described previously except that targets are initially presented at the 5% probability level—i.e., it is a stimulus that 95% of the normal population is able to detect. This screening procedure is referred to as the C-20-5 test procedure. If the stimulus is detected, then no further testing is performed at that location and its sensitivity is designated as being within normal limits. If the stimulus is missed, the 5% probability level is presented again. If it is missed again, then a stimu-

lus at the 2% probability level is prese... stimulus is missed, then the stimulus at t... bility level is presented. Different gray... are used to indicate locations with a sens... better than the 5% probability level (th... the 5% probability level is seen on the f... presentation) or is worse than the 5% pr... (stimulus missed both times at the 5... level), worse than the 2% probability le... missed at the 2% probability level), or w... 1% probability level (stimulus missed at... ability level). Figure 18–12 presents an e... results produced by the C-20-5 test proce...

The C-20-5 screening procedure has... tivity than the C-20-1 screening strategy... of early glaucomatous visual field... specificity is not as high. Thus, it is mo... screening in a clinical setting where the... likelihood of encountering ocular patho... importance of detecting early, subtle ab... greater. Note that the results from the... procedures may look different even... might be quite consistent. This is be... stimulus presented by the C-20-1 test p... stimulus at the 1% probability level) is t... lus presented by the C-20-5 test proced... stimuli are missed (again, the stimul... probability). Thus a location with very... on the C-20-5 test procedure is the e... location with very light shading on th... procedure. An example of consistent... C-20-5, the C-20-1, and the full-threshol... dure is presented in Fig. 18–13 for a... glaucomatous visual field loss.

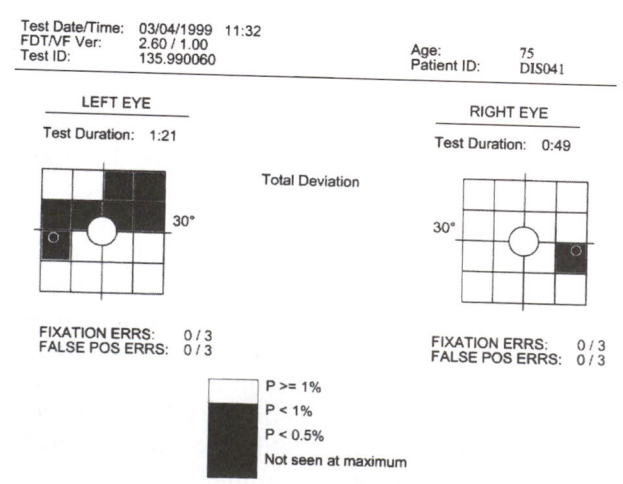

Figure 18–11. The printed output for the C-20-1 screening program for the FDT perimeter (Viewfinder shoftware program). The left and right eyes of a glaucoma patient are presented.

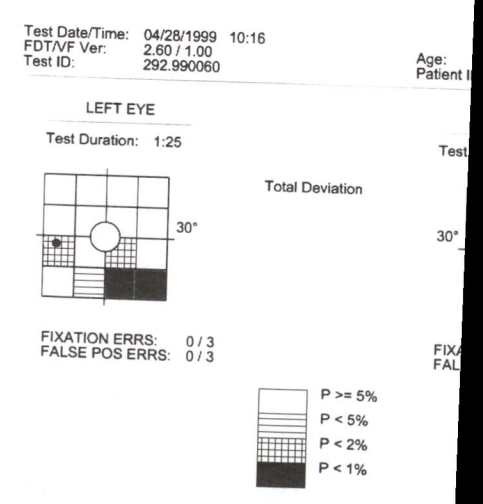

Figure 18–12. The printed output for the C-2... gram for the FDT perimeter (Viewfinder software... and right eyes of a glaucoma patient are presente...

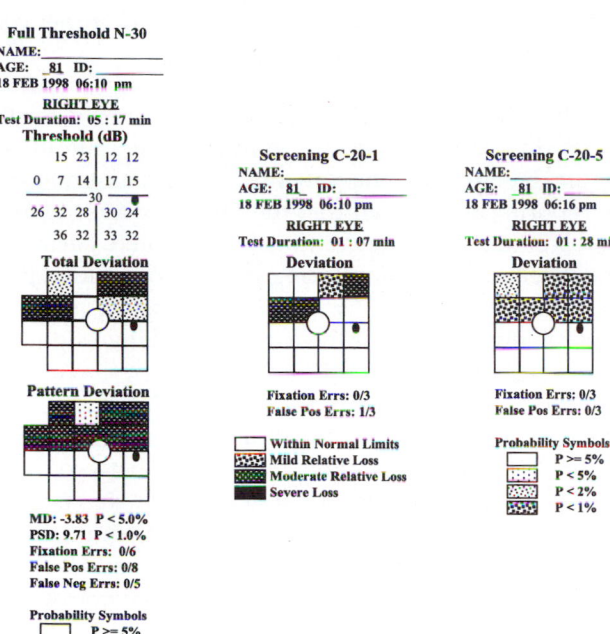

Full Threshold N-30
NAME: _____
AGE: **81** ID: _____
18 FEB 1998 06:10 pm
RIGHT EYE
Test Duration: 05 : 17 min
Threshold (dB)

```
      15 23 | 12 12
   0  7 14 | 17 15
  ----------30------
  26 32 28 | 30 24
  36 32    | 33 32
```

Total Deviation

Pattern Deviation

MD: -3.83 P < 5.0%
PSD: 9.71 P < 1.0%
Fixation Errs: 0/6
False Pos Errs: 0/8
False Neg Errs: 0/5

Probability Symbols
P >= 5%
P < 5%
P < 2%
P < 1%
P < 0.5%

Screening C-20-1
NAME: _____
AGE: 81 ID: _____
18 FEB 1998 06:10 pm
RIGHT EYE
Test Duration: 01 : 07 min
Deviation

Fixation Errs: 0/3
False Pos Errs: 1/3

Within Normal Limits
Mild Relative Loss
Moderate Relative Loss
Severe Loss

Screening C-20-5
NAME: _____
AGE: 81 ID: _____
18 FEB 1998 06:16 pm
RIGHT EYE
Test Duration: 01 : 28 min
Deviation

Fixation Errs: 0/3
False Pos Errs: 0/3

Probability Symbols
P >= 5%
P < 5%
P < 2%
P < 1%

Figure 18-13. A comparison of results for the N-30 full-threshold procedure (*left*), the C-20-1 screening procedure (*middle*), and the C-20-5 screening procedure (*right*). All tests were performed on the same eye on the same day.

Frequency-doubling technology perimetry is a relatively new test procedure that has initially been introduced with two full-threshold test procedures, two screening procedures, a statistical analysis package, and a software package and cable for permanently storing patient data on a PC. In addition, a primer for frequency-doubling technology perimetry is available, which provides background information on the test procedures and analysis package as well as a large series of examples obtained in patients with a variety of ocular and neurological visual disorders. In its present form, frequency-doubling technology

perimetry is a useful and efficient technique for detecting visual field loss produced by glaucoma and other ocular disorders.[73-84] With further refinement of the procedure—in conjunction with additional investigations—the capabilities of frequency-doubling technology perimetry to monitor progression of glaucomatous visual field loss will be identified. Additional features under development include new analysis procedures (glaucoma change probability, Bebie curves), a new "smart" threshold estimation strategy to reduce test time, and a 24-2 stimulus-presentation pattern with smaller targets to enhance the ability to detect subtle changes.

HIGH-PASS RESOLUTION PERIMETRY

High-pass resolution perimetry (HRP) was developed by Lars Frisen.[87-89] It consists of a series of "ring" targets of varying size that are generated on a video monitor by performing a "high-pass" spatial frequency filtering of a target incorporating a light circular center and a dark annular surround, as shown in Fig. 18-14. The target is filtered so that only high spatial frequencies are represented in the stimulus. With standard visual acuity optotypes as well as the line gratings used for detection and resolution perimetry (discussed further on), the targets can be detected at a size much smaller than they can be resolved (i.e., discriminating one target from another on the basis of fine detail). HRP optotypes, on the other hand, have been designed so that the detection and resolution thresholds occur at the same target size. The underlying basis of the HRP stimulus design is that it corresponds more closely to the center-surround arrangement of retinal ganglion cell receptive fields, and it may therefore be better than conventional automated perimetry in revealing glaucomatous damage.[87-89]

In this view, Frisen has compared HRP thresholds with estimates of retinal ganglion cell density from the literature and has found good correlations

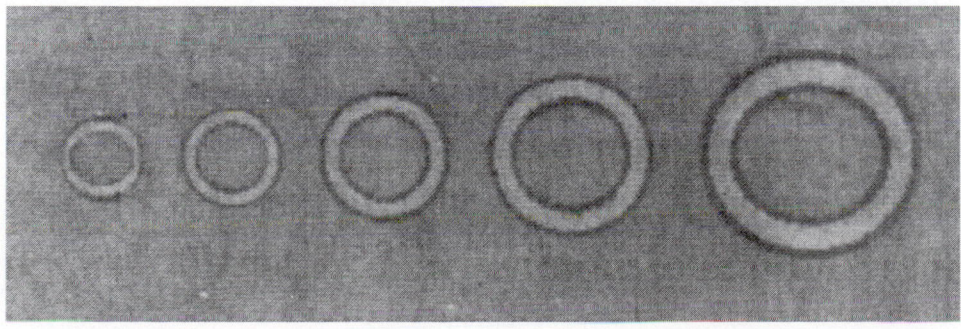

Figure 18-14. The ring stimulus used in high-pass resolution perimetry (HRP). (Reproduced with permission from Frisen L. *Doc Ophthalmol Proc Ser.* 1987;49:441-446. Reproduced with kind permission from Kluver Academic Publishers.)

between this density and HRP thresholds as a function of eccentricity and age; this has prompted him to provide estimates of neural capacity, functional channels, and adjusted neural channels based on HRP threshold values.[90-92] In particular, he has reported that it primarily reflects the function of P cells.[92] The calculations of neural capacity and functional channels are based on several assumptions, sparse and variable data on retinal ganglion cell counts, and correlations between HRP thresholds and the densities of retinal ganglion cells. It is therefore not clear whether these values accurately reflect the proportion of retinal ganglion cells damaged by glaucoma. However, it has been reported that the neural capacity index for the HRP correlates highly with mean deviation (MD) on the Humphrey field analyzer and global defect (GD) on the Octopus. The local deviation index on the HRP correlates highly with pattern standard deviation on the Humphrey field analyzer and with loss variance (LV) on the Octopus.[93-95] Reliability indices on the HRP and the Humphrey field analyzer also are highly correlated.[96]

In the HRP, stimulus contrast is held constant and target size is varied to determine the smallest ring stimulus that can be detected at different visual field locations. A total of 14 target sizes in equal 0.1-log unit (1-dB) steps are available, giving the instrument an operating range of 14 dB. The main advantages of the HRP include its relatively quick examination time, its ease of use, the interactive feedback the test procedure provides to patients, and the high degree of patient preference for the HRP over conventional perimetric techniques. In addition, the HRP has excellent test-retest reliability and—unlike conventional automated perimetry, where variability increases considerably in damaged visual field locations, the HRP shows only minimal increases in variability for visual field locations with reduced sensitivity.[97,98] The low variability of the HRP makes it possible to determine progression of visual field loss earlier than for conventional automated perimetry on the Humphrey field analyzer. In a well-designed prospective longitudinal investigation of glaucoma patients, Chauhan and colleagues[99] found that in the majority of patients undergoing progressive glaucomatous visual field loss on both the HRP and conventional automated perimetry on the Humphrey field analyzer, the progression was detected an average of approximately 1 1/2 years earlier on the HRP. The biggest disadvantage of the HRP at the present time is its limited commercial distribution and representation, particularly in North America. In addition, the HRP requires a near correction of +6 diopters greater than the patient's distance correction, requiring a special trial lens set and placing a greater emphasis on proper centration and alignment of the patient.

Although there have been a few investigations that have reported slightly poorer performance for the HRP in comparison to conventional automated perimetry in glaucoma patients,[100,101] the vast majority of reports have shown that the HRP performs as well as or better than conventional automated perimetry for detection and monitoring of glaucomatous visual field loss.[90,93-96,99,102,103] Frisen has published an excellent review of many of the early clinical investigations of the HRP.[90] Several investigations have also reported good correlations between HRP measurements and the thickness of the retinal nerve fiber layer.[104-106] Similarly, good correlations between HRP measures and neuroretinal rim area have been reported,[107] although this has not been found by all investigators.[108] In addition to glaucoma, HRP has also been reported to be useful for a variety of neuroophthalmologic conditions.[98,109-111]

An example of HRP results is presented in Fig. 18–15 for the right eye of a patient with

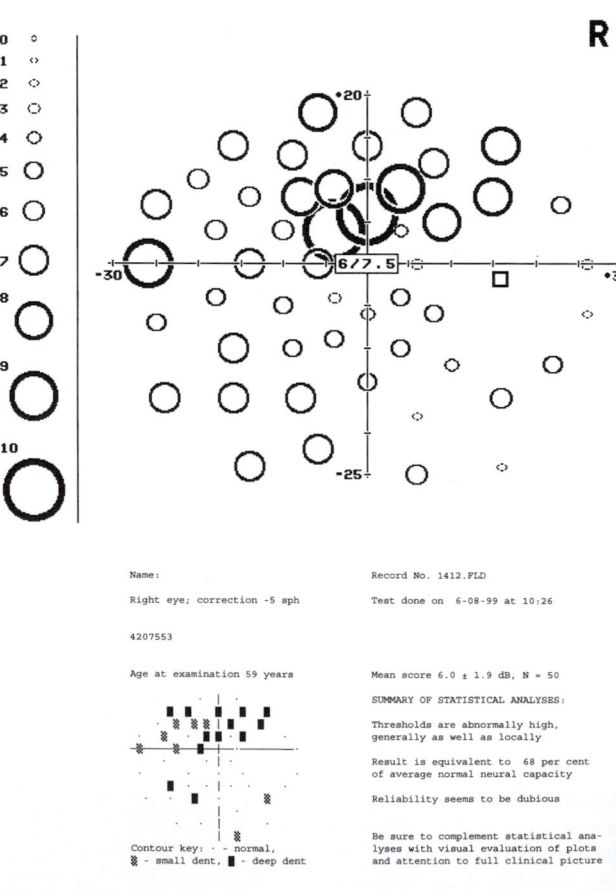

Figure 18–15. An example of HRP results indicating a superior visual field defect for the right eye of a glaucoma patient. (Courtesy of Dr. Balwantray Chauhan, Dalhousie University.)

predominantly a superior arcuate glaucomatous visual field loss. The visual field representation at the top show the smallest ring that was detected at each visual field location tested, and the superior arcuate deficit can be readily appreciated by means of the larger circles. Below this is a small visual field map giving the relative depth of the visual field loss at each location and a summary of the statistical analyses. Figure 18–16 shows a more detailed breakdown of the statistical analyses. For comparison, results obtained for the same eye on the Humphrey field analyzer are presented in Fig. 18–17, and it can be appreciated that there is good agreement between the two test results.

Thus, there is now an abundance of evidence indicating that HRP is a useful clinical test procedure that produces results equal to or better than conventional automated perimetry and that patients prefer over conventional automated perimetry.

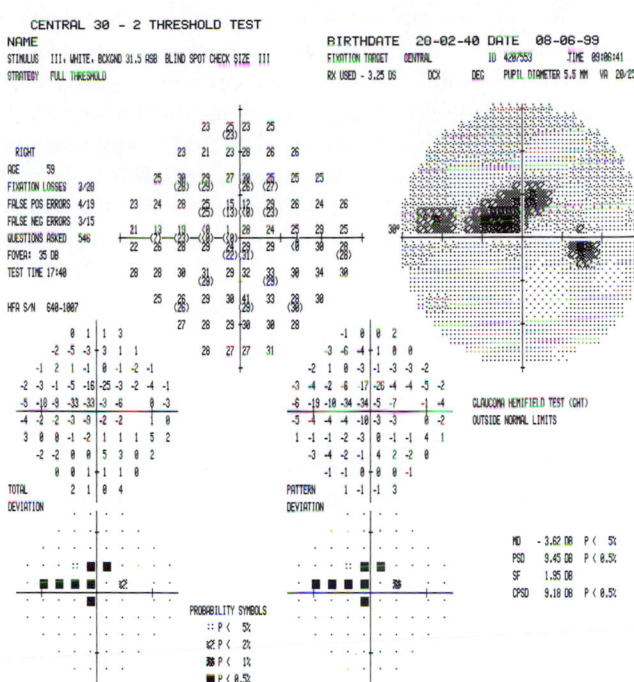

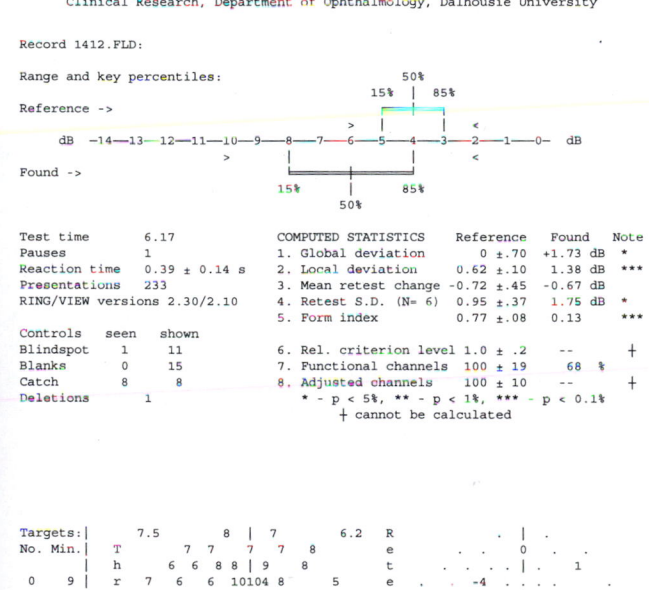

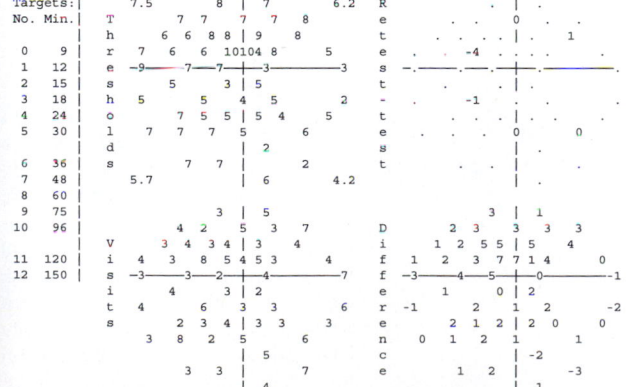

Figure 18–16. Additional statistical comparison and quantitative information for HRP results for the patient shown in Fig. 18–15. (Courtesy of Dr. Balwantray Chauhan, Dalhousie University.)

Figure 18–17. Humphrey field analyzer results for the same patient whose HRP results are shown in Figure 18–15. (Courtesy of Dr. Balwantray Chauhan, Dalhousie University.)

FLICKER PERIMETRY

The ability to detect a rapidly flickering stimulus is believed to be mediated by magnocellular (M-cell) mechanisms. Because of this, flicker perimetry has received considerable attention as a new test procedure for detecting early glaucomatous damage. Tyler[112] was one of the first investigators to examine flicker sensitivity in patients with glaucoma and those at risk of developing glaucoma. His findings revealed deficits in flicker sensitivity, particularly for high temporal frequencies (rapid flicker), in glaucoma patients and in a high percentage of ocular hypertensive eyes. However, his measures were obtained for only a couple of locations in the central visual field. Subsequent investigators have employed a stimulus display similar to those employed by conventional automated perimetry, obtaining measures at 40 to 80 locations.[19,46,100,113–125] Studies by a number of investigators have now shown that flicker perimetry is able to detect early damage that is not detected by conventional automated perimetry[19,46,100,113–123] and that it can be predictive of future glaucomatous visual field loss on conventional automated perimetry.[46]

Several methods have been employed to perform flicker perimetry. One procedure has been developed and validated by Lachenmayr and colleagues.[100,113–117]

This procedure employs light-emitting diodes (LEDs) that are matched in luminance to a uniform background of 50 cd/m². Thus, the LEDs are on continuously and are at the same luminance level as the background. Stimuli are then briefly flickered at 100% contrast and the patient is instructed to press a response button if flicker is detected. The temporal frequency of the flicker is varied to determine the highest rate at which flicker can be detected (critical flicker fusion or CFF). Because the average luminance of the flickering stimulus is matched to the background, stimuli flickering at rates above the CFF will appear to be steady and identical in appearance to when they are not flickering. Measures of CFF are thus obtained for a number of visual field locations. Lachenmayr and associates have shown that this method is more sensitive than conventional automated perimetry and is more highly correlated with retinal nerve fiber layer and neuroretinal rim measurements of the optic nerve.[117]

Another method of performing flicker perimetry uses a fixed rate of flicker and varies the contrast or modulation of the flickering stimulus.[46,118–120] It has been referred to as temporal modulation perimetry (TMP). As with Lachenmayr's procedure, this technique employs stimuli that are matched in luminance to the background; the stimulus then undergoes flicker above and below the background but maintains an average luminance that is equal to the background. This method thus measures contrast thresholds for a fixed rate of flicker, in comparison to Lachenmayr's procedure, which employs a fixed contrast and varies the flicker rate to measure CFF. Investigations using this method of flicker perimetry have also reported that it is more sensitive than conventional automated perimetry and that it is predictive of future glaucoma-tous visual field loss for conventional automated perimetry.[46] A direct comparison of the two techniques revealed that the TMP flicker-perimetry technique provided slightly better ability to distinguish early glaucoma patients from age-matched normals than CFF flicker perimetry, although both procedures were found to be effective.[120] An example of results obtained for both procedures in comparison to conventional automated perimetry (Humphrey field analyzer 30-2 program) is presented in Fig. 18–18 for a patient with early glaucomatous visual field loss.

A third method of performing flicker perimetry has been to present a stimulus that has a fixed rate of flicker and a fixed contrast level and to vary its luminance.[121–125] This procedure is thus similar to conventional automated perimetry in that a luminance threshold is determined, but the patient's task is to detect whether the stimulus is flickering rather than whether he or she can see the stimulus. This method has been implemented in a commercial perimeter, the Medmont M600 (Medmont Pty. Ltd., Camberwell, Victoria, Australia), and has been used to study a variety of ocular disorders.[123–125] It also has been reported to detect early losses that are not evident with conventional automated perimetry.[124,125] Unlike the other two flicker-perimetry techniques, in which only one stimulus attribute (flicker) is changing, two stimulus characteristics (flicker and luminance) are here being changed simultaneously. Thus, the patient is instructed to respond only if flicker is detected and not to respond if he or she detects only a bright spot of light that is not flickering. This can be confusing for some patients, especially if they are used to performing conventional automated perimetry, and can lead to a greater number of false-positive responses.

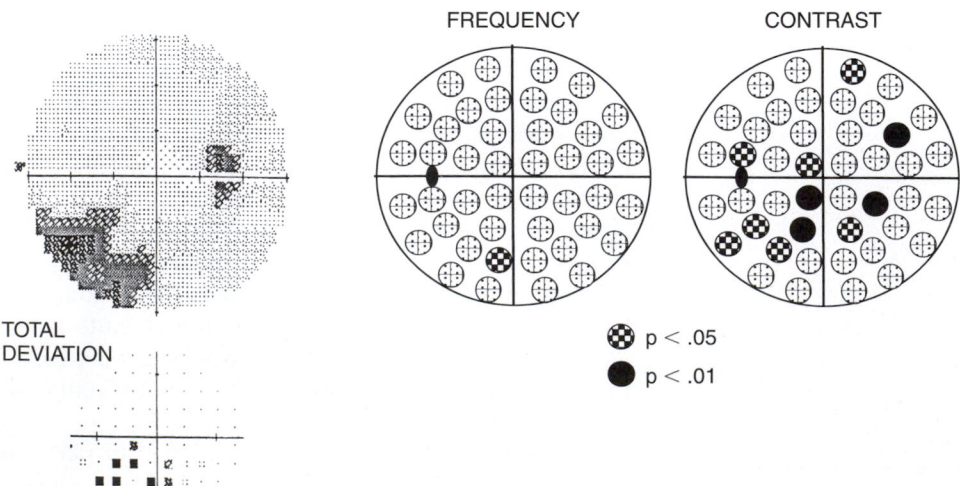

FREQUENCY   CONTRAST

TOTAL
DEVIATION

⬙ p < .05
⬤ p < .01

Figure 18–18. An example of results for critical flicker fusion (frequency) and temporal contrast modulation (contrast) forms of flicker perimetry in comparison to Humphrey field analyzer results (*left*). The lightly stippled circles indicate locations within normal limits, the checkered circles indicate locations that are worse than the normal 5% probability level, and the black circles indicate locations that are worse than the normal 1% probability level. (Reproduced with permission from Yoshiyama KK, Johnson CA. *Invest Ophthalmol Vis Sci.* 1997;38: 2270–2277. Copyright ©1997 Association for Research in Vision and Ophthalmology.)

Flicker perimetry has several advantages over conventional automated perimetry. With it, normal aging effects appear to be more gradual than for conventional automated perimetry, especially for older ages.[116] Also, flicker perimetry is more resistant to optical degradation (blur, cataract, etc.) than conventional automated perimetry.[115]

MOTION PERIMETRY

The ability to detect motion has been a visual function of interest for detection of glaucoma because of the reports that M cells and large-diameter fibers may be preferentially damaged early in glaucoma. Because motion sensitivity is believed to be mediated by M-cell mechanisms, early glaucomatous losses may be reflected in a degradation of motion perception. Evidence from many investigators indicates that this procedure is effective in detecting glaucomatous visual field loss, and that these deficits precede those found with conventional automated perimetry.[56,126–136]

There are several different methods of performing motion perimetry. The procedure employed by Fitzke, Johnson, and others involves detection of the direction of motion of a single small dot or line stimulus.[127–131] This procedure determines the minimum displacement of the stimulus necessary to detect movement. Several investigations have reported that motion-displacement thresholds are elevated in glaucoma patients, often in visual field locations with normal sensitivity for conventional automated perimetry.[127–131] In addition, motion-displacement thresholds have been reported in some patients at risk of developing glaucoma who have normal visual fields for conventional perimetry. Figure 18–19 presents a comparison of the number of abnormal visual field locations for conventional automated perimetry and motion-displacement perimetry in a group of patients with early glaucomatous visual field loss. It can be observed that in nearly all cases, there are a greater number of abnormal visual field locations for motion stimuli than for conventional automated perimetry (luminance threshold testing).

Another method of performing motion perimetry uses a random pattern of light and dark dots, similar to the "snow" pattern observed on a television set that is tuned to a blank channel. A small portion of this display is then moved in a particular direction, as shown in Fig. 18–20. There have been a number of different procedures for measuring motion sensitivity using this type of stimulus display. One variation presents the total display of dots undergoing random or Brownian motion and then briefly presents a subgroup of dots that move coherently in the same direction. The patient's task is to determine the direction of motion of the dot subgroup, and the minimum percentage of dots (coherence) needed to accurately detect the direction of motion is determined. This procedure thus yields a coherence threshold for detection of motion. A 100% coherence stimulus will have all of the dots moving in the same direction. Similarly, a 50% coherence stimulus will have half of the dots moving in the same direction and half moving in random directions.

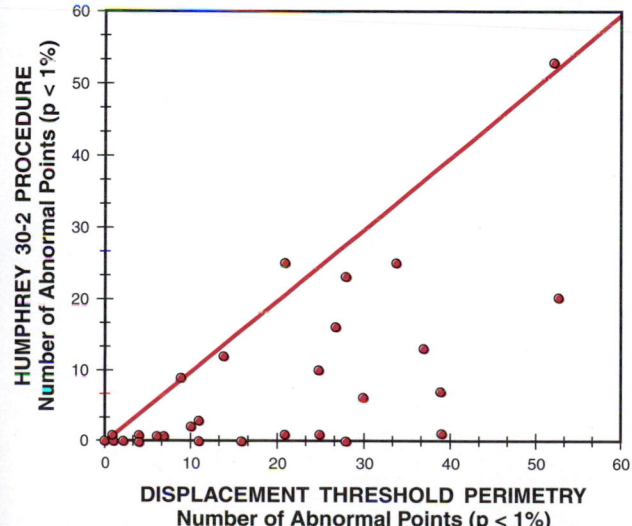

GLAUCOMA PATIENTS, SUSPECTS & OH's

DISPLACEMENT THRESHOLD PERIMETRY
Number of Abnormal Points (p < 1%)

Figure 18–19. A comparison of the number of locations that were worse than the normal 1% probability level of displacement threshold perimetry (abscissa) and standard automated perimetry (ordinate) for glaucoma patients and glaucoma suspects. (Reproduced with permission from Johnson CA, Marshall D, Eng KM. In: Mills RP, Wall M, eds. *Motion Perimetry in Optic Neuropathies: Perimetry Update 1994/95*. Amsterdam: Kugler; 1995:103–110.)

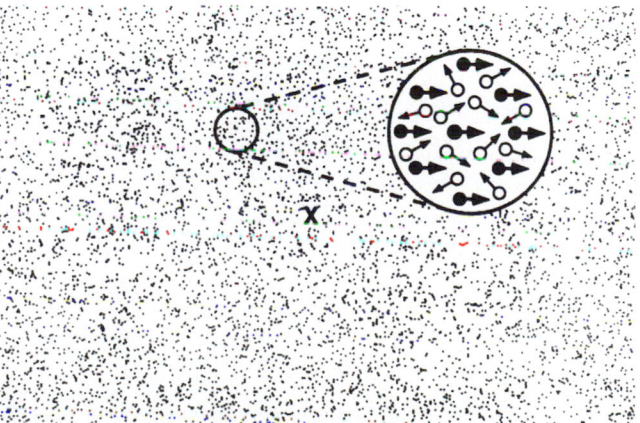

Figure 18–20. The stimulus used for random dot-motion coherence perimetry. (Reproduced with permission from Wall, M. In: Mills RP, Wall M, eds. *Motion Perimetry in Optic Neuropathies: Perimetry Update 1994/95*. Amsterdam: Kugler; 1995:111–117.)

Motion perimetry has several advantages. First, motion is a very salient stimulus for peripheral vision, thereby making this a test that is relatively easy for patients to perform. Second, like flicker perimetry, motion perimetry is highly resistant to optical degradation produced by blur or scattered light from cataract or corneal opacities. Third, large changes in pupil size do not appear to have much effect on motion-perimetry thresholds. Finally, motion perimetry is less affected by background luminance and contrast than other visual functions. Thus, there are several factors that make motion perimetry a robust test procedure for clinical testing.

At the present time, a commercial version of motion perimetry is not available.

DETECTION AND RESOLUTION ACUITY PERIMETRY

Acuity perimetry has been performed in the past by several methods. The Tubinger perimeter[137–139] included a series of circular and square targets whereby

luminance thresholds for detection (ability to detect the presence of a stimulus) and resolution (ability to distinguish a circular stimulus from a square stimulus) could be independently determined. Studies employing these procedures reported that the information derived was useful for the evaluation and differential diagnosis of various ocular disorders.[137–140] Phelps and associates developed an instrument to generate interference fringes on the retina to measure visual resolution in the peripheral visual field.[141,142] They reported that acuity perimetry was a useful technique for the early detection of glaucomatous visual loss.

Recently, Thibos and colleagues have developed another method of performing acuity perimetry.[143–146] They separated the tasks of detection acuity (ability to distinguish a patterned stimulus from a uniform field) and resolution acuity (ability to distinguish one patterned stimulus from another, e.g., determining whether a grating stimulus is oriented vertically or horizontally). Detection acuity is defined by the smallest grating stripes that can be detected from a uniform background; it is limited by the optics of the eye. Resolution acuity is defined as

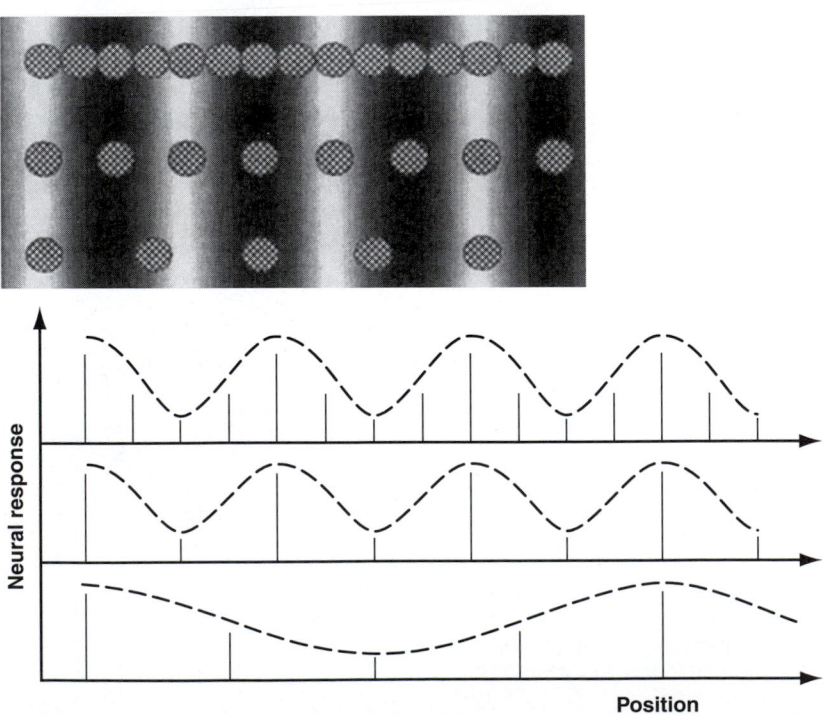

Figure 18–21. An illustration of oversampling (*top*), appropriate sampling (*middle*), and undersampling (*bottom*) of a grating by retinal ganglion cell receptive fields. When the grating is oversampled or sampling is at the Nyquist limit (two samples per light/dark cycle), the grating is accurately represented. When the grating is undersampled (i.e., the pattern is finer than the spacing betwen sampling elements), the pattern is not accurately represented and "aliasing" occurs. (Reproduced with permission from Thibos LN. *Optom Vis Sci.* 1998;75:399–406.)

the smallest grating whose orientation can be accurately determined; it is limited by the density of underlying visual mechanisms as defined by sampling theory. For a grating to be accurately represented, there must be two or more samples per cycle (light/dark bar pair) of the grating. This is shown in Fig. 18−21.

The top diagram shows a grating being sampled by many mechanisms; the grating is therefore accurately represented. The middle diagram shows the minimum requirement of two samples per grating cycle; the grating is again accurately represented. The bottom diagram shows the case in which the grating is finer than the underlying sampling density; less than two samples per cycle are obtained and the grating is not accurately represented. Note that a grating pattern is still represented, but one that is of a different size than that of the actual grating. This phenomenon is known as *aliasing*. Figure 18−22 shows aliasing on a two-dimensional basis and illustrates how the orientation of the grating is misrepresented. This forms the basis of the resolution-acuity test procedure. By determining the smallest grating for which orientation can be accurately distinguished, the underlying sampling density can be derived. Thibos and associates have presented convincing evidence that resolution acuity in the peripheral visual field is limited by the sampling density of receptive fields of retinal ganglion cells, particularly P-cell ganglion cells.[143,144,146] Thus, ganglion cell dropout from glaucomatous damage should produce a reduction in resolution acuity.

This technique has recently been put into a form that is more like conventional automated perimetry. Using Quadravision (a system consisting of four high-resolution 21-in. monitors), it is possible to test both detection and resolution acuity perimetry at locations corresponding to a 24-2 stimulus-presentation pattern. Figures 18−23 and 18−24 present examples of the results of detection and resolution acuity perimetry, respectively, for a patient with early glaucomatous visual field loss. A normative database, a STATPAC-like analysis, has been derived for detection and resolution acuity perimetry, so that total- and pattern-deviation probability plots can be generated for these procedures.

At present, there is only limited information concerning the clinical performance of acuity perimetry.[146] It has been shown that resolution-acuity perimetry is able to detect glaucomatous visual field loss, but more information is needed concerning its sensitivity and specificity in relation to conventional automated perimetry. The approach is appealing because it is solidly based on sampling

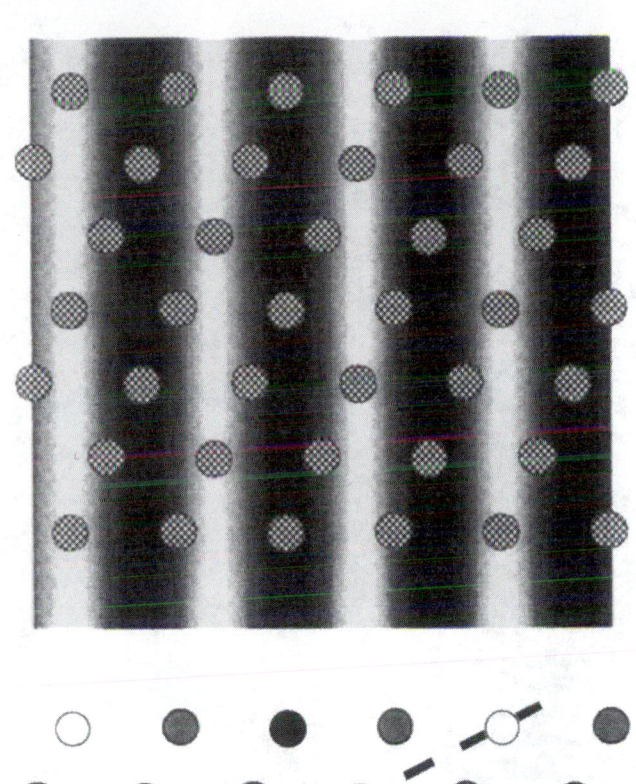

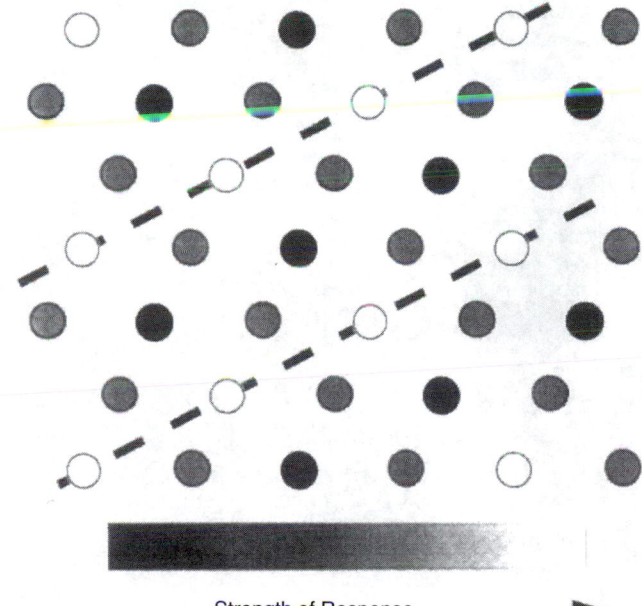

Strength of Response

Figure 18−22. An illustration of the misrepresentation of pattern orientation under conditions in which aliasing occurs. (Reproduced with permission from Thibos LN. *Optom Vis Sci.* 1998;75: 399−406.)

theory. One potential disadvantage is that the redundancy that is present in the P-cell system may make this test less sensitive than other techniques. However, the resolution-acuity procedure could certainly be applied to ganglion cell subgroups with minimal redundancy, such as the short-wavelength-sensitive

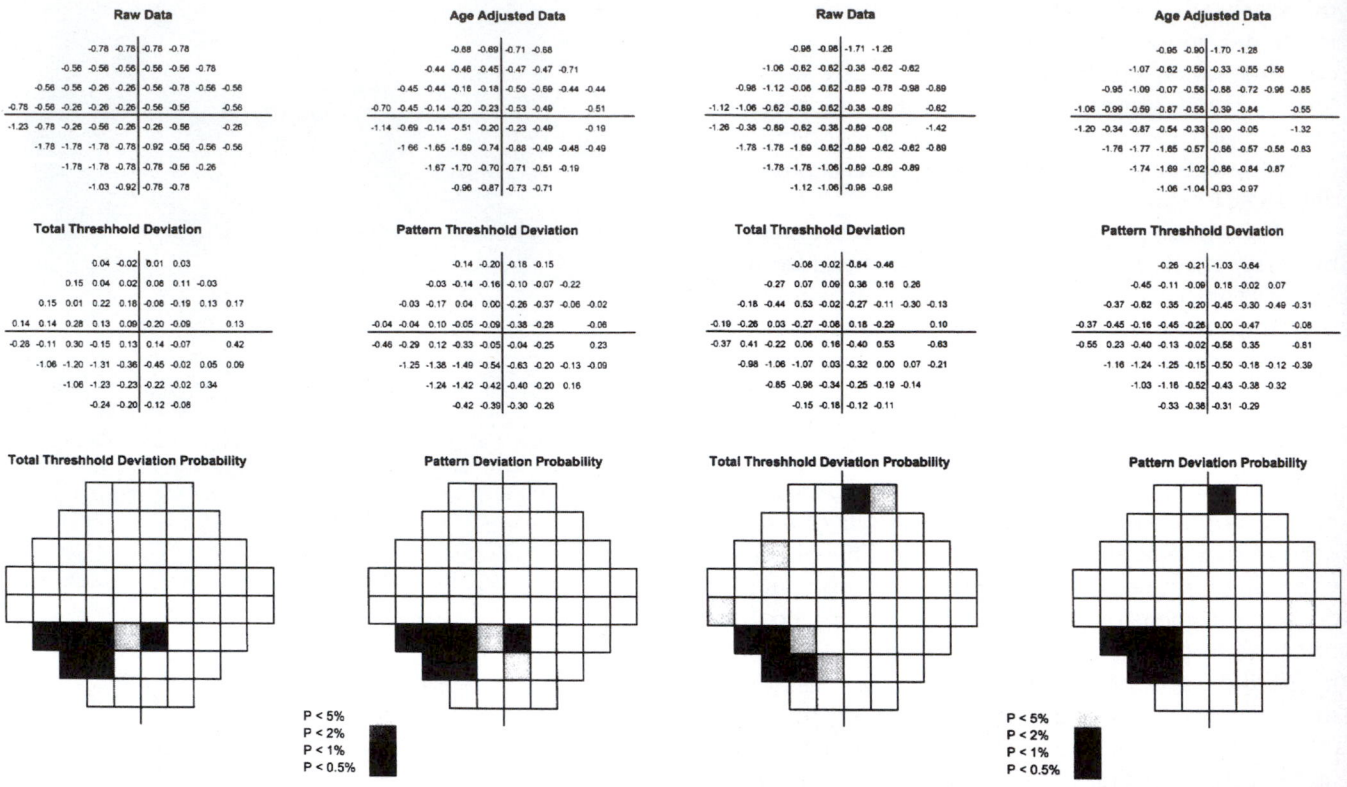

Figure 18–23. An example of total-deviation and pattern-deviation results for the right eye of a glaucoma patient using detection acuity perimetry. An inferior nasal step is shown. Open squares indicate locations that are within normal limits; successively darker gray levels reflect locations that are worse than the normal 5, 2, 1, and 0.5% probability levels, respectively.

Figure 18–24. An example of total-deviation and pattern-deviation results, using resolution acuity perimetry, for the right eye of a glaucoma patient. An inferior nasal step is shown. Open squares indicate locations within normal limits; successively darker gray levels reflect locations that are worse than the normal 5, 2, 1, and 0.5% probability levels, respectively.

pathways. Currently, a commercial device for performing detection and resolution perimetry is not available, although it could readily be implemented on a computer system with a large high-resolution monitor.

CONCLUSIONS

Several of the new perimetric test procedures have been shown to be effective for the early determination of visual function losses and for monitoring patients over time. In particular, short-wavelength automated perimetry (SWAP), frequency-doubling technology (FDT) perimetry, and high-pass resolution perimetry (HRP) have all been shown to be effective clinical tools that offer additional capabilities beyond those that can be achieved with conventional automated perimetry. SWAP has been shown to be able to detect

glaucomatous visual field loss approximately 3 to 5 years earlier than conventional automated perimetry and can also indicate more rapid progression than conventional automated perimetry. FDT perimetry is able to perform very rapid screening for glaucomatous visual field loss, is highly portable, and may be more sensitive than conventional automated perimetry in some cases of early glaucomatous damage. HRP is a rapid, easy to perform test procedure that has excellent capabilities for detecting glaucomatous visual field loss; it is highly reproducible and can determine progression of glaucomatous visual field loss approximately 1 to 2 years earlier than conventional automated perimetry. At the present time, these new techniques are able to supplement conventional automated perimetry by providing some additional capabilities. In the future, as these techniques are further refined, they may possibly become the standard for visual field testing.

ACKNOWLEDGMENTS

Preparation of the chapter was supported in part by a National Eye Institute Research Grant (EY-03424).

REFERENCES

1. Fankhauser F. Developmental milestones of automated perimetry. *ACTA: XXIV International Congress of Ophthalmology*, I. Philadelphia: Lippincott; 1983:147–150.

2. Anderson DR, Patella VM. *Automated Static Perimetry*, 2nd ed. St. Louis: Mosby; 1999.

3. Drance SM, Anderson DR. *Automated Perimetry in Glaucoma: A Practical Guide*. New York: Grune & Stratton; 1985.

4. Lieberman MF, Drake MV. Computerized perimetry: A simplified guide. Thorofare, NJ: Slack; 1992.

5. Livingstone M, Hubel D. Segregation of form, color, movement and depth: Anatomy, physiology and perception. *Science*. 1988;240:740–749.

6. Livingstone M, Hubel D. Psychophysical evidence for separate channels for the perception of form, color, movement and depth. *J Neurosci*. 1987;7:3416–3468.

7. Lennie P. Parallel visual pathways: A review. *Vision Res*. 1980;20:561–594.

8. Shapley R. Visual sensitivity and parallel retinocortical chanels. *Annu Rev Psychol*. 1990;41:635–658.

9. Martin PR, White AJ, Goodchild AK, Wilder HD, Sefton AE. Evidence that blue-on cells are part of the third geniculocortical pathway in primates. *Eur J Neurosci*. 1997;9:1536–1541.

10. Merigan WH, Maunsell JHR. How parallel are the primate visual pathways? *Annu Rev Neurosci*. 1993;16:369–402.

11. Lee BB. Macaque ganglion cells and spatial vision. *Prog Brain Res*. 1993;95:33–43.

12. Lee BB, Martin PR, Valberg A. Sensitivity of macaque ganglion cells to luminance and chromatic flicker. *J Physiol (Lond)*. 1989;414:223–243.

13. Van Essen DC, Andersen CH, Felleman DJ. Information processing in the primate visual system: An integrated systems perspective. *Science*. 1992;255:419–423.

14. Quigley HA, Dunkelburger GR, Green WR. Chronic human glaucoma causing selectively greater loss of large optic nerve fibers. *Ophthalmology*. 1988;95:357–363.

15. Quigley HA, Sanchez RM, Dunkelburger GR, Henaut NL, Baginski TA. Chronic glaucoma selectively damages large optic nerve fibers. *Invest Ophthalmol Vis Sci*. 1987;28:913–918.

16. Glovinsky Y, Quigley HA, Dunkelburger GR. Retinal ganglion cell loss is size dependent in experimental glaucoma. *Invest Ophthalmol Vis Sci*. 1991;32:484–491.

17. Dandona L, Hendrickson A, Quigley HA. Selective effects of experimental glaucoma on axonal transport by retinal ganglion cells to the dorsal lateral geniculate nucleus. *Invest Ophthalmol Vis Sci*. 1991;32: 1593–1599.

18. Chaturvedi N, Hedley-Whyte ET, Dreyer EB. Lateral geniculate nucleus in glaucoma. *Am J Ophthalmol*. 1993; 116:182–188.

19. Johnson CA. The Glenn Fry Lecture: Early losses of visual function in glaucoma. *Optom Vis Sci*. 1995;72: 359–370.

20. Sample PA, Madrid ME, Weinreb RN. Evidence for a variety of functional defects in glaucoma-suspect eyes. *J Glaucoma*. 1994;3(suppl):S5–S18.

21. Johnson CA. Selective versus nonselective losses in glaucoma. *J Glaucoma*. 1994;1(suppl):S32–S44.

22. Feree CE, Rand G. Effect of brightness of preexposure and surrounding field on breadth and shape of the color fields for stimuli of different sizes. *Am J Ophthalmol*. 1924;7:843–850.

23. Hedin A, Verriest G. Is clinical colour perimetry useful? *Doc Ophthalmol Proc Ser*. 1980;26:161–184.

24. Stiles WS. *Mechanisms of Color Vision*. New York: Academic Press; 1978.

25. Marre M. Clinical examination of the three color vision mechanisms in acquired color vision defects. *Mod Prob Ophthalmol*. 1972;11:224–227.

26. Zisman F, King-Smith PE, Bhargava SK. Spectral sensitivities of acquired color defects analyzed in terms of color opponent theory. *Mod Prob Ophthalmol*. 1978;19: 254–257.

27. King-Smith PE, Lubow M, Benes SC. Selective damage to chromatic mechanisms in neuro-ophthalmologic diseases: I. Review of published evidence. *Doc Ophthalmol*. 1984;58:241–250.

28. Hart WM, Hartz RK, Hagen RW, Clark KW. Color contrast perimetry. *Invest Ophthalmol Vis Sci*. 1984;25: 400–413.

29. Hart WM, Gordon MO. Color perimetry of glaucomatous visual field defects. *Ophthalmology* 1984;91: 338–346.

30. Kitahara K, Tamaki R, Noji J, Kandatsu A, Matsuzaki H. Extrafoveal Stiles pi mechanisms. *Doc Ophthalmol Proc Ser*. 1982;35:397–404.

31. Heron G, Adams AJ, Husted R. Central visual fields for short wavelength sensitive pathways in glaucoma and ocular hypertension. *Invest Ophthalmol Vis Sci*. 1988;29:64–72.

32. Johnson CA, Adams AJ, Twelker JD, Quigg JM. Age-related changes in the central visual field for short-wavelength-sensitive pathways. *J Opt Soc Am A*. 1988; 5:2131–2139.

33. Sample PA, Weinreb RN, Boynton RM. Isolating color vision loss of primary open angle glaucoma. *Am J Ophthalmol*. 1988;106:686–691.

34. Johnson CA, Adams AJ, Lewis RA. Automated perimetry of short-wavelength sensitive mechanisms in glaucoma and ocular hypertension. Preliminary findings. In: Heijl A, ed. *Perimetry Update 1988/89*. New York: Kugler and Ghedini; 1989:31–37.

35. Sample PA, Weinreb RN. Color perimetry for assessment of primary open angle glaucoma. *Invest Ophthalmol Vis Sci*. 1990;31:1869–1875.

36. de Jong LAMS, Snepvangers CE, van den Berg TJTP, Langerhorst CT. Blue-yellow perimetry in the detection of early glaucomatous damage. *Doc Ophthalmol.* 1990;75:303–314.

37. Adams AJ, Johnson CA, Lewis RA. S cone pathway sensitivity loss in ocular hypertension and early glaucoma has nerve fiber bundle pattern. In: Drum B, Moreland J, Serra A, eds. *Proceedings of the 10th Symposium of the International Research Group on Colour Vision Deficiencies.* Amsterdam: Kluwer; 1991:535–542.

38. Weinreb RN, Sample PA: Short-wavelength visual field testing in eyes with primary open angle glaucoma. In: Krigelstein GK, ed. *Glaucoma Update IV.* Berlin: Springer-Verlag; 1991:146–155.

39. Flanagan JG, Trope GE, Popick W, Grover A. Perimetric isolation of the SWS cones in OHT and early POAG. In: Mills RP, Heijl A, eds. *Perimetry Update 90/91.* Amsterdam: Kugler; 1991:331–337.

40. Tamaki R, Kitahara K, Kandatsu A, Nishio Y. The vulnerability of the blue cone system in glaucoma. In: Mills RP, Heijl A, eds. *Perimetry Update 90/91.* Amsterdam: Kugler; 1991:343–345.

41. Johnson CA, Adams AJ, Casson EJ. Short-wavelength-sensitive perimetry (SWSP) can predict which glaucoma suspects will develop visual field loss. *Progress in Biomedical Optics: Proceedings of Ophthalmic Technologies II.* Bellingham, WA: SPIE, 1992;1644:230–236.

42. Sample PA, Weinreb RN: Progressive color visual field loss in glaucoma. *Invest Ophthalmol Vis Sci.* 1992;33:240–243.

43. Johnson CA, Adams AJ, Casson EJ, Brandt JD. Blue-on-yellow perimetry can predict the development of glaucomatous visual field loss. *Arch Ophthalmol.* 1993;111:645–650.

44. Johnson CA, Adams AJ, Casson EJ, Brandt JD. Progression of early glaucomatous visual field loss for blue-on-yellow and standard white-on-white automated perimetry. *Arch Ophthalmol.* 1993;111:651–656.

45. Johnson CA, Adams AJ, Casson EJ. Blue-on-yellow perimetry: A five-year overview. In: Mills RP, ed. *Perimetry Update 1992/93.* New York: Kugler; 1993:459–466.

46. Casson EJ, Johnson CA, Shapiro LR. Longitudinal comparison of temporal-modulation perimetry with white-on-white and blue-on-yellow perimetry in ocular hypertension and early glaucoma. *J Optom Soc Am A.* 1993;10:1792–1806.

47. Sample PA, Martinez GA, Weinreb RN. Color visual fields: A 5-year prospective study in eyes with primary open angle glaucoma. In: Mills RP, ed. *Perimetry Update 1992/93.* New York: Kugler; 1993:467–473.

48. Sample PA, Taylor JDN, Martinez G, Lusky M, Weinreb RN. Short wavelength color visual fields in glaucoma suspects at risk. *Am J Ophthalmol* 1993;115:225–233.

49. Sample PA, Weinreb RN. Variability and sensitivity of short wavelength color visual fields in normal and glaucoma eyes. In: *Technical Digest, Topical Meeting on Noninvasive Assessment of the Visual System.* Washington, DC: Optical Society of America; 1993:292–295.

50. Sample PA, Martinez GA, Weinreb RN. Short-wavelength automated perimetry without lens density testing. *Am J Ophthalmol.* 1994;118:632–641.

51. Johnson CA, Brandt JD, Khong AM, Adams AJ. Short-wavelength automated perimetry in low-, medium-, and high-risk ocular hypertensives: Initial baseline results. *Arch Ophthalmol.* 1995;113:70–76.

52. Felius J, de Jong LAMS, van den Berg TJTP, Greve EL. Functional characteristics of blue-on-yellow perimetric thresholds in glaucoma. *Invest Ophthalmol Vis Sci.* 1995;36:1665–1674.

53. Demirel S, Johnson CA. Isolation of short wavelength sensitive mechanisms in normal and glaucomatous visual field regions. *J Glaucoma.* 2000;9:63–73.

54. Sample PA, Johnson CA, Haegerstrom-Portnoy G, Adams AJ. The optimum parameters for short-wavelength automated perimetry. *J Glaucoma.* 1996;5:375–383.

55. Demirel S, Johnson CA. Short wavelength automated perimetry (SWAP) in ophthalmic practice. *J Am Optom Assoc.* 1996;67:451–456.

56. Sample PA, Bosworth CF, Weinreb RN. Short-wavelength automated perimetry and motion automated perimetry in patients with glaucoma. *Arch Ophthalmol.* 1997;115:1129–1133.

57. Yamagishi N, Anton A, Sample PA, Zangwill L, Lopez A, Weinreb RN. Mapping structural damage of the optic disk to visual field defect in glaucoma. *Am J Ophthalmol.* 1997;123:667–676.

58. Polo V, Abecia E, Pablo EC, Pinella I, Larrosa JM, Honrubia FM. Short-wavelength automated perimetry and retinal nerve fiber layer evaluation in suspected cases of glaucoma. *Arch Ophthalmol.* 1998;116:1295–1298.

59. Teesalu P, Airaksinen PJ, Tuulonen A. Blue-on-yellow visual field and retinal nerve fiber layer in ocular hypertension and glaucoma. *Ophthalmology.* 1998;105:2077–2081.

60. Mueller AJ, Plummer DJ, Dua R, Taskintuna I, Sample PA, Grant I, Freeman WR. Analysis of visual dysfunctions in HIV-positive patients without retinitis. *Am J Ophthalmol.* 1996;122:5421–5549.

61. Plummer DJ, Marcotte TD, Sample PA, Woldson T, Heaton RK, Grant I, Freeman WR. Neuropsychological impairment-associated visual field deficits in HIV infection. *Invest Ophthalmol Vis Sci.* 1999;40:435–442.

62. Lobefalo L, Verotti A, Mastropasqua L, Della Loggia G, Cherubini V, Morgese G, Gallenga PE, Chiarelli F. Blue-on-yellow and achromatic perimetry in diabetic children without retinopathy. *Diabetes Care.* 1998;21:2003–2006.

63. Hudson C, Flanagan JG, Turner GS, Chen HC, Young LB, McLeod D. Short-wavelength sensitive visual field loss in patients with clinically significant diabetic macular oedema. *Diabetologia.* 1998;41:918–928.

64. Keltner JL, Johnson CA. Short-wavelength automated perimetry in neuro-ophthalmologic disorders. *Arch Ophthalmol.* 1995;113:475–481.

65. Johnson CA, Keltner JL. Short-wavelength automated perimetry (SWAP) in optic neuritis. In: Mills RP, Wall

M, eds. *Perimetry Update 94/95*. Amsterdam: Kugler; 1995:91–96.

66. Fujimoto N, Adachi-Usami E. Use of blue-on-yellow perimetry to demonstrate quadrantanopia in multiple sclerosis. *Arch Ophthalmol.* 1998;116:828.

67. Sample PA, Esterson FD, Weinreb RN, Boynton RM. The aging lens: In vivo assessment of light absorption in 84 human eyes. *Invest Ophthalmol Vis Sci.* 1988;29:1306–1311.

68. Moss ID, Wild JM, Whitaker DJ. The influence of age-related cataract on blue-on-yellow perimetry. *Invest Ophthalmol Vis Sci.* 1995;36:764–773.

69. Wild JM, Hudson C. The attenuation of blue-on-yellow perimetry by the macular pigment. *Ophthalmology.* 1995;102:911–917.

70. Wild JM, Cubbidge RP, Pacewy IE, Robinson R. Statistical aspects of the normal visual field in short wavelength automated perimetry. *Invest Ophthalmol Vis Sci.* 1998;39:54–63.

71. Kwon YH, Park HJ, Jap A, Urgulu S, Caprioli J. Test-retest variability of blue-on-yellow perimetry is greater than white-on-white perimetry in normal subjects. *Am J Ophthalmol.* 1998;126:29–36.

72. Maddess T, Henry GH. Performance of nonlinear visual units in ocular hypertension and glaucoma. *Clin Vis Sci.* 1992;7:371–383.

73. Johnson CA, Samuels SJ. Screening for glaucomatous visual field loss with frequency doubling perimetry. *Invest Ophthalmol Vis Sci.* 1997;28:413–425.

74. Cello KE, Nelson-Quigg JM, Johnson CA. Frequency doubling technology (FDT) perimetry for detection of glaucomatous visual field loss. *Am J Ophthalmol.* 2000;129:314–322.

75. Sponsel WE, Arango S, Trigo Y, Menash J. Clinical classification of glaucomatous visual field loss by frequency doubling perimetry. *Am J Ophthalmol* 1998;125:830–836.

76. Johnson CA, Demirel S. The role of spatial and temporal factors in frequency doubling perimetry. In: Wall M, Heijl A, eds. *Perimetry Update, 1996/1997*. Amsterdam: Kugler; 1997:13–19.

77. Johnson CA, Cioffi GA, Van Buskirk EM. Frequency doubling technology perimetry using a 24-2 stimulus presentation pattern. *Optom Vis Sci.* 1999;76:571–581.

78. Kondo Y, Yamamoto T, Sato Y, Matsubara M, Kitazawa Y. A frequency-doubling perimetric study in normal-tension glaucoma with hemifield defect. *J Glaucoma.* 1998;7:261–265.

79. Quigley HA. Identification of glaucoma-related visual field abnormality with the screening protocol of frequency doubling technology. *Am J Ophthalmol.* 1998;125:819–829.

80. Johnson CA, Cioffi GA, Van Buskirk EM. Evaluation of two screening tests for frequency doubling technology perimetry. In: Wall M, Wild J, eds. *Perimetry Update 1998/1999*. Amsterdam: Kugler; 1999:103–109.

81. Nearing RK, Wall M, Withrow K. Sensitivity and specificity of frequency doubling perimetry in neuro-ophthalmologic disorders: Arvo abstract. *Invest Ophthalmol Vis Sci (Suppl).* 1999;38:S390.

82. Johnson CA. The frequency doubling illusion as a screening procedure for detection of glaucomatous visual field loss. ARVO abstract. *Invest Ophthalmol Vis Sci. (Suppl).* 1995;36:S335.

83. Chauhan BC, Johnson CA. Test-retest variability characteristics of frequency doubling perimetry and conventional perimetry in glaucoma patients and normal controls. *Invest Ophthalmol Vis Sci.* 1999;40:648–656.

84. Adams CW, Bullimore MA, Wall M, Fingeret M, Johnson CA. Normal aging effects for frequency doubling technology perimetry. *Optom Vis Sci.* 1999;76:582–587.

85. Tyrrell RA, Owens DA. A rapid technique to assess the resting states of the eyes and other threshold phenomena: The modified binary search (MOBS). *Behav Res Methods Instr Comp.* 1988;20:137–141.

86. Johnson CA, Wall M, Fingeret M, Lalle P. *A Primer for Frequency Doubling Technology Perimetry*. Skaneateles, NY: Welch Allyn; 1998.

87. Frisen L. Vanishing optotypes: New type of acuity test letters. *Arch Ophthalmol.* 1986;104:1194–1198.

88. Frisen L. High-pass resolution targets in peripheral vision. *Ophthalmology.* 1987;94:1194–1198.

89. Frisen L. A computer-graphics visual field screener using high-pass spatial frequency resolution targets and multiple feedback devices. *Doc Ophthalmol Proc Ser.* 1987;49:441–446.

90. Frisen L. High-pass resolution perimetry: A clinical review. *Doc Ophthalmol.* 1993;83:1–25.

91. Frisen L. Acuity perimetry: Estimation of neural channels. *Int Ophthalmol.* 1988;12:169–174.

92. Frisen L. High-pass resolution perimetry: Evidence for parvocellular channel dependence. *Neuroophthalmology.* 1992;12:257–264.

93. Birt CM, Shin DH, McCarty B, Kim C, Lee DT, Chung HS. Comparison between high-pass resolution perimetry and differential light sensitivity perimetry in patients with glaucoma. *J Glaucoma.* 1998;7:111–116.

94. Meyer JH, Funk J. High-pass resolution perimetry and light-sense perimetry in open angle glaucoma. *German J Glaucoma.* 1995;4:222–227.

95. Chauhan BC, LeBlanc RP, McCormick TA, Rogers JB. Comparison of high-pass resolution perimetry and pattern discrimination perimetry to conventional perimetry in glaucoma. *Can J Ophthalmol.* 1993;28:306–311.

96. Chauhan BC, Mohandas RN, Whelan JH, McCormick TA. Comparison of reliability indices in conventional and high-pass resolution perimetry. *Ophthalmology.* 1993;100:1089–1094.

97. Chauhan BC, House PH. Intratest variability in conventional and high-pass resolution perimetry. *Ophthalmology.* 1991;98:79–83.

98. Wall M, LeFante J, Conway M. Variability of high-pass resolution perimetry in normals and patients with idiopathic intracranial hypertension. *Invest Ophthalmol Vis Sci.* 1991;32:3091–3095.

99. Chauhan BC, House PH, McCormick TA, LeBlanc RP. Comparison of conventional and high-pass resolution perimetry in a prospective study of patients with

glaucoma and healthy controls. *Arch Ophthalmol.* 1999; 117:24–33.

100. Lachenmayr BJ, Drance SM, Douglas GR, Mikelberg FS. Light-sense, flicker and resolution perimetry in glaucoma: A comparative study. *Graefes Arch Clin Exp Ophthalmol.* 1991;229:246–251.

101. Sample PA, Ahn DS, Lee PC, Weinreb RN. High-pass resolution perimetry in eyes with ocular hypertension and primary open-angle glaucoma. *Am J Ophthalmol.* 1992;113:309–316.

102. Graham SL, Drance SM. Interpretation of high-pass resolution perimetry with a probability plot. *Graefes Arch Clin Exp Ophthalmol.* 1993;233:140–149.

103. Martinez GA, Sample PA, Weinreb RN. Comparison of high-pass resolution perimetry and standard automated perimetry in glaucoma. *Am J Ophthalmol.* 1995; 119:195–201.

104. Airaksinen PJ, Tuulonen A, Valimaki J, Alanko HI. Retinal nerve fiber layer abnormalities and high-pass resolution perimetry. *Acta Ophthalmol.* 1990;68:687–689.

105. Shirakashi M, Abe H, Sawaguchi S, Funaki S. Measurement of thickness of retinal nerve fiber layer by scanning laser polarimetry and high-pass resolution perimetry in patients with primary open-angle or normal-tension glaucoma. *Acta Ophthalmol.* 1997;75:641–644.

106. Shirakashi M, Funaki S, Funaki H, Yaoeda K, Abe H. Measurement of retinal nerve fibre layer by scanning laser polarimetry and high-pass resolution perimetry in normal tension glaucoma with relatively high or low intraocular pressure. *Br J Ophthalmol.* 1999;83: 353–357.

107. Tomita G, Maeda M, Sogano S, Kitazawa Y. An analysis of the relationship between high-pass resolution perimetry and neuroretinal rim area in normal-tension glaucoma. *Acta Ophthalmol.* 1993;71:196–200.

108. Chauhan BC, LeBlanc RP, McCormick TA, Mohandas RN, Wijsman K. Correlation between the optic disc and results obtained with conventional, high-pass resolution and pattern discrimination perimetry in glaucoma. *Can J Ophthalmol.* 1993;28:312–316.

109. Wall M. High-pass resolution perimetry in optic neuritis. *Invest Ophthalmol Vis Sci.* 1991;32:2525–2529.

110. Wall M, Conway MD, House PH, Allely R. Evaluation of sensitivity and specificity of spatial resolution and Humphrey automated perimetry in pseudotumor cerebri patients and normal subjects. *Invest Ophthalmol Vis Sci.* 1991;32:3306–3312.

111. Lindblom B, Hoyt WF. High-pass resolution perimetry in neuro-ophthalmology: Clinical impressions. *Ophthalmology.* 1992;99:700–705.

112. Tyler CW. Specific deficits of flicker sensitivity in glaucoma and ocular hypertension. *Invest Ophthalmol Vis Sci.* 1981;100:135–146.

113. Lachenmayr BJ, Tothbacher H, Gleissner M. Automated flicker perimetry versus quantitative static perimetry in early glaucoma. In: Heijl A, ed. *Perimetry Update 1988/1989. Proceedings of the Eighth International Perimetric Society Meeting, Vancouver, 1988.* Amsterdam: Kugler & Ghedini; 1989:359–386.

114. Lachenmayr BJ, Drance SM, Chauhan BC, House PH, Lalani S. Diffuse and localized glaucomatous field loss in light-sense, flicker and resolution perimetry. *Graefes Arch Clin Exp Ophthalmol.* 1991;229:267–273.

115. Lachenmayr BJ, Gleissner M. Flicker perimetry resists retinal image degradation. *Invest Ophthalmol Vis Sci.* 1992;33:3539–3542.

116. Lachenmayr BJ, Kojetinski S, Ostermaier N, Angstwurm K, Vivell PM, Schamberger M. The different effects of aging on normal sensitivity in flicker and light-sense perimetry. *Invest Ophthalmol Vis Sci.* 1994; 35:2741–2748.

117. Lachenmayr BJ, Airaksinen PJ, Drance SM, Wijsman K. Correlation of retinal nerve-fiber-layer loss, changes at the optic nerve head and various psychophysical criteria in glaucoma. *Graefes Arch Clin Exp Ophthalmol.* 1991; 229:133–138.

118. Casson EJ, Johnson CA. Temporal modulation perimetry in glaucoma and ocular hypertension. In: Mills RP, ed. *Perimetry Update 1992/1993. Proceedings of the Xth International Perimetry Society Meeting, Kyoto, Japan. 1993.* Amsterdam/New York: Kugler; 1993.

119. Casson EJ, Johnson CA, Nelson-Quigg, JM. Temporal modulation perimetry: The effects of aging and eccentricity on sensitivity in normals. *Invest Ophthalmol Vis Sci.* 1993;34:3096–3101.

120. Yoshiyama KK, Johnson CA. Which method of flicker perimetry is most effective for detection of glaucomatous visual field loss? *Invest Ophthalmol Vis Sci.* 1997; 38:2270–2277.

121. Austin MW, O'Brien CJ, Wishart PK. Flicker perimetry using a luminance threshold strategy at frequencies from 5–25 Hz in glaucoma, ocular hypertension and normal controls. *Curr Eye Res.* 1994;13:717–723.

122. Feghall JG, Bocquet X, Charlier J, Odom JV. Static flicker perimetry in glaucoma and ocular hypertension. *Curr Eye Res.* 1991;10:205–212.

123. Zhang L, Drance SM, Douglas GR. The ability of Medmont M600 automated perimetry to detect threats to fixation. *J Glaucoma.* 1997;6:259–262.

124. McKendrick AM, Badcock DR, Heywood J, Vingrys AJ. Effects of migraine on visual function. *Aust N Z J Ophthalmol.* 1998;26:S111–S113.

125. Vingrys AJ, Pesudova K. Localized scotomata detected with temporal modulation perimetry in central serous chorioretinopathy. *Aust N Z J Ophthalmol.* 1999;27: 109–116.

126. Bullimore MA, Wood JM, Swenson K. Motion perception in glaucoma. *Invest Ophthalmol Vis Sci.* 1993;34: 3526–3533.

127. Fitzke FW, Poinoosawmy D, et al. Peripheral displacement thresholds in normals, ocular hypertensives and glaucoma. *Doc Ophthalmol Proc Ser.* 1987;49:447–452.

128. Fitzke FW, Poinoosawmy D, et al. Peripheral displacement thresholds in glaucoma and ocular hypertension. In: Heijl A, ed. *Perimetry Update 1988/1989.* Amsterdam: Kugler; 1989:399–405.

129. Poinoosawmy D, Wu JX, et al. Discrimination between progression and non-progression visual field loss in

low tension glaucoma using MDT. In: Mills RP, ed. *Perimetry Update 1992/93.* Amsterdam: Kugler; 1992: 109–114.

130. Westcott MC, Fitzke FW, Hitchings RA. Abnormal motion displacement thresholds are associated with fine scale luminance sensitivity loss in glaucoma. *Vis Res.* 1998;38:3171–3180.

131. Johnson CA, Marshall D, Eng K. Displacement threshold perimetry in glaucoma using a Macintosh computer system and a 21 inch monitor. In: Mills RP, Wall M, eds. *Perimetry Update 1994/95.* Amsterdam: Kugler; 1995:103–110.

132. Wall M, Ketoff KM. Random dot motion perimetry in patients with glaucoma and in normal subjects. *Am J Ophthalmol.* 1995;120:587–596.

133. Wall M, Jennisch CS, Munden PM. Motion perimetry identifies nerve fiber bundlelike defects in ocular hypertension. *Arch Ophthalmol.* 1997;115:26–33.

134. Wall M, Jennisch CS. Random dot motion stimuli are more sensitive than light stimuli for detection of visual field loss in ocular hypertension patients. *Optom Vis Sci.* 1999;76:550–557.

135. Bosworth CF, Sample PA, Gupta N, Bathija R, Weinreb RN. Motion automated perimetry identifies early glaucomatous field defects. *Arch Ophthalmol.* 1998;116: 1153–1158.

136. Bosworth CF, Sample PA, Weinreb RN. Perimetric motion thresholds are elevated in glaucoma suspects and glaucoma patients. *Vis Res.* 1997;37:1989–1997.

137. Aulhorn E, Harms H. Visual perimetry. In: Jameson D, Hurvich LM, eds. *Visual Psychophysics: Handbook of Sensory Physiology VII/4.* New York: Springer-Verlag; 1972.

138. Johnson CA, Keltner JL, Balestrery FG. Acuity profile perimetry: Description of technique and preliminary clinical trials. *Arch Ophthalmol.* 1979;97:684–689.

139. Johnson CA, Keltner JL. Static and acuity profile perimetry in optic neuritis. *Doc Ophthalmol Proc Ser.* 1981;26:305–312.

140. Keltner JL, Johnson CA, Cowley IJ. Acuity profile perimetry in a unique case of bilateral central serous retinopathy. *Ann Ophthalmol.* 1980;12:726–731.

141. Phelps CD. Acuity perimetry and glaucoma. *Trans Am Ophthalmol Soc.* 1984;82:753–791.

142. Phelps CD, Blondeau P, Carney B. Acuity perimetry: A sensitive test for the detection of glaucomatous optic nerve damage. *Doc Ophthalmol Proc Ser.* 1985;42: 359–363.

143. Thibos LN, Cheney FE, Walsh DJ. Retinal limits to the detection and resolution of gratings. *J Opt Soc Am A.* 1987;4:1524–1529.

144. Thibos LN, Walsh DJ, Cheney FE. Vision beyond the resolution limit: Aliasing in the periphery. *Vis Res.* 1987;27:2193–2197.

145. Wang YZ, Thibos LN, Bradley A. Effects of refractive error on detection acuity and resolution acuity in peripheral vision. *Invest Ophthalmol Vis Sci.* 1997;38: 2134–2143.

146. Thibos LN. Acuity perimetry and the sampling theory of visual resolution. *Optom Vis Sci.* 1998;75:399–406.

Chapter 19

AN APPROACH TO THE DIAGNOSIS OF GLAUCOMA

Thomas L. Lewis
Murray Fingeret

Reaching an early diagnosis may be the most important step in the management of a patient with glaucoma. An early diagnosis permits timely intervention with treatment that has the best prognosis for long-term control of the disease.[1-5] The greatest clinical challenge, therefore, is timing the initiation of treatment so as to start as early as possible in patients with true glaucoma, but without overtreating. The clinician must be as sure as possible that the clinical evidence is sufficient to warrant committing patients to a lifetime of treatment for their disease.[6]

The timing of when a patient is labeled as having some form of glaucoma is critical for several reasons. On the one hand, making this decision too hastily can result in the treatment of patients presenting with normal fluctuation or who are merely glaucoma suspects. Prior to the 1970s, it was a common practice to treat all patients with elevated intraocular pressure (IOP), even though the majority of these patients never develop glaucoma.[7,8] The side effects from the treatment of glaucoma are significant, making the overdiagnosis and treatment of the disease inappropriate.

Conversely, waiting until a glaucoma patient has absolute, reproducible visual function loss before treatment is begun dramatically reduces the potential benefit of the therapeutic regimen.[1,9,10] In some glaucoma patients, as much as 50% of the ganglion cell axons may be destroyed with the patient presenting with normal visual fields.[11] There is a narrow window of opportunity in which an early yet not premature diagnosis of glaucoma can be made and treatment initiated prior to the occurrence of an excessive amount of tissue damage from the glaucomatous process.

It is difficult to make a timely differential diagnosis in a patient with a subtle presentation of glaucoma. This is especially true in a patient you are examining for the first time. Having the advantage of prior clinical information to establish baseline parameters is of great value in diagnosing the disease. This is because the most important clinical observation to be made in the early diagnosis of glaucoma patients is change in any of the key clinical parameters that are typically altered by the disease, i.e., IOP, the optic nerve, the nerve fiber layer, and visual function.[12,13] The only possible way to observe change is through multiple examinations. Change over time beyond the point of normal variation or fluctuation confirms the diagnosis and allows treatment to begin.

There are times, however, when it is not possible or appropriate to allow enough time to pass to observe changes in these parameters. You may find, on a single visit, that the potential risk of damage to the optic nerve is such that treatment must be strongly considered.

RELATIVE RISK

The most effective way of assuring the proper diagnosis of glaucoma is by collecting a complete matrix of clinical information and then determining the probability of whether or not the patient will develop the disease. It is only through proper testing that the true relative risk for glaucoma will surface. Unfortunately, there is no single clinical test with a 100% specificity and sensitivity for glaucoma.[3] Therefore, a combination of tests, analyzed collectively, is necessary to arrive at the proper diagnosis.

Years of clinical studies have uncovered different risk factors for glaucoma. It is clear that the prevalence of the disease is greater among patients with certain clinical characteristics as opposed to others. For example, patients with elevated IOPs have a greater prevalence for glaucoma than individuals with pressures below 21 mmHg.[14–21] Patients with ocular hypertension, therefore, are at greater risk of developing glaucoma than those with statistically normal IOP. It is important to understand what this really means from a clinical perspective.

Simply because one clinical finding or characteristic places a patient at greater risk of developing glaucoma does not mean that all individuals with this finding or characteristic will get the disease. Using ocular hypertension as an example, a study that followed patients for an average of 16 years, one group with ocular hypertension and the other normotensive, found that 5.5% of the ocular hypertensive patients developed glaucoma whereas 0.25% of the normotensive patients were diagnosed with the disease.[22] This clearly points out that the risk of glaucoma is greater with ocular hypertension (more than 20 times in the study), but that not everyone with ocular hypertension develops the disease. In fact, a vast majority (94.5%) of patients, over a period of 16 years, did not. Similar data exist for other risk factors for glaucoma.

It is, therefore, the relative risk for the development of glaucoma that is important to determine in a timely manner in dealing with a glaucoma suspect. A complete analysis of the patient will permit the clinician to assess this risk.

PATIENT PROFILE

An effective way to determine the probability of a patient developing glaucoma is to create a profile that identifies his or her risk factors for the disease. Initially, it may be valuable to display this profile on a clinical form (Table 19–1), which helps you analyze all the appropriate risk factors and visualize the profile of the patient. With experience, you will be able to develop the same perspective mentally without committing it to paper.

The patient profile form forces the clinician to develop an appropriate clinical examination regimen for the early differential diagnosis of glaucoma. It ensures that all the necessary clinical tests are completed and properly analyzed. With incomplete clinical data, the clinician is not able to effectively diagnose the more difficult presentations of glaucoma.

DIAGNOSTIC PUZZLE

Each patient presents a diagnostic challenge to the clinician. Subconsciously, the clinician handles each new patient as a "puzzle," so that he or she must collect all the necessary pieces in order to solve it. Glaucomas are

TABLE 19–1. PATIENT PROFILE

Factors	Low Risk	Moderate Risk	High Risk
Age	_____	_____	_____
Gender	_____	_____	_____
Race	_____	_____	_____
Family history	_____	_____	_____
High blood pressure	_____	_____	_____
Low blood pressure	_____	_____	_____
Heart disease	_____	_____	_____
Atherosclerosis	_____	_____	_____
Local vasospasms	_____	_____	_____
Migraine headache	_____	_____	_____
Corticosteroid use	_____	_____	_____
Refractive error	_____	_____	_____
Intraocular pressure	_____	_____	_____
Anterior chamber angle	_____	_____	_____
Optic nerve	_____	_____	_____
Nerve fiber layer	_____	_____	_____
Visual fields	_____	_____	_____
Color vision	_____	_____	_____
Afferent pupillary defect	_____	_____	_____
Retinal vein occlusion	_____	_____	_____
Ocular trauma	_____	_____	_____
Exfoliation syndrome	_____	_____	_____
Pigmentary dispersion syndrome	_____	_____	_____
Rubeosis irides	_____	_____	_____
Ocular inflammation	_____	_____	_____

a group of diseases to which the concept of a diagnostic puzzle is very relevant. If all the pieces of the puzzle are collected, it is much easier to determine a given patient's relative risk of developing glaucoma, to feel comfortable in making an early definitive diagnosis, and to follow the patient properly once treatment has been initiated.

The following clinical findings or patient characteristics are important pieces of the puzzle for glaucoma.

Risk Factors

There are a variety of risk factors—general, systemic, and ocular in nature—that apply to glaucoma. These risk factors vary for the different types of glaucoma. Risk factors can be causal or non-causal for the disease. This distinction is important in planning treatment. In reality, the most important risk factors clinically are those that are treatable.[23]

In primary open-angle glaucoma (POAG), the general risk factors usually include a family history,[24–30,32] an advanced age,[14,16,19–21,25,28,31–33] and being black.[17,32–36] Systemic factors that were once considered as risks for glaucoma were high[37] or low blood pressure[38] and diabetes mellitus.[36,39,40–42] However, more recent studies have brought into question the relationship of systemic hypertension[21,28,32,37,40,41,43] and diabetes mellitus[14,21,32,41,44] with POAG. These conditions may play a role in POAG but do not have an independent effect.[32] Clearly, systemic blood pressure and IOP have a relationship, but no association seems to exist between glaucoma and systemic hypertension. More recent evidence indicates that the duration of the systemic hypertension may be a consideration.[45] Systemic hypertension may have a protective effect in individuals younger than 60 years of age, and an adverse effect on glaucoma among those 70 years of age or older.[42,45] Low perfusion pressures[28,42,45,46] and nocturnal systemic hypotension do seem to be associated with the progression of glaucoma.[46,47]

Ocular risk factors include elevated IOP[48] the presence of nerve fiber layer dropout,[21,49] large physiological cups,[21,50] high myopia,[57] glaucoma in one eye,[10,52] and retinal vein occlusions.[53–56] Controversy exists as to whether nerve fiber dropout or large cupping is a risk factor or a sign of the disease.

The risk factors for normal-tension glaucoma are primarily vascular in nature, related to either a poor perfusion of blood to the optic nerve or local vasospastic events.[57–58] In addition to being elderly and being a woman,[59] systemic risk factors for normal-tension glaucoma are low blood pressure,[60,61] occlusive vascular diseases,[60] and a history of migraine headaches.[62,63] Nocturnal systemic hypertension may be especially important.[47,61,64] Ocularly, one might observe flame-shaped hemorrhages[19,61,63,65,66] on or near the optic nerve as well as a significant difference in IOP in the erect as compared with the supine position.[67]

In narrow-angle glaucoma, the major risk factor clearly is an anatomically shallow anterior chamber and/or narrow angle. This type of angle is influenced by familial factors,[68] increasing age,[69] and moderate to high hyperopia.[69] Women are three times more likely to have narrow angles than men.[70] Orientals[73–75] and Eskimos[71,72] are predisposed to narrow angles.

Certain ocular conditions are risk factors for the secondary development of glaucoma. A few of the more important ones may include pigmentary dispersion syndrome,[76] exfoliation syndrome,[77] ocular trauma,[78] retinal neovascular diseases,[79] uveitis,[80] and a history of systemic or ocular use of steroids.[81]

Within the past 10 years, six loci on chromosomes that include genes for various forms of glaucoma have been mapped.[82,83] This has reinforced the idea that the glaucomas are polygenic in nature and has initiated the use of DNA samples for genome-wide screening of families with the disease.

The presence of one or more of these risk factors would increase the probability of a patient developing one of the various forms of glaucoma. The more risk factors, the greater the probability.

Intraocular Pressure

The measurement of IOP through tonometry is an essential step in collecting information for the proper diagnosis of glaucoma. However, relying too heavily on a single tonometric reading can lead to overdiagnosis and, even more important, result in missing glaucoma patients with large diurnal variations in IOP or normal-tension glaucoma.[84]

The clinical interpretation of tonometry is complicated by two problems. The first is the issue of what a "normal" IOP is for a specific patient. The second is that IOP constantly fluctuates by several millimeters of mercury on a moment-to-moment basis,[85] and by as much as 10 mmHg or more in certain glaucoma patients from day to day.[86] Because of this, a single tonometric reading may represent such a small sample that it gives a very misleading representation of the patient's true pressure.

It is clear that a statistically abnormal IOP (above 21 mmHg) increases the risk (7 to 22 times) for the development of glaucoma.[87] The higher the pressure, the greater the risk of damage.[84] However, a vast majority of individuals with ocular hypertension will never develop glaucoma.[88–91] Among people with ocular hypertension, glaucoma will develop in about 1% per year.[89] Most clinicians will attempt to lower IOP if it exceeds 30 mmHg because of the risk of a secondary retinal vein occlusion[92] and because of the probability (33.3%) of damage to the optic nerve with pressure this high.[93]

Unfortunately, the only way to determine whether or not a certain level of IOP has exceeded the normal value for a given patient is to look for tissue damage in the optic nerve. The level of pressure that causes damage varies significantly from individual to individual and even in the same person as he or she grows older.[10,85] With age, there seems to be an increased susceptibility to optic nerve damage from levels of IOP that were previously well tolerated.[14,91] There is no single level of IOP above which all patients develop glaucoma and below which all patients are free of the disease.[48] Pressures below 21 mmHg do not ensure immunity from glaucoma.[94]

The fact that IOP is constantly fluctuating is an important concept in understanding the clinical value of tonometry. Fluctuation of IOP is due to a multitude of factors, some of which occur normally within the body every day,[95–97] and some of which are external influences, such as temperature,[98] exercise,[99] and fluid intake.[100] The short-term fluctuation in IOP that occurs diurnally can be problematic for the early diagnosis of glaucoma. The highest IOP can be reached at any time of the day, not necessarily just in the early morning.[86] It is essential, therefore, to record the time of day at which tonometry is performed. Diurnal pressure changes of more than 10 to 15 mmHg have been observed in glaucoma patients.[101] In fact, normal individuals have shown fluctuations as much as 10 mmHg. Any diurnal pressure swing of more than 6 mmHg should be considered suspicious. In a glaucoma suspect with suspicious optic nerves or visual fields but yet a low IOP on a single tonometric reading, a large diurnal fluctuation should be considered and assessed clinically. Even after treatment has begun, periodic evaluation of diurnal fluctuation in IOP is important.[102,103]

Long-term fluctuation can also occur in IOP. Several studies have indicated that a gradual increase in pressure over time may be more important in causing damage to the optic nerve than the absolute level of pressure at any given moment.[104] The presence of change in IOP over time is an important risk factor for glaucoma regardless of the baseline IOP for that patient.

Asymmetry in IOP between the eyes is another significant risk factor for glaucoma,[105] especially if the difference in pressures is more than 4 mmHg.[106] Asymmetry in IOP can cause asymmetrical damage even in normal-tension glaucoma,[106,107] and should also alert the clinician to a possible secondary cause for the glaucoma, i.e., trauma, exfoliation, or inflammation.[108]

All things considered, the clinician should not rely too heavily on a single tonometric reading, since such a reading by itself is a very poor indicator of glaucoma.[17,23,109] It is not possible to develop a magical cut-off point for IOP that differentiates normal from abnormal patients.[89] In fact, as an indicator of glaucoma, the sensitivity (50 to 70%) and specificity (90%) of tonometry[31] at a cut-off pressure of 21 mmHg is not impressive.[17,84] Because of the significant variation in IOP, 1/3 to 1/2 of all glaucoma patients show an IOP below 21 mmHg on a single pressure reading.[17,110] Therefore, if you rely too heavily on tonometry for the detection of glaucoma, you will miss a significant number of patients with the disease.

Using tonometry to develop baseline pressure levels, to monitor long-term and short-term fluctuation, and to look for symmetry between the two eyes makes evaluating IOP a useful component in the clinical work-up for the diagnosis and management of glaucoma (Table 19–2). The current status of our understanding of the role of IOP in the etiology of glaucoma indicates that it is a major, but not decisive, risk factor in the early disease process.[111] The chance of developing glaucoma in an individual eye is additionally modified by other risk factors, some of which are not yet validated on a prospective basis of epidemiological proof. Intraocular pressure alone cannot be relied on for the diagnosis of glaucoma, and it is not the sole determinant of visual field survival in patients receiving therapy.[112] However, IOP is one of the few risk factors, or perhaps the only risk factor amenable to treatment, and therefore remains the focus of patient management.

Biomicroscopy

For the diagnosis and treatment of glaucoma, it is essential to assess the anterior portion of the eye and the anterior chamber angle. Biomicroscopy in combination with gonioscopy allows the clinician to differentiate open from closed angles and also, in many instances, primary from secondary glaucomas. This information is critical in designing an appropriate management plan for a glaucoma patient.

With the biomicroscope, the clinician should assess the cornea for the presence of edema or

TABLE 19–2. VALUE OF TONOMETRY IN DIAGNOSING GLAUCOMA

Developing a baseline
Monitoring short-term fluctuation
Monitoring long-term fluctuation
Asymmetry

pigment on the back surface; the anterior chamber for pigment, cells, flare, keratic precipitates, and hyphema; the iris for pigment, defects in the pupillary ruff, exfoliation flakes, transillumination defects, rubeosis irides, iris atrophy, and posterior synechiae; and the crystalline lens for thickening, pigmentation, or exfoliation flakes.

Gonioscopy may reveal a narrow or closed angle, pigmentation, exfoliation, anterior synechiae, angle recession, or neovascularization. The openness of the angle, the curvature of the iris, the degree of pigmentation in the angle, and the presence of abnormal material or anatomy should be recorded.[113] If a closed angle is observed, indentation gonioscopy should be performed to determine whether the closure is synechial or appositional. This will influence the patient's treatment.

There is debate as to whether provocative testing is of any value in identifying those patients with narrow angles that are most likely to close. The provocative tests currently available are hampered by high false-positive and false-negative results.[114] If you wish to perform a provocative test, the choice might be a combined dark room–prone test, with a rise in pressure of 8 mmHg or more considered positive.[115]

Biomicroscopy and gonioscopy should be performed frequently on patients with a history of ocular trauma and/or with diabetic retinopathy, retinal vein occlusions, and other diseases that can lead to neovascularization of the retina.

Clinical Assessment of the Optic Nerve

A stereoscopic, magnified view of the optic nerve through a dilated pupil is critical for the early diagnosis of glaucoma. This can be achieved through a variety of techniques that include the biomicroscope in association with a Hruby lens, goniolenses, fundus contact lenses, and high plus lenses (i.e., 60 D, 78 D, 90 D). Stereophotography is critical for documentation of the appearance of the optic nerve for two reasons. One obvious reason is medicolegal. The other is that the permanent record created by ocular photography allows the best opportunity for the observation of subtle changes in the optic nerve tissue over time. Without photography, these changes are difficult to document clinically. Over the past 20 years, glaucoma specialists have moved from a detailed drawing, description, or both of the optic nerve head to photography, stereophotography, red-free photography, and, currently, computer-aided video analysis and confocal laser scanning tomography.[116–121]

Stereoscopic assessment of the optic nerve should stress five points: the integrity of the neuroretinal rim (NRR) with respect to thickness and color; the size

and shape of the disk and cup; the symmetry of the optic cupping between the two eyes; the size and shape of peripapillary atrophy; and the integrity of the surrounding retinal nerve fiber layer (Table 19–3). It is critical for the clinician to direct his or her attention to changes in the NRR tissue and not solely to the cup portion of the optic nerve.[122] The cup-to-disc ratio is dependent on the overall size of the disc and has a wide normal range.[123] The earliest disc changes in glaucoma cannot be adequately identified by estimates of cup-to-disc ratio.[124,125]

A majority of glaucoma patients incur some degree of both focal and diffuse damage to the optic nerve during the course of the disease (Table 19–4).[125] The most specific optic nerve findings for glaucoma

TABLE 19–3. CHANGES IN THE OPTIC NERVE AND NERVE FIBER LAYER IN GLAUCOMA

Optic Nerve
Enlargement of cup
Narrowing of rim
Asymmetry of cupping between the two eyes
Notching of the neuroretinal rim
Disc hemorrhages
Acquired parapapillary atrophy
Baring of the circumlinear vessel

Nerve Fiber Layer
Diffuse loss
Focal loss: wedges, slits

TABLE 19–4. CORRELATION OF STRUCTURAL DAMAGE AND FUNCTIONAL CHANGES IN GLAUCOMA

Diffuse Glaucomatous Damage	Focal Glaucomatous Damage
Optic Nerve	
Concentric enlargement of the cup	Vertical elongation of cup
Diffuse nerve fiber loss	Notching of rim
	Wedge or slit defects in nerve fiber layer
	Hemorrhages
Visual Function	
Generalized depression of threshold	Paracentral scotoma
Generalized contraction of isopter	Nasal steps
Color vision defects	
Decreased latency and amplitude of pattern electroretinograms	
Decrease in spatial and temporal contrast sensitivity	

include focal changes in the NRR (87%) usually in the form of a notch (Fig. 19–1).[126] Notches occur most frequently on the inferior rim, followed by the superior rim.[127] Temporal rim pallor is seen infrequently.[127] Vertical elongation of the cup also occurs from focal damage to the optic nerve.[125,127–129]

Even though focal damage is specific for glaucoma, more commonly one sees a generalized thinning of the NRR due to diffuse damage to the optic nerve (Fig. 19–2).[122,125,130] In some cases, this can be reflected through baring of the circumlinear vessels on the surface of the nerve.[131] In normal-tension glaucoma, the NRR may be significantly thinner.[132] In more advanced glaucoma cases, bean-pot enlargement of the cup can result in bayonetting of the large blood vessels as they cross the inner edge of the NRR.[127] Asymmetrical cup-to-disc ratios between the two eyes of more than 0.2 are highly significant for the diagnosis of glaucoma.[21,50]

Pallor of the NRR, although not specific for glaucoma, is quite commonly found and is indicative of the death of ganglion cell axons.[133,134] The color of the NRR can be misleading, since it is influenced by the technique used to examine the optic nerve and by media changes.[135] Parapapillary chorioretinal atrophy is associated with glaucoma, especially normal-tension glaucoma.[21,136–138] It correlates with NRR loss,[139–141] RNFL dropout,[139,141] disc hemorrhages[138] and visual field damage,[139,140] but not with IOP.[142] As NRR damage approaches the edge of the disc, parapapillary atrophy becomes more prevalent.[139] Parapapillary atrophy does not correlate with IOP or the size of the optic disc.[143]

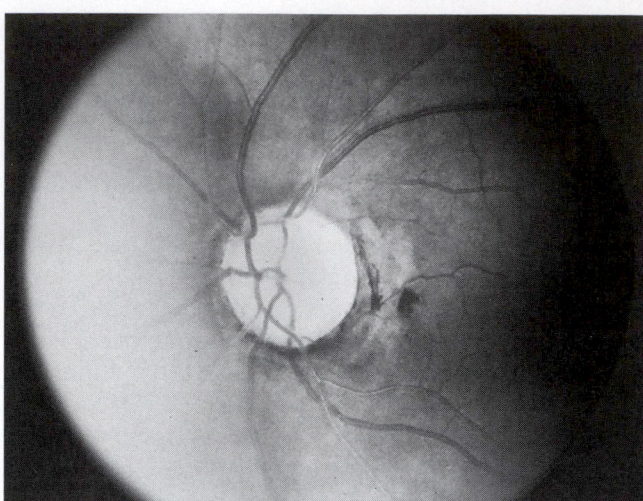

Figure 19–2. Generalized damage to neuroretinal rim. Left eye of glaucoma patient with symmetrical thinning and pallor of the neuroretinal rim. Peripapillary atrophy is present around the entire optic nerve head but more extensive temporally.

Associated findings in glaucoma may include the presence of large, elongated laminar dots in the center of the optic nerve[144] as well as splinter- or flame-shaped hemorrhages on or near the disc.[19,145,146] These hemorrhages, which are more commonly found in normal-tension glaucoma,[61,65,147–149] may represent infarction of the blood supply to the optic nerve and therefore could be a clinical sign of impending nerve damage and visual field loss.[146,150–154] They have been shown to be associated with RNFL defects and parapapillary atrophy[138] and to precede clinical changes in the retinal nerve fiber layer and visual fields in some glaucoma patients.[65,151,155,156]

Proper assessment of the optic nerve is very sensitive (70 to 90%)[157,158] and specific (80 to 97%)[157,158] for the early diagnosis of glaucoma. There are a few glaucoma patients who will show visual function loss prior to presenting with clinically observable damage to the optic nerve, especially individuals with a large optic disc and large physiological cup.[13,158] Early intervention to lower IOP may reverse optic nerve changes in some patients.[159]

Clinical Assessment of the Nerve Fiber Layer

Evaluation of the retinal nerve fiber layer (RNFL) within two disc diameters of the optic nerve is essential for the proper diagnosis and management of glaucomas. Various techniques can be used to perform this evaluation, including indirect ophthalmoscopy and procedures similar to those used to evaluate the optic nerve. Detection of subtle RNFL loss is difficult and clinically challenging. The use of red-free light for

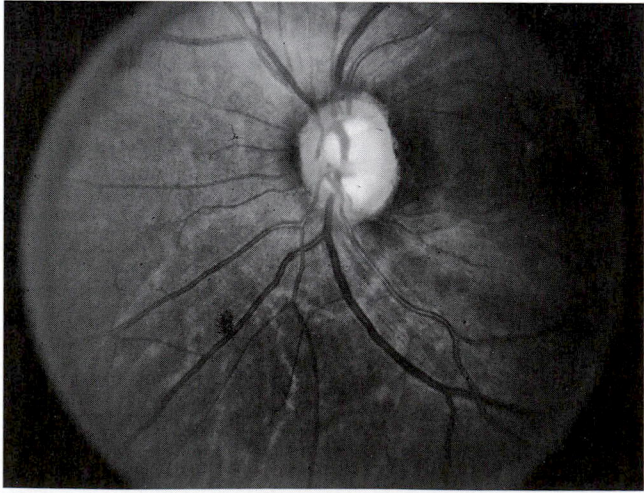

Figure 19–1. Focal damage to the neuroretinal rim. Left eye of a glaucoma patient with a notch at the inferior rim at 6 o'clock, and thinning of the neuroretinal rim. Narrow wedges of nerve fiber layer dropout are present at 1 and 6 o'clock.

both the evaluation and photographing of the RNFL is helpful in accentuating the reflection of light off of this tissue and in observing any defects that might exist.[160] Recently, scanning laser polarimetry[161–164] and optical coherence tomography[165,166] have been introduced to measure changes in RNFL thickness.

Nerve fiber defects can occur focally in the form of slits or wedges (Fig. 19–3) or diffusely around the optic nerve (see Table 19–4).[167] The predominant pattern of RNFL damage distinguishing glaucomatous field loss is diffuse rather than focal. The presence of RNFL defects is highly specific (80 to 90%) and sensitive (85 to 97%) for glaucoma,[167–170] especially in view of the fact that slit-like defects are found in normal people and are neither common nor reliable for glaucoma.[171,172]

The clinical importance of RNFL dropout is that it seems to occur early in the disease in many glaucoma patients, usually preceding visual field loss.[168–170,173] In fact, it may be the earliest recognizable sign of glaucoma.[174] When approximately 50% of axons in a given area have been destroyed at the level of the lamina cribrosa, the retrograde degeneration appears clinically on the surface of the retina.[175] Studies have shown RNFL defects to be present up to 5 years before detectable visual field loss occurred clinically.[169,176,177] In addition, there is a very strong correlation between the type of RNFL defect (focal or diffuse) and the type and location of subsequent visual field loss.[178] Therefore, there appears to be great value in assessing the RNFL for the presence of glaucomatous damage and for the progression of this damage once it has begun.

Evaluation of Visual Function

Assessment of visual function can be accomplished through a variety of psychophysical and electrophysiological tests.[179,180] These include evaluation of visual fields, color vision, contrast sensitivity, pattern electroretinograms, and visual evoked potentials. Visual field testing is the most practical diagnostic procedure to perform clinically in a private practice setting.

There continues to be concern regarding the specificity of the changes seen in psychophysical and electrophysiological testing as it relates to glaucoma. This is because of the significant overlap between the findings in normal people, glaucoma suspects, and glaucoma patients. In addition, changes similar to those seen in glaucoma can also be found in a variety of other conditions, including aging, cataracts, and other media changes.[181] One clear result of data from psychophysical testing is that nerve fibers mediating central visual function are adversely affected in glaucoma, even early in the disease process.[182]

Glaucoma can produce morphological damage to the optic nerve focally, diffusely, or in combination. Diffuse changes such as concentric enlargement of the cup and generalized thinning of the NRR and RNFL are often difficult to distinguish from normal patients, as well as to quantify. Functionally, this type of damage manifests itself by general depression of the visual field, color vision defects, changes in contrast sensitivity, and altered electrodiagnostic tests (see Table 19–4). The value of psychophysical and electrodiagnostic testing may lie in improving the specificity and diagnostic value of evaluating diffuse damage.

Yellow-blue and blue-green defects in color vision have been identified in certain glaucoma patients.[183–185] As many as 20% of glaucoma suspects[186] may have defects in color vision, yet 25% of advanced glaucoma patients may not.[187,188] Loss of

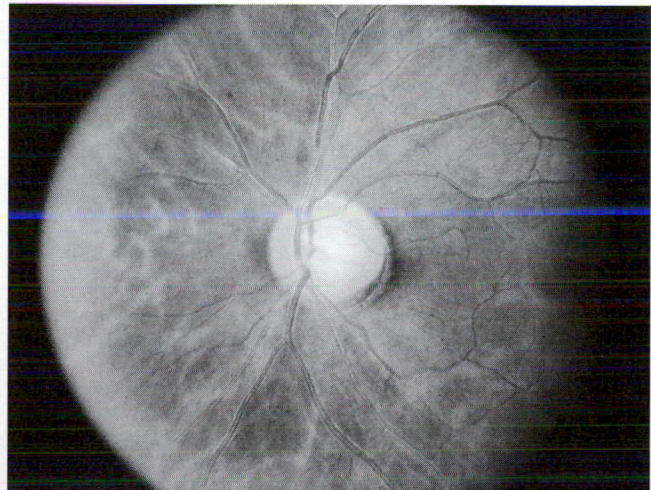

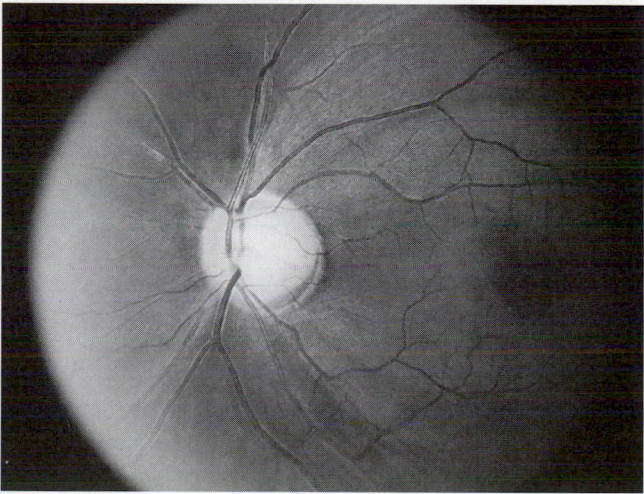

Figure 19–3. Focal nerve fiber layer dropout. Color and companion red-free photography of the left eye of a glaucoma patient with several slit-like defects in the nerve fiber layer between 12 and 2 o'-clock and a large wedge defect between 5 and 7 o'clock. (*See also Color Plate 40.*)

color vision is often associated more with glaucoma patients who have higher levels of IOP.[189,190]

The most practical procedure to perform clinically, which is sensitive for acquired defects of color vision, is a desaturated D-15 test done monocularly under proper illumination.[191] Two or more cross-over defects with this test indicate failure. Color vision tests should be conducted on all glaucoma suspects, as the results represent an additional piece of information to assess their relative risk of developing the disease. Defects in color vision, if they occur, usually correlate well with the extent of the visual field loss.[192] Abnormalities of color vision may be present before changes in the visual field and assist the clinician in making an earlier diagnosis of loss of visual function.[184,186,188]

Visual field testing has been the standard method of assessing loss of visual function in glaucoma. Automated perimetry has become a practical form of visual field testing and shows its greatest value clinically in the diagnosis and management of glaucoma.[193,194] Changes in retinal sensitivity are uncovered at an earlier stage with automated than with manual perimetry.[195] Threshold visual fields in the central 30° should be performed on all glaucoma suspects. Threshold perimetry, with a statistical analysis of the data, has a 93% sensitivity and 84% specificity for glaucoma.[196] Screening tests with automated perimeters may have some value in detecting the presence of field abnormalities in those patients who otherwise present with minimal risks for glaucoma.[197]

The location of the earliest visual field loss may depend on the type of glaucoma. Individuals with very high IOPs may present primarily with diffuse damage to the optic nerve and a general depression of sensitivity of the visual field.[189,198] This may be difficult to differentiate from similar changes occurring in otherwise normal individuals because of small pupils, uncorrected refractive error, media changes,[199] or age.[200] If the damage to the optic nerve is primarily focal in nature, the glaucoma patient would present with the classic field defects of increased fluctuation in isolated areas of the visual field,[201] paracentral scotomas 5 to 20° from fixation, and either central or peripheral nasal steps (Fig. 19–4).[199,202] These defects occur more frequently in a superior than an inferior hemisphere of the visual field.[3,203] Between 75 and 90% of the earliest visual field defects appear in the central 30° of the visual field.[202] Visual-field defects such as generalized constriction, enlargement of the blind spot, and baring of the blind spot—which have traditionally been associated with glaucoma—are in reality not specific for the disease and should not be used as criteria for a definitive diagnosis or for ongoing management.[199]

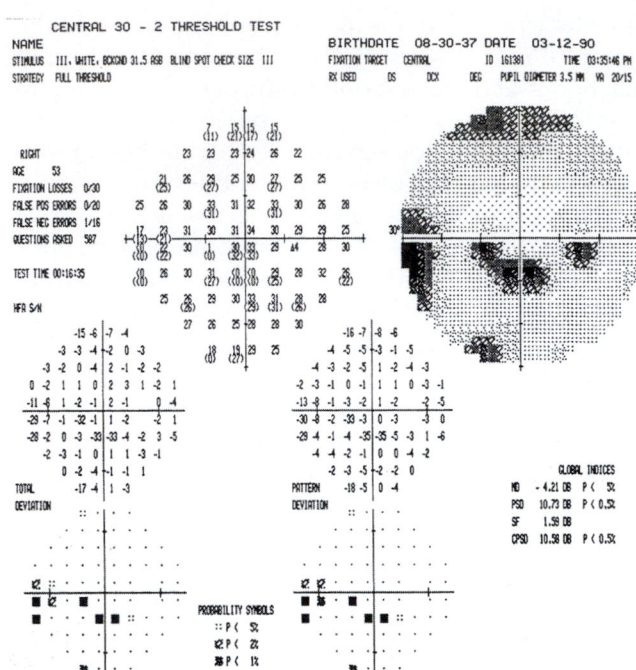

Figure 19–4. Visual field defects. Automated visual field printout of the right eye of a glaucoma patient showing an extensive inferior arcuate scotoma and a nasal field defect in the central visual field.

It is not uncommon, in early glaucoma, for the nasal hemisphere to show incongruity between the superior and inferior quadrants (see Fig. 19-4).[3,204,205] Visual field defects in glaucoma are often limited to a single altitudinal hemifield, with the corresponding hemifield remaining unaffected for up to 10 years.[3] Normal-tension glaucoma usually causes focal types of field defects that are somewhat unique in being closer to fixation and denser.[59,206–211] Asymmetry in the sensitivity between the two eyes of more than a few decibels on repeated testing may be clinically significant.[212] Glaucoma patients with asymmetrical nerve damage and/or visual field loss may show an afferent pupillary defect.[213]

The most important aspect of visual field testing in glaucoma is to detect the field loss as early as possible. This has been aided by the introduction of automated perimetry.[214] Quigley's studies have shown that a significant portion of the optic nerve is already destroyed before traditional methods of assessing visual function become abnormal.[11] Once damage has reached this level, progression of visual field loss occurs more rapidly, since there is less of a buffer or redundancy in the number of ganglion cells and their receptive fields.[8]

If glaucoma can be identified prior to visual field defects through observation of the changes in the optic nerve, treatment of the disease has the best chance of slowing down or preventing any further damage.[3,215] If glaucoma is not treated until the patient has absolute reproducible visual field defects, damage to the optic nerve may be so significant that, even with a dramatic reduction of IOP, the disease continues to progress.[216]

Summary

Collecting all the pieces of the puzzle (clinical data, patient characteristics) allows one more opportunities to make the diagnosis. With the data available from a complete work-up, the clinician is able to analyze the information and assess the probability of the patient developing glaucoma. If the patient does have several risk factors, it is important to determine whether or not damage from glaucoma has already occurred. If it has, treatment must be initiated.

An analysis of each piece of clinical data in isolation from any other does not give complete insight into the relative risk of the patient for glaucoma.[12,217] The simultaneous analysis of multiple pieces of the puzzle has been shown to be much more effective in predicting which patients will eventually develop the disease.[218–220] As an example, if you were to examine 1000 patients over the age of 40, you might find 7 to 8% with IOPs over 21 mmHg, 5 to 6% with cup-to-disc ratios of greater than 0.5, 2 to 5% with visual-field loss, but only 0.5 to 1% with glaucoma. Even though each of these findings is a risk factor for glaucoma, their prevalence in the general population would exceed the prevalence of glaucoma. This is true for all of the risk factors discussed. By analyzing multiple risk factors in an individual, the probability of identifying those patients with the greatest chance of progressing to glaucoma increases dramatically.[14,42,216,217,220]

MANAGEMENT OF THE PATIENT

The reason for making as early a definitive diagnosis of glaucoma as possible is to initiate appropriate treatment. The process used to reach the decision to treat or not is complex and varies among clinicians. Many factors must be weighed before committing a patient to a life of drugs and/or surgery. These would include the cumulative risk of the patient to develop some form of glaucoma, the patient's age, the patient's level of anxiety about the disease, the doctor's level of concern, the likelihood of patient compliance with treatment, and the ability of the patient to be able to afford the care on a long-term basis.[219] Ultimately, the decision to treat will be made by weighing the benefits versus the risk to the patient.

CONCLUSION

The early differential diagnosis of glaucoma is the most critical step in the proper management of the disease. Early diagnosis is possible if the clinician collects all the appropriate clinical data and properly analyzes the patient's characteristics. This allows a determination of the relative risk or probability of the patient developing glaucoma.

REFERENCES

1. Hattenhauer MG, Johnson DH, Ing HH, Herman DC, et al. The probability of blindness from open-angle glaucoma. *Ophthalmology*. 1998;105:2099–2104.
2. Graham PA. The definition of pre-glaucoma: A prospective study. *Trans Ophthalmol Soc UK*. 1968;88:153–165.
3. Hart WM, Becker B. The onset and evolution of glaucomatous visual field defects. *Ophthalmology*. 1982;89:268–279.
4. Mao LK, Stewart WC, Shields MB. Correlation between intraocular pressure control and progressive glaucomatous damage in primary open-angle glaucoma. *Am J Ophthalmol*. 1991;111:51–55.
5. Chauhan BC, Drance SM. The relationship between intraocular pressure and visual field progression in glaucoma. *Graefes Arch Clin Exp Ophthalmol*. 1992;230:521–526.
6. Phelps CD. The "no treatment" approach to ocular hypertension. *Surv Ophthalmol*. 1980;25:175–182.
7. Drance SM. Review: The medical management of open angle glaucoma. *Can J Ophthalmol*. 1978;13:123–127.
8. Quigley HA. Glaucoma's optic nerve damage: Changing clinical perspectives. *Ann Ophthalmol*. 1982;14:611–612.
9. Chandler PA. Long-term results in glaucoma therapy. *Am J Ophthalmol*. 1975;80:62–69.
10. Grant WM, Burke JF. Why do some people go blind from glaucoma? *Am J Ophthalmol*. 1982;89:991–998.
11. Quigley HA, Addicks EM, Green WR. Optic nerve damage in human glaucoma: III. Quantitative correlation of nerve fiber loss and visual field defects in glaucoma, ischemic optic neuropathy, papilledema, and toxic optic neuropathy. *Arch Ophthalmol*. 1982;100:135–146.
12. Krupin T, Rosenberg LF, Ruderman JM. Update: Diagnostic concept in open-angle glaucoma. *Curr Opin Ophthalmol*. 1991;2:120–127.
13. Motolko M, Drance SM. Features of the optic disc in pre-glaucomatous eyes. *Arch Ophthalmol*. 1981;99:1992–1994.
14. Armaly MF, Krueger DE, Maunder L, Becker B, et al. Biostatistical analysis of the collaborative glaucoma study: I. Summary report of the risk factors for glaucomatous visual field defects. *Arch Ophthalmol*. 1980;98:2163–2172.
15. Hoskins HD. The management of elevated intraocular pressure with normal optic discs and visual fields: II. An approach to early therapy. *Surv Ophthalmol*. 1977;21:479–493.

16. Leibowitz HM, Krueger DE, Maunder LR, Milton RC, et al. The Framingham Eye Study Monograph. *Surv Ophthalmol*. 1980; 112:821–829.

17. Sommer A, Tielsch JM, Katz J, Quigley HA, et al. Relationship between intraocular pressure and primary open angle glaucoma among white and black Americans: The Baltimore Eye Survey. *Arch Ophthalmol*. 1991;109:1090–1095.

18. Davanger M, Ringvold A, Blika S. The probability of having glaucoma at different IOP levels. *Acta Ophthalmol*. 1991; 69:565–568.

19. Klein BE, Klein R, Sponsel WE, Franke T, et al. Prevalence of glaucoma: The Beaver Dam Eye Study. *Ophthalmology*. 1992;99:1499–1504.

20. Leske MC, Connell AMS, Schachat AP, Hyman L, and the Barbados Eye Study Group. The Barbados Eye Study. Prevalence of open angle glaucoma. *Arch Ophthalmol*. 1994;112:821–829.

21. Quigley HA, Enger C, Katz J, Sommer A, et al. Risk factors for the development of glaucomatous visual field loss in ocular hypertension. *Arch Ophthalmol*. 1994;112:644–649.

22. Jenson JE. Glaucoma screening: A 16-year follow-up of ocular normotensives. *Acta Ophthalmol*. 1984;62:203–209.

23. Anderson DR. Glaucoma: The damage caused by pressure. XLVI Edward Jackson Memorial Lecture. *Am J Ophthalmol*. 1989;108:485–495.

24. Paterson G. A nine-year follow-up of studies on first-degree relatives of patients with glaucoma simplex. *Trans Ophthalmol Soc UK*. 1970;90:515–525.

25. Leske MC. The epidemiology of open-angle glaucoma: A review. *Am J Epidemiol*. 1983;118:166–191.

26. Rosenthal AR, Perkins ES. Family studies in glaucoma. *Br J Ophthalmol*. 1985;69:664–667.

27. Tielsch JM, Katz J, Sommer A, Quigley HA, Javitt JC. Family history and risk of primary open-angle glaucoma: The Baltimore Eye Survey. *Arch Ophthalmol*. 1994;112:69–73.

28. Leske MC, Roberts LW, Wu S-Y. Open-angle glaucoma and ocular hypertension: The Long Island Glaucoma Case-Control Study. *Ophthalmol Epidemiol*. 1996;3: 85–96.

29. Nemesure B, Leske MC, He Q, Mendell N. Analyses of reported family history of glaucoma: A preliminary investigation. *Ophthalmol Epidemiol*. 1996;3:135–141.

30. Wolfs RCW, Klaver CCW, Ramrattan RS, van Duijn CM, et al. Genetic risk of primary open-angle glaucoma. Population-based familial aggregation study. *Arch Ophthalmol*. 1998;116:1640–1645.

31. Hollows FC, Graham PA. Intraocular pressure, glaucoma and glaucoma suspects in a defined population. *Br J Ophthalmol*. 1966;50:570–586.

32. Leske MC, Connell AMS, Wu S-Y, Hyman LG, Schachat AP, and the Barbados Eye Study Group. Risk factors for open-angle glaucoma: The Barbados Eye Study. *Arch Ophthalmol*. 1995;113:918–924.

33. Tielsch JM, Sommer A, Katz J, Royall RM, et al. Racial variation in the prevalence of primary open-angle glaucoma: The Baltimore Eye Survey. *JAMA*. 1991;266: 369–374.

34. Martin MJ, Sommer A, Gold EB, Diamond EL. Race and primary open-angle glaucoma. *Am J Ophthalmol*. 1985;99:383–387.

35. Leske MC, Connell AMS, Wu S-Y, Hyman L, Schachat AP, and the Barbados Eye Study Group. Distribution of intraocular pressure: The Barbados Eye Study. *Arch Ophthalmol*. 1997;115:1051–1057.

36. Wu S-Y, Leske MC, and the Barbados Eye Study Group. Associations with intraocular pressure in the Barbados Eye Study. *Arch Ophthalmol*. 1997;115:1572–1576.

37. Leske MC, Podgor MJ. Intraocular pressure, cardiovascular risk variables and visual field defects. *Am J Epidemiol*. 1983;118:280–287.

38. Francois J, Neetens A. The deterioration of the visual field in glaucoma and the blood pressure. *Doc Ophthalmol*. 1970;28:70–132.

39. Becker B. Diabetes mellitus and primary open-angle glaucoma. *Am J Ophthalmol*. 1971;70:1–16.

40. Morgan RW, Drance SM. Chronic open angle glaucoma and ocular hypertension: An epidemiological study. *Br J Ophthalmol*. 1975;59:211–215.

41. Katz J, Sommer A. Risk factors for primary open angle glaucoma. *Am J Prev Med*. 1988;4:110–114.

42. Wilson MR, Hertzmark E, Walter AM, Childs-Shaw K, Epstein DC. A case-control study of risk factors in open angle glaucoma. *Arch Ophthalmol*. 1987;105:1066–1071.

43. Kahn HA, Leibowitz HM, Ganley JP. The Framingham Eye Study: II. Association of ophthalmic pathology with single variables previously measured in the Framingham Heart Study. *Am J Epidemiol*. 1977; 106:33–41.

44. Tielsch JM, Katz J, Quigley HA, Javitt JC, Sommer A. Diabetes, intraocular pressure, and primary open-angle glaucoma in the Baltimore Eye Survey. *Ophthalmology*. 1995;102:48–53.

45. Tielsch JM, Katz J, Sommer A, Quigley HA, Javitt JC. Hypertension, perfusion pressure and primary open-angle glaucoma. *Arch Ophthalmol*. 1995;113:216–221.

46. Hayreh SS, Zimmerman B, Podhajsky P, Alward WLM. Nocturnal arterial hypotension and its role in optic nerve head and ocular ischemic disorders. *Am J Ophthalmol*. 1994;114:603–624.

47. Graham SL, Drance SM, Wijsman K, Douglas GR, Mikelberg FS. Ambulatory blood pressure monitoring in glaucoma: The nocturnal dip. *Ophthalmology*. 1995; 102:61–69.

48. Sommer A. Intraocular pressure and glaucoma. *Am J Ophthalmol*. 1989;107:186–188.

49. Hoyt WF, Frisen L, Newman NW. Fundoscopy of the nerve fiber layer defects in glaucoma. *Invest Ophthalmol*. 1973;12:814–829.

50. Yablonski ME, Zimmerman TJ, Kass MA, Becker B. Prognostic significance of optic disc cupping in ocular hypertensive patients. *Am J Ophthalmol*. 1980;89:585–590.

51. Perkins ES, Phelps CD. Open-angle glaucoma, ocular hypertension, low tension glaucoma and refraction. *Arch Ophthalmol*. 1982;100:1464–1467.

52. Kass MA, Kolker AE, Becker B. Prognostic factors in

glaucomatous visual field loss. *Arch Ophthalmol.* 1976; 94:1274–1276.

53. David R, Zangwill L, Badarna M, Yassur Y. Epidemiology of retinal vein occlusion and its association with glaucoma and increased intraocular pressure. *Ophthalmologica.* 1988;197:69–74.

54. Rath EZ, Frank RN, Shin DH, Kim C. Risk factors for retinal vein occlusions: A case-control study. *Ophthalmology.* 1992;99:509–514.

55. Appiah AA, Greenridge KC. Factors associated with retinal-vein occlusions in Hispanics. *Ann Ophthalmol.* 1987;19:307–312.

56. The Eye Disease Case-Control Study Group. Risk factors for central retinal vein occlusions. *Arch Ophthalmol.* 1996;114:545–554.

57. Drance SM, Douglas GR, Wijsmank K, et al. Response of blood flow to warm and cold in normal and low-tension glaucoma patients. *Am J Ophthalmol.* 1988;105:35–39.

58. Gasser P. Ocular vasospasm: A risk factor in the pathogenesis of low-tension glaucoma. *Int Ophthalmol.* 1989; 13:281–290.

59. Levene R. Low tension glaucoma: A critical review and new material. *Surv Ophthalmol.* 1980;24:621–664.

60. Drance SM, Sweeney VP, Morgan RW, Feldman F. Studies of factors involved in the production of low tension glaucoma. *Arch Ophthalmol.* 1973;89:457–465.

61. Ishida K, Yamamoto T, Kitazawa Y. Clinical factors associated with progression of normal-tension glaucoma. *J Glaucoma.* 1998;7:372–377.

62. Phelps CD, Corbett JJ. Migraine and low-tension glaucoma. *Invest Ophthalmol Vis Sci.* 1985;26:1105–1108.

63. Yamazaki Y, Hayamizu F, Miyamoto S, Nakagami T, et al. Optic disc findings in normal tension glaucoma. *Jpn J Ophthalmol.* 1997;41:260–267.

64. Meyer JH, Brandi-Dohrn J, Funk J. Twenty four hour blood pressure monitoring in normal tension glaucoma. *Br J Ophthalmol.* 1996;80:864–867.

65. Kitazawa Y, Shirato S, Yamamoto T. Optic disc hemorrhage in low-tension glaucoma. *Ophthalmology.* 1986; 93:853–857.

66. Chumbley LC, Brubaker RF. Low-tension glaucoma. *Am J Ophthalmol.* 1994;97:730–737.

67. Hyams SW, Frankel A, Keroub C, Antal J. Postural changes in intraocular pressure with particular reference to low tension glaucoma. *Glaucoma.* 1984;6:178–181.

68. Low RF. Primary angle-closure glaucoma: Inheritance and environment. *Br J Ophthalmol.* 1972;56:13–20.

69. Fontana SC, Brubaker RF. Volume and depth of the anterior chamber in the normal aging human eye. *Arch Ophthalmol.* 1980;98:1803–1808.

70. Alsbirk PH. Corneal diameter in Greenland Eskimos: Anthropometric and genetic studies with special reference to primary angle-closure glaucoma. *Acta Ophthalmol.* 1975;53:635–646.

71. Alsbirk PH. Primary angle-closure glaucoma: Oculometry, epidemiology, and genetics in a high risk population. *Acta Ophthalmol Suppl.* 1976;127:5–31.

72. Drance SM, Morgan RW, Bryett J, Fairclough M. Ante-

rior chamber depth and gonioscopic findings among the Eskimos and Indians in the Canadian Arctic. *Can J Ophthalmol.* 1973;8:255–259.

73. Fujita K, Negishi C, Fujikik K, et al. Epidemiology of primary angle closure glaucoma: Report 1. *Jpn J Clin Ophthalmol.* 1983;37:625–629.

74. Foster PJ, Baasanhu J, Alsbirk PH, Munkhbayar D, et al. Glaucoma in Mongolia. *Arch Ophthalmol.* 1996;114: 1235–1241.

75. Congdon NG, Youlin Q, Quigley HA, Hung PT, et al. Biometry and primary angle-closure glaucoma among Chinese, white and black populations. *Ophthalmology.* 1997;104:1489–1495.

76. Sugar HS. Pigmentary glaucoma: A 25-year review. *Am J Ophthalmol.* 1966;62:499–507.

77. Sugar HS. The pseudoexfoliation syndrome. *Metab Pediatr Syst Ophthalmol.* 1982;6:227–236.

78. Jones WL. Post-traumatic glaucoma. *J Am Optom Assoc.* 1987;58:708–715.

79. Brown GC, Magargal L, Schachat A, Shah H. Neovascular glaucoma: Etiologic considerations. *Ophthalmology.* 1984;91:315–319.

80. Posner A, Schlossman A. Syndrome of unilateral recurrent attacks of glaucoma with cyclitic symptoms. *Arch Ophthalmol.* 1948;39:517–535.

81. Schwartz B. The response of ocular pressure to corticosteroids. *Int Ophthalmol Clin.* 1966;6:929–987.

82. Raymound V. Molecular genetics of the glaucomas: Mapping of the first five "GLC" loci. *Am J Hum Genet.* 1997;60:272–277.

83. Wirtz MK, Samples JR, Rust K, Lie J, et al. GLC1F, a new primary open-angle glaucoma locus, maps to 7q35-q36. *Arch Ophthalmol.* 1999;117:237–241.

84. Sommer A. Glaucoma screening: Too little, too late? *J Gen Intern Med.* 1990;5(suppl):533–537.

85. Leydhecker W. The intraocular pressure: Clinical aspects. *Ann Ophthalmol.* 1976;8:389–399.

86. Katavisto M. The diurnal variations of ocular tension in glaucoma. *Acta Ophthalmol (Copenh).* 1964;78(suppl): 3–130.

87. Sponsel WE. Tonometry in question: Can visual screening tests play a more decisive role in glaucoma diagnosis and management? *Surv Ophthalmol.* 1989;33(suppl): 291–300.

88. Armaly MF. Ocular pressure and visual fields: A 10-year follow-up study. *Arch Ophthalmol.* 1969;81:25–40.

89. Kitazawa Y, Horie T, Aoki S, Suzuki M, Nishioka K. Untreated ocular hypertension: A long-term prospective study. *Arch Ophthalmol.* 1977;95:1180–1184.

90. Linner E. Ocular hypertension: The clinical course during ten years without therapy: Aqueous humor dynamics. *Acta Ophthalmol.* 1976;54:707–720.

91. Perkins ES. The Bedford glaucoma survey: II. Rescreening of normal population. *Br J Ophthalmol.* 1973;57: 186–192.

92. Ellenberg G, Freedman J. Retinal vein occlusion and ocular hypertension. *Ann Ophthalmol.* 1982;14:920–922.

93. Schappert-Kemmijser J. A five-year follow-up of subjects with IOP of 20–30 mm Hg without anom-

alies of optic nerve and visual field typical for glaucoma at first investigation. *Ophthalmologica*. 1971;162: 289–295.

94. Cotton T, Ederer F. The distribution of intraocular pressures in the general population. *Surv Ophthalmol*. 1980; 25:123–129.

95. Kass MA, Sears ML. Hormonal regulation of intraocular pressure. *Surv Ophthalmol*. 1977;22:153–176.

96. Shiose Y. The aging effect on intraocular pressure in an apparently normal population. *Arch Ophthalmol*. 1984; 102:883–887.

97. Shiose Y. Statistical analysis of systemic effect on intraocular pressure. *Glaucoma*. 1984;6:231–235.

98. Blumenthal M, Blumenthal R, Peritz E, Best M. Seasonal variation in intraocular pressure. *Am J Ophthalmol*. 1970;69:608–610.

99. Marcus DF, Krupin T, Podos SM. The effect of exercise on intraocular pressure: I. Human beings. *Invest Ophthalmol*. 1970;9:749–752.

100. Galin MA, Davidson R, Pasmanik S. An osmotic comparison of urea and mannitol. *Am J Ophthalmol*. 1963; 55:244–247.

101. Kitazawa Y, Horie T. Diurnal variation of intraocular pressure and its significance in the medical treatment of primary open-angle glaucoma. In: Krieglstein GK, Leydhecker W, eds. *Glaucoma Update*. New York: Springer; 1979:169–176.

102. Horie T, Kitazawa Y. The clinical significance of diurnal pressure variation in primary open-angle glaucoma. *Jpn J Ophthalmol*. 1979;23:310–333.

103. Jonas JB, Gusek GC, Naumann GOH. Optic disc, cup and neuroretinal rim size, configuration, and correlations in normal eyes. *Invest Ophthalmol Vis Sci*. 1988;29:1151–1158.

104. Schwartz B, Talusan AG. Spontaneous trends in ocular pressure in untreated ocular hypertension. *Arch Ophthalmol*. 1980;98:105–111.

105. Davanger M. The difference in ocular pressure in the two eyes of the same person: In individuals with healthy eyes and in patients with glaucoma simplex. *Acta Ophthalmol*. 1965;43:299–313.

106. Crichton A, Drance SM, Douglas GR, Schulzer M. Unequal intraocular pressure and its relation to asymmetric visual field defects in low-tension glaucoma. *Ophthalmology*. 1989;96:1312–1314.

107. Cartwright MJ, Anderson DR. Correlation of asymmetric damage with asymmetric intraocular pressure in normal-tension glaucoma (low-tension glaucoma). *Arch Ophthalmol*. 1988;106:898–900.

108. Alexander LJ. Diagnosis and management of primary open-angle glaucoma. In: Classe JG, ed. *Optometry Clinics: Glaucoma*. Norwalk, CT: Appleton & Lange; 1991:19–102.

109. Leske MC, Rosenthal J. Epidemiologic aspect of open-angle glaucoma. *Am J Epidemiol*. 1979;109:250–272.

110. Kahn HA, Milton RC. Alternative definitions for open-angle glaucoma: Effect on prevalence and association in the Framingham Eye Study. *Arch Ophthalmol*. 1980; 98:2172–2177.

111. Krieglstein GK. Glaucoma: Editorial overview. *Curr Opin Ophthalmol*. 1990;1:103–104.

112. Sponsel WE. Quantification and monitoring of visual field defects and a prospective, randomized comparison of pilocarpine and timolol using computerized perimetry (summary). *Surv Ophthalmol*. 1989;33(suppl): 427–428.

113. Greenidge KC. Angle-closure glaucoma. *Int Ophthalmol Clin*. 1990;30:177–185.

114. Wand M. Provocative tests in angle-closure glaucoma: A brief review with commentary. *Ophthalmic Surg*. 1974;5:32–37.

115. Harris LS, Galin MA. Prone provocative testing for narrow-angle glaucoma. *Arch Ophthalmol*. 1972;87: 493–496.

116. Caprioli J, Miller JM. Videographic measurements of optic nerve topography in glaucoma. *Invest Ophthalmol Vis Sci*. 1988;29:1294–1298.

117. Mikelberg FS, Parfitt CM, Swindale NV, Graham SL, et al. Ability of the Heidelberg retina tomograph to detect early glaucomatous field loss. *J Glaucoma*. 1995;4: 242–247.

118. Hatch WV, Flanagan JG, Etchells, Williams-Lyn DE, Trope GE. Laser scanning tomography of the optic nerve head in ocular hypertension and glaucoma. *Br J Ophthalmol*. 1997;81:871–876.

119. Uchida H, Brigatti L, Caprioli J. Detection of structural damage from glaucoma with confocal laser image analysis. *Invest Ophthalmol Vis Sci*. 1996;37:2393–2401.

120. Zangwill LM, van Horn S, DeSouza Lima M, Sample PA, Weinreb RN. Optic nerve head topography in ocular hypertensive eyes using confocal scanning laser ophthalmoscopy. *Am J Ophthalmol*. 1996;122:520–525.

121. Kamal DS, Viswanathan AC, Garway-Heath DF, Hitchings RA, et al. Detection of optic change with the Heidelberg retina tomograph before confirmed visual field change in ocular hypertensives converting to early glaucoma. *Br J Ophthalmol*. 1999;83:290–294.

122. Airaksinen PJ, Drance SM, Schulzer M. Neuroretinal rim area in early glaucoma. *Am J Ophthalmol*. 1985; 99:1–4.

123. Bengtsson B. The variation and covariation of cup and disc diameters. *Acta Ophthalmol*. 1976;54:804–818.

124. Lichter PR. Variability of expert observers in evaluating the optic disc. *Trans Am Ophthalmol Soc*. 1976;74: 532–572.

125. Pederson JE, Anderson DR. The mode of progressive disc cupping in ocular hypertension and glaucoma. *Arch Ophthalmol*. 1980;98:490–495.

126. Trobe JD, Glaser JS, Cassady J, Herschler J, Anderson DR. Nonglaucomatous excavation of the optic disc. *Arch Ophthalmol*. 1980;98:1046–1050.

127. Read RM, Spaeth GL. The practical clinical appraisal of the optic disc in glaucoma: The natural history of cup progression and some specific disc-field correlations. *Trans Am Acad Ophthalmol Otolaryngol*. 1974;78:255–274.

128. Kirsch R, Anderson DR. Clinical recognition of glaucomatous cupping. *Am J Ophthalmol*. 1973;75:442–454.

129. Sommer A, Pollack I, Maumenee AE. Optic disc parameters and onset of glaucomatous field loss: I. Method

and progressive change in disc morphology. *Arch Ophthalmol.* 1979;97:1444–1448.

130. Balazsi AG, Drance SM, Schulzer M, Douglas GR. Neuroretinal rim area in suspected glaucoma and early chronic open-angle glaucoma. *Arch Ophthalmol.* 1984; 102:1011–1014.

131. Herschler J, Osher R. Baring of the circumlinear vessels: An early sign of optic nerve damage. *Arch Ophthalmol.* 1980;98:865–869.

132. Caprioli J, Spaeth G. Comparison of the optic nerve in high- and low-tension glaucoma. *Arch Ophthalmol.* 1985;103:1145–1149.

133. Schwartz B. Cupping and pallor of the optic disc. *Arch Ophthalmol.* 89;1973:272–277.

134. Schwartz B. Optic disc changes in ocular hypertension. *Surv Ophthalmol.* 1980;25:148–154.

135. Sorenson PN. The colour of the optic disc variation with location of illumination. *Acta Ophthalmol.* 1980;58: 1005–1010.

136. Buus DR, Anderson DR. Peripapillary crescents and halos in normal-tension glaucoma and ocular hypertension. *Ophthalmology.* 1989;96:17–19.

137. Araie M, Sekine M, Suzuki Y, Koseki N. Factors contributing to the progression of visual field damage in eyes with normal tension glaucoma. *Ophthalmology.* 1994;101:1440–1444.

138. Sugiyama K, Tomita G, Kitazawa Y, Onda E, Shinohara H. The associations of optic disc hemorrhage with retinal nerve fiber layer defect and peripapillary atrophy in normal-tension glaucoma. *Ophthalmology.* 1997;104: 1926–1933.

139. Jonas JB, Naumann COH. Parapapillary chorioretinal atrophy in normal and glaucoma eyes. II. Correlations. *Invest Ophthalmol Vis Sci.* 1989;30:919–926.

140. Tezel G, Kass MA, Kolker AE, Wax MB. Comparative optic disk analysis in normal pressure glaucoma, primary open angle glaucoma, and ocular hypertension. *Ophthalmology.* 1996;103:2105–2113.

141. Jonas JB, Fernández MC, Naumann GOH. Glaucomatous parapapillary atrophy: Occurrence and correlations. *Arch Ophthalmol.* 1992;110:214–222.

142. Jonas JB, Papastathopoulos KI. Pressure-dependent changes of the optic disk in primary open-angle glaucoma. *Am J Ophthalmol.* 1995;119:313–317.

143. Jonas JB, Stuermer J, Papastathopoulos KI, Meier-Gibbons F, Dichtl A. Optic disc size and optic nerve damage in normal pressure glaucoma. *Br J Ophthalmol.* 1995;79:1102–1105.

144. Miller KM, Quigley HA. The clinical appearance of the lamina cribrosa as a function of the extent of glaucomatous optic nerve damage. *Ophthalmology.* 1988;95: 135–138.

145. Kottler MS, Drance SM. Studies on hemorrhages on the optic disc. *Can J Ophthalmol.* 1976;11:102–105.

146. Shihab ZM, Lee PF, Hay P. The significance of disc hemorrhage in open-angle glaucoma. *Ophthalmology.* 1982;89:211–213.

147. Drance SM, Fairclough M, Butler DM, Kottler MS. The importance of disc hemorrhage in the prognosis of

chronic open angle glaucoma. *Arch Ophthalmol.* 1977;95:226–228.

148. Bengtsson B, Holmin C, Krakau CET. Disc hemorrhage and glaucoma. *Acta Ophthalmol.* 1981;59:1–14.

149. Jonas JB, Xu L. Optic disk hemorrhages in glaucoma. *Am J Ophthalmol.* 1994;118:1–8.

150. Diehl DLC, Quigley HA, Miller NR, Sommer A, Burney EN. Prevalence and significance of optic disc hemorrhage in a longitudinal study of glaucoma. *Arch Ophthalmol.* 1990;108:545–550.

151. Drance SM. Disc hemorrhages in glaucomas. *Surv Ophthalmol.* 1989;33:331–337.

152. Siegner SW, Netland PA. Optic disc hemorrhages and progression of glaucoma. *Ophthalmology.* 1996;103: 1014–1024.

153. Heijl A. Frequent disk photography and computerized perimetry in eyes with optic disk haemorrhage. *Acta Ophthalmol.* 1986;64:274–281.

154. Rasker MT, van den Enden A, Bakker D, Hoyng PFJ. Deterioration of visual fields in patients with glaucoma with and without optic disc hemorrhages. *Arch Ophthalmol.* 1997;115:1257–1262.

155. Zeyen TG, Caprioli J. Progression of disc and field damage in early glaucoma. *Arch Ophthalmol.* 1993; 111:62–65.

156. Airaksinen PJ, Mustonen E, Alanko HI. Optic disc hemorrhages precede retinal nerve fiber layer defects in ocular hypertension. *Acta Ophthalmol (Copenh).* 1981;59: 627–641.

157. Drance SM. Correlation between optic disc changes and visual field defects in chronic open-angle glaucoma. *Trans Am Acad Ophthalmol Otolaryngol.* 1976;81: 224–225.

158. Hoskins HD, Gelber EC. Optic disc topography and visual field defects in patients with increased intraocular pressure. *Am J Ophthalmol.* 1975;80:284–290.

159. Schwartz B, Takamoto T, Nagin P. Measurements of reversibility of optic disc cupping and pallor in ocular hypertension and glaucoma. *Ophthalmology.* 1985;92: 1396–1407.

160. Miller NR, George TW. Monochromatic (red free) photography and ophthalmoscopy of the peripapillary retinal nerve fiber layer. *Invest Ophthalmol Vis Sci.* 1978; 17:1121–1124.

161. Weinreb RN, Shakiba S, Zangwill L. Scanning laser polarimetry to measure the nerve fiber layer of normal and glaucomatous eyes. *Am J Ophthalmol.* 1995;119: 627–636.

162. Tjon-Fo-Sang M, Lemig HG. The sensitivity and specificity of nerve fiber layer measurements in glaucoma as determined with scanning laser polarimetry. *Am J Ophthalmol.* 1997;123:62–69.

163. Weinreb RN, Zangwill L, Berry CC, Bathija R, Sample PA. Detection of glaucoma with scanning laser polarimetry. *Arch Ophthalmol.* 1998;116:1583–1589.

164. Shirakashi M, Funaki S, Funaki H, Yaoeda K, Abe H. Measurement of retinal nerve fiber layer by scanning laser polarimetry and high pass resolution perimetry in normal tension glaucoma with relatively high or

low intraocular pressure. *Br J Ophthalmol.* 1999;83: 353–357.

165. Schuman JS, Hee MR, Puliafito CA, Wong C, et al. Quantification of nerve fiber layer thickness in normal and glaucomatous eyes using optical coherence tomography. *Arch Ophthalmol.* 1995;113:586–596.

166. Pieroth L, Schuman JS, Hertzmark MA, Hee MR, et al. Evaluation of focal defects of the nerve fiber layer using optical coherence tomography. *Ophthalmology.* 1999;106:570–579.

167. Airaksinen PJ, Drance SM, Douglas GR, Mawson DK. Diffuse and localized nerve fiber loss in glaucoma. *Am J Ophthalmol.* 1984;98:566–571.

168. Sommer A, Quigley HA, Robin AL, Miller NR, et al. Evaluation of nerve fiber layer assessment. *Arch Ophthalmol.* 1984;102:1766–1771.

169. Sommer A, Katz J, Quigley HA, Miller NR, et al. Clinically detectable nerve fiber atrophy precedes the onset of glaucomatous field loss. *Arch Ophthalmol.* 1991; 109:77–83.

170. Quigley HA, Miller NR, George T. Clinical evaluation of nerve fiber layer atrophy as an indicator of glaucomatous optic nerve damage. *Arch Ophthalmol.* 1980; 98:1564–1568.

171. Quigley HA. Examination of the retinal nerve fiber layer in the recognition of early glaucoma damage. *Trans Am Ophthalmol Soc.* 1986;84:920–966.

172. Jonas JB, Schiro D. Localized wedge shaped defects of the retinal nerve fiber layer in glaucoma. *Br J Ophthalmol.* 1994;78:285–290.

173. Caprioli J. Correlation of visual function with optic nerve and nerve fiber layer structure in glaucoma. *Surv Ophthalmol.* 1989;33(suppl):319–330.

174. Drance SM, Airaksinen PJ. Signs of early damage in open-angle glaucoma. In: Weinstein GW, ed. *Open Angle Glaucoma.* New York: Churchill Livingstone; 1986:17–29.

175. Quigley HA, Addicks EM. Quantitative studies of retinal nerve fiber layer defects. *Arch Ophthalmol.* 1982; 100:807–814.

176. Sommer A, Miller NR, Pollack I, Maumenee AE, George T. The nerve fiber layer in the diagnosis of glaucoma. *Arch Ophthalmol.* 1977;95:2149–2156.

177. Quigley HA, Katz J, Derick RJ, Gilbert D, Sommer A. An evaluation of optic disk and nerve fiber layer examinations in monitoring progression of early glaucoma damage. *Ophthalmology.* 1992;99:19–28.

178. Airaksinen PK, Drance SM, Douglas GR, Schulzer M, Wijsman K. Visual field and retinal nerve fiber layer comparison in glaucoma. *Arch Ophthalmol.* 1985;103: 205–207.

179. Flammer J, Drance SM. Correlation between color vision scores and quantitative perimetry in suspected glaucoma. *Arch Ophthalmol.* 1984;102:38–39.

180. Stamper RL. Psychophysical changes in glaucoma. *Surv Ophthalmol.* 1989;33(suppl):309–318.

181. Balazsi AG, Rootman J, Drance SM, Schulzer M, Douglas GR. The effect of age on the nerve fiber population in human optic nerve. *Am J Ophthalmol.* 1984;97: 760–766.

182. Marx MS, Bodis-Wollner I, Lustgarten JS, Podos SM. Electrophysiological evidence that early glaucoma affects foveal vision. *Doc Ophthalmol.* 1987;67:281–301.

183. Adams AJ, Heron G, Husted R. Clinical measures of central vision function in glaucoma and ocular hypertension. *Arch Ophthalmol.* 1987;105:782–787.

184. Drance SM, Lakowski R, Schulzer M, Douglas GR. Acquired color vision changes in glaucoma: Use of 100-hue test and Pickford anomaloscope as predictors of glaucomatous field change. *Arch Ophthalmol.* 1981;99: 829–831.

185. Sample PA, Weinreb RN, Boynton RM. Acquired dyschromatopsia in glaucoma. *Surv Ophthalmol.* 1986; 31:54–64.

186. Lakowski R, Drance SM. Acquired dyschromatopsias: The earliest functional losses in glaucoma. *Doc Ophthalmol Proc Ser.* 1979;19:159–165.

187. Airaksinen PJ, Lakowski R, Drance SM, Prince M. Color vision and retinal nerve fiber layer in early glaucoma. *Am J Ophthalmol.* 1986;101:208–213.

188. Lakowski R, Bryett J, Drance SM. A study of colour vision in ocular hypertensives. *Can J Ophthalmol.* 1972;7: 86–95.

189. Flammer J. Psychophysics in glaucoma: A modified concept of disease. In: Greve EL, Leydhecker W, eds. *2nd European Glaucoma Symposium.* The Hague: W. Junk Publishers; 1985:11–17.

190. Yamazaki Y, Drance SM, Lakowski R, Schulzer M. Correlation between color vision and highest intraocular pressure in glaucoma patients. *Am J Ophthalmol.* 1988; 106:397–399.

191. Adams AJ, Rodic R, Husted R, Stampler RL. Spectral sensitivity and color discrimination changes in glaucoma and glaucoma-suspect patients. *Invest Ophthalmol Vis Sci.* 1982;23:516–524.

192. Flammer J, Drance SM. Correlation between color vision scores and quantitative perimetry in suspected glaucoma. *Arch Ophthalmol.* 1984;102:38–39.

193. Keltner JL, Johnson CA. Screening for visual field abnormalities with automated perimetry. *Surv Ophthalmol.* 1983;28:175–183.

194. Keltner JL, Johnson CA. Effectiveness of automated perimetry in following glaucomatous visual field progression. *Ophthalmology.* 1982;87:247–254.

195. Heijl A, Drance SM. A clinical comparison of three computerized automatic perimeters in the detection of glaucoma defects. *Arch Ophthalmol.* 1981;99:832–836.

196. Enger C, Sommer A. Recognizing glaucomatous field loss with the Humphrey STATPAC. *Arch Ophthalmol.* 1987;105:1355–1357.

197. Kosok O, Sommer A, Auer C. Screening with automated perimetry using a threshold-related three-level algorithm. *Ophthalmology.* 1986;93:882–886.

198. Drance SM, Douglas GR, Airaksinen PJ, Schulzer M, Hitchings RA. Diffuse visual field loss in chronic open angle and low-tension glaucoma. *Am J Ophthalmol.* 1987;104:577–580.

199. Aulhorn E, Harms H. Early visual field defects in glau

coma. In: Leydhecker W, ed. *Glaucoma Symposium, Tutzig Castle, 1966*. Basel, Switzerland: Karger; 1967:151–186.

200. Jaffe GJ, Alvarado JA, Juster RP. Age-related changes of the normal visual field. *Arch Ophthalmol.* 1986;104: 1021–1025.

201. Werner EB, Drance SM. Early visual field disturbances in glaucoma. *Arch Ophthalmol.* 1977;95:1173–1176.

202. Bryars JH, Cowan EC, Linton D. The earliest visual field changes in glaucoma simplex. *Trans Ophthalmol Soc UK.* 1974;97:1050–1051.

203. Nicholas SP, Werner EB. Location of early glaucomatous visual field defects. *Can J Ophthalmol.* 1980;15:131–133.

204. Duggan C, Sommer A, Auer C, Burkhard K. Automated differential threshold perimetry for detecting glaucomatous visual field loss. *Am J Ophthalmol.* 1985;100:420–423.

205. Mikelberg FS, Schulzer M, Drance SM, Lau N. The rate of progression of scotomas in glaucoma. *Am J Ophthalmol.* 1986;101:1–6.

206. Caprioli J, Spaeth GL. Comparison of visual field defects in the low-tension glaucomas with those in the high-tension glaucomas. *Am J Ophthalmol.* 1984;97:730–737.

207. Hitchings RA, Anderton SA. A comparative study of visual field defects seen in patients with low-tension glaucoma and chronic simple glaucoma. *Br J Ophthalmol.* 1983;67:818–821.

208. Glicklich RE, Steinmann WC, Spaeth GL. Visual field change in low-tension glaucoma over a five-year follow-up. *Ophthalmology.* 1989;96:316–320.

209. Araie M, Yamagami J, Suzuki Y. Visual field defects in normal-tension and high-tension glaucoma. *Ophthalmology* 1993;100:1808–1814.

210. Koseki N, Araie M, Yamagami J, Suzuki Y. Sectorization of central 10-degree visual field in open angle glaucoma: An approach for its brief evaluation. *Graefes Arch Clin Exp Ophthalmol.* 1995;233:621–626.

211. Araie M, Kitazawa M, Koseki N. Intraocular pressure and central visual field of normal tension glaucoma. *Br J Ophthalmol.* 1997;81:852–856.

212. Feuer WJ, Anderson DR. Static threshold asymmetry in early glaucomatous field loss. *Ophthalmology.* 1989;96: 1285–1297.

213. Kohn AN, Moss AP, Podos SM. Relative afferent pupillary defects in glaucoma without characteristic field loss. *Arch Ophthalmol.* 1979;97:294–296.

214. Heijl A, Drance SM, Douglas GR. Automated perimetry (Competer): Ability to detect early glaucomatous field defects. *Arch Ophthalmol.* 1980;98:1560–1563.

215. Chandler PA, Grant MW. Ocular hypertension versus open-angle glaucoma. *Arch Ophthalmol.* 1977;95:585–586.

216. Wilson R, Walker AM, Ducker DF, Crick RP. Risk factors for rate of progression of glaucomatous visual field loss. *Arch Ophthalmol.* 1982;100:737–741.

217. Hart WM, Yablonski M, Kass MA, Becker B. Multivariate analysis of the risk of glaucomatous visual field loss. *Arch Ophthalmol.* 1979;97:1455–1458.

218. Ford VJ, Zimmerman TJ. How to follow "ocular hypertension." *Ann Ophthalmol.* 1982;14:309–310.

219. Kass MA. When to treat ocular hypertension. *Surv Ophthalmol.* 1983;26(suppl):229–232.

220. Drance SM, Schulzer M, Douglas GR, Sweeney VP. Use of discriminant analysis: II. Identification of persons with glaucomatous visual field defects. *Arch Ophthalmol.* 1981;99:1019–1022.

Part III

TREATMENT AND MANAGEMENT

Chapter 20

PHARMACOLOGY OF ANTIGLAUCOMA MEDICATIONS

Kristine A. Erickson
Alison Schroeder

Medical intervention is typically the first choice for the treatment of primary open-angle glaucoma (POAG). The basis for medical treatment lies in its ability to reduce the intraocular pressure (IOP), delaying the loss of nerve fibers that follows periods of elevated IOP. In most cases, changes on the optic nerve head occur in response to an elevated intraocular pressure (>22 mmHg). However, it has become increasingly clear that optic nerve cupping can occur with pressures in the normal range.

Although lowering the IOP with medical treatment is often effective, no medical treatment to date is curative. Medical treatment often fails with time owing to disease progression, lack of compliance, or subsensitivity to the treatment regimens. This chapter describes the basic pharmacology, toxicology, and mechanism of IOP reduction of specific drugs used in the treatment of glaucoma (Table 20–1). For the most part, the literature covered includes reports published within the past 20 years. The earlier sections deal with the older forms of therapy and the methods by which the medications reduce IOP, while the remaining portions deal with newer advances in glaucoma therapy. For a more comprehensive treatment of this subject, the reader is referred to the excellent summary of Grant.[1]

INTRAOCULAR PRESSURE AND GLAUCOMA

The increased IOP associated with glaucoma is due to a resistance in the aqueous outflow pathways (a reduction of outflow facility) in the chamber angle. The pressure rises in accordance with the modified Goldmann equation[2]:

$$F = C(Pi - Pe) + U$$

where

$$F = \text{aqueous flow}$$
$$C = \text{facility of outflow}$$
$$Pi = \text{intraocular pressure}$$
$$Pe = \text{episcleral venous pressure}$$
$$U = \text{uveoscleral outflow}$$

Drugs that are used in the treatment of POAG exert their therapeutic effects by decreasing aqueous outflow resistance, reducing aqueous humor formation, or increasing uveoscleral flow.

TABLE 20–1: MECHANISM OF INTRAOCULAR PRESSURE REDUCTION ACHIEVED BY CLASSES OF DRUGS COMMONLY USED TO TREAT PRIMARY OPEN-ANGLE GLAUCOMA

Drug Class	Available Strength	Duration	Therapeutic Effect
Cholinergics (Direct Acting)			Increased aqueous outflow
Pilocarpine	0.25–10%	4–6 h	
Aceclidine			
Carbachol	0.75–3%	8 h	
Cholinergics: Cholinesterase Inhibitors (Indirect Acting)			
Physostigmine	0.25–0.5%	12–36 h	
Demecarium	0.125–0.25%	Days–weeks	
Edrophonium			
Echothiophate	0.03–0.25%	Days–weeks	
Isoflurophate	0.025%	Days–weeks	
Adrenergic Agonists			Decreased outflow resistance
Epinephrine	0.5–2%	12–24 h	
Dipivefrin	0.1%	12 h	
Apraclonidine	0.5%; 1%	6–8 h	Decreased aqueous inflow
Brimonidine	0.2%; 0.5%	6–8 h	
Beta-Adrenergic Receptor Blockers			Decreased aqueous production
Timolol	0.25–0.5%	12–24 h	
Levobunolol	0.5%	12–24 h	
Betaxolol	0.25–0.5%	12 h	
Carteolol	1%	12 h	
Metipranolol	0.3%	12–24 h	
Carbonic Anhydrase Inhibitors			Decreased aqueous inflow
Acetazolamide	125–500 mg	4–6 h	
Methazolamide	25–50 mg	4–6 h	
Dichlorophenamide	50 mg	6 h	
Dorzolamide	2%	6–12 h	
Brinzolamide	1%	6 h–12 h	
Prostaglandins			
Latanoprost	0.005%	24 h	Increased uveoscleral outflow

CLASSIC TREATMENT OF PRIMARY OPEN-ANGLE GLAUCOMA

Drugs That Increase Aqueous Outflow Facility

Cholinergic Agents

One of the oldest drugs used in the treatment of glaucoma is pilocarpine, whose use was first described by Weber.[3] Cholinergic agents lower intraocular pressure by increasing the facility of aqueous humor outflow through the conventional outflow routes via contraction of the ciliary muscle. The precise mechanism by which contraction of the ciliary muscle reduces resistance to the outflow of aqueous humor has not yet been defined. In human and other primate eyes, the "scleral spur" to which the ciliary muscle is attached is intimately related to aqueous outflow channels. Severing the attachment of the ciliary muscle to the scleral spur prevents the change in resistance to aqueous outflow that normally occurs in response to parasympa-

thetic innervation or to the action of cholinergic or anticholinesterase agents.[4] In excised eyes, with the attachment to the scleral spur intact, mechanically manipulating the ciliary muscle by pulling on the zonules attached to the lens reversibly reduces resistance to aqueous outflow. This can be prevented by detaching the ciliary muscle, suggesting that this resistance is subject to physical modulation and that it is the potentiation of contraction of ciliary muscle that is important in the treatment of glaucoma by means of cholinergic agents.[5] With continuing therapy, there may be a decrease in the effectiveness of cholinergic agents with time.[6] Lütjen-Drecoll and Kaufman[7,8] have described microscopic structural alterations that may account for a decrease in the effectiveness of cholinergic agents in the treatment of glaucoma. This effect is thought to occur by a contraction of the longitudinal portion of the ciliary muscle.[9,10]

The muscarinic cholinergic agents can be classified according to their action at the neuromuscular junction. Direct-acting agents (pilocarpine, carbachol, and aceclidine) bind muscarinic receptors (thought to be M3[11,12]) on the ciliary muscle. The indirect-acting agents (eserine, echothiophate iodide, and demecarium) act by binding to acetylcholinesterase in the junctional cleft, thereby preventing degradation of acetylcholinesterase.

Until the advent of beta blockers, muscarinic agents were the treatment of choice in POAG. Their efficacy is comparable to or even better than that of beta blockers; however, they produce a number of undesirable side effects. Muscarinic agents are still used mainly in adjunctive therapy.

Pilocarpine is generally administered as an aqueous solution but may also be given as a sustained-release medication by a device (Ocusert) placed into the cul-de-sac of the eye. Because of the low concentration of the drug in the eye at any given time with Ocusert, the side effects of pilocarpine on miosis and accommodation are reduced.

Contraindications. Cholinergics are contraindicated in patients with hypersensitivity to any component of the formulation and where cholinergic effects such as constriction are undesirable (e.g., acute iritis, some forms of secondary glaucoma, pupillary-block glaucoma, acute inflammatory disease of the anterior chamber). Cholinesterase inhibitors are contraindicated in patients with hypersensitivity to any component of the formulation or with an active uveal inflammation, any inflammatory disease of the iris or ciliary body, or glaucoma associated with iridocyclitis. Demecarium and isofluoride are contraindicated in pregnancy; echothiophate iodide is contraindicated in most cases of angle-closure glaucoma.

Ocular Side Effects. Much has been learned about the ophthalmic toxicology of muscarinic agents from testing in animals and humans, from observations in accidental poisonings, and in connection with medical uses of both direct-acting agents and anticholinesterases in the treatment of glaucoma, accommodative strabismus, and myasthenia gravis (Table 20–2).

Clinical examination of the cornea and conjunctiva after application of anticholinesterase eyedrops, such as are used in the treatment of glaucoma, usually reveals only hyperemia of the conjunctiva from dilation of conjunctival blood vessels. The cornea usually shows no abnormality. There are scattered reports of cases of the development of pseudopemphigoid in the treated eye after several years of treatment with miotics, including echothiophate iodide and pilocarpine eyedrops.[13–15] Long-term administration of pilocarpine has been associated with conjunctival changes, including hyperemia and the appearance of follicles.[16] A diffuse corneal haze

has also been noted during therapy with pilocarpine gel, probably secondary to the chlorobutanol used as a preservative in the gel.[17] Band keratopathy has also been associated with long-term administration of pilocarpine drops containing the preservative phenyl mercuric nitrate.[18]

Rarely, disturbances of the lacrimal apparatus have been reported after treatment with topical miotics. Also, a case has been reported of bilateral stenosis of the tear ducts after use of echothiophate iodide eyedrops twice a day for 13 years.[19] Excessive tearing from stimulation of the lacrimal glands has been noted in anticholinesterase poisoning.[20]

Cholinergic agents affect the iris in several ways, usually producing miosis but sometimes causing dilation of the pupil. Certain concentrations of anticholinesterases and direct-acting agonists, such as aceclidine, in contact with the eye may cause the pupil to become extremely miotic but may affect accommodation only moderately.[21,22] In systemic poisoning by

TABLE 20–2. SIDE EFFECTS ASSOCIATED WITH THE USE OF TOPICAL CHOLINERGIC DRUGS

Ocular Side Effects
- Transient stinging and burning
- Corneal clouding
- Persistent bullous keratopathy
- Transient conjunctival hyperemia
- Miosis
- Brow ache
- Ciliary spasm
- Blurred vision
- Shallowing of the anterior chamber
- Iritis
- Pupillary cysts
- Accommodation

Rare:
- Anterior and posterior subcapsular lens opacities
- Retinal detachment

Systemic Side Effects
- Salivation
- Diaphoresis
- GI disturbances
- Diarrhea
- Nausea
- Vomiting
- Headache
- Tremor
- Exacerbation of asthma
- Cardiac arrhythmia

Rare:
- Tachycardia
- Hypotension
- Pulmonary edema
- Bradycardia
- Paralysis of respiratory muscles

anticholinesterases, the pupils may become extremely small. Paradoxically, however, in some cases of severe poisoning, the pupils are found to be dilated.[23,24]

According to Romano and Jackson,[25] Wilkie et al.,[26] and Drance,[27] when miosis is maintained for weeks or months by daily anticholinesterase eyedrops, there is a gradual shallowing of the anterior chamber. In rare instances, angle-closure glaucoma has resulted. The mean decrease of axial depth for a group of patients receiving echothiophate iodide was 0.2 and 0.44 mm at 1 week and 8 weeks, respectively. None of these patients developed glaucoma. When the administration of echothiophate iodide was discontinued, their axial depth gradually returned toward normal.[26]

Iritis is an infrequent complication in humans from contact of the eye with anticholinesterases. Iritis usually is associated with conjunctival hyperemia and consists of dilation of the iris vessels with cells in the anterior chamber. It has usually been associated with the use of anticholinesterase eyedrops, but in one case it has been described in both eyes from a spray of the insecticide bromophos.[1] The development of cysts of the pupillary border of the iris is a common complication of repeated application of anticholinesterases to the human eye. In adults, the cysts usually develop only in response to strong miosis; but in children, they commonly develop in association with moderate miosis.[28-31] Rarely, the pupillary cysts interfere with vision, particularly in association with extreme miosis.[32,33] Simultaneous use of phenylephrine eyedrops can enlarge the pupil slightly and reduce the tendency to form cysts.[29-31,34,35] The ciliary processes have rarely been reported to have cysts in association with pupillary cysts from miotics.[36]

The ciliary body, which consists of the ciliary muscle and ciliary processes, has two main functions that are affected by cholinergic agents. One is accommodation, i.e., focusing of the eye, and the other is an action on the aqueous outflow system, which facilitates aqueous outflow and reduces intraocular pressure. Both are muscular functions. Also, there are responses of the nonmuscular portions of the ciliary body to cholinergic agents, to be described further on.

Anticholinesterase drugs used as eyedrops in the treatment of glaucoma can cause changes in the transparency of the crystalline lens, leading to a decrease in vision in some patients.[1] Most have agreed that careful slit-lamp examination of the lens after several months of daily administration of anticholinesterase eyedrops reveals anterior and posterior subcapsular vacuoles or small opacities in about half of the patients studied. It is generally accepted that anticholinesterase drugs — including echothiophate iodide, demecarium bromide, paraoxon, and isoflurophate — produce a much higher incidence of anterior and posterior subcapsular changes than do pilocarpine or carbachol eyedrops or than occurs in untreated controls. Not all observers have been wholly in agreement.[37-39] It appears that eyes that have been treated with pilocarpine prior to shifting to anticholinesterase eyedrops are somewhat protected from the effects of anticholinesterases on the lens.[40-44] The reason for this is unknown.

A review by Alpar[45] lists case reports in which retinal detachment occurred after initiation of treatment of glaucoma with miotics, especially with anticholinesterase miotics. However, retinal detachment has also been noted after treatment with shorter-acting miotics such as pilocarpine.[46] The results of a survey of 91 retinal surgeons and examination of data obtained from the National Registry of Drug-Induced Ocular Side Effects strongly suggest the possibility of miotic-induced retinal detachment in patients with preexisting retinal pathology, including high myopia, lattice degeneration of the retina, and a previous history of retinal detachment.[47]

Systemic Side Effects. Acute poisoning with anticholinesterase agents produces the cholinergic crisis syndrome, consisting of sweating, gastrointestinal (GI) disturbances, bradycardia, and paralysis of respiratory muscles. Acute poisoning with direct-acting muscarinic agonists can also be life-threatening and involves the cardiovascular system but not the diaphragm. The incidence of acute toxicity associated with the repeated application of pilocarpine eyedrops, which consists of sweating, salivation, nausea, tremor, and decreased blood pressure, is reviewed by Grant.[1]

Delayed peripheral neurotoxicity from organophosphorus esters has been a well-known clinical entity for over 50 years, particularly from the contamination of food or drink by tri-ortho-cresyl phosphate. The anticholinesterases diisopropyl fluorophosphate (DFP) and mipafox have caused delayed neurotoxicity involving axonal degeneration with secondary demyelination but without clinically evident involvement of the eyes.[48,49]

Caution should be exercised in using cholinergic agents in patients with asthma. The administration of pilocarpine in the subconjunctival sac has been associated with reports of bronchoconstriction in patients with asthma.[50,51]

Adrenergic Agonists

Epinephrine has been used for a number of years in the treatment of glaucoma. Although it has served as a mainstay therapeutic agent, its primary use today is as an adjunctive therapy. Nonselective adrenergic agonists, such as epinephrine, stimulate both alpha- and beta-adrenergic receptors. They exert their therapeutic effect on intraocular pressure by reducing resistance to aqueous outflow. The mechanism of action is mediated through stimulation of the beta-adrenergic receptors.[52-54] Autoradiographic studies of human outflow tissue in situ show the presence of beta-adrenergic receptors with a predominance of the beta$_2$ subtype.[55,56] These in vitro studies are consistent with findings from clinical studies demonstrating that epinephrine-induced increases in total outflow facility are blocked by the coadministration of timolol.[4,52,56] In the intact monkey eye, epinephrine and cyclic AMP analogues increase outflow facility.[1,53-61] Further, perfusion of the human anterior ocular segment in vitro leads to an increase in outflow facility associated with a rise in cyclic AMP; both effects can be blocked by ICI118551, indicating that the response is due to beta$_2$ receptors.[56] In addition, adrenergic agonists are known to affect a number of ocular physiologic parameters, including smooth muscle tone in the iris and ciliary body, aqueous humor production, and intra- and extraorbital vascular tone. The incidence of cardiovascular stimulation after topical ocular treatment is a potential major side effect that limits the therapeutic use of epinephrine. The addition of two pivalyl groups to epinephrine developed the prodrug formulation dipivefrin; the pivalyl groups are then cleaved from the compound when it passes through the cornea, allowing free epinephrine to reach intraocular sites.[62] This development has allowed smaller concentrations of epinephrine to be administered, thus limiting the external sensitivity and risk of adverse systemic effects.

Epinephrine is available as either a hydrochloride or a borate salt. These drugs are therapeutically equal when given in equivalent doses of epinephrine. However, the borate salt may cause less discomfort upon administration.[63]

Contraindications. Adrenergic agonists are contraindicated for patients with a hypersensitivity to any components of the formulation. They should not be used in patients with narrow or shallow angles (e.g., angle-closure glaucoma) or aphakia, or in cases where the nature of the glaucoma has not been clearly established. Patients with narrow angles may be predisposed to an attack of angle-closure glaucoma. In addition, epinephrine should not be used in patients wearing soft contact lenses, as discoloration of the lenses may occur.

Ocular Side Effects. Allergic contact sensitivity to epinephrine is common. It is characterized by itching, burning, epiphora, and hyperemia of the conjunctiva and lids (Table 20-3).[1] Although changing to another salt form of epinephrine will often reduce these side effects, the associated side effects will cause discontinuation of the drug in 20 to 50% of patients.[64] Adrenomelanin deposits occur on the conjunctiva or lids owing to the accumulation of metabolic by-products of epinephrine. Although these deposits are benign and symptomless, they resemble malignant melanomas.[65] In cases of preexisting epithelial defects, a similar corneal discoloration, called *black cornea*, can occur.[1] The occurrence of dacryoliths has also been attributed to the buildup of epinephrine breakdown products after chronic topical treatment with 1% epinephrine.[66] Actual epithelial toxicity is rare. However, Grant[1] and others[14,15] have summarized several reports of corneal and conjunctival epithelial toxicity, including pseudopemphigoid.

Drug preservatives themselves can have toxic effects. The corneal endothelium appears to be susceptible to commercial preparations of epinephrine. The long-term use of epinephrine drops containing preservative caused a slight decrease in the number of corneal endothelial cells. However, the number stayed within the normal range.[67] Dipivefrin-induced abnormalities have also been noted and include symblepharon,[68] conjunctival shrinkage,[65] and follicular conjunctivitis.[69,70]

Experimentally, epinephrine dramatically reduces blood flow to the ciliary processes in the cynomolgus monkey[71] and the albino rat[72] but not to the ciliary muscle,[71] as observed by a functional resin-casting method.

As reviewed by Grant, epinephrine-induced retinal toxicity was not recognized until the 1960s.[1] A reduction in visual acuity can occur with long-term administration of epinephrine. Generally, this is reversible within several months of discontinuing epinephrine.

Chronic use of epinephrine, especially after intraocular surgery, has been associated with cystoid macular edema.[1] Retinal and choroidal blood flow, as measured by laser Doppler methods, is decreased by topically applied 2% epinephrine, which may be the mechanism underlying epinephrine-induced maculopathy. An alternative explanation involves the interaction of epinephrine and the release of prostaglandins by ocular tissues. In rabbit eyes, topical administration of 1.5% epinephrine resulted in a breakdown of the blood-aqueous and blood-retinal barriers 2 to 3 months after initiation of treatment, which could be blocked by coadministration of indomethacin.[73] Chronic treatment with epinephrine was associated with elevated PGE levels in both the aqueous and vitreous humors in rabbit eyes after 5 months of treatment.[74]

Systemic Side Effects. Hypertension and heart palpitations occur in some patients after the administration

TABLE 20–3: SIDE EFFECTS ASSOCIATED WITH THE USE OF TOPICAL ADRENERGIC DRUGS

A. Epinephrine and Dipivefrin

Ocular Side Effects

Transient local symptoms:
Burning, stinging
Eye pain/ache
Brow ache
Conjunctiva hyperemia

Frequent (25%):
Allergic contact sensitivity of the cornea, conjunctiva, and lids

Prolonged administration:
Conjunctival or cornea pigmentation
Ocular irritation
Localized adrenochrome deposits in conjunctiva, cornea, lids

Macular abnormalities
Reversible cystoid macular edema may result in aphakic eye

Systemic Side Effects

Severe headache
Hypertension
Palpitations
Cardiac arrhythmia
Tachycardia
Extrasystoles
Faintness
Trembling
Diaphoresis

B. Apraclonidine and Brimonidine

Ocular Side Effects

Hyperemia
Burning and stinging
Conjunctival blanching
Discomfort
Upper lid elevation
Mydriasis
Foreign-body sensation
Dryness
Itching
Blurred visual acuity
Allergic reactions
Conjunctival hemorrhage
Hypotony
Eyelid erythema
Ocular ache / pain

Ocular Side Effects (*cont.*)
Eyelid edema
Conjunctival edema
Blepharitis
Irritation
Abnormal vision
Lid crusting

Systemic Side Effects

Central nervous system:
Insomnia
Dream disturbance
Irritability
Decreased libido
Somnolence
Dizziness
Depression
Anxiety

Gastrointestinal:
Abdominal pain
Diarrhea
Stomach discomfort
Vomiting

Other:
Abnormal taste
Oral dryness
Nasal dryness
Headache
Upper respiratory symptoms
Clammy or sweaty palms
Body heat sensation
Shortness of breath
Increased pharyngeal secretion
Extremity pain
Paraesthesia
Pruritus
Muscular pain

Cardiovascular:
Bradycardia
Vasovagal attack
Palpitations
Orthostatic episode
Edema
Arrhythmia

of topical epinephrine. Grant presents an extensive review.[1] The combination of beta blockers and epinephrine can lead to serious complications.[75] A hypertensive crisis that is immediately followed by cardiac slowing and possible cardiac arrest is sometimes observed. Despite the potential for adverse cardiovascular effects, the use of intraocular epinephrine has become standard practice in cataract surgery and no untoward effects on the cardiovascular system have been noted.[76–78]

Drugs That Decrease Aqueous Humor Inflow

Adrenergic Beta-Receptor Blocking Drugs

The advent of timolol to the treatment armamentarium brought an efficacy in reducing IOP comparable to that of pilocarpine without the disturbing side effects of miosis and accommodation. This made timolol the treatment of choice in glaucoma and the "gold standard" against which other glaucoma drugs have been judged. After the introduction of timolol other beta blockers began to appear. Today, a number of beta blockers are used in the treatment of glaucoma, and they can be classified according to their selectivity for beta receptors (Table 20–4). Timolol, betaxolol, and levobunolol are the most efficacious of the beta blockers and continue to be widely used in the treatment of POAG. Timolol, levobunolol, and metipranolol are nonselective beta blockers (e.g., they bind $beta_1$ and $beta_2$ receptors with nearly equal affinity), whereas betaxolol is somewhat selective for the $beta_1$ receptor. Carteolol is unique in that it is nonselective but also has intrinsic sympathomimetic activity. All of the drugs in this class work by decreasing the inflow of aqueous humor; they have virtually no effect on aqueous outflow. The mechanism of the reduction in aqueous inflow is incompletely understood; however, studies show that it probably involves $beta_2$ receptors.[79,80] Further, the flow rate of aqueous humor into the eye is subject to a diurnal rhythm, which decreases at night.[81,82] The intraocular pressure is thus lowest at night, with a minimum pressure evident at about 3:00 A.M.,[81,83] after which intraocular pressure peaks at about 7:00 A.M. in response to increased flow of aqueous humor. Recent studies suggest that the mechanism underlying the diurnal rhythm in IOP involves the homologous desensitization of the beta receptor mediated by beta-adrenergic receptor kinase (BARK) and beta arrestin.[84] These findings are the scientific basis for the lack of efficacy of beta blockers at night. Since beta receptors are uncoupled and therefore ineffective at night, beta blockers are not effective when given before bedtime. Therefore, once daily formulations such as Timoptic XE should be given in the morning, upon rising.

There is an extensive literature on the tendency of beta blockers to cause cardiovascular and respiratory problems.[7,85,86] Theoretically, the selectivity of a beta blocker for $beta_1$ or $beta_2$ receptors would make it a better choice for use in patients with asthma and cardiovascular insufficiency, respectively. However, the drugs currently in use do not have selectivity sufficient to prevent their binding of all beta receptors at therapeutic concentrations.

In addition to receptor selectivity, several other pharmacologic parameters will determine the profile of side effects associated with a given beta blocker. Beta blockers with some intrinsic sympathomimetic activity (ISA), such as carteolol, are less likely to cause cardiovascular insufficiency, bronchospasm, or adverse changes in serum lipids.[87] The degree of lipid solubility should influence how many drugs need to be given topically to reach therapeutic levels in the anterior chamber. Also, the degree of plasma protein binding would influence how much free drug was available to the systemic circulation. Beta blockers also differ in their activity as membrane-stabilizing (and anesthetic) agents. All of these factors will influence the degree of local and systemic toxicity.

A recent area of investigation has involved the development of prodrugs of timolol and levobunolol that might allow greater corneal permeability; therefore, the required topical dose of the drug could be reduced, minimizing possible systemic toxicity.[88,89] Timoptic XE (a formulation of timolol that forms a gel upon contact with the ocular surface) administered once a day was shown to be as effective in lowering IOP as the equivalent concentration of topical timolol administered twice a day. The safety profile is similar to that of equivalent concentrations of timolol.[90] Interestingly, a study of 371 patients found timolol hemihydrate (Betimol) to have an ocular hypotensive efficacy and safety profile equivalent to that of timolol maleate for up to 1 year.[91]

A recent study has found that a new combination formulation containing timolol hyaluronate and pilocarpine hyaluronate improves the bioavailability of the drugs and extends the duration of their action in rabbits.[92]

Contraindications. Beta blockers are contraindicated for patients with a hypersensitivity to any component of the formulation. Additionally, beta blockers should not be administered to individuals with bronchial asthma, a history of bronchial asthma, or severe chronic obstructive pulmonary disease, sinus bradycardia, a secondary or tertiary atrioventricular (AV) block, overt cardiac failure, or cardiogenic shock.

Ocular Side Effects. The most frequent ocular complaint (Table 20–5) with the administration of beta blockers is a burning sensation on instillation or transient discomfort. Timoptic XE is associated with a higher incidence of transient blurred vision (30%) than timolol because of the physical characteristics of the formulation.[90] A factor that may influence corneal irritation is the degree of membrane stabilization of the beta blocker; those producing less corneal desensitization cause less corneal irritation. However, other potentially more serious complications have been noted. The pattern of intraocular side effects may be

---

TABLE 20–4: CLASSIFICATION OF BETA BLOCKERS USED IN THE TREATMENT OF GLAUCOMA

Timolol (mixed β_1, β_2 blocker)
Levobunolol (mixed β_1, β_2 blocker)
Metipranolol (mixed β_1, β_2 blocker)
Betaxolol ("cardioselective" or β_1 blocker)
Carteolol (mixed β_1, β_2 blocker with intrinsic sympathomimetic activity)

TABLE 20–5. SIDE EFFECTS ASSOCIATED WITH THE USE OF TOPICAL BETA BLOCKERS

Ocular Side Effects
 Relatively common:
  Transient burning, tearing, stinging
  Blurred vision
 Conjunctivitis
 Blepharitis
 Keratitis
 Blepharoptosis
 Visual disturbances
 Photophobia
 Eye dryness
 Reduction in tear breakup time
 Transient corneal irritation
 Corneal sensitivity (rare)
 Corneal anesthesia
 Possible toxicity to corneal endothelium
 Cataractogenesis
 Changes in retinal blood flow
 Cystoid macular edema
 Choroidal detachment

Systemic Side Effects
 Bronchial constriction
 Cardiovascular effects:
  Bradycardia
  Decreased cardiac contractility
  Prolongation of atrioventricular conduction
 Increased serum lipids
 Alopecia (rare)
 Arthropathy
 Exacerbation of myasthenia gravis
 CNS effects:
  Depression
  Sexual dysfunction
  Emotional lability
Psoriasis

---

mediated in part by the pigment-binding characteristics of the beta blockers.[93] Those drugs that bind more avidly to pigment may produce an enhanced toxicity due to the buildup of a substantial drug reservoir within the eye.

There have been reports of timolol-induced reduction in tear secretion, causing discomfort sufficient to stop treatment. Further, with the exception of levobunolol,[94,95] beta blockers, including timolol, metipranolol, befunolol, bupranolol, carteolol, pindolol, and betaxolol, also reduce tear breakup time.[94–96] Timoptic XE has also been shown to be associated with conjunctivitis in 1 to 5% of patients.[90] In addition, beta blockers have been shown to reactivate latent herpesvirus type 1 (HSV-1) corneal ulcers in rabbit and mouse eyes.[97,98] Changes in the morphology and physiology of the corneal endothelium have been noted after administration of beta blockers. However, there have been conflict-

ing reports on the toxicity of beta-blocker administration to the corneal endothelium.

The ocular pulse pressure is affected differently by the various beta blockers. Carteolol 2% reduced pulse pressure, timolol 0.5% and betaxolol 0.5% had no effect on pulse pressure, and levobunolol (0.5%) significantly increased the amplitude of the ocular pulse.[99]

Retinal circulation is affected by beta-blocker administration. As measured by fluorescein angiography, timolol decreased the arteriovenous passage time and the dye bolus velocity in normal human subjects, implying that timolol increased retinal perfusion.[100] Similarly, topical timolol increased the rate of blood flow in the retinae of normotensive and hypertensive human eyes as measured by bidirectional laser Doppler velocimetry and monochromatic fundus photography.[101–103] These changes in retinal blood flow are maintained for at least a 2-week period of chronic topical treatment[104] and may relate to isolated reports of beta blocker–induced cystoid macular edema.[105]

Yoshida et al.[106] have found, by laser Doppler, that retinal blood flow increased significantly compared to baseline in human eyes following 2 weeks of treatment with betaxolol. However, timolol was found to reduce retinal blood flow significantly. Similarly, Kiel and Patel[107] found that betaxolol lowered mean arterial pressure slightly but significantly. Further, Kiel found that timolol increased choroidal vascular resistance. Turacli et al.[108] found that betaxolol improved ocular hemodynamics by lowering the resistivity index of the ophthalmic artery, which resulted in improvement of visual fields in patients with normal-tension glaucoma. In contrast, Schmetterer et al.[109] and Ishikawa et al.[110] found no effect on retinal blood flow with betaxolol.

Systemic Side Effects. As of 1985, the U.S. Food and Drug Administration and the National Registry of Drug-Induced Ocular Side Effects had tabulated a total of 450 case reports of serious cardiovascular or respiratory complications, 32 of which resulted in death after administration of topical timolol. Of the 212 patients for whom medical history was provided, 92% had either cardiovascular or respiratory problems.[111] Therefore, a careful medical history is necessary, in order to eliminate the possibility of exacerbating an underlying condition, before prescribing a topical beta blocker for the treatment of glaucoma.

In addition to the contraindications noted below, beta blockers should not be used in combination with calcium channel blockers, since sudden death has been reported after the systemic administration of a beta blocker and verapamil.[112,113]

Beta blockers may cause bronchial constriction as a consequence of binding to beta$_2$ receptors in the bronchi. Beta blockers that are nonselective (such as timolol) may compromise ventilation in patients with obstructive lung disease, asthma, or bronchospasm. The National Registry of Drug-Induced Ocular Side Effects has received over 200 reports of topical timolol-induced respiratory problems. Sixteen fatal attacks of status asthmaticus have occurred following application of topical timolol.[14]

Betaxolol, a beta$_1$ selective blocker, lowers intraocular pressure to therapeutically acceptable levels but apparently has less effect on pulmonary function than timolol.[114,115] In general, betaxolol is well tolerated in patients with underlying obstructive lung disease.[116–119] However, betaxolol has only a limited selectivity, and the therapeutic intraocular dose may actually be high enough to bind both beta$_1$ and beta$_2$ receptors. There have been scattered reports of respiratory problems following the use of topical betaxolol.[120–123] Collectively, these observations dictate that caution should be exercised even with the use of selective beta$_1$ antagonists in patients with respiratory disease.[122,124]

Cardiovascular effects of beta blockers include decreases in cardiac rate and contractility, and prolongation of AV conduction. Topical timolol has been associated with serious cardiac decompensation when used in the treatment of glaucoma.[111] Although betaxolol is beta$_1$-selective, it was thought to be an "oculoselective drug" owing to its high lipid solubility and its affinity for binding to plasma proteins.[125] However, instances of potentially dangerous cardiac decompensation associated with the use of topical betaxolol have been reported.[122,126,127] It appears that the beta blockers with ISA are associated with fewer cardiovascular problems. In one study, befunolol (which has ISA) was administered topically to patients with glaucoma for 1 week. No significant changes in mean, maximum, or minimum blood pressure, heart rate, or PR intervals compared with baseline values were noted as measured by continuous electrocardiography.[128]

Topical beta blockers have been associated with central nervous system side effects, including depression, sexual dysfunction, and emotional lability.[129–136] There is some evidence that the incidence and severity of these effects may be lower with the selective beta$_1$ blocker betaxolol.[137,138] However, at least one case report documents the occurrence of betaxolol-induced severe depression.[139] Topical beta blockers can also can cause elevated serum lipids, hair loss, and skin disorders.[129–136,138]

Oral Carbonic Anhydrase Inhibitors

Carbonic anhydrase inhibitors—including acetazolamide, methazolamide, ethoxzolamide, and dichlor-phenamide—have been used in the treatment of glaucoma, usually when maximum topical medical therapy has failed. They have been administered orally because the highly polar nature of the compounds has prevented topical penetration through the cornea.[140] Even though systemically administered carbonic anhydrase inhibitors are effective in lowering IOP, the constellation of side effects associated with their use has limited their clinical usefulness in the treatment of glaucoma.

Inhibition of carbonic anhydrase in the ciliary processes of the eye reduces aqueous humor secretion, presumably by slowing the formation of bicarbonate ions, with subsequent reduction in sodium and fluid transport. The result is a reduction in IOP.[141] A major reason for the systemic side effects of oral carbonic anhydrase inhibitors is that they have to be administered in high concentrations, as approximately 99% inhibition of the enzyme is necessary for the effects on aqueous inflow to be significant.

Contraindications. Carbonic anhydrase inhibitors are contraindicated for patients with any hypersensitivity to these agents. Cross-sensitivity between antibacterial sulfonamides and sulfonamide derivative diuretics, including acetazolamide and various thiazides, has been reported. Additionally, they should be avoided in patients with depressed sodium or potassium serum levels, marked kidney and liver disease or dysfunction, hyperchloremic acidosis, suprarenal gland failure, cirrhosis, decreased sodium and potassium levels, and adrenocortical insufficiency/failure. Dichlorphenamide should not be used for patients with severe pulmonary obstruction who are unable to increase alveolar ventilation since acidosis may be increased. Long-term use should be avoided in chronic, noncongestive angle-closure glaucoma, since organic closure of the angle may occur while worsening glaucoma is masked by lowered IOP.

Ocular Side Effects. Ocular toxicity (Table 20–6) with orally administered carbonic anhydrase inhibitors is rare. Infrequently, acute myopia is noted. An alteration of the hydration of the lens and the resulting change in refractive power may underlie the myopia. In almost all cases, the myopia is reversible within 2 days of discontinuing treatment.[1] In rare instances, the myopia has been more complicated. Further details can be found in reviews by Grant[1] and Berson.[142]

Systemic Side Effects. Oral administration of acetazolamide results in side effects ranging from minimal

TABLE 20–6: SIDE EFFECTS ASSOCIATED WITH THE USE OF CARBONIC ANHYDRASE INHIBITORS

Orally Administered

Ocular Side Effects
Acute myopia
Increased corneal thickness
  after cataract extraction

Systemic Side Effects
Paresthesia
Fatigue
Weight loss
Anorexia
Impotence
Depression
Blood dyscrasias
  Thrombocytopenia
  Agranulocytosis
  Aplastic anemia
Respiratory difficulties
Osteomalacia
Rash
Alopecia

Topically Administered

Ocular Side Effects
Transient burning and stinging
Tearing
Blurred vision
Photophobia
Transient myopia
Allergic sensitivity
Superficial punctate keratopathy
Dryness
Iridocyclitis
Postmarketing hypersensitivity

Systemic Side Effects
Bitter taste
Headache
Nausea
Fatigue
Rash
Urolithiasis
Dizziness
Paresthesia

discomfort to life-threatening events. Detailed reviews of systemic toxicity have been published.[1]

Tingling in the extremities or the face occurs commonly with acetazolamide treatment. However, it is transient and is generally not severe enough to discontinue treatment. Of greater consequence is the malaise syndrome consisting of fatigue, weight loss, anorexia, impotence, and depression. It is this side effect that most often causes patients to discontinue treatment.[143] The malaise syndrome is probably a consequence of acidosis, which can be relieved by treatment with sodium bicarbonate and titration of the drug dosage.[1,143] Cotreatment with salicylates is also contraindicated, since the combination of salicylates and acetazolamide can produce a serious acidosis.[1] The most serious side effect of acetazolamide is the rare but life-threatening occurrence of blood dyscrasias; thrombocytopenia, agranulocytosis, and aplastic anemia have all been reported. The dyscrasias that occur are not dose-related and are idiosyncratic in nature.[144] Grant[1] points out that most of the blood dyscrasia results from an acute immunologic sensitivity reaction. The collective consensus appears to be that routine blood chemistries would not be predictive of this complication.[1,145]

Other complications resulting from the use of oral acetazolamide include respiratory difficulties in patients with chronic obstructive lung disease, osteomalacia with bone demineralization, skin rashes, hair loss, and excessive hair growth.

NEW DEVELOPMENTS IN THE MEDICAL TREATMENT OF GLAUCOMA

During the past 5 years, an explosion of new pharmaceuticals has emerged on the marketplace; these new agents promise to expand and enhance our ability to safely and effectively lower IOP in the treatment of glaucoma. With the exception of latanoprost (Xalatan), all of these new additions lower pressure by decreasing aqueous humor inflow. However, while not ideal (i.e., glaucoma is a disease of outflow, not inflow), they at least provide alternatives to beta blockers, which are contraindicated in many patients with cardiovascular and chronic obstructive pulmonary disease. Additionally, they provide an alternative strategy in lowering IOP and are additive to beta blockers. One of the new medications (CoSopt) is actually a combination therapy: a carbonic anhydrase inhibitor and a beta blocker in one drop. Latanoprost is an entirely novel therapeutic agent, as it lowers intraocular pressure by increasing uveoscleral outflow. A summary of the characteristics of some of the new agents follows.

Alpha-Adrenergic Agonists

Clonidine, Apraclonidine (Iopidine)

Clonidine is a relatively selective alpha$_2$-adrenergic agonist that is used clinically as an antihypertensive agent. The hypotensive effect is mediated by activation of alpha$_2$ receptors in the central nervous system.[146] Topically, clonidine reduces IOP[147–151] and aqueous humor flow[152] by binding alpha$_2$ receptors in the ciliary body that inhibit adenylate cyclase.[80] Apraclonidine (Iopidine) is a *para*-amino derivative of clonidine that is incapable of penetrating the blood-brain barrier. Therefore, the use of topical apraclonidine should prevent the systemic hypotension that can occur with the use of topical clonidine. Apraclonidine is as effective as clonidine in lowering IOP[153,154] and has been used clinically in preventing the large elevations in intraocular pressure that may occur after argon laser iridotomy,[155,156] argon laser trabeculoplasty,[156,157] and neodymium-YAG posterior capsulotomy.[156,158] Before the advent of brimonidine (see below), it was used in the treatment of POAG,[159,160] particularly in cases where a patient on maximally tolerated medical therapy was awaiting surgery. However, long-term use of apraclonidine is limited by the frequent occurrence of tachyphylaxis.

After administration of apraclonidine, maximal IOP reduction, comparable to that due to timolol, occurs by 6 hours. The half-life is 8 hours, necessitating t.i.d. dosing. Unlike with beta blockers, IOP reduction is achieved both during the day and at night. Apraclonidine is additive to other glaucoma drugs and will reduce IOP in patients on maximal medical therapy. On the average, it will reduce IOP an additional 5 mmHg beyond the reduction achieved with timolol.[159–161]

Contraindications. Clonidine and apraclonidine should be avoided in patients receiving monoamine oxidase inhibitors and in those who are hypersensitive to any component of the formulations.

Ocular Side Effects. Possible ocular side effects of clonidine or apraclonidine reported to date may relate to their effects on hemodynamics. In adult humans, ocular perfusion pressure is decreased bilaterally after unilateral topical application of 0.125% clonidine. However, the decrease to the treated eye is greater, suggesting a local as well as a systemic effect on hemodynamics.[162] Approximately 15% of patients discontinue apraclonidine because of allergic reactions. Additional ocular side effects of apraclonidine in 1% of patients include conjunctival blanching, upper lid elevation, mydriasis, burning, foreign-body sensation, hypotony, and blurred vision.[161]

Systemic Side Effects. Caution should be exercised in the use of clonidine to avoid systemic toxicity, especially in children. A recent report documented clonidine poisoning in a 2-year-old after the child ingested clonidine from a discarded patch used as an aid in smoking cessation.[163] To date, it appears that apraclonidine obviates much of the systemic toxicity of clonidine. A number of studies have demonstrated minimal if any effects of apraclonidine on resting heart rate or mean arterial blood pressure when applied locally to the eye.[155–159,164–166]

Some of the systemic side effects that have occurred in less than 1% of patients include abdominal pain, diarrhea, stomach discomfort, emesis, dry mouth, bradycardia, vasovagal attack, palpitations, asthenia, peripheral arrhythmia, insomnia, somnolence, dizziness, dream disturbance, irritability, decreased libido, paresthesia, headache, and taste abnormalities.[161]

Brimonidine Tartrate (Alphagan)

Brimonidine, a relatively selective alpha$_2$-adrenergic agonist, is tenfold more selective for the alpha$_2$ receptors than apraclonidine. As such, it is thought to produce fewer of the hemodynamic side effects (i.e., conjunctival blanching and reduction in retinal blood flow) than apraclonidine. The peak IOP-lowering effect (27.2%) occurs 2 hours after dosing.[167] The recommended dosing is three times daily. Initially, brimonidine was developed as a 0.5% eyedrop for use after laser surgery. However, clinically, this concentration resulted in systemic drug effects, including decreased systolic blood pressure of 18.3 to 24 mmHg and decreased diastolic blood pressure. As a result, a 0.2% eyedrop, which avoided the systemic blood pressure effects, was developed for glaucoma treatment.[168] The advantage of brimonidine over apraclonidine is that there appears to be a lower incidence of allergic reactions, and tachyphylaxis does not occur.

Contraindications. Brimonidine should be avoided in patients receiving monoamine oxidase inhibitors and in those who are hypersensitive to any component of the formulation.

Ocular Side Effects. It is thought that the lower potential for hapten formation is responsible for the lowered allergic response with brimonidine relative to apraclonidine.[167] However, the potential for allergic reaction is still rather high. Treatment with brimonidine has induced ocular hyperemia, burning and stinging, blurring, foreign-body sensation, conjunctival follicles, SPK, and ocular allergic reaction in 10 to 30% of patients. Less common side effects include corneal erosion, photophobia, eyelid erythema, ocular pain, dryness, tearing, edema, blepharitis, and abnormal vision.[167]

The IOP-lowering effects of brimonidine are comparable to those of timolol but without the cardiopulmonary disease contraindications, and the allergic response is significantly less than that with apraclonidine (12.7% versus 23%).[169–174]

Topical Carbonic Anhydrase Inhibitors

Dorzolamide (Trusopt)

Dorzolamide (2% dorzolamide hydrochloride) was developed as a long-awaited carbonic anhydrase inhibitor that can be administered topically rather than systemically. It inhibits carbonic anhydrase type II, reduces IOP by 21.8 to 26.2% depending on b.i.d. or t.i.d. dosing, respectively, and is used alone or as an adjunctive therapy.[175] Although it is administered topically, the potential for systemic absorption exists. Therefore its use is contraindicated with oral carbonic anhydrase inhibitors.[141]

Contraindications. Concurrent administration of oral carbonic anhydrase inhibitors should be avoided. In addition, dorzolamide should be avoided in patients who are hypersensitive to any component of the formulation or who are allergic to sulfa drugs.

Ocular Side Effects. The most common ocular side effects (see Table 20–6) of dorzolamide include ocular burning and stinging in 33% of patients, superficial punctate keratitis in 10 to 15%, allergic reactions in 10%, and blurred vision, tearing, dryness, and photophobia in 1 to 5%.[141]

Systemic Side Effects. Most of the systemic side effects that occur with oral carbonic anhydrase inhibitors apparently do not occur with topical dorzolamide. However, treatment with dorzolamide resulted in a bitter taste in 25% of patients, and headache, nausea, fatigue, skin rashes, urolithiasis, and dizziness occurred in less than 1%. Because dorzolamide and its metabolites are excreted predominately by the kidneys, it is not recommended for use in patients with renal failure. In addition, dorzolamide is contraindicated in patients with an allergy to sulfa drugs.[141]

Brinzolamide (Azopt)

Brinzolamide (1% brinzolamide ophthalmic solution) was recently approved as a new topical carbonic anhydrase inhibitor. Brinzolamide inhibits carbonic anhydrase II in the ciliary processes and presumably decreases aqueous humor secretion by slowing the formation of bicarbonate ions, with a subsequent reduction in sodium and fluid transport. Following topical administration, brinzolamide inhibits aqueous humor formation and reduces elevated intraocular pressure. Brinzolamide reduces IOP by 15 to 20% (4.1 to 5.6 mmHg), and is used alone or as an adjunctive therapy to beta blockers (providing an additional 3.2- to 4.1-mmHg reduction).[176]

Contraindications. Brinzolamide is a sulfonamide, and although it is administered topically, it is absorbed systemically. Therefore the same types of adverse reactions that are attributable to sulfonamides may occur with topical administration of brinzolamide. Concurrent administration of oral carbonic anhydrase inhibitors should be avoided. In addition, brinzolamide should be avoided in patients who are hypersensitive to any component of the formulation or are allergic to sulfa drugs. Concurrent administration of high-dose salicylate therapy should also be avoided.

Ocular Side Effects. The most common ocular side effects (see Table 20–6) of brinzolamide include blurred vision and ocular stinging. Brinzolamide may cause superficial punctate keratitis in patients with dry eyes; therefore it should be avoided in these patients.[176] Brinzolamide has been found to produce less burning and stinging than dorzolamide upon topical administration, possibly owing to a more physiologic pH (pH 7.5 versus 5.6, respectively).

Systemic Side Effects. Treatment with brinzolamide produced a bitter metallic taste in 5.7% percent of patients, and headache and gastrointestinal disturbances in 1 to 5%. Because brinzolamide and its metabolites are excreted predominately by the kidneys, it is not recommended for use in patients with renal failure. In addition, brinzolamide is contraindicated in patients with hepatic failure or an allergy to sulfa drugs.[176]

CoSopt

CoSopt, new to the glaucoma therapy market, is made up of two components: dorzolamide hydrochloride (2%) and timolol maleate (0.5%). An advantage of CoSopt is that it simplifies therapy, thereby increasing adherence, by combining the two active agents into a medication that is administered twice daily. Dorzolamide is an inhibitor of human carbonic anhydrase II. Timolol maleate is a $beta_1$- and $beta_2$- (nonselective) adrenergic blocking agent. The combined effect of the two agents administered as CoSopt b.i.d. results in an additional reduction in intraocular pressure beyond that provided by either component alone, but the reduction is not as great as when dorzolamide t.i.d. and timolol b.i.d. are administered together.[175] Although CoSopt is administered topically, it is absorbed systemically. Therefore the same types of adverse reactions that are attributable to sulfonamides and/or systemic administration of beta-adrenergic blocking agents may occur with topical administration.[175]

Contraindications. CoSopt is contraindicated in patients with bronchial asthma or a history of bronchial asthma, severe chronic obstructive pulmonary disease, sinus bradycardia, second- or third-degree AV block, overt cardiac failure, or cardiogenic shock.[175]

Ocular Side Effects. In clinical studies, local ocular adverse effects (see Tables 20–5 and 20–6), primarily conjunctivitis and lid reactions, were reported with chronic administration of CoSopt. Approximately 5% of patients discontinued therapy with CoSopt because of adverse reactions. The most frequently reported adverse events were ocular burning and/or stinging in up to 30%. Conjunctival hyperemia, blurred vision, superficial punctate keratitis, or eye itching was reported in 5 to 15% of patients. The following ocular adverse events were reported in 1 to 5% of patients: blepharitis, cloudy vision, conjunctival discharge, conjunctival edema, conjunctival follicles, conjunctival injection, conjunctivitis, corneal erosion, corneal staining, cortical lens opacity, eye dryness, eye debris, eye discharge, eye/eyelid pain, eye tearing, eyelid edema, eyelid erythema, eyelid exudate/scales, foreign-body sensation, glaucomatous cupping, lens nucleus coloration, lens opacity, nuclear lens opacity, postsubcapsular cataract, visual field defect, and vitreous detachment.[175]

Systemic Side Effects. Up to 30% of patients experienced taste perversion. The following adverse events were reported in 1 to 5% of patients: abdominal pain, back pain, bronchitis, cough, dizziness, dyspepsia, headache, hypertension, influenza, nausea, pharyngitis, sinusitis, upper respiratory infection, and urinary tract infection.[175]

Prostaglandins

Latanoprost (Xalatan)
Prostaglandins were discovered in the eye in the course of a search for mediators of ocular inflammation. Prostaglandins D_2, E_2, and $F_{2\alpha}$ are synthesized by ocular tissues[177] and are actively transported out of the eye.[178] Aside from playing a role in intraocular inflammation, there is some evidence that prostaglandins play an endogenous role in normal physiologic processes.[178] Some prostaglandins may actually act to attenuate an inflammatory response.[179] Prostaglandin (PG) $F_{2\alpha}$ causes a dramatic reduction in intraocular pressure in monkey eyes[179–186] and in normal[187,188] and glaucomatous[189] human eyes—a response that is apparently mediated by increased nonconventional outflow.[181,183–185] Prostaglandin E_2 also apparently reduces intraocular pressure in human eyes.[190] However, the potential for an irritative response is apparently greater with PGE_1 and PGE_2 than with $PGF_{2\alpha}$.[186]

Latanoprost, a $PGF_{2\alpha}$ analogue that has recently been introduced for the treatment of glaucoma, is a prodrug metabolized by corneal esterases. Latanoprost (0.005%) reduces IOP by about 27% when administered once daily in the morning and, interestingly, by about 35% when administered once daily in the evening.[191] After dosing, the peak effect occurs in about 2 hours. There is apparently no tachyphylaxis. Latanoprost reduces IOP by enhancing uveoscleral outflow.

Contraindications. Latanoprost is contraindicated in patients with known hypersensitivity to benzalkonium chloride or any other ingredient in this product.

Ocular Side Effects. The ocular side effects (Table 20–7) associated with latanoprost are foreign-body sensation, punctate epithelial keratopathy, stinging, conjunctival hyperemia, blurred vision, itching, burning, and iris pigmentation.[191] Additionally, in a 6-month study comparing latanoprost with timolol in open-angle glaucoma and ocular hypertension, 10% of patients developed increased iris pigmentation. All of these patients had hazel irides.[192] Latanoprost increases the amount of brown pigment in the iris by increasing the number of melanosomes within melanocytes rather than causing a proliferation of melanocytes. The increase in brown pigment does not progress following discontinuation of treatment, but the resultant color change may be permanent. Recently Johnstone[193] found that patients receiving unilateral topical latanoprost developed hypertrichosis, involving ipsilateral

TABLE 20–7: SIDE EFFECTS ASSOCIATED WITH THE USE OF LATANOPROST IN THE TREATMENT OF PRIMARY OPEN-ANGLE GLAUCOMA

Ocular Side Effects
Hyperemia
Transient stinging
Blurred vision
Itching
Burning
Foreign-body sensation
Punctate epithelial keratopathy
Iris pigmentation
Macular edema
Iritis

Pseudodentrites
Herpes simplex keratitis

Systemic Side Effects
Respiratory tract infection/cold/flu
Muscle/joint/back pain
Chest pain/angina pectoris
Rash/allergic skin reaction

terminal eyelashes and regional intermediate hairs of the upper and lower eyelid as well as the vellus hair of the lower eyelid skin. These changes consisted of increased number, length, thickness, curvature, and pigmentation. More recently, reports of cystoid macular edema and iritis have appeared.[194] Typically, these serious side effects are rare and have occurred in eyes with a previous history of extensive surgery or previous incidence of iritis.

Systemic Side Effects. Latanoprost is perhaps unique among the glaucoma medications in that it is not associated with serious effects on cardiovascular and pulmonary function. Systemic side effects that have been reported include flu-like symptoms, muscle aches and pains, and headache.[191]

CONCLUSIONS

Within our current abilities to treat glaucoma, several generalizations can be made. First, effective lowering of IOP can now be accomplished safely and successfully in patients with severe heart disease or chronic obstructive pulmonary disease with latanoprost or dorzolamide. Additionally, intolerance or side effects of glaucoma medications should be less common problems with the advent of new therapeutics with different pharmacological profiles. Further, maximum medical therapy can now be optimized by inclusion of a number of drugs from different classes. This may prove to delay the need for surgery significantly.

TABLE 20–8. OPTIONS AVAILABLE FOR LOWERING INTRAOCULAR BLOOD PRESSURE IN GLAUCOMA

Class	Generic	Trade Name	Concentration	Size, mL	Dosage	Top Color
Nonselective beta blockers	Timolol maleate	Timoptic, generic	0.25%, 0.5%	2.5, 5, 10, 15	q.d., b.i.d.	Light blue (0.25%) / Yellow (0.5%)
	Timolol maleate	Timoptic XE	0.25%, 0.5%	2.5, 5	q.d.	Yellow
	Timolol hemihydrate	Betimol	0.25%	5, 10, 15	q.d. b.i.d.	White
	Levobunolol HCl	Betagan, generic	0.25%, 0.5%	2.5, 5, 10, 15	q.d., b.i.d.	Light blue (0.25%)/ Yellow (0.5%)
	Carteolol HCl	Ocupress	1.0%	5, 10	q.d., b.i.d.	White
	Metipranolol	Optipranolol	0.3%	5, 10	b.i.d.	White
Selective beta blockers	Betaxolol HCl	Betoptic S	0.25%	2.5, 5, 10, 15	q.d., b.i.d.	Light blue
	Betaxolol HCl	Betoptic	0.5%	2.5, 5, 10, 15	q.d., b.i.d.	Dark blue
Combination beta blocker/CAI*	Timolol maleate and dorzolamide	CoSopt	0.5%, 2%	5, 10	b.i.d.	Yellowish
Topical CAI	Dorzolamide HCl	Trusopt	2%	5, 10	b.i.d., t.i.d.	Orange
	Brinzolamide HCl	Azopt	1%	5, 10, 15	b.i.d., t.i.d.	Orange
Prostaglandin	Latanoprost	Xalatan	0.005%	2.5	q.d	White (with tabs)
Alpha₂ agonist	Apraclonidine HCl	Iopidine	0.5%	5, 10	b.i.d., t.i.d.	White
	Brimonidine tartrate	Alphagan	0.2%	5, 10, 15	b.i.d., t.i.d.	Purple
Sympathomimetic	Epinephrine HCl	Epifrin	0.5%, 1%, 2%	5, 10, 15	b.i.d.	White
		Glaucon	1%, 2%	10	q.d., b.i.d.	White
	Epinephrine bitartrate	Epitrate	2%	7.5	q.d., b.i.d.	White
	Epinephrine borate	Epinal	0.5%,1%	7.5	q.d., b.i.d.	White
	Dipivefrin HCl	Propine	0.1%	5, 10, 15	b.i.d.	Purple
Muscarinics	Isoptocarbachol	Carbachol	0.75%, 1.5%, 2.25%, 3%	15, 30	q.i.d., b.i.d.	Green
	Pilocarpine HCl	Ocusert	P20, P40	8	Weekly	Green
		Pilocar	0.5%, 1%, 2%, 3%, 4%, 6%	15	q.i.d.	Green
		Pilopine-HS gel	4%	4 g	q.h.s.	Green
		Isoptocarpine	0.25%, 0.5%, 1–6%, 8%, 10%	15, 30	q.i.d.	Green
	Pilocarpine nitrate	Pilagan	1%, 2%, 4%	15	q.i.d.	Green
	Demecarium bromide	Humorsol	0.125%, 0.25%,	5	q.d., b.i.d.	Green
	Echothiophate iodide	Phospholine Iodide	0.03%, 0.06%, 0.125%, 0.25%	5	q.d., b.i.d.	Green

*CAI, carbonic anhydrase inihibiter.

However, although the last few years have brought a welcome expansion in the options available for lowering IOP in glaucoma (Table 20–8), POAG remains an incurable disease. With current medical and surgical treatments, we are able, at best, to delay the progressive visual loss associated with glaucoma. Although the lowering of IOP seems to be instrumental in preventing the loss of ganglion cells, it apparently is not sufficient. There is a growing recognition of the importance of finding methods to prevent ganglion cell loss and thus preserve visual function. Early work in this area pointing to the feasibility of this approach includes studies by Netland[195–197] and Dryer et al.[198,199] Netland showed that increases in retinal blood flow might delay the visual field loss associated with low-tension glaucoma.[195–197] Dryer et al. demonstrated that retinal glutamate levels are elevated in glaucoma and that glutamate receptor antagonists can effectively prevent optic neuropathy in animal models of glaucoma.[198,199] It is likely that breakthroughs in this area will be made within the next decade, so that, in addition to treating pressure, medical treatment will be aimed at maintaining the health of ganglion cells.

ACKNOWLEDGMENTS

The preparation of this manuscript was supported in part by grants from the National Eye Institute (EYO 7321), Research to Prevent Blindness, and the Massachusetts Lions Eye Research Fund.

REFERENCES

1. Grant WM. *Toxicology of the Eye*, 3rd ed. Springfield, IL: Charles C Thomas; 1986.
2. Goldmann H. Weitere Mitteilungber den Abfluss des Kammerwassers beim Menschen. *Ophthalmologica.* 1946;112:344.
3. Weber A. Die Ursache des Glaukoms. *Graefes Arch Clin Exp Ophthalmol.* 1877;23:1.
4. Kaufman PL, Wiedman T, Robinson JR. Cholinergics. In: Sears ML, ed. *Handbook of Experimental Pharmacology 69.* Berlin: Springer-Verlag; 1984;150–191.
5. Grant WM. Experimental aqueous perfusion in enucleated human eyes. *Arch Ophthalmol.* 1963;69:783.
6. Grant WM. Additional experiences with tetraethyl pyrophosphate in treatment of glaucoma. *Arch Ophthalmol.* 1950;44:362.
7. Lütjen-Drecoll E, Kaufman PL. Echothiophate-induced structural alterations in the anterior chamber angle of the cynomolgus monkey. *Invest Ophthalmol Vis Sci.* 1979;18:918.
8. Lütjen-Drecoll E, Kaufman PL. Biomechanics of echothiophate-induced anatomic changes in monkey aqueous outflow system. *Graefes Arch Clin Exp Ophthalmol.* 1986;224:564.
9. Lütjen-Drecoll E, Kaufman PL, Eichhorn M. Long-term timolol and epinephrine in monkeys. I. Functional morphology of the ciliary process. *Trans Ophthalmol Soc UK.* 1986;105:180.
10. Lütjen-Drecoll E, Kaufman PL. Long-term timolol and epinephrine in monkeys: II. Morphological alterations in trabecular meshwork and ciliary muscle. *Trans Ophthalmol Soc UK.* 1986;105:196.
11. Pang I, Matsumoto S, Tamm E, DeSantis L. Characterization of muscarinic receptor involvement in human ciliary muscle cell function. *J Ocul Pharmacol.* 1994;10:125–136.
12. Zhang X, Schroeder A, Erickson KA. Effect of continuous administration of cholinergic agent on [^{3}H]4-DAMP binding and m3 mRNA expression in cultured human ciliary muscle cells. *J Ocul Pharm Ther.* 1998;15:153.
13. Patten JT, Cavanagh HD, Allansmith MR. Induced ocular pseudopemphigoid. *Am J Ophthalmol.* 1976;82:272.
14. Fraunfelder FT, Meyer SM. Ocular toxicology update. *Aust N Z J Ophthalmol.* 1984;12:391.
15. Pouliquen Y, Patey A, Foster CS, et al. Drug-induced cicatricial pemphigoid affecting the conjunctiva: Light and electron microscopic features. *Ophthalmology.* 1986;93:775.
16. Cvetkovic D, Parunovic A, Kontic D. Conjunctival changes in local long-term medical glaucomatous therapy. *Fortschr Ophthalmol.* 1986;83:407.
17. Johnson DH, Kenyon KR, Epstein DL, et al. Corneal changes during pilocarpine gel therapy. *Am J Ophthalmol.* 1986;101:13.
18. Brazier DJ, Hitchings RA. Atypical band keratopathy following long-term pilocarpine treatment. *Br J Ophthalmol.* 1989;73:294.
19. Wood JR, Anderson RL, Edwards JJ. Phospholine iodide toxicity and Jones' tubes. *Ophthalmology.* 1980;87:346.
20. Ecobichon DJ, Ozere RL, Reid E, et al. Acute fenitrothion poisoning. *Can Med Assoc J.* 1977;116:377.
21. Moylan-Jones RJ, Thomas DP. Cyclopentolate in treatment of sarin miosis. *Br J Pharmacol.* 1973;48:309.
22. Erickson-Lamy K, Schroeder A. Dissociation between the effect of aceclidine on outflow facility and accommodation. *Exp Eye Res.* 1990;50:143.
23. Leuzinger S, Pasi A, Dolder R. Synoptische Auswertung von Alkylphosphatvergiftungen. *Schweiz Med Wochenschr.* 1971;101:563.
24. Dixon EM. Dilatation of the pupils in parathion poisoning. *JAMA.* 1957;163:444.
25. Romano J, Jackson H. Clinical observations on the use of phospholine iodide in glaucoma. *Br J Ophthalmol.* 1964;48:480.
26. Wilkie J, Drance SM, Schulzer M. The effects of miotics on anterior chamber depth. *Am J Ophthalmol.* 1969;68:78.
27. Drance SM. The effects of phospholine iodide on the lens and anterior chamber depth. In: Leopold IH, ed. *Symposium on Ocular Therapy.* St. Louis: CV Mosby; 1969:25–31.
28. Hill K, Stromberg AE. Echothiophate iodide in the management of esotropia. *Am J Ophthalmol.* 1962;53:488.

29. Chin NB, Gold AA, Breinin GM. Iris cysts and miotics. *Arch Ophthalmol.* 1964;71:611.

30. Catros A, Cahn R, Guyader M. Effets secondaires des myotiques forts dans le traitement du strabisme accommodatif de l'enfant. *Bull Soc Ophtalmol Fr.* 1969; 69:370.

31. Chamberlain W. Anticholinesterase miotics in the management of accommodative esotropia. *J Pediatr Ophthalmol.* 1975;12:151.

32. Swan KC. Iris pigment nodules complicating miotic therapy. *Am J Ophthalmol.* 1954;37:886.

33. Funder W. Pigmentzysten nach Mintacolgebrauch. *Klin Monatsbl Augenheilkd.* 1955;126:218.

34. Abraham SV. The use of an echothiophate-phenylephrine formulation (echophenyline-B3) in the treatment of convergent strabismus with special reference to cysts. *J Pediatr Ophthalmol.* 1967;4:29.

35. Haddad HM, Rivera H. Echophenyline-B3 and phospholine iodide 0.3% in the management of esotropia. *J Pediatr Ophthalmol.* 1967;4:24.

36. Kraft H. Auftreten von zystischen Veranderungen an den Ziliarörperforätzen bei langer dauerndem Gebrauch von cholinesterasehemmenden Medikamenten. *Klin Monatsbl Augenheilkd.* 1962;140:584.

37. Cinotti AA, Patti JC. Lens abnormalities in an aging population of nonglaucomatous patients. *Am J Ophthalmol.* 1968;65:25.

38. Thoft RA. Incidence of lens changes in patients treated with echothiophate iodide. *Arch Ophthalmol.* 1968;80:317.

39. Abraham SV, Teller JJ. Influence of various miotics on cataract formation. *Br J Ophthalmol.* 1969;53:833.

40. Shaffer RN, Hetherington J Jr. Anticholinesterase drugs and cataracts. *Trans Am Ophthalmol Soc.* 1966;64:204.

41. Shaffer RN, Hetherington J Jr. Anticholinesterase drugs and cataracts. *Trans Am Ophthalmol Soc.* 1966;62:613.

42. Levene RZ. Echothiophate iodide and lens changes. In: Leopold IH, ed. *Symposium on Ocular Therapy.* St. Louis: CV Mosby; 1969:45–52.

43. Nordmann J, Gerhard JPA. Propos de la cataracte par miotiques. *Bull Soc Ophtalmol Fr.* 1969;69:649.

44. Nordmann J, Gerhard JP. La phospholine et le cristallin. *Bull Soc Ophtalmol Fr.* 1970;70:745.

45. Alpar JJ. Miotics and retinal detachment: A survey and case report. *Ann Ophthalmol.* 1979;11:395.

46. Puustärvi T. Retinal detachment during glaucoma therapy. *Ophthalmologica.* 1985;190:40.

47. Beasley H, Fraunfelder FT. Retinal detachments and topical ocular miotics. *Ophthalmology.* 1979;86:95.

48. Duffy FH, Burchfiel JL. Long-term effects of the organophosphate sarin on EEG's in monkeys and humans. *Neurotoxicology.* 1980;1:667.

49. Koelle GB. Anticholinesterase agents. In: Goodman LS, Gilman A, eds. *The Pharmacologic Basis of Therapeutics.* New York: Macmillan; 1975:445–466.

50. Bruchhausen D, Haschem J, Dardenne MU. Veänderungen des Bronchialwiderstandes bei Asthmatikern nach Applikation von Pilocarpin in den Konjunktivalsack. *Dtsch Med Wochenschr.* 1969;94:1651.

51. Bruchhausen D, Haschem J, Baack G, et al. Medikamenöse Provokation von Bronchospasmen bei Asthmatikern. *Verh Dtsch Ges Inn Med.* 1971;77:1321.

52. Kaufman PL, Robinson JC. Epinephrine, norepinephrine and timolol effects on outflow facility in the cynomolgus monkey. *Invest Ophthalmol Vis Sci ARVO Suppl.* 1989;30:444.

53. Kaufman PL. The effects of drugs on the outflow of aqueous humor. In: Drance SM, ed. *Applied Pharmacology in the Medical Treatment of Glaucomas.* New York: Grune & Stratton; 1984:429–458.

54. Neufeld AH, Bartels SP. Receptor mechanisms for epinephrine and timolol. In: Lütjen-Drecoll E, ed. *Basic Aspects of Glaucoma Research.* Stuttgart: FK Schattauer; 1982:113–122.

55. Lütjen-Drecoll E, Rohen JW. Reactive changes in primate trabecular meshwork cells following surgical and pharmacological stimulation. *Proc Int Soc Eye Res.* 1980;1:4.

56. Erickson-Lamy KA, Nathanson JA. Epinephrine increases facility of outflow and cyclic AMP content in the human eye in vitro. *Invest Ophthalmol Vis Sci.* 1992; 33:2672–2678.

57. Thomas JV, Epstein DL. Timolol and epinephrine in primary open angle glaucoma: Transient additive effect. *Arch Ophthalmol.* 1981;99:91.

58. Erickson-Lamy KA, Ostovar B, Hunnicutt EJ, et al. Epinephrine increases facility of outflow and trabecular meshwork cAMP content in the human eye in vitro. *Invest Ophthalmol Vis Sci.* 1990;31:184.

59. Gharagozloo NZ, Relf SJ, Brubaker RF. Aqueous flow is reduced by the alpha-adrenergic agonist apraclonidine hydrochloride (ALP 2145). *Ophthalmology.* 1988; 95:1217.

60. Crawford K, Kaufman PL, Gabelt BT. Prostaglandins and aqueous humor dynamics. In: Shields MB, Pollack IP, eds. *Perspectives in Glaucoma: Transactions of First Scientific Meeting of the American Glaucoma Society.* Thorofare, NJ: Slack; 1988:259–267.

61. Kaufman PL, Crawford K, Gabelt BT. The effects of prostaglandins on aqueous humor dynamics. *Ophthalmol Clin North Am.* 1989;2:141.

62. Epstein DL. Primary open angle glaucoma. In: Epstein DL, ed. *Chandler and Grant's Glaucoma*, 3rd ed. Philadelphia: Lea & Febiger; 1986:138.

63. Agents for glaucoma. In: Bartlett JD, Ghormley NR, Jaanus SD, Rowsey JJ, Zimmerman TJ, eds. *Ophthalmic Drug Facts.* St. Louis: Wolters Kluwer; 1995: 162–167.

64. Bartlett JD, Novack GD, Hiett JA, Jaanus SD, Sharir M, Antiglaucoma drugs. In: Bartlett JD, Jaanus SD, eds. *Clinical Ocular Pharmacology*, 3rd ed. Boston: Butterworth-Heinemann; 1995:204–208.

65. Soong HK, McKenney MJ, Wolter JR. Adrenochrome staining of senile plaque resembling malignant melanoma. *Am J Ophthalmol.* 1986;101:380.

66. Bradbury JA, Rennie IG, Parsons MA. Adrenaline dacryolith: Detection by ultrasound examination of the nasolacrimal duct. *Br J Ophthalmol.* 1988;72:935.

67. Waltman SR, Yarian D, Hart W Jr, et al. Corneal endothelial changes with long term topical epinephrine therapy. *Arch Ophthalmol.* 1977;95:1357.

68. Blanchard DL. Adrenergic-associated symblepharon. *Glaucoma.* 1987;9:18.

69. Liesegang TJ. Bulbar conjunctival follicles associated with dipivefrin therapy. *Ophthalmology.* 1985;92:228.

70. Coleiro JA, Sigurdsson H, Lockyer JA. Follicular conjunctivitis on dipivefrin therapy for glaucoma. *Eye.* 1988;2:440.

71. Funk R, Rohen JW. SEM studies of the functional morphology of the ciliary process vasculature in the cynomolgus monkey: Reactions after application of epinephrine. *Exp Eye Res.* 1988;47:653.

72. Seki R. Scanning electron microscopic observations on vascular casts of ciliary processes in normal and topical epinephrine-treated rats. *Jpn J Ophthalmol.* 1988;32:288.

73. Miyake K, Kayazawa F, Manabe R, et al. Indomethacin and the epinephrine-induced breakdown of the blood-ocular barrier in rabbits. *Invest Ophthalmol Vis Sci.* 1987;28:482.

74. Miyake K, Shirasawa E, Hikita M, et al. Synthesis of prostaglandin E in rabbit eyes with topically applied epinephrine. *Invest Ophthalmol Vis Sci.* 1988;29:332.

75. Brummett RE. Warning to otolaryngologists using local anesthetics containing epinephrine: Potential serious reaction occurring in patients treated with beta adrenergic receptor blockers. *Arch Otolaryngol* 1984;110:561.

76. Fiore PM, Cinotti AA. Systemic effects of intraocular epinephrine during cataract surgery. *Ann Ophthalmol* 1988;20:23.

77. Yamaguchi H, Matsumoto Y. Stability of blood pressure and heart rate during intraocular epinephrine irrigation. *Ann Ophthalmol.* 1988;20:58.

78. Dupeyron G, Eledjan JJ, Poupard P, et al. Perfusion d'adrenaline intra-camerulaire dans la chirugie extra-capsulaire du cristallin interet et limites de la methode. *Bull Soc Ophtalmol Fr.* 1985;85(5):631.

79. Gregory DS, Bausher LP, Bromberg BB, et al. The beta adrenergic receptor and adenyl cyclase of rabbit ciliary processes. In: Sears ML, ed. *New Directions in Ophthalmic Research.* New Haven, CT: Yale University Press; 1981:127–148.

80. Mittag TW, Tormay A. Drug responses of adenylate cyclase in iris-ciliary body determined by adenine labelling. *Invest Ophthalmol Vis Sci.* 1985;26:396.

81. Sears ML. Regulation of aqueous flow by the adenylate cyclase receptor complex in the ciliary epithelium. *Am J Ophthalmol.* 1985;100:194–198.

82. Topper JE, Brubaker RF. Effects of timolol, epinephrine, and acetazolamide on aqueous flow during sleep. *Invest Ophthalmol Vis Sci.* 1985;26:1315–1319.

83. Kitazawa Y, Horie T. Diurnal variation of intraocular pressure in primary open-angle glaucoma. *Am J Ophthalmol.* 1975;79(4):557–566.

84. Wan XL, Sears J, Chen S, Sears M. Circadian aqueous flow mediated by beta-arrestin induced homologous desensitization. *Exp Eye Res.* 1997;64(6):1005–1011.

85. Novack GD, Leopold IH. The toxicity of topical ophthalmic beta blockers. *J Toxicol Cutan Ocul Toxicol.* 1987;6:283.

86. Novack GD. Ophthalmic beta-blockers since timolol. *Surv Ophthalmol.* 1987;31:307.

87. James IM. Pharmacologic effects of beta-blocking agents used in the management of glaucoma. *Surv Ophthalmol.* 1989;33:453.

88. Chang SC, Bundgaard H, Buur A, et al. Improved corneal penetration of timolol by prodrugs as a means to reduce systemic drug load. *Invest Ophthalmol Vis Sci.* 1987;28:487.

89. Potter DE, Shumate DJ, Bundgaard H, et al. Ocular and cardiac antagonism by timolol prodrugs timolol and levobunolol. *Curr Eye Res.* 1988;7:755.

90. Timoptic XE (timolol maleate ophthalmic gel forming solution, 0.25% and 0.5%). Product insert. West Point, PA: Merck & Co, Inc; 1993.

91. Dubiner HB, Hill R, Kaufman H, Keates EU, Zimmerman TJ, Mandell AI, Mundorf TK, Bahr RL, Schwartz LW, Towey AW, Hurvitz LM, Starita RJ, Sassani JW, Ropo A, Gunn R, Stewart WC. Timolol hemihydrate vs timolol maleate to treat ocular hypertension and open-angle glaucoma. *Am J Ophthalmol.* 1996;121(5):522–528.

92. Bucolo C, Spadaro A, Mangiafico S. Pharmacological evaluation of a new timolol/pilocarpine formulation. *Ophthalm Res.* 1998;30(2):101–106.

93. Aula P, Kalla T, Huupponen R, et al. Timolol binding to bovine ocular melanin in vitro. *J Ocul Pharmacol.* 1988;4:29.

94. Strempel I. Influence of β-blockers on the tear film stability. *Ophthalmologica.* 1987;195:61.

95. Strempel I. The influence of topical β-blockers on the breakup time. *Ophthalmologica.* 1984;189:110.

96. Strempel I. Different β-blockers and their short-time effects on "breakup time." *Ophthalmologica.* 1986;192:11.

97. Haruta Y, Rootman DS, Hill JM. Recurrent HSV-1 corneal epithelial lesions induced by timolol iontophoresis in latently infected rabbits. *Invest Ophthalmol Vis Sci.* 1987;29:387.

98. Hill JM, Shimomura Y, Dudley JB, et al. Timolol induces HSV-1 ocular shedding in the latently infected rabbit. *Invest Ophthalmol Vis Sci.* 1987;28:585.

99. Bucci MG, Pescosolido N, Mariotti SP, et al. Comportamento dell'ampiezza del polso oculare dopo instillazione di β-bloccanti. *Boll Ocul.* 1990;69:285.

100. Wolf S, Schulte K, Berg B, et al. Einflub von β-Blockern auf die retinale Ämodynamik. *Klin Monatsbl Augenheilkd* 1989;195:229.

101. Grunwald JE. Effect of topical timolol on the human retinal circulation. *Invest Ophthalmol Vis Sci.* 1986;27:1713.

102. Grunwald JE. Topical timolol and the human retinal circulation. *Surv Ophthalmol.* 1989;33(suppl):415.

103. Grunwald JE. Effect of timolol maleate on the retinal circulation of human eyes with ocular hypertension. *Invest Ophthalmol Vis Sci.* 1990;31:521.

104. Grunwald JE. Effect of two weeks of timolol maleate treatment on the normal retinal circulation. *Invest Ophthalmol Vis Sci.* 1991;32:39.

105. Hesse RJ, Swan JL II. Aphakic cystoid macular edema secondary to betaxolol therapy. *Ophthalm Surg.* 1988; 19:562.

106. Yoshida A, Ogasawara H, Fujio N, Konno S, Ishiko S, Kitaya N, Kagokawa H, Nagaoka T, Hirokawa H. Comparison of short- and long-term effects of betaxolol and timolol on human retinal circulation. *Eye.* 1998;12(5):848–853.

107. Kiel JW, Patel P. Effects of timolol and betaxolol on choroidal blood flow in the rabbit. *Exp Eye Res.* 1998; 67(5):501–507.

108. Turacli ME, Ozden RG, Gurses MA. The effect of betaxolol on ocular blood flow and visual fields in patients with normotension glaucoma. *Eur J Ophthalmol.* 1998; 8(2):62–66.

109. Schmetterer L, Strenn K, Findl O, Breiteneder H, Graselli U, Agneter E, Eichler HG, Wolzt M. Effects of antiglaucoma drugs on ocular hemodynamics in healthy volunteers. *Clin Pharmacol Ther.* 1997;61(5):583–595.

110. Ishikawa Y, Kiuchi Y, Takamatsu M, Mishima H. Effects of beta adrenergic blockers on retinal circulation. *Acta Soc Ophthalmol Jpn.* 1996;100(10):798–802.

111. Nelson WL, Fraunfelder FT, Sills JM, et al. Adverse respiratory and cardiovascular events attributed to timolol ophthalmic solution 1978–1985. *Am J Ophthalmol.* 1986;102:606.

112. Brown JH, McGeown MG. Chronic renal failure associated with topical application of paraphenylenediamine. *BMJ.* 1987;294:155.

113. Collignon P. Cardiovascular and pulmonary effects of β-blocking agents: Implications for their use in ophthalmology. *Surv Ophthalmol.* 1989;33(suppl):455.

114. Bleckmann H, Dorow P. Cardioselective β-blockers locally applied and histamine provocation in patients suffering from obstructive airways disease. *Fortschr Ophthalmol.* 1986;84:346.

115. D'Andrea A, Ando F, De Natale R, et al. Studio della funzionalita respiratoria in soggetti glaucomatosi sottoposti a terapia con β-bloccanti. *Boll Ocul.* 1989;68:423.

116. Brooks AMV, Gillies WE, West RH. Betaxolol eye drops as a safe medication to lower intraocular pressure. *Aust N Z J Ophthalmol.* 1987;15:125.

117. Brooks AMV, Burdon JGW, Gillies WE. The significance of reactions to betaxolol reported by patients. *Aust N Z J Ophthalmol.* 1989;15:353.

118. Ofner S, Smith TJ. Betaxolol in chronic obstructive pulmonary disease. *J Ocul Pharmacol.* 1987;3:171.

119. Weinreb RN, Van Buskirk EM, Cherniack R, et al. Long-term betaxolol therapy in glaucoma patients with pulmonary disease. *Am J Ophthalmol.* 1988;106:162.

120. Nelson WL, Kuritsky JN. Early postmarketing surveillance of betaxolol hydrochloride Sept 1985–Sept 1986. *Am J Ophthalmol.* 1987;4:592.

121. Berger WE. Betaxolol in patients with glaucoma and asthma. *Am J Ophthalmol.* 1987;4:600.

122. Harris LS, Greenstein SH, Bloom AF. Respiratory difficulties with betaxolol. *Am J Ophthalmol.* 1986;102:274.

123. Roholt PC. Betaxolol and restrictive airway disease. *Arch Ophthalmol.* 1987;105:1172.

124. Goldberg I. Betaxolol. *Aust N Z J Ophthalmol.* 1989;17:9.

125. Atkins JM, Pugh BR Jr, Timewell RM. Cardiovascular effects of topical β-blockers during exercise. *Am J Ophthalmol.* 1985;99:173.

126. Ball S. Congestive heart failure from betaxolol. *Arch Ophthalmol.* 1987;105:320.

127. Zabel RW. MacDonald IM. Sinus arrest associated with betaxolol ophthalmic drops. *Am J Ophthalmol.* 1987; 104:431.

128. Dorigo MT, Crivellari MP, Fracasso G, et al. Valutazione della frequenza cardiaca mediante registrazione elettrocardiografica (Holter) dopo instillazione di befunololo. *Boll Ocul.* 1988;67:309.

129. Lynch MG, Whitson JT, Brown RH, et al. Topical β-blocker therapy and central nervous system side effects. *Arch Ophthalmol.* 1988;106:908.

130. Waal HJ. Propranolol-induced depression. *BMJ.* 1967; 2:50.

131. Hinshelwood RD. Hallucinations in propranolol. *BMJ.* 1969;1:445.

132. Petrie WM, Maffucci RJ, Woosley RL. Propranolol and depression. *Am J Psychiatry.* 1982;139:92.

133. Cove-Smith JR, Kirk CA. CNS-related side-effects with metoprolol and atenolol. *Eur J Clin Pharmacol.* 1985;28:69.

134. Westerlund A. Central nervous system side-effects with hydrophilic and lipophilic β-blockers. *Eur J Clin Pharmacol.* 1985;28:73.

135. Betts TA, Alford C. β-Blockers and sleep: A controlled trial. *Eur J Clin Pharmacol.* 1985;28:65.

136. Davidorf FH. Did I tell you the story about Jim the neurologist? *Contemp Ophthalm Forum.* 1987;5:4.

137. Shaivitz SA. Timolol and myasthenia gravis. *JAMA* 1979;242:1611.

138. de Vries J, van de Merwe SA, Jan de Heer L. From timolol to betaxolol. *Arch Ophthalmol.* 1989;107:634.

139. Orlando RG. Clinical depression associated with betaxolol. *Am J Ophthalmol.* 1986;102:275.

140. Kass MA. Topical carbonic anhydrase inhibitors. *Am Ophthalmol.* 1989;107:280.

141. Trusopt (dorzolamide hydrochloride ophthalmic solution). Product insert. West Point, PA: Merck & Co, Inc. 1994.

142. Berson FG. Carbonic anhydrase inhibitors of the eye: A review. *J Toxicol Cutan Ocul Toxicol.* 1982;1:169.

143. Epstein DL, Grant WM. Management of carbonic anhydrase inhibitor side effects. *Symp Ocul Ther.* 1979 11:51.

144. Fraunfelder FT, Meyer SM, Bagby GC Jr, Dreis MW. Hematologic reactions to carbonic anhydrase inhibitors. *Am J Ophthalmol.* 1986;100:79.

145. Mogk LG, Cyrlin MN. Blood dyscrasias and carbonic anhydrase inhibitors. *Ophthalmology.* 1988;95:768.

146. Schneeweiss A. *Drug Therapy in Cardiovascular Diseases.* Philadelphia: Lea & Febiger; 1986:793–794.

147. Harrison R, Kaufmann CS. Clonidine: Effects of a topically administered solution on intraocular pressure and blood pressure in open-angle glaucoma. *Arch Ophthalmol.* 1977;95:1368.

148. Hodapp E, Kolker AE, Kass MA. The effect of topical clonidine on intraocular pressure. *Arch Ophthalmol.* 1981;99:1208.

149. Kaskel D, Becker H, Rudolf H. Frühwirkungen von Clonidin, Adrenalin, und Pilocarpin auf den Augeninnendruck und Episkleralvenendruck des gesunden menschlichen Auges. *Graefes Arch Clin Exp Ophthalmol.* 1980;213:251.

150. Krieglstein GK, Langham ME, Leydhecker W. The peripheral and central neural actions of clonidine in normal and glaucomatous eyes. *Invest Ophthalmol Vis Sci.* 1978;17:149.

151. Ralli R. Clonidine effect on the intraocular pressure and eye circulation. *Acta Ophthalmol.* 1975;125:37.

152. Lee DA, Topper JE, Brubaker RF. Effect of clonidine on aqueous humor flow in normal human eyes. *Exp Eye Res.* 1984;38:239.

153. Abrams DA, Robin AL, Pollack IP, et al. The safety and efficacy of topical 1% ALO 2145 (p-aminoclonidine hydrochloride) in normal volunteers. *Arch Ophthalmol.* 1987;105:1205.

154. Gharagozloo NZ, Relf SJ, Brubaker RF. Aqueous flow is reduced by alpha-adrenergic agonist apraclonidine hydrochloride (ALO 2145). *Ophthalmology.* 1988; 95:1217.

155. Robin AL, Pollack IP, de Faller JM. Effects of topical 1% ALO 2145 (p-aminoclonidine hydrochloride) on the acute intraocular pressure rise after argon laser iridotomy. *Arch Ophthalmol.* 1987;105:1208.

156. Brown RH, Stewart RH, Lynch MG, et al. ALO 2145 reduces the intraocular pressure elevation after anterior segment laser surgery. *Ophthalmology.* 1988;95:378.

157. Robin AL, Pollack IP, House B, et al. Effects of ALO 2145 on intraocular pressure following argon laser trabeculoplasty. *Arch Ophthalmol.* 1987;105:646.

158. Pollack IP, Brown RH, Crandall AS, et al. Prevention of the rise in intraocular pressure following neodymium-YAG posterior capsulotomy using topical 1% apraclonidine. *Arch Ophthalmol.* 1988;106:754.

159. Jampel HD, Robin AL, Quigley HA, et al. Apraclonidine hydrochloride: A one-week dose response study. *Arch Ophthalmol.* 1988;106:1069.

160. Morrison JC, Robin AL. Adjunctive glaucoma therapy: A comparison of apraclonidine and dipivefrin when added to timolol maleate. *Ophthalmology.* 1989;96:3.

161. Iopidine (apraclonidine ophthalmic solution, 0.5%). Product monograph. Alcon Ophthalmic. Ft. Worth, TX: Alcon Laboratories, Inc; 1996.

162. Marquardt R, Pillunat LE, Stodtmeister R. Ocular hemodynamics following local application of clonidine. *Klin Monatsbl Augenheilkd.* 1988;193:637.

163. Corneli HM, Banner WW, Vernon DD, et al. Toddler eats clonidine patch and nearly quits smoking for life. *JAMA.* 1989;261:42.

164. Coleman AL, Diehl DLC, Jampel HD, et al. Topical timolol decreases plasma high-density lipoprotein cholesterol level. *Arch Ophthalmol.* 1990;108:1260.

165. Abrams DA, Robin AL, Pollack IP. et al. The safety and efficacy of topical 1% ALO 2145 (p-aminoclonidine monohydrochloride) in normal volunteers. *Arch Ophthalmol.* 1987;105:1205.

166. Robin AL. Short-term effects of unilateral 1% ALO 2145 (p-aminoclonidine hydrochloride) therapy. *Arch Ophthalmol.* 1988;106:912.

167. Alphagan (brimonidine tartrate ophthalmic solution). Product monograph. Irvine, CA: Allergan, Inc; 1996.

168. Greenfield DS, Liebmann JM. Ritch R. Brimonidine: a new alpha²-adrenoreceptor agonist for glaucoma treatment. *J Glaucoma.* 1997;6(4):250–258.

169. Nordlund JR, Pasquale LR, Robin AL, Rudikoff MT, Ordman J, Chen KS, Walt J. The cardiovascular, pulmonary, and ocular hypotensive effects of 0.2% brimonidine. *Arch Ophthalmol.* 1995;113(1):77–83.

170. Adkins JC, Balfour JA. Brimonidine. A review of its pharmacological properties and clinical potential in the management of open-angle glaucoma and ocular hypertension. *Drugs Aging.* 1998;12(3):225–241.

171. Schuman JS, Horwitz B, Choplin NT, David R, Albracht D, Chen K. A 1-year study of brimonidine twice daily in glaucoma and ocular hypertension: A controlled, randomized, multicenter clinical trial. Chronic Brimonidine Study Group. *Arch Ophthalmol.* 1997; 115(7):847–852.

172. Wilensky JT. The role of brimonidine in the treatment of open-angle glaucoma. *Surv Ophthalmol.* 1996;41 (suppl 1):S3–S7.

173. Schuman JS. Clinical experience with brimonidine 0.2% and timolol 0.5% in glaucoma and ocular hypertension. *Surv Ophthalmol.* 1996;41(suppl 1):S27–S37.

174. Walters TR. Development and use of brimonidine in treating acute and chronic elevations of intraocular pressure: A review of safety, efficacy, dose response, and dosing studies. *Surv Ophthalmol.* 1996;41:S19–S26.

175. CoSopt (dorzolamide hydrochloride–timolol maleate ophthalmic solution): Two proven agents, one simple solution. Product monograph. West Point, PA: Merck & Co, Inc; 1998.

176. Azopt (brinzolamide ophthalmic solution, 1%). Product monograph. Ft. Worth, TX: Alcon Laboratories, Inc; 1998.

177. Goh Y. The metabolism and actions of prostaglandins in the eye. *Folia Ophthalmol Jpn.* 1989;40:2589.

178. Bito LZ. Prostaglandins and other eicosanoids: Their ocular transport pharmacokinetics and therapeutic effects. *Trans Ophthalmol Soc.* 1986;105:162.

179. Yamane A, Tokura T, Sano T, et al. Experimental studies on the relationship of prostaglandin to the occurrence of corneal edema and neovascularization in anterior segmental ischemia in the rabbit eyes. *Folia Ophthalmol Jpn.* 1987;38:1579.

180. Kaufman PL. Effects of intracamerally infused prostaglandins on outflow facility in cynomolgus monkey eyes with intact or retrodisplaced ciliary muscle. *Exp Eye Res.* 1986;43:819.

181. Crawford K, Kaufman PL. Pilocarpine antagonizes prostaglandin $F_{2\alpha}$-induced ocular hypotension in monkeys: Evidence for enhancement of uveoscleral outflow by prostaglandin $F_{2\alpha}$. *Arch Ophthalmol.* 1987; 105:1112.

182. Kerstetter JR, Brubaker RF, Wilson SE, et al. Prostaglandin $F_{2\alpha}$1-isopropylester lowers intraocular pressure without decreasing aqueous humor flow. *Am J Ophthalmol.* 1988;105:30.

183. Crawford K, Kaufman PL, Gabelt BT. Effects of topical $PGF_{2\alpha}$ on aqueous humor dynamics in cynomolgus monkeys. *Curr Eye Res.* 1987;6:1035.

184. Nilsson SFE, Samuelsson M, Bill A, et al. Increased uveoscleral outflow as a possible mechanism of ocular hypotension caused by prostaglandin $F_{2\alpha}$ 1-isopropylester in the cynomolgus monkey. *Exp Eye Res.* 1989; 48:707.

185. Gabelt BT, Kaufman PL. Prostaglandin $F_{2\alpha}$ increases uveoscleral outflow in the cynomolgus monkey. *Exp Eye Res.* 1989;49:389.

186. Camras CB, Friedman AH, Rodrigues MM, et al. Multiple dosing of prostaglandin $F_{2\alpha}$ or epinephrine on cynomolgus monkey eyes. *Invest Ophthalmol Vis Sci.* 1988;29:1428.

187. Lee PY, Shao H, Xu L, Qu CK. The effect of prostaglandin $F_{2\alpha}$ on intraocular pressure in normotensive human subjects. *Invest Ophthalmol Vis Sci.* 1988;29:1474.

188. Villumsen J, Alm A. Prostaglandin $F_{2\alpha}$ isopropylester eye drops: Effects in normal human eyes. *Br J Ophthalmol.* 1989; 73:419.

189. Villumsen J, Alm A, Öderstöm M. Prostaglandin $F_{2\alpha}$ isopropylester eye drops: Effect on intraocular pressure in open-angle glaucoma. *Br J Ophthalmol.* 1989; 73:975.

190. Flach AJ, Eliason JA. Topical prostaglandin E_2 effects on normal human intraocular pressure. *J Ocul Pharmacol.* 1988;4:13.

191. Xalatan (latanoprost solution 0.005%): A new direction in glaucoma therapy. Product monograph. Kalamazoo, MI: Pharmacia & Upjohn; 1996.

192. Watson P, Stjernschantz J. A six month, randomized, double-masked study comparing latanoprost with timolol on open-angle glaucoma and ocular hypertension. *Ophthalmology.* 1996;103(1):126.

193. Johnstone MA. Hypertrichosis and increased pigmentation of eyelashes and adjacent hair in the region of the ipsilateral eyelids of patients treated with unilateral topical latanoprost. *Am J Ophthalmol.* 1997;124(4): 544–547.

194. Heier JS, Steinert RF, Frederick AR Jr. Cystoid macular edema associated with latanoprost use (letter). *Arch Ophthalmol.* 1998;116(5):680–682.

195. Netland PA, Chaturvedi N, Dreyer EB. Calcium channel blockers in the management of low-tension and open-angle glaucoma. *Am J Ophthalmol.* 1993;115:608.

196. Netland PA, Grosskreutz CL, Feke GT, et al. Color Doppler ultrasound analysis of ocular circulation after topical calcium channel blocker. *Am J Ophthalmol.* 1995;119(6):694–700.

197. Netland PA, Erickson KA. Calcium channel blockers in glaucoma management. *Ophthalmol Clin North Am.* 1995;8:327–334.

198. Dreyer EB, Zurakowski D, Schumer RA, Podos SM, Lipton SA. Elevated glutamate levels in the vitreous body of humans and monkeys with glaucoma. *Arch Ophthalmol.* 1996;114(3):299–305.

199. Vorwerk CK, Lipton SA, Zurakowski D, Hyman BT, Sabel BA, Dreyer EB. Chronic low-dose glutamate is toxic to retinal ganglion cells: Toxicity blocked by memantine. *Invest Ophthalmol Vis Sci.* 1996;37(8): 1618–1624.

Color Plates

Illustrations on the color plates are also represented in black and white with their relevant discussions in each chapter.

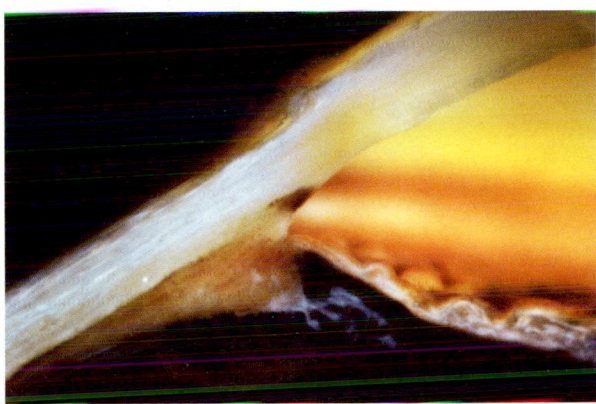 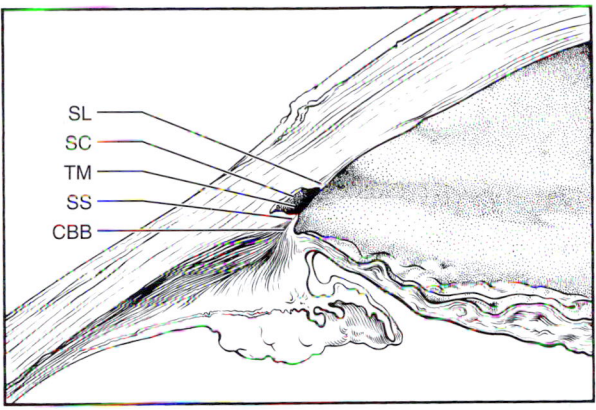

Plate 1 (Fig. 3–17). Macroscopic photograph and corresponding sketch identifying structures visible in a sagittal section of the normal anterior chamber angle. The anterior chamber is artifactually deepened due to posterior sagging of the iris following removal of the crystalline lens.

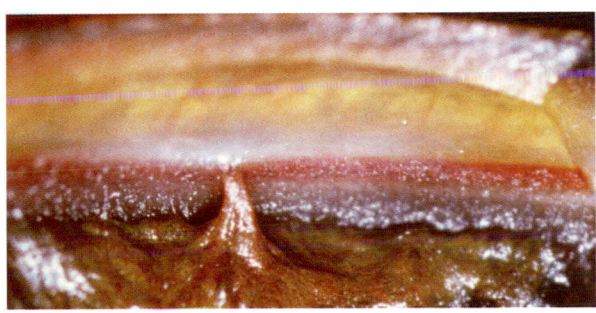 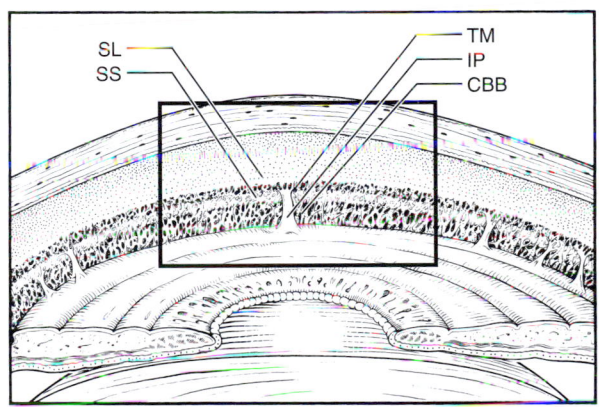

Plate 2 (Fig. 3–18). Macroscopic photograph and corresponding sketch of angle structures viewed from the perspective shown in the adjacent sketch. Schlemm's canal is filled with blood in this specimen, demonstrating its relationship to the other angle structures. An iris process is also shown. Compare the view of the angle structures in this figure with the corresponding sagittal view shown in Fig. 3–17.

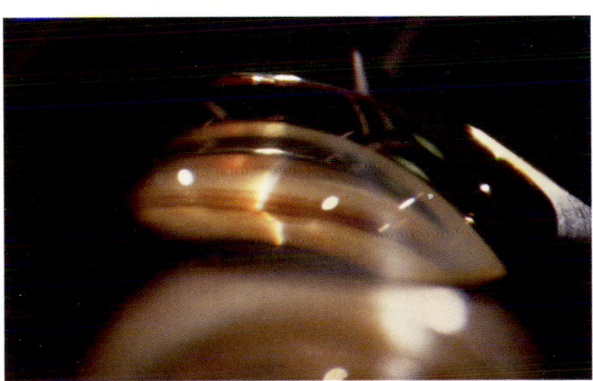 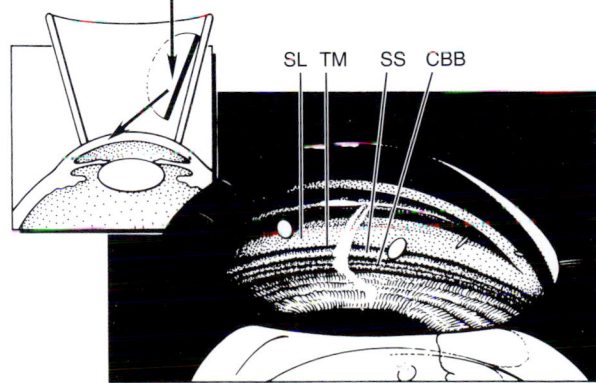

Plate 3 (Fig. 3–19). Goniophotograph of a normal open angle, and corresponding sketch representing a view analogous to that shown in Fig. 3–18. Inset in sketch depicts the placement of the gonioscope onto the cornea and the manner in which the angle structures are viewed. Key: SL = Schwalbe's line; SC = Schlemm's canal; TM = trabecular meshwork; SS = scleral spur; CBB = ciliary body band; IP = iris process. (Photograph courtesy of Rodney Gutner, O.D.)

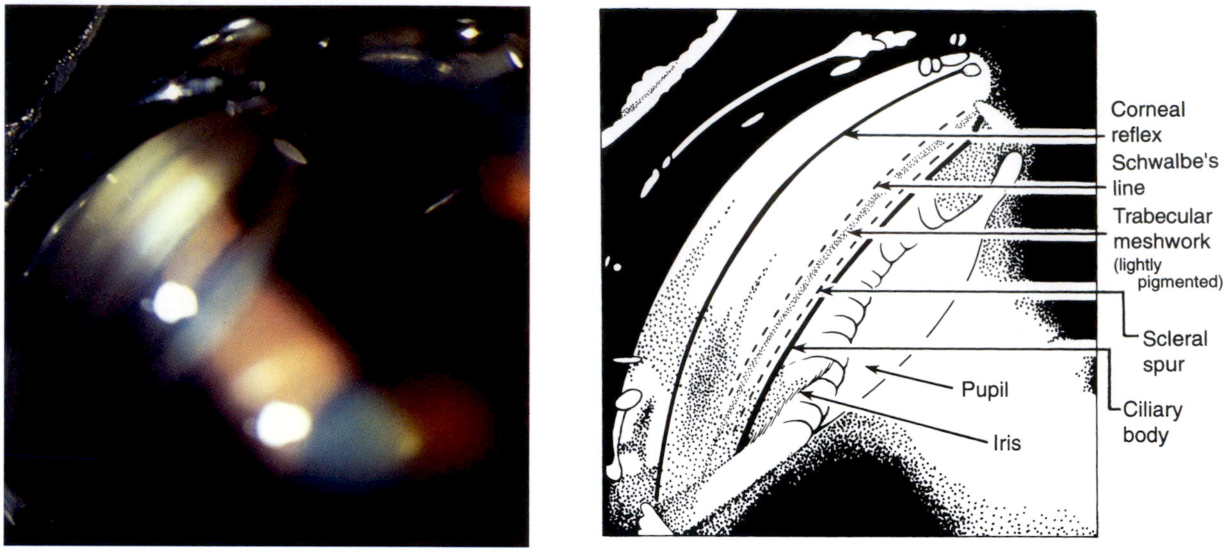

A

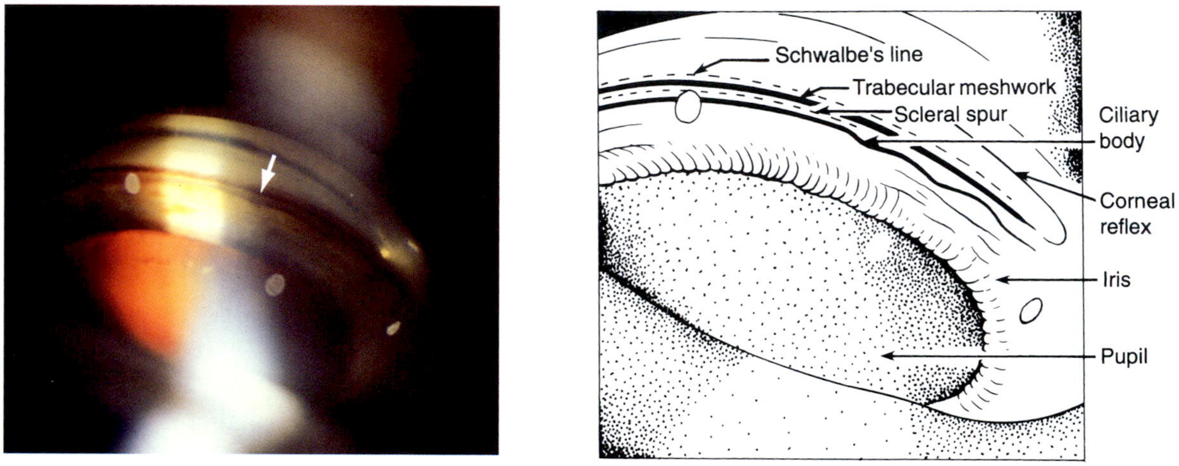

Corneal reflex
Schwalbe's line
Trabecular meshwork (lightly pigmented)
Scleral spur
Pupil
Ciliary body
Iris

B

Schwalbe's line
Trabecular meshwork
Scleral spur
Ciliary body
Corneal reflex
Iris
Pupil

Plate 4 (Fig. 11–8). Normal angle anatomy. Note ciliary body, scleral spur, trabecular meshwork, and Schwalbe's line. The patient in *A* has very little pigmentation in the trabecular meshwork. The patient in *B* has a heavily pigmented trabecular meshwork. There may be considerable variation in the clinical appearance of the normal angle. (Courtesy of Tony Litwak, O.D.)

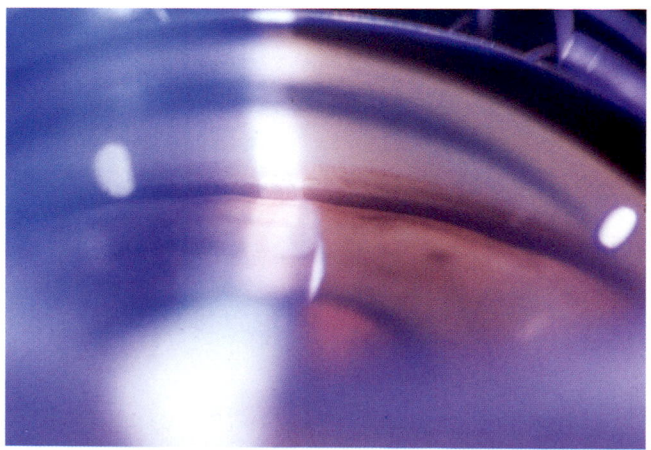

Plate 5 (Fig. 11–9). An image of the normal angle anatomy. All structures are visible. (Courtesy of Kelly Dignam, O.D.)

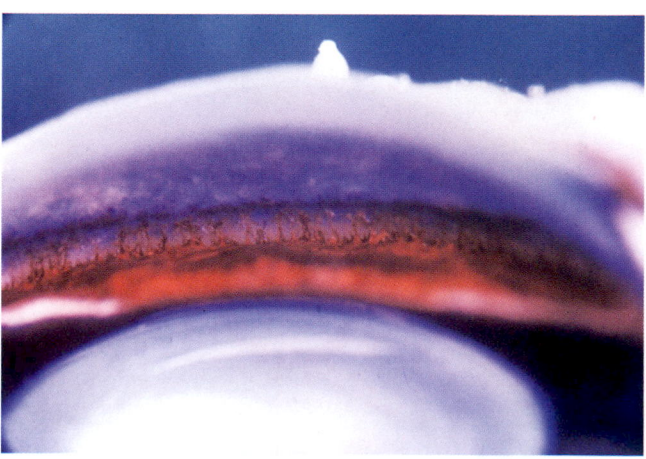

Plate 6 (Fig. 11–10). Iris processes are visible, obscuring some detail of other anterior angle structures. (Courtesy of Kelly Dignam, O.D.)

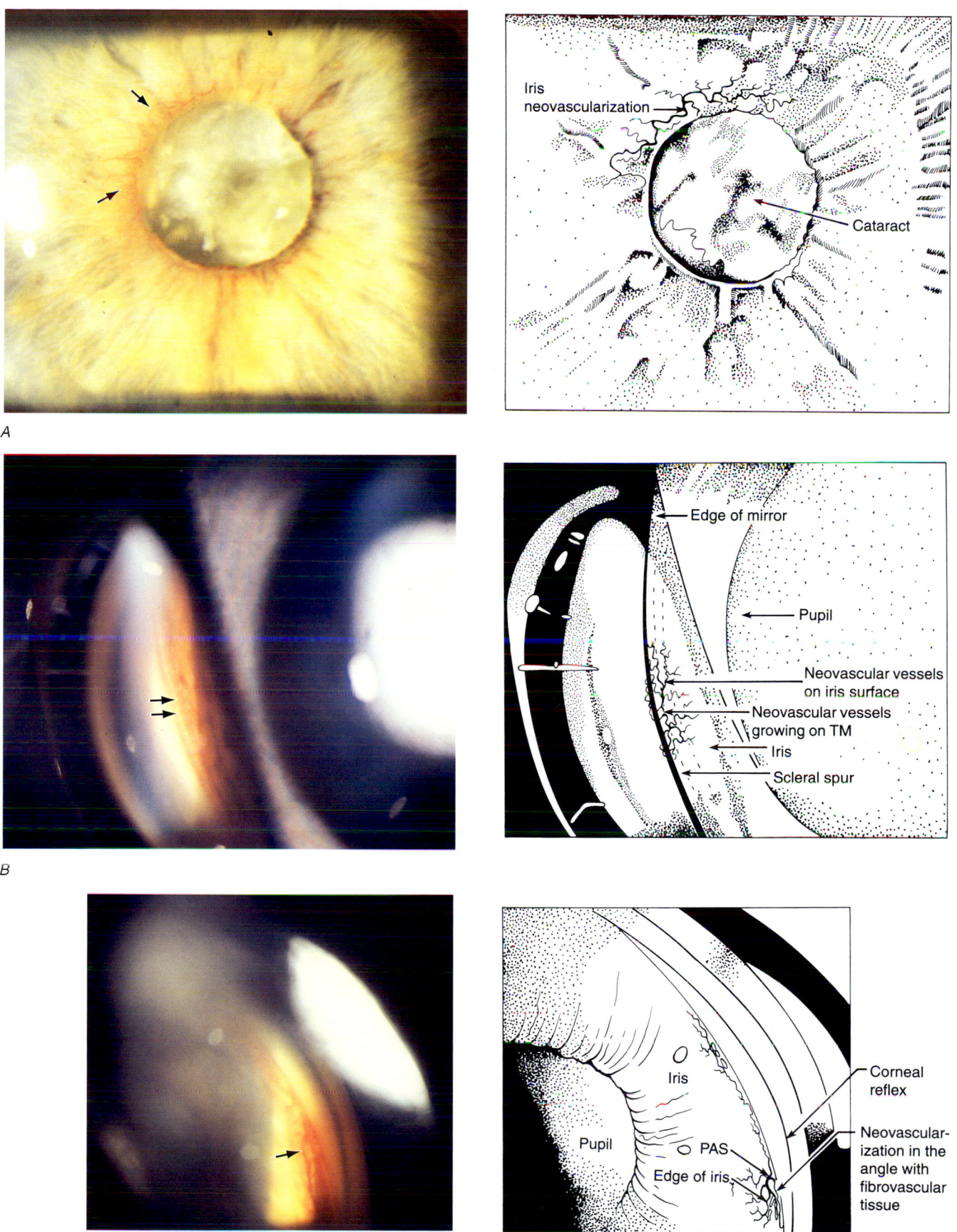

Plate 7 (Fig. 11–18). Iris neovascularization *(arrows)*. Neovascular vessels typically occur at the pupillary margin of the iris (*A*) after an ischemic event to the retina. These vessels may grow into the angle (*B*) along with fibrovascular tissue forming PAS (*C*) and neovascular glaucoma. (Courtesy of Tony Litwak, O.D.)

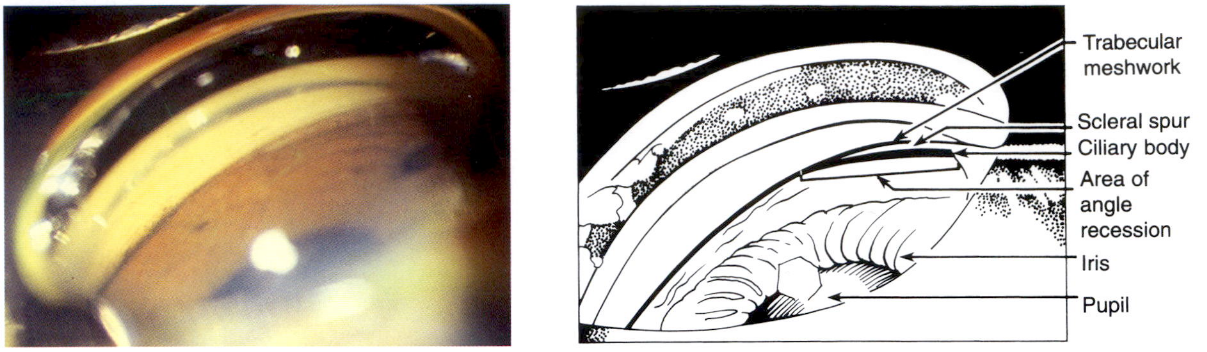

A

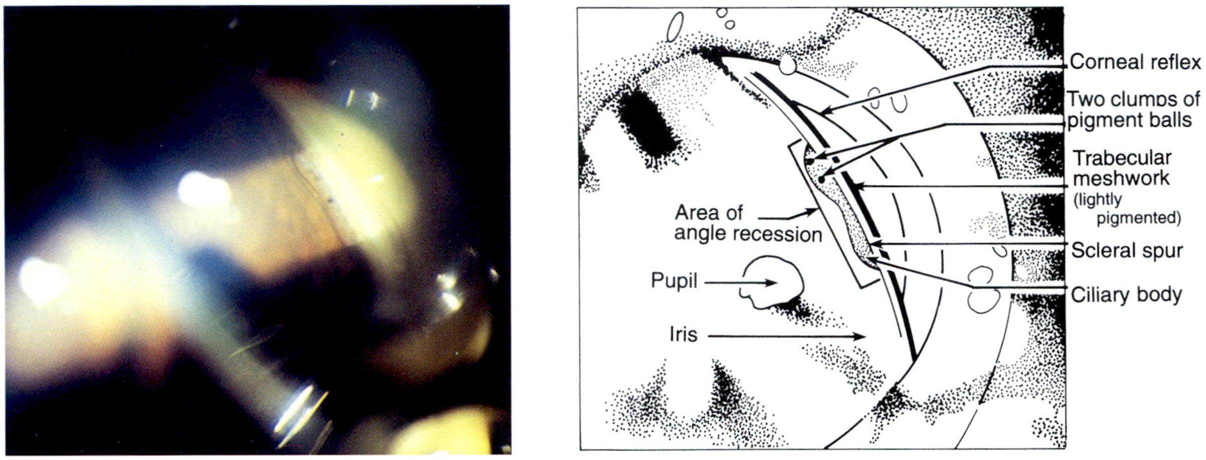

Trabecular meshwork

Scleral spur
Ciliary body

Area of angle recession

Iris

Pupil

B

Corneal reflex

Two clumps of pigment balls

Trabecular meshwork (lightly pigmented)

Scleral spur

Ciliary body

Area of angle recession

Pupil

Iris

Plate 8 (Fig. 11–20). Angle recession after blunt trauma. *A.* Note visibility of scleral spur and ciliary body in area of angle recess. *B.* Angle recession or clumps of pigment in the angle are indicators of possible damage to the trabecular meshwork and development of traumatic glaucoma. (Courtesy of Tony Litwak, O.D.)

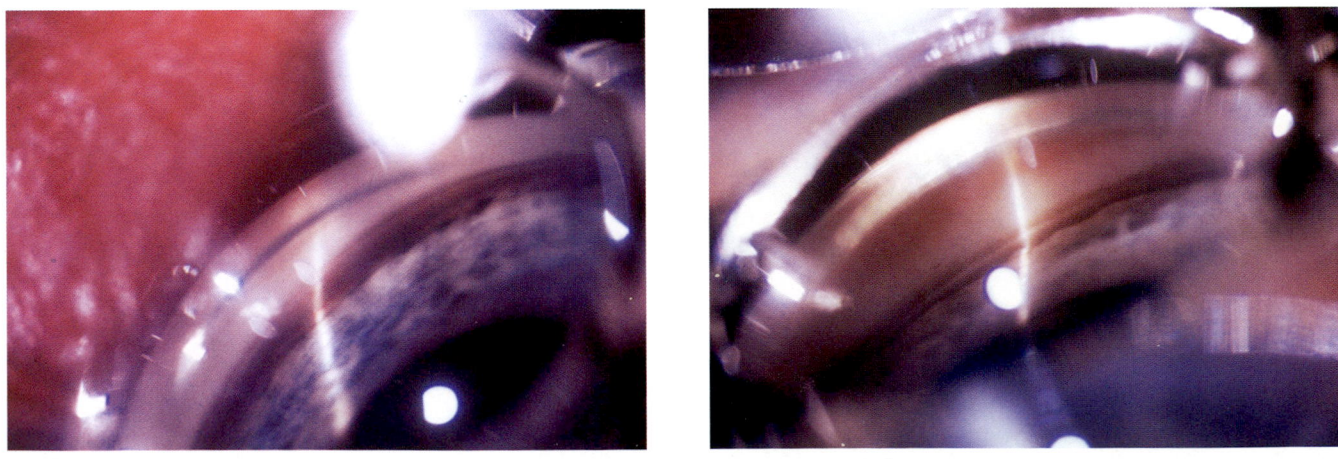

A

B

Plate 9 (Fig. 11–21). *A.* An angle recession is seen in the superior view of this patient, who suffered trauma. Note the extent to which the ciliary body is visible, especially in comparison to the fellow eye. *B.* The fellow eye of this patient. Note the normal-appearing angle with a visible ciliary body. (Courtesy of Kelly Dignam, O.D.)

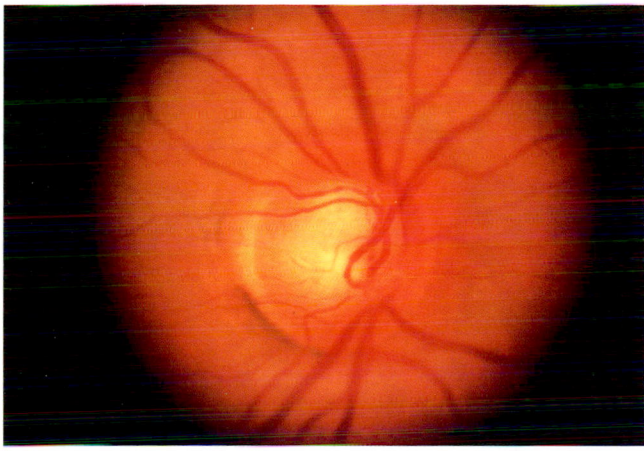

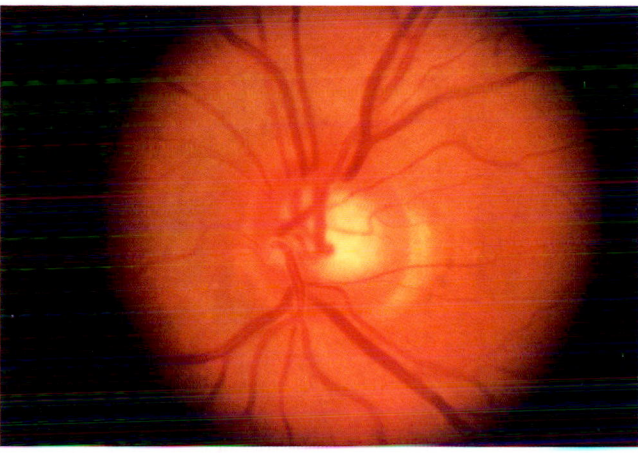

Plate 10 (Fig. 12–1A). Optic nerve head asymmetry is present as well as a slightly enlarged optic disc area: OD>OS. Extensive cupping is judged to be 0.70/0.75 OD, with inferior overpass cupping and superior baring of the circumlinear vessel.

Plate 11 (Fig. 12–1B). Cupping OS is judged to be 0.65/0.60, with a slight temporal slope. Peripapillary atrophy is also present, with zone β approximately 5% of the disc area OD; zone α 5%; and zone β 5% of the disc area OS. No defects in the nerve fiber layer, hemorrhages, or areas of vasoconstriction are seen OD or OS.

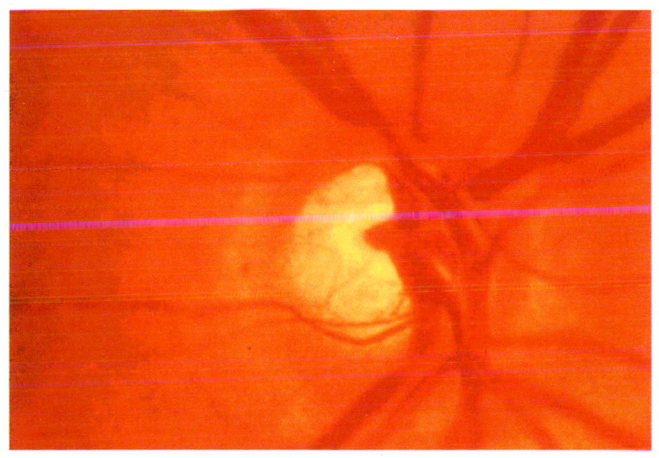

A

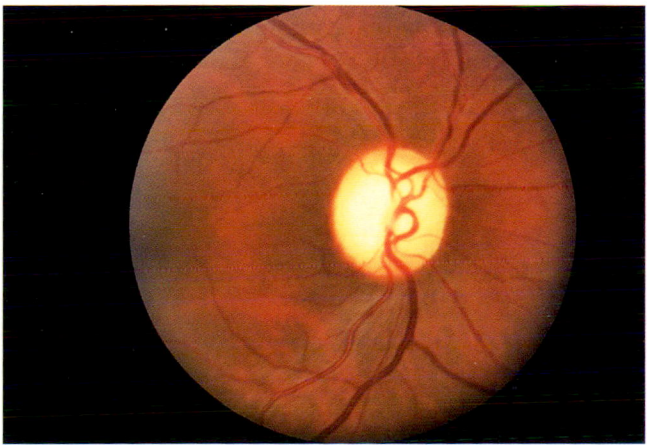

B

Plate 12 (Fig. 12–2). Cup-to-disc asymmetry is present, but it is related to the significant asymmetry in optic disc size. The left optic nerve (B) is twice the size of the right optic nerve (A).

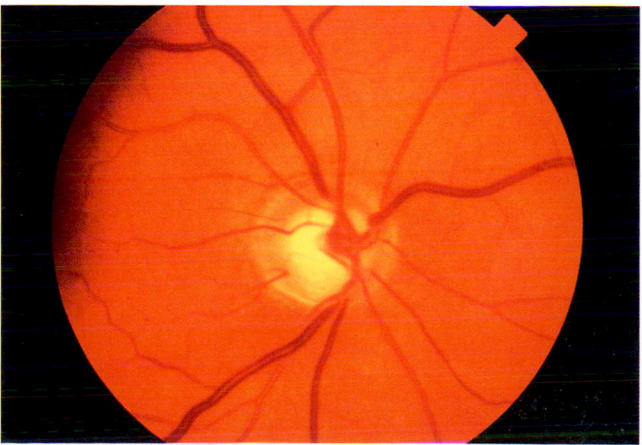

Plate 13 (Fig. 12–12). Pallor of the optic nerve due to pituitary adenoma. Pallor is greater than the extent of cupping.

Plate 14 (Fig. 12–13). A focal notch is present at 7 o'clock. This notch is associated with a wedge defect of the nerve fiber layer.

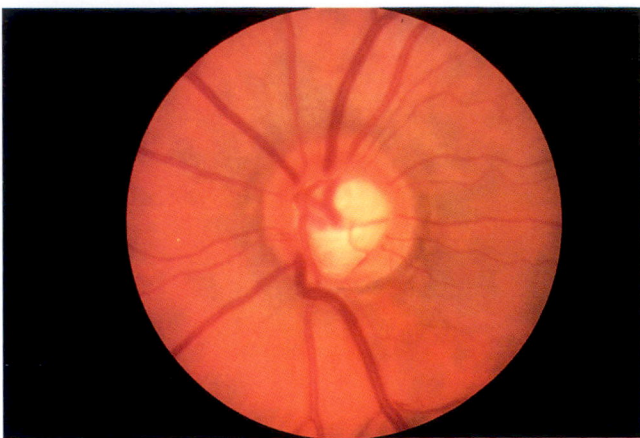

Plate 15 (Fig. 12–14). This focal notch at 5 o'clock is accompanied by a resolving hemorrhage of the nerve fiber layer and a wedge defect of the nerve fiber layer.

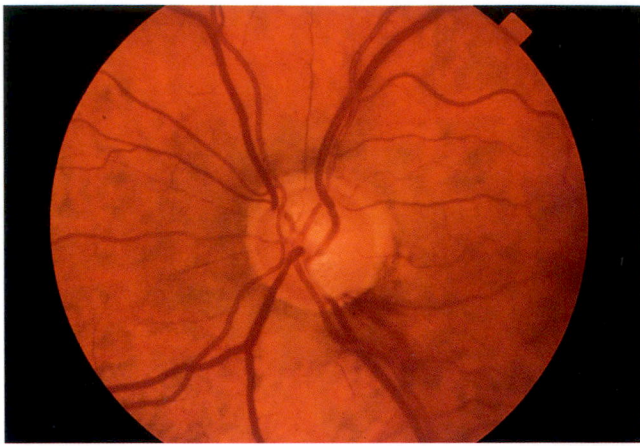

Plate 18 (Fig. 12–17). An extensive hemorrhage of the nerve fiber layer is present at 5 o'clock. This flame-shaped hemorrhage is associated with severe loss of the neuroretinal rim.

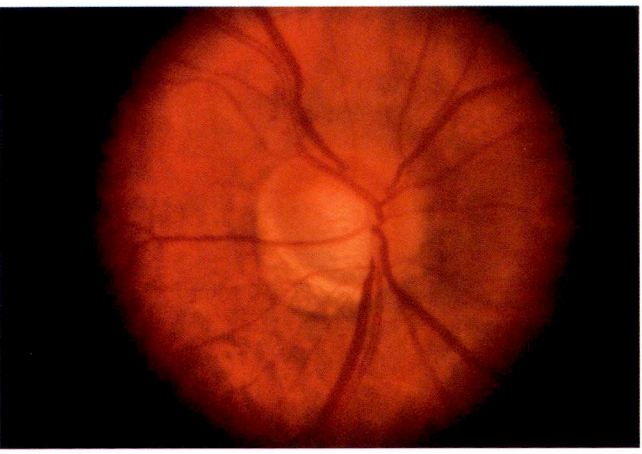

Plate 16 (Fig. 12–15). An acquired pit of the optic nerve (APON) is present at 6 o'clock. APON appears as a focal gray defect at the disc margin. This defect is associated with a dense arcuate scotoma with threat to fixation.

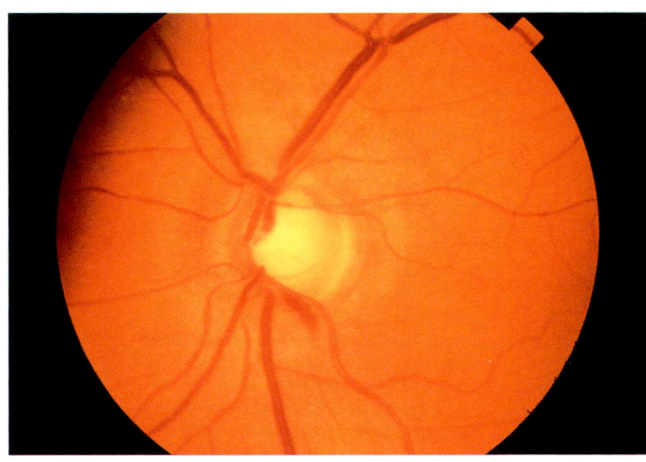

Plate 19 (Fig. 12–18). A hemorrhage of the nerve fiber layer can recur or develop in other sectors of the optic nerve. This finding can be followed by a change in the visual field, nerve fiber layer, or vascular caliber.

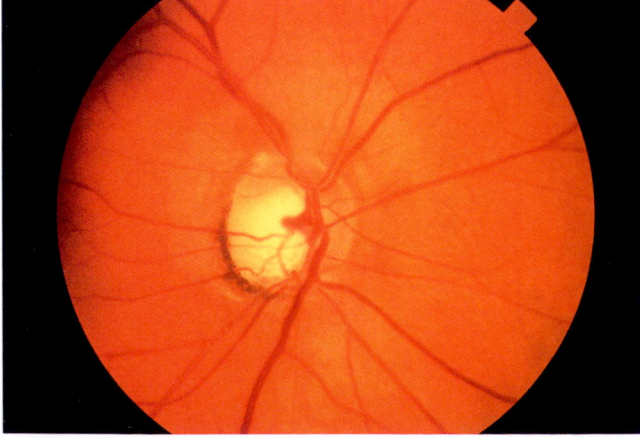

Plate 17 (Fig. 12–16). APON can appear as an enlarged laminar pore, although it is usually more extensive in size. The defect is present at 7 o'clock.

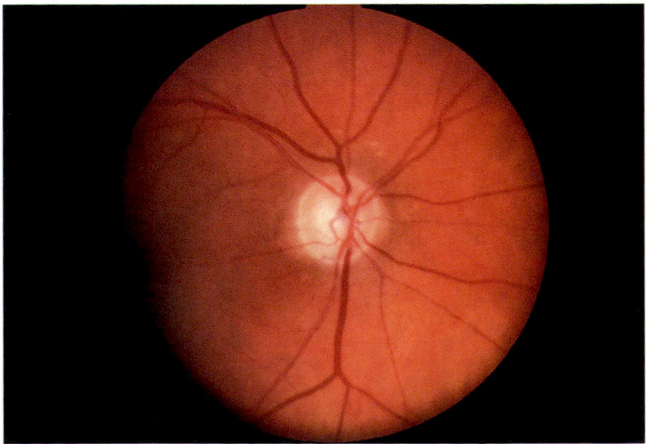

Plate 20 (Fig. 12–19). Focal arteriolar narrowing at 4 and 6 o'clock is observed as an irregularity in vessel diameter at the margin of the optic disc.

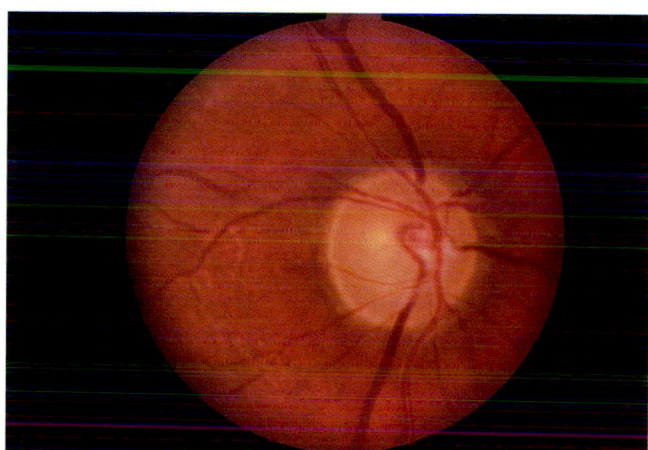

Plate 21 (Fig. 12–20). Vascular sheathing can occur in association with focal arteriolar narrowing. Focal vasoconstriction may be obvious (10 o'clock) or more subtle (11 o'clock).

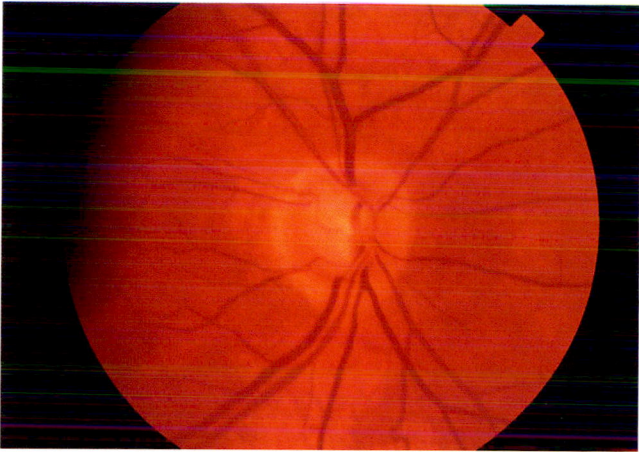

Plate 24 (Fig. 12–23). Bayonetting of retinal vessels is present at 6 o'clock. The vein overlying the disc margin turns back beneath the rim and then turns again to lie along the floor of the cup, forming a "Z" pattern.

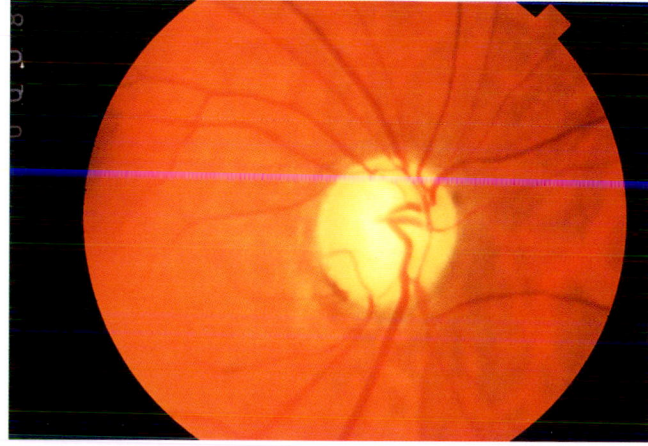

Plate 22 (Fig. 12–21). Severe vascular attenuation can occur in association with glaucoma and other optic neuropathies.

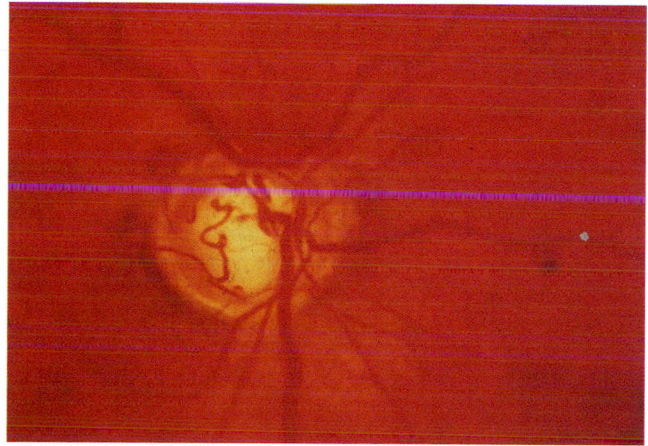

Plate 25 (Fig. 12–24). Disc collateral vessels in a patient with advanced open-angle glaucoma and no history of retinal vascular occlusion.

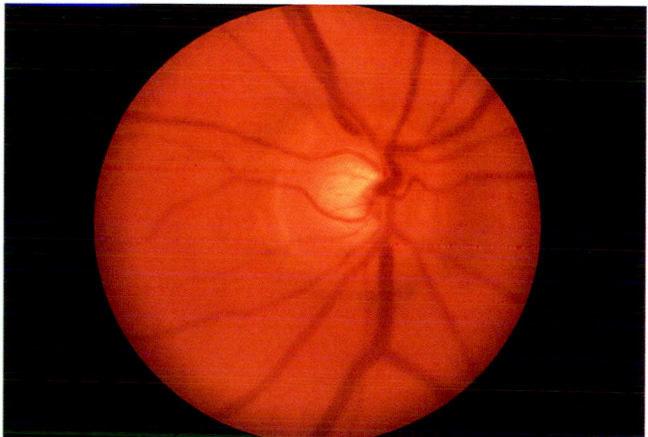

Plate 23 (Fig. 12–22). Baring of the circumlinear vessels occurs when cupping progresses.

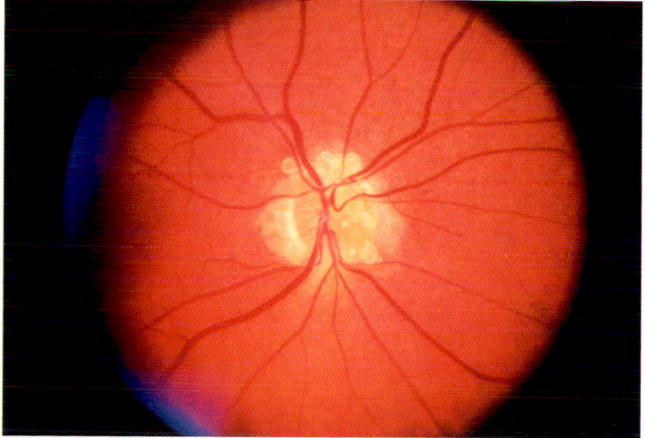

Plate 26 (Fig. 12–25). Optic disc drusen appear as refractile globular deposits on the surface or within the disc substance. Defects or hemorrhages of the nerve fiber layer can occasionally be associated.

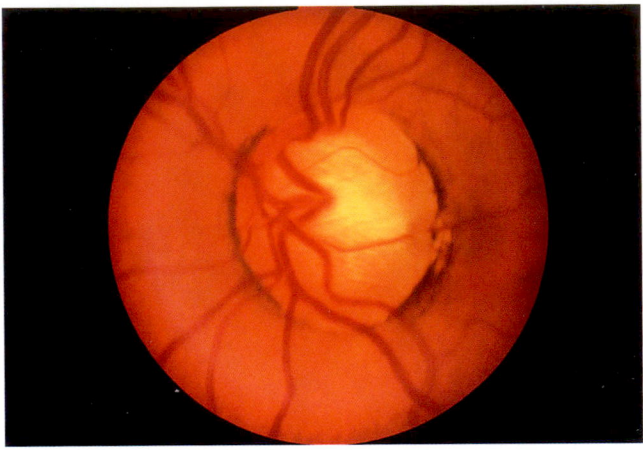

Plate 27 (Fig. 12–26). A congenital pit in the optic disc is generally observed temporally on the disc margin as a localized depression. This is in contrast to acquired optic disc pits, which are more common superiorly or inferiorly.

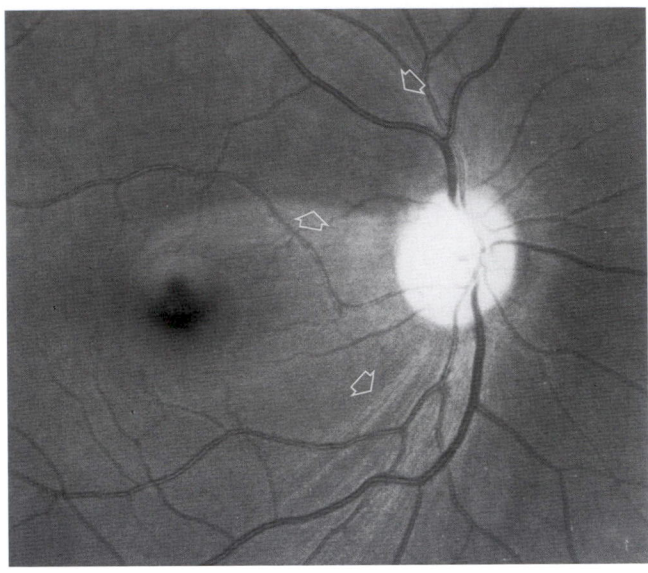

Plate 30 (Fig. 13–1). Generalized loss of axons with a narrow, localized defect inferotemporally *(arrow)* and an even deeper and wider localized sector-shaped dropout of axon bundles superotemporally *(arrows)*.

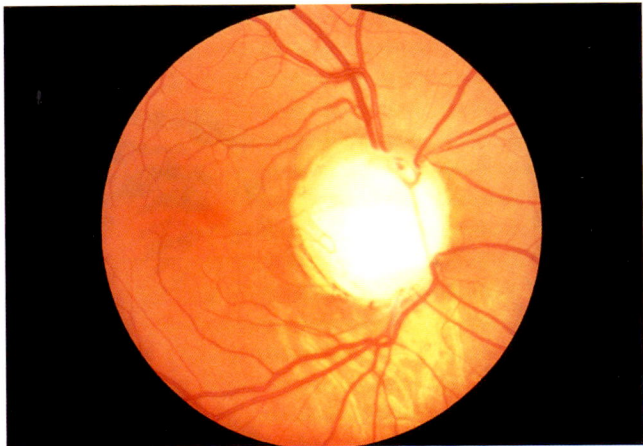

Plate 28 (Fig. 12–27). An optic nerve coloboma may occur with incomplete closure of the embryonic fissure.

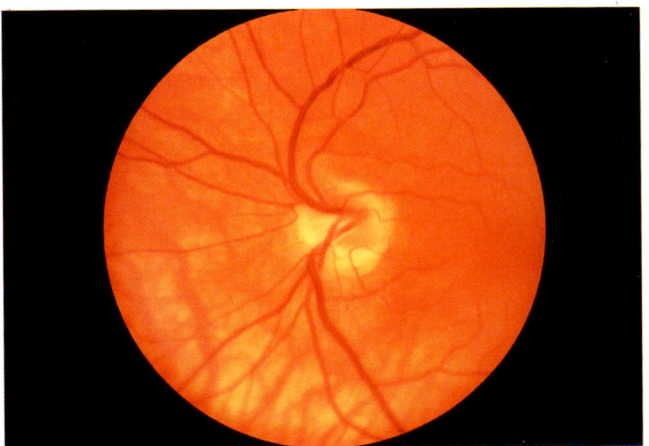

Plate 29 (Fig. 12–28). Tilted optic disc demonstrates relative crowding of the superior nerve fibers and inferior scleral crescent.

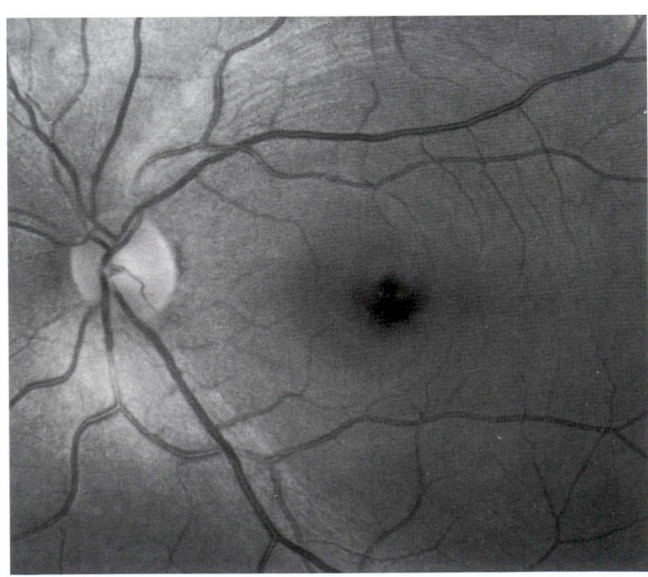

Plate 31 (Fig. 13–3). Normal nerve fiber layer showing typical pattern of the arcuate, papillomacular, and nasal bundles.

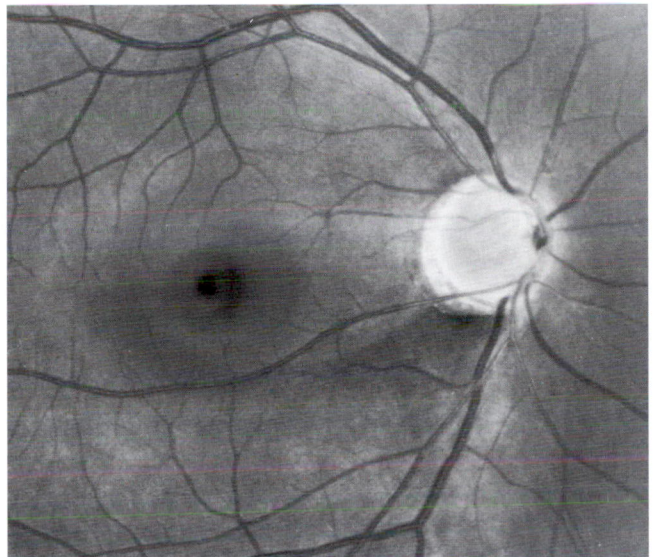

Plate 32 (Fig. 13–4). Diffuse or generalized loss of nerve fibers inferiorly. Note the mottled appearance of the pigment epithelium and sharp wall images of the small retinal vessels.

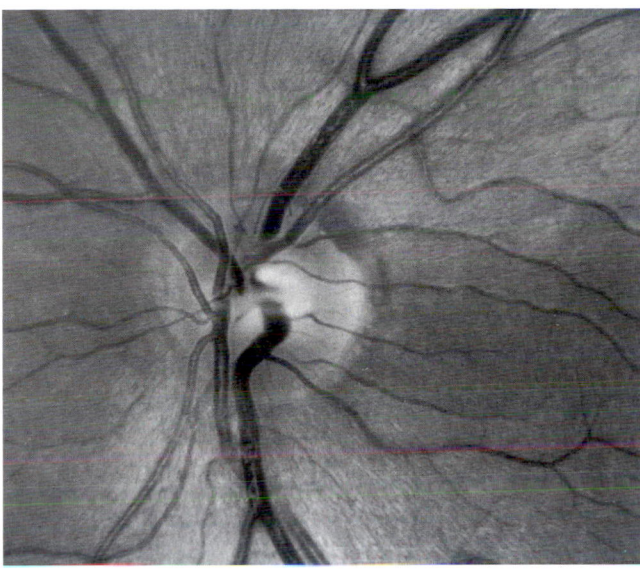

Plate 33 (Fig. 13–5). Normal retinal nerve fiber layer. The margins of the small vessels appear blurred and cross-hatched, as they are within the healthy nerve fiber layer.

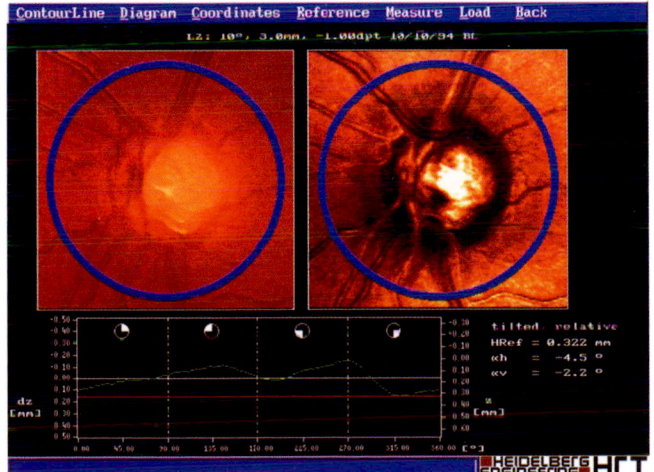

Plate 34 (Fig. 14–3). The reference ring is illustrated in blue on this HRT printout of a glaucomatous patient. The absolute mean height and the tilt of the retinal surface are determined relative to the reference ring. The mean height of the reference ring is set to zero and all height values are measured relative to this zero position. (Courtesy of Dr. S. Hosking.)

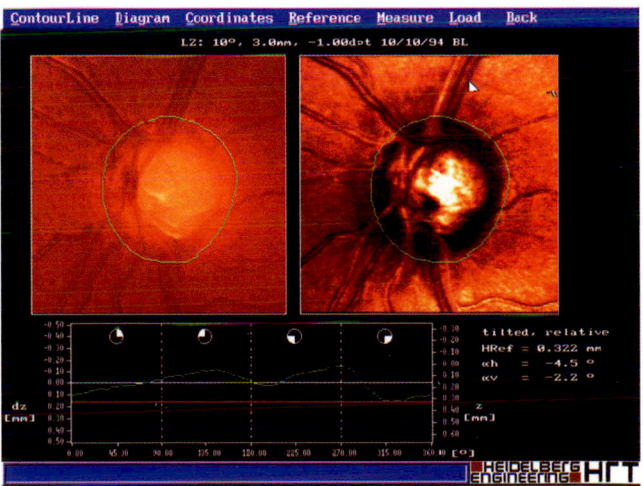

Plate 35 (Fig. 14–4). HRT printout showing a contour line drawn around the optic nerve head and identifying an area of interest for subsequent analysis. On the bottom of the printout is a plot of the height values along this contour line. (Courtesy of Dr. S. Hosking.)

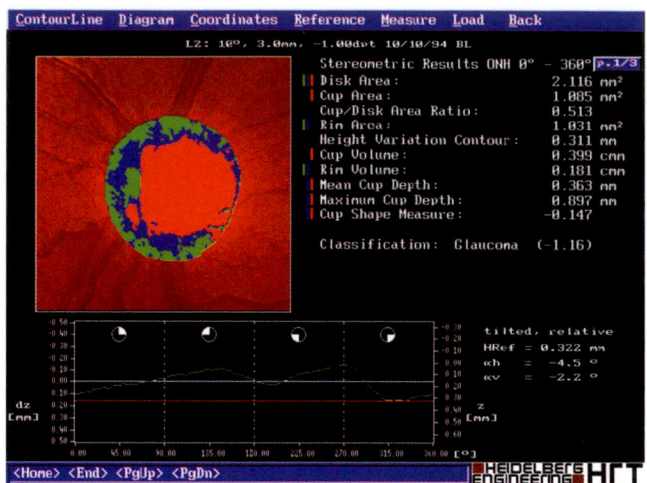

Plate 36 (Fig. 14–6). HRT printout of a glaucomatous patient showing the global analysis of the optic nerve head as defined by the contour line. The "cup" is illustrated in red and defined as the height values distal to the reference plane. The "rim" is illustrated in green and blue and defined by the height values proximal to the reference plane. The stereometric parameters generated for assessment of the optic nerve head are defined in Table 14-1. (Courtesy of Dr. S. Hosking.)

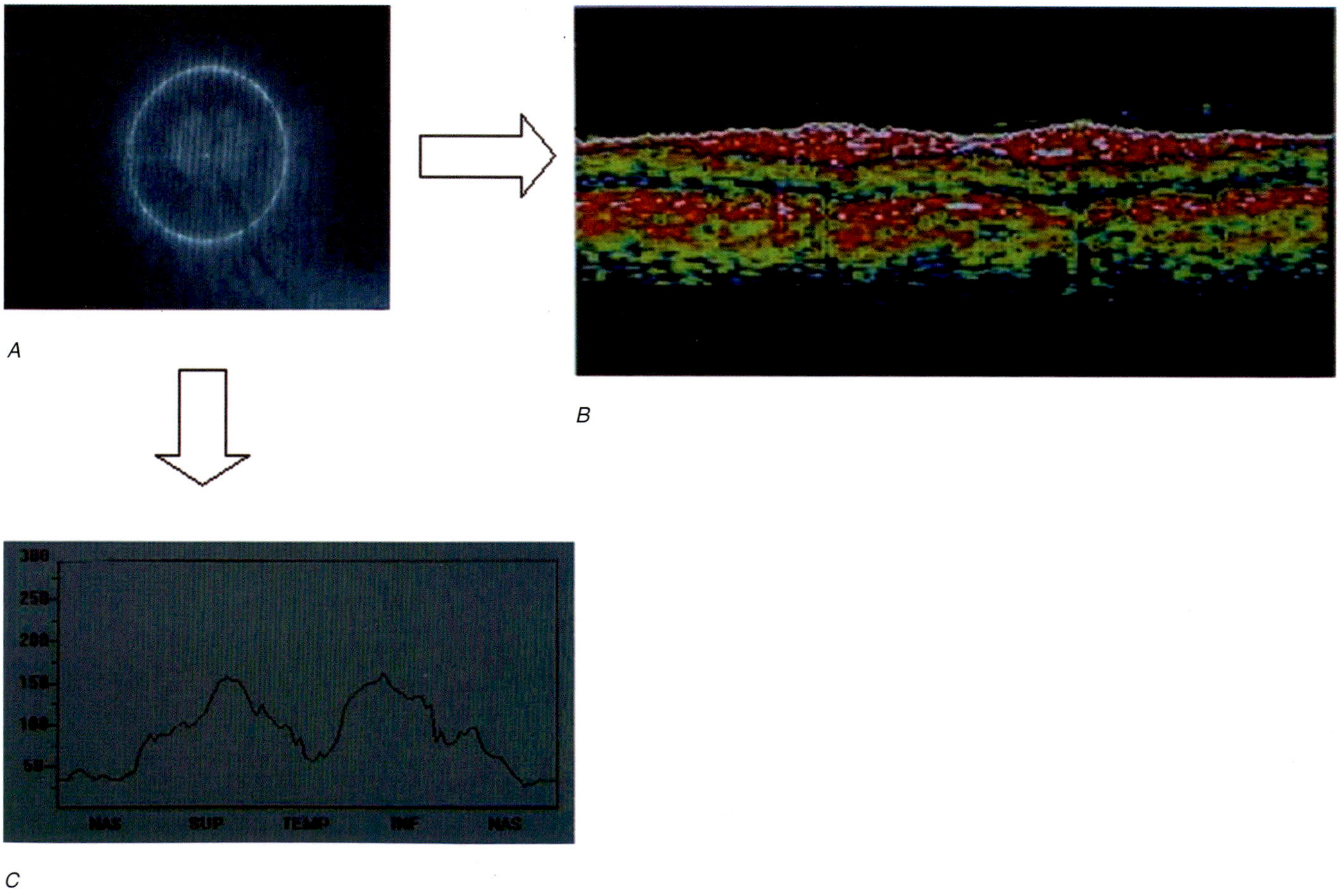

A

B

C

Plate 37 (Fig. 14–11). OCT tomogram sampled from a peripapillary circle (A), showing the retinal thickness around the optic nerve head. The retina is illustrated as a typically four-banded retina (B). The brightest inner band has been related to the nerve fiber layer and the outermost bright band to the retinal pigment epithelium/choriocapillaris. The in-between layers are considered as the plexiform layer and the photoreceptor layer. The thickness of the nerve fiber layer is illustrated as a line graph (C). (Courtesy of Dr. T. Simpson.)

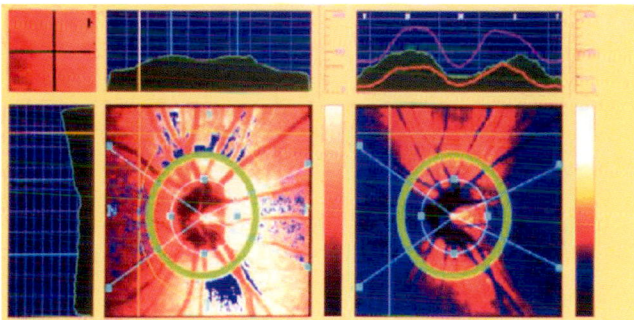

Plate 38 (Fig. 14−13). Retardation map of a normal subject produced by the GDx/Nerve Fiber Analyzer. The line plot in the top right of the image shows a thickness of the nerve fiber layer that falls within the confidence intervals for normality. (Reproduced with permission from Laser Diagnostics Technologies, Inc.)

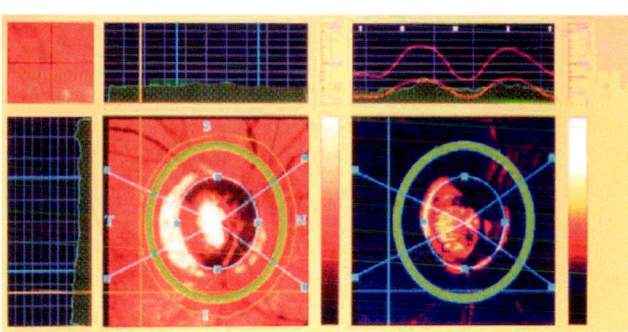

Plate 39 (Fig. 14−14). Retardation map of a patient with glaucoma as produced by the GDx/Nerve Fiber Analyzer. The line plot in the top right of the image shows a thickness of the nerve fiber layer that falls outside the confidence intervals for normality. (Reproduced with permission from Laser Diagnostics Technologies, Inc.)

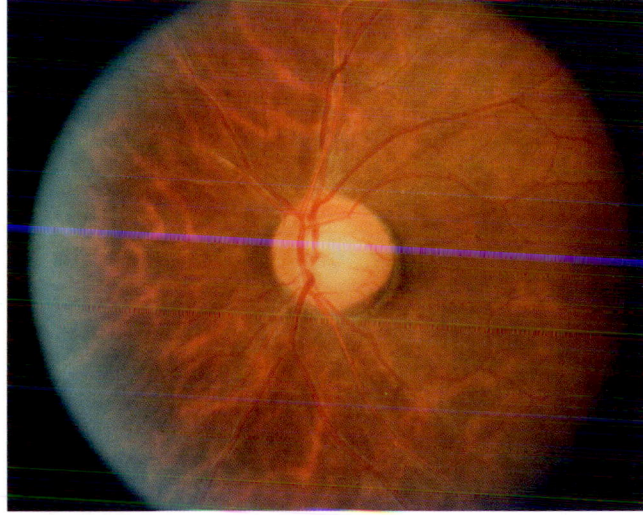

A

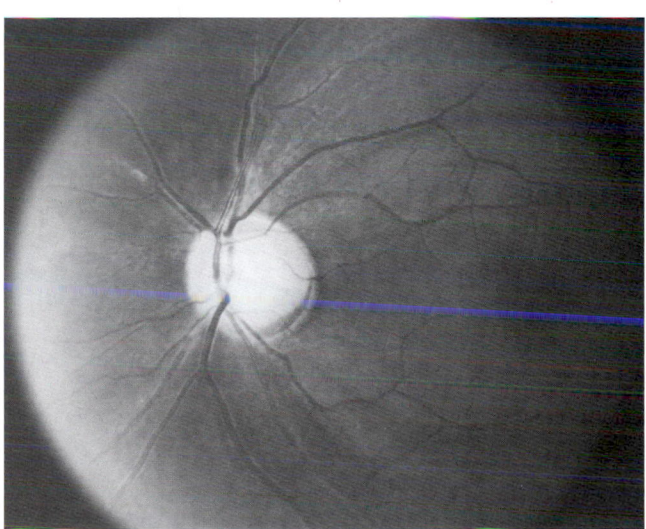

B

Plate 40 (Fig. 19−3). Focal nerve fiber layer dropout. Color and companion red-free photography of the left eye of a glaucoma patient with several slit-like defects in the nerve fiber layer between 12 and 2 o'clock and a large wedge defect between 5 and 7 o'clock.

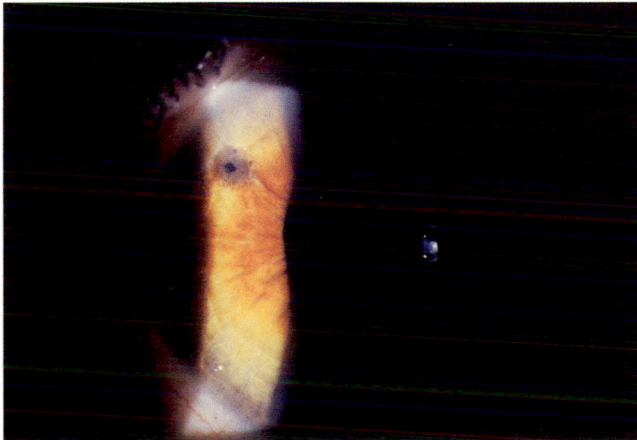

Plate 41 (Fig. 22−4). Postoperative photograph of a patent laser peripheral iridectomy. To be certain that the iridectomy is patent, the lens capsule should be seen through the iridectomy opening.

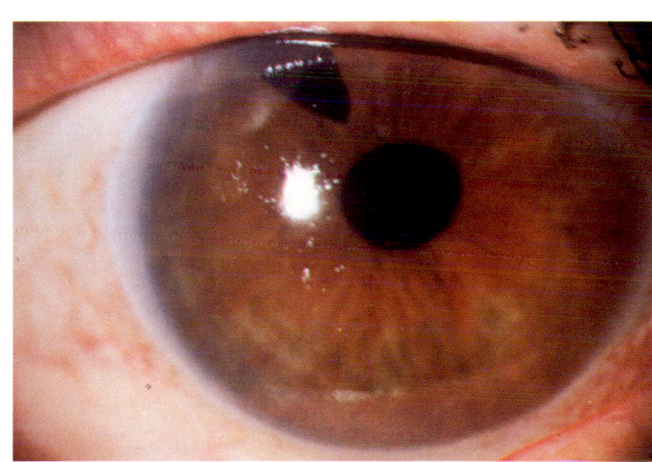

Plate 42 (Fig. 22−5). Photograph of a patent surgical iridectomy.

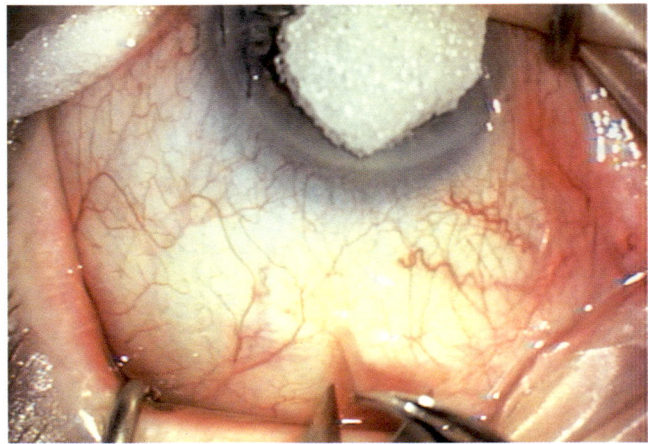

Plate 43 (Fig. 23–1). Exposure of the surgical site. Note the traction suture in the peripheral cornea.

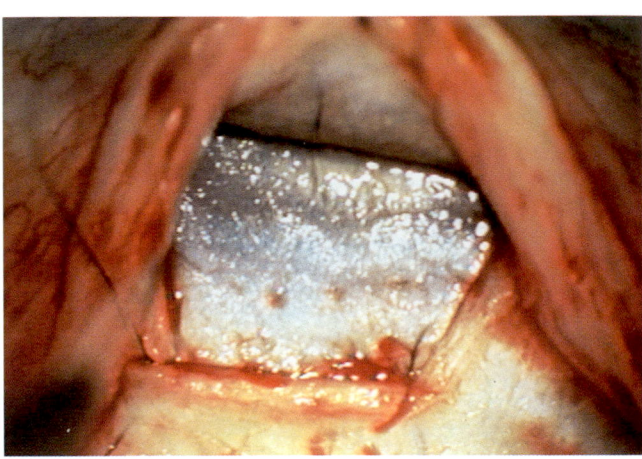

Plate 46 (Fig. 23–4). Exposure of the surgical limbus prior to use of intra-operative antimetabolites.

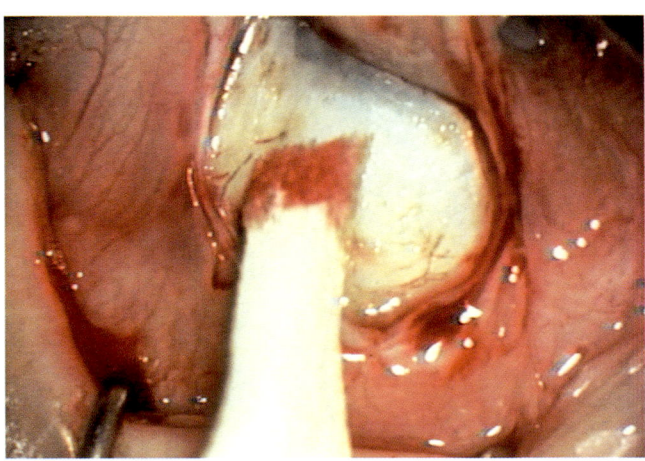

Plate 44 (Fig. 23–2). Dissection of Tenon's capsule has been completed.

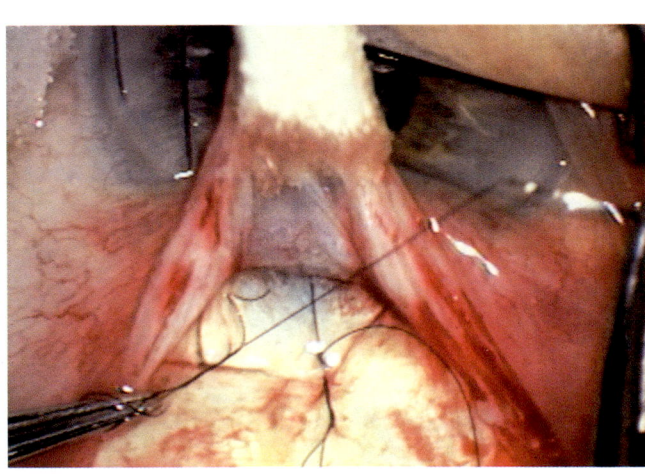

Plate 47 (Fig. 23–5). Placement of releasable sutures to prevent hypotony in the early postoperative period.

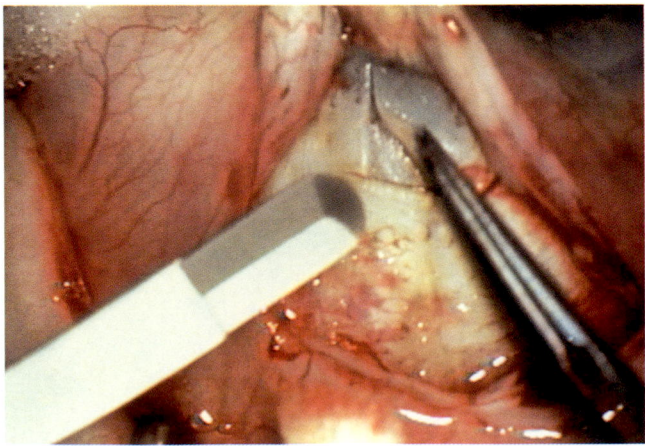

Plate 45 (Fig. 23–3). Lamellar scleral flap of approximately 50% scleral thickness.

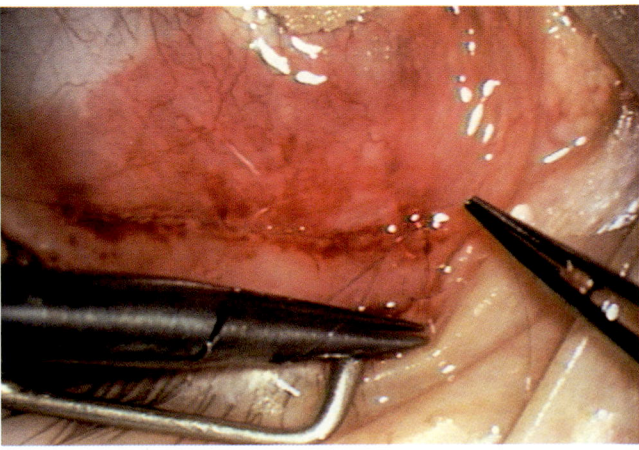

Plate 48 (Fig. 23–6). Conjunctival closure at completion of case.

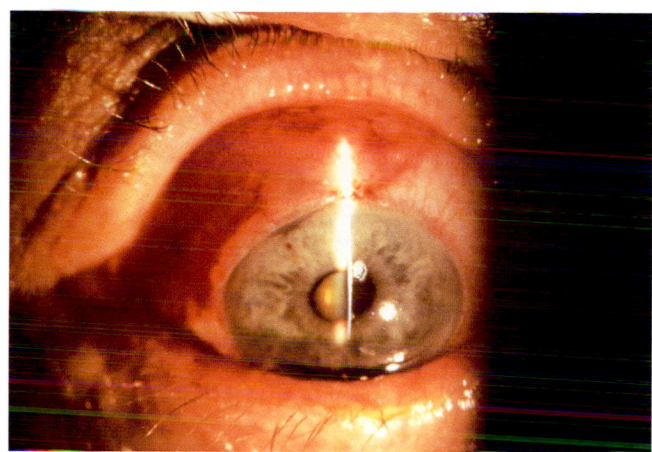

Plate 49 (Fig. 23–7). Fornix-based trabeculectomy in the early postoperative period. Subconjunctival hemorrhages are common.

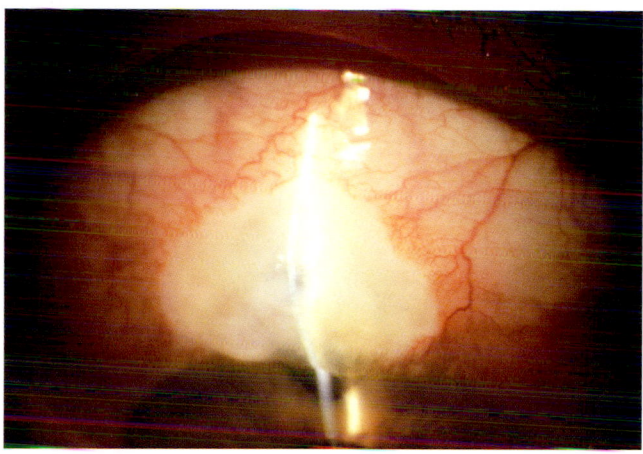

Plate 52 (Fig. 23–10). Thin, moderately elevated macrocystic bleb with surrounding conjunctival injection.

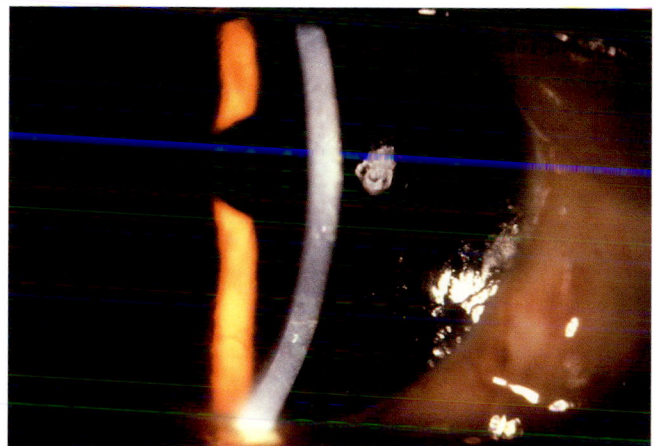

Plate 50 (Fig. 23–8). Punctate keratitis associated with postoperative injections of 5-fluorouracil.

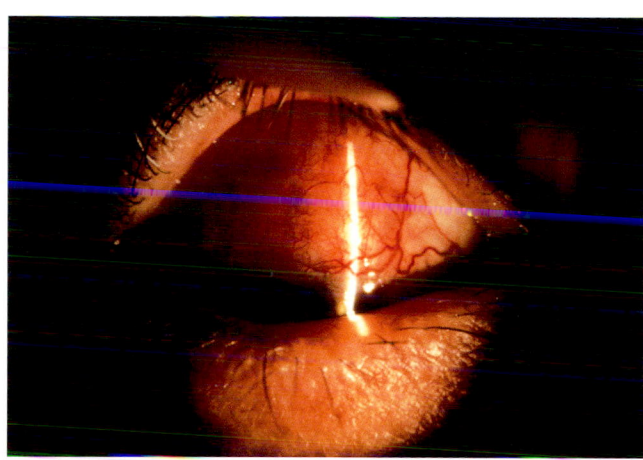

Plate 53 (Fig. 23–11). High, thick focal bleb with telangiectatic vessels. This filter is failing.

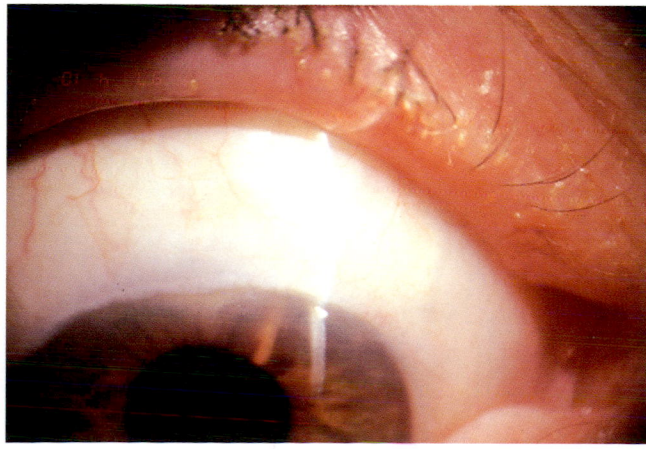

Plate 51 (Fig. 23–9). Diffuse, succulent, low-lying bleb with minimal vascularity and absence of conjunctival injection.

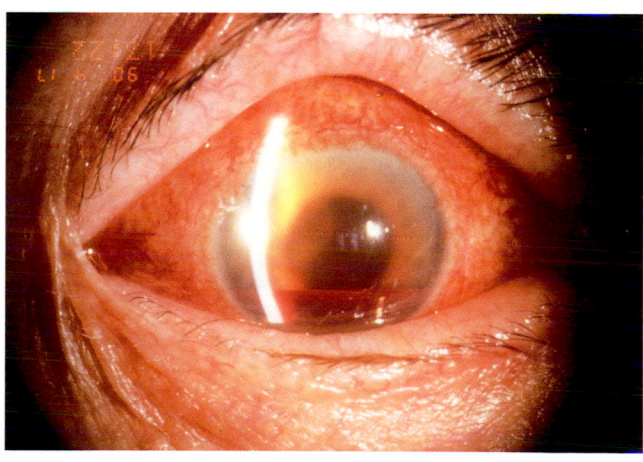

Plate 54 (Fig. 23–12). Hyphema following trabeculectomy.

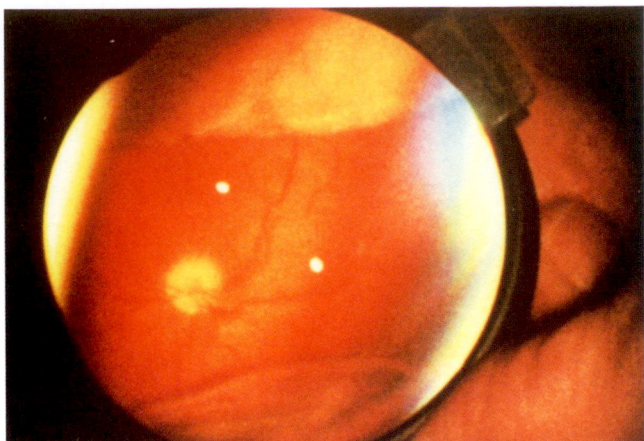

Plate 55 (Fig. 23–13). Choroidal detachment.

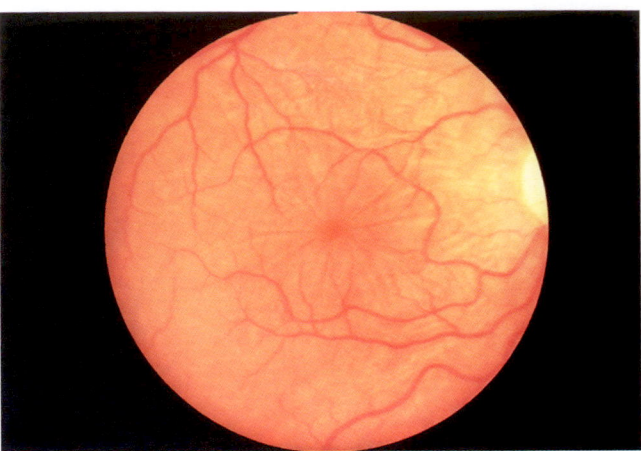

Plate 57 (Fig. 23–16). Hypotony maculopathy in a young, myopic male with pigmentary dispersion glaucoma.

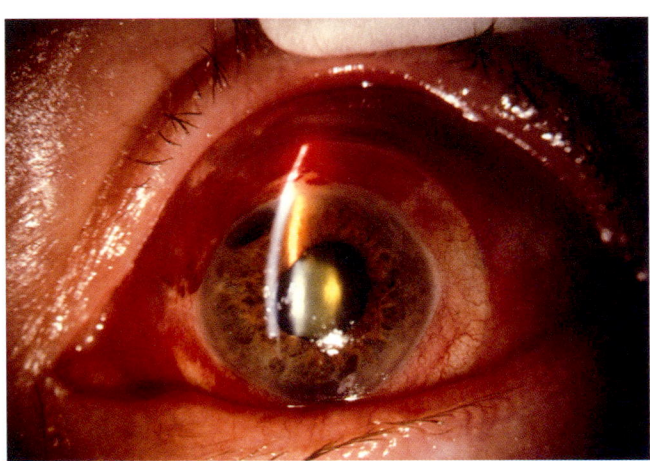

Plate 58 (Fig. 23–17). Bandage soft contact lens inserted to manage hypotony secondary to overfiltration.

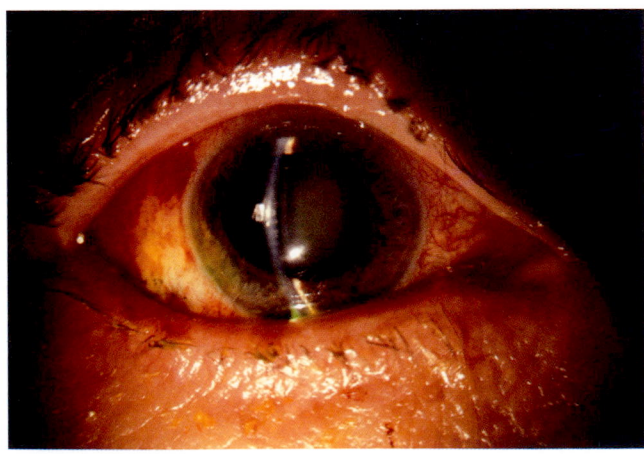

Plate 56 (Fig. 23–15). Shallow anterior chamber following filtering surgery, with peripheral iris-corneal touch.

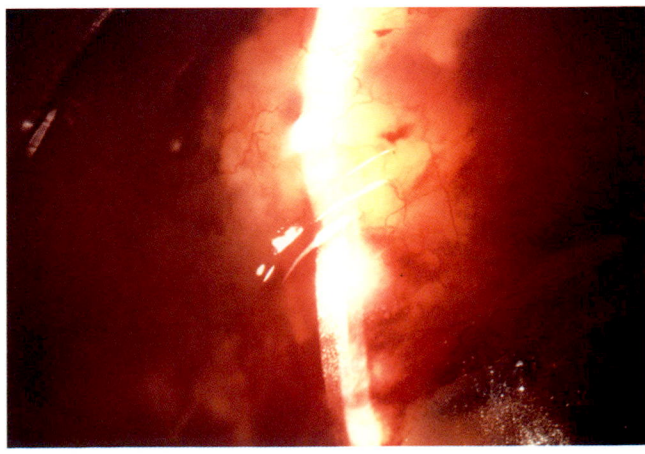

Plate 59 (Fig. 23–18). Edge of bandage soft contact lens demonstrating moderate compression of the bleb.

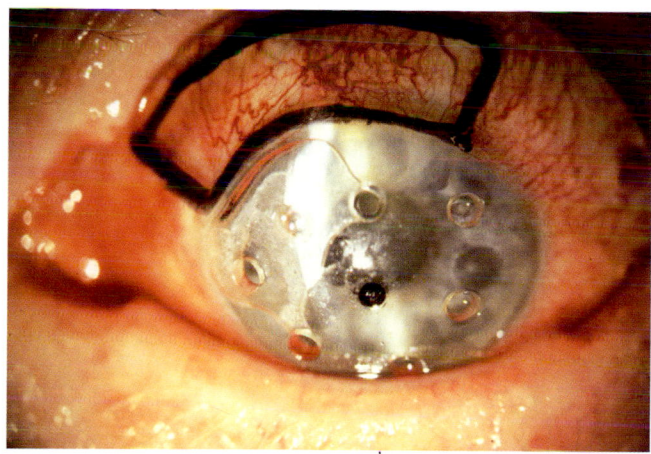

Plate 60 (Fig. 23–19). Simmons shell with tamponade portion centered over filtration site.

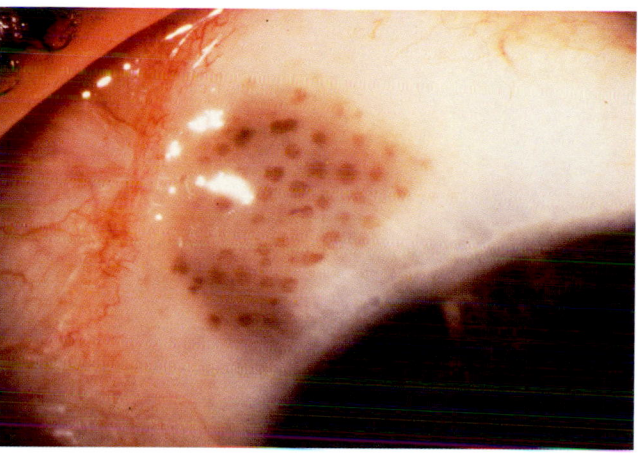

Plate 63 (Fig. 23–22). Nd:YAG laser revision of overfiltering bleb. (Courtesy of Mary Lynch, M.D.)

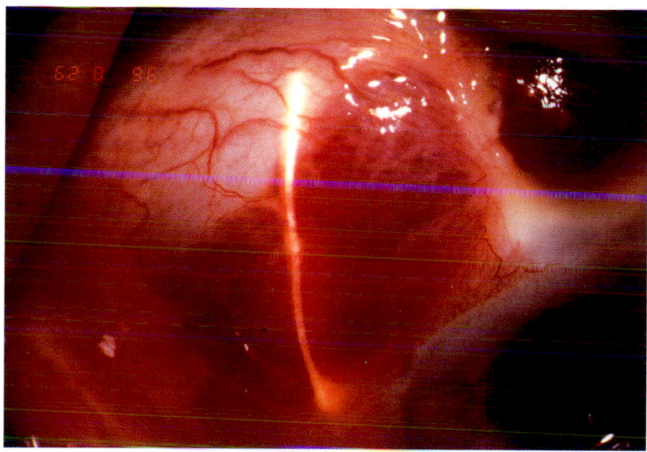

Plate 61 (Fig. 23–20). Subconjunctival hemorrhage following autologous blood injection.

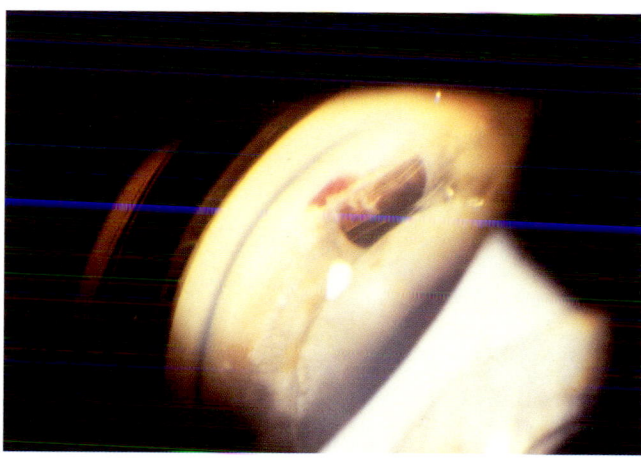

Plate 64 (Fig. 23–23). Clot adjacent to internal osteum following trabeculectomy for glaucoma associated with an anterior chamber intraocular lens.

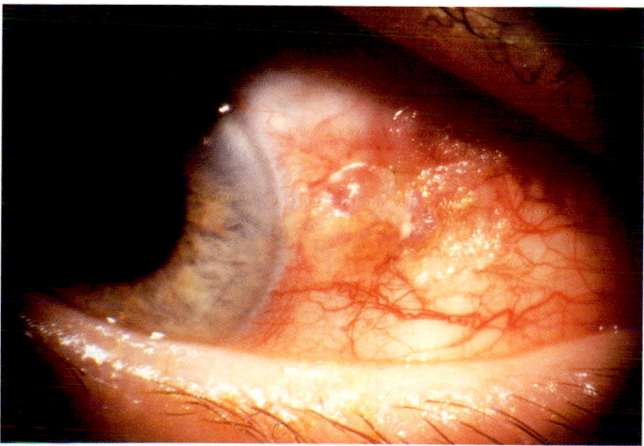

Plate 62 (Fig. 23–21). Cyanoacrylate repair of late wound leak.

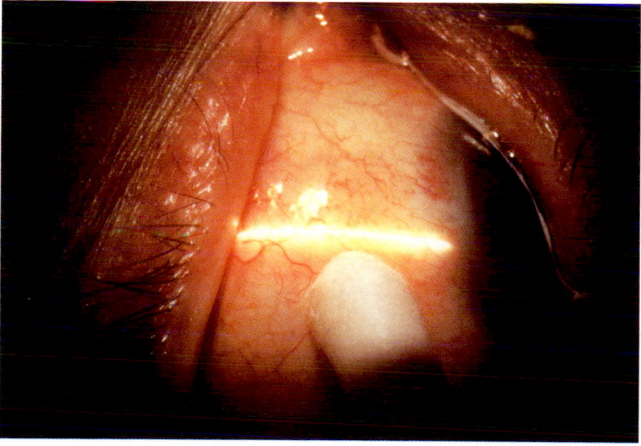

Plate 65 (Fig. 23–24). Use of cotton swab adjacent to the scleral flap to perform focal compression—i.e., the Traverso maneuver.

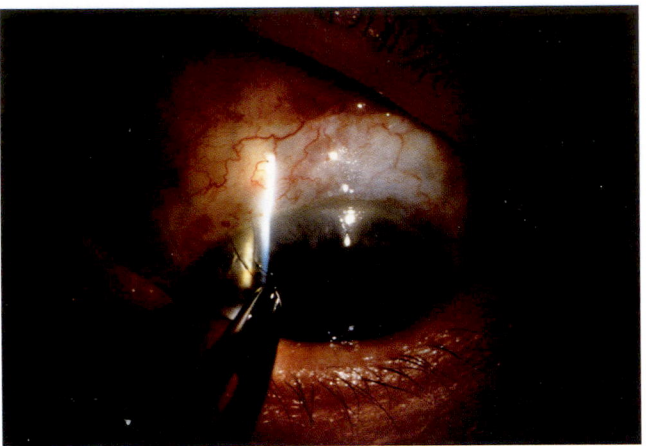

Plate 66 (Fig. 23–25). Removal of tight scleral flap suture in the postoperative period.

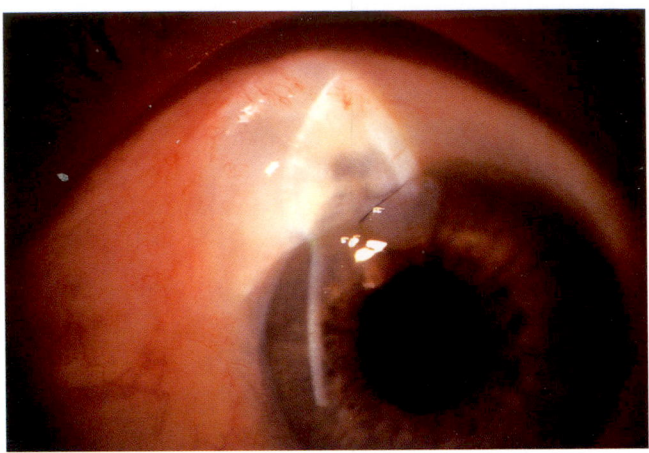

Plate 69 (Fig. 23–28). Suture bleb revision for symptomatic bleb with corneal extension.

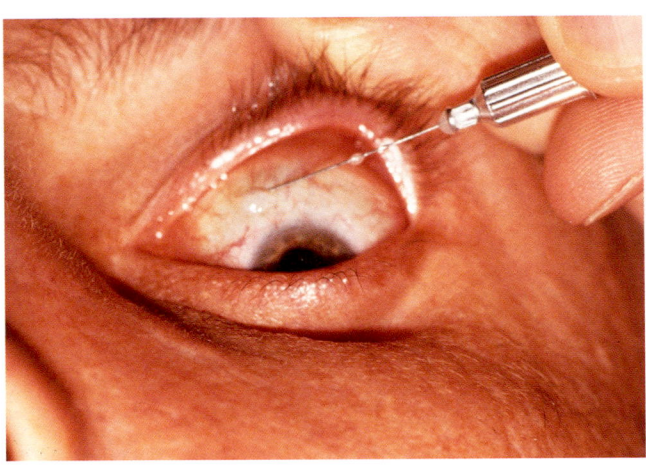

Plate 67 (Fig. 23–26). Adjunctive postoperative 5-fluorouracil injection.

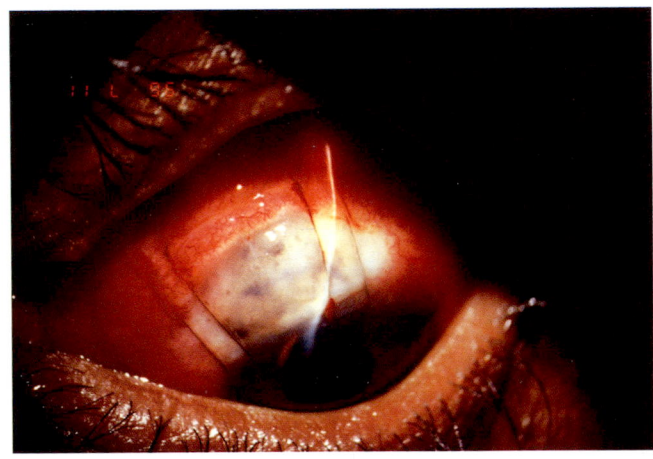

Plate 70 (Fig. 23–29). Compression suture used in hypotony secondary to overfiltration. This technique can be used in bleb dysesthesias.

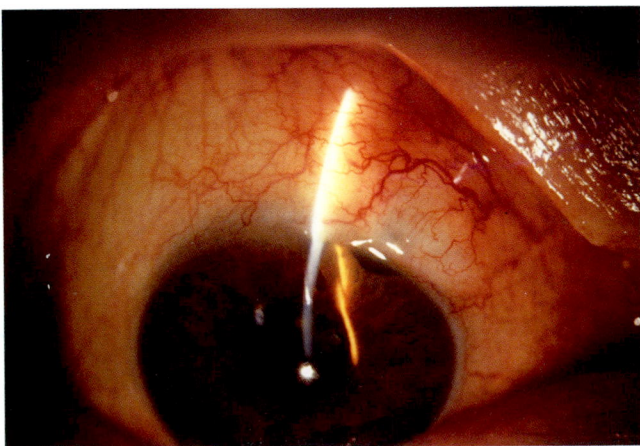

Plate 68 (Fig. 23–27). Tenon cyst formation accompanied by high bleb, vascularization of the bleb, and conjunctival telangiectasia.

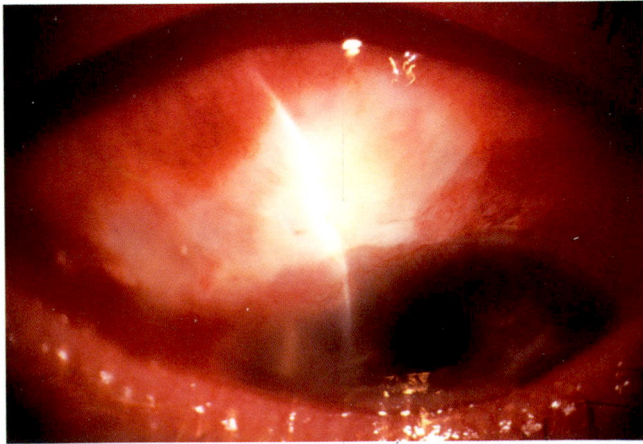

Plate 71 (Fig. 23–30). Blebitis in a thin, pale, avascular bleb. A wound leak was present. Infiltrates were limited to the bleb substance.

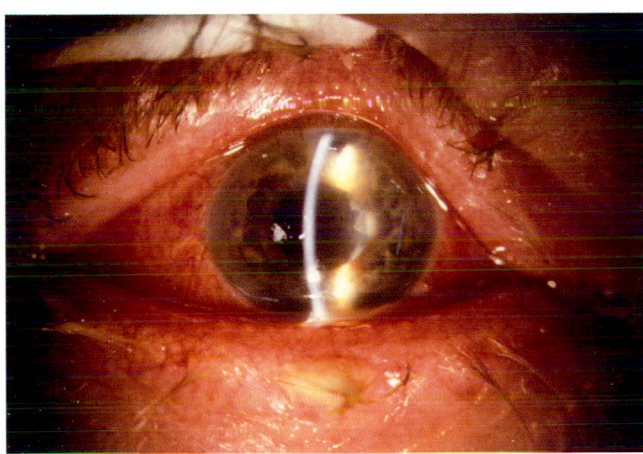

Plate 72 (Fig. 23−31). Bleb-related endophthalmitis associated with severe anterior chamber inflammation. Prognosis for visual recovery is generally poor.

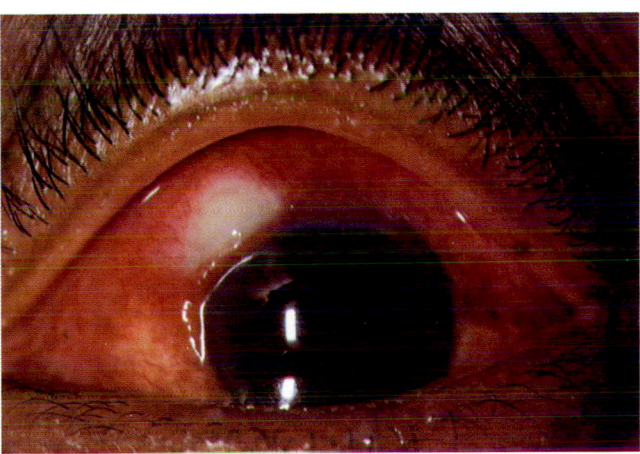

Plate 75 (Fig. 24−3). An infected bleb associated with endophthalmitis. This complication is associated with thin-walled blebs that occur as a result of the use of antifibrotic agents. The eye is hyperemic; the bleb is filled with pus and appears white.

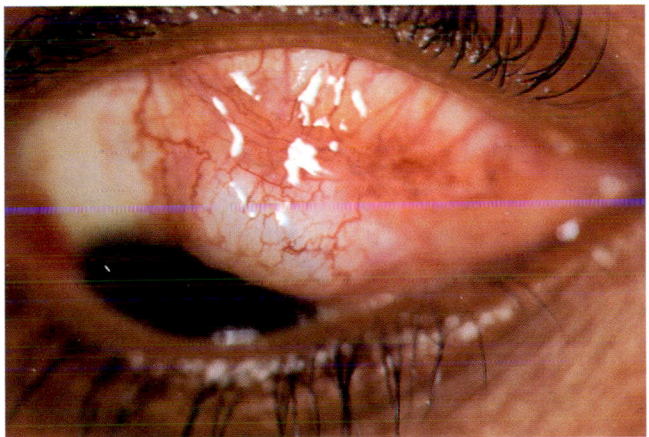

Plate 73 (Fig. 24−1). An example of failure of standard filtering surgery. The bleb is tense, opaque, encapsulated, elevated, and vascularized.

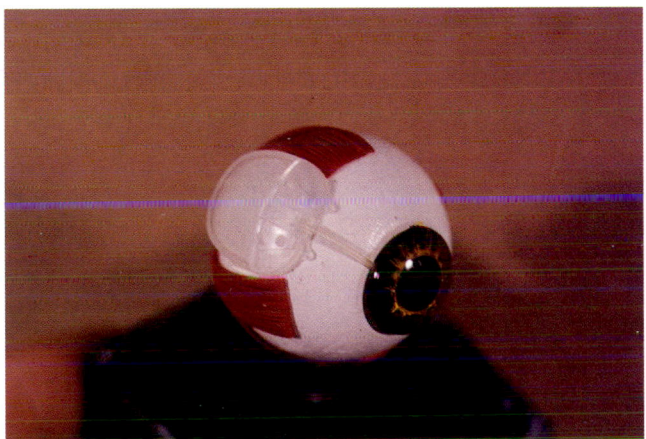

Plate 76 (Fig. 24−5). Photograph of an aqueous tube-shunt device placed on a model eye showing the positioning of the filtration plate relative to the extraocular muscles.

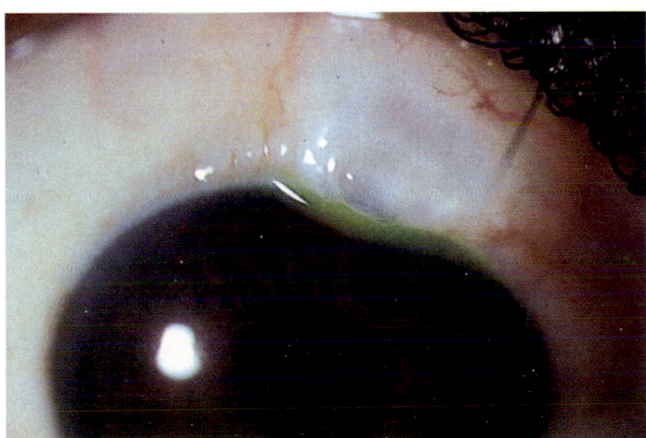

Plate 74 (Fig. 24−2). An example of successful filtration surgery done with mitomycin C. The filtering bleb has thin walls; it is avascular and translucent, with microcysts at the outer edge.

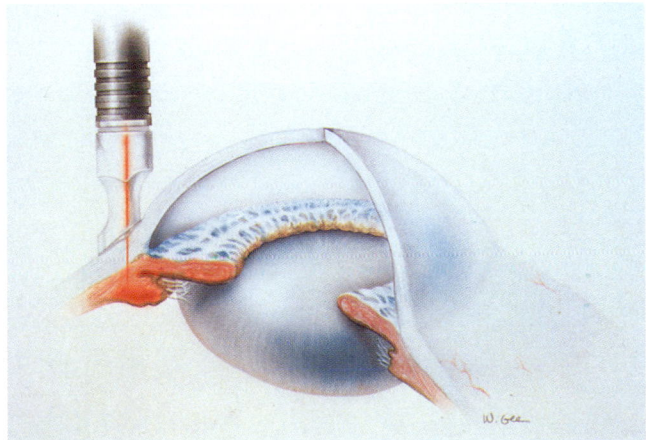

Plate 77 (Fig. 24−7). Drawing of a contact type of transscleral laser cyclophotocoagulation. Laser energy is delivered by the handpiece through the sclera to the ciliary epithelium. (Reproduced, with permission, from IRIDEX Corporation, Mountain View, California).

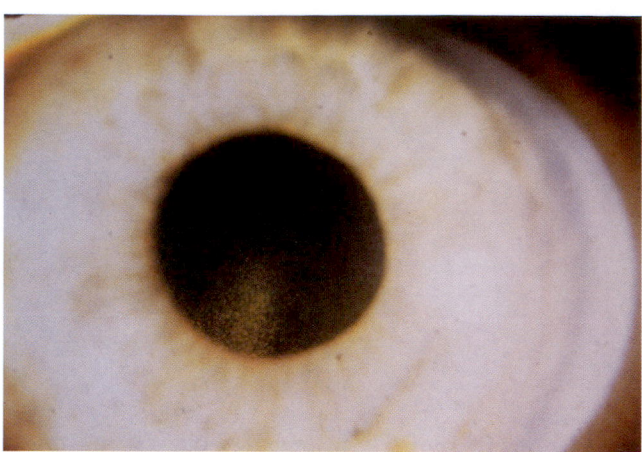

Plate 78 (Fig. 26–1). Krukenberg spindle.

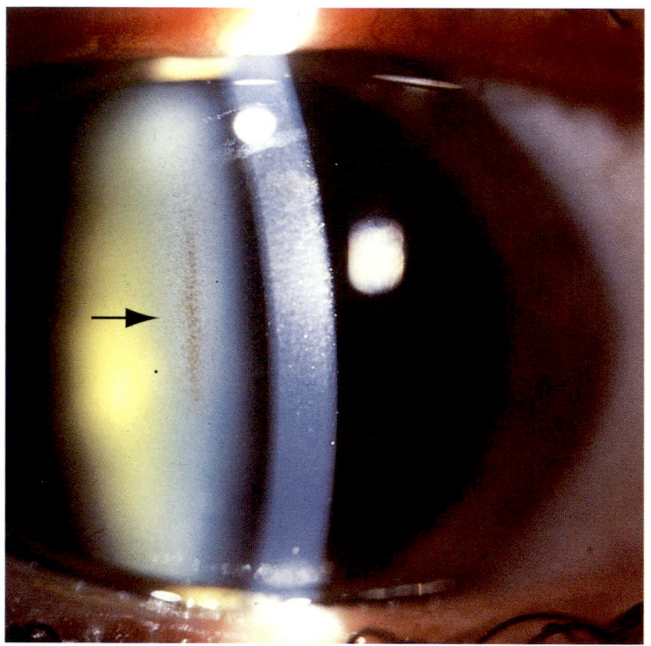

Plate 79 (Fig. 26–2). Typical pattern of fine pigment deposition on the corneal endothelial surface *(arrow)* (Krukenberg spindle) associated with pigment dispersion syndrome. Note the vertical orientation.

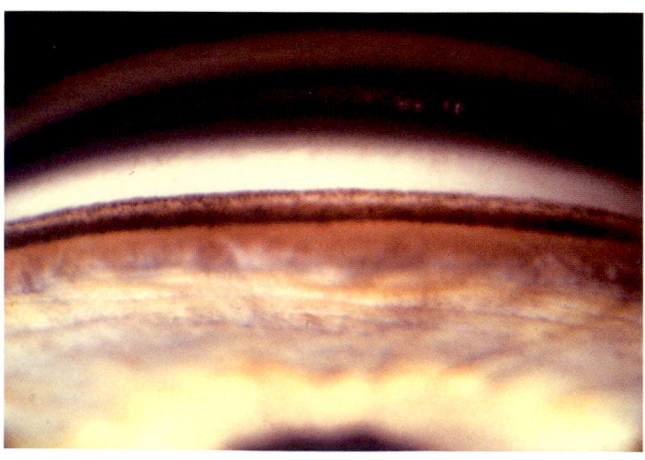

Plate 80 (Fig. 26–3). Dense, homogeneous trabecular meshwork pigmentation in pigmentary glaucoma.

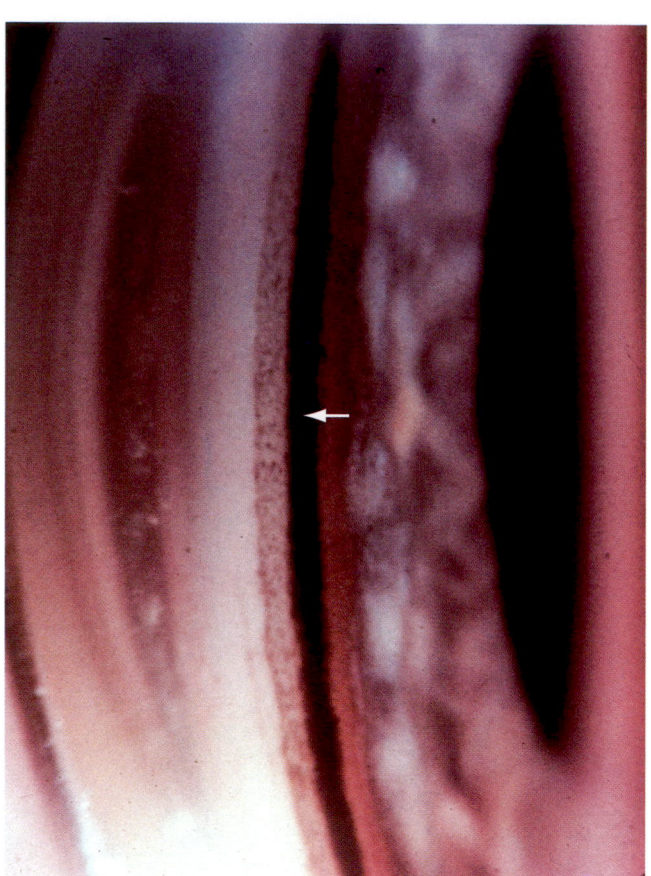

Plate 81 (Fig. 26–4). Dense trabecular meshwork pigmentation noted in an individual with pigmentary glaucoma.

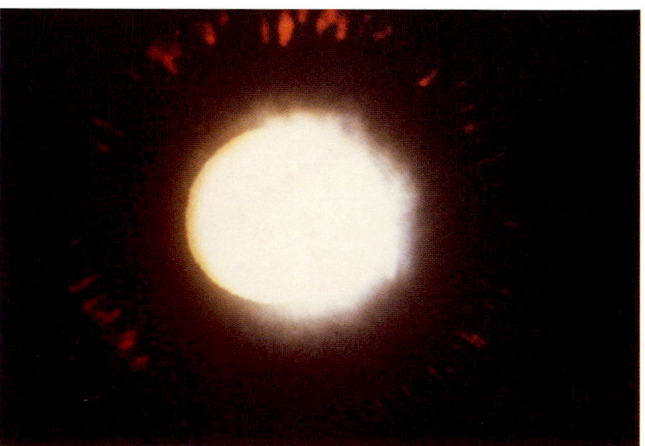

Plate 82 (Fig. 26–6). The transillumination defects found in PDS are located in the midperipheral iris and result from mechanical contact between the iris pigment epithelium and packets of anterior zonular bundles.

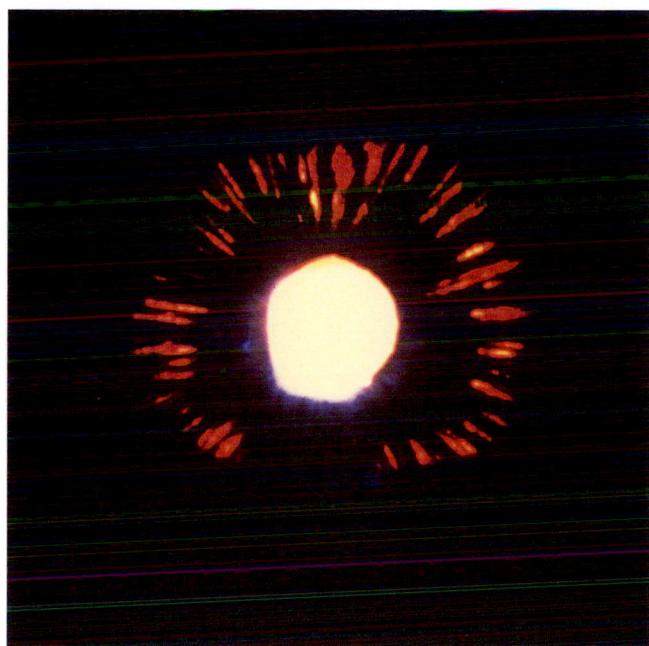

Plate 83 (Fig. 26–7). Iris transillumination defects, associated with pigment dispersion syndrome, occur in the midperiphery and are circumferential in appearance.

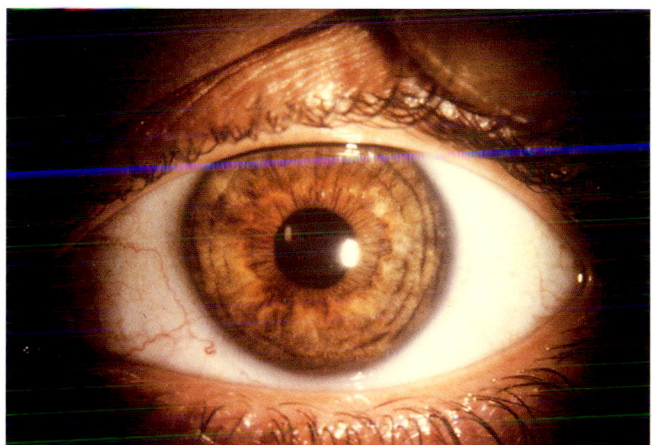

Plate 84 (Fig. 26–9). In cases with more pronounced pigment liberation, pigment granules may accumulate in iris furrows, where they are visible as concentric rings.

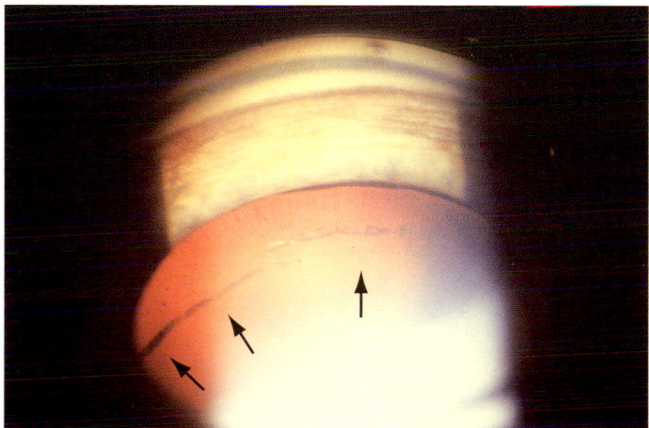

Plate 85 (Fig. 26–10). Pigment on the posterior lens capsule (arrows).

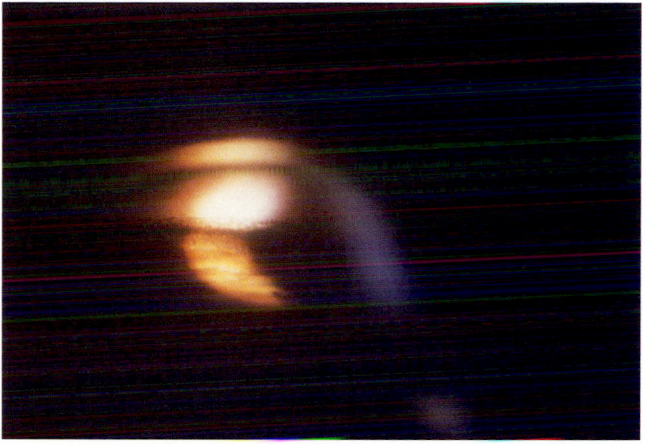

C

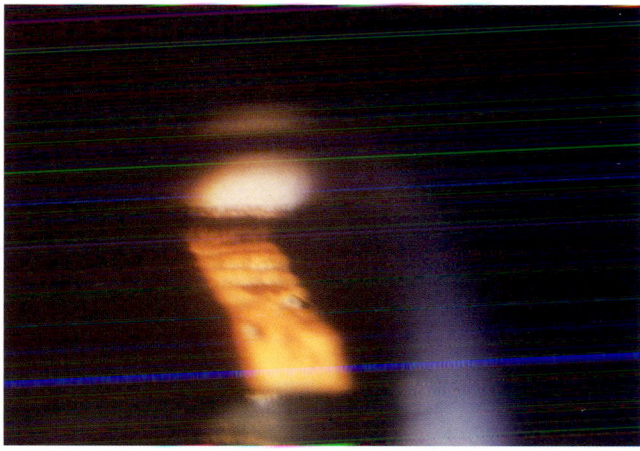

D

Plate 86 (Fig. 26–15) *C*. Prior to laser iridectomy, gonioscopy demonstrates a concave iris configuration. *D*. Following laser iridectomy, the iris assumes a flat configuration.

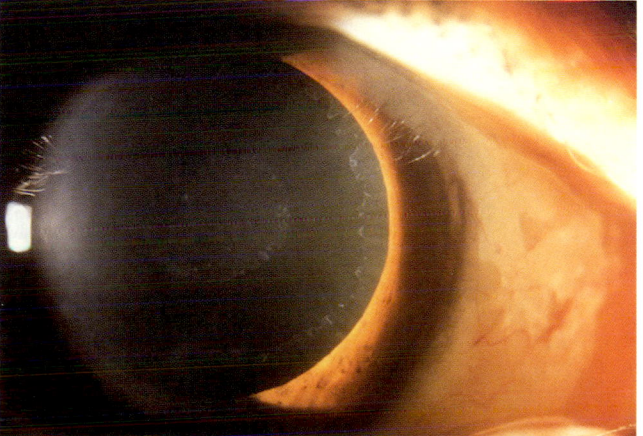

Plate 87 (Fig. 27–1). The classic appearance of the lens in an eye with exfoliation syndrome. The central gray zone, intermediate clear zone, and peripheral granular zone are visible.

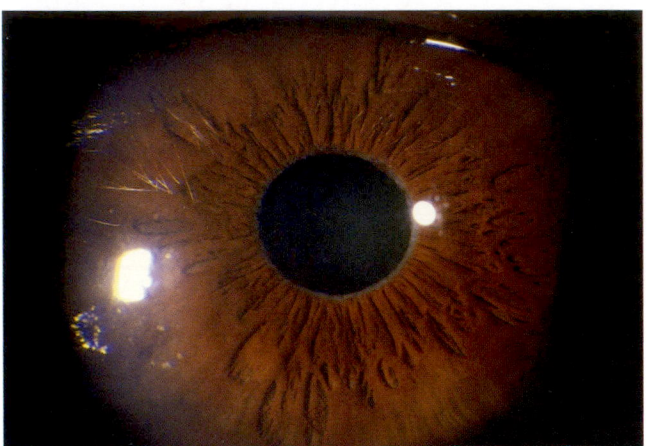

Plate 88 (Fig. 27–2). Exfoliation material on the pupillary border. Note the absent pupillary ruff.

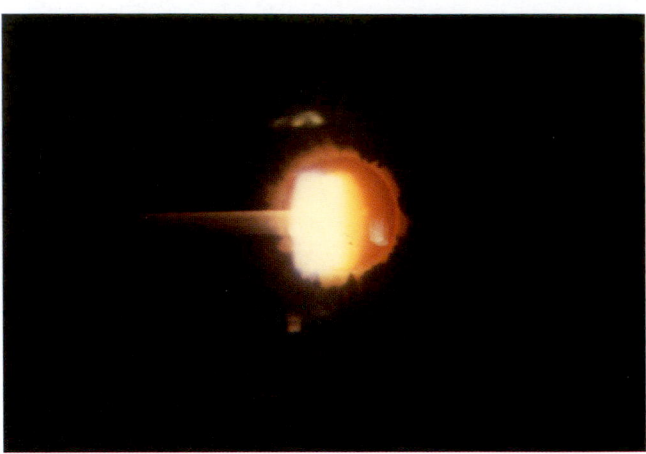

Plate 91 (Fig. 27–6). Typical diffuse iris sphincter region transillumination in an eye with exfoliation syndrome.

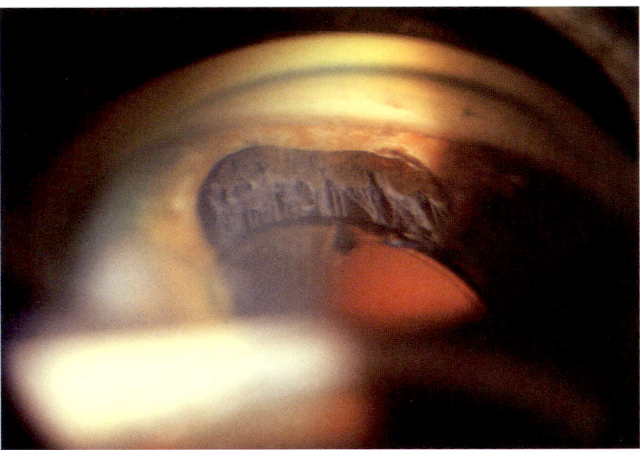

Plate 89 (Fig. 27–3). Dense accumulations of exfoliation material on the zonules and ciliary body. The zonules are distorted, fragmented, and absent in areas. Complications at the time of cataract extraction are significantly greater than in normal eyes.

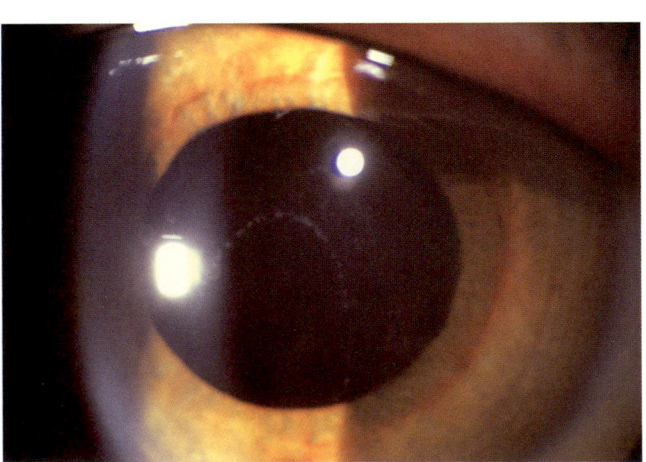

Plate 90 (Fig. 27–5). Particles of exfoliation material on the anterior hyaloid face in an aphakic eye.

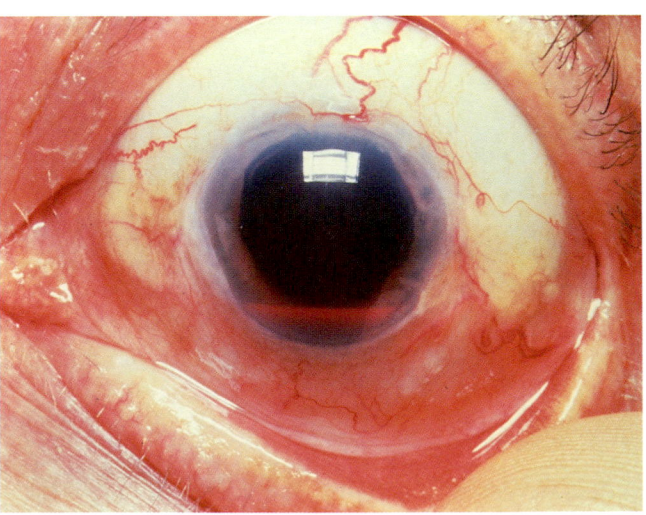

Plate 92 (Fig. 28–2). Hyphema following blunt trauma to the globe. (*Courtesy of Rodney Gutner, OD.*)

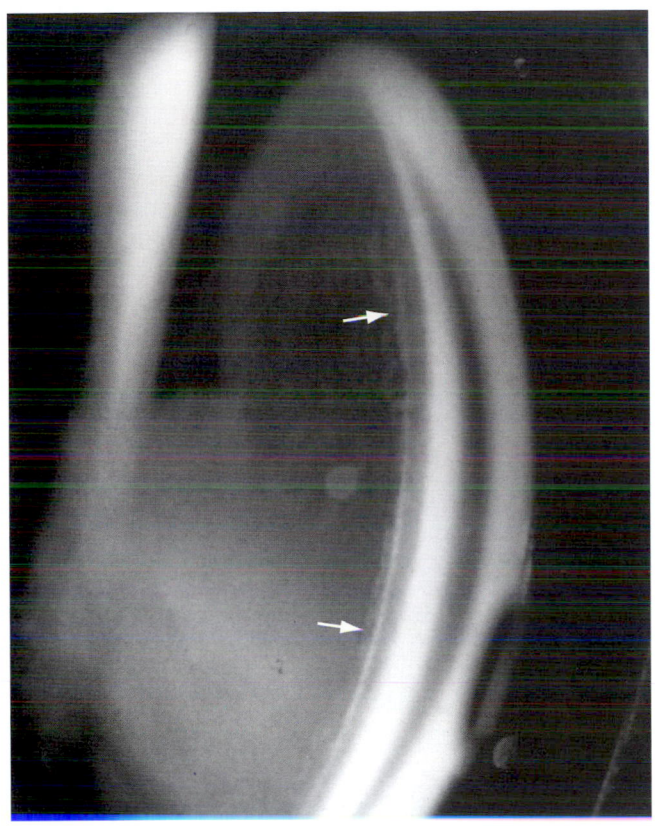

Plate 93 (Fig. 28–3). Moderate angle recession *(arrows)* following blunt trauma. Note the variation in color and depth of the angle at the ciliary recess. The arrows point to the edge of the iris.

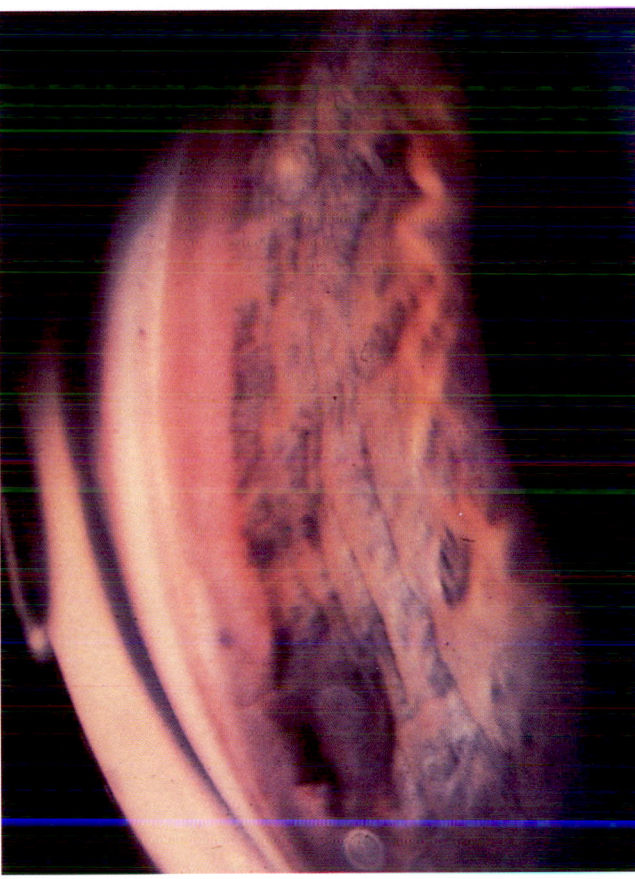

Plate 94 (Fig. 28–4). Severe angle recession. Note how wide open the angle appears.

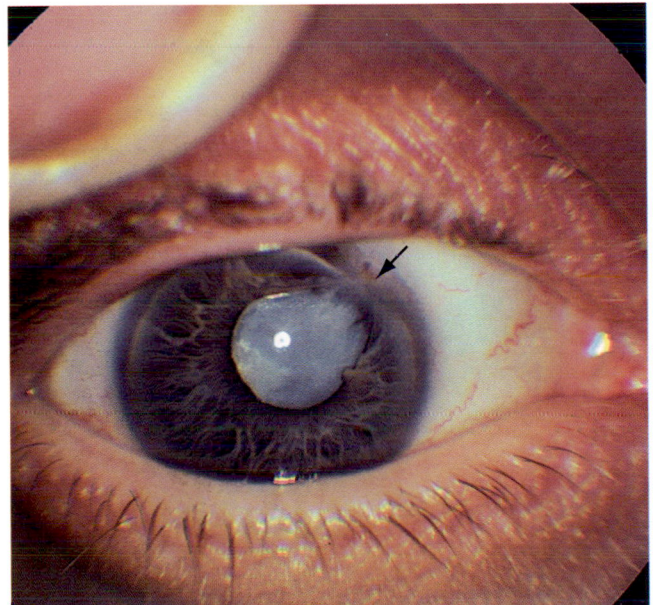

Plate 95 (Fig. 28–5). Formation of peripheral anterior synechiae *(arrow)* following trauma to the anterior segment.

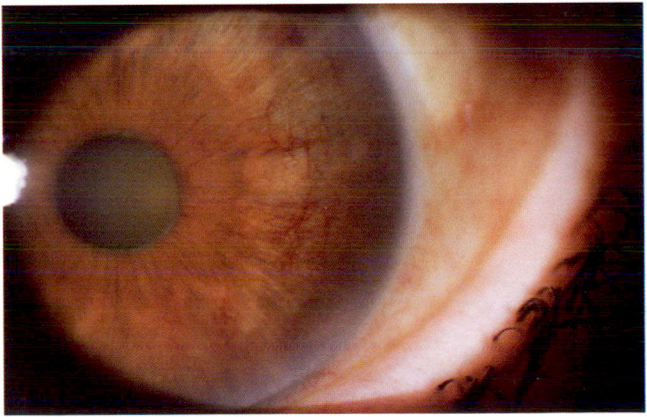

Plate 96 (Fig. 28–7). Early neovascular changes seen at the pupillary zone and midperiphery of the iris.

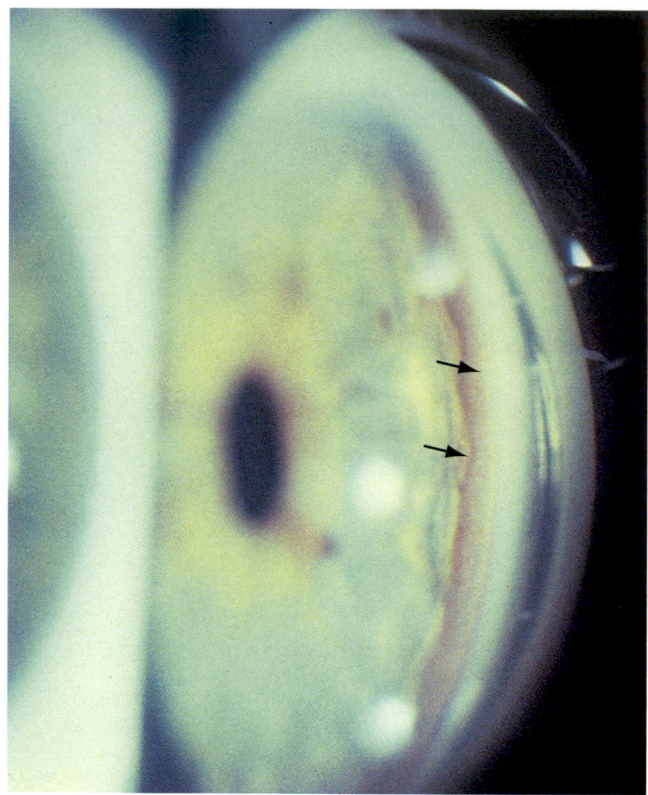

Plate 97 (Fig. 28–8). Moderate neovascular glaucoma. New blood vessels are seen in the angle *(arrows)*. *(Courtesy of Rodney Gutner, OD.)*

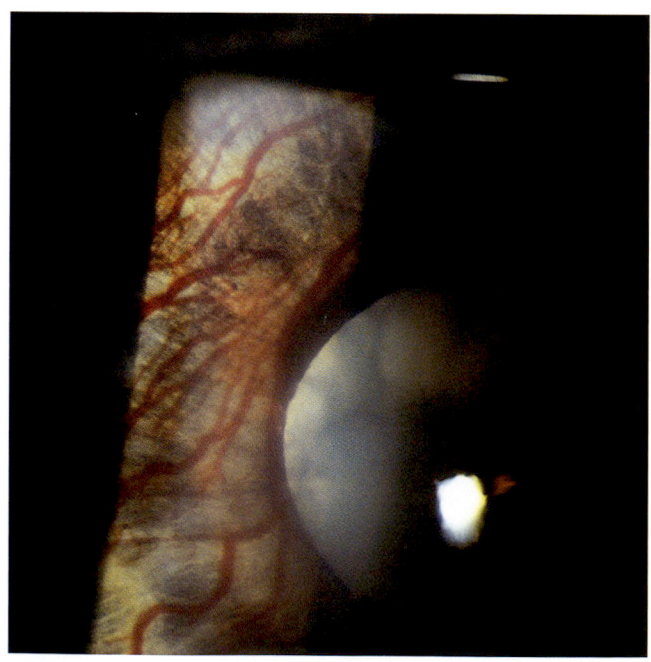

Plate 98 (Fig. 28–9). End-stage neovascular glaucoma with significant vessel development on the iris surface.

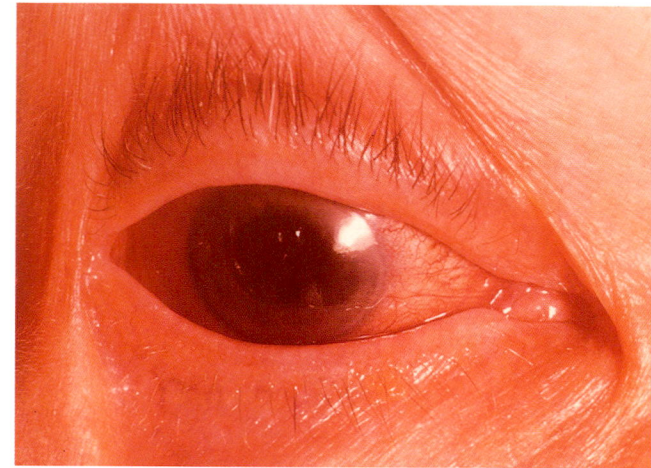

Plate 99 (Fig. 29–9). An angle-closure attack typically presents with a red eye, cloudy cornea, and a middilated pupil.

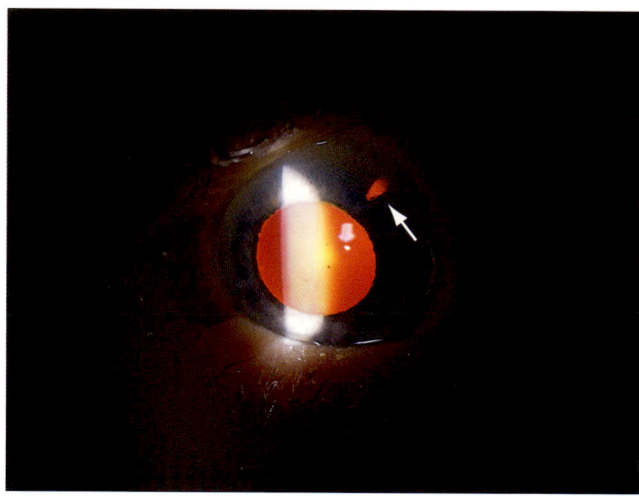

Plate 100 (Fig. 29–10). A laser peripheral iridotomy *(arrow)*. (Courtesy of Mitchell Dul, O.D.)

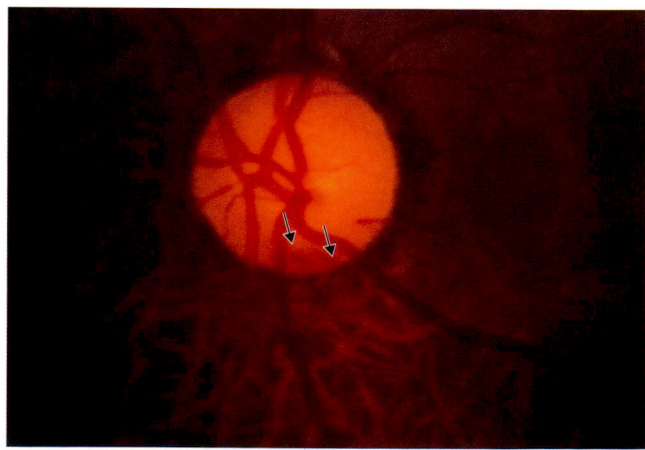

Plate 101 (Fig. 30–2). Optic disc of a patient with NTG illustrates two splinter disc hemorrhages *(arrows)* along the inferior neural rim.

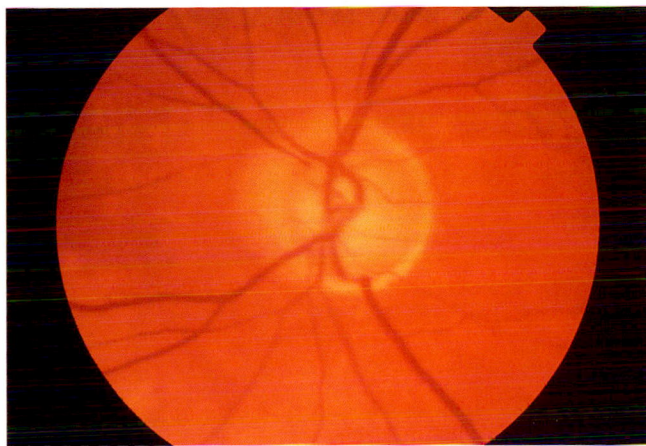

Plate 102 (Fig. 30–3). An inferiorly located acquired pit of the optic nerve head gives a moth-eaten appearance to the optic nerve head.

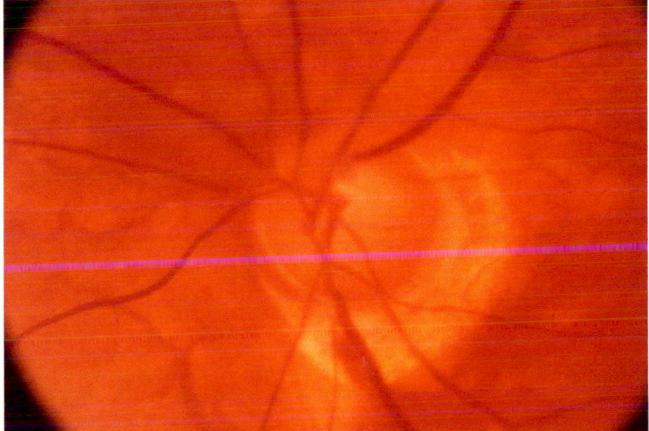

Plate 103 (Fig. 30–5). Appearance of the optic nerve in an eye with senile sclerotic NTG; there is a pale, moth-eaten disc with surrounding areas of peripapillary atrophy and choroidal sclerosis.

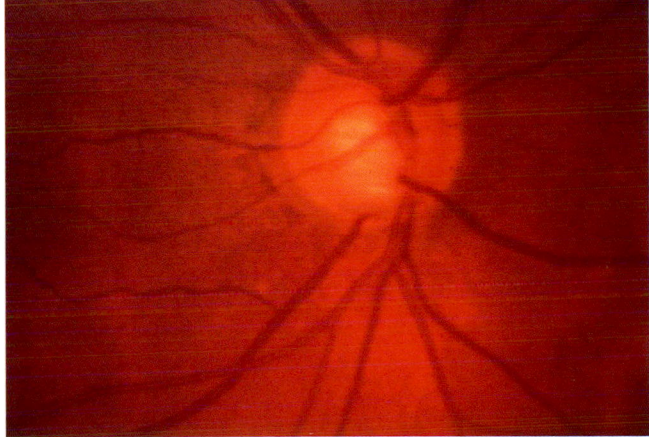

Plate 104 (Fig. 30–6). Photograph of the optic nerve in an eye with focal ischemic NTG characterized by discrete areas of neural rim loss.

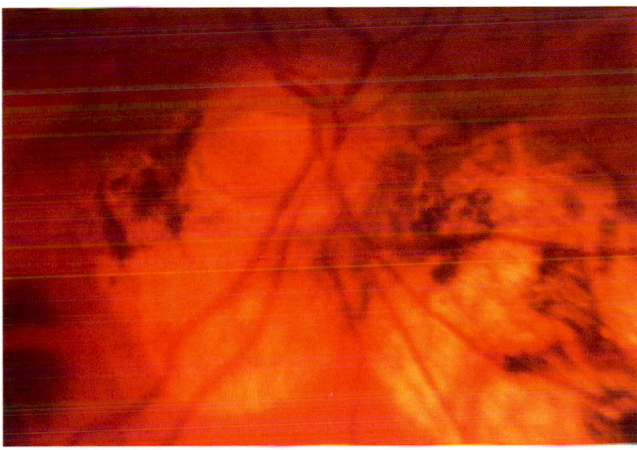

Plate 105 (Fig. 30–7). Photograph of the optic nerve in an eye with myopic NTG characterized by high axial myopia. The optic nerve is tilted and has an oblique insertion.

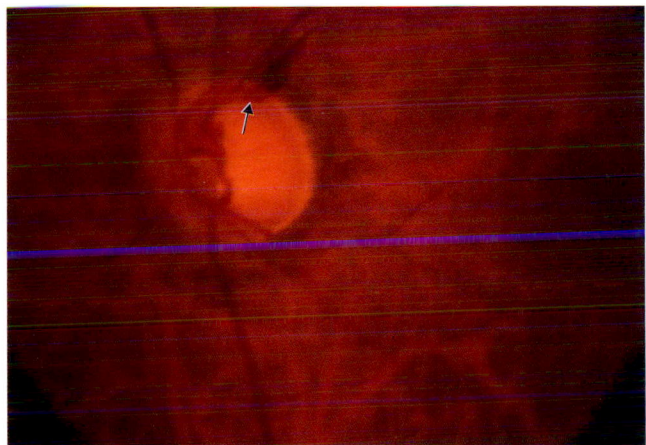

Plate 106 (Fig. 30–8). Miscellaneous NTG represents those eyes that do not satisfy criteria for inclusion in other subgroups. Note the fresh splinter hemorrhage along the superotemporal aspect of the optic disc.

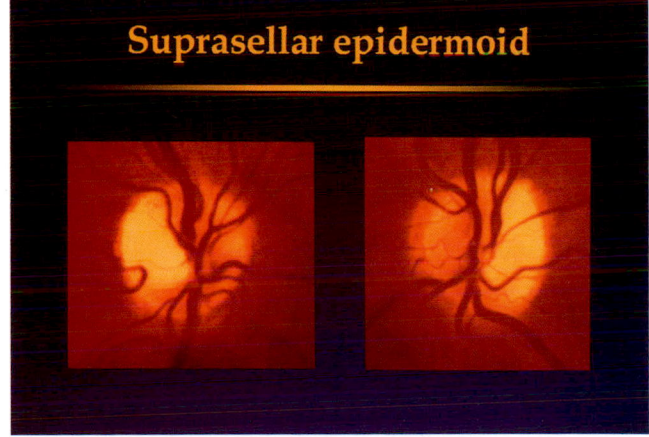

Plate 107 (Fig. 30–9). *A.* Optic nerve photographs of a patient with a suprasellar epidermoid tumor show an absence of focal defects in the neuroretinal rim and moderate temporal pallor.

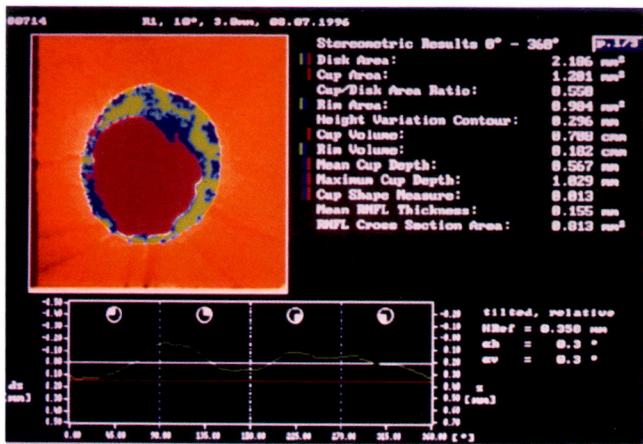

Plate 108 (Fig. 30–11). Confocal scanning laser ophthalmoscopy (CSLO) image of a patient with NTG shows loss of the inferior neuroretinal rim (green) and associated stereometric parameters. There is a focal depression in the double-hump pattern of the height-variation diagram corresponding to the decreased height of the inferotemporal quadrant (*below*).

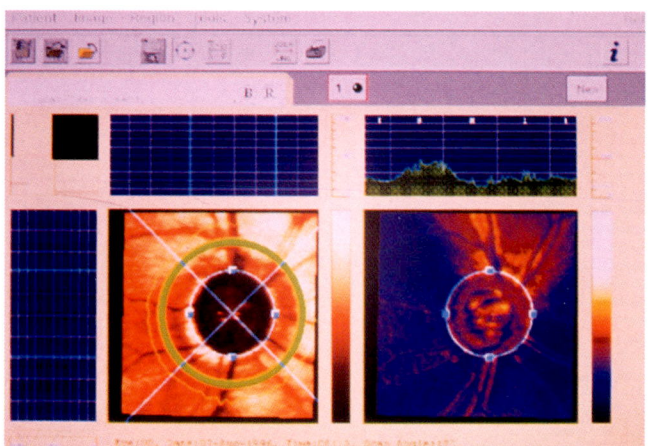

Plate 109 (Fig. 30–12). Scanning laser polarimetry (SLP) image (NFA II) of the patient illustrated in Fig. 30-11 demonstrates advanced loss of the inferior retinal nerve fiber layer. Retardation in the inferior region of the linear polar cross-section diagram is reduced compared with the superior region, indicating thinning of this area.

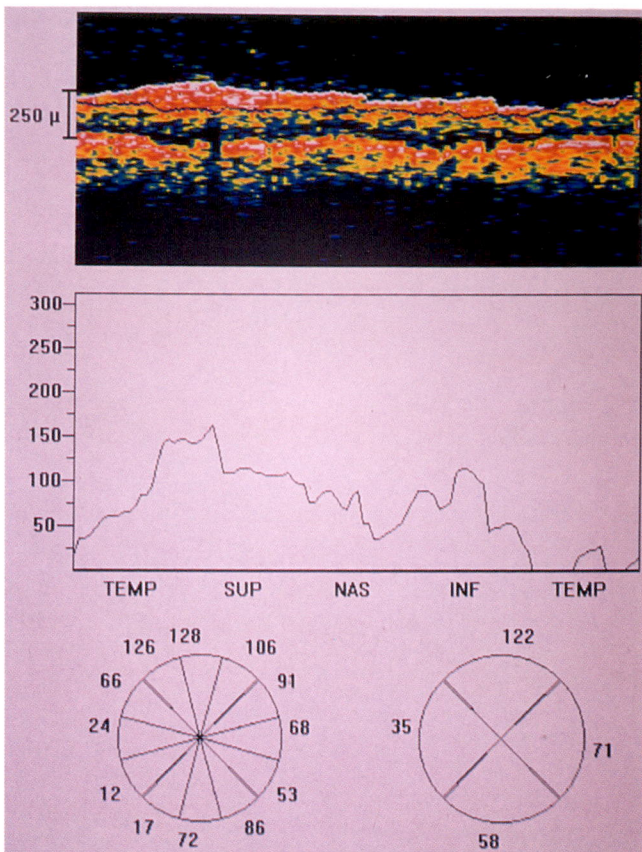

Plate 110 (Fig. 30–13). Circular optical coherence tomography (OCT) scan of the patient illustrated in Fig. 30-11 demonstrates the inferior defect in the retinal nerve fiber layer (RNFL) in cross-section as a region of localized thinning. The mean height of the inferior RNFL quadrant is reduced (58 μm), compared with the mean height of the superior quadrant (122 μm).

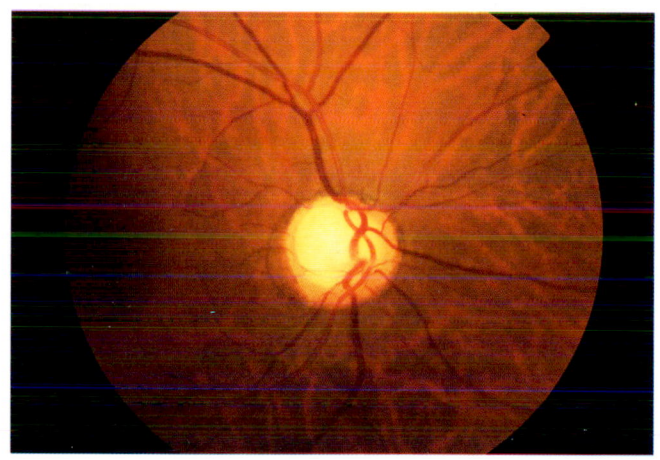

A

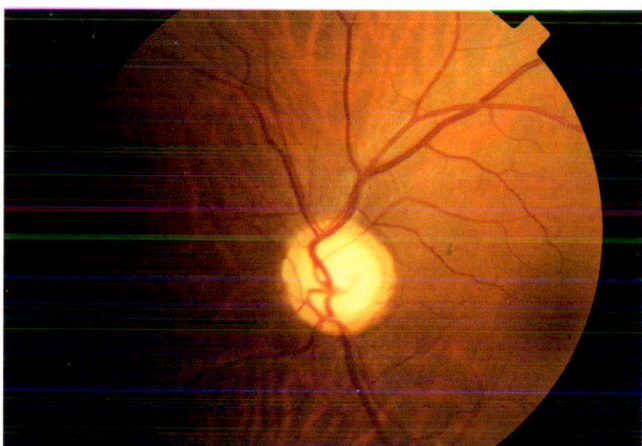

B

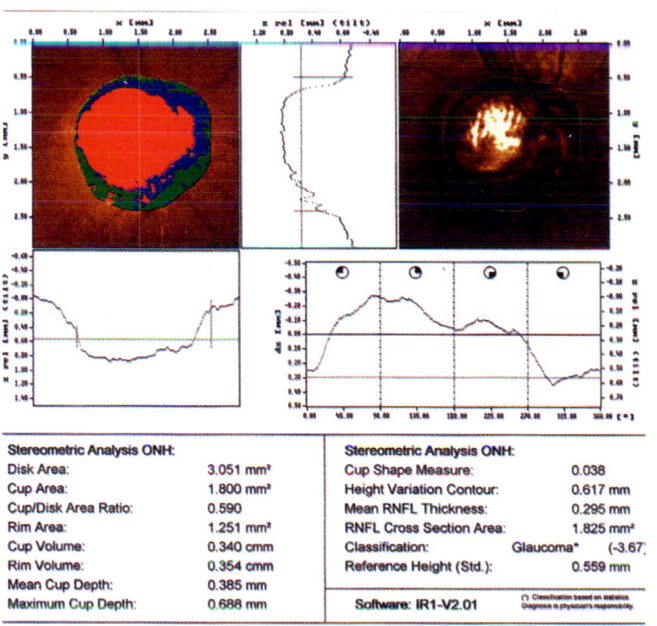

Stereometric Analysis ONH:		Stereometric Analysis ONH:	
Disk Area:	3.051 mm²	Cup Shape Measure:	0.038
Cup Area:	1.800 mm²	Height Variation Contour:	0.617 mm
Cup/Disk Area Ratio:	0.590	Mean RNFL Thickness:	0.295 mm
Rim Area:	1.251 mm²	RNFL Cross Section Area:	1.825 mm²
Cup Volume:	0.340 cmm	Classification:	Glaucoma* (-3.67)
Rim Volume:	0.354 cmm	Reference Height (Std.):	0.559 mm
Mean Cup Depth:	0.385 mm		
Maximum Cup Depth:	0.688 mm	Software: IR1-V2.01	(*) Classification based on statistics. Diagnosis is physician's responsibility.

OD

C

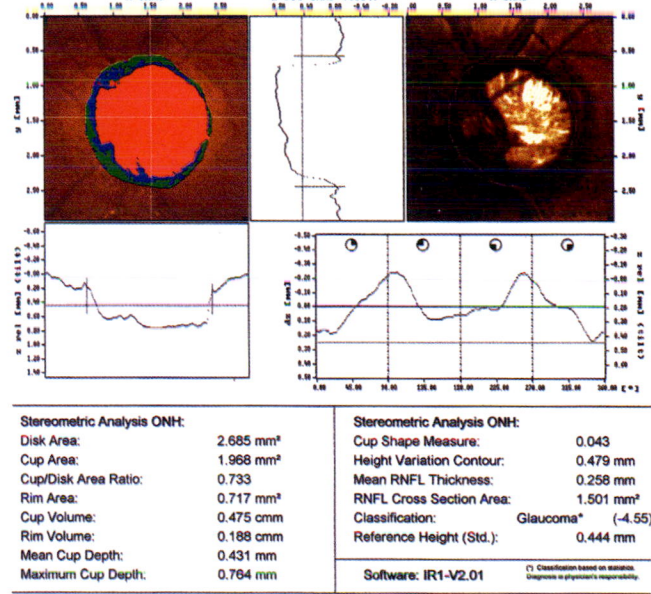

Stereometric Analysis ONH:		Stereometric Analysis ONH:	
Disk Area:	2.685 mm²	Cup Shape Measure:	0.043
Cup Area:	1.968 mm²	Height Variation Contour:	0.479 mm
Cup/Disk Area Ratio:	0.733	Mean RNFL Thickness:	0.258 mm
Rim Area:	0.717 mm²	RNFL Cross Section Area:	1.501 mm²
Cup Volume:	0.475 cmm	Classification:	Glaucoma* (-4.55)
Rim Volume:	0.188 cmm	Reference Height (Std.):	0.444 mm
Mean Cup Depth:	0.431 mm		
Maximum Cup Depth:	0.764 mm	Software: IR1-V2.01	(*) Classification based on statistics. Diagnosis is physician's responsibility.

OS

D

Plate 111 (Case One).

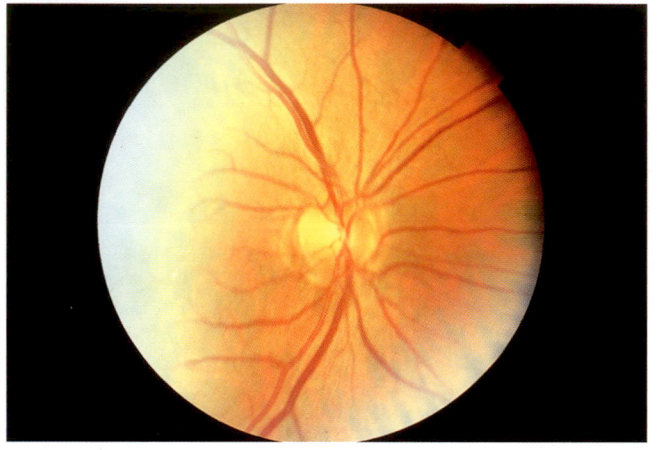

A

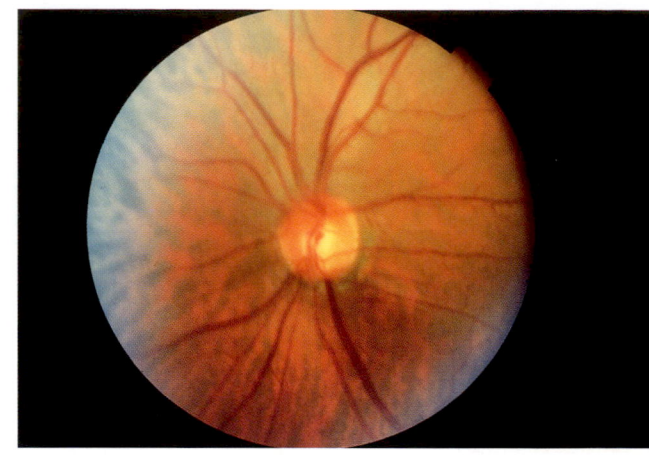

B

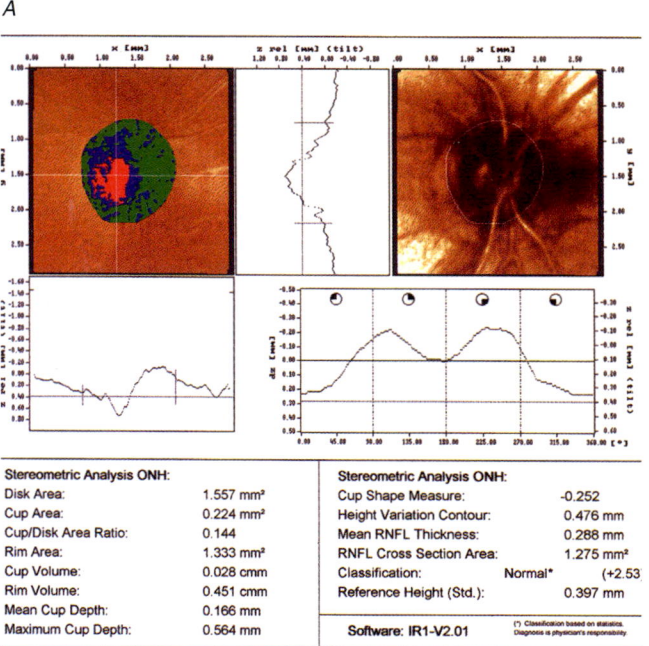

Stereometric Analysis ONH:

Disk Area:	1.557 mm²	Cup Shape Measure:	-0.252
Cup Area:	0.224 mm²	Height Variation Contour:	0.476 mm
Cup/Disk Area Ratio:	0.144	Mean RNFL Thickness:	0.288 mm
Rim Area:	1.333 mm²	RNFL Cross Section Area:	1.275 mm²
Cup Volume:	0.028 cmm	Classification: Normal* (+2.53)	
Rim Volume:	0.451 cmm	Reference Height (Std.):	0.397 mm
Mean Cup Depth:	0.166 mm		
Maximum Cup Depth:	0.564 mm	Software: IR1-V2.01	(*) Classification based on statistics. Diagnosis is physician's responsibility.

OD

C

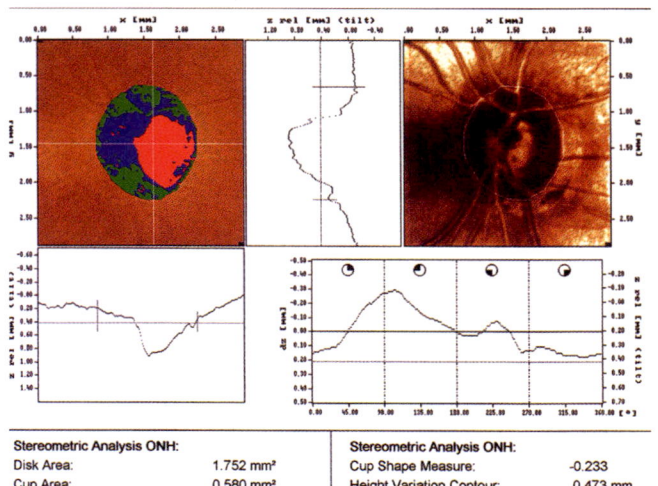

Stereometric Analysis ONH:

Disk Area:	1.752 mm²	Cup Shape Measure:	-0.233
Cup Area:	0.580 mm²	Height Variation Contour:	0.473 mm
Cup/Disk Area Ratio:	0.331	Mean RNFL Thickness:	0.216 mm
Rim Area:	1.173 mm²	RNFL Cross Section Area:	1.017 mm²
Cup Volume:	0.126 cmm	Classification: Normal* (+0.30)	
Rim Volume:	0.269 cmm	Reference Height (Std.):	0.419 mm
Mean Cup Depth:	0.214 mm		
Maximum Cup Depth:	0.695 mm	Software: IR1-V2.01	(*) Classification based on statistics. Diagnosis is physician's responsibility.

OS

D

Plate 112 (Case Two).

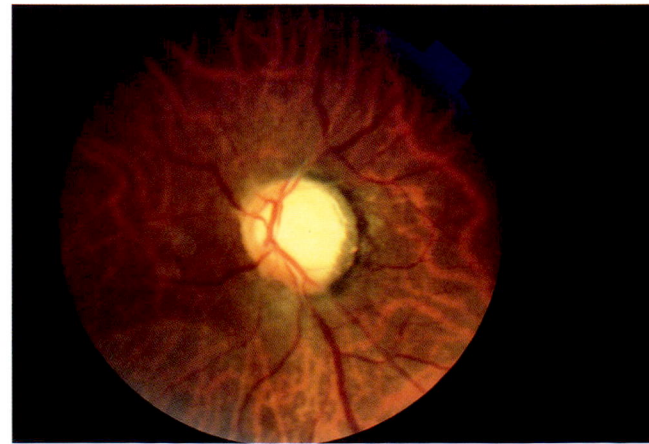

A

B

Plate 113 (Case Three).

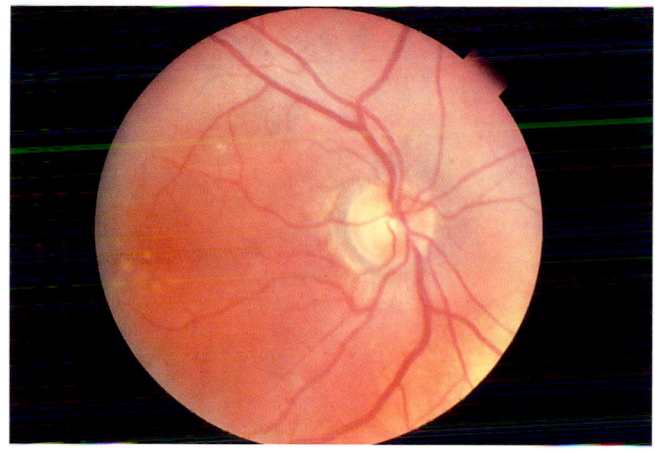

A

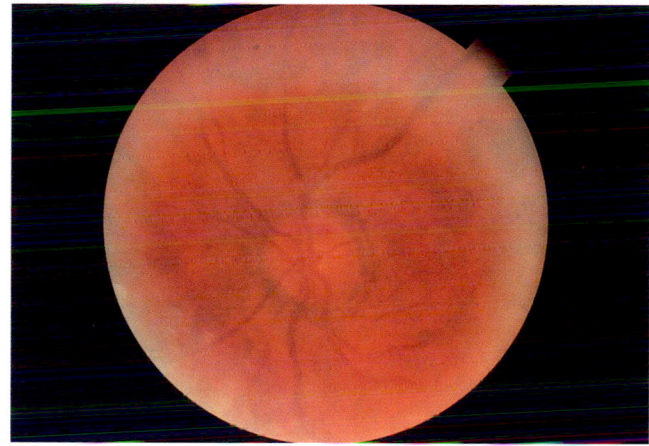

B

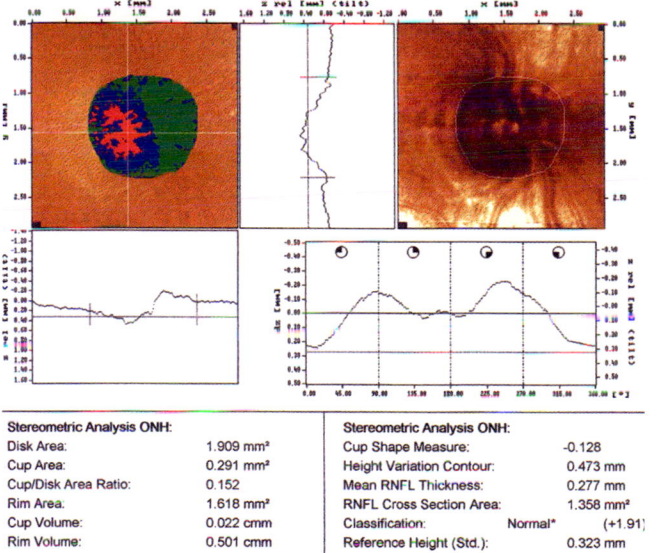

Stereometric Analysis ONH:		Stereometric Analysis ONH:	
Disk Area:	1.909 mm²	Cup Shape Measure:	-0.128
Cup Area:	0.291 mm²	Height Variation Contour:	0.473 mm
Cup/Disk Area Ratio:	0.152	Mean RNFL Thickness:	0.277 mm
Rim Area:	1.618 mm²	RNFL Cross Section Area:	1.358 mm²
Cup Volume:	0.022 cmm	Classification: Normal*	(+1.91)
Rim Volume:	0.501 cmm	Reference Height (Std.):	0.323 mm
Mean Cup Depth:	0.152 mm		
Maximum Cup Depth:	0.406 mm	Software: IR1-V2.01	(*) Classification based on statistics. Diagnosis is physician's responsibility.

OD

C

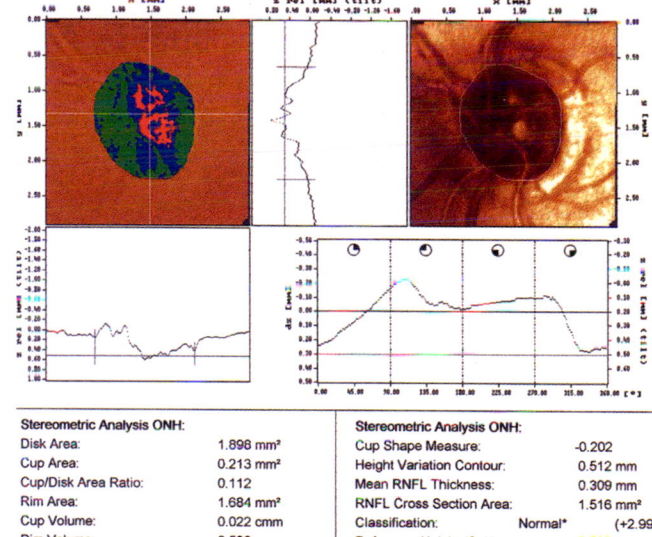

Stereometric Analysis ONH:		Stereometric Analysis ONH:	
Disk Area:	1.898 mm²	Cup Shape Measure:	-0.202
Cup Area:	0.213 mm²	Height Variation Contour:	0.512 mm
Cup/Disk Area Ratio:	0.112	Mean RNFL Thickness:	0.309 mm
Rim Area:	1.684 mm²	RNFL Cross Section Area:	1.516 mm²
Cup Volume:	0.022 cmm	Classification: Normal*	(+2.99)
Rim Volume:	0.538 cmm	Reference Height (Std.):	0.507 mm
Mean Cup Depth:	0.184 mm		
Maximum Cup Depth:	0.649 mm	Software: IR1-V2.01	(*) Classification based on statistics. Diagnosis is physician's responsibility.

OS

D

Plate 114 (Case Four).

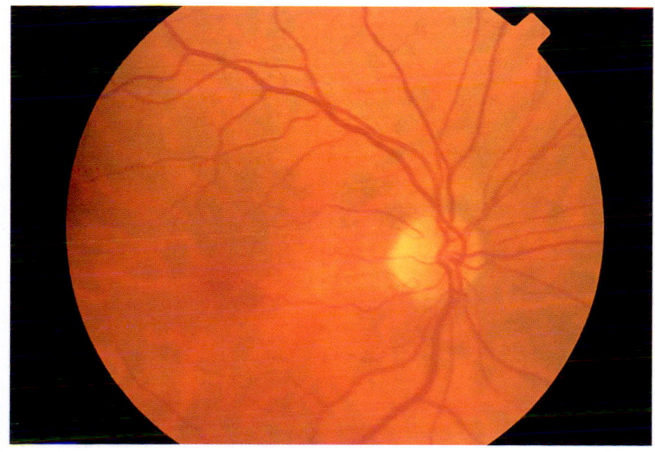

A

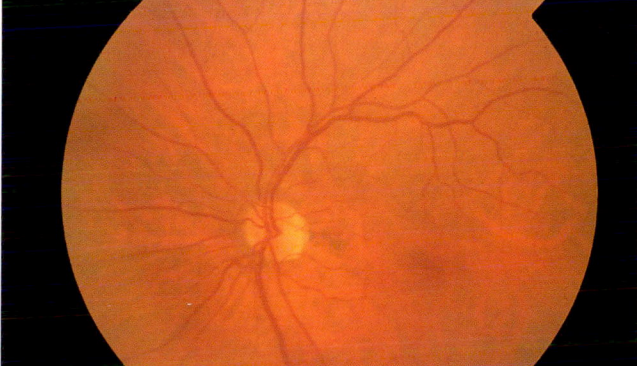

B

Plate 115 (Case Five).

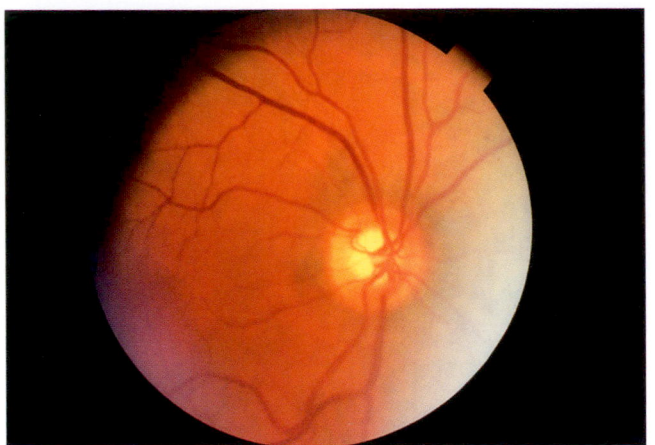

A

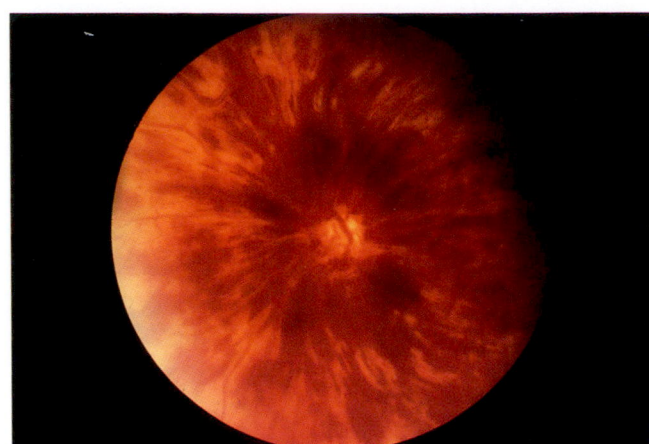

B

Plate 116 (Case Six).

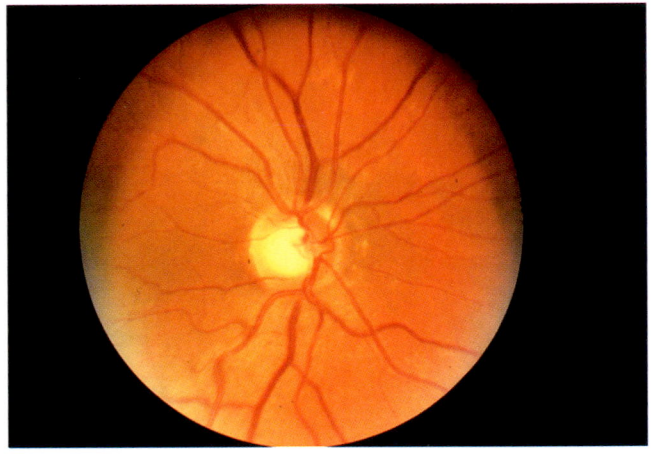

A

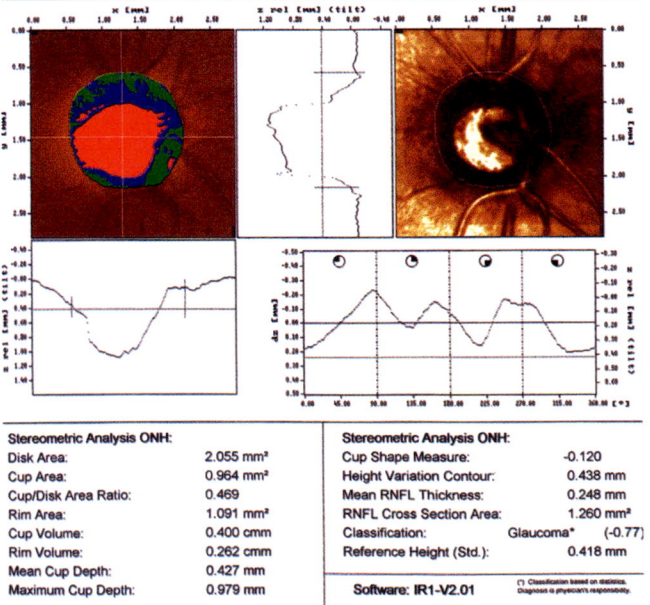

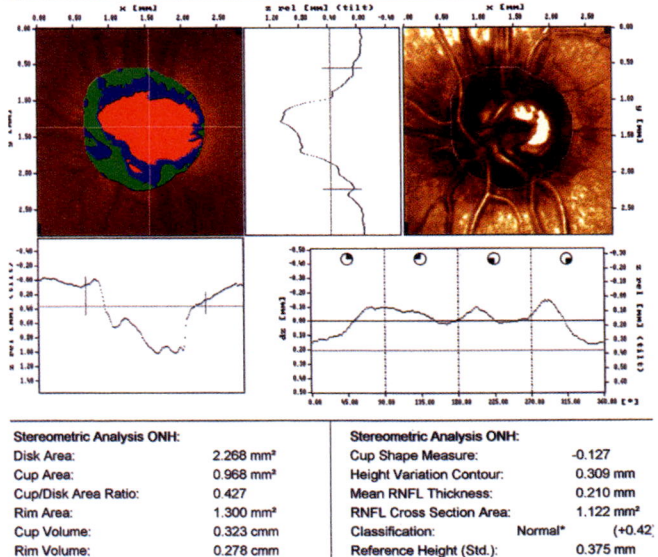

B

Stereometric Analysis ONH:		Stereometric Analysis ONH:	
Disk Area:	2.055 mm²	Cup Shape Measure:	-0.120
Cup Area:	0.964 mm²	Height Variation Contour:	0.438 mm
Cup/Disk Area Ratio:	0.469	Mean RNFL Thickness:	0.248 mm
Rim Area:	1.091 mm²	RNFL Cross Section Area:	1.260 mm²
Cup Volume:	0.400 cmm	Classification: Glaucoma* (-0.77)	
Rim Volume:	0.262 cmm	Reference Height (Std.):	0.418 mm
Mean Cup Depth:	0.427 mm		
Maximum Cup Depth:	0.979 mm	Software: IR1-V2.01	(*) Classification based on statistics. Diagnosis is physician's responsibility.

OD

C

Stereometric Analysis ONH:		Stereometric Analysis ONH:	
Disk Area:	2.268 mm²	Cup Shape Measure:	-0.127
Cup Area:	0.968 mm²	Height Variation Contour:	0.309 mm
Cup/Disk Area Ratio:	0.427	Mean RNFL Thickness:	0.210 mm
Rim Area:	1.300 mm²	RNFL Cross Section Area:	1.122 mm²
Cup Volume:	0.323 cmm	Classification: Normal* (+0.42)	
Rim Volume:	0.278 cmm	Reference Height (Std.):	0.375 mm
Mean Cup Depth:	0.345 mm		
Maximum Cup Depth:	0.842 mm	Software: IR1-V2.01	(*) Classification based on statistics. Diagnosis is physician's responsibility.

OS

D

Plate 117 (Case Seven).

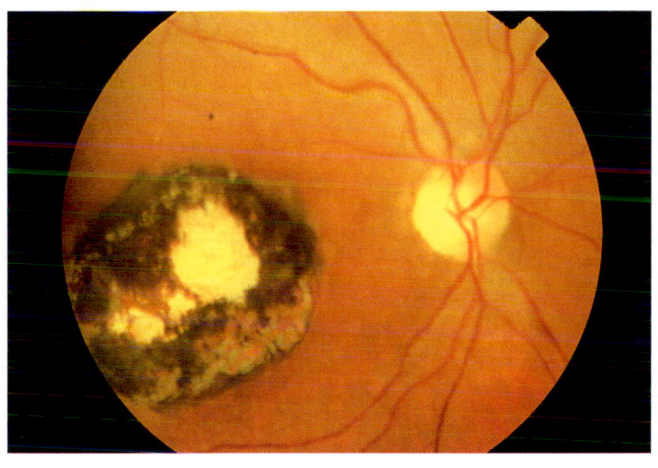

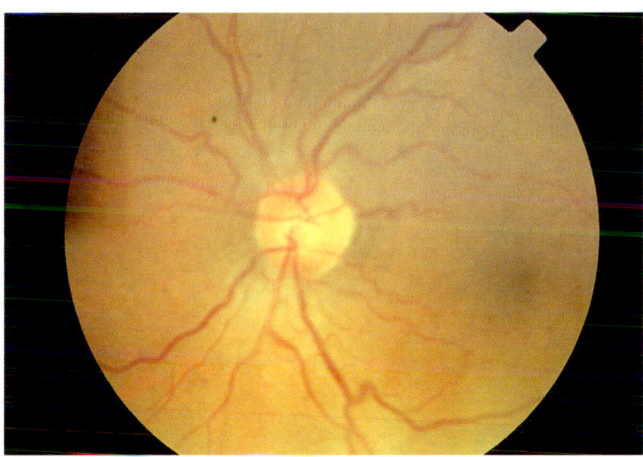

A

B

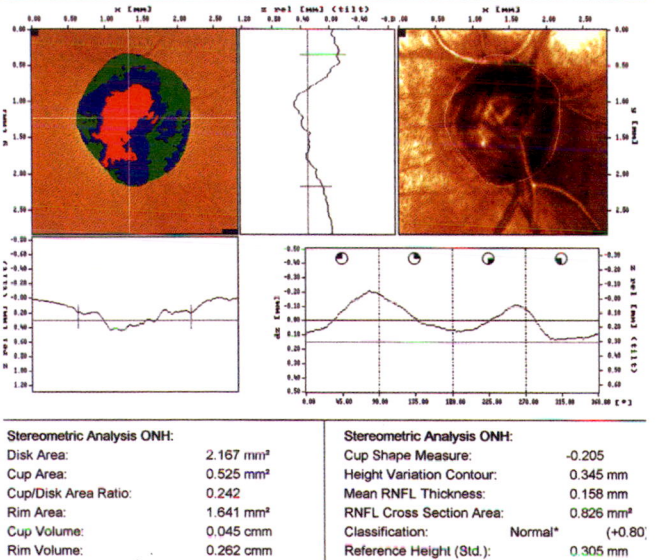

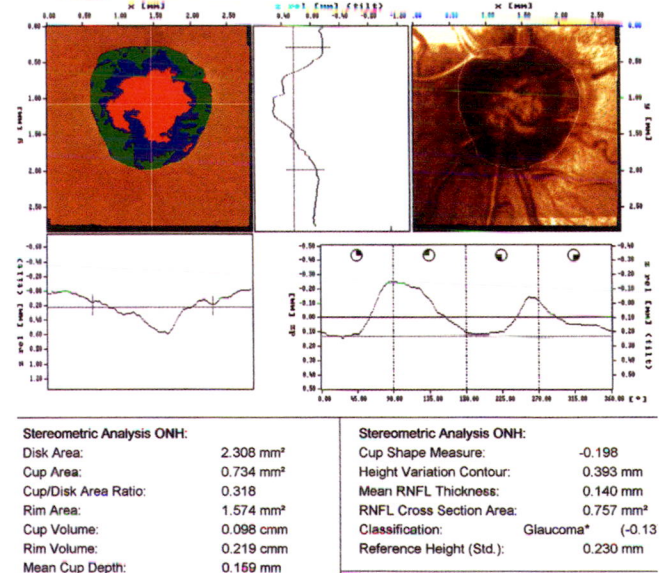

Stereometric Analysis ONH:		Stereometric Analysis ONH:	
Disk Area:	2.167 mm²	Cup Shape Measure:	-0.205
Cup Area:	0.525 mm²	Height Variation Contour:	0.345 mm
Cup/Disk Area Ratio:	0.242	Mean RNFL Thickness:	0.158 mm
Rim Area:	1.641 mm²	RNFL Cross Section Area:	0.826 mm²
Cup Volume:	0.045 cmm	Classification: Normal* (+0.80)	
Rim Volume:	0.262 cmm	Reference Height (Std.):	0.305 mm
Mean Cup Depth:	0.126 mm		
Maximum Cup Depth:	0.377 mm	Software: IR1-V2.01	(*) Classification based on statistics. Diagnosis is physician's responsibility.

OD

Stereometric Analysis ONH:		Stereometric Analysis ONH:	
Disk Area:	2.308 mm²	Cup Shape Measure:	-0.198
Cup Area:	0.734 mm²	Height Variation Contour:	0.393 mm
Cup/Disk Area Ratio:	0.318	Mean RNFL Thickness:	0.140 mm
Rim Area:	1.574 mm²	RNFL Cross Section Area:	0.757 mm²
Cup Volume:	0.098 cmm	Classification: Glaucoma* (-0.13)	
Rim Volume:	0.219 cmm	Reference Height (Std.):	0.230 mm
Mean Cup Depth:	0.159 mm		
Maximum Cup Depth:	0.473 mm	Software: IR1-V2.01	(*) Classification based on statistics. Diagnosis is physician's responsibility.

OS

C

D

Plate 118 (Case Eight).

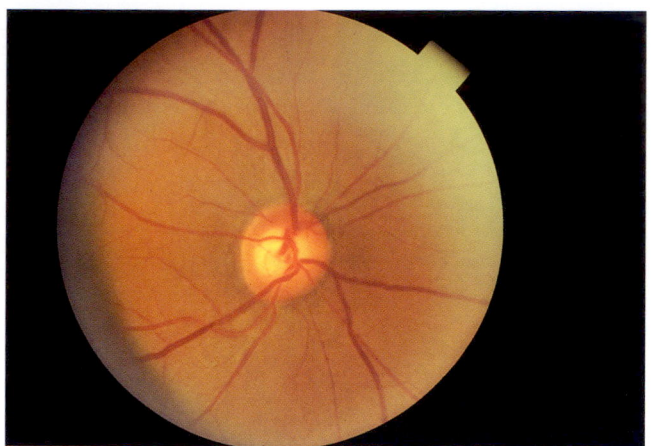

A

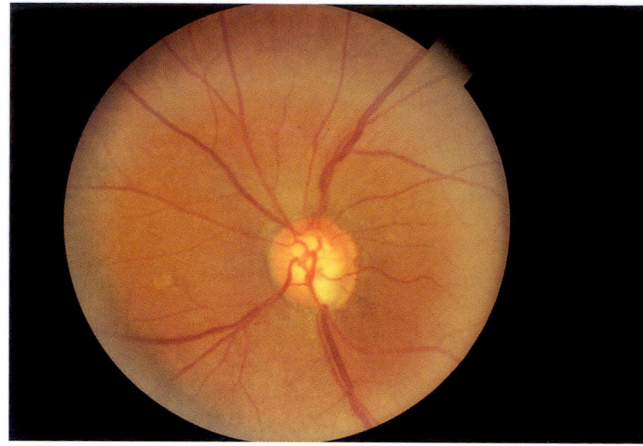

B

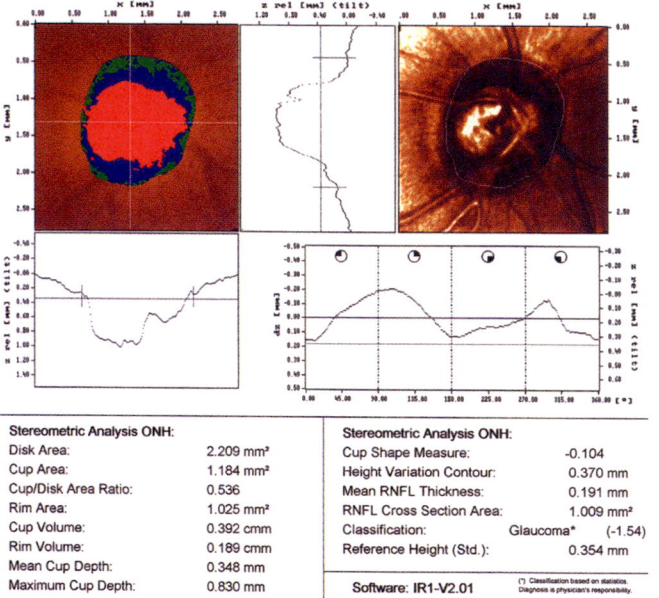

Stereometric Analysis ONH:		Stereometric Analysis ONH:	
Disk Area:	2.209 mm²	Cup Shape Measure:	-0.104
Cup Area:	1.184 mm²	Height Variation Contour:	0.370 mm
Cup/Disk Area Ratio:	0.536	Mean RNFL Thickness:	0.191 mm
Rim Area:	1.025 mm²	RNFL Cross Section Area:	1.009 mm²
Cup Volume:	0.392 cmm	Classification:	Glaucoma* (-1.54)
Rim Volume:	0.189 cmm	Reference Height (Std.):	0.354 mm
Mean Cup Depth:	0.348 mm		
Maximum Cup Depth:	0.830 mm	Software: IR1-V2.01	(*) Classification based on statistics. Diagnosis is physician's responsibility.

OD

C

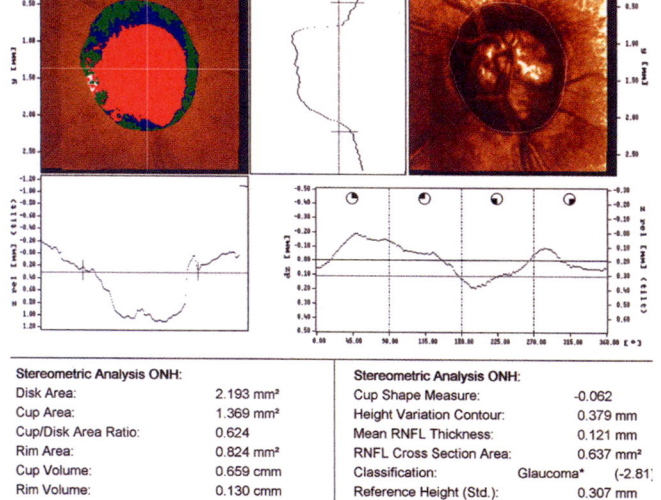

Stereometric Analysis ONH:		Stereometric Analysis ONH:	
Disk Area:	2.193 mm²	Cup Shape Measure:	-0.062
Cup Area:	1.369 mm²	Height Variation Contour:	0.379 mm
Cup/Disk Area Ratio:	0.624	Mean RNFL Thickness:	0.121 mm
Rim Area:	0.824 mm²	RNFL Cross Section Area:	0.637 mm²
Cup Volume:	0.659 cmm	Classification:	Glaucoma* (-2.81)
Rim Volume:	0.130 cmm	Reference Height (Std.):	0.307 mm
Mean Cup Depth:	0.488 mm		
Maximum Cup Depth:	1.007 mm	Software: IR1-V2.01	(*) Classification based on statistics. Diagnosis is physician's responsibility.

OS

D

Plate 119 (Case Nine).

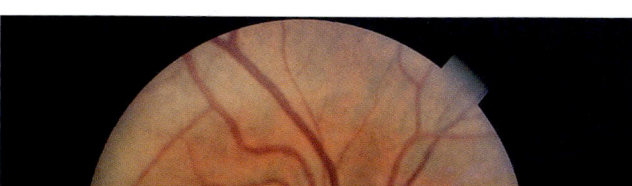

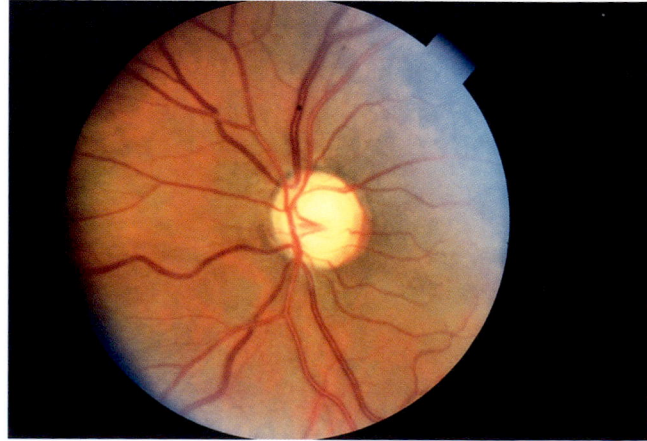

A

B

Plate 120 (CaseTen).

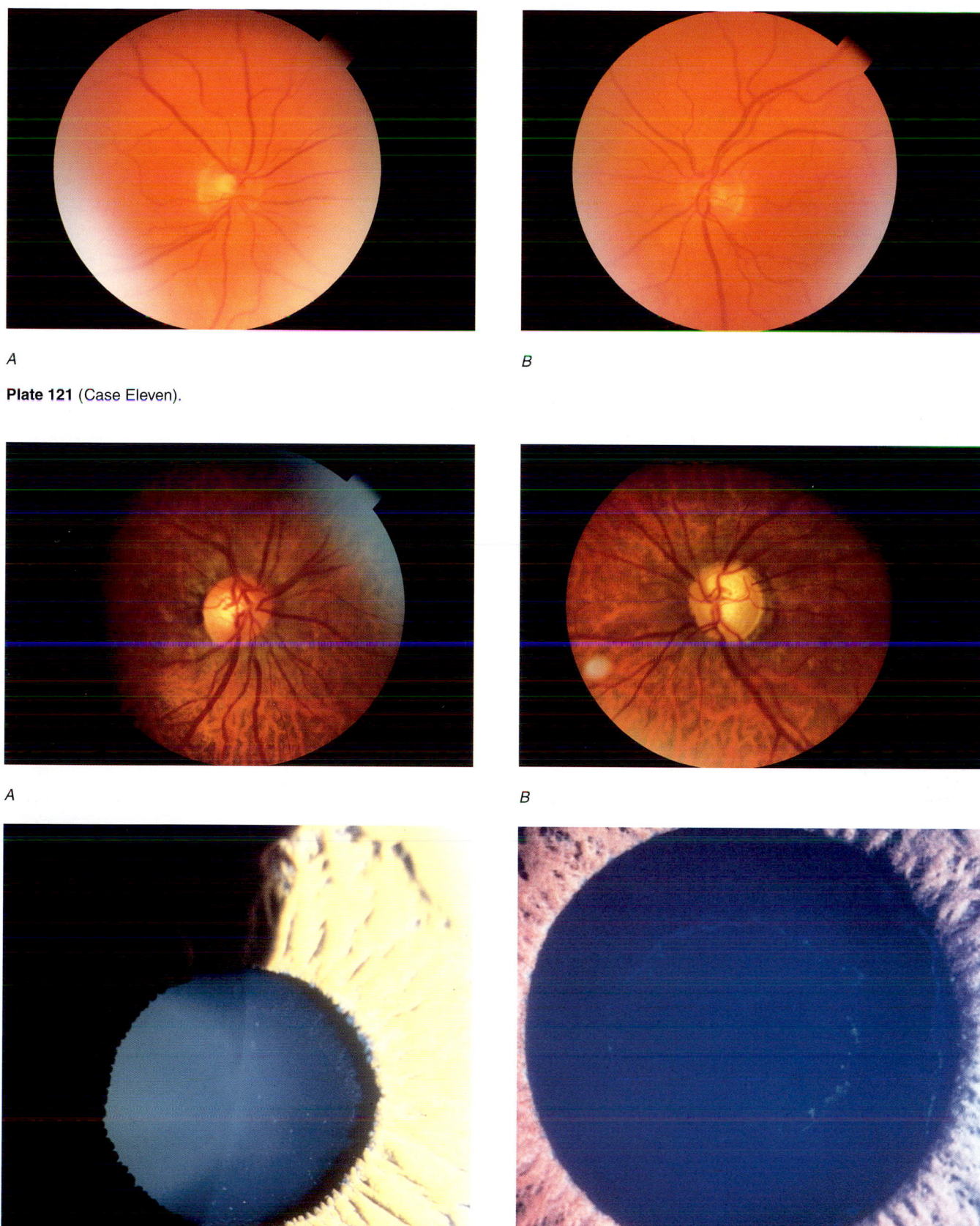

A

B

Plate 121 (Case Eleven).

A

B

C

D

Plate 122 (Case Twelve).

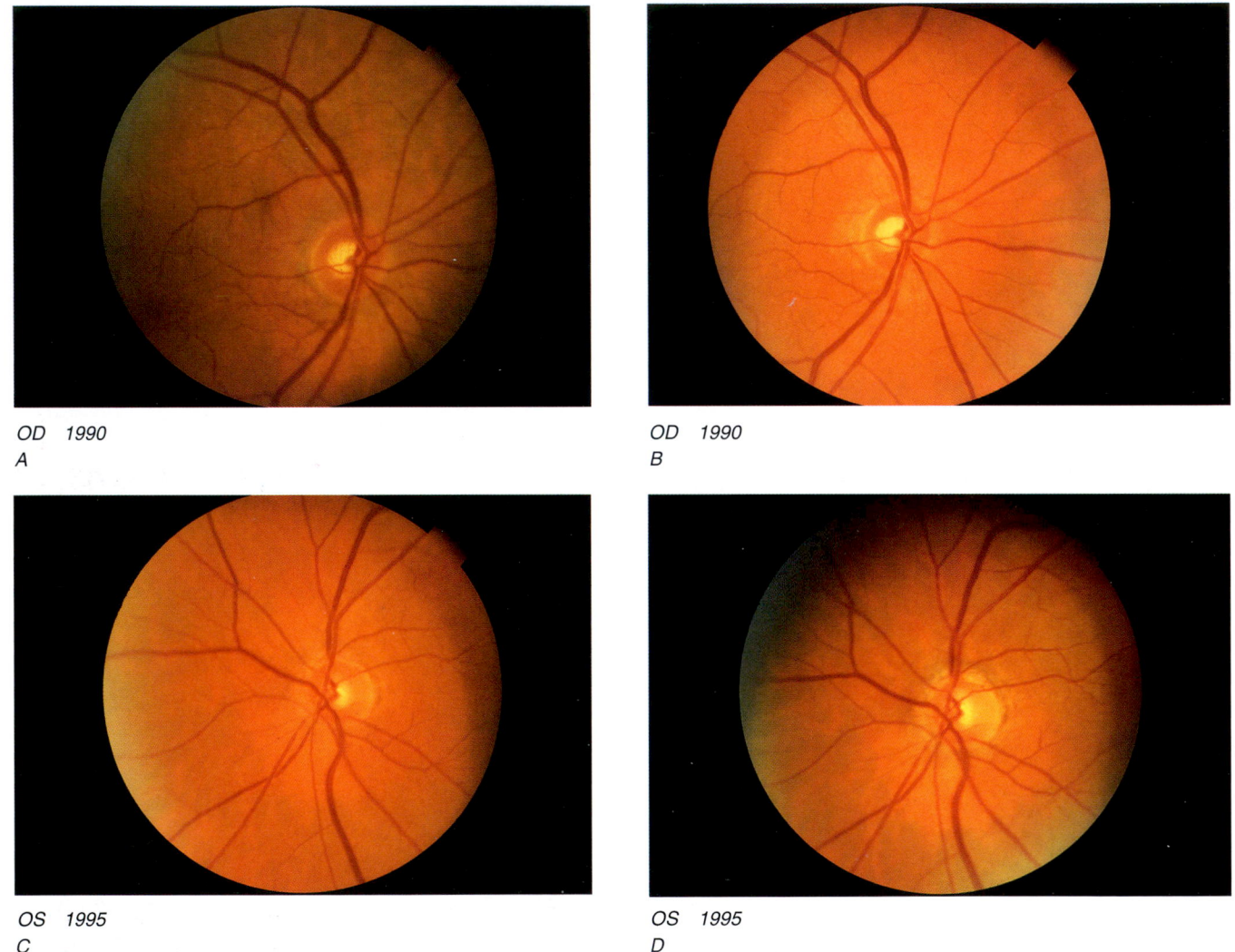

OD 1990
A

OD 1990
B

OS 1995
C

OS 1995
D

Plate 123 (Case Thirteen).

Chapter 21

MEDICAL MANAGEMENT OF GLAUCOMA

Murray Fingeret

The treatment and management of primary open-angle glaucoma (POAG) and ocular hypertension is a challenging, rewarding, and at times frustrating endeavor that will often span the lifetime of the patient. The treatment rendered will vary depending on many factors, including examination findings, ocular history, family history, medical history, and extent of damage at the time of diagnosis. Ocular hypertension is defined as intraocular pressure (IOP) greater than or equal to 22 mmHg, and occurs in 4 to 10% of patients over 40 years of age.[1,2] Approximately 1% of patients with ocular hypertension develop glaucomatous damage (detectable injury to the optic nerve or loss of visual field) every year.[2,3] In addition, up to 50% of individuals with glaucoma present with IOP in the "normal" range.[1] Ideally, one would like to diagnose glaucoma at an early stage and treat only those patients who have developed glaucoma or will do so. Unfortunately, current diagnostic methods do not always allow the differentiation between the "preglaucomatous" and nonglaucomatous individual at an early stage, since they often appear similar. As a result, controversy exists among "experts" as to when therapy should be initiated for individuals with elevated IOP but without obvious glaucomatous damage (ocular hypertension). In addition, there is a reluc-

tance to diagnose individuals with glaucoma when the IOP is not elevated.

Some years ago, before the term *ocular hypertension* was coined, one simplistic approach was to treat all individuals with statistically elevated IOP (>21 mmHg) regardless of the appearance of the optic nerve or visual field. This led to a great deal of overtreatment, with all the associated side effects, expense, and inconvenience. Several clinicians noted that many of these patients had normal optic nerves and visual fields. This observation, that not every patient with elevated IOP had glaucomatous damage, led to the evolution of a different management strategy in the 1970s. With this new strategy, IOP was used as a guideline, with emphasis on the careful monitoring of the visual field and optic nerve for glaucomatous damage. Unless the IOP was significantly elevated, usually around 30 mmHg, treatment was withheld until damage to the optic nerve and/or visual field was documented. It was during this period that the term *ocular hypertension* (OHTN) was coined. This approach had shortcomings but was workable as long as state-of-the-art equipment was available, along with cooperative patients who understood the risks involved. A variant of this latter strategy is to follow the patient as a glaucoma suspect at regular intervals, with deferment of treatment until the risk of glaucomatous damage exceeds an arbitrary level or damage is noted on either conventional tests (optic nerve analysis, automated perimetry) or more contemporary testing (short-wavelength automated perimetry, optic nerve and nerve fiber analysis). IOP in the latter strategy does not drive the diagnosis but rather is one of several risk factors analyzed. The level of acceptable risk before therapy is initiated changes over time, just as other patient factors may vary with age.

The controversy over when therapy for OHTN should be initiated was brought to light by a series of studies published in the late 1980s and early 1990s. On one side are two prospective studies done by Epstein and Kass showing that, in certain situations, early initiation of therapy for OHTN will reduce the chance for developing glaucomatous visual field loss.[5,6] These studies suggested the need to adopt an aggressive approach to OHTN, with early initiation of therapy if the risk for glaucomatous damage is significant. On the other side of the debate was a prospective study done by Schulzer and Drance in which therapy for OHTN was seen to be of little benefit.[7] These and other studies brought little closure on the issue, leading to the development of the Ocular Hypertension Treatment Study (OHTS).[8] The OHTS is a long-term, randomized, multicenter clinical trial sponsored by the National Eye Institute in which individuals with OHTN are randomized to either a treatment or a nontreatment group. Recruitment was completed in 1996 and 5-year follow-up is ongoing. Results from the OHTS study unfortunately will not be available until after the year 2001. Until then, we must base our treatment decisions for OHTN on anecdotal evidence, experience, and the conflicting studies in the literature. Still, once the decision to treat is made, a management strategy is necessary that incorporates the careful monitoring of the optic nerve and visual fields to identify any signs of progression of the disease.

The current approach to the treatment of glaucoma is mainly palliative. Most clinicians have seen the rare case in which glaucomatous defects are reversed with treatment, but those are exceptions. At present, there are no drugs for reversal of the basic histopathologic abnormalities, whether in the outflow pathways or at the level of the retinal ganglion cell. The medications used either decrease aqueous production or improve outflow, all through poorly understood mechanisms (see Chap. 20). Pharmaceutical agents developed over the past decade for reduction of the IOP provide the clinician with a number of options for initiating treatment and managing individuals with glaucoma. The medications used exert an ocular hypotensive effect but may also cause ocular and/or systemic side effects. Therefore it becomes the clinician's responsibility to choose those medications that offer maximal efficacy and safety with minimal side effects.

PHARMACEUTICAL AGENTS USED FOR TREATMENT

Adrenergic Antagonists

The topical adrenergic antagonists consist of timolol maleate 0.25% and 0.50% (Timoptic) and generics, timolol hemihydrate 0.25% and 0.5% (Betimol), levobunolol 0.25% and 0.5% (Betagan) and generics, carteolol 1.0% (Ocupress), metipranolol 0.3% (Optipranolol), and betaxolol 0.25% suspension and 0.5% solution (Betoptic S, Betoptic). These are commonly referred to as beta blockers for their specific action of beta-adrenergic receptor blockade, which results in decreased aqueous production. Beta blockers are usually the first medications prescribed for individuals diagnosed with open-angle glaucoma because of their effectiveness in reducing IOP and their few ocular side effects. Most beta blockers reduce the IOP by approximately 16 to 25%. However, not every person will show a reduction in IOP with beta-blocker therapy. It is for this reason that a uniocular trial should be performed whenever any medication is prescribed, looking for the ocular hypotensive response (using the contralateral eye as a control) and any possible side effects.

When used topically, beta blockers may reduce the heart rate and decrease pulmonary function, causing symptoms that can go unnoticed.[9,10] Some patients may not notice fatigue or breathlessness during normal activity but will do so during periods of exercise or strenuous effort (e.g., going up a flight of stairs). Thus patients using topical beta blockers must be alert to their potential systemic side effects, since the topical medication may be absorbed into the circulatory system, affecting beta receptors located throughout the body.[11] An eyedrop absorbed through the nasolacrimal drainage system is similar to an intravenous injection, since any medication, no matter how small, entering the systemic circulation may cause effects, both wanted and unwanted.[12] One way to reduce systemic absorption is with nasolacrimal (eyelid closure) or punctal occlusion for a period of 3 minutes. Either method of occlusion will reduce systemic absorption by approximately 50%.[13,14] It is the cardiac and pulmonary side effects that usually lead to the modification or discontinuation of topical beta blockers. Other less common but significant side effects include diarrhea, nausea and cramps, depression, anxiety, and confusion.[15,16]

Timolol, carteolol, metipranolol, and levobunolol are nonselective beta blockers. These drugs act at both the beta$_1$ and beta$_2$ receptors and are usually administered every 12 hours. In selected individuals, once-daily use may be implemented, but the IOP must be measured 20 to 24 hours after instillation to ensure adequate efficacy. Timolol also comes in an extended-release form that is used once per day (Timoptic XE), preferably in the morning. The contraindications for nonselective beta blockers include cardiovascular disease, second- and third-degree heart block, congestive heart failure, hypotension, asthma, chronic obstructive pulmonary disease (COPD), and emphysema.[17] Baseline blood pressure and pulse measurements are needed—in addition to a review of the medical history—before beginning treatment with a topical beta blocker. The ocular side effects of nonselective beta blockers include burning, stinging,[18,19] hyperemia, punctate keratitis,[20] and corneal hypoesthesia.[21] These side effects may be bothersome but are not usually of sufficient magnitude to necessitate discontinuing the medication.

Carteolol is a unique nonselective beta blocker, having additional intrinsic sympathomimetic activity (ISA). ISA allows the adrenergic system to be blocked at certain receptors and stimulated at others. One advantage of ISA is that carteolol does not appear to affect the heart rate or cholesterol level, while timolol reduces both, including the high-density lipoprotein (HDL) level in healthy individuals as well as those with glaucoma.[14,22] Reduced HDL levels may increase the risk of cardiovascular disease. Therefore one indication for the use of carteolol may be a history of cardiovascular disease in an individual with glaucoma.

Betaxolol (Betoptic) is a cardioselective beta blocker that is not as efficacious in reducing IOP as many of the nonselective beta blockers. This relatively selective beta$_1$ blocker has minimal affinity for the beta$_2$ receptors of the pulmonary and gastrointestinal tissues, permitting its use with caution in situations where nonselective beta blockers are contraindicated (i.e., past history of asthma or COPD).[23] In addition, while betaxolol is specific for the beta$_1$ receptors, its affinity to those receptors is less than that of timolol. This makes betaxolol a safer drug to use than nonselective beta blockers when there is concern about its possible systemic effects on the cardiovascular, pulmonary, or central nervous system. Betaxolol does not usually exert a significant effect on the cardiovascular system,[22] and studies have shown that it can be used safely in patients with pulmonary dysfunction.[23,25,26] Still, betaxolol is not the initial drug of choice for individuals with pulmonary problems. It may be used in patients having a relative contraindication when other medications

have not performed as required if it is approved by the patient's internist. Cases of exacerbation of asthma and decreased forced expiratory volume have been reported with betaxolol when it was used in individuals without a history of pulmonary problems.[27,28] Insomnia and depressive neurosis have also rarely been reported.[24] There have been reports that betaxolol may have both blood flow–enhancing properties and neuroprotective capabilities.[29–31] While not as potent as timolol or levobunolol in reducing IOP,[32] betaxolol may show a greater additive effect with the adrenergic agonist dipivefrin (Propine).[33–35]

Betaxolol comes in a 0.25% suspension (Betoptic S) and a 0.5% solution (Betoptic). Comparative studies between the 0.25% suspension and 0.5% solution have shown an equal clinical efficacy in reducing IOP. Each is used every 12 hours. Ocular side effects of betaxolol 0.5% solution (Betoptic) include stinging and burning, which is more intense than that of betaxolol 0.25% suspension or timolol.[23,24] Corneal anesthesia has not been reported with betaxolol, as it has been with timolol.

A dissipation phenomenon of the beta blockers, studied most extensively with timolol, is known as "short-term escape" and "long-term drift."[36,37] When therapy with a topical beta blocker is initiated, there is often a large initial decrease in IOP that lasts from several days to a few weeks. Short-term escape then occurs, resulting in a small rise in IOP. After 2 to 4 weeks of use, the IOP usually stabilizes at a level below that which existed before treatment. IOP control may then last, varying with the patient, from weeks to years. Long-term drift is a slow steady rise in IOP after months to years of treatment. Many studies have attempted to identify the mechanism responsible for this decreased efficacy. One study suggests there may be a change in the number of beta-adrenergic receptors with continued exposure to adrenergic blockade.[38] Another explanation may be that open-angle glaucoma, being a slowly progressive disorder, is getting worse and becoming more difficult to control. Also, we assume that topical beta blockers, like any other medication, will always reduce the IOP when instilled in the eye. Unfortunately, this is not always the case, as 10 to 15% of individuals will not show a reduction in IOP when beta blockers are instilled. One reason for a lack of response may be that the patient is using a systemic beta blocker for hypertension. In this situation, the IOP may already be reduced because the eye's beta receptors are already blocked. Therefore no further blockade occurs when a topical beta blocker is utilized. In other individuals who are not using systemic beta blockers, for reasons not entirely clear, the topical beta blockers show no IOP-reducing effect at all.

Adrenergic Agonists

The topical adrenergic agonists used for glaucoma therapy include epinephrine, dipivefrin (Propine), apraclonidine (Iopidine) and brimonidine (Alphagan). Epinephrine and dipivefrin are alpha- and beta-adrenergic agonists that are only mildly effective in reducing IOP. Their use has declined as more effective agents have become available. Epinephrine is one of the oldest IOP-reducing agents, and although the mechanism of action is obscure, it is believed that alpha- and beta-receptor stimulation promotes increased outflow facility.[39] Epinephrine is available in three solution forms: epinephrine borate (0.5, 1.0, and 2.0%), epinephrine hydrochloride (0.25, 0.5, 1.0, and 2.0%), and epinephrine bitartrate (1.0 and 2.0%). The most common forms are 1% borate and 2% hydrochloride, both used twice a day. The bitartrate forms contain approximately one-half the concentration labeled on the bottle and are rarely used except in eyedrops formulated in combination with pilocarpine 1, 2, 3, 4, and 6% solutions.

Ocular side effects that limit epinephrine's long-term use include hyperemia, allergic follicular conjunctivitis, tearing, adrenochrome deposits, and, in aphakia or pseudophakia, cystoid macular edema.[40,41] Discoloration of soft contact lenses has also been observed.[42] Because of its potential mydriatic effect, epinephrine should be avoided in individuals with narrow angles. Systemic side effects include hypertension, arrhythmia, tachycardia, headache, and brow ache.[43] Caution should be exercised in treating patients with arteriosclerosis, cardiovascular disease, or hyperthyroidism and those who are using tricyclic antidepressants.[43]

Dipivefrin (Propine) is a prodrug form of epinephrine. It comes in a 0.1% solution instilled twice daily. Dipivefrin and epinephrine are not as potent as the other antiglaucoma agents in reducing the IOP, though they usually improve in efficacy over the first months of treatment.

One advantage of dipivefrin as compared with epinephrine is that it penetrates the cornea extremely well, being converted to epinephrine after entering the eye. The chemical makeup of dipivefrin allows increased corneal penetration, so that a smaller concentration of the drug may be used, which, in turn, reduces the systemic side effects while providing a reduction in IOP similar to that of epinephrine. Still, with newer, more efficacious classes of medications available, dipivefrin and epinephrine are rarely used today.

Alpha-Adrenergic Agonists

Apraclonidine HCl (Iopidine) is a relatively selective alpha$_2$-adrenergic agonist that was initially available in a 1% concentration for use prior to and immediately after anterior segment laser procedures to prevent postoperative IOP spikes. A 0.5% concentration subsequently became available for use as a t.i.d. dosage for the treatment of open-angle glaucoma. Apraclonidine lowers intraocular pressure by approximately 20 to 25% by reducing aqueous production, and its effects appear to be additive to those of other glaucoma medications.[44] As with all medications, several shortcomings have been recognized. Allergic blepharoconjunctivitis is common and similar to that seen with epinephrine. A red, itchy eye develops from 20 to 50% of the time, depending upon which study is reviewed.[44,45] The frequency of allergy may decrease with a b.i.d. dosage;[44] it may occur as early as the initial instillation or not be seen until after months of use. Another problem with apraclonidine is tachyphylaxis, in which tolerance develops and the medication no longer reduces the IOP. Tachyphylaxis has been reported to occur in up to 50% of cases.[46] Although apraclonidine is recommended for short-term use, many patients may tolerate the medication without the appearance of allergy or tachyphylaxis and thus be able to use the drug indefinitely.

Apraclonidine does not readily cross the blood-brain barrier, so that few systemic side effects occur, even if the drug is absorbed systemically. Apraclonidine's excellent safety profile is one distinct advantage. Apraclonidine, like topical carbonic anhydrase inhibitors and brimonidine, is approved as a t.i.d. medication, though some individuals can be controlled on a b.i.d. basis. Apraclonidine may, in select individuals, have alpha$_1$-receptor stimulation, which leads to several side effects, including mydriasis, conjunctival vasoconstriction, and eyelid retraction.

Brimonidine (Alphagan) is a relatively selective alpha$_2$ agonist. It was approved by the FDA in September 1996 and released in a 0.2% solution utilizing a t.i.d. dosage. Its efficacy and side effects are similar to those of apraclonidine, with a few differences.[47] Brimonidine has a dual mechanism for decreasing the IOP: reducing the amount of aqueous produced as well as enhancing uveoscleral outflow.[48] This drug being more lipophilic than apraclonidine, crosses the blood-brain barrier and can therefore cause central nervous system (CNS) side effects such as fatigue. Its history of inducing allergic conjunctivitis and tachyphylaxis appears to be less significant than that of apraclonidine. Many individuals who have developed an allergy on apraclonidine may use brimonidine without incident. Brimonidine appears to be similar in efficacy to timolol at its peak effect (providing an IOP reduction of approximately 25%), though it does reduce the IOP as well at the trough measurement.[47,4]

In addition, there appears to be a mild contralateral effect, and brimonidine, like apraclonidine, may be used to prevent IOP spikes after laser surgery.[50] Although this drug is approved as a t.i.d. medication, some individuals may be controlled on a b.i.d. dosage, especially if brimonidine is used in conjunction with a topical beta blocker.

Prostaglandin Analogues

Latanoprost 0.005% (Xalatan) is a topical prostaglandin approved in 1996. When given in a low concentration, it is at least as effective in reducing the IOP as timolol.[51–54] Latanoprost may reduce the IOP up to 35% when it is used just once a day,[52–54] with an efficacy that lasts for 24 hours.[55] Its effect is greatest when it is given at night,[55] and its mechanism of action is the enhancement of uveoscleral outflow. This novel approach leads to a drug that is additive to most other glaucoma medications, though its efficacy when used with miotics varies. Systemic side effects are rare, but several ocular side effects have been reported. An increase in conjunctival hyperemia occurs in up to 30% of individuals.[53] Increased iris pigmentation has been observed, especially in lightly pigmented eyes that are mixed in color, such as green-brown or blue-brown eyes (concentric heterochromia). The darkening of the iris is due to an increase in the number of melanosomes (pigment granules) within melanocytes of the iris stroma. The darkening has been observed in up to 16% of treated individuals and appears to be permanent.[53,54] Although it is apparently not harmful to the eye, iris darkening may be bothersome. Patients need to be informed about this potential side effect before therapy is initiated, and the color of the iris must be documented in the record. If a color change is noted, treatment may be discontinued. Although the iris will not revert to the original color, no further evidence of color change has been noted upon discontinuation of the medication. Another ocular side effect associated with latanoprost is punctate epithelial keratopathy, which occurs three times more frequently than in patients treated with timolol. The keratopathy is likely due to the fact that latanoprost has a benzalkonium chloride concentration of 200 mg/mL, which is higher than the concentration typically used in other ophthalmic preparations.[52] Other corneal side effects include the development of pseudodendrites that disappear with cessation of latanoprost and the exacerbation of herpes simplex keratitis in individuals who have had prior infections. There have also been reports of eyelashes increasing in length and thickness with the use of latanoprost.[56] Finally, there are reported cases of reactivation of anterior uveitis and cystoid macular edema, especially in individuals with a prior history of anterior uveitis or those who have had complicated intraocular surgery.[57,58]

Cholinergic Agonists

The topical cholinergic agonists and anticholinesterase medications are classified as miotics. These agents stimulate the longitudinal fibers of the ciliary muscle, resulting in the mechanical opening of the trabecular meshwork and in increased aqueous outflow. The cholinergic agonists are direct-acting agents that mimic acetylcholine and stimulate the cholinergic receptors within the ciliary muscles. The sphincter muscle of the iris is also stimulated, leading to reduced pupil size (miosis), which has no bearing on the reduction of the IOP. The cholinergic agents available for topical use include pilocarpine and carbachol, which rarely elicit systemic side effects in the concentrations used to treat POAG. However, ocular side effects are common. Those most frequently reported include pain in the globe and orbit, brow ache, blurred vision, secondary accommodative spasm, miosis, hyperemia, visual field constriction, and dimness of vision. One common side effect associated with miotics is a myopic shift, which is most pronounced in young individuals. The shift in myopia is usually constant and can be corrected with spectacles.

Miotics have declined in use as newer classes of glaucoma agents with fewer side effects and more desirable dosage schedules have become available. If a miotic is used, pilocarpine is the agent of choice; it is produced in a variety of forms and concentrations. The solution form is manufactured in 0.5 to 10% concentrations, usually administered four times per day, with 2% and 4% most commonly prescribed. Concentrations greater than the 4% strength do little to produce further IOP reduction, but they increase the risk of systemic and ocular side effects. When pilocarpine is used in combination with other glaucoma agents such as timolol, the 4% form may be used on a b.i.d. dosage schedule with efficacy comparable to that of a q.i.d. dosage.[59]

Pilocarpine 4% is available in a gel form (Pilopine HS Gel) and is administered at bedtime. One advantage of the gel form is that side effects occur while the patient is asleep. Pilopine HS Gel may also be beneficial for those patients suspected of poor compliance, elderly patients who have difficulty with eyedrop insertion, or individuals necessitating miotic use but intolerant to the ocular side effects. Care must be taken that only a small amount (about 1/8 in.) is applied into the inferior cul-de-sac. The gel is best applied by placing a small, measured amount on the end of the finger and using the fingertip to place it into the inferior cul-de-sac (Fig. 21–1). An excessive amount may be applied if the gel is placed directly from the tube into the eye. As with any medication being used once a day, the IOP must be measured at trough or 20 to 24 hours after instillation (before the next dosage cycle) to ensure that there is not a spike in the IOP.

Pilocarpine is also available in wafer form for sustained release. Known as Ocuserts, these wafers are supplied with release rates of 20 mg/h (roughly equal to that of 1% drops) and 40 mg/h (roughly equal to 2% drops); they are inserted into the inferior or superior cul-de-sac on a weekly basis. Ocuserts may be useful in the elderly who have poor dexterity in instilling eyedrops or in young patients requiring miotic therapy. Foreign-body sensation is one side effect of Ocuserts that may limit their usefulness.

Another indication for pilocarpine is in pigment dispersion syndrome (PDS) or pigmentary glaucoma (see Chap. 26), since, in addition to producing miosis, the drug's action moves the iris forward, reducing iris-zonule touch. By reducing iris-zonule touch, the amount of pigment being liberated may be reduced. Unfortunately, most individuals with PDS or pigmentary glaucoma (PG) are young and do not usually tolerate the ocular side effects. For young individuals with PDS or PG, Ocuserts offer an alternative form of miotic therapy.

The ocular side effects associated with miotics are usually the reason for poor patient compliance. One method to improve compliance is by having the patient slowly adapt to the ocular side effects. In this situation, the dosage and concentration of pilocarpine are started at the lowest possible level, with a gradual buildup to full strength and dosage over a few weeks' time. For example, miotic therapy is begun with the 1% concentration once a day for 4 days; it is then increased to twice a day for 4 days, three times a day for 4 days, and finally to four times a day. The IOP and side effects are evaluated at this time, and the concentration may be increased to the 2% strength if further IOP reduction is required, provided that the side effects are tolerable. During this buildup phase, the IOP may not be properly controlled throughout the day. Therefore this regimen cannot be used for patients with markedly elevated IOP or advanced glaucoma. The objective of a slow pilocarpine buildup is improved long-term patient compliance.

Caucasians with mild glaucoma may be adequately controlled with pilocarpine 1%, whereas many blacks require at least the 2% strength for proper IOP reduction. If greater IOP reduction is

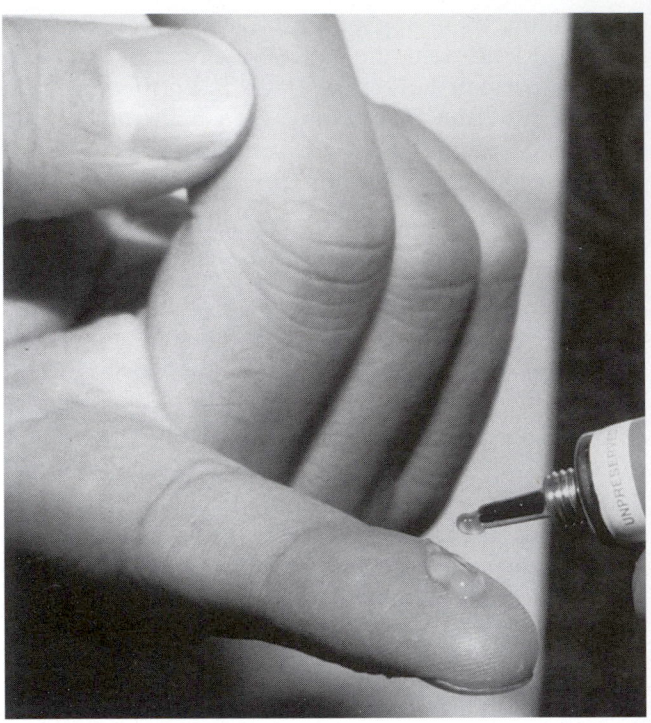

A

B

Figure 21–1. *A.* One method for patients to instill ointment into their eyes is by first placing it onto the fingertip. *B.* The ointment is then placed from the fingertip directly into the inferior cul-de-sac.

needed, the medication may be increased to 4% strength. There is rarely a benefit to using a concentration greater than the 4%, since the severity of side effects correlates with the strength of the concentration used, and IOP reduction plateaus at around the 4% strength. Finally, patient compliance tends to be worse for pilocarpine than for any other topical glaucoma medication because of the increased dosage schedule (four times per day) and frequent reports of ocular side effects.

Carbachol solution, another miotic medication, is available in 0.75, 1.50, 2.25, and 3.0% concentrations. The most common concentration prescribed is 3% administered three times a day. Carbachol 3% is a close equivalent to pilocarpine 4% and is used when pilocarpine 4% is not effective or tolerated. One concern is that carbachol penetrates the cornea poorly in some individuals, so that the resultant IOP is higher than it would be with pilocarpine 4%.

Anticholinesterases

The anticholinesterase agents are especially strong miotics because their endogenous acetylcholine action is enhanced by inhibiting cholinesterase enzymes. Because of their severe side effects, these agents are held in reserve for patients who do not respond to the direct-acting cholinergic agents and who show a progression of their glaucoma on all other glaucoma medications. Thus anticholinesterase agents are rarely used in the care of patients with glaucoma. Candidates for the use of anticholinesterases include pseudophakic/aphakic patients and poorly controlled postsurgical patients. Echothiophate (Phospholine Iodide) 0.125% administered twice a day is the most commonly used anticholinesterase agent; the concentrations of 0.03, 0.06, and 0.25% are less commonly utilized. Anticholinesterase solutions cannot be used with dipivefrin (Propine), because dipivefrin requires esterase to convert it to epinephrine.

The ocular side effects of echothiophate include miosis, anterior subcapsular cataracts, pupillary cysts, irritation, conjunctival injection, lacrimation, and retinal detachment. Systemic side effects deserve particular attention. Repeated administration can cause depressed serum and erythrocyte cholinesterase levels, resulting in urinary incontinence, diarrhea, profuse sweating, muscle weakness, rhinorrhea, abdominal cramps, apnea, and bradycardia. Individuals receiving anticholinesterase who are exposed to carbamate or organophosphate-based pesticides or insecticides should be warned of the additive effects from absorption of the insecticides via the respiratory tract or skin.[60] The most serious possible drug interaction with echothiophate involves succinylcholine, a muscle relaxant given before or during general anesthesia. In order to avoid the risk of prolonged respiratory paralysis, it is vital that, in attending to patients on echothiophate, surgeons be aware of the patient's use of this drug before any surgical procedure is scheduled.[60]

Other anticholinesterase agents that are available but are rarely used for glaucoma treatment include demecarium bromide (Humorsol) in 0.125% solution and isoflurophate (Floropryl) in 0.025% ointment.

Carbonic Anhydrase Inhibitors

Another class of pharmaceutical agents used for the treatment of primary open-angle glaucoma is the carbonic anhydrase inhibitors (CAI), which are available as topical or oral agents. In their oral form, CAIs are the most potent of the ocular hypotensive drugs; both forms work by inhibiting the enzyme carbonic anhydrase, which results in decreased production of aqueous humor.

Topical Carbonic Anhydrase Inhibitors

Systemic CAIs have long been recognized for their superior ability to reduce IOP. Unfortunately, when they are taken orally, a host of side effects including nausea, vomiting, depression, gastrointestinal upset, and loss of libido may occur. Topical preparations had been investigated for many years; as a result, dorzolamide 2% (Trusopt) was released in the spring of 1995 and brinzolamide 1% (Azopt) in the spring of 1998.

Carbonic anhydrase isoenzymes II and IV are critical for the secretion of aqueous humor, as they accelerate the reversible conversion of carbon dioxide and bicarbonate. The formation of bicarbonate is linked to the secretion of Na^+, which is related to the formation of aqueous humor. When 99% of the carbonic anhydrase isoenzyme is inhibited by either a topical or systemic CAI, the formation of bicarbonate and Na^+ is affected, leading to reduced secretions of aqueous humor and lowered IOP.

The topical CAIs are dosed t.i.d., though some individuals may be adequately controlled on a b.i.d. basis.[61] Dorzolamide and brinzolamide reduce IOP by about 16 to 22%[62,63]; they are available as a topical solution (dorzolamide) or a suspension (brinzolamide).[64] Although they are close to the oral preparations in efficacy, the topical forms are preferred because of their better safety profile. CAIs are additive to other glaucoma medications, including beta blockers, miotics, and adrenergics.[65] Systemic side effects are rare with topical CAIs, but headache and a metallic taste are common complaints. Ocular side effects, while infrequent, include irritation, itching, and hyperemia. Brinzolamide 1% (Azopt) performs similarly to dorzolamide, with added comfort upon instillation.[64]

Topical CAIs, because of their safety profile and efficacy, have become commonly used second-line medications for the therapy of glaucoma. In situations where a beta blocker is contraindicated, topical CAIs may become the primary medications. They are extremely safe to use, with the only contraindication being a history of allergy to sulfa-containing drugs.

Oral Carbonic Anhydrase Inhibitors

The use of oral CAIs has diminished since the introduction of their topical cousins. Their use is often limited to advanced cases, where maximal topical medical therapy has failed to reduce the IOP to a desired level or glaucomatous progression is seen on maximum medications. The most commonly used agents are acetazolamide (Diamox) and methazolamide (Neptazane), with the frequent reporting of systemic side effects often limiting their long-term use. These side effects, which are in part related to the concentration and dosage used, include paresthesias, tingling sensations, anorexia, weight loss, diarrhea, nausea and vomiting, fatigue, loss of libido, bone marrow toxicity, malaise, and metallic taste.[66] Acetazolamide can also cause an increased propensity for kidney stone formation.

An allergy to sulfa drugs contraindicates the use of CAIs. A rare blood dyscrasia, aplastic anemia, has been reported secondary to CAI use.[67] This idiosyncratic reaction may occur after only one dose, though it is usually seen during the first 2 to 3 months of use; it is fatal 50% of the time even with treatment. A routine complete blood count (CBC) may allow earlier diagnosis but would not affect the final outcome and is not ordinarily recommended. A CBC may be warranted before treatment in certain elderly patients with the appearance of or past history of anemia. This anemia should be treated and corrected before the initiation of CAI therapy.

Methazolamide (Neptazane), the oral CAI of choice because of its lesser tendency to promote the formation of kidney stones, is available in 25- and 50-mg tablets. Therapy with methazolamide usually begins with a 25-mg tablet twice a day. The dosage regimen is increased by 25-mg steps until satisfactory control of IOP is achieved, up to a maximum dose of 50 mg three times a day. At lower body weights, increasing methazolamide from 100 to 150 mg per day may not have a clinically significant IOP-lowering effect. Acetazolamide (Diamox) tablets are held in reserve if the maximum dosage of metha-

zolamide is not sufficient to reduce the IOP to the desired level or if the patient cannot tolerate methazolamide. Acetazolamide is available in 250-mg tablets and in 500-mg time-release capsules (Diamox Sequels). The dosage may be increased up to 250 mg four times a day in tablet form or 500 mg twice a day in capsule form.

A reduced dosage and concentration of an oral CAI is often useful, allowing it to be tailored to each patient's needs. Reductions in dosage levels may diminish unwanted side effects while still maintaining proper IOP control. The medication may also be given at specific times of the day to flatten a daily spike in IOP. Mild gastrointestinal upset secondary to the medication may be alleviated by taking the tablets or capsules with meals or using a sodium bicarbonate tablet.[66]

Combination Medications

CoSopt (dorzolamide 2% and timolol maleate 0.5%) is the first new combination product for glaucoma in 30 years. Introduced in 1998, it offers the advantage of combining two glaucoma medications in one bottle. This allows an effective reduction of IOP with a reduced dosage, which should improve compliance. CoSopt reduces IOP from 18 to 31%, with the side effects and contraindications associated with both dorzolamide and timolol.[68-70] CoSopt is best used as a second- or third-line agent after at least a single medication, usually a beta blocker, has been tried and found to be effective but not to achieve the target pressure.

WHEN TO BEGIN TREATMENT

Review Diagnostic Findings

The clinical evaluation of the glaucoma patient or glaucoma suspect involves assessments in several areas: IOP, the optic nerve and nerve fiber layer, the visual field, and the anterior chamber angle. Other diagnostic tests may be useful, as well as performing a risk-factor assessment and taking a careful history.

Open-angle glaucoma is a distinctive optic neuropathy. In patients who present with elevated IOP, one eye tends to have a higher reading. Still, many individuals may present with open-angle glaucoma without an elevated IOP.[71] It has been estimated that up to 35% of patients with POAG never have an IOP reading above 21 mmHg.[71] Thus the IOP, while easily measured, needs to be evaluated with caution and viewed as a risk factor, but it is not the parameter that defines the condition (see Chaps. 1 and 2). The higher the IOP, the greater the chance for developing open-angle glaucoma; but individuals may nevertheless develop POAG with IOP measurements in the "normal" range.

A dilated, binocular stereoscopic examination of the optic nerve and surrounding tissue is necessary to detect subtle changes in the nerve and nerve fiber layer that may precede visual field loss. Serial stereo color photography permits the comparison of the optic nerve depth, the size of the optic cup, and the integrity of the rim tissue from one examination to the next. The appearance of the optic nerve is most useful for establishing the diagnosis of open-angle glaucoma, with automated visual fields emphasized for following progression or change over time. The problem in relying on optic nerve evaluation alone for the diagnosis of glaucoma is in differentiating a large physiological cup from glaucomatous cupping. One guide is that physiological cupping tends to be symmetrical, with a large optic disk accompanied by full visual fields and healthy neuroretinal rim tissue.

The visual field helps establish the patient's level of visual function. The more sensitive the visual field examination, the more readily visual field defects can be detected, resulting in earlier diagnosis and treatment. Automated static perimetry is capable of detecting early visual field changes indicative of glaucoma. Still, perimetry by any method has its limitations. The optic nerve and nerve fiber layer may be damaged early in glaucoma, sometimes before visual field changes are evident.[72,73] Because visual field changes often occur after damage to the optic nerve, they are not always required to establish a diagnosis of glaucoma. When seen, they confirm that damage has occurred.

Evaluation of the anterior chamber angle using the goniolens is necessary to differentiate POAG from secondary open-angle forms as well as chronic angle-closure glaucoma. Gonioscopy must be performed on all narrow- and open-angle glaucoma suspects to determine the type of glaucoma that exists, since this will affect the treatment regimen.

Occasionally, a complete diagnostic evaluation may not be accomplished because of circumstances beyond the patient's or clinician's control. Examples include poor visual field results in patients with limited ability to execute the test procedure or noncommunicating (aphasic) patients. Media opacities, such as corneal leukomas, dense cataracts, and vitreous hemorrhage, may cause diffuse visual field defects that mask glaucomatous visual field loss. In addition, media opacities may make it difficult to visualize the optic nerve. Also, there may be situations when a visual field defect resembles or masks a glaucomatous field defect. For example, panretinal photocoagulation creates tiny retinal burns that produce visual field defects. When these defects are located within the arcuate bundle area, visual field defects similar to those of glaucoma may be seen. In addition, central nervous system or optic nerve disorders such as cerebrovascular accidents, optic nerve drusen, or retrobulbar optic neuritis may also cause visual field loss. Difficulty in assessing either the optic nerve or visual fields makes therapeutic decisions more difficult. The decision may then depend on IOP, family history, medical history, other risk factors, and past examination findings.

Review of Risk Factors

The risk factors for glaucoma play a critical role in the decision of when to initiate therapy.[74-78] These risk factors include age, race, family history, medical history (e.g., diabetes mellitus, untreated or poorly controlled high blood pressure), refractive error (myopia), and secondary glaucoma findings.[77,78] For a more detailed discussion of risk factors, see Chap. 2.

Treatment Guidelines

The goal of treatment in open-angle glaucoma is to stabilize the optic nerve and visual function, preventing any change over time. To prevent any loss of visual function, the one risk factor that can be affected is the IOP. Although not every case of open-angle glaucoma is due to elevated IOP, currently the only therapeutic option is to reduce IOP to a level below which optic nerve and visual field damage should not occur or progression of existing damage may be prevented. This level of IOP (target IOP) is different for each individual. The objective of therapy is to reduce the IOP to that level using the least expensive, most benign method, allowing the patient to retain maximal visual function for the remainder of his or her life. In years to come, other therapeutic options may become available, such as agents to improve blood flow or neuroprotective medications.

There are general guidelines to follow in initiating therapy. Based on the diagnostic evaluation, an evaluation of the risk factors, and consideration of the risk-to-benefit ratio of treatment, the decision to initiate medical therapy is made. Since primary open-angle glaucoma is a bilateral, often asymmetrical condition, both eyes are often treated unless an etiology is discovered that would support unilateral glaucoma (i.e., angle recession) or the pressure elevation is strikingly asymmetrical, with the more involved eye possibly requiring additional therapy.

Glaucoma Suspect

Glaucoma suspects are a group of individuals who have a risk of developing glaucoma or in whom there is a suspicion that glaucoma is developing. This group may include individuals with elevated IOP (ocular hypertension), those with a visual field defect consistent with glaucoma without other signs, or those with an optic nerve appearance consistent with glaucoma without any other signs.

Different models have evolved to indicate when therapy for ocular hypertension is indicated. Some practitioners, being conservative, opt to wait for obvious optic nerve or visual field damage, while others may initiate therapy in select cases when the IOP is elevated but definitive glaucoma damage has not been identified. In the latter situation, the risk factors for developing glaucoma are reviewed along with the examination data (optic nerve, visual fields, biomicroscopy, gonioscopy). The benefits of therapy are evaluated against the risks, and treatment is considered when the benefits are predominant. This model takes into account the patient's ocular history, medical history, family history, occupation, and mental status in addition to the IOP, optic nerve findings, and integrity of the visual field. The model has evolved as new instrumentation, surgical modalities, and medications became available. Murray's rule is one such model used in deciding which glaucoma suspects/ocular hypertensives may require treatment. It was developed on the basis of listening, reading, observing, and working with many individuals. In this model, the risks (family history, race, systemic health, ocular status), signs (optic nerve appearance, visual fields, gonioscopy, biomicroscopic signs of secondary glaucoma), and other pertinent data (IOP) are carefully weighed in deciding whether treatment is indicated. The clinical information is analyzed by the best computer possible, the human brain, and an outcome is arrived at (treat, do not treat, follow). This rule is meant to be a clinical guide and not a doctrine or "cookbook." Each case must always be weighed individually and decided on its merits. It may seem contradictory that, although the diagnostic limitations of the IOP are well known, it is nevertheless the IOP on which this rule largely depends.

Murray's Rule

1. The base starting point is 30 mmHg, which has historically been the "chickening out" point, where most practitioners initiate therapy even when there are no signs of glaucoma (see Fig. 21–2). The Baltimore Eye Study revealed the significance of this mark in indicating that the risk for developing glaucoma increased as the IOP approached 30 mmHg.[71]

MURRAY'S RULE
Initiating Therapy in Ocular Hypertension
Based upon the Highest Measured IOP, Associated Risk Factors and Ocular Signs

Consider therapy if highest IOP measurement 30 mm Hg or greater

Add 1.0 mm Hg to the Base IOP for the following:
• Apparent healthy looking optic nerves with C/D ratio not greater than 0.2 in greatest dimension

Subtract 1.5 mm Hg from the Base IOP for the following:
• Race- African American
• Family History of Glaucoma
• IOP Asymmetry of 5 mm Hg or greater between the eyes
• Monocular
• Cup disc asymmetry of 0.2 or greater
• Cup disc ratio greater than or equal to 0.6
• Individuals less than 50 years of age
• Secondary glaucoma findings
        Pigment dispersion syndrome
        Pseudoexfoliation
        Angle recession
        Steroid responder

Subtract 0.5 mm Hg from the Base IOP for the following:
• 50–59 years old
• Systemic vascular conditions
        examples- diabetes, hypertension, carotid artery disease, atherosclerosis
• Patients unable to perform a visual field test

Figure 21–2. Murray's rule, a checklist that aids clinicians in determining whether therapy may be indicated for ocular hypertension.

2. Optic nerves with small, healthy optic cups (C/D in greatest dimension not greater than 0.2) and a wide, even area of neuroretinal rim allow a margin of +1 mmHg. The starting base would now be 31 mmHg.

3. The following risk factors are significant and demand consideration in deciding who may develop open-angle glaucoma.[71,75,78] When any of these exist, 1.5 mmHg is subtracted from the base starting point.

   a. African American race
   b. Family history of glaucoma
   c. IOP asymmetry between the eyes of 5 mmHg or greater
   d. Ocular status—uniocular, with only one functioning eye for any reason
   e. Cup-to-disc asymmetry between the eyes of 0.2 or greater
   f. Cup-to-disc ratio greater than or equal to 0.6
   g. Age below 50 years
   h. Secondary glaucoma findings (e.g., pigment dispersion syndrome, pseudoexfoliation)

4. The following risk factors and conditions must also be considered in determining who may develop glaucoma, but they do not carry the risk of the factors listed above. Where any of these exists, 0.5 mmHg is subtracted from the base starting point.

   a. Age between 50 and 60 years
   b. Systemic vascular conditions such as diabetes, hypertension, carotid artery disease, or atherosclerosis
   c. Inability to perform a test such as perimetry

For this model, only 1.5 or 0.5 is allotted per category even if several factors from the same category are identified. An example would be an individual who had diabetes and hypertension. In this situation, only 0.5 mmHg would be subtracted from the base points. Also, when half numbers are found, they are rounded up to the higher number. In addition to this model, other factors must be considered, such as the risks versus benefits of therapy, the age and health of the individual, the anxiety of both the patient and the doctor, the patient's mental status, his or her occupation, how compliant the patient is expected to be, and the level of family support. Any of these variables may influence the decision regarding when therapy for ocular hypertension is indicated. Murray's rule is meant to provide guidance and organization for practitioners as they weigh the different pieces of information utilized in determining when therapy should be instituted. It is used with common sense, recognizing the limitations of any "guideline" and always keeping the patient's best interests in mind.

Treatment for open-angle glaucoma becomes mandatory when visual field and/or optic nerve head changes occur that are consistent with glaucoma, independent of the level of IOP. If the pressure is always low (below 17 mmHg) after diurnal IOP testing is performed, a normal-tension glaucoma evaluation is indicated (see Chap. 30). Another indication for instituting therapy is when IOP measurements are greater than 21 mmHg, along with a history of a retinal occlusive vascular disorder. Treatment is then indicated bilaterally, even if the optic nerve and visual fields in the uninvolved eye appear healthy, since the objective is to reduce the IOP to prevent a branch or central retinal vein occlusion from occurring in the contralateral eye.

The individual presenting with elevated IOP in one eye only also requires evaluation. After a careful examination to rule out secondary causes for the IOP elevation, a decision must be made as to whether the eye without elevated IOP also requires therapy. Bear in mind that POAG is a bilateral and asymmetrical condition, so that it is not unusual to find one eye with a lower IOP that may still require therapy.

A different clinical scenario is one in which the patient refuses treatment because of his or her feelings of apprehension. This problem is especially acute if there is already glaucomatous damage. Such apprehension may, for example, be due to complications resulting from previous treatment of the other eye. In such a situation, patient education is crucial for proper care, with all findings and the patient's wishes carefully documented in the record. Finally, another consideration is the patient diagnosed at an early age e.g., before (the age of 40) who requires aggressive management, considering that he or she will have the disease for many years.

INITIATING THERAPY

The objective of instituting therapy is to control the glaucomatous disease process and prevent further damage. Associated with any treatment regimen is an inherent risk of complications and undesired side effects due to the medications or procedures. The relative likelihood of achieving the desired benefits in the face of the possible risks of complications is known as the "risk-to-benefit ratio," Glaucoma is not exempt from this association. As is evident from Chap. 20, in the review of glaucoma medication pharmacology, the topical and oral antiglaucoma agents all have potential ocular and systemic side effects, so that the risk-to-benefit ratio must be considered for each individual before treatment is begun.

Uniocular Trial

Once the decision to treat is made, topical medications are begun in one eye only (uniocular trial) for a short period of time. If the IOP is markedly elevated with advanced damage in both eyes and treatment must be urgently instituted bilaterally, one approach may be to use an oral carbonic anhydrase inhibitor (CAI) temporarily while a uniocular trial is performed. If the trial is positive, the topical medication is used in both eyes and the CAI withdrawn. The uniocular therapeutic trial is a useful tool in determining how each individual may react to a given medication. It is designed to determine both the efficacy of a particular medication in reducing the IOP and any side effects that may be related to the drug. The uniocular trial should also be considered whenever a medication is added or changed; it is also required because a given glaucoma medication is not effective in every individual. The trial is performed by instilling a medication in one eye only, preferably the eye with the higher IOP, and using the fellow eye as an untreated control. The intraocular pressure is evaluated 2 to 3 weeks after starting therapy, preferably at the same time of day as during the pretrial checks. Assuming that the diurnal variation is equal in both eyes (which is not always the case),[79] the IOP reduction is evaluated, as is the difference between the two eyes. Also, when topical beta blockers are used, the contralateral eye's IOP may be lowered with unilateral instillation.[80,81] If a 20% or greater decrease in IOP is noted in the treated eye as compared with the untreated eye, the trial is positive and the patient should then use the medication in both eyes. In addition, the side effects, both ocular and systemic, are evaluated to determine whether the medication can safely be tolerated by the patient.

Choosing a Medication

Ocular Considerations

Certain ocular conditions may coexist with glaucoma, prohibiting the use of specific antiglaucoma medications.

Uvea. A history of or an active inflammatory process of the uvea, particularly an anterior uveitis, precludes the use of topical cholinergic agonists or topical prosta-

glandins. Miotics may enhance the formation of posterior synechiae, increase ciliary spasm, and exacerbate a quiescent inflammation. Open anterior chamber angles must be confirmed before pilocarpine is used in open-angle glaucoma, since its use may narrow the angle, potentially leading to the development of chronic angle-closure glaucoma. Topical prostaglandins may reactivate anterior uveitis or create an anterior uveitis in eyes having had intraocular surgery and a difficult postoperative course.[82]

Lens. Patients under 40 years of age with active accommodation will not tolerate the accommodative spasm induced by cholinergic stimulation of the ciliary muscle. Miotics should also be avoided in patients with cataracts located centrally along the visual axis, so as to prevent loss of visual acuity. Use of adrenergic agonists should be avoided in aphakic and pseudophakic patients owing to the increased risk of cystoid macular edema. Topical prostaglandins may be associated with cystoid macular edema, especially in postoperative eyes having a difficult postsurgical course.[82] Phospholine iodide is contraindicated in phakic patients because of the increased risk of developing cataracts.

Retina. Miotics should be used with caution in patients with a history of peripheral retinal holes or tears owing to the risk of inducing a retinal detachment by the strong contraction of the ciliary muscle on the peripheral retina. This problem can be significant in highly myopic individuals, who are more likely to have peripheral retinal degeneration.

Systemic Considerations

Although glaucoma is a disease confined to the eye, its treatment, especially with topical beta blockers, warrants systemic health considerations. Patients must be educated about the potential systemic side effects secondary to topical medications, since most individuals will recognize a side effect due to a tablet taken orally without realizing that similar side effects may be due to eyedrops. It is important to review an individual's medical history, both past and present, and, when necessary, to consult the patient's primary care physician regarding the use of topical medications. Also, all patients should be taught to either occlude the punctum or close their eyes for 3 minutes after eyedrop instillation to prevent any medication from entering the systemic circulation.

Pulmonary System. Topical beta blockers may have specific effects on the pulmonary system. If the beta$_2$ receptors found in the pulmonary smooth muscle are blocked by a topical beta$_2$ antagonist, bronchoconstriction may result. This can lead to detrimental effects, especially if a patient suffers from chronic obstructive pulmonary disease (COPD), asthma, or emphysema. Timolol, a nonselective beta blocker, has been shown to decrease FEV1 in patients with documented asthma or COPD.[23,83] Few published data are available for the other nonselective beta blockers. Also, the cardioselectivity of betaxolol does not exclude it from causing pulmonary side effects, and it must be used with caution in cases of relative contraindication to nonselective beta blockers. Given the different therapeutic alternatives now available (alpha-adrenergic agonists, topical CAIs, prostaglandins), other therapeutic options should be explored in patients with pulmonary problems before considering even a cardioselective beta blocker.

Cardiovascular System. Systemic beta blockers have been used for many years for the treatment of cardiovascular disease, so it stands to reason that systemic absorption of topical beta blockers may have a secondary effect on the cardiovascular system. Beta blockers have been reported to cause heart block in susceptible individuals, bradycardia, arrhythmia, hypotension, and exacerbation of congestive heart failure.[83] Although the resting pulse rate may not be affected, reduction of exercise-induced tachycardia has been shown with timolol and levobunolol.[84–86] Because of its reduced affinity for beta$_1$-receptor binding as compared with timolol, betaxolol has demonstrated less cardiac blockade than timolol.[87,88] One reason a topical beta blocker may not be effective in reducing the IOP is that the person may also be taking an oral beta blocker. In this situation, the IOP may already be maximally reduced from beta blockade. When a patient on a topical beta blocker is to discontinue its use and has been on it for a period of time, tapered withdrawal is recommended, since one report has documented reflex tachycardia after abrupt withdrawal of timolol.[89]

The adrenergic agonists also warrant consideration with regard to cardiovascular response.[43] Patients with coronary insufficiency and increased arterial blood pressure as well as those on myocardium-sensitizing drugs should avoid the use of adrenergic agonists. Also, any patient with significant cardiovascular disease or an increased propensity for arrhythmia should avoid the use of adrenergic agonists and antagonists. If any of these medications is to be used, the patient should be closely followed by his or her internist or cardiologist. Also, medications used for the treatment of hypertension or cardiac disease may interact with ocular medications. CAIs and other diuretics

may upset the potassium balance, affect the required digitalis dosage, or induce cardiac arrhythmia.

Kidneys. CAIs may have significant effects on electrolyte balance and kidney function. Metabolic acidosis, potassium depletion (hypokalemia), and an increased propensity for the formation of kidney stones are side effects that can be significant, especially in those with a history of renal disease.[66] CAIs should be avoided in these individuals.

Endocrine System. At high dosages, CAIs may induce a metabolic acidosis that may exaggerate hypokalemia in patients using long-term corticosteroids. In addition, diabetics undergoing an attack of acute angle-closure glaucoma should avoid all oral hyperosmotic agents if possible.[90] Oral hyperosmotic agents other than isosorbide (Ismotic) undergo metabolism by the liver. Isosorbide is not metabolized and, if required, may be used with caution in diabetic patients.[91]

Starting Therapy

The First Drug

Before starting therapy, make sure all findings are carefully documented in detail, establishing a baseline diagnostic record and ruling out any secondary forms of glaucoma (Fig. 21–3). Start with the lowest dosage and strength of the selected medication, using a uniocular trial. A nonselective beta blocker, used twice daily, is generally the drug of first choice in patients without contraindications to its use. The lowest concentration is used initially and is often effective in whites with a mild form of glaucoma; the 0.5% strength is usually required in black individuals. If compliance is a factor, consider using a once-daily medication.[92,93] For patients in whom beta blockers are contraindicated, either a topical CAI, alpha$_2$ agonist, or topical prostaglandin may be the initial drug.

Document baseline exam
Establish diagnosis
Rule out secondary forms
Start with lowest dosage and strength
Uniocular trial
Counsel patient on potential side effects
Teach instillation technique of drops/ointment
Eyelid closure/punctal occlusion for 3 minutes
Always inquire about compliance at each examination

Figure 21–3. Steps in the initiation of therapy in open-angle glaucoma.

Patient Education

Patient education plays an integral role in the management of individuals with glaucoma. Each person must be aware that open-angle glaucoma is an asymptomatic, chronic, and progressive disease that is controlled by a lifelong medication and/or surgical regimen. Up to the time of diagnosis, the individual usually has not experienced any symptoms. This will change, since most medications cause problems that will test the patient's resolve and make him or her question the need to continue with therapy. The patient must understand that failure to adhere to the treatment regimen can result in loss of vision. In addition, therapy involves a financial cost to the patient, both from medications and from the frequent follow-up examinations.[94] These financial constraints may affect the patient's adherence with therapy.

Noncompliance affects many glaucomatous individuals adversely. Education is one way to improve compliance. Reassure each patient that he or she will not have to contemplate changes or restrictions in lifestyle. Calm the patients' fears and let them know that they can use their eyes, read all they want, exercise as before, and continue to drink in moderation.

Communication with the patient's general physician is important, letting him or her know what medications are being used and keeping him or her informed of any change in the treatment regimen. Also, ask the patient's physician to contact you if there is a change in the patient's health status or medication profile.

The side effects of antiglaucoma medications should be discussed with the patient prior to their use, with verbal and written dosage schedules provided (Fig. 21–4). Explain that systemic side effects may be due to the eyedrops and ask patients to record side effects when they occur and to contact you in that event. In-office education and training on proper eyedrop instillation will help most individuals. Many elderly people have problems putting drops into their eyes and need training to do so (Fig. 21–5). Teach the patient to squeeze the bottle from the bottom, not the side, and document all forms of patient education in the chart (Fig. 21–6). Remind patients to occlude the punctum with a finger or close the eyelids for 3 minutes after eyedrop instillation to reduce systemic absorption and increase the therapeutic index (Fig. 21–7).[13] Try to incorporate the dosage schedule into the patient's daily routine. If possible, patients should refrigerate all medications and feel for the cold sting when a drop hits the eye. If multiple medications are used, a separation of 5 minutes between drops prevents dilution or washout of the first eyedrop. A record is kept in the chart when prescriptions are written, the number of refills, and the size of the bottle. This record may be helpful in the treatment of patients requiring refills too frequently, as they may be instilling the medications improperly, or for individuals who rarely require refills, possibly indicating poor compliance. Be careful with the number of refills and size of bottle given to patients with questionable compliance who may not return for future examinations. Compliant patients are usually given multiple prescriptions for each medication, so that a separate bottle may be left in the office, at home, or wherever it will be accessible when the time for drop instillation occurs. Larger-size bottles (10 or 15 mL) are more cost-effective than the 5-mL size, so the larger bottle, when available, may be prescribed for compliant individuals.

Frequently, patients have difficulty in pronouncing the names of medications. Also, several of these names sound the same, so when medical regimens are reviewed during follow-up visits, some confusion occurs. To avoid confusion for both the patient and the clinician, the topical medications may also be identified by the color of the bottle or bottle cap (Fig. 21–8). For instance, timolol (Timoptic) 0.5% may be identified as "the yellow bottle" or pilocarpine as "the green-capped drop." A summary of the most common bottle and cap colors is given in Table 21–1.

Although there are no studies yet linking smoking with glaucoma, several do link it with macular degeneration.[95,96] It appears that a disturbance in blood flow regulation develops due to smoking,[97,98] which may also relate to the development of glaucoma. In

TABLE 21–1. COMMON BOTTLE AND CAP COLORS OF GLAUCOMA MEDICATIONS

Timolol, levobunolol, betaxolol 0.25%	Light blue cap
Timolol, levobunolol 0.50%	Yellow cap
Betaxolol 0.5%	Dark blue cap
Metipranolol 0.3%	White cap
Carteolol 1.0%	Yellow cap
Pilocarpine (all concentrations)	Green cap
Carbachol (all concentrations)	Green cap
Phospholine iodide (all concentrations)	Clear glass bottle
Dipivefrin	Purple cap
Epinephrine (all concentrations)	Brown bottle or white cap/red label
Apraclonidine	White cap
Brimonidine	Purple cap
Dorzolamide	Orange cap
Brinzolamide	Orange cap
Timolol and dorzolamide	Orange and yellow cap
Latanoprost	Clear top

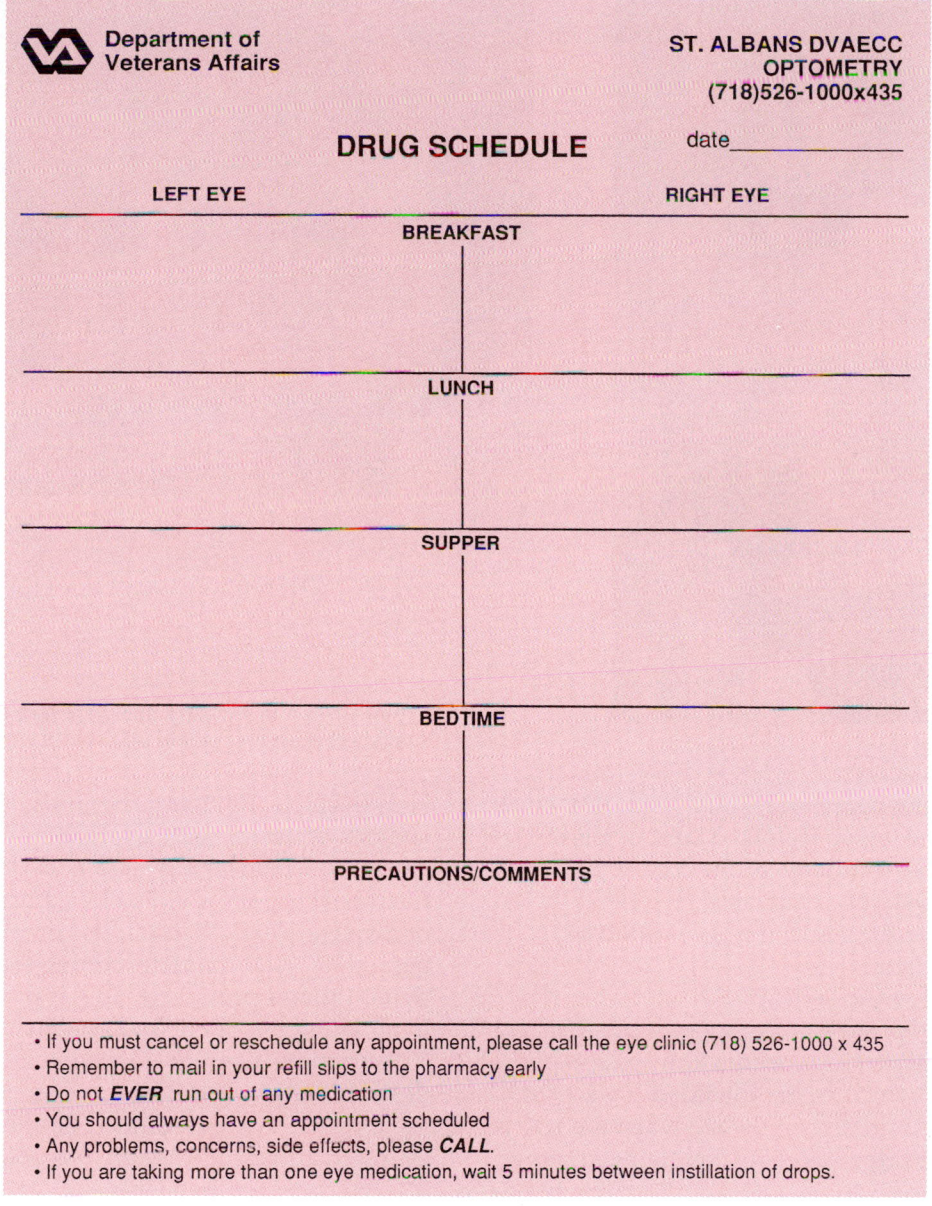

Figure 21-4. Patient information dosage schedule.

regard to exercise, there are several studies showing that it may reduce the IOP and be helpful for any individual with glaucoma or ocular hypertension.[99,100] Weight loss and a healthy diet may also help individuals with glaucoma.[101,102] Thus any patient diagnosed with glaucoma may benefit from counseling in regard to smoking cessation, weight loss, diet, and exercise. Although many individuals have heard it before, telling them one more time and documenting this conversation in the chart can do no harm and may help some individuals to understand their glaucoma better.

Treatment Schemes

Goals for Therapy

The more advanced the damage associated with glaucoma, the more the IOP must be reduced to stabilize the optic nerve and prevent further visual field loss. The goal for therapy is to provide a low enough IOP throughout the day that optic nerve damage and visual field loss are arrested, using the least expensive, safest medications possible. With this in mind, an individualized therapeutic plan is designed, taking into account the patient's medical history, prior

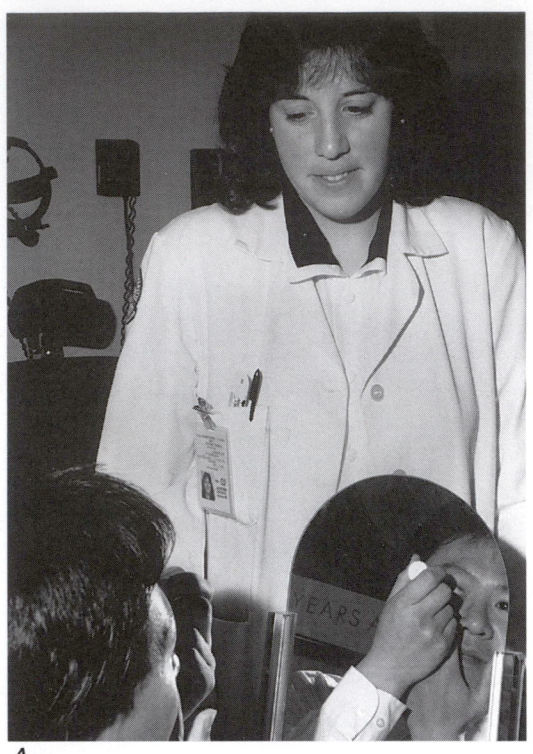

A

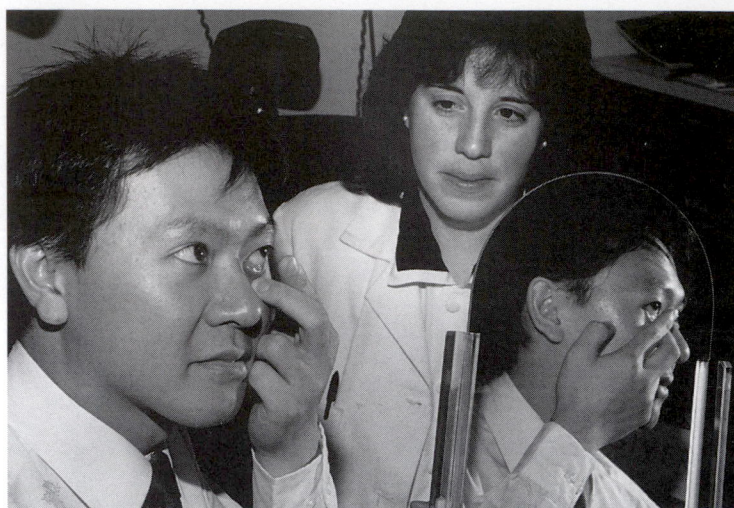

B

Figure 21–5. On initiating therapy, instruction is required in the proper technique for eyedrop (*A*) and ointment instillation (*B*).

damage to the optic nerve and visual field, IOP level, ocular history, and other factors. Many of these factors, including the condition of the visual field and optic nerve, must be evaluated periodically to determine whether the glaucoma is controlled.

Functional Groups/Target IOP

A functional group scheme, proposed by Richardson,[103] provides general guidelines toward establishing a target IOP, which is the intended level of IOP when treatment is initiated. In theory, when the IOP is consistently at the target level, further damage should

be prevented. By using the initial range of IOP measurements along with evaluation of the optic nerve and visual field along with a risk-factor assessment, functional groups are developed based upon the level of damage. The IOP in the less involved eye is another parameter useful in determining the target IOP. Functional groups provide a simple picture that is useful in initiating treatment and establishing a target IOP.

Another way of formulating target IOPs was described in the text of Hodapp et al.[104] In this model, the target IOP is determined on the basis of the highest pretreatment IOP as well as the extent of damage

PROCEDURE FOR PROPER EYE DROP ADMINISTRATION
1) BASIC INSTRUCTIONS FOR EYE DROP INSTILLATION GIVEN ☐
2) ADVISED PT TO:
   1. EYELID CLOSURE FOR 3 MINUTES ☐
   2. WAIT 5 MINUTES BETWEEN DIFFERENT DROPS ☐
3) REVIEWED TIME SCHEDULE OF MEDICATIONS/GIVEN DOSAGE SCHEDULE ☐
4) RETURN DEMONSTRATION DONE:
   GOOD UNDERSTANDING OF TECHNIQUE ☐
   NEEDS REINFORCEMENT ☐
5) STRESSED NECESSITY:
   1. TO KEEP APPOINTMENTS ☐
   2. DO NOT RUN OUT OF MEDICATIONS ☐
   3. TO TAKE DROPS AS ORDERED ☐

SIGN: _____

Figure 21–6. A stamp placed on the patient's record documents that patient education has been performed.

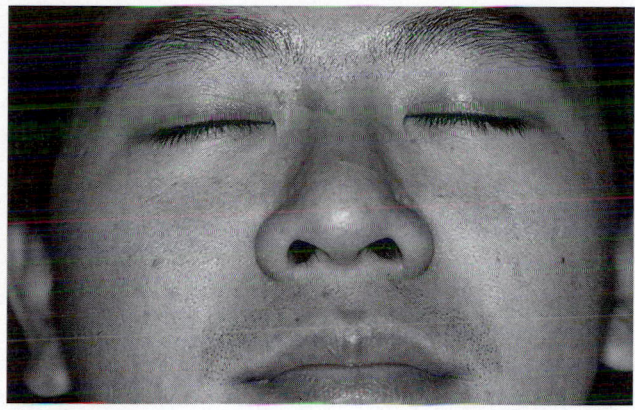

A

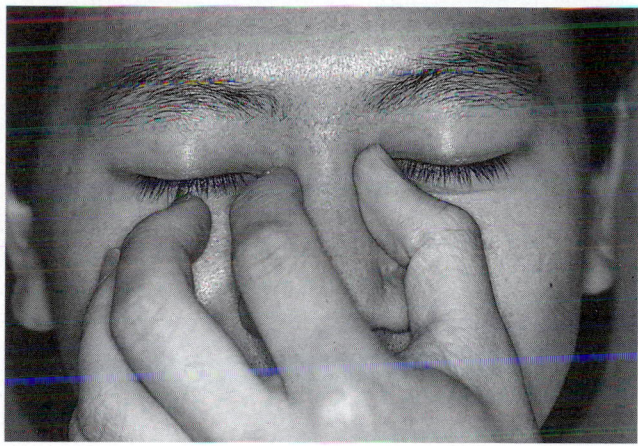

B

Figure 21–7. On instillation of topical medications, eyelid closure (*A*) or punctal occlusion (*B*) will reduce systemic absorption of the medication.

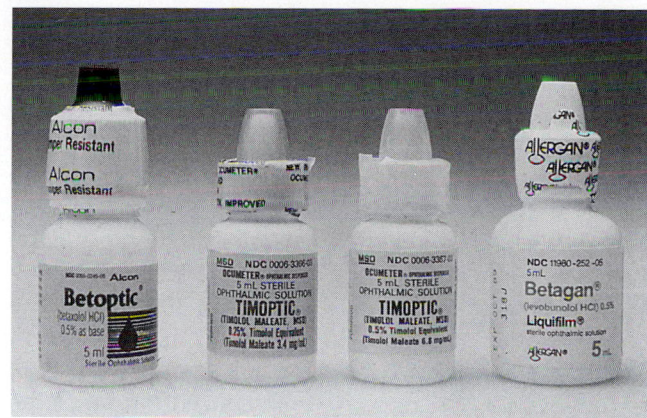

Figure 21–8. Ophthalmic medications may be identified by the color of the bottle or bottle cap.

to the optic nerve and visual field. The higher the IOP and the greater the amount of damage, the more the IOP needs to be lowered. The amount of reduction is determined by a percentage, not absolute numbers. A small cup with an IOP around 25 mmHg with mild visual field loss requires an initial IOP reduction of 25% to get to the expected target. An IOP in the mid-30s with moderate visual field loss and/or moderate optic nerve damage may require a 45 to 50% reduction. Advanced damage, with or without IOP elevation, may require a pressure reduction up to 60% to reach the required level.

Another way to think about the target IOPs is with regard to the number of medication(s) utilized to reach the needed level. A 20 to 30% reduction in IOP may be achieved with one medication, but a greater drop would require two or more drugs. Thus, for moderate to advanced glaucoma, the clinician will know at the outset that two or more drugs will

be required to control the condition; he or she will then have to decide which combination of medication(s) would best achieve the desired goal. Medications are still started one at a time, using a uniocular trial. One key point is that the target IOP is an arbitrary determination. Only careful observation of the optic nerve and visual fields will ensure that the condition is stable.

One difficulty with any system used to determine the target IOP lies in deciding whether the optic nerve or visual field has suffered mild, moderate, or advanced damage. For the visual fields, damage in one hemifield not involving fixation is labeled as mild. When both hemifields are involved, fixation is involved, or a great many points in one hemifield are affected, the damage is moderate. Advanced damage occurs when extensive injury is seen in both hemifields. The grading of optic nerve damage is more difficult and subjective than that of damage to the visual fields because one does not always know where the optic nerve damage began. Thus the grading is subjective and relies on the extent of damage to the neuroretinal rim as well as the cup/disc ratio.

The tendency for many clinicians is to add medications until the IOP is as low as possible, but this approach may unnecessarily increase patient morbidity and expense. Rather, establish a target IOP level based upon risk factors, the highest untreated IOP, and damage to the optic nerve and visual fields and modify the therapeutic regimen as needed to meet this goal. The target IOP may not be obtainable because of excessive side effects or poor patient response. A decision must then be made regarding how aggressive therapy must be to meet the target IOP. Care must be taken to not overtreat, but, at the same time, if signs of progression occur, the therapeutic regimen must be reevaluated. This includes increasing the concentration and/or dosage of the medications, adding an additional medication, or considering a surgical procedure. Finally, with increasing damage, the target IOP must be reset to a lower level.

At the follow-up visit, the side effects and proximity to the target IOP are assessed. Compare the pretreatment IOP level to the level after therapy. Is the IOP low enough? If the difference between the post-treatment and target IOP is small, increasing the concentration or dosage (if available) may be appropriate, while a large difference may require a change in the medication, an increase in concentration, or the addition of another medication. Second-line medications that may be added to a topical beta blocker include topical CAIs, topical prostaglandins, and alpha₂ agonists. Third-line treatments include any of the drugs not previously utilized as well as argon laser trabeculoplasty. The selection of a medication is based upon individual characteristics, and often any of the available agents may be appropriate. Still, when a large reduction in IOP is needed (40% decrease or greater), utilizing one medication that reduces aqueous production or inflow, such as a beta blocker, along with another that improves outflow (such as a topical prostaglandin, a miotic, or an alpha agonist) is often efficacious.

Dosage and Follow-up Schedule

The first follow-up visit after initiation of therapy is scheduled in 2 to 4 weeks. The return examination should include history (time of last medication instillation, symptoms, side effects, or changes in systemic health), visual acuity, pulse (if on beta blocker), slit-lamp evaluation, IOP measurement, and an abbreviated optic nerve assessment. Most important is the assessment of the patient's acceptance of the treatment regimen and reinforcement of education about the chronic nature of glaucoma. Any reports of side effects must be evaluated. When side effects occur, a decision must be made as to whether the medication must be eliminated or the concomitant management for these side effects is possible. For example, the sting of an eyedrop can be better tolerated if the medication has been refrigerated before it is used.

Decreased visual acuity, confirmed with a pinhole, necessitates a visual field and dilated fundus examination to rule out new pathology. A dilated fundus exam is also indicated at least yearly in all glaucomatous individuals and in patients with new complaints of photopsia after miotic therapy has been initiated to rule out an acute retinal tear or detachment.

The IOP is evaluated relative to the level before treatment as well as the desired level with treatment (target IOP). Alterations in the medication regimen are

Select target pressure based on prior damage, IOP level, history
Maintain IOP below that level with intervention as needed
Monitor visual fields, optic nerve for progression
Reset target pressure (lower) with increasing damage
Minimize side effects of medications
Recognize failure in medications early
Move to advanced therapy as needed (laser, surgery)

Figure 21–9. Open-angle glaucoma management.

made if the target IOP is not met (Fig. 21–9). Early in the course of therapy, several visits with modifications in the treatment regimen may be required until the target IOP is met. Evaluating the IOP at the end of the dosage schedule (trough) is a better indicator of control than an IOP measurement taken just after instillation. Whenever a medication is added, deleted, or changed, a new dosage schedule is written and given to the patient with a follow-up examination scheduled for approximately 2 to 4 weeks later. Occasionally, a new medication does little to lower IOP, and this is usually obvious when the medication is added as part of a uniocular trial. In this case, if compliance is not the problem, the new medication can be discontinued and a stronger concentration tried, if available, or a medication from another class can be tried. Because medications are not always effective, two medications should rarely be started at the same time.

Biomicroscopy should be performed at every visit to check for allergic reactions, toxicity, and changes in the color of the iris as well as to verify compliance with miotics (small fixed pupil). Visual fields may be examined with a dilated pupil, often at the same time as the yearly dilated fundus examination. Dilation will reduce the peripheral field constriction due to a small pupil. It is not imperative that all pupils be dilated before visual field exams are done, but it is important that the pupil size be consistent from field to field. Dilation is not required if the lens is clear or the pupil in a dark room is 3 mm or larger. When they are using miotics, patients should discontinue them 2 days prior to their visit if dilation is planned. Dilation with a mydriatic and cycloplegic solution is then necessary, especially with darkly pigmented eyes, to provide maximum mydriasis and to prevent the formation of posterior synechiae. After the examination, the patient is instructed to resume miotic therapy and may need to return shortly for additional IOP assessment if the IOP is elevated.

Continual evaluation of the patient's history, IOP, optic nerves, gonioscopy, and visual fields is required, since all can change with time. Patients should be reexamined at 2 to 4 weeks, 6 to 8 weeks, and then 3 to 4 months after treatment is initiated; however, those who are poorly controlled must be seen more often to get their disease under control. Once patients are stable, a visit every 3 to 4 months is appropriate.

A glaucoma flowchart is used to keep track of each visit, documenting the IOP and time of the visit, when tests were performed, medications or procedures utilized, and changes in the treatment plan. The use of a flowchart, in addition to the patient record, allows the recording of all findings related to the glaucoma examination (Figs. 21–10 and 21–11). A flowchart simplifies follow-up, provides maximum management efficiency, and allows one to see trends in the IOP, optic nerve, or visual field.[105]

Modifying the Therapeutic Regimen

Once a drug has been started, its effect must be evaluated. If the medication is effective but the IOP is still higher than desired, the medication must be increased in either strength or dosage, if possible, or a second medication must be added. This is the "step

method" of management (Fig. 21–12). A medication is modified or another class of medication is added (step), and this is always with a uniocular trial. Each time the IOP is too high (above the target IOP) or progression is seen, another step is taken until all medical alternatives are exhausted. Side effects due to medications may be another reason to discontinue one medication (step) and go on to the next. Many years ago, surgery of any type was not performed until all medical options were exhausted. Thus, patients on maximally tolerated medical therapy would be taking or would at least have tried three or four medications. Now surgery is considered before all medical options are exhausted, on an individual basis.

There is no typical treatment scheme utilized by each clinician, but rather the medical regimen is tailored for each individual patient. Topical beta blockers are often the first class of medications used, though there is no rule that precludes the use of an-

Name_____			**Glaucoma Flowsheet**				When? Where? What?	
Address_____		Type					Previous DX_____	
SS#_____			V				Previous TX_____	
DOB_____		C/D	R				MH_____	
TEL #_____			L					
Date	IOP	VF	DFE	GON	PIX	Comments/Exam Results	Meds/Start/Δ	Referral

Figure 21–10. Example of flowsheet for open-angle glaucoma.

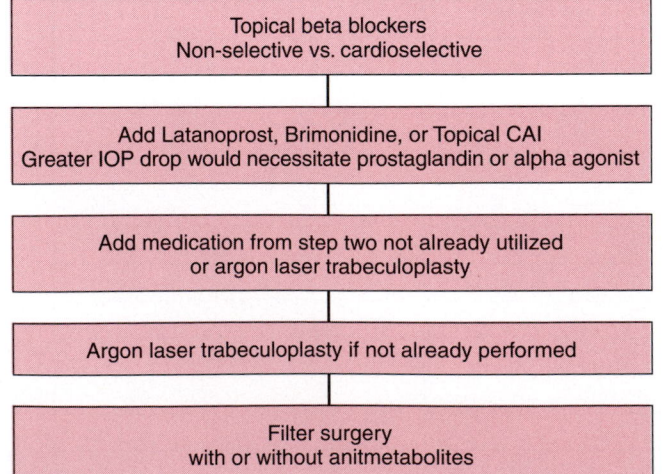

Name **Jack Straw** *s/p cat. extraction* **Glaucoma Flowsheet**

Address **Wichita** *ē FILTER OD 1984*

SS# *1 - - - - - 1* Type **COAG**

DOB **2-22-20** C/D R .55/.60

TEL # *(-) - -* L .5/.5

V 20/20⁻ cc 20/20⁻

When? Where? What?

Previous DX **HIP, MANHATTAN VA**

Previous TX **T 1/2 x 2 OD   x 5 yrs**

MH ⊕ HTN

Date	IOP	VF	DFE	GON	PIX	Comments/Exam Results	Meds/Start/Δ	Referral
1-11-90	13/23 11³⁰ AM							
1-30-90	13/20 1⁵⁰ PM		✓		✓		START T 1/2 x 2 OU	
2-22-90		✓				pt called to say VF done @ HIP – pt told to bring copy (DR. 니미미)		
2-14-90	12/14 8⁴⁵							
3-14-90	12/18 8³⁰ AM	–				pt had D/C T 1/2 for last 2 weeks		
3-19-90		✓	@ HIP - HUMPHREY			VF < sup arc / early sup arc		
4-16-90	10/14 12 NOON							
5-22-90	11/14 9³⁰					D/C T 1/2 due to palpitations,	START B 1/2 x 2 OS only	

89 SEP 33 PM 12:10

Figure 21–11. Example of a sample completed flowsheet.

Topical beta blockers
Non-selective vs. cardioselective

Add Latanoprost, Brimonidine, or Topical CAI
Greater IOP drop would necessitate prostaglandin or alpha agonist

Add medication from step two not already utilized
or argon laser trabeculoplasty

Argon laser trabeculoplasty if not already performed

Filter surgery
with or without anitmetabolites

Figure 21–12. Flowchart for the management of open-angle glaucoma.

other class for front-line therapy. If, after using one medication, further IOP reduction is required, either because of progressing damage or because the IOP remains above the target goal, a decision is made to add or substitute either a topical prostaglandin, topical CAI, or alpha agonist to the first medication. If the IOP needs further reduction, either a new medication is added or substituted (one not utilized previously) or argon laser trabeculoplasty (ALT) is performed. Some clinicians do not have patients take more than two medications, feeling that compliance is reduced with more than two, and use ALT as the next modality. Finally, filtering surgery is considered if damage continues after medications and ALT have been utilized. For individuals who present initially with advanced glaucomatous damage, filtering surgery may be the only modality that will achieve a safe target pressure. Another situation in which to consider either laser or filtering surgery initially is in treating individuals whose compliance is questionable, for whatever reason.

Rather than thinking in terms of the number of medications that a patient may be able to effectively take and still be compliant in the therapeutic regimen, another model is to use the number of drug instillations performed per day. Each time a patient takes a drop of a medication, this is considered an instillation. For example, an individual taking timolol twice per day in each eye along with latanoprost once at bedtime is using three instillations per eye. Patients who take four or less instillations per day usually show excellent compliance, with five instillations producing borderline results. When six or more instillations of all glaucoma medications are required per day, compliance appears to suffer. As we have more medications with q.d. or b.i.d. dosage, along with combination medications, we have greater flexibility in tailoring a treatment regimen, so that no more than 4 or 5 drops are taken in each eye per day.

Argon laser trabeculoplasty (ALT) has become an effective method for reducing the IOP and is often viewed as an alternative to adding another medication (see Chap. 22). By applying focal laser burns to the trabecular meshwork in open-angle glaucoma, ALT may reduce the IOP. ALT is similar to adding a medication, since it rarely replaces medications already in use. The use of ALT delays the time interval before another medication or filtering surgery becomes necessary and, in rare instances, ALT may be the treatment of choice if poor compliance is likely to hinder adequate medical management.

Oral CAIs are rarely used to treat glaucoma. Although they reduce the IOP significantly, their numerous side effects limit their usefulness, and topical CAIs have taken their place. If oral CAIs are to be added to the topical regimen, the patient must be educated on the proper dosage and frequency of administration. Starting with methazolamide (Neptazane) 25 mg two times a day, the dosage is increased in 25-mg steps should the IOP-lowering effect not be adequate. The dosage should not exceed 50 mg three times a day. Occasionally, though it is not recommended, an increase in the dose of methazolamide to a maximum of 100 mg three times a day may demonstrate a greater ocular hypotensive effect, but these patients must be monitored carefully for side effects. In sensitive individuals, acetazolamide (Diamox) 250-mg tablets may be substituted for methazolamide, starting at 125 mg (one-half tablet) four times a day and building to 250 mg four times a day as needed. If this is still unsuccessful, Diamox Sequels (500 mg) may reduce IOP further.

LONG-TERM MANAGEMENT

POAG requires monitoring and follow-up throughout the patient's life. Tolerance may develop to any medication over time, leading to inadequate control, IOP elevation, and progression. When glaucoma appears stable, examinations are scheduled for every 3 to 4 months. The return visit should consist of a history, IOP evaluation, determination of visual acuity, pulse measurement (for beta blockers), slit-lamp examination, and undilated optic nerve examination. The history includes time of last medication, symptoms, any changes in health, and noted side effects. Gonioscopy should also be done yearly. An extended visit is scheduled at least yearly for a dilated fundus exam, photography, and visual field testing. The visual fields and optic nerves should be compared with previous slides and fields, looking for change. Depending on the stage of the disease, follow-up examinations may need to be scheduled more frequently than on a quarterly basis.

It may take several visits to determine whether progression has occurred by observing changes in the diagnostic data. For example, automated visual field testing must be repeated to differentiate long-term fluctuation or ptosis-induced superior field depression from true glaucomatous visual field loss. The management regimen should not be altered on the basis of a solitary diagnostic finding. If progression in damage to the visual fields or optic nerves is noted, the treatment regimen must be adjusted as well. Also, the fields or optic nerves may be stable, but if the IOP rises to unacceptable levels (above the target IOP), the treatment regimen may have to be modified. Once extensive damage to the optic nerve has occurred, leaving it completely cupped with visual fields constricted to a few degrees, the central 10-degree visual field is used for follow-up. When central vision is lost, the IOP and optic nerves become the only parameters to monitor.

The ocular and systemic side effects of medications must be continually assessed using the history from a well-educated patient. Still, subtle side effects may occur that are not always appreciated by the patient. If side effects are a problem, one must determine whether the medication's dosage or concentration can be reduced or whether the medication must be discontinued and another substituted (Table 21–2).

FAILURE OF THERAPY

One of the most frustrating aspects of the treatment of glaucoma is the failure of medications to control the

TABLE 21–2. GLAUCOMA MEDICATIONS MODIFICATIONS

IOP Control	Medication Tolerance	Management Adjustments
IOP goal reached	Tolerated well	Continue treatment
IOP goal reached	Tolerated poorly	1. Lower concentration if possible and recheck IOP 2. Lower dosage if possible 3. Switch medications
Borderline control	Tolerated well	1. Follow visual field, optic nerve, IOP closely without modifications in medications 2. Increase concentration 3. Increase dosage 4. Add another medication
Poor control	Tolerated well	1. Increase concentration 2. Increase dosage 3. Add another medication 4. Repeat steps 1, 2, and/or 3 until IOP at desired range (do only one step at a time)
Borderline or poor control	Tolerated poorly	1. Stop present medications 2. Switch to other medications 3. Consider ALT or surgery

Key: IOP, intraocular pressure; ALT, argon laser trabeculoplasty.

disease adequately. Maintaining the IOP at a level appropriate to prevent optic nerve and visual field deterioration is a goal that is not always achieved with medications, because of either the progressive nature of the condition, its severity, poor response to medications, or noncompliance on the part of the patient.

When advancing visual field loss occurs in the presence of an acceptable IOP and apparent compliance, progressive optic neuropathy may not be associated with glaucoma. Optic nerve or retinal disorders that mimic glaucomatous field loss or cupping must then be ruled out. The differential diagnosis of optic nerve disease other than glaucoma includes optic nerve drusen, cerebral tumors, ischemic optic neuropathy, and orbital or optic nerve neoplasms.

Poor IOP control may result from the development of tolerance (tachyphylaxis) to a medication. Timolol and other beta blockers may demonstrate a "long-term drift" phenomenon in which a gradual rise of IOP is noted after months or years of use. This gradual increase in IOP may eventually exceed the target IOP, necessitating a switch to a higher concentration of medication, the addition of another medication, or implementation of a laser/surgical procedure to achieve greater control. The IOP may also rise because of the slow development of peripheral anterior synechiae. This occurs in already narrow angles, and when 180 degrees or greater of the angle is occluded, chronic angle-closure glaucoma has developed. This condition is associated with the use of miotic agents. Indentation gonioscopy is the best tool to identify it (see Chap. 29).

When the IOP rises above the target goal for a patient under treatment, one response is to add an additional medication. The medication(s) being utilized must be evaluated to determine whether they are still effective or should be discontinued. The IOP elevation may be due to a worsening of the glaucoma or to the fact that the medication has lost some of its efficacy over time (long-term drift). Beta blockers are best known for developing long-term drift, though this possibility should be considered for any medication. One method to determine whether a drug is still effective is by performing a reverse uniocular trial, in which a medication is withdrawn from one eye only. The patient then returns in a few weeks, after the drug has washed out from the eye. The IOP is measured in each eye, comparing the IOP in the treated to that in the untreated eye as well as to previous IOP measurements. A rise in IOP in the untreated eye with no change in the treated eye provides evidence that the medication is working and that it should be continued, with an additional one added. If little difference is seen between IOP measurements in the treated and untreated eyes, the medication has probably lost its efficacy and should be discontinued, with another started in its place. Finally, the reverse uniocular trial must be done with care in individuals with advanced disease, since a small rise in IOP may be deleterious.

Noncompliance

Noncompliance represents the single most common and frustrating reason for failure of therapy.[106,107] All patients miss a dosage occasionally, but the goal is to minimize the number of dosages missed. Studies have shown that the more complex the therapeutic regimen, the greater the likelihood of poor compliance.[108,109] Toxicity, length of treatment, and side effects of medication also contribute to poor compliance.[109,110] There are many varieties of noncompliance; these include taking too many or too few doses, missing doses, spacing doses improperly, ineffective self-administration, or discontinuing the medication prematurely. Individuals who miss appointments often comply poorly with medications and must be managed differently from compliant individuals. Patients must also be reminded that taking additional dosages will not help their condition and may lead to additional side effects. Studies on compliance performed by Kass demonstrated the difficulty of predicting which individuals would be compliant and showed that there is little correlation with the age, sex, race, or occupation of the patient and his or her compliance.[108,110] In addition, patients tend to be compliant on the day of their examination, so the IOP measurement or pupil size is not a useful indicator of compliance.[110]

One way of reducing noncompliance is by educating the patient as to the nature of glaucoma; the proper use of the medications, including eyedrop instillation; establishing good patient-doctor rapport; and incorporating the drug regimen into the patient's daily routine. In particular, the doctor-patient relationship is important in terms of improving compliance. If the doctor is viewed as an empathetic, caring individual, there is a greater likelihood that all of his or her instructions will be followed. Patient education is also important in the sense that each individual with glaucoma needs to understand how devastating the condition may be. Patients who know the name of the disease as well as its consequences will do better in the long run. Glaucoma is a chronic, lifelong condition without symptoms, and medications will not immediately alleviate its potential consequences. Thus, patient education is paramount, so that patients will understand why medications are needed. In addition, the more complex the treatment regimen is, the greater the chance that some dosages will be missed. One may attempt to simplify the regimen as much as possible, recognizing that every time a drug is added, compliance may suffer (Tables 21–3 and 21–4).

Five steps can be used to optimize patient compliance. First, explain what glaucoma is and how it is treated, and lay out the course of therapy. Patient education should not stop after the initial diagnosis, but rather is needed throughout the patient's lifetime. Second, teach the patient how to instill medications and

TABLE 21–3 TYPES OF POOR PATIENT COMPLIANCE

Missed dosages
Cessation of therapy
Improper spacing of medications
Ineffective self-administration
Increased number of dosages

TABLE 21–4. FIVE STEPS TO IMPROVE COMPLIANCE

Explain what glaucoma is
Teach eyedrop instillation
Keep therapeutic regimen simple
Discuss medication(s)
Describe potential adverse reactions

check to ensure the patient can get the drug into the eye. Include a discussion on punctal occlusion/eyelid closure. Third, simplify the treatment scheme and tailor it to the patient's schedule. Fourth, educate the patient about the medication: how it works, cap color, and treatment goals. Fifth, describe potential adverse reactions and what the patient should do if any occur. Involve the patient in any treatment decisions and explain the patient's condition to his or her family physician, also outlining the proposed treatment.

If compliance cannot be improved, then ALT or surgery must be considered, even if the IOP can be reduced to acceptable levels with medication alone.

Comanagement and Referral

Several components are comprised in the comanagement and referral process in regard to glaucoma. In difficult cases, the practitioner may request a consultation with a glaucoma specialist to confirm the diagnosis. Such a consultation may involve additional diagnostic testing that is not available in the practitioner's office (i.e., optic nerve imaging or short-wavelength perimetry) or evaluation of the diagnostic tests. The patient may also be referred to a glaucoma specialist because of poorly controlled, persistently elevated IOP that is not responding to medical treatment. In addition, if there are any medical conditions or concurrent medical treatments that may produce adverse interactions with glaucoma medications, a visit to the internist may be helpful. Once progression occurs or the IOP no longer responds to topical medications, a consultation with a glaucoma specialist may be another therapeutic option. Certainly it is inadvisable to wait until significant visual field loss or nerve damage has occurred before making the referral. If one waits too long, it may be difficult to halt or diminish the rate of progression by any possible means.

The last component of the referral process is the examination by the comanager. The most important portion of the examination is the history. A detailed but concise letter sent to the comanager prior to the patient's appointment should outline the patient's previous diagnosis, including date of onset and date(s) and type(s) of previous treatment, with a list of the medications used or laser/surgical procedures performed. A copy of the flowchart (see Fig. 21–10) used by the referring practitioner greatly simplifies the clinical summary. The current status of the patient's optic disc, visual field, and gonioscopy findings must be included. Photographs, preferably stereo slides of the disc, will allow direct comparison, so that progressive disc damage will be apparent. With automated perimeters, include a copy of the patient's visual fields on a floppy disc, when possible, thus allowing new data to be added and returned so that direct comparisons and analyses can be made by both doctors involved in the patient's care. The impression and recommendations should be returned in a summary letter to the referring doctor to be added to the patient's file for future reference.

MANAGEMENT OF SPECIFIC TYPES OF GLAUCOMA

Normal-Tension Glaucoma

The case of low-tension, normal-tension, or pressure-independent glaucoma represents a clinical dilemma in that glaucomatous optic nerve damage and visual field defects exist in an eye with "normal" IOPs after being assessed diurnally (see Chap. 30). This condition remains a therapeutic enigma in that the underlying cause for optic nerve damage remains unclear. It may be a variant of POAG with the optic nerve sensitive to a lower IOP, or it may be due to some other factors such as reduced blood flow to the optic nerve. The target pressure should be set so that a 25 to 30% reduction is obtained. Medical therapy, while similar to that for POAG, may have little impact on IOP because of the difficulty in reducing IOP into the teens. A medication that reduces IOP by 20% may show a nice reduction when the IOP is in the 30s but lower IOP by only 1 or 2 mmHg when it is in the teens. Conflicting opinions exist on whether adrenergic agonists or topical beta blockers should be used in "pressure-independent glaucoma" because they may decrease vascular perfusion to the optic nerve, thereby contributing to potential optic nerve ischemia. Still, many experienced practitioners use these medicines if significant IOP reduction can be achieved without side effects. All patients with normotensive glaucoma should be evaluated by an internist with a careful workup of the cardiovascular and neurological systems. If progression is seen with IOPs consistently in the teens, filtration surgery may be a viable option.

Pigmentary Glaucoma

Pigmentary glaucoma is usually found in young, myopic males with signs of pigment dispersion syn-

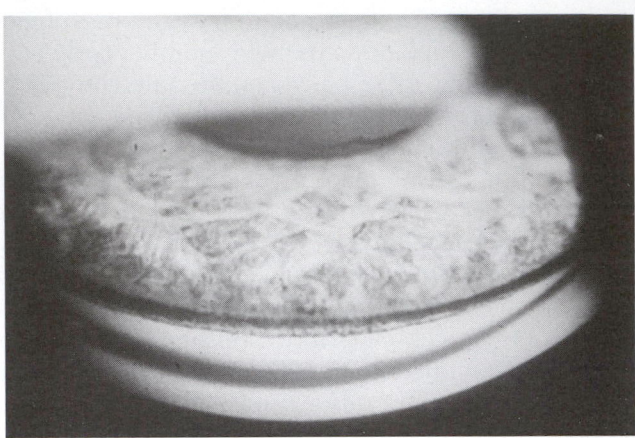

Figure 21–13. The gonioscopic appearance of a deeply pigmented trabecular meshwork associated with pigment dispersion syndrome.

drome (PDS) along with elevated IOPs (Figs. 21–13 and 21–14). The liberation of pigment from the posterior midperipheral iris results in iris transillumination defects, Krukenberg spindle formation on the corneal endothelium, and deposition of pigment debris into the trabecular meshwork (see Chap. 27). Wide fluctuations in IOP can occur. The decision to treat pigmentary glaucoma is often based upon observing the signs of pigmentary dispersion syndrome along with elevated IOP, rather than waiting for nerve and field damage. Usually, when ocular hypertension is seen along with signs of PDS, treatment is indicated.

Medical management is similar to that for POAG, with the chance that the IOP may decrease over time owing to a reduction in the liberation of pigment and

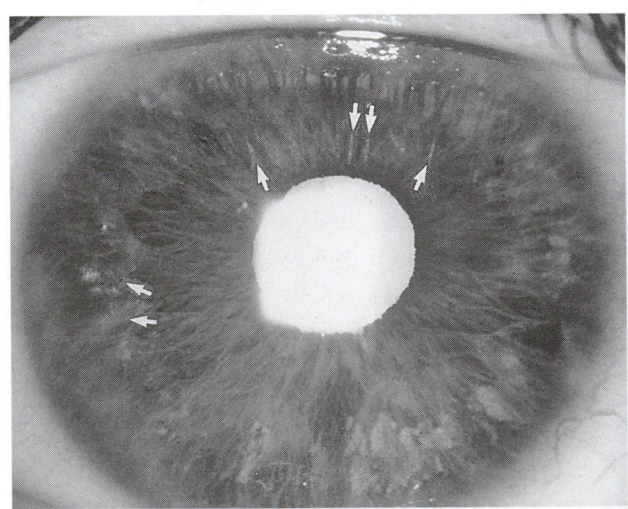

Figure 21–14. Transillumination defects of the iris associated with pigment dispersion syndrome.

thus of pigmentation in the trabecular meshwork. Miotics are the theoretical drugs of choice for pigmentary glaucoma, with prostaglandins an alternative. Miotics create pupillary constriction and move the lens forward. The forward lens movement decreases the rubbing of the zonules on the iris, with a diminished release of pigment as a result. Unfortunately, miotics are poorly tolerated by young individuals, though Ocuserts represent an alternative. Beta blockers and adrenergic agents may also be used instead to reduce IOP. Topical prostaglandins may be useful agents in pigmentary glaucoma, since they enhance outflow through the uveoscleral area, flushing pigment from the eye. It is important to monitor the optic nerves and visual fields rather than IOP in pigmentary glaucoma, since IOP spikes can occur, especially with exercise or pharmacologic pupillary dilation. Pigmentary glaucoma does show an excellent response to ALT, so that this is also a useful option.

Pseudoexfoliative Glaucoma

Patients with pseudoexfoliative glaucoma often have higher IOPs and greater visual field loss at the time of diagnosis than do POAG patients (see Chap. 27). Medical management of pseudoexfoliative glaucoma is similar to that of other forms of open-angle glaucoma, though the results are not always easily achieved (Fig. 21–15). Excellent results are often obtained with ALT, with filtration surgery reserved for difficult cases.

Spikes in IOP are often seen after pupillary dilation in individuals with pseudoexfoliative glaucoma, requiring that postdilation IOP measurements be obtained whenever dilation is performed. If a spike is seen, it is temporary and may not require additional therapy, depending on the status of the optic nerve, ocular history, and level of the spiking pressure.

Posttraumatic Glaucoma

Hyphema

Medical management of acute hyphema includes cycloplegia, bed rest, and head elevation to promote resorption of the hemorrhage (Fig. 21–16). Aminocaproic acid (Amicar), an antifibrinolytic agent, may prevent rebleeding and its associated complications. One goal in the management of a hyphema is to prevent rebleeding, since rebleeds are usually larger than the initial hyphema, leading to complications and a poorer prognosis. The systemic side effects of aminocaproic acid have limited its use in many cases.

Antiglaucoma medications should include the topical beta blockers, adrenergic agonists, and CAIs if necessary. In African Americans with sickle cell disease, CAIs cannot be used because they may promote sickling of the red blood cells, thus elevating IOP further. Therefore all black patients should have their hemoglobin checked and a sickle cell test performed prior to CAI administration when a hyphema is present. Miotic agents should also be avoided to prevent the formation of posterior synechiae and exacerbation of the inflammatory response. Reduction of IOP is important in large hyphemas, minimizing the chance of corneal blood staining and unrecognized nerve damage. Elevated IOP causes decompensation of the corneal endothelium, permitting released

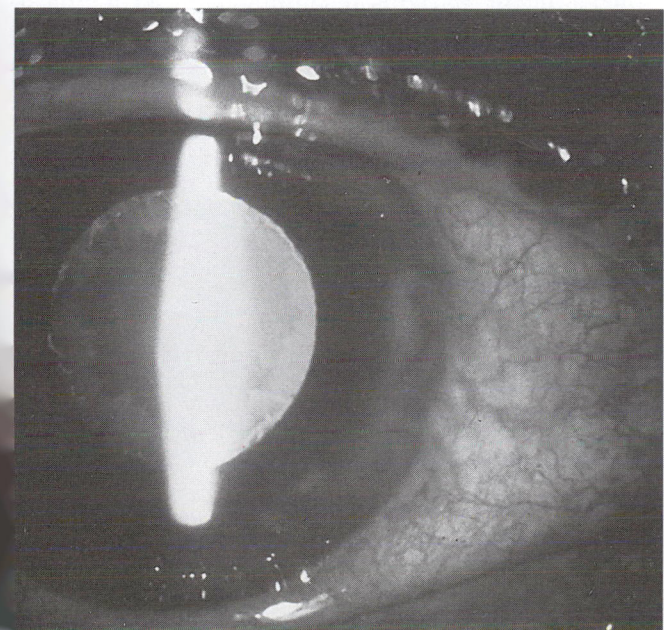

Figure 21–15. Pseudoexfoliation of the lens, seen in retroillumination.

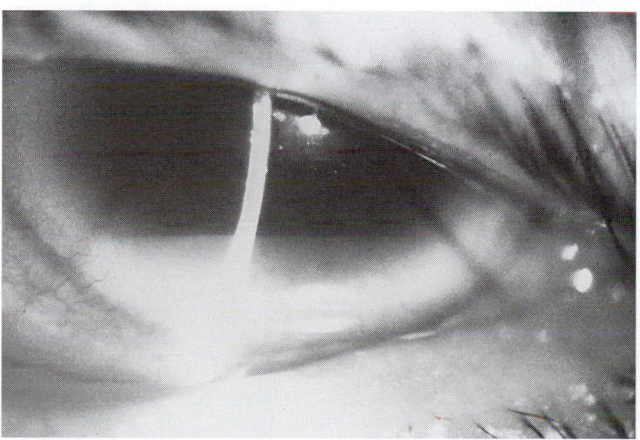

Figure 21–16. A hyphema, due to trauma, with associated corneal edema.

hemoglobin to penetrate the cornea. If stromal penetration occurs, it may take months for the blood stain to clear. If a large hyphema does not improve promptly (within 12 to 24 hours) with medical management, as shown by the clearing of blood from the anterior chamber and lowering of the IOP, prompt surgical treatment is needed to break up the clot and relieve pupillary block. Any delay can affect the final visual outcome.

Angle-Recession Glaucoma

Medically, angle-recession glaucoma responds to drugs much as POAG does, except that miotics show little effect (see Chap. 28). Also, ALT has not been shown to be of benefit. It is important to follow angle-recession patients, like glaucoma suspects, on a regular basis so as to detect increases in IOP as they occur, making it possible to initiate medical therapy at the earliest possible stage (Fig. 21–17).

Ghost-Cell Glaucoma

Symptoms of ghost-cell glaucoma include ocular pain and blurred vision, along with corneal edema if the IOP is elevated (see Chap. 29). Careful monitoring is needed if a mild IOP elevation is noted, while medical intervention is warranted for high IOP. If the IOP cannot be controlled, vitrectomy may be necessary.

Hemolytic Glaucoma

The management of hemolytic glaucoma is similar to that for ghost-cell glaucoma, using medications to control elevated IOP (see Chap. 28).

Neovascular Glaucoma

Medically, topical beta blockers, alpha$_2$ agonists, and CAIs may be employed to reduce the IOP in neovascular glaucoma (Fig. 21–18). In addition, topical steroids and cycloplegic agents may quiet the inflammatory component and relieve ciliary muscle spasm, providing increased comfort. Pilocarpine should be avoided, since it may increase the inflammatory response. Surgical intervention for intractable elevated IOP includes filtering procedures, cycloablative procedures, or a Molteno implant (see Chaps. 23 and 24).

Steroid-Induced Glaucoma

Treatment for steroid-induced glaucoma includes discontinuing the steroid, if possible, and using antiglaucoma topical medications to reduce the IOP (see Chap. 28). If steroid use is necessary because of an ongoing ocular condition, then a steroid may be selected that does not easily penetrate into the eye. If continued steroid use is necessary for uveitis, switching to a different steroid (fluorometholone or rimexolone) may minimize the ocular hypertensive effect. When a potent steroid is absolutely required, a topical beta blocker and/or CAI may be used concomitantly to reduce the IOP. The steroid is tapered or discontin-

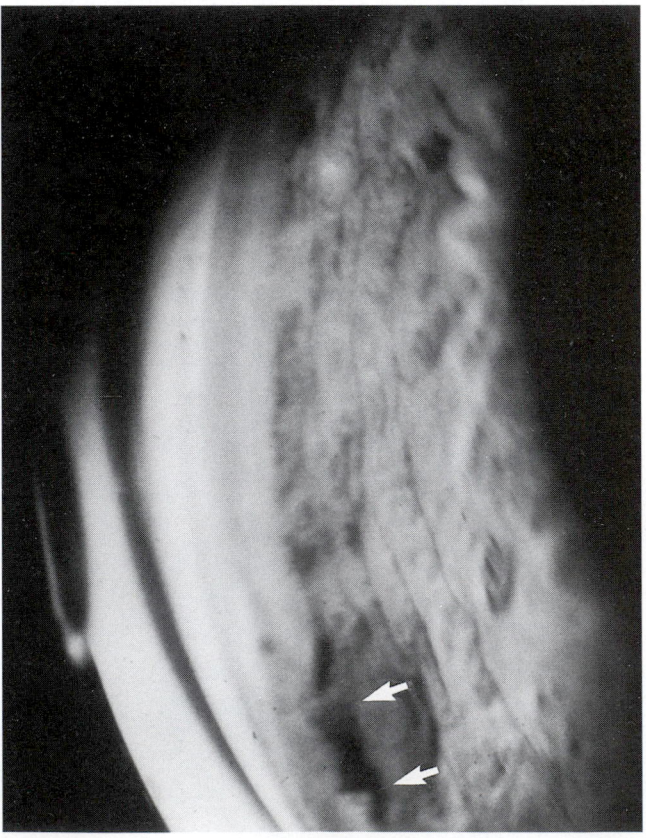

Figure 21–17. The gonioscopic appearance of angle recession. Note how wide open the angle appears.

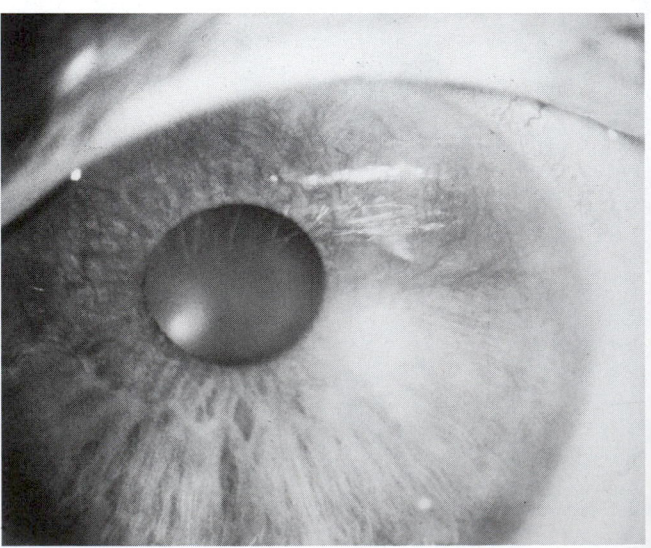

Figure 21–18. Rubeosis iridis associated with diabetic retinopathy.

ued as soon as possible, with the IOP monitored over weeks to months until it returns to pretreatment levels.

Acute Angle-Closure Glaucoma

The goal of treatment in acute angle-closure glaucoma is to move the iris out of the anterior chamber angle to break the attack. This will prevent the formation of peripheral anterior synechiae and allow unrestricted outflow of aqueous (Fig. 21–19). Typically, miotics are used to move the iris. However, an IOP greater than 45 to 50 mmHg causes ischemia of the iris sphincter muscle, rendering miotic agents ineffective (see Chap. 28). The IOP must first be lowered, either by temporarily opening the angle via indentation gonioscopy or by instilling a topical beta blocker, topical prostaglandin, oral hyperosmotic agent, or CAI (two 250-mg tablets of acetazolamide) followed by a miotic once the IOP drops below 40 mmHg.

Indentation gonioscopy with a Zeiss or Posner four-mirror lens may be effective in breaking an acute angle-closure attack by mechanically opening the angle when oral agents are not available or warranted.[111] Indentation of the cornea followed by release, done in 15-second intervals, is continued for 5 minutes. This push-release method is employed to prevent a possible occlusion of the central retinal artery.[111] If indentation gonioscopy is unsuccessful, an oral hyperosmotic agent may be used.

Osmotics must be used with care in the elderly. Nausea from the attack may be aggravated by the agent, leading to vomiting. When oral agents are precluded due to nausea, a faster-acting dose of intra-venous acetazolamide 500 mg or mannitol may be of benefit. A prochlorperazine (Compazine) suppository may be used to reduce the nausea prior to administering glycerin or isosorbide, but care is required, since prochlorperazine may induce some pupillary dilation. The treatment regimen for oral glycerin is to have the patient drink a 50% solution in a dose of 1.5 g/kg of body weight (about 4 to 6 fluid ounces). In the case of diabetics, metabolically inactive isosorbide in 45% solution (Ismotic) is used. Pouring the solution over ice will diminish the pungent taste and thin the solution for easier consumption and faster absorption (Fig. 21–20). After the patient has drunk isosorbide or glycerin, one drop of a topical beta blocker and an alpha agonist is administered. The IOP is then checked every 30 minutes and, upon its reaching about 40 mmHg or less, one drop of pilocarpine 2% is administered at 30-minute intervals for 1 hour. Increasing systemic symptoms attributed to an ongoing angle-closure attack can be due to pilocarpine overdosage and its secondary parasympathomimetic side effects if used in excessive amounts. Once an acceptable reduction in IOP is seen, gonioscopy is repeated to confirm the reopening of the angle. Referral for laser peripheral iridotomy is made as soon as possible once the attack is broken, with the patient maintained on a mild miotic such as pilocarpine 1% in each eye to prevent repeated angle closure. If the IOP and/or angle configuration does not return to normal, iridotomy, gonioplasty, or surgical iridectomy should be performed within several hours of the onset of the attack.

Chronic Angle-Closure Glaucoma.

The first-line treatment of chronic angle-closure glaucoma, which appears similar to open-angle glaucoma in that the IOP is elevated with nerve and field damage but a closed angle is present, includes medical therapy. Medical therapy must be tailored for this specific form of glaucoma, utilizing medications that reduce aqueous production or improve uveoscleral outflow, along with a laser peripheral iridotomy. In cases where control is difficult to achieve, filtering surgery may be required.

CONCLUSION

Treatment of glaucoma is a challenging endeavor that taxes a clinician's diagnostic and therapeutic skills. The doctor must establish the diagnosis, review the patient's medical and ocular history, and select a medication and target pressure. For all of these decisions, there are numerous choices that can be difficult

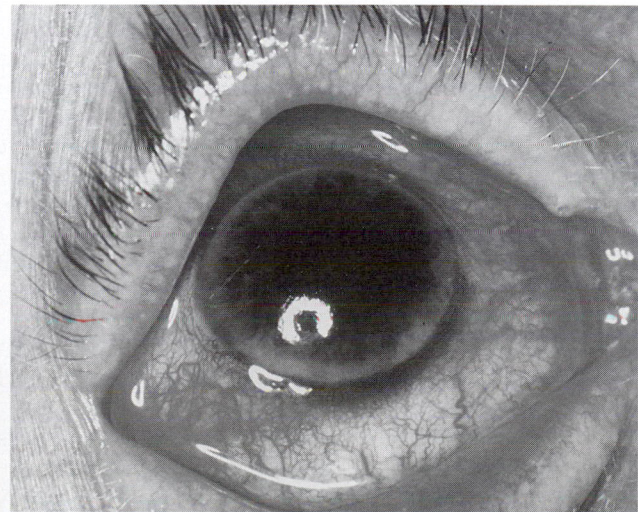

Figure 21–19. Angle-closure glaucoma as seen with a red eye and a dilated, fixed pupil.

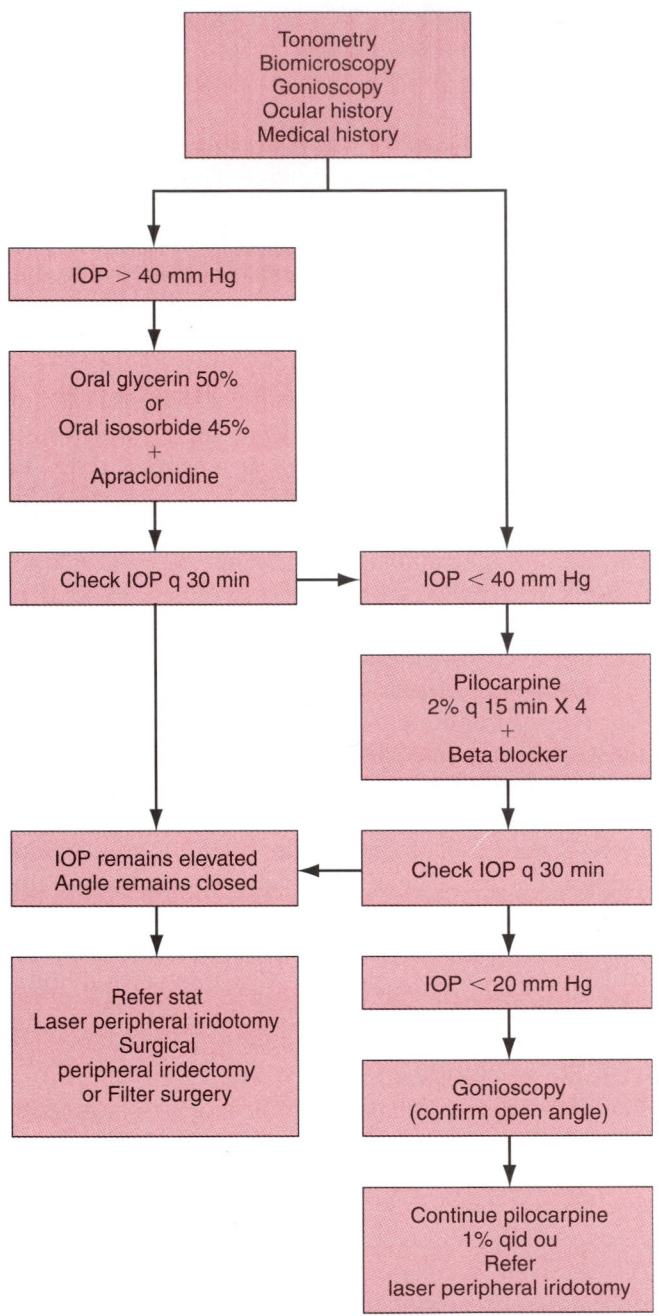

Figure 21–20. Angle-closure glaucoma flowchart.

to make. In addition, the patient must be educated regarding glaucoma: what it is, how it is managed, and potential side effects from the medications used. Periodic monitoring is required to look for medication intolerance, IOP stability, and signs of glaucomatous progression. Finally, the doctor must establish a relationship with the patient built on trust and confidence so that if problems do arise, the doctor will be alerted. For all of this, the best that one can usually

hope for is to "break even" and preserve the patient's vision. The treatment of glaucoma is a difficult task with few thanks, and the preservation of the patient's vision may be the doctor's only reward.

REFERENCES

1. Sommer A, Tielsch JM, Katz J, et al. Relationship between intraocular pressure and primary open angle glaucoma among white and black Americans: The Baltimore Eye Survey. *Arch Ophthalmol*. 1991;109(8):1090–1095.
2. Leske MC, Connell AM, Wu SY, Hyman L, et al. Distribution of intraocular pressure: The Barbados Eye Study. *Arch Ophthalmol*. 1997;115(8):1051–1057.
3. Armaly MF. On the distribution of applanation pressure: I. Statistical features and the effect of age, sex and family history of glaucoma. *Arch Ophthalmol*. 1965;73:11–18.
4. Kass MA. When to treat ocular hypertension. *Surv Ophthalmol*. 1983;28(suppl):229–232.
5. Epstein DL, Krug JH, Hertzman E, et al. A long term clinical trial of timolol therapy versus no treatment in the management of glaucoma suspects. *Ophthalmology*. 1989;96:1460–1467.
6. Kass MA, Gordon MO, Hoff MR, et al. Topical timolol administration reduces the incidence of glaucomatous damage in ocular hypertensive individuals. *Arch Ophthalmol*. 1989;107:1590–1598.
7. Schulzer M, Drance SM, Douglas GR. A comparison of treated and untreated glaucoma suspects. *Ophthalmology*. 1991;98(3):301–307.
8. Kass MA. The Ocular Hypertension Treatment Study. *J Glaucoma*. 1994;3:97–100.
9. Diggory P, Heyworth P, Chau G, et al. Improved lung function tests on changing from topical timolol: Nonselective beta-blockade impairs lung function tests in elderly patients. *Eye*. 1993;7(pt 5):661–663.
10. Diggory P, Cassels Brown A, Vail A, Abbey LM, Hillman JS. Avoiding unsuspected respiratory side effects of topical timolol with cardioselective or sympathomimetic agents. *Lancet*. 1995;345(8965):1604–1606.
11. Bartlett JD, Novack GD, Hiett JA, et al. Antiglaucoma drugs. In: Bartlett JD, Jaanus SD, eds. *Clinical Ocular Pharmacology*, 3rd ed. Boston: Butterworth-Heinemann; 1995:183–247.
12. Passo MS, Palmer EA, Van Buskirk EM. Plasma timolol in glaucoma patients. *Ophthalmology*. 1984;91(11):1361–1363.
13. Zimmerman TJ, Kooner KS, Kandarakis AS, Ziegler LP. Improving the therapeutic index of topically applied ocular drugs. *Arch Ophthalmol*. 1984;102:551–553.
14. Freedman SF, Freedman NJ, Shields MB, et al. Effects of ocular carteolol and timolol on plasma high density lipoprotein cholesterol level. *Am J Ophthalmol*. 1993;116(5):600–611.
15. Forte EJ, Weber PA. Psychologic effects of topical timolol maleate. *Contemp Ophthalmol Forum*. 1987;5:11–18.

16. Lynch MA, Whitson JT, Brown RH, et al. Topical beta blocker therapy and central nervous system side effects. *Arch Ophthalmol*. 1988;106:908–911.

17. Burggraf GW, Munt PW. Topical timolol therapy and cardiopulmonary function. *Can J Ophthalmol*. 1980;15:159–160.

18. McMahon CD, Shaffer RN, Hoskins HD Jr. Adverse effects experienced by patients taking timolol. *Am J Ophthalmol*. 1979;88:736–738.

19. Cinotti A, Cinotti D, Grant W, et al. Levobunolol vs. timolol for open angle glaucoma and ocular hypertension. *Am J Ophthalmol*. 1985;99:11–17.

20. Nielsen-Angelo K. Timolol topically and diabetes mellitus. *JAMA*. 1980;244:1567.

21. Van Buskirk EM. Corneal anesthesia after timolol maleate therapy. *Am J Ophthalmol*. 1979;88:739–743.

22. Yamamoto T, Kitazawa Y, Noma A, et al. The effects of the beta-adrenergic blocking agents, timolol and carteolol, on plasma lipids and lipoproteins in Japanese glaucoma patients. *J Glaucoma*. 1996;5(4):252–257.

23. Schoene RB, Abuan T, Ward RL, Beasley CH. Effects of topical betaxolol, timolol and placebo on pulmonary function in asthmatic bronchitis. *Am J Ophthalmol*. 1984;97:86–92.

24. Berry DP, Van Buskirk EM, Shields MB. Betaxolol and timolol: A comparison of safety and side effects. *Arch Ophthalmol*. 1984;102:42–45.

25. Ofner S, Smith TJ. Betaxolol in chronic obstructive pulmonary disease. *J Ocul Pharmacol*. 1987;3:171–173.

26. Van Buskirk EM, Weinreb RN, Berry DP, et al. Betaxolol in patients with glaucoma and asthma. *Am J Ophthalmol*. 1986;101:531–534.

27. Dunn TL, Gerber MJ, Shen AS, et al. The effect of topical ophthalmic instillation of timolol and betaxolol on lung function in asthmatic subjects. *Annu Rev Respir Dis*. 1986;133:264–268.

28. Harris LS, Greenstein SH, Bloom RF. Respiratory difficulties with betaxolol. *Am J Ophthalmol*. 1986;102:274.

29. Hester RK, Chen Z, Becker EJ, et al. The direct vascular relaxing action of betaxolol, carteolol and timolol in porcine long posterior ciliary artery. *Surv Ophthalmol*. 1994;38(suppl):S125–S134.

30. Hoste AM, Sys SU. The relaxant action of betaxolol on isolated bovine retinal microarteries. *Curr Eye Res*. 1994;13:483–487.

31. Osborne NN, Cazevielle C, Carvalho AL, et al. In vivo and in vitro experiments show that betaxolol is a retinal neuroprotective agent. *Brain Res*. 1997;751:113–123.

32. Allen RC, Hertzmark E, Walker AM, Epstein DL. A double masked comparison of betaxolol vs. timolol in the treatment of open angle glaucoma. *Am J Ophthalmol*. 1986;101:535–541.

33. Cyrlin MN, Thomas JV, Epstein DL. Additive effect of epinephrine to timolol therapy in primary open angle glaucoma. *Arch Ophthalmol*. 1982;100:414–418.

34. Allen RC, Epstein DL. Additive effect of betaxolol and epinephrine in primary open angle glaucoma. *Arch Ophthalmol*. 1986;104:1178–1184.

35. Allen RC, Robin AL, Long D, et al. A combination of levobunolol and dipivefrin for the treatment of glaucoma. *Arch Ophthalmol*. 1988;106:904–907.

36. Steinert RF, Thomas JV, Boger WP. Long term drift and continued efficacy after multi-year timolol therapy. *Arch Ophthalmol*. 1981;99:100–103.

37. Boger WP III. Short term "escape" and long term "drift." *Surv Ophthalmol*. 1983;28(suppl):235–240.

38. Neufeld AH, Zawistowski KA, Page ED, Bromberg BB. Influences on the density of beta adrenergic receptors in the cornea and iris-ciliary body of the rabbit. *Invest Ophthalmol Vis Sci*. 1978;17:1069–1075.

39. Townsend DJ, Brubaker RF. Immediate effect of epinephrine on aqueous in the normal human eye as measured by fluorophotometry. *Invest Ophthalmol Vis Sci*. 1980;19:256–266.

40. Durkee D, Bryant BG. Drug therapy in glaucoma. *Am J Hosp Pharmacol*. 1979;35:682–690.

41. Kolker AE, Becker B. Epinephrine maculopathy. *Arch Ophthalmol*. 1968;79:552–562.

42. Sugar J. Adrenochrome deposits in hydrophilic lenses. *Arch Ophthalmol*. 1974;91:11–12.

43. Ballin N, Becker B, Goldman ML. Systemic effects of epinephrine applied topically to the eye. *Invest Ophthalmol*. 1966;5:125–129.

44. Robin AL. Short-term effects of unilateral 1% apraclonidine therapy. *Arch Ophthalmol*. 1988;106:912–918.

45. Nagasubramanian S. Comparison of apraclonidine and timolol in chronic open angle glaucoma. *Ophthalmology* 1993;100:1318–1322.

46. Araujo S, Bond JB, Wilson RP. Long term effect of apraclonidine. *Br J Ophthalmol*. 1995;79:1098–1101.

47. Nordlund JR, Pasquale LR, Robin AL. The cardiovascular, pulmonary and ocular hypotensive effects of 0.2% brimonidine. *Arch Ophthalmol*. 1995;113:77–83.

48. Toris CB, Gleason ML, Camras CB. Effects of brimonidine on aqueous humor dynamics in human eyes. *Arch Ophthalmol*. 1995;113:1514–1517.

49. LeBlanc RP for the Brimonidine Study Group. Twelve-month results of an ongoing randomized trial comparing brimonidine tartrate 0.2% and timolol 0.5% given twice daily in patients with glaucoma or ocular hypertension. *Ophthalmology*. 1998:105(10):1960–1967.

50. Barnebey HS, Robin AL, Zimmerman TJ. The effect of brimonidine in decreasing elevations in intraocular pressure after laser trabeculoplasty. *Ophthalmology*. 1993;100:1083–1088.

51. Alm A, Stjernschantz J, the Scandinavian Latanoprost Study Group. Effects on intraocular pressure and side effects of 0.005% latanoprost applied once daily, evening or morning. *Ophthalmology*. 1995;102:1744–1752.

52. Watson P, Stjernschantz J, The Latanoprost Study Group. A six-month, randomized double-masked study comparing latanoprost with timolol in open-angle glaucoma and ocular hypertension. *Ophthalmology*. 1996;103:126–136.

53. Camras CB, The United States Latanoprost Study Group. Comparison of latanoprost and timolol in patients with ocular hypertension and glaucoma: A

Chapter 22

LASER PROCEDURES IN THE THERAPY OF GLAUCOMA

Elliot B. Werner

PROCEDURES TO RELIEVE PUPIL BLOCK: LASER IRIDECTOMY

The primary and secondary pupil-block angle-closure glaucomas all have in common an increased resistance to aqueous flow at the pupillary margin. As a result, the pressure in the posterior chamber is increased sufficiently to cause the iris to bow forward until it occludes the trabecular meshwork and obstructs the outflow of aqueous. Most pupil-block glaucomas are urgent situations, with iridectomy being the primary treatment modality.[1,2] Medical therapy may be used to lower intraocular pressure (IOP) temporarily and prepare the eye for iridectomy, but definitive therapy should not be delayed (see Chap 29).[3,4]

Treatment of pupil block is designed to equalize the pressure in the posterior and anterior chambers by creating a hole in the iris. This is now usually accomplished with laser energy, although incisional surgery may be used in rare cases.

Indications

Laser iridectomy is indicated in any angle-closure glaucoma where pupil block is present.[5,6] Prophylactic laser iridectomy is also indicated when the risk of developing pupil block seems very high. Once pupil block has been diagnosed, iridectomy should generally be performed without delay. In most cases, a patent iridectomy will either cure the glaucoma or facilitate management. In all cases, an iridectomy will eliminate pupil block. Table 22–1 summarizes the diseases in which iridectomy is indicated and likely to be beneficial. Iridectomy for angle-closure glaucomas without pupil block is not rational because the procedure will be of no benefit to the patient.

The decision to perform a prophylactic iridectomy is often difficult. Prophylactic iridectomy in the fellow eye of a patient with pupillary-block angle-closure is generally accepted as appropriate treatment.[7] In cases of bilateral asymptomatic, anatomically narrow angles, the indication for prophylactic iridectomy is less clear.[8] Here the clinician is not treating a disease but trying to assess the risk of future development of pupil block and the potential benefit of iridectomy in preventing it. Table 22–2 summarizes the situations in which prophylactic iridectomy should be considered.

In patients with asymptomatic, anatomically narrow angles, the depth of the central anterior chamber is a good guideline and should be measured. If the central anterior chamber is less than 2.1 mm, the risk of angle closure is extremely high and iridectomy should be advised.[9–11]

TABLE 22–1. INDICATIONS FOR LASER IRIDECTOMY IN PRIMARY AND SECONDARY PUPIL-BLOCK GLAUCOMAS

Primary pupil-block angle-closure glaucomas
 Acute angle closure
 Intermittent angle closure
 Chronic angle closure

Secondary pupil-block angle-closure glaucomas
 Aphakic or pseudophakic pupil block
 Lens-induced angle-closure glaucoma*
  Lens subluxation
  Phacomorphic angle closure
 Iris bombé due to extensive posterior synechiae

*In general, definitive therapy for lens-induced glaucomas is lens extraction. However, iridectomy is often valuable on a temporary basis.

TABLE 22–2. SITUATIONS IN WHICH PROPHYLACTIC IRIDECTOMY SHOULD BE CONSIDERED

Asymptomatic, anatomically narrow angles
 Slit-like or very narrow angles on gonioscopy
 Moderate hyperopia
 Shallow central depth of anterior chamber

Fellow eye of patient with primary pupil-block angle closure
 Absolute indication, since risk of subsequent angle closure
  is very high

Patient with primary open-angle glaucoma and coincidentally narrow angles
 Especially if using miotic therapy
 Prior to laser trabeculoplasty in narrow-angle eyes

Nanophthalmos
 High hyperopia
 Small axial length

Contraindications

Laser iridectomy is a relatively safe procedure with few contraindications. Corneal edema or opacities that obscure the iris are the major contraindications. A flat anterior chamber in which the iris is in contact with the cornea is another contraindication. In such situations, it is impossible to perform the iridectomy without also hitting the cornea with the laser beam. If there was great difficulty in treating the first eye or a serious complication ensued, the clinician might hesitate in treating the second eye. Finally, if because of physical or psychiatric problems the patient is unable to be positioned in the laser delivery system or to cooperate with the treatment, an alternative to laser iridectomy should be considered.

Technique

Iridectomies may be created with either thermal argon (Fig. 22–1) or disruptive Nd:YAG (Fig. 22–2) laser. The laser energy is usually delivered through the optics of a slit lamp using a fiberoptic system between the laser tube and the slit lamp. Once the iridectomy has been created, the results are the same regardless of which technique has been used.[12–15]

One major advantage of the argon laser is that bleeding does not occur during the procedure. In

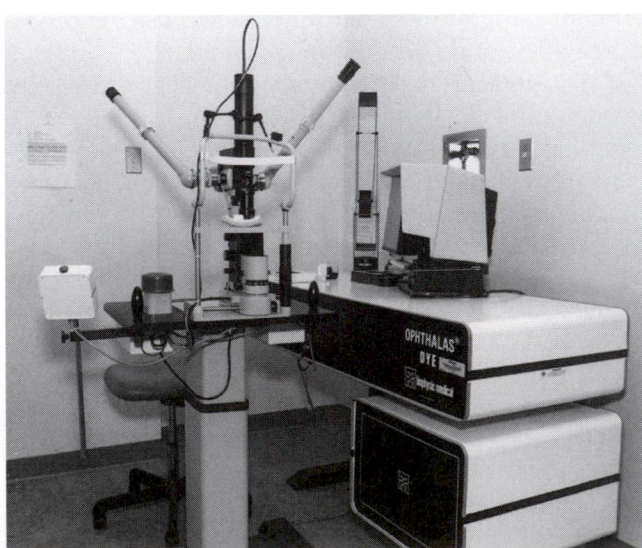

Figure 22–1. Photograph of an argon laser showing the console containing the laser tube on the right and the slit-lamp delivery system to the left.

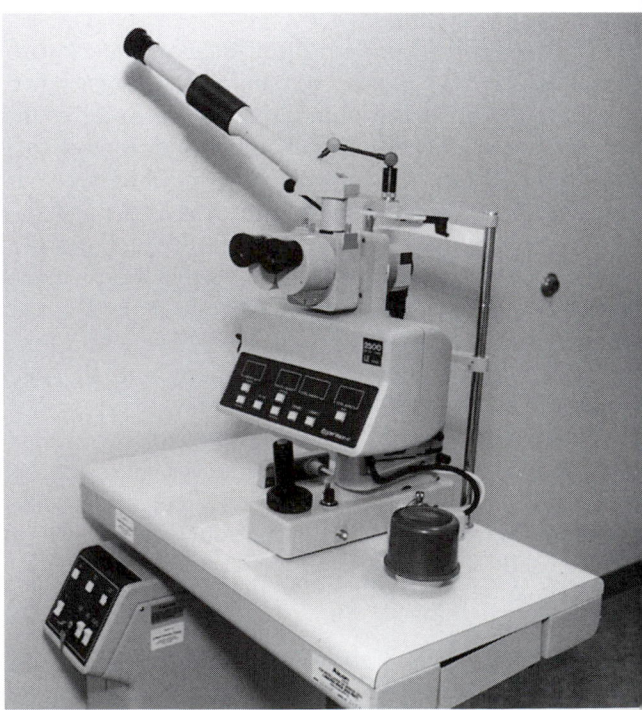

Figure 22–2. Photograph of a Nd:YAG laser. The laser tube is located in the small console just below the oculars of the slit-lamp delivery system.

many patients, it is more difficult to create an iridectomy with the argon laser alone. Late closure of the opening in the iris is more likely in argon laser iridectomy. Iridectomy with the Nd:YAG laser is usually quicker and less likely to be complicated by late closure. In thick, dark brown irides, such as are found in many African-American or Oriental patients, a combined technique in which the surface of the iris is first treated with the argon laser and subsequently penetrated with the Nd:YAG laser works well. In patients with blue or lightly pigmented irides, most clinicians now employ the Nd:YAG laser.[14,15] Whether the argon or Nd:YAG laser is used, virtually all surgeons perform laser iridectomy through an Abraham (Fig. 22–3) or similar contact lens.[16] This is a planoconcave lens with a small high plus convex lens glued onto the front surface. The Abraham lens allows better focusing of the laser energy onto the iris, keeps the eyelids open, and helps control eye movement during the procedure.

The iridectomy is usually placed in the upper nasal quadrant so that the upper lid will cover it (Fig. 22–4). This helps prevent glare or diplopia. Nasal placement also directs the laser beam away from the macula and reduces the risk of inadvertent damage to the central retina.

In phakic patients, patency of the iridectomy is determined by visualizing the anterior surface of the

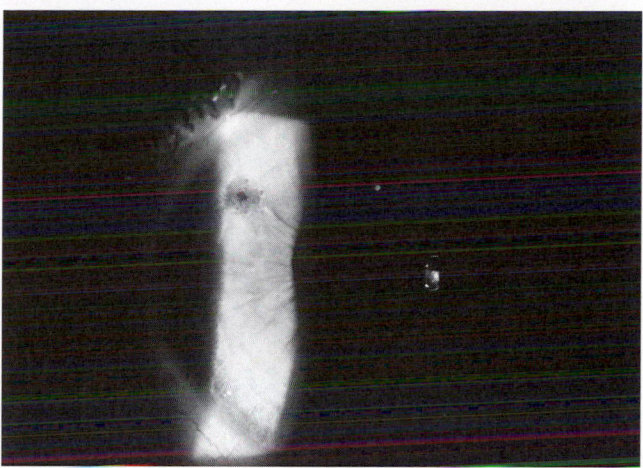

Figure 22–4. Postoperative photograph of a patent laser peripheral iridectomy. To be certain that the iridectomy is patent, the lens capsule should be seen through the iridectomy opening. (*See also Color Plate 41*)

lens through the iridectomy with the slit lamp. Transillumination alone is not a reliable indicator of patency. In aphakic or pseudophakic patients, patency is determined by visualizing the vitreous face or intraocular lens surface through the iridectomy.

Complications

Intraoperative complications include failure to penetrate the iris, corneal burns, hemorrhage, and inadvertent retinal damage.[17] Failure to penetrate the iris may result from corneal edema or a corneal opacity that prevents delivery of adequate laser energy to the iris. Some irides are very thick or vascular and are extremely difficult to penetrate. If the iris begins to bleed or if large amounts of pigment are released into the aqueous, the surgeon may be unable to visualize the iris well enough to complete the procedure. If an iridectomy cannot be created during the initial attempt with the laser, the patient may be brought back in 24 or 48 hours for another attempt. Sometimes, in very difficult cases, it may be necessary to resort to an incisional iridectomy (Fig. 22–5).

Corneal burns sometimes result if the laser beam is not aimed and focused properly or if the iris is very close to the cornea. These burns rarely cause permanent scarring or difficulty, but they may obscure the iris and prevent the surgeon from completing the procedure.

Hemorrhage from the iris is a common occurrence with the Nd:YAG laser. The amount of hemorrhage is usually small and rarely causes permanent sequelae. Blood in the anterior chamber may, however, prevent completion of the procedure and may be associated with a marked increase in IOP postoperatively.

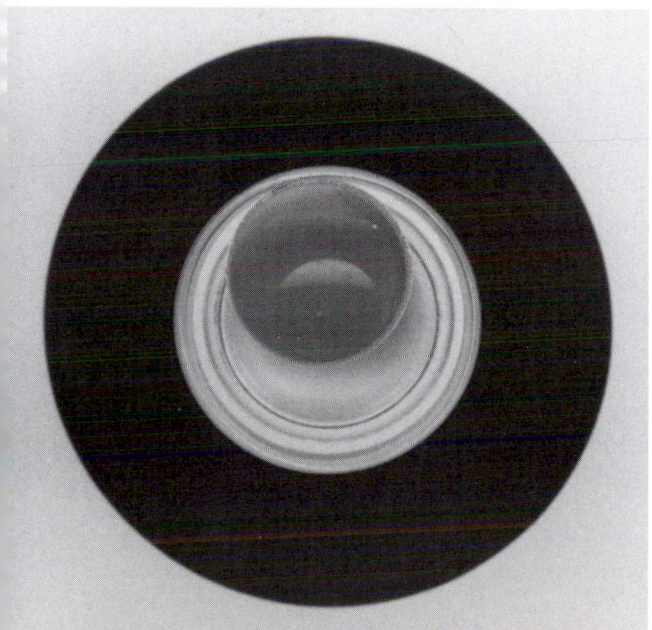

Figure 22–3. Photograph of an Abraham lens. The convex button glued onto the front surface of the planoconcave contact lens concentrates and focuses the laser energy onto the iris during the peripheral iridectomy.

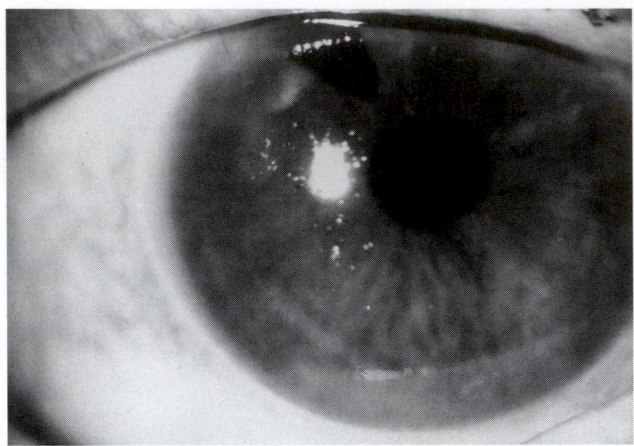

Figure 22–5. Photograph of a patent surgical iridectomy. (*See also Color Plate 42*)

Inadvertent retinal damage from a misdirected laser beam is fortunately rare. If the iridectomy is made in the nasal portion of the iris and the delivery system is directed nasally, damage to the macula will be avoided even if the retina is accidentally coagulated.

Postoperative complications include increased IOP, iritis, posterior synechiae, corneal abrasion, and late closure of the iridectomy.[17] A significant number of patients undergoing laser iridectomy will suffer a marked increase in IOP within the first 2 hours of the procedure. The frequency and severity of this complication can be reduced by the preoperative and postoperative use of apraclonidine drops.[18] All patients should be monitored during the immediate postoperative period. If the IOP increases, the patient may be treated with beta-adrenergic blocking agents, alpha$_2$-adrenergic agonists, carbonic anhydrase inhibitors, or hyperosmotic agents as needed until the pressure returns to normal. This complication rarely causes permanent sequelae but acute intraocular pressure elevation may be associated with optic nerve infarction or retinal vessel occlusions. In patients with very advanced glaucoma, progressive loss of visual field may occur even when the IOP is elevated for only a short time.

Most patients will have some degree of iritis following laser iridectomy.[19] Routine treatment with topical corticosteroids for 3 to 5 days postoperatively will usually prevent any major problems. Some patients will, however, have a prolonged inflammatory response or develop an iritis when the corticosteroid drops are stopped.[20,21] Even in the presence of a mild anterior chamber reaction, some patients will form posterior synechiae following laser iridectomy.

Corneal abrasions may result in some patients from the contact lens used during the treatment. This is treated like any other corneal abrasion but may contraindicate the use of topical corticosteroids for several days postoperatively.

Late closure of the iridectomy is a common complication with the argon laser, occurring in anywhere from 10 to 35% of patients. It is much less common with the Nd:YAG laser.[15,22] If an iridectomy is going to close, it will usually do so within the first 6 weeks. When late closure occurs, the procedure must be repeated. Usually the previously made iridectomy can be reopened. Alternatively, a new site on the iris may be chosen.

Postoperative Management

As is true of any surgical procedure, the extent of the postoperative follow-up depends on the occurrence of complications and the patient's course. In an uncomplicated iridectomy in which there has been no postoperative increase in IOP, the patient should be treated with topical corticosteroids for 3 to 5 days and seen within a week. If there are no problems, the patient should be seen again 6 to 8 weeks postoperatively. At this point gonioscopy should be performed to see if the configuration of the anterior chamber angle has changed as a result of the iridectomy. The pupil should also be dilated in order to examine the retina. In patients with pupil block, this may never have been done because of the risk of angle closure. Naturally, postoperative management will need to be modified if the patient has complications or a severe preexisting glaucoma.

PROCEDURES TO INCREASE AQUEOUS OUTFLOW: LASER TRABECULOPLASTY

Indications

In any patient with uncontrolled glaucoma where the IOP is sufficiently high to pose a major risk of future vision loss, laser treatment to increase aqueous outflow, if successful, will usually result in better control of IOP. Laser trabeculoplasty can be performed only in patients with an open anterior chamber angle and achieves its best results in primary open-angle glaucoma and a few secondary open-angle glaucomas, such as pseudoexfoliation and pigmentary glaucoma.

Laser trabeculoplasty is indicated in any patient with an open anterior chamber angle in whom IOP is not low enough to prevent progressive cupping of the optic nerve and loss of visual field.[23] Determining when laser trabeculoplasty is indicated requires careful follow-up of glaucoma patients. Stereoscopic optic disc photographs and visual field examinations should be obtained at frequent and regular intervals

In general, younger patients, patients with minimal or absent trabecular meshwork pigment, and those with normal or minimally elevated IOP are less likely to respond to laser trabeculoplasty. Certain types of glaucomas are more likely to respond to laser trabeculoplasty than others, as shown in Table 22–3.

Contraindications

Contraindications include corneal edema or opacities that prevent clear visualization of the anterior chamber angle, angle closure glaucoma, and a physical or psychiatric illness that prevents adequate patient cooperation. Relative contraindications include diseases in which laser trabeculoplasty is unlikely to be effective, such as those listed in Table 22–3, as well as patients under the age of 35.[24,25]

Technique

Although several different types of lasers have been used experimentally, the vast majority of surgeons perform trabeculoplasty with an argon laser. A variety of contact lenses have been devised for use during trabeculoplasty. All use gonioscopic mirrors to visualize the anterior chamber angle. The Ritch four-mirrored lens is widely used (Fig. 22–6). The laser beam is aimed at the anterior half of the pigmented trabecular meshwork (Fig. 22–7). The number of laser applications and the extent of the angle treated vary from surgeon to surgeon. Some prefer to treat only 180 degrees of the angle initially, while others treat 360 degrees. There is no evidence that one technique is safer or

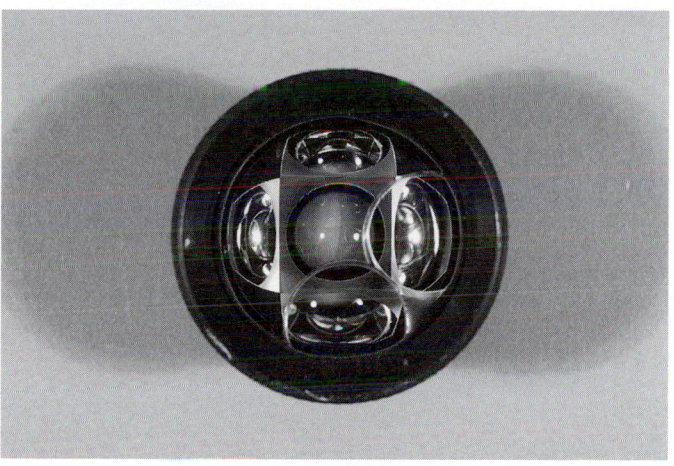

Figure 22–6. Photograph of the Ritch four-mirrored lens. The four mirrors are designed to allow visualization of different angle configurations during laser trabeculoplasty.

more effective than the other. Treatments of less than 40 applications are unlikely to be successful. The ideal number seems to be between 80 and 100 applications if 360 degrees of the angle are treated. The number of applications and their location on the trabecular meshwork seem to be more important in obtaining a good result than the extent of the angle treated.[25,26]

Laser trabeculoplasty lowers intraocular pressure by increasing the facility of aqueous outflow.[27] The mechanism by which this occurs is unknown, but there is evidence suggesting that laser energy alters and increases the metabolic and mitotic activity of the trabecular endothelial cells. This may result in more efficient movement of aqueous through the trabecular meshwork.[28]

Complications

Serious complications following laser trabeculoplasty are unusual. The reported complications include corneal abrasion, corneal burns, hemorrhage, peripheral anterior synechiae, iritis, a transient or permanent increase in IOP, syncope, allergic or toxic reactions to the eyedrops, and failure to lower IOP.

The most common complication is a transient increase in IOP during the immediate postoperative period, sometimes to very high levels. The use of apraclonidine drops preoperatively can reduce the frequency and severity of this complication.[29] Treatment is the same as outlined for complications of laser iridectomy.

The other common complication is failure to lower the IOP. The response to trabeculoplasty is not usually apparent for 6 to 8 weeks postoperatively. Some patients will show a very marked response in the first

TABLE 22–3. EXPECTED RESPONSE TO LASER TRABECULOPLASTY IN VARIOUS TYPES OF GLAUCOMA

Good (>67% initial success)
  Primary open-angle glaucoma
  Pseudoexfoliation glaucoma
  Pigmentary glaucoma

Fair (33–67% initial success)
  Aphakic or pseudophakic patient
  Angle-recession glaucoma
  Following failed filtering surgery
  Inactive uveitis
  Postiridectomy secondary open-angle glaucoma

Poor (<33% initial success)
  Active uveitis
  Neovascular glaucoma
  Congenital, juvenile glaucoma
  Mesodermal dysgenesis
  Elevated episcleral venous pressure
  Irido-corneal-endothelial syndrome
  Steroid glaucoma
  Rheumatoid scleritis

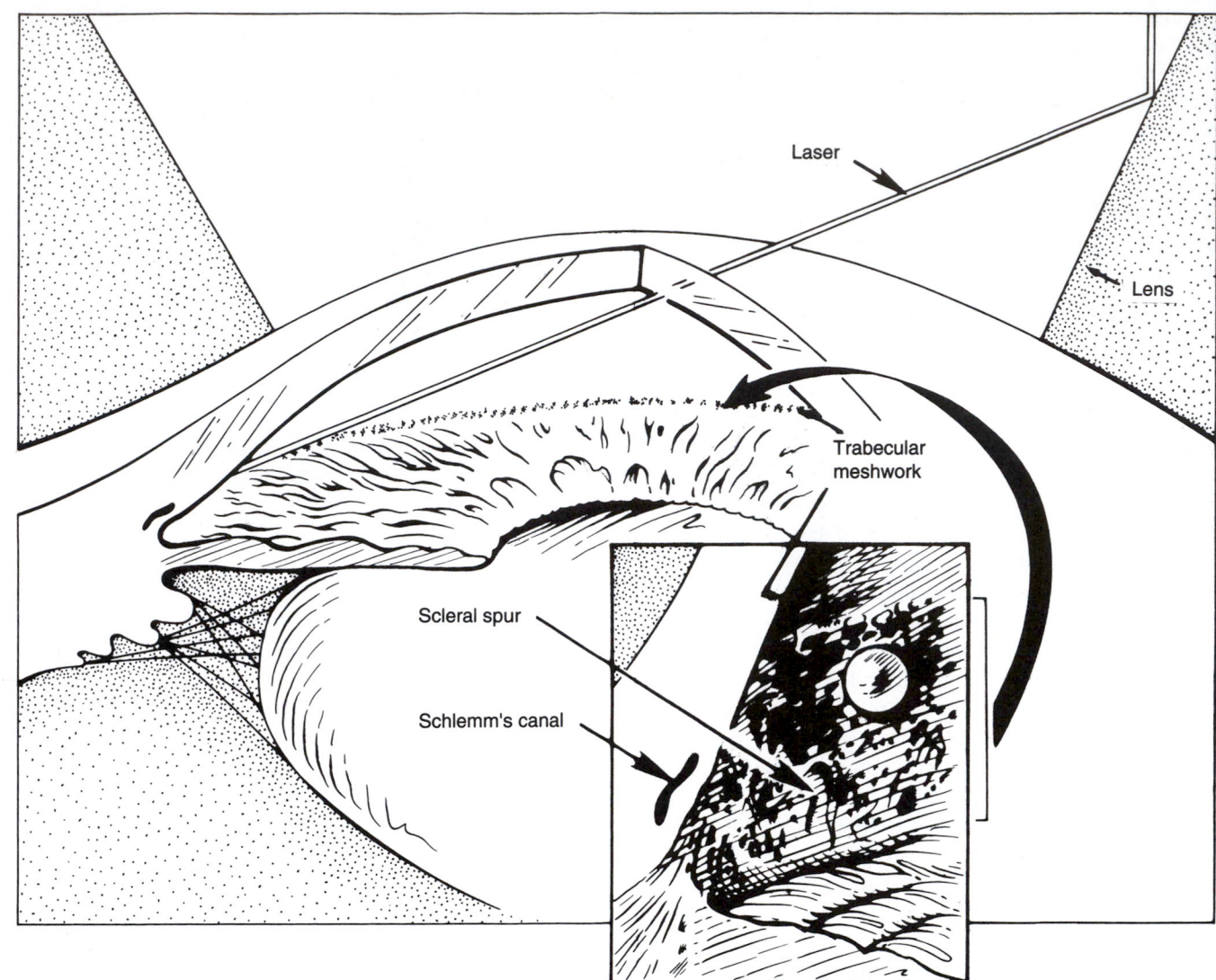

Figure 22–7. In argon laser trabeculoplasty, the laser beam strikes the Goldmann three-mirrored lens. The beam is reflected onto the anterior portion of the pigmented trabecular meshwork. A small bubble of blanching of the trabecular meshwork after each application indicates that the proper power setting has been used.

week or two, only to have no significant change in pressure 8 weeks later. Other patients may show very little effect in the first 2 weeks and still have a successful result later on. Some patients show no effect at all.

In primary open-angle glaucoma, one can expect a satisfactory decrease in IOP in about 70 to 80% of patients. In many patients, however, the effect is not permanent. Late-term failures occur in about 10% of patients each year, so that by 5 years after trabeculoplasty, less than 50% of patients will still have adequate control of IOP:[30,31] The other complications of laser trabeculoplasty are similar to those following laser iridectomy and are managed in a similar manner.

Postoperative Management

Patients should be checked 1 and 2 hours following trabeculoplasty to be sure that there is no postoperative increase in IOP. Topical corticosteroids are used for 5 days after the treatment to minimize the iritis. The patient's glaucoma therapy is usually continued without change. Barring any complications, patients are usually seen about 2 and 8 weeks postoperatively. If the IOP response is satisfactory, the patient is then followed like any other patient with chronic glaucoma. Stereo disc photographs and visual fields should be obtained at regular intervals. If progression of the disease continues, additional therapy or filtering surgery will be needed. Some patients may require less medication to control IOP after trabeculo-plasty.

In the event of late failure, the options are to increase the medical therapy, repeat the trabeculoplasty, or perform filtering surgery. There is evidence that good results can be obtained following a repeat trabeculoplasty in patients who have had a good result for at least a year following the initial treatment.[32] Repeat trabeculoplasty is not indicated if the initial effect was not satisfactory or if the duration of the lowered IOP was less than 1 year. In any case, the results following repeat trabeculoplasty are not nearly as good as those following the initial treatment.

A new form of trabeculoplasty, selective laser trabeculoplasty (SLT), is performed similarly to argon laser trabeculoplasty (ALT). By using a different wavelength, one can target melanized trabecular meshwork cells selectively, leaving the other trabecular cells intact. This modification is meant to prevent the extensive tissue damage common with ALT. Still, the procedure is new, with few data available on the outcomes. The advantage to SLT is that it is repeatable[33] if IOP elevates. Still, the procedure should not be repeated until 6 months have passed since the last treatment.

REFERENCES

1. American Academy of Ophthalmology Preferred Practice Patterns Glaucoma Panel. *Primary Angle Closure Glaucoma.* San Francisco: American Academy of Ophthalmology; 1996.

2. David R, Tessler Z, Yassur Y. Long-term outcome of primary acute angle-closure glaucoma. *Br J Ophthalmol.* 1985;69:261–262.

3. Schwartz GF, Steinmann WC, Spaeth GL, Wilson RP. Surgical and medical management of patients with narrow anterior chamber angles: Comparative results. *Ophthalm Sur.* 1992;23:108–112.

4. Higginbotham EJ. Laser peripheral iridotomy for pupillary block glaucoma. *Ophthalmology.* 1994;101:1749–1756.

5. Abraham RK, Miller GL. Outpatient argon laser iridectomy for angle closure glaucoma: A two-year study. *Trans Am Acad Ophthalmol Otolaryngol.* 1975;79:529–538.

6. Panek WC: Role of laser treatment in glaucoma. *Focal Points Clinical Modules for Ophthalmologists.* Vol. 9, No. 1, March 1993. San Francisco: American Academy of Ophthalmology; 1993:1–2.

7. Edwards RS. Behaviour of the fellow eye in acute angle-closure glaucoma. *Br J Ophthalmol.* 1982;66:576–579.

8. Wilensky JT, Kolker AE, Ritch R. Should patients with anatomically narrow angles have prophylactic iridectomy? *Surv Ophthalmol.* 1996;41:31–36.

9. Lee DA, Brubaker RF, Ilstrup DM. Anterior chamber dimensions in patients with narrow angles and angle-closure glaucoma. *Arch Ophthalmol.* 1984;102:46–50.

10. Panek WC, Christenson RE, Lee DA, et al. Biometric variables in patients with occludable anterior chamber angles. *Am J Ophthalmol.* 1990;110:185–188.

11. Wilensky JT, Anderson R, Ritch R, et al. Follow-up of angle-closure glaucoma suspects. *Am J Ophthalmol.* 1993;115:338–346.

12. Tomey KF, Traverso CE, Shammas IV. Nd:YAG laser iridotomy in the treatment and prevention of angle closure glaucoma. *Arch Ophthalmol.* 1987;105:476–481.

13. Morsman CD, Lusky M, Bosem ME, Weinreb RN. Anterior chamber angle configuration before and after iridotomy measured by Scheimpflug video imaging. *J Glaucoma.* 1994;3:114–116.

14. Moster MR, Schwartz LW, Spaeth GL, et al. Laser iridectomy: A controlled study comparing argon and neodymium:YAG. *Ophthalmology.* 1986;93:20–24.

15. Del Priore LV, Robin AL, Pollack IP. Neodymium:YAG and argon laser iridotomy. Long-term follow-up in a prospective, randomized clinical trial. *Ophthalmology.* 1988;95:1207–1211.

16. Abraham RK. Protocol for single session argon laser iridectomy for angle-closure glaucoma. *Int Ophthalmol Clin.* 1981;21:145–159.

17. Ritch R, Liebmann JM. Laser iridotomy and peripheral iridoplasty. In: Ritch R, Shields MB, Krupin T, eds. *The Glaucomas,* 2nd ed. St. Louis: CV Mosby; 1996:1549–1573.

18. Zimmerman TJ, Price RE. Apraclonidine for intraocular pressure control. *Ocul Therapeut Mgt.* 1990;1:1–12.

19. Shields MB. *Textbook of Glaucoma,* 4th ed. Baltimore: Williams & Wilkins; 1997:490–501.

20. Choplin NT, Bene CH. Cystoid macular edema following laser iridotomy. *Ann Ophthalmol.* 1983;15:172–173.

21. Cohen JS, Bibler L, Tucker D. Hypopyon following laser iridotomy. *Ophthalm Surg.* 1984;15:604–606.

22. Schwartz LW, Moster MR, Spaeth GL, Wilson RP, Poryzees E. Neodymium-YAG laser iridectomies in glaucoma associated with closed or occludable angles. *Am J Ophthalmol.* 1986;102:41–44.

23. Gieser SC, Savage JT, Wilensky JT. Laser trabeculoplasty for primary open-angle glaucoma. *Ophthalmology.* 1996;103:1708–1712.

24. Reiss GR, Wilensky JT, Higginbotham EJ. Laser trabeculoplasty. *Surv Ophthalmol.* 1991;35:407–428.

25. Weinreb RN, Tsai CS. Laser trabeculoplasty. In: Ritch R, Shields MB, Krupin T, eds. *The Glaucomas,* 2nd ed. St. Louis: CV Mosby; 1996:1549–1573.

26. Grayson DK, Ritch R, Camras C, et al. Influence of treatment protocol on the long-term efficacy of argon laser trabeculoplasty. *J Glaucoma.* 1993;2:7–12.

27. Brubaker RF, Liesegang TJ. Effect of trabecular photocoagulation on the aqueous humor dynamics of the human eye. *Am J Ophthalmol.* 1983;96:139–147.

28. Van Buskirk EM. Pathophysiology of laser trabeculoplasty. *Surv Ophthalmol.* 1989;33:264–272.

29. Shields MB. *Textbook of Glaucoma,* 4th ed. Baltimore: Williams & Wilkins; 1997:470–477.

30. Shingleton BJ, Richter CU, Bellows AR, Hutchinson T, Glynn RJ. Long-term efficacy of argon laser trabeculoplasty. *Ophthalmology.* 1987;94:1513–1517.

31. Spaeth GL, Baez KA. Argon laser controls one-third of cases of progressive, uncontrolled open-angle glaucoma for five years. *Arch Ophthalmol.* 1992;110:491–494.

32. Richter CU, Shingleton BJ, Bellows AR, et al. Retreatment with argon laser trabeculoplasty. *Ophthalmology.* 1987;94:1085–1089.

33. Damji KF, Shah KC, Bains KS, Rock W, et al. A randomized clinical trial of selective laser trabeculoplasty. *Br J Ophthalmol.* 1999;34:257–265.

Chapter 23

FILTERING SURGERY

Howard S. Barnebey
Kathy C. Yang-Williams

INDICATIONS FOR SURGICAL INTERVENTION

Consideration of surgical intervention for glaucoma involves many factors, including the clinical findings of optic nerve damage or functional changes such as progressive visual field loss. In the past, surgery for glaucoma was reserved for patients who were unresponsive to medical therapy and had reached maximally tolerated medical therapy. The definition of "maximally tolerated medical therapy" (MTMT) is evolving. Sensitivity to medications causes certain patients to seek alternative interventions, such as laser or incisional surgery. Other patients are simply unresponsive to medications or may elect to consider incisional surgery because of lifestyle or health factors that prevent them from instilling their medications appropriately.

In trabeculectomy, the most common form of glaucoma filtering surgery, a new channel is created for aqueous to flow out of the eye. Migdal and Hitching have studied the impact of primary filter surgery or trabeculectomy (surgery being the first modality used to treat glaucoma) and its success in controlling IOP in the Moorefields Primary Treatment Trial (MPTT).[1] They found that acceptable intraocular pressure (IOP) was achieved more frequently in patients who underwent primary trabeculectomy than in those who were treated with medications or laser trabeculoplasty. Further, primary trabeculectomy resulted in a lower mean diurnal IOP than was achieved in either of the other two treatment arms of the study. Primary trabeculectomy seemed to decrease IOP in a greater proportion of patients than delayed trabeculectomy. These results suggest that trabeculectomy could be considered earlier for selected patients—i.e., those who have difficulty with medical treatment, who are poorly controlled with medicine, or who require an IOP of 15 mmHg or less.

Jay and Allan found similar results when they evaluated patients with open-angle glaucoma randomized to either initial surgery or medical treatment.[2] These investigators found that intraocular pressures in both patient groups were controlled, but patients who were treated with medications first tended to have more visual field loss than those who were initially treated with surgery. The investigators concluded that visual field damage was more likely to occur during unsuccessful medication trials.

The ongoing Collaborative Initial Treatment of Glaucoma Study is designed to clarify the question of whether it is appropriate to consider incisional surgery as a primary intervention.[3] This multicenter, randomized, controlled clinical trial will evaluate the efficacy of different interventions for glaucoma and other outcomes measures, including visual function and quality-of-life issues.

Obviously, it falls to the clinician to educate the patient about the treatment options available as well as the risks and benefits of these procedures. Therefore, it is incumbent upon the practitioner to be familiar with filtering procedures for glaucoma, with the reasons for their consideration, and with the potential complications that may be encountered.

PREOPERATIVE CONSIDERATIONS

Preoperative Counseling

Patients who undergo incisional surgery for glaucoma should be counseled about the normal postoperative course, including the frequency of follow-up appointments. Generally patients are seen on the first postoperative day, weekly for the first month, biweekly for the second month, and monthly for the third to sixth months following surgery. Of course, the frequency of follow-up will be tailored specifically for the patient, since each patient responds differently to trabeculectomy.

With remodeling of the ocular surface, there is generally a need for an update in spectacle correction following surgery. As the IOP varies within the early postoperative period, the vision will also fluctuate. Patients need to be counseled that this is to be expected. Refractive changes can be associated with a myopic shift secondary to an anterior displacement of the lens iris diaphragm, induced astigmatism related to sutures, cycloplegia following use of anticholinergic agents, and so on. A retrospective case review documented the recovery of visual acuity in 93% of patients following trabeculectomy with and without antimetabolite therapy. A majority of these patients recovered vision by the eighth postoperative week; however, a small number of patients experienced delayed recovery of vision.[4] One study found that recovery of vision following surgery was similar after trabeculectomy with 5-fluorouracil (5-FU) or mitomycin C (MMC).[4]

Other transient symptoms that patients experience following trabeculectomy include tenderness at the surgical site, foreign-body sensation, and photophobia. The patient may complain about injection or redness of the eye related to subconjunctival hemorrhage.

It is important to emphasize to the patient that the primary goal is to stabilize the IOP at an acceptable level and to prevent further pressure-induced damage to vision. Incisional surgery brings greater risk in cases with advanced visual field loss involving split fixation or advanced damage to the optic nerve head. Patients need to be counseled that the recovery to best vision may be prolonged, and this is especially important in one-eyed patients.[4]

Preoperative Use of Antiglaucoma Medications

Although antiglaucoma medications are important in the preoperative period, there are certain medications that should be discontinued shortly before surgery. For example, cholinesterase inhibitors such as physostigmine, demecarium bromide, and echothiophate iodide should be discontinued 4 weeks before surgery owing to risk for disruption of the aqueous-blood barrier and facilitation of postoperative inflammation. Consideration should also be given to patients treated with cholinesterase inhibitors because of the potential for interaction with medications such as succinylcholine. Patients undergoing surgery with general anesthesia using this group of medications are at risk for apnea. Direct-acting miotics such as pilocarpine should be discontinued 3 to 7 days preoperatively for the same reason. It is important to balance the risk of increased preoperative IOP and potential for exaggerated postoperative inflammation in these patients.

A newer prostaglandin analogue, latanoprost 0.005% (Xalatan, Pharmacia-Upjohn, Columbus, OH) has been shown to disrupt the blood-aqueous barrier in the early postoperative period following cataract surgery.[5] Whether this activity has any bearing on the final outcome of trabeculectomy has yet to be determined. However, in a procedure where inflammatory modulators can precipitate fibroblast activity, it may be prudent to have patients stop their use of this medication several days before surgery. This is more significant for patients undergoing combined procedures.

Other medications can adversely affect the outcome of incisional surgery by increasing the risk of postoperative bleeding and hyphema. Epinephrine-derived compounds as well as antiplatelet or anticoagulant therapy should be discontinued 2 to 7 days before surgery to minimize this risk. For patients with unstable systemic conditions, changes to these medications are best made after conferring with their primary care physicians or an appropriate specialist. Medications that are aqueous suppressants (including beta-blocking adrenergic and alpha-adrenergic agents and topical or oral carbonic anhydrase inhibitors) can be continued until the morning of surgery.

Patients with active disease of the ocular surface—e.g., meibomitis or blepharoconjunctivitis—should be treated with appropriate antibiotic therapy prior to surgery because of the increased risk of endophthalmitis.

Previous Use of Glaucoma Medications

There has been concern that the previous use of antiglaucoma medications may have some adverse effect on the outcome of trabeculectomy. An investigation of cumulative duration (described as the number of medications times the length of use for each) has shown this to be a significant risk factor for loss of IOP control in combined glaucoma-cataract procedures.[6] Another study evaluated patients with varying treatment regimens and found that duration of treatment had no effect when topical medications were used for less than 3 years; however, beyond 3 years, there was a significant risk for loss of IOP control. Further, the number of antiglaucoma medications seemed to play a role in the final outcome of the procedure, with patients on multiple medical therapies having a greater risk for treatment failure.[7]

The means by which topical antiglaucoma medications affect wound healing in glaucoma is not exactly known. Broadway et al. have suggested that these medications may have their effect through indirect pathways related to subclinical inflammation and irritation to the tissues, with resultant fibroblast proliferation.[8] An investigation into the effect of topical medications on the integrity of the conjunctival tissue has shown that the conjunctival tissue in eyes treated for at least a year does show a substantial change in populations of goblet cells as well as other conjunctival cell types.[9] Other studies have shown similar findings, with the greatest degree of abnormality in cell populations and conjunctival epithelial metaplasia occurring in eyes subjected to multiple medications.[10,11] These findings are supported by recent data suggesting that treatment with multiple agents produces histological changes in inflammatory cell and fibroblast populations and is partly related to the response of the ocular surface to the application of benzalkonium chloride.[12]

Cataract Surgery following Filtering Procedures

Cataract surgery following incisional surgery requires careful evaluation and follow-up in order to reduce the risk of bleb failure. Although the techniques used in cataract extraction induce less inflammation than older methods do, there is still some postoperative inflammation with risk for bleb failure. Not infrequently, patients who have had filtering surgery have abnormal pupillary function related to the chronic use of miotic agents, pseudoexfoliation, diabetes, uveitis, or iris neovascularization. This increases the risk for postoperative bleeding, since manipulation of the iris may be necessary if the pupil is insufficiently dilated for the procedure.[13]

The risk for increase in intraocular pressure following cataract surgery may place a patient with advanced optic nerve damage at risk for further compromise. Reports have documented IOP eleva-

tion of 30 mmHg in 4 to 14% of patients on the first postoperative day following cataract surgery.[14–16,19] However, a recent retrospective review of patients with filtering blebs who underwent temporal corneal phacoemulsification procedures found smaller increases in IOP in the immediate postoperative period, with no patients having an elevation greater than 30 mmHg.[17] Postoperative fluctuations in IOP are also a consideration in patients with advanced glaucoma, and elevations in postoperative IOP have been associated with increased risk of bleb failure.[13]

Special consideration should be given to patients with certain secondary glaucomas. For example, there is a significant risk of loss of zonular support in patients with pseudoexfoliative glaucoma and potential for lens subluxation intraoperatively or postoperatively. Patients with uveitic or neovascular glaucoma may require more frequent corticosteroid therapy or a longer period of treatment than usual with postoperative medications because of an exaggerated inflammatory response.[13,18]

In any case, inflammation and its associated chemical mediators can induce fibrosis and reduce the effectiveness of the filtering bleb. External fibrosis can lead to shrinkage of the bleb. Reports have documented loss of bleb function following cataract surgery, with subsequent elevation in IOP.[14,19,20] Adjunctive antimetabolite injections or initiation of ocular massage may be required in the early postoperative period to maintain the function of the bleb. However, ocular massage should be deferred for the first week following cataract surgery because of the risk of dislocating the intraocular lens. If necessary, focal decompression or aqueous suppressants can be used during this period for improved IOP control.

COMBINED TRABECULECTOMY, PHACOEMULSIFICATION, AND INTRAOCULAR LENS IMPLANTATION

Patients with symptomatic cataracts as well as poorly controlled glaucoma may consider combined surgery as a management option. For example, patients with advanced nerve head damage who are at significant risk for further neuroretinal rim loss secondary to IOP elevation following cataract extraction alone would be good candidates. However, there have been reports that phacoemulsification with posterior chamber intraocular lens implantation alone can decrease IOP and reduce the number of antiglaucoma medications required postoperatively following cataract extraction. Anders et al. found that combined phacotrabeculectomy significantly decreased IOP and number of glaucoma medications compared to phacoemulsification alone, although there was a small change also noted in patients undergoing phacoemulsification alone.[21] This is supported by a recent investigation by Kim et al., who found uncomplicated phacoemulsification to produce a significant decrease in IOP in glaucoma patients, with decreased numbers of medications required for IOP control.[22]

Other investigations found that combined glaucoma and cataract extraction helped to improve visual acuity as well as IOP control, with fewer medications needed.[23] After 1 year, phacotrabeculectomy resulted in a similar postoperative IOP and bleb appearance compared with trabeculectomy alone.[24] The most common complications following combined procedures included hyphema, posterior capsular opacification (PCO), corneal edema, choroidal detachments, and cystoid macular edema.[23]

There has been considerable discussion regarding the best course of management for patients with cataract and glaucoma. A staged procedure may be appropriate in certain cases, while in others a combined one- or two-site phacotrabeculectomy may prove a better option. A retrospective case-control study of patients undergoing trabeculectomy with or without temporal corneal phacoemulsification (two-site procedure) showed that combined surgery reduced IOP less in long-term follow-up than trabeculectomy alone.[25] A prospective study compared one- to two-site procedures and found that both produced similar improvements in visual acuity and IOP control.[26] However, more patients required antiglaucoma therapy and also a larger number of medications in the one-site than the two-site group at the last follow-up appointment (16.5 ± 4.5 months following surgery). These investigators suggested that the two-site procedure may result in less conjunctival and scleral manipulation and therefore less trauma to the trabeculectomy site.

The role of antimetabolite therapy as an adjunct to combined glaucoma and cataract procedures has been debated. Some reports document no substantial difference in outcome for patients receiving antimetabolite therapy as compared with those who do not.[27–31] However, a recent report documented a substantial reduction in IOP in a placebo-controlled, double-masked evaluation of combined glaucoma and cataract procedures with and without MMC.[32] Fewer bleb revisions were required in patients treated with MMC as compared with those on placebo; however, wound leaks and hypotony occurred more frequently as a complication in this group. Further, the use of intraoperative MMC was found to inhibit lens epithelial cell proliferation and reduce the need for posterior

capsulotomy in patients undergoing combined procedures.[33] A comparison between combined procedure in case-matched patients with and without adjunctive 5-FU concluded that adjunctive 5-FU significantly improved the success rate of trabeculectomy combined with clear corneal cataract extraction.[34] Our experience favors the use of intraoperative antimetabolites when combined surgery is performed.

Risk factors for filtration failure following combined glaucoma and cataract surgery have been identified.[31] Those patients requiring an additional surgical procedure and glaucoma therapy were found to have risk factors including black race, diabetes, preoperative IOP greater than or equal to 20 mmHg, and more than two preoperative medications. A second group, albeit with a more stringent criterion for filtration failure, included patients in whom more than one glaucoma medication was required postoperatively or there was no filtering bleb. Risk factors for filtration failure under this definition included black race, preoperative IOP greater than or equal to 20 mmHg, and more than one preoperative medication. These clinicians concluded that the judicious use of MMC was recommended in primary phacotrabeculectomy and should be limited to patients with one or more risk factors for filtration failure. A follow-up report documented that patients with prognostic factors for filtration failure did have better postsurgical outcomes with the use of adjunctive MMC.[35] Patients without these risk factors did not benefit from the antimetabolite therapy in primary glaucoma and cataract procedures.

Conclusions about the use of MMC in primary and secondary combined procedures have been reported.[36] MMC was not found to significantly increase the success rate in primary triple procedures but did so in secondary cases. Previous failed glaucoma surgery was determined to be a risk factor for filtration failure in secondary combined procedures.

A recent report has documented that even the implanted intraocular lens has some influence on the surgical outcome. Lemon et al. evaluated silicone and polymethylmethacrylate (acrylic) lenses implanted during primary glaucoma triple procedures with MMC.[37] Although both types of intraocular lenses were associated with decreased IOP and use of fewer glaucoma medications, acrylic lenses were associated with higher postoperative IOP and more frequent postoperative IOP spike. Removal of releasable sutures occurred earlier in the postoperative period in patients with acrylic intraocular lenses.

Early postoperative increases in IOP can be managed with digital compression, but the potential risk for lens dislocation is greater for patients undergoing combined procedures if ocular manipulation is required.

Lens decentration occurs infrequently with focal compression but can result in pupillary capture with optical aberration or chronic inflammation.

TRABECULECTOMY

Wound Healing in Glaucoma Filtering Surgery

Modulation of wound healing in glaucoma filtering surgery is directed toward minimizing tissue healing in the episclera and sclera while retaining normal healing of the conjunctiva. Minimizing tissue manipulation during surgery as well as maintaining hemostasis can reduce inflammation and fibrosis.

Skuta suggested that wound healing could be classified as three separate phases.[38] The first phase, *inflammation*, involves the response to tissue insult, including clot formation, cellular migration, and recruiting of fibroblasts, leukocytes, and other growth factors. In the second phase, *proliferation*, vascular formation, migration of monocytes, and division of fibroblasts increases the cellular components of the healing tissue. In the final phase, the new cells undergo a process of *remodeling*, where the collagenous elements are altered.

The degree of wound healing following filtering surgery must be strictly controlled. If wound healing is insufficient, there may be hypotony due to excessive outflow through the scleral passage or a wound leak due to incomplete closure of the conjunctival tissue. At the opposite extreme, if wound healing is excessive, there is a potential for bleb failure due to restricted outflow from fibrous tissue. Wound healing involves a fine balance between external and internal factors that ultimately affect the function of the filtering bleb.

Risk Factors for Bleb Failure in Filtering Surgery

Previous filtering surgery can reduce the success rate of subsequent procedures because of the presence of fibrotic elements in the tissue bed. Often, an adjacent site is chosen for repeat trabeculectomy; however, this is not always possible if patients have undergone other, more invasive procedures such as vitrectomy or retinal detachment surgery or intracapsular cataract extraction with significant scarring at the limbus. The Fluorouracil Filtering Surgery Study found that history of cataract extraction or prior surgery did influence the outcome of trabeculectomy.[39,40] Further, it appeared that the length of time from last surgery affecting conjunctiva also was significant. Coleman et al. found that concomitant intraocular procedures performed in conjunction with glaucoma surgery, such as vitrectomy, substantially increase the risk of postoperative complications (e.g., endophthalmitis, retinal detachment, bleb revision, or cyclophotocoagulation).[41] The benefit of adjunctive MMC in such patients has also been debated, with one study showing an increased success rate[42] but another showing no significant impact.[43]

Certain patient populations are at significant risk for bleb failure based on the nature of their healing response. This would include patients of African-American descent[44] and also younger patients. However, a study evaluating risk factors associated with possible complications following partial or full-thickness glaucoma procedures did not find that black race was significantly associated with increased risk of endophthalmitis, retinal detachment, bleb revision, or cyclophotocoagulation. Another case-matched study comparing the outcome of trabeculectomy with 5-FU found no significant difference in average IOP for African Americans compared to Caucasians, although variability in IOP was more significant in African Americans, as was the need for multiple glaucoma medications following surgery.[45] The Fluorouracil Filtering Surgery Study found that race and age did not affect the outcome of trabeculectomy with 5-FU.[39,40]

Other risk factors that have been associated with bleb failure following surgery include uveitis, aphakia,[46] and secondary angle closure.[39,40] The presence of preexisting conditions that predispose the eye to an exaggerated inflammatory response can also influence surgical outcome.[47] Antimetabolites have helped to increase surgical success in uveitic glaucoma by decreasing excessive scar tissue formation.[48] Investigators have shown that trabeculectomy with adjunctive MMC can decrease IOP in patients with a history of ocular inflammation, although complications can frequently occur and may require further glaucoma surgery for acceptable IOP control.[49] Patients with uveitic glaucoma may require systemic steroid therapy following filtration surgery and may benefit from the immunosuppressive effects of adjunctive 5-FU or MMC. An exaggerated inflammatory response is also a concern in patients with neovascular glaucoma undergoing filtering surgery.[47] Tsai et al. found that glaucoma filtering surgery with 5-FU in patients with neovascular glaucoma carried a poor prognosis for long-term IOP control.[50] The risk of hyphema and microhyphema is greater for patients with active iris or angle neovascularization.

Patients with angle-recession glaucoma are more likely to suffer from bleb failure due to preexisting changes in the drainage pathway than are patients with primary open-angle glaucoma.[51] However, the use of antimetabolite agents can significantly

TABLE 23-1. RISK FACTORS ASSOCIATED
WITH BLEB FAILURE

Previous surgery—e.g., filtering surgery,
   cataract extraction
Concomitant vitrectomy
African-American race
Young age
Uveitis
Aphakia
Neovascularization
Angle recession
Secondary angle closure

improve the success rate of incisional surgery in
these patients.[52,53]

Careful consideration of preexisting risk factors
(Table 23–1) is necessary in determining likelihood of
success following glaucoma filtering procedures.
These factors may play a role in the type of surgery
performed (i.e., the selection, duration, and concentration of adjunctive chemotherapy), frequency of follow-up, and prognosis for long-term IOP control.

SURGICAL TECHNIQUE
FOR TRABECULECTOMY

1. Exposure: The globe is rotated inferiorly to provide a good view of the sclera and conjunctival
   fornix. A traction suture is placed in the peripheral cornea or under the superior rectus muscle
   (Fig. 23–1). We use a 6-0 Vicryl suture on a
   spatulated needle in the peripheral cornea.

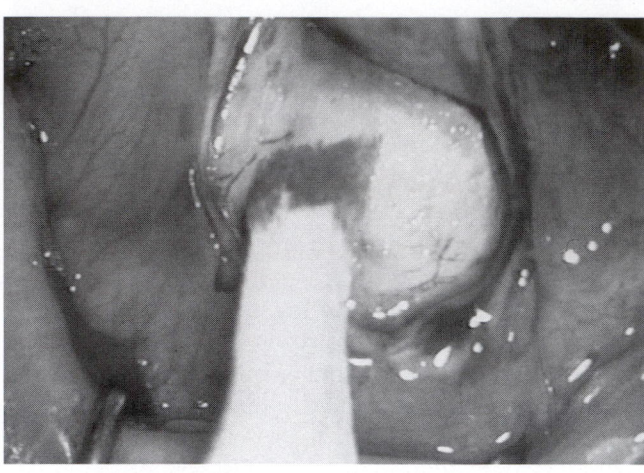

Figure 23-2. Dissection of Tenon's capsule has been completed.
(*See also Color Plate 44.*)

2. Conjunctival incision: This may be placed either at the limbus to create a fornix-based conjunctival flap, or 8 to 9 mm posterior to the
   limbus, in the conjunctival fornix, to create a
   limbus-based flap. We prefer to create a limbus-based flap, since antimetabolites are used
   intraoperatively and we want to minimize any
   leaks close to the actual site of the trabeculectomy. Dissection of Tenon's capsule is important to maintain an appropriate thickness of
   the bleb wall, especially with the use of antimetabolites (Fig. 23–2).
3. Scleral flap: A lamellar flap of sclera is fashioned, approximately one-half thickness of the
   sclera with the base of the flap at the limbus
   (Figs. 23–3 and 23–4). The actual dimensions
   and shape of the flap vary from surgeon to surgeon; however, these factors have no influence

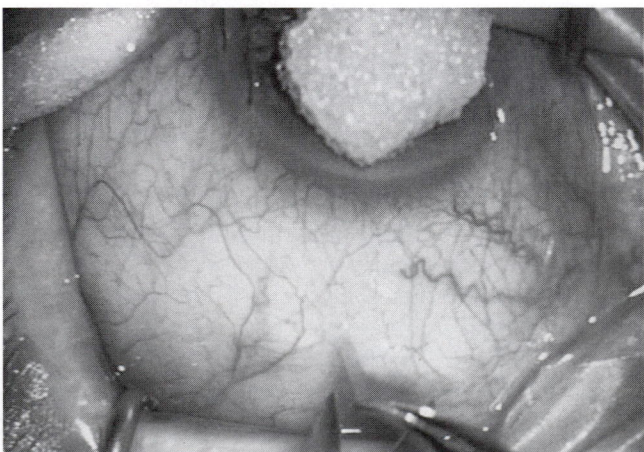

Figure 23-1. Exposure of the surgical site. Note the traction suture in the peripheral cornea. (*See also Color Plate 43.*)

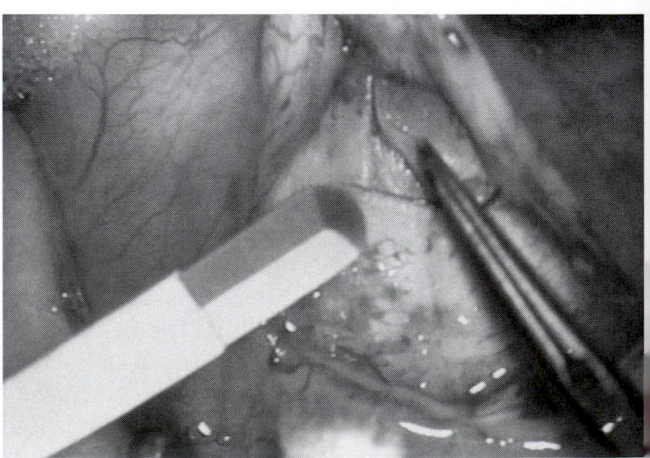

Figure 23-3. Lamellar scleral flap of approximately 50% scleral
thickness. (*See also Color Plate 45.*)

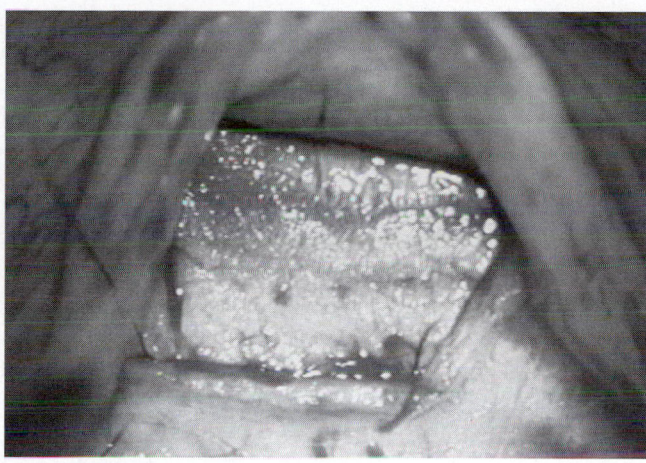

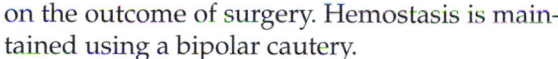

Figure 23–4. Exposure of the surgical limbus prior to use of intraoperative antimetabolites. (*See also Color Plate 46.*)

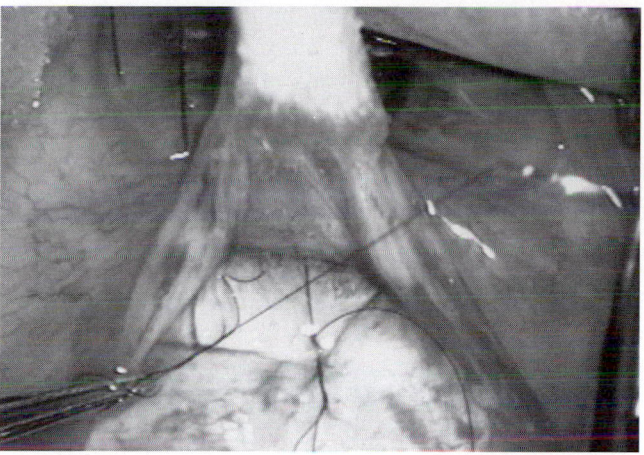

Figure 23–5. Placement of releasable sutures to prevent hypotony in the early postoperative period. (*See also Color Plate 47.*)

on the outcome of surgery. Hemostasis is maintained using a bipolar cautery.

4. Application of antimetabolites: If antimetabolites are used, these are applied either before creation of the scleral flap or immediately thereafter. Sponges are made from Mericel wicks or Weck-cel wicks. These pledgets are soaked in the selected antimetabolite (5-FU or MMC) and placed either directly on the scleral surface or under the newly created scleral flap for a brief period of time (2 to 5 minutes). The underlying conjunctival tissue is laid over the flap with care to ensure that this free edge of tissue is not touching the antimetabolite sponge.

5. Excision of trabecular meshwork: The limbal portion of the scleral flap actually extends into clear cornea. An incision parallel to the limbus is made with a sharp blade into the anterior chamber next to the location of the trabecular meshwork. A block of trabecular meshwork is removed posterior to the corneal incision, either with a specially designed punch or freehand with fine Vannas scissors. This opening is located directly under the base of the scleral flap and is smaller than the lateral margins of the lamellar scleral flap.

6. Iridectomy: A small peripheral iridectomy is created through the trabecular-corneal opening under the scleral flap. This prevents the iris from closing and blocking the opening in the early postoperative period should the anterior chamber become shallow.

7. Scleral flap closure: The scleral flap is repositioned back to the original location and secured tightly with interrupted 9-0 or 10-0 nylon sutures. This particular aspect of the operation

tends to be the most critical and requires fastidious attention to detail, since small flow through the scleral flap is desired but not too much, where hypotony would be a significant concern. The sutures may be fashioned as releasable sutures (Fig. 23–5) or traditional interrupted sutures. Should the IOP become too high postoperatively, the scleral flap can be loosened either by removing the releasable sutures or by lasering the sutures transconjunctivally.

8. Conjunctival closure: The original incision is carefully reapproximated with a fine suture. Often Tenon's layer is closed independently of the conjunctiva, thus creating a two-layer closure. The important point is to suture the conjunctiva together so there is no leakage of fluid (Fig. 23–6).

9. Injections: After removing the traction suture, antibiotics and steroids are administered in the

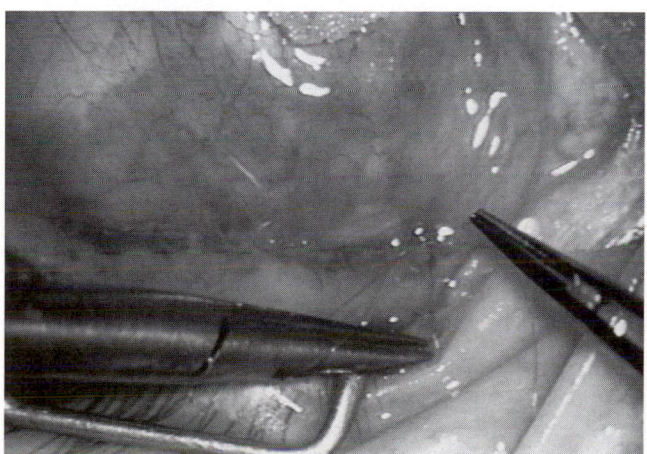

Figure 23–6. Conjunctival closure at completion of case. (*See also Color Plate 48.*)

sub-Tenon space. Often an antibiotic drop and a cycloplegic drop are instilled before placing a patch and shield over the eye.

Surgical Variations in Trabeculectomy

Limbus-versus Fornix-Based Scleral Flap in Trabeculectomy

Limbus-based trabeculectomy actually involves a conjunctival incision in the conjunctival fornix, with the conjunctiva and Tenon's capsule dissection directed anteriorly toward the limbus. Blebs fashioned in this style are generally more cystic[54] and elevated than the fornix-based flaps and are perhaps more easily checked for early signs of failure than comparatively lower-lying fornix-based blebs. Studies have shown that limbus- and fornix-based conjunctival flaps are equally successful in terms of complication rates and effect on outcome, whether performed alone[55] or in combination with cataract extraction.[56] Reichert et al. reported similar findings; however, IOP was lower in patients with limbus-based trabeculectomy.[57] These clinicians also documented a higher incidence of posterior capsular rupture in combined cataract and limbus-based glaucoma procedures.

This type of trabeculectomy reduces the risk of corneal exposure to the antimetabolite and poses a lower risk of wound leak along the posterior conjunctival incision line. However, it can be difficult to dissect the conjunctiva toward the limbus in patients who have extensive scarring of the limbal conjunctiva.

A fornix-based trabeculectomy could be considered in cases when access to the surgical site is limited by the orbital structure or where prior conjunctival surgery was associated with scarring (Fig. 23–7). A fornix-based trabeculectomy produces a bleb that is generally more diffuse and lower-lying. This technique has an advantage because of the improved access to the surgical site and a shorter conjunctival incision.[58,59] El Sayyad et al. found that fornix-based flaps were as successful as limbus-based flaps in controlling IOP in long-term follow-up and that these blebs were less likely to develop wound leaks.[54] This was also true when fornix-based trabeculectomy was combined with cataract extraction.[60] Hemostasis is more easily maintained. However, because of the bleb's proximity to the limbus, significantly more postoperative astigmatism can be induced. Patients with fornix-based flaps must take extra precautions in performing ocular massage, since there is an increased vulnerability of the surgical site to wound leak as well as weakness in the attachments between the cornea and conjunctiva.

Use of Antimetabolites in Filtering Surgery

Advances in trabeculectomy have been associated with increasing the success rate of filtering surgery. One of the major efforts involves modulation of wound healing, since fibrosis following glaucoma procedures can lead to bleb failure. Antimetabolites such as MMC and 5-FU have been used to reduce fibroblast proliferation especially in eyes with significant risk factors for failure. In vitro studies of these and other agents have demonstrated the local effects of these medications on sub-Tenon fibroblasts.[61,62] A more recent report has investigated the mechanism of effect for 5-FU and MMC. The investigators have determined that these antimetabolites induce apoptosis, a gene-directed programmed cell death in human Tenon's capsule fibroblasts.[63]

Antifibrotic agents such as 5-FU interfere with fibroblast replication. This chemotherapeutic agent can be applied intraoperatively beneath or on top of the scleral flap or postoperatively through subconjunctival injections. The Fluorouracil Filtering Surgery Study showed that postoperative injections of subconjunctival 5-FU increased the rate of IOP control at 1, 3, and 5 years after surgery.[39,40,64] The postsurgical outcome was significantly improved for patients at risk for bleb failure, including those with prior cataract surgery or previous failed glaucoma filtering surgery. A retrospective case review showed that adjunctive 5-FU improved IOP control and decreased the number of antiglaucoma medications required as compared with control eyes.[65] Other studies found similar results for patients receiving postoperative injections of 5-FU.[66–68] Intraoperative 5-FU has been associated with better IOP control compared with postoperative subconjunctival injections of 5-FU, although there is a greater risk for hypotony with

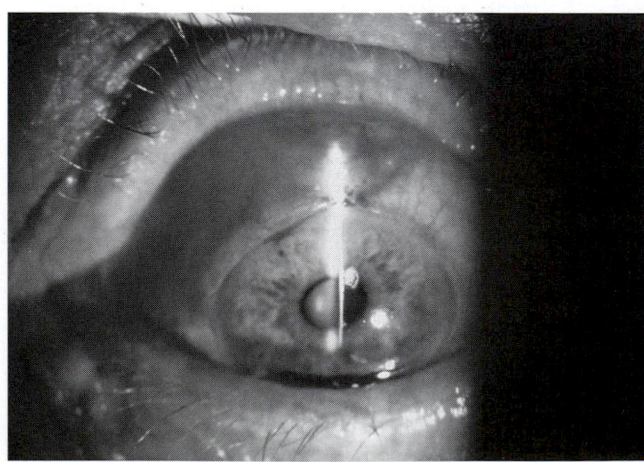

Figure 23–7. Fornix-based trabeculectomy in the early postoperative period. Subconjunctival hemorrhages are common. (*See also Color Plate 49.*)

the intraoperative administration of this agent.[69,70] Other investigators have concurred with these findings, concluding that intraoperative 5-FU resulted in good IOP control with fewer corneal epithelial defects.[71-73] This antimetabolite can be also used intraoperatively in primary trabeculectomy instead of MMC to reduce the risk of postoperative hypotony.[74]

The use of 5-FU can be associated with hypotony, wound leaks, keratitis (Fig. 23–8), corneal epithelial defects, progression of cataract, and slower recovery of vision.[39,40,64-66,69,70,73,75] Intraoperative 5-FU may be preferred over postoperative injections of 5-FU owing to the reduced risk of ocular perforation and lower incidence of toxic corneal epitheliopathy.

MMC is a biological material produced by *Streptomyces caespitosus*, a fungus, which has antineoplastic effects. Chen first described its use in ocular surgery in 1983.[76] In animal studies, subconjunctival MMC was found to decrease IOP and increase bleb duration after full-thickness surgery in rabbits.[77] These effects also have been documented in human eyes; however, the benefit of MMC in glaucoma filtering procedures has been debated. Various reports regarding its success and failure in different patient populations as well as its associated complications—such as wound leak, chronic hypotony, and endophthalmitis—have been published. In an editorial comment, Higginbotham posed the question: "Is it worth the risk?"[78] She felt that the benefits of trabeculectomy with MMC outweighed the risks, although she urged surgeons to exercise caution in selecting the concentration and exposure time for this chemotherapy.

The use of MMC has been evaluated in primary and secondary glaucoma filtering surgery for patients with primary open-angle and secondary glaucomas.

In one population, MMC trabeculectomy was shown to control IOP for up to 50% of patients after 3 years, with a 30% risk for complications and a 15% chance of surgical revision being required for correction of postoperative complications.[79] A prospective study evaluated the success of primary trabeculectomy with a single dose and high-duration application of MMC in 89 eyes. Investigators found that 75% of patients did not require reoperation and had IOP readings below 15 mmHg at 1 year and 64% at 2 years.[44] Another study of primary MMC trabeculectomy in white patients documented good control in 92% of patients using a less stringent criterion.[80] Judicious use of MMC in primary trabeculectomy has been suggested because of the risk of hypotony and endophthalmitis.

In other populations, MMC has been shown to influence the outcome of trabeculectomy. As previously discussed, this may be a more pertinent issue in patient populations with greater risk of bleb failure. Other populations have benefited from the adjunctive use of intraoperative MMC, including those with normal-tension glaucoma and pediatric glaucoma; however, further studies are necessary.[81-83]

Surgical variations in the application of MMC include the duration and location of application, the type of applicator, and the concentration of MMC solution. MMC applied after dissection of the scleral bed was found to control IOP better than episcleral application (before scleral bed dissection).[84] Flynn et al. found a substantial difference in the absorption and swelling characteristics of commercially available microsurgical sponges.[85] These investigators concluded that exposure to MMC and varying success rates reported in the literature can be related to this intraoperative factor. A survey of glaucoma subspecialists from the United States and Japan found that the dosages of MMC given intraoperatively and the duration of application were quite varied and were influenced by the number and type of previous procedures, the presence of conjunctival scarring, age, race, refractive error, and phakic status.[74] Dosages ranged from 0.1 to 0.5 mg/mL and for 5 seconds to 7 minutes. Surgeons were found to adjust the concentration and duration of treatment with MMC according to risk factors for bleb failure, with longer duration for patients with neovascular glaucoma and shorter duration for patients undergoing primary trabeculectomy or combined procedures. Increasing concentrations of the MMC solution applied during fornix-based trabeculectomy in an Indian population were associated with decreased IOP.[86] Another study documented differences in short- and long-term IOP control with two concentrations of MMC.[87] These investigators did not control for duration of application, although the duration of MMC

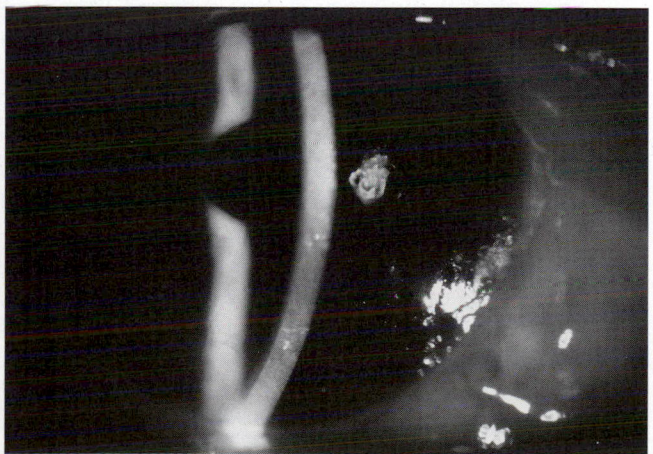

Figure 23–8. Punctate keratitis associated with postoperative injections of 5-fluorouracil. (*See also Color Plate 50.*)

application was not found to be significant in another report.[43] Obviously, there is a fine balance between IOP control and potential for postoperative complications when surgical parameters related to use of MMC are considered.

This antimetabolite has effects locally as well as on other ocular tissues. Cataract progression was related to increased exposure to mitomycin therapy.[86] An association between MMC and decreased corneal endothelial cell density has been documented.[88] Scleritis has been associated infrequently with MMC trabeculectomy.[89] Other reports have documented cases of central retinal vein occlusion associated with MMC trabeculectomy, although it is unclear that the use of MMC was the primary cause of the vascular event.[90]

MMC and 5-FU have been compared in a number of studies. Skuta et al. compared postoperative subconjunctival injections of 5-FU with intraoperative MMC in patients at high risk for surgical failure. These investigators found that eyes treated with MMC had lower IOP readings and that fewer antiglaucoma medications were required postoperatively.[91] A follow-up report documented that additional glaucoma filtering surgery was later required in 15% of eyes.[92] Other reports have shown a similar increase in IOP control following MMC trabeculectomy.[93] In addition to superior IOP reduction, fewer corneal epithelial defects are observed following trabeculectomy with MMC than following multiple postoperative subconjunctival injections of 5-FU.[91,93] With the exception of corneal epitheliopathy, other postoperative complications (including flat anterior chamber, hypotony, choroidal detachment, bleb failure, hyphema, and cataract progression) occurred with equal frequency following MMC or 5-FU trabeculectomy.[93,94] However, other reports have documented a higher incidence of wound leak following trabeculectomy with antimetabolites,[95,190] more often associated with MMC.[96]

Scleral Flap Sutures

Scleral flap sutures allow the surgeon to titrate the effect of the trabeculectomy and reduce the incidence of postoperative hypotony. These sutures may be releasable or interrupted. Both types are placed at the time of surgery and then cut or removed as necessary as wound healing occurs. The sutures effectively slow the egress of fluid by tightening the scleral flap until sufficient healing has occurred. Blok et al. have described a series of patients who underwent trabeculectomy procedures augmented by varying numbers of interrupted scleral flap sutures.[97] Complications related to a shallow or flat anterior chamber occurred less frequently with increased numbers of flap sutures. Laser suture lysis was used to treat postoperative elevation of IOP. In a retrospective

chart review, Kolker et al. reported similar findings for patients with both interrupted scleral flap sutures and releasable sutures.[98] The depth of the anterior chamber was reduced less frequently with releasable sutures, and fewer surgical interventions for anterior chamber reformation were required. Similar conclusions were reached by a recent randomized prospective study that compared releasable sutures with conventional interrupted sutures.[99] Other investigators have also found that releasable sutures were associated with fewer postoperative complications and resulted in better immediate postoperative IOP control.[100,101] Since the releasable suture is externalized on the corneal or conjunctival surface, the potential for infection along the suture track should be considered; case reports have documented this occasional occurrence.[102,103]

There is a certain window of opportunity in which the sutures can be released. However, the advent of antimetabolite therapy has expanded this window, so that sutures can be released with significant pressure-lowering effect even months after surgery. Tezel et al. found that intraoperative antimetabolite agents would extend the interval during which IOP could be lowered through the release of sutures after trabeculectomy with either MMC or 5-FU.[104] Even when releasable sutures were removed after the third postoperative week, a significant effect was observed. This was true for patients undergoing trabeculectomy as well those undergoing trabeculectomy and cataract extraction without the use of metabolites.

Postoperative Medications

Postoperative medications after trabeculectomy generally include anti-inflammatory, antibiotic, and cycloplegic agents. The prophylactic antibiotic is usually administered four times daily and is generally discontinued after the first postoperative week.

The anti-inflammatory is administered more frequently in the immediate postoperative period, with dosage schedules up to every 1 hour depending on the nature and potential of the inflammatory response. The corticosteroid is tapered according to the patient's healing response. If the eye is hypotonous, steroids may be tapered more quickly in order to encourage fibrosis. In general, the postoperative use of corticosteroids has been associated with fewer subsequent glaucoma surgeries, fewer antiglaucoma medications, and lower IOP by comparison with untreated eyes.[105–107] In other patients with a history of ocular inflammation—i.e., uveitic glaucoma—topical steroid therapy may be augmented by oral steroid medications; however, there is no benefit of oral prednisone in addition to topical therapy for glaucoma not related to inflammatory processes.[106,107] There may be a concern for steroid-induced increase in IOP related to the frequent dosage of the corticosteroid,[108] although some investigations have shown that a postoperative increase in IOP also occurs in controls.[107]

More recently, nonsteroidal anti-inflammatory drugs (NSAIDs) have been used to successfully control postoperative inflammation. A prospective study compared diclofenac 0.1% and prednisolone acetate 1% and found the NSAID medication to be equally effective in controlling postoperative inflammation.[109] There was no significant difference in the IOP outcome following trabeculectomy with either agent.

Cycloplegic agents in the postoperative period help to enhance the blood-brain barrier and reduce postoperative inflammation and leakage of plasma proteins. A strong cycloplegic such as atropine 1% can be administered from one to four times daily. The cycloplegic is also of benefit in hypotonous eyes and can help to prevent shallowing of the anterior chamber. Although cycloplegic agents are usually discontinued after the first week following surgery, the duration of treatment may be prolonged if the eye develops hypotony.

Patient Counseling: Postoperative

Following trabeculectomy, patients are instructed to avoid vigorous activity, straining, and lifting of objects weighing more than 25 pounds. There is an increased risk of suprachoroidal hemorrhage in the postoperative period with Valsalva maneuver, including coughing, choking, sneezing, and nose-blowing. This is of particular concern in aphakic patients, elderly patients with high preoperative IOP, or those who have undergone vitrectomy. Precautions should be taken to prevent inadvertent rupture of the globe in the immediate postoperative period; this may include the use of a perforated metal shield, spectacle correction, or sunglasses. Patients are also asked to refrain from getting water into the eye—i.e., swimming or shower during the first week following surgery.

In general, anti-inflammatory agents are taken for approximately 6 weeks after surgery; however, the frequency of dosage is tapered on an individual basis. Patients with an exaggerated postoperative inflammatory response generally will remain on steroid therapy for an extended period. Alternatively, patients with ocular hypotony may have their steroid eyedrops tapered more quickly in an effort to induce scar formation.

Postoperative Assessment

The characteristics of a filtering bleb vary significantly. A bleb may vary in extent, height, thickness, vascularity, or color (Table 23–2). Blebs can be described as focal, localized, or diffuse (Fig. 23–9). A focal bleb is well circumscribed, with well-defined borders. Other blebs can extend several clock-hours around the

TABLE 23–2. POSTOPERATIVE EVALUATION

External Appearance
  Ptosis
  Lid edema
  Lid ecchymosis
Cornea
  Epithelial defects
  Dellen
  Toxic keratopathy
  Abrasions or foreign-body tracking related to sutures
  Microcystic edema
  Descemet or stromal folds
Conjunctiva
  Hyperemia
  Chemosis
  Telangiectasia adjacent to bleb
  Subconjunctival hemorrhage
Bleb
  Extent
  Elevation or height
  Thickness
  Pallor
  Vascularity
  Telangiectasia of conjunctival vessels
  Conjunctival epithelial defects overlying bleb
  Presence or absence of Seidel
  Transudation or "ooze"

Anterior Chamber
  Presence or absence of cells or flare
  Hyphema
  Hypopyon
  Central and peripheral depth
Iris
  Iris contour
  Regularity of pupil
  Patency of peripheral iridotomy
  Sphincter abnormalities—e.g., hemorrhage following pupillary stretching, sphincterectomies
Lens
  Centration of intraocular implant
  Transparency of posterior capsule
  Opacities of the crystalline lens
IOP
  Before and after focal decompression or ocular massage
Retina
  Macula: edema, folds or striae, epiretinal membrane
  Hemorrhages: dot, blot, nerve fiber layer
  Periphery: retinal tear or detachment, choroidal detachment, suprachoroidal hemorrhage

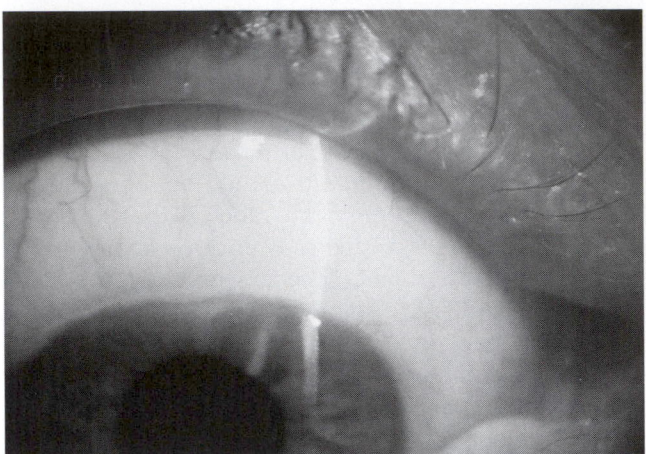

Figure 23–9. Diffuse, succulent, low-lying bleb with minimal vascularity and absence of conjunctival injection. (*See also Color Plate 51.*)

limbus or circumferentially. Smaller cystic blebs were found to fail more quickly than larger blebs following MMC trabeculectomy.[110] The height of the bleb is also important because a high bleb may directly cause discomfort or indirectly affect the tear film. Rarely, pain can occur secondary to transient air-bubble formation. A flat bleb is of concern, since the height of the bleb generally decreases with loss of filtering function.

A bleb may also be described as thick or thin—a characteristic that generally describes the visibility of the underlying flap (Fig. 23–10). Thinner blebs occur more frequently following full-thickness procedures compared to partial-thickness procedures.[111,112] These blebs may be at greater risk for wound leak.[96] The bleb may be described as macrocystic. A macrocystic bleb exhibits grape-like lobules within its substance. This type of bleb is more common with use of postoperative corticosteroids.[107]

Instillation of sodium fluorescein allows for the assessment of several features of the filtering bleb, including the presence or absence of conjunctival epithelial defects, microcysts, and transudation—the slow "ooze" of aqueous through the functioning intact conjunctival tissue. Microcysts form because of transconjunctival fluid movement and are generally present on the surface of well-functioning blebs. Transudation must be distinguished from a wound leak that manifests as a "Seidel sign." A moistened fluorescein strip or a 2% sodium fluorescein solution should be applied directly to the bleb and the tear film evaluated for a rapid diffusion of fluorescein around a dark stream of fluid. A Seidel sign indicates that the integrity of the bleb surface has been compromised and a leak is present. If an eye is hypotonous, the entire conjunctival surface must be evaluated for a wound leak, since wound leaks are not always located over the bleb. Because of changes in the ocular surface as a result of filtering surgery, distal conjunctival tissue that is thinner or fibrosed may also be vulnerable to epithelial breakdown.

The bleb should also be assessed for the extent and nature of vascular changes. The conjunctival vasculature may be attenuated or absent in eyes that have been treated with antimetabolites. A comparison of eyes following antimetabolite trabeculectomy has documented an increased incidence of wound leak in eyes with ischemic (nonvascularized) blebs as compared with those that have vascularized blebs.[113] Conjunctival blood vessels may appear smooth in their course or twisted. Telangiectasia of the conjunctival blood vessels can occur in eyes that are progressing toward bleb failure secondary to inflammatory mediators (Fig. 23–11). Injection of these blood vessels is also of concern as an indicator of inflammation or infection.

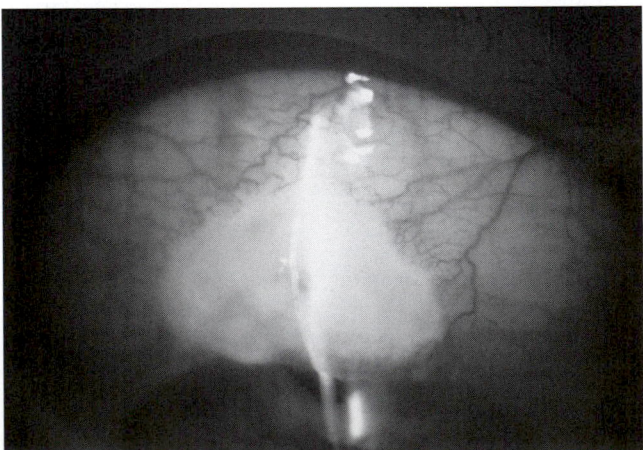

Figure 23–10. Thin, moderately elevated macrocystic bleb with surrounding conjunctival injection. (*See also Color Plate 52.*)

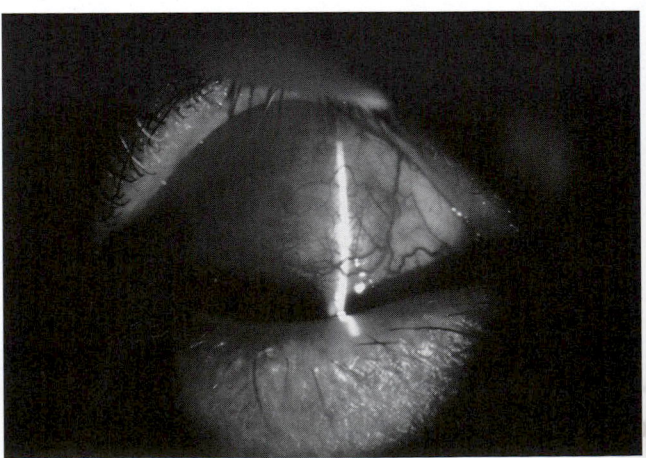

Figure 23–11. High, thick focal bleb with telangiectatic vessels. This filter is failing. (*See also Color Plate 53.*)

Careful assessment of the surrounding conjunctival vasculature is also helpful.

Other aspects of the ocular surface to be described include the appearance of the conjunctiva—e.g., areas of elevation associated with an extensive bleb. Subconjunctival hemorrhages are common following filtering surgery; however, the position of the hemorrhage may be significant if it is adjacent to or beneath the scleral flap.

The cornea must be evaluated for epithelial defects that may occur following surgery. Punctate keratitis can occur because of antimetabolite therapy and preservative toxicity from postoperative medications. Epithelial defects can result from thinning of the tear film due to moderate or high blebs.

Stromal folds or folds in Descemet's membrane may be present. Microcystic edema may also develop when pressures are significantly elevated following surgery. If the IOP is very low, the epithelial mosaic is easily seen with fluorescein. This pattern is observed when the corneal epithelium infolds as a result of hypotony.

The anterior chamber should be evaluated for cell and flare. Other significant findings would include the presence of a blood clot caused by trauma to iris vessels or to vascular rupture within the ostium. If sufficient bleeding occurs, a hyphema may be present (Fig. 23–12). If the pressure were acceptable on the first postoperative day, it would be reasonable to defer any manipulation of the surgical site for a day or two in order to reduce the risk for rebleeding. The presence of excessive inflammatory material may give rise to fibrotic membranes or even a hypopyon.

Fundus assessment should include an evaluation of the peripheral retina for retinal detachment or tear. Other significant findings would include choroidal detachment or suprachoroidal hemorrhage. The macula should be carefully inspected for signs of macular edema, epiretinal membrane formation, and macular folds. If there is a significant decrease in IOP following surgery, dot and blot hemorrhages may be present in the posterior pole or midperiphery. These hemorrhages develop because of the acute decompression of the eye after trabeculectomy. This condition has been termed *rebound or decompression retinopathy* and has been reported in a number of patients following glaucoma filtering surgery.[114]

Decreased Intraocular Pressure following Filtering Surgery

Qualitatively, hypotony has been described as the condition of low IOP that is able to produce structural alterations within the retina as well as visual disturbances (Table 23–3). Although the definition of hypotony varies from study to study, reports of hypotony (IOP ≤ 5 mmHg) in the literature range from 0 to 38%.[80] Hypotony is a significant complication that has been associated with delayed visual recovery following filtering surgery.[4] In addition, excessively low IOP can be associated with a number of other postoperative complications, including a shallow anterior chamber, serous choroidal detachment, cataract, progression of visual field loss, and hypotony maculopathy.[115]

Certain risk factors have been associated with hypotony, which has been shown to occur more frequently with longer application times for antimetabolites,[116] use of MMC in primary trabeculectomy,[116] young age, and myopia.

Inadvertent Eye Rubbing

Patients may inadvertently reduce IOP by rubbing the eye. This often occurs in response to foreign-body sensation or irritation related to the incision site, elevation of the bleb, or the presence of sutures. Eye rubbing may occur while tears are being blotted from the eyes or the eyes are dabbed after the instillation of postoperative eyedrops. Bleb rupture has been reported following MMC trabeculectomy as a result of the blotting of tears.[117] Often, the patient is unaware that this pattern of

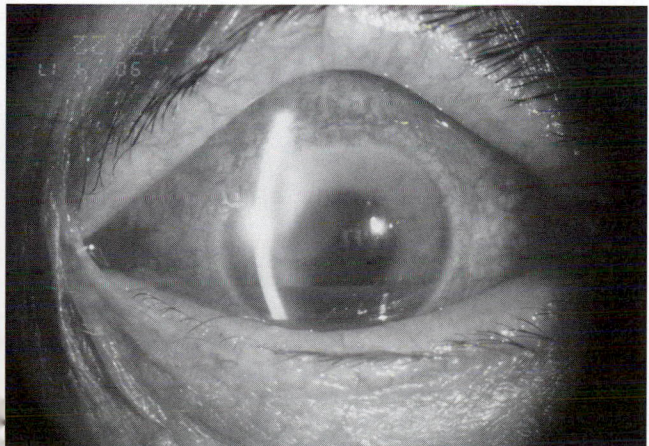

Figure 23–12. Hyphema following trabeculectomy. (*See also Color Plate 54.*)

TABLE 23–3. ETIOLOGY OF HYPOTONY
Inadvertent eye rubbing
Concomitant use of glaucoma medications
Aqueous hyposecretion
Cyclodialysis cleft
Choroidal detachment
Overfiltration
Wound leak

behavior has developed until questioned specifically about it. Hypotony related to inadvertent eye rubbing quickly resolves once the offending behavior has been recognized and discontinued.

Concomitant Use of Glaucoma Medications

Hypotony may also occur in postoperative trabeculectomy patients related to the use of antiglaucoma medications after surgery. A series of case reports has documented the occurrence of hypotony after filtering surgery related to the use of dorzolamide.[118] Patients undergoing glaucoma surgery must be adequately counseled regarding the discontinuation of usual glaucoma medications in the operative eye. Decreased IOP may result from crossover effects if the patient is being treated with a beta-blocking agent or an alpha-adrenergic agonist in the contralateral eye. Temporary discontinuation of the medication is suggested to rule out an additional IOP-lowering effect when postoperative hypotony is a concern. Special consideration should be given to treatment of the fellow eye when oral carbonic anhydrase inhibitors are discontinued.

Aqueous Hyposecretion

Ciliary body shutdown can develop after filtration surgery due to intraocular inflammation and breakdown of the blood-aqueous barrier. Reduced aqueous production can be related to the degree of postoperative uveitis. Therefore, eyes with substantial postoperative inflammation and hypotony should be aggressively treated with topical corticosteroids every 1 or 2 hours. In patients with uveitis, systemic corticosteroids may be required for additional anti-inflammatory effect.

Cyclodialysis Cleft

Cyclodialysis occurs when the ciliary body becomes disinserted from its origin at the scleral spur. Most commonly, this separation occurs as a result of trauma or eye surgery. Cyclodialysis clefts have been reported following glaucoma and cataract surgery.[119,120] Other associated conditions have included choroidal detachment, hypotony maculopathy, and hyperopic shift of refractive error. Cyclodialysis clefts occur very infrequently and are often difficult to observe. More recent technology has permitted the diagnosis of these clefts in hypotonous eyes by ultrasound biomicroscopy.[121,122] Initial treatment in eyes with suspected cyclodialysis involves the use of cycloplegic agents to encourage the reapposition of the ciliary body to the scleral tissues.[123] If this procedure is unsuccessful, surgical correction can be considered. Cyclodialysis clefts, although rare, should be considered in the differential diagnosis of hypotony following filtering surgery.

Ciliochoroidal Detachment

Ciliochoroidal detachments occur due to the imbalance between the fluid pressure within the eye and the choroidal vasculature. In a hypotonous eye, this allows fluid to accumulate in the potential space between the choroid and the sclera. As the IOP increases, this hydrostatic differential is reduced, with gradual resolution of the choroidal detachment.

Ciliochoroidal detachments occur more commonly in hypotonous eyes and may mask a suprachoroidal hemorrhage. A choroidal detachment can be differentiated from a retinal detachment by its smooth, opaque appearance (Fig. 23–13). A retinal detachment undulates with eye movement, and pigmented cells or a retinal break may be observed. However, a choroidal detachment can demonstrate a shallow overlying retinal detachment.[124] Adjunctive testing including ultrasound B-scan can aid in the differential diagnosis between choroidal detachment, retinal detachment, and suprachoroidal hemorrhage.

Clinically, it is important to compare the depth of the peripheral anterior chamber in the involved eye with that in the fellow eye in order to detect subtle shallowing of the anterior chamber. Patients can become symptomatic and may describe a "shadow" or "veil" that passes through their vision with eye movements.

Because ciliochoroidal detachment can be related to decreased aqueous production and cyclitis, it is important to manage patients with hypotony and ciliochoroidal detachment adequately with appropriate dosages of topical and/or systemic corticosteroids and cycloplegic agents.

Choroidal detachments may require surgical intervention in the event of prolonged apposition of choroidal detachments, or "kissing choroidals," that

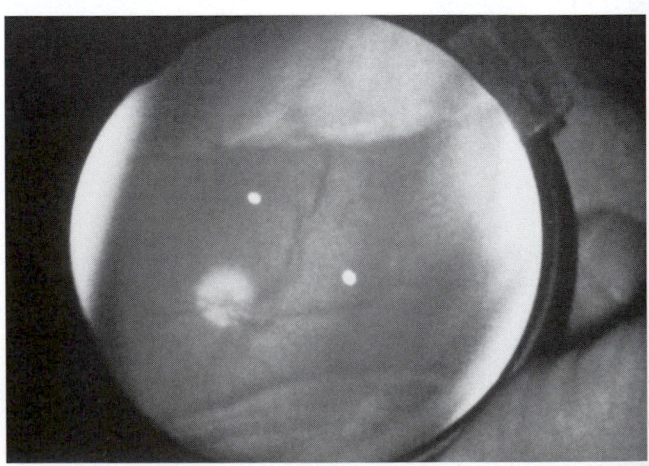

Figure 23–13. Choroidal detachment. (*See also Color Plate 55.*)

would predispose the eye to fibrous retinal adhesions or if the anterior chamber flattened. Posterior sclerotomies allow for drainage of the suprachoroidal fluid.

Overfiltration

Overfiltration may occur if the outflow of aqueous exceeds aqueous production. This may occur as a result of decreased resistance to outflow. Hypotony secondary to a scleral fistula as created during trabeculectomy can result in a diffuse, extensive bleb and a low IOP without wound leak.

Wound Leak

A wound leak may develop early or late in the postoperative period. Wound leaks may also occur years after filtration surgery. Risk factors increasing the chance of a conjunctival defect include use of an antimetabolite during filtration surgery, thin bleb,[113] and thinned or scarred conjunctiva secondary to prior ocular surgery. Wound leaks can result from excessive manipulation of the conjunctiva during surgery. Reports documenting the incidence of wound leak following trabeculectomy with 5-FU or MMC have ranged from 5 to 30%, although a more recent study has documented rates of 3.7% of patients with MMC trabeculectomy and 1.4% of patients with 5-FU trabeculectomy.[96] Histopathology of tissue following wound leak associated with antimetabolite filtering surgery has documented breakdown of the conjunctival epithelium with thinning and stromal necrosis.[95]

The bleb should be evaluated for a wound leak at each appointment, since wound leaks may develop even in eyes that are not hypotonous.[96] The conjunctiva should be evaluated for a positive Seidel sign in areas that are peripheral to the bleb. If the pressure is very low, there may be insufficient aqueous to produce a Seidel sign. In this case, very gentle pressure should be exerted against the globe after instillation of sodium fluorescein to perform a "pressure Seidel test." The manipulation of the eyeball may cause aqueous to leak more visibly from a subtle defect.

It is important to instill fluorescein from a moistened sterile strip or from a 2% droperette to evaluate for a wound leak. Commercial preparations including sodium fluorescein and topical anesthetic agents may be too viscous and lead to false-negative results. If a leak is observed, the position and extent of the leak should be evaluated. A defect may occur along the conjunctival incision site, along the suture track, or in the bleb itself. Small wound leaks must be differentiated from normal transudation of aqueous or "bleb sweat." In the early postoperative period, limbal wound leaks create a risk for conjunctival and episcleral adhesions due to flattening of the bleb and possi-

ble bleb failure. Further, any wound leak places the eye at risk for bleb infection.

COMPLICATIONS OF HYPOTONY

Flat Anterior Chamber

The depth of the anterior chamber can be classified in three stages (Fig. 23–14). If the peripheral iris is in contact with the corneal endothelium, this is classified as stage I (Fig. 23–15). Further shallowing creates increased iridocorneal contact with the pupillary border, which is classified as stage II. Grade III shallowing of the anterior chamber is observed when the crystalline lens or intraocular implant is in contact with the corneal endothelium.

When the crystalline lens and cornea are in apposition, there is significant risk for permanent corneal decompensation and rapid cataract formation. This situation can result from conditions related to ocular hypotony, including overfiltration, wound leak, or extensive choroidal detachment. In such instances, the anterior chamber must be reformed immediately in the office or the operating room. In the office, the anterior chamber can be reformed by the injection of a balanced salt solution or a viscoelastic agent through a preexisting paracentesis track. The side port can be reestablished by the introduction of a 30-gauge needle. Caution must be taken not to overfill the anterior chamber with viscoelastic material, as a significant elevation in IOP can result.

A retrospective case review found that a flat anterior chamber was significantly associated with a higher preoperative IOP.[125] Prevention of a flat ante-

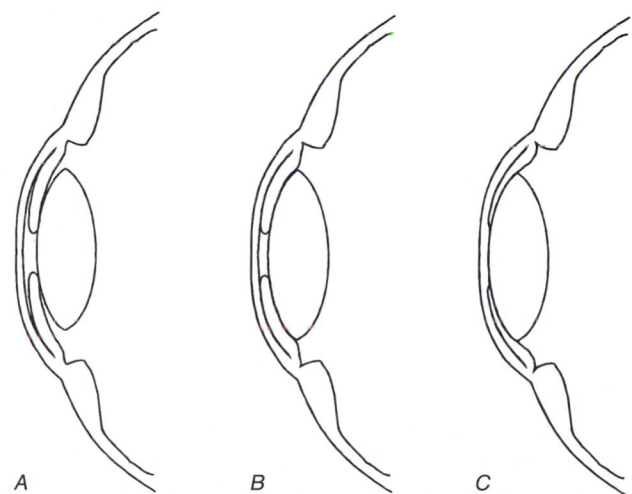

Figure 23–14. *A.* Grade I: Peripheral iris and corneal endothelium in apposition. *B.* Grade II: Apposition of the iris and corneal endothelium at the pupillary margin. *C.* Grade III: Lens-corneal touch.

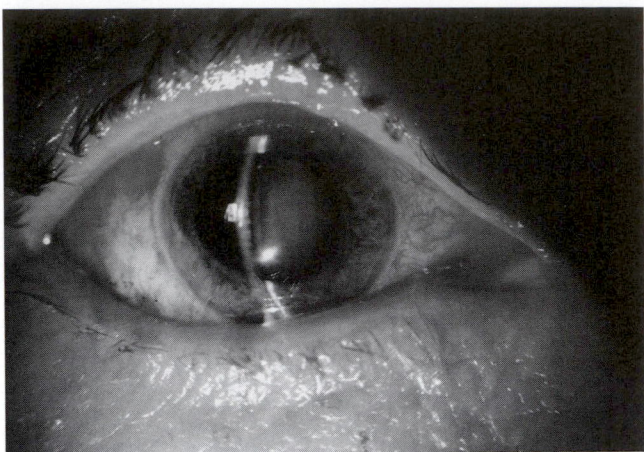

Figure 23–15. Shallow anterior chamber following filtering surgery, with peripheral iris-corneal touch. (*See also Color Plate 56.*)

rior chamber has been suggested to reduce the potential for postoperative complications. Wand has suggested that intraoperative use of an intracameral viscoelastic agent would significantly reduce the incidence of flat anterior chamber following partial- and full-thickness glaucoma procedures.[126]

If the anterior chamber is flat due to a wound leak—i.e., conjunctival buttonhole—repair of the conjunctival defect is recommended immediately, before the tissue has the opportunity to atrophy or thin. Anterior chamber reformation is generally temporary in the presence of extensive choroidal detachments. If there is no wound leak and the anterior chamber remains flat even after reformation with a viscoelastic agent, a surgical procedure is required. Posterior sclerotomies are created to drain the choroidal effusions and then the anterior chamber is reformed in the operating room. In the absence of cornea-lens touch, careful monitoring of the patient is generally recommended for the first 2 postoperative weeks, since gradual deepening of the anterior chamber does occur. Reformation of the anterior chamber should be considered for those patients who have a shallow anterior chamber in the absence of other complications, since this condition is unlikely to resolve without intervention.[127]

Other Complications

Hypotony has been associated with other complications including structural alterations to the retina and choroid, cataract, progression of visual field loss, and bleb failure.

Macular folds occurring with hypotony and edema of the optic nerve head were first described by Dellaporta in 1955.[128] Stereoscopic evaluation of the macula demonstrates choroidal folds oriented generally in a radial pattern that may be accompanied by retinal striae (Fig. 23–16). This pattern is attributed to the infolding of the sclera, a condition that can be differentiated from cystoid macular edema by the absence of leakage following fluorescein angiography in patients with hypotony maculopathy. A study evaluating risk factors for hypotony maculopathy found that these retinal changes were more common in younger patients and those with myopia.[129] These findings were irrespective of the surgical technique and were equally prevalent in patients having intraoperative MMC and postoperative 5-FU.

Hypotony maculopathy is clinically significant because of its related visual symptoms. This condition has been associated with loss of visual acuity after trabeculectomy.[115,129,130] Cataract surgery has been reported to resolve hypotony maculopathy in a series of case reports,[131] but this finding was not observed in another study.[13] Surgical revision of the bleb with increased IOP can be used to treat persistent cases. Vitrectomy with perfluorocarbon gas has been used successfully to flatten the retina in selected cases.[132] Even following the resolution of hypotony maculopathy, the retinal pigment epithelium may demonstrate permanent change and pigment mottling.

Cataract has been described as a complication of prolonged hypotony.[125,130,133,236] Cataract formation occurs more often than hypotony maculopathy, and progression may occur after the appearance of a flat anterior chamber.[125] Lens opacification can cause decreased visual acuity following trabeculectomy.[130,133] This finding has been attributed to the changes in aqueous humor dynamics in hypotonous eyes.[133]

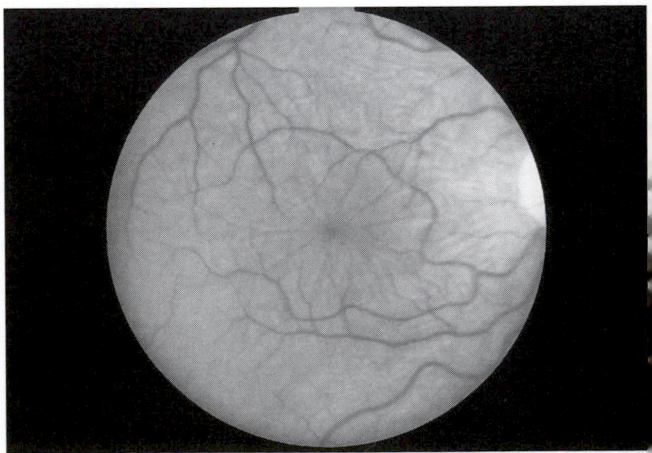

Figure 23–16. Hypotony maculopathy in a young, myopic male with pigmentary dispersion glaucoma. (*See also Color Plate 57.*)

Another potential cause of a decline in visual acuity has been called "wipeout" or "snuff out" syndrome, referring to the loss of central field following incisional surgery.[130–134] This was found to occur in eyes with advanced visual field defects splitting fixation and was also associated with advanced age.[135] The diagnosis was made only after other possible causes of vision loss, including cataract and hypotony maculopathy, were eliminated.

Bleb failure has also been associated with chronic hypotony. Without the appropriate outflow of aqueous to maintain the function of the bleb, there is sufficient opportunity for fibrosis, with eventual loss of bleb function.

MANAGEMENT OF HYPOTONY

Injection of Viscoelastic

Viscoelastic agents can be used in the reformation of the anterior chamber with lens-corneal touch, but they can also be used in the early postoperative period to occlude the internal fistula temporarily and reduce outflow of aqueous (Table 23–4). This can be helpful when immediate postoperative hypotony is related to overfiltration. The effect is transient and usually lasts only 1 or 2 days.

Pressure Patch

A pressure patch is an appropriate management for hypotony related to overfiltration or a very small bleb leak. The patch provides sufficient tamponade effect to encourage reepithelialization of the conjunctival defect. "Torpedo" patching can be used to create more focal pressure in the area of concern. A small section of a sterile eye pad is moistened with sterile saline and then placed directly over the area where the wound leak has occurred. The pressure patch is then taped in place according to usual procedure.

TABLE 23–4. MANAGEMENT OF HYPOTONY

Injection of viscoelastic

Pressure patch

Bandage soft contact lens

Simmons shell

Autologous blood injection

Chemical cauterization

Cyanoacrylate

Fibrin tissue glue

Laser bleb revision

Cryotherapy

Bleb revision with repair

Bandage Soft Contact Lens

Bandage soft contact lenses can be used to control IOP in patients with hypotony secondary to overfiltration[136] (Fig. 23–17). These lenses have an oversized diameter varying from 20.5 mm (Megasoft lens, Procornea, Netherlands) to 22.0 mm (Flexlens, Paragon Vision Services, Mesa, AZ) These bandage contact lenses have been used successfully in the reversal of flat anterior chambers as well as wound leaks.[137] This technique is appropriate only where the wound leak will have sufficient compression from the edge of the contact lens.

The contact lens should be evaluated for centration, extent of coverage of the bleb, and degree of centration. A lens that centers poorly due to a moderate to high filtering bleb can be recentered manually before a pressure patch is put in place. The pressure patch effectively slows outflow and reduces the height of the bleb, so that the contact lens will center. An antibiotic drop should be prescribed for prophylaxis while the contact lens is in place, and any other postoperative medications should be instilled as usual over the contact lens. If hypotony develops secondarily to a wound leak, then the addition of an aqueous suppressant may be considered in order to reduce the outward-driving fluid forces in the area of the wound leak.

Compression of the therapeutic soft lens is assessed at the edge of the contact lens (Fig. 23–18). The edge of the lens should indent the conjunctival tissue in order to have any therapeutic benefit. If there is no compressive effect, then a moderate to high minus–power lens can be inserted. These lenses have a thicker edge profile, which may provide the needed compression. Once inserted, the bandage soft contact lens is worn for at least 5 to 7 days. If the patient develops substantial corneal edema or epithelial breakdown related to

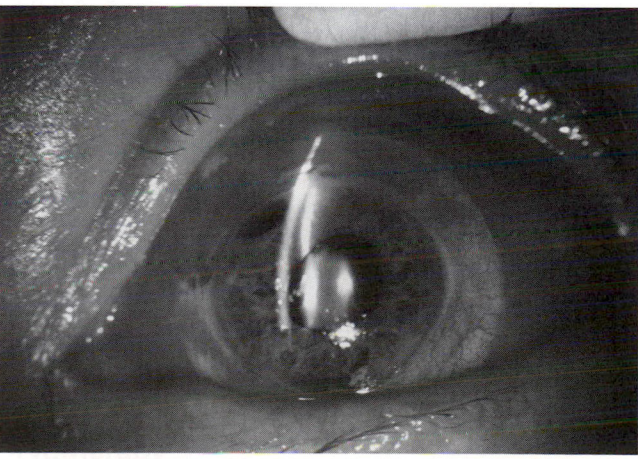

Figure 23–17. Bandage soft contact lens inserted to manage hypotony secondary to overfiltration. (*See also Color Plate 58.*)

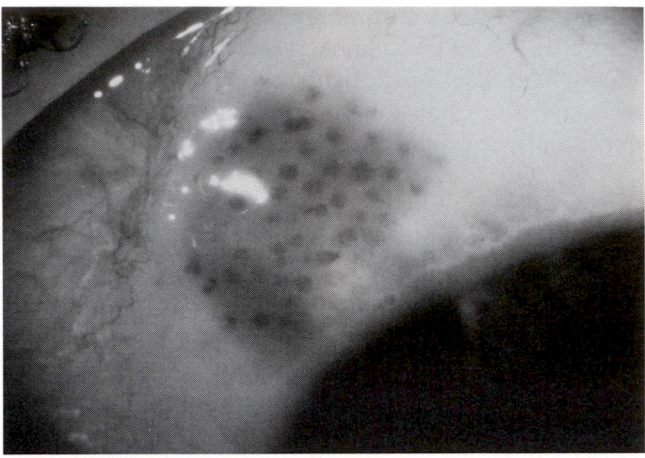

Figure 23–22. Nd:YAG laser revision of overfiltering bleb. (Courtesy of Mary Lynch, M.D.) (*See also Color Plate 63.*)

and has been employed in the treatment of inadvertent bleb following cataract surgery.[166] This type of treatment has sealed wound leaks as well.[167] Caution should be used in treating overfiltering or leaking blebs with this technique, since there is significant risk that wound leak will develop elsewhere if the conjunctiva is thin or weak.

Bleb Revision with Repair

Surgical revision following trabeculectomy can be performed to resolve hypotony secondary to overfiltration or wound leak. Wound leaks can be corrected by in-office suturing with 9-0 or 10-0 nylon suture. The conjunctival tissue must be sufficiently thick and mobile to allow for suture repair. However, wound leaks tend to occur where the conjunctival tissue is thin, and suture repair may cause wound leaks to develop in adjacent areas of the bleb. A clothesline suture has been suggested to repair an inadvertent buttonhole following trabeculectomy. A 10.0 nylon suture is placed between the buttonhole and flap to create a barrier to outflow, as an alternative to autograft.[168]

More invasive procedures may involve autologous conjunctival grafts. Conjunctival resection from a site adjacent to the bleb has been described.[169,170] Free autologous conjunctival patch graft can be used to patch wound leaks that are unresponsive to other, less invasive techniques.[171] The leaking cystic blebs were excised before placing the patch grafts. This technique can also be used without resection of the conjunctival tissue. Buxton et al. reported good success with free conjunctival autograft in the revision of leaking blebs.[172] They found this technique particularly helpful for patients in whom significant conjunctival scarring prevented local revision. Concerns

should include wound dehiscence with the creation of new bleb leaks and loss of bleb function with a subsequent increase in IOP.

When hypotony is related to overfiltration, scleral flap revision can be considered. Sutures can be placed along the scleral flap, a procedure that allows the surgeon to titrate the effect and maintain bleb function.[173,174] However, if the scleral flap is thin or perforated, a donor scleral patch graft may be sutured in place[175,176] to reduce the aqueous outflow. A series of case reports detailed the successful resolution of hypotony and late leaks following endophthalmitis using a scleral patch with conjunctival advancement or autograft.[177]

INCREASED INTRAOCULAR PRESSURE FOLLOWING FILTERING SURGERY

Aqueous Misdirection

Aqueous misdirection should be suspected when the IOP is elevated in the presence of a shallow or flat anterior chamber (Table 23–5). This condition is believed to result from the misdirection of aqueous posteriorly, so that the ensuing fluid pressure causes an anterior shift of the lens-iris diaphragm with collapse of the anterior chamber.

Aqueous misdirection can be treated initially by a cycloplegic agent to deepen the anterior chamber and by hyperosmotics or carbonic anhydrase inhibitors. If these measures are unsuccessful, laser treatment can be performed. A Nd:YAG laser is used to photodisrupt the anterior vitreous face to allow aqueous to diffuse from the posterior hyaloid space. This procedure is more appropriate in the management of pseudophakic or aphakic patients because of the risk of damage to the posterior capsular membrane in a phakic eye. Trans-pars plana vitrectomy is the definitive treatment for aqueous misdirection that is unresponsive to medical therapy. The goal of this procedure is the removal of sufficient vitreous to allow aqueous flow into the anterior chamber. Reports have documented the success of vitrectomy in reliev-

TABLE 23–5. ETIOLOGY OF INCREASED INTRAOCULAR PRESSURE FOLLOWING FILTERING SURGERY

Steroid response
External obstruction
Internal obstruction
Encapsulated bleb
Aqueous misdirection

ing aqueous misdirection.[178,179] Possible complications include serous choroidal detachment, suprachoroidal hemorrhage, retinal detachment, and cataract formation. Lensectomy has been suggested for pseudophakic or phakic patients with significant corneal edema, dense cataract, and persistent shallow anterior chamber following vitrectomy.[179]

Aqueous misdirection must be differentiated from pupillary block due to obstruction of the peripheral iridectomy by posterior synechiae, blood, fibrin, or vitreous.

Pupillary Block

Pupillary block can occur following filtration surgery but is unlikely to be the cause of elevated IOP in the presence of a shallow anterior chamber if the peripheral iridectomy is determined to be patent. The clinician must differentiate between a centrally deep anterior chamber with midperipheral iris convexity associated with pupillary block and an anterior shift of the lens-iris diaphragm related to aqueous misdirection. If the distinction is unclear and it is not apparent that the peripheral iridectomy is functioning, then a peripheral iridotomy should be performed to relieve a suspected pupillary block. If the IOP remains elevated and the anterior chamber angle does not appreciably deepen, other conditions including aqueous misdirection should be considered.

Suprachoroidal Hemorrhage

Suprachoroidal hemorrhage is a potential cause of elevated IOP with shallowing of the anterior chamber. This condition may occur intra- or postoperatively. Intraoperatively, suprachoroidal hemorrhage is a concern owing to the risk of expulsion of the intraocular contents. This condition should be considered if there is a sudden increase in the intraoperative IOP coupled with the appearance of an expanding choroid. Intraoperative suprachoroidal hemorrhage should be treated by compression of the wound and completion of scleral sutures.

Postoperative suprachoroidal hemorrhage is uncommon but may result in a severe, boring eye pain within the first days following surgery. Risk factors include advanced age, arteriosclerosis, previous ocular surgery, inflammation, and clotting disorders. Givens and Shields found that suprachoroidal hemorrhages were more common in eyes that were aphakic and that had undergone prior vitrectomy procedures.[180] Rockwood et al. found that aphakia was indeed a risk factor; however, concurrent vitrectomy rather than prior vitrectomy was significant.[181] However, the Fluorouracil Filtering Surgery Study Group did not confirm these findings. These investigators found that of the risk factors discussed, only preoperative IOP was strongly associated with suprachoroidal hemorrhage.[182] Suprachoroidal hemorrhage is a concern in hypotonous eyes and may occur because of venous congestion of the vortex veins due to scleral collapse or shearing of feeding arterioles with arterial choroidal bleeding.

Suprachoroidal hemorrhage occurs more commonly in particular types of glaucomas, such as nanophthalmos and Sturge-Weber syndrome. In nanophthalmos, this increased risk is related to thicker sclera. Suprachoroidal hemorrhage is a surgical risk factor in Sturge-Weber syndrome due to a potential rupture of a choroidal hemangioma. Patients should be counseled about activities that induce a Valsalva maneuver (such as coughing, straining at stool, or heavy lifting) that could precipitate a suprachoroidal hemorrhage.

Suprachoroidal hemorrhage may be preceded by choroidal detachment; however, the choroidal detachment may persist even after the resolution of the hemorrhage. Surgical drainage should be considered in cases with persistent severe ocular pain, increased IOP, evidence of retinal gliosis due to kissing choroidal hemorrhages, or a prolonged flat chamber. A suprachoroidal hemorrhage is drained through a sclerostomy 3 to 4 mm posterior to the limbus while the anterior chamber is deepened with constant infusion through a limbal paracentesis.

Suprachoroidal hemorrhage can resolve with good visual outcome; however, loss of vision can also occur in some cases.[180,181]

Annular Peripheral Choroidal Detachment

Annular peripheral choroidal detachment (APCD) has been reported in a number of patients with flat anterior chambers following filtering surgery. This condition must be differentiated from aqueous misdirection. Assessment of APCD is most easily accomplished by the use of ultrasound sonography, since peripheral retinal examination with scleral indentation is contraindicated in the immediate postoperative period due to the risk of wound dehiscence. APCD can be difficult to observe, since the detachment does not generally extend past the equator. APCD was found to respond to steroids and cycloplegics, although the condition took longer to resolve with medical therapy than with surgical drainage of suprachoroidal fluid.[183]

APCD should be considered in addition to other previously discussed potential causes for a flat anterior chamber with elevated IOP following filtering surgery.

External Obstruction

External obstruction of the filtration fistula may occur in the immediate postoperative period related to the

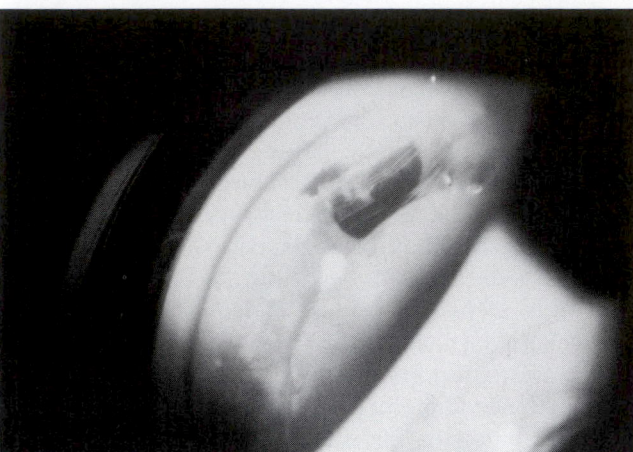

Figure 23–23. Clot adjacent to internal osteum following trabeculectomy for glaucoma associated with an anterior chamber intraocular lens. (*See also Color Plate 64.*)

TABLE 23–6. MANAGEMENT OF INCREASED INTRAOCULAR PRESSURE FOLLOWING FILTERING SURGERY

External Obstruction
    Ocular massage and focal compression
    Laser suture lysis
    Adjunctive antimetabolite injections
    Needling
Internal Obstruction
    Ab interno revision
    Gonioscopic laser revision
Encapsulated Bleb
    Topical anti-inflammatories
    Aqueous suppressants
    Ocular massage
    Needle revision with or without adjunctive
       antimetabolite injection
    Surgical revision

presence of fibrinoid material or hemorrhage (Fig. 23–23). This condition must be differentiated from increased IOP secondary to a tight scleral flap. In the late postoperative period, external obstruction may occur due to the development of an episcleral membrane overlying the scleral flap.

Clinically, the bleb appears low in height or even flat and demonstrates no microcystic response of the conjunctiva. Conjunctival vasculature may be present, although with varying degrees of conjunctival injection or engorgement. The conjunctiva may be mobile and easily moved over the scleral surface using a cotton-tipped applicator. Loss of bleb function should be suspected when the IOP is tending to increase in subsequent visits.

If the loss of bleb function is related to accumulation of cellular material under the scleral flap, then ocular massage (discussed below) can dislodge the fibrotic strands before permanent bleb failure results. If the elevating IOP is related to a tight scleral flap, then suture release or suture lysis can be considered. Appropriate interventions may help to restore bleb function if they are initiated in a timely fashion. However, surgical revision will be required if other, more conservative therapies are unsuccessful.

Ocular Massage and Focal Compression
Ocular massage and focal compression are used for several purposes (Table 23–6). These techniques can be used to evaluate the function of a bleb, assess the appropriateness of suture release, disrupt intraflap hemorrhage or fibrosis, or treat an encapsulated bleb.

The "Traverso maneuver" involves the use of a cotton swab adjacent to the flap to deform it and allow fluid to escape (Fig. 23–24).[184] This method is in direct contrast to ocular massage that involves direct compression against the globe 180 degrees from the flap location. In the early postoperative period, the Traverso maneuver helps to disrupt early intraflap fibrosis; however, there is a concern for subconjunctival or anterior chamber hemorrhage due to bleeding vessels beneath the scleral flap. In an encapsulated bleb, ocular massage will weaken scar tissue. Ocular massage can reduce the IOP to acceptable levels following filtering surgery. In a small patient population, digital

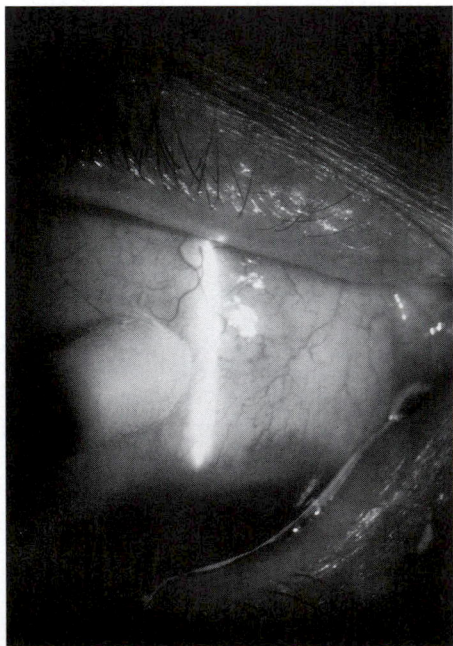

Figure 23–24. Use of cotton swab adjacent to the scleral flap to perform focal compression—i.e., the Traverso maneuver. (*See also Color Plate 65.*)

compression was found to have an extended IOP-lowering effect in over 50% of patients, with duration of effect lasting more than 90 minutes.[185]

A survey of American glaucoma subspecialists showed that most physicians employed ocular massage in selected patients following glaucoma surgery; however, there was no standardized method, duration, or timing for ocular compression.[186] In our practice, we generally recommend ocular massage from one to five cycles of 10 seconds each with frequency varying from one to four times daily. Patients with focal blebs should perform digital compression more frequently, since localized blebs seem to recover from this procedure more often than diffuse blebs.[185] After instructing patients about the proper hygiene, positioning, and direction of compression, written instructions and a schedule should be provided. Patients should be advised to perform no more massage than is necessary, since the IOP can increase to over 100 mmHg with massage.[187] If done incorrectly, this procedure can be more harmful than beneficial. In fact, transiently elevated IOP decreases the pattern electroretinogram in ocular hypertensive patients as compared with controls and results in a greater delay in recovery.[188] If ocular massage is found to be ineffective, it should be discontinued because of the risk of complications associated with the procedure. These infrequent complications include iris incarceration,[189] wound leak,[190] bleb rupture,[191] and choroidal rupture with subretinal hemorrhage.[192]

In glaucoma patients who have previously undergone cataract surgery or combined procedures, ocular massage is generally discontinued for the first week postoperatively in order to reduce the risk of lens decentration or subluxation.

Assessment of Tight Scleral Sutures

If there is a concern for an elevated IOP following filtering surgery in an eye with a formed chamber, digital compression can be used to determine whether the increased IOP is related to a tight scleral flap. It is important to establish that the elevation in IOP is not caused by an internal obstruction such as iris prolapse. Gonioscopy should be performed before ocular massage is attempted.

Focal pressure can be applied to the globe in an area adjacent to the scleral flap. If the bleb suddenly elevates with pressure, then the most likely cause for the elevated pressure is a tight flap or fibrous adhesions within the scleral bed. Resistance to deformation can occur when a clot or fibrous tissue develops between the scleral flap and bed. Repeated focal massage may be necessary to prevent its reformation or the use of subconjunctival tissue plasminogen activator considered.[190]

Clinically, the bleb should be evaluated qualitatively and quantitatively after digital compression. The bleb may elevate only minimally or extensively after ocular massage. The fluid may diffuse in a generalized or limited fashion. Significant chemosis of the conjunctiva may be noted. The IOP should be measured before and after ocular massage is performed.

If the IOP drops significantly and the outflow of aqueous is diffuse, then the bleb may be immature and suture release may produce ocular hypotony. It is important to evaluate the bleb margin after ocular massage for a moderate circumscribed elevation that would indicate sufficient maturation of the bleb. Removal of one or more releasable sutures may be appropriate if there is a trend towards increasing IOP in successive postoperative visits (Fig. 23–25).

Laser Suture Lysis

Once it has been established that the IOP is elevated secondary to a tight scleral suture, release of the scleral flap suture can be attempted. However, if the suture becomes fibrosed, it will be difficult to remove the stitch without breaking the suture. In eyes where scleral flap sutures have been placed subconjunctivally, laser suture lysis will also be required. This procedure can be used where appropriate to titrate the IOP in the immediate postoperative period.[194–196]

Suture lysis has been performed with several types of laser including argon, krypton, and frequency-doubled Nd:YAG.[197] This procedure can be more difficult if the conjunctival flap is edematous or the flap sutures are obscured by subconjunctival hemorrhage. Several laser gonioprisms (e.g., Hoskins,[198] Mandelkorn,[199] Ritch[200]) have been used to help in visualizing flap sutures; however, wound leaks remain a serious concern, and the filtering bleb should be

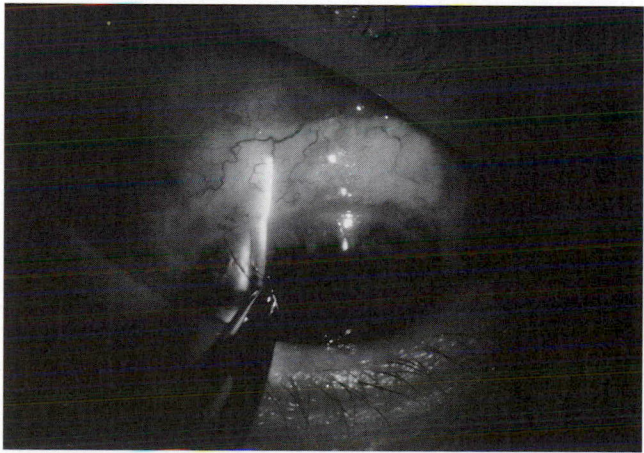

Figure 23–25. Removal of tight scleral flap suture in the postoperative period. (*See also Color Plate 66.*)

evaluated for the Seidel sign immediately after the procedure.[97] Schwartz and Weiss reported two cases of bleb leak with hypotony following argon laser suture lysis.[201] Others have suggested that krypton suture lysis may reduce the risk for wound leak, since less energy is required and krypton laser energy is not absorbed by blood.[59,202,203]

Suture lysis is of clinical benefit for a limited amount of time following trabeculectomy. If fibrosis occurs within the scleral bed, laser suture lysis will be of no benefit. However, if laser suture lysis is performed too early in the postoperative period, there is a significant risk of hypotony or shallowing of the anterior chamber.[97] Clinicians should remember that there is a nonlinear response of IOP to suture lysis when multiple sutures are treated.

Laser suture lysis is generally recommended within the first 2 weeks following trabeculectomy with 5-FU and within 1 to 3 months following trabeculectomy with MMC. The suture lysis should be deferred for approximately 2 to 4 weeks following trabeculectomy with MMC to allow for sufficient maturation of the bleb. A study evaluating the efficacy of late suture lysis using argon laser determined that it was effective even when performed up to 21 weeks after trabeculectomy with MMC.[204] The investigators concluded that MMC extended the period of effect for argon laser suture lysis.[196,204]

In addition to the risks of hypotony, a flat anterior chamber, and wound leak following laser suture lysis, other complications may occur. These include aqueous misdirection, iris incarceration, and a high bleb.[205,206]

Adjunctive Antimetabolite Injections

Adjunctive 5-FU has been suggested to prevent fibrosis in external scarring (Fig. 23–26). In a study that

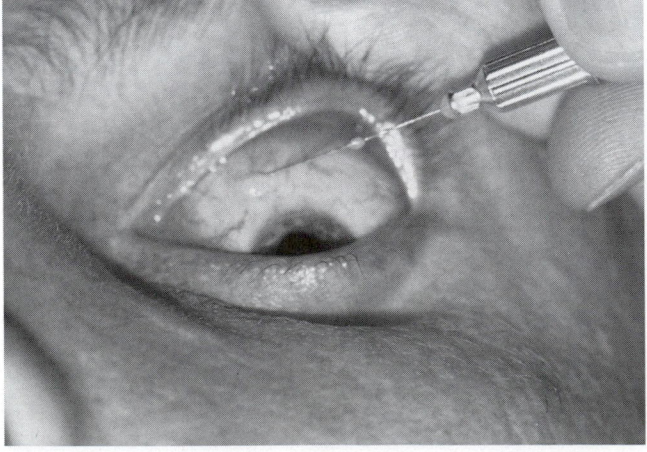

Figure 23–26. Adjunctive postoperative 5-fluorouracil injection. (*See also Color Plate 67.*)

compared the success rate following needle revision with and without adjunctive 5-FU, the outcomes were similar even though the antimetabolite injections were given to those patients deemed to be at greater risk for bleb failure.[207] Comparatively, a study evaluating the benefit of postoperative 5-FU in posttrabeculectomy patients with or without MMC showed that adjunctive 5-FU was helpful in reducing bleb failure in both subgroups.[208] These investigators found that postoperative 5-FU injections were of greater benefit in eyes that had a significant decrease in IOP with ocular massage—i.e., eyes with a functional filtering bleb. If the conjunctival vasculature overlying the bleb appears to be telangiectatic or engorged and accompanied by a decrease in bleb height or increase in IOP, there is risk of bleb failure. A 0.1-mL volume of 50 mg/mL 5-FU can be given approximately 180 degrees away from the bleb. This procedure is performed following the instillation of a topical anesthetic. Possible complications of this procedure include coalesced corneal epithelial defects or conjunctival wound leaks.

Needling

Once the potential for bleb failure has been recognized, additional interventions such as needle revision with or without an adjunctive antimetabolite can be considered. When ocular massage does not prevent the development of external fibrosis, bleb revision can help to restore bleb function.

Reports of needle revision and adjunctive antimetabolite injection have been promising. These investigations have documented successful restoration of bleb function in a significant number of patients and have shown this procedure to reduce the number of additional surgical procedures required. However, the means by which this procedure succeeds is unknown. The bleb revision involves mechanical disruption of fibrous tissue, the use of antimetabolite agents, and also the creation of a partial- or full-thickness perforation by the needle. Maintaining sterile technique, a 27- or 30-gauge needle is used to lift the scleral flap and lyse intraflap adhesions. As the fibrotic tissue is disrupted, aqueous is free to flow out of the eye and a diffuse bleb will form.

As previously discussed, Ewing and Stamper found that needle revision procedures with and without 5-FU had similar outcomes.[207] Shin et al. reported success in approximately 80% of their patient population after multiple needling procedures. These clinicians found that patients who underwent needle revision of a filtering bleb required fewer IOP-lowing medications postoperatively.[209] MMC-augmented needle revision of filtering blebs has been described in several studies[210,211] and may have advantages over needle revision with 5-FU because of reduced risk for corneal epithelial defect.[207] Higher pretreatment IOP and previous surgery with conjunctival scarring were found to affect the outcome of the procedure adversely,[210] while Caucasian heritage and long duration since prior filtering operation were positively correlated with success.[211]

Complications related to needling bleb revision included wound leak, choroidal detachment, hyphema, and corneal abrasion. Care should be taken to prevent sight-threatening complications such as suprachoroidal hemorrhage, hypotony, or endophthalmitis.

Internal Obstruction

Obstruction of the internal osteum may occur from various sources, including viscoelastic material, blood, or capsular material. Iris, vitreous, or ciliary body prolapse into the osteum can be problematic. A fibrotic membrane derived from the sclera or cornea can occlude the surgical fistula internally.

Management of Internal Obstruction

Obstruction of the osteum by blood or viscoelastic is generally self-limiting and will often resolve within the first few postoperative days. The formation of internal membranes can be more problematic, since surgical revision will be required to restore filtration. A diathermy probe or spatula can be inserted into the anterior chamber to lyse the fibrotic strands of the internal membrane. This method has significant disadvantages owing to the need for hospitalization and anesthesia, increased risk of damage to the crystalline lens, infection, and bleeding. Alternatively, the fibrotic membrane, iris strands, or lens capsule can be ruptured indirectly by the use of laser. Nd:YAG[212-214] and argon[215,216] lasers have been successfully used to reopen filtration fistulas. However, treatments were successful only when good bleb function was present before the internal membrane developed and when filtration following the procedure was not limited by external scarring.

Vitreous prolapse can be treated by Nd:YAG laser; however, photodisruption is generally not successful for broad vitreal bands and may place the patient at risk for retinal tears or detachment. Anterior vitrectomy is generally preferred for patients with internal obstruction secondary to vitreous prolapse.

Encapsulated Bleb

An encapsulated bleb or Tenon's cyst develops within the first few weeks after filtering surgery in 3.6 to 28%[217-220,223,224] of patients following trabeculectomy. One study found that fewer encapsulated blebs developed after MMC trabeculectomy.[221] Clinically, the bleb

appears as a high, tense, dome-like structure with sharply defined vascularized conjunctiva overlying the cyst (Fig. 23–27). The conjunctiva appears to be tightly stretched and may demonstrate engorgement of the vessels.

Encapsulated blebs were observed more commonly in male patients[219,222] and patients with a history of prior encapsulated bleb and/or previous use of beta-blocking or sympathomimetic agents.[219,223] Surgical history also plays a role, with encapsulated cysts occurring more frequently in patients with prior laser trabeculoplasty and prior ocular surgery affecting the conjunctiva.[219,228] The Advanced Glaucoma Intervention Study found that prior history of laser trabeculoplasty increased the risk of encapsulated filtering bleb, although this was not a statistically significant finding.[222] Intraoperative factors such as surgical glove powder[224] and surgical technique (limbus versus fornix-based flap) have been suggested as risk factors.[217] The use of antimetabolite therapy may decrease the frequency of encapsulated filtering blebs.[221,224]

Management of Encapsulated Bleb

Topical anti-inflammatory medications inhibit further fibrosis, but with minimal effects. Conservative therapies may include digital compression or ocular massage in an effort to stretch the fibrotic wall of Tenon's cyst. Aqueous suppressants are also recommended to treat elevated IOP. These therapies can be successfully used to manage an encapsulated bleb and reduce the need for surgical intervention.[217,220,225,226]

If ocular massage and aqueous suppressants are unsuccessful, bleb revision is required. Needle revision with or without adjunctive antimetabolite injection has been reported to treat encapsulated filtering blebs

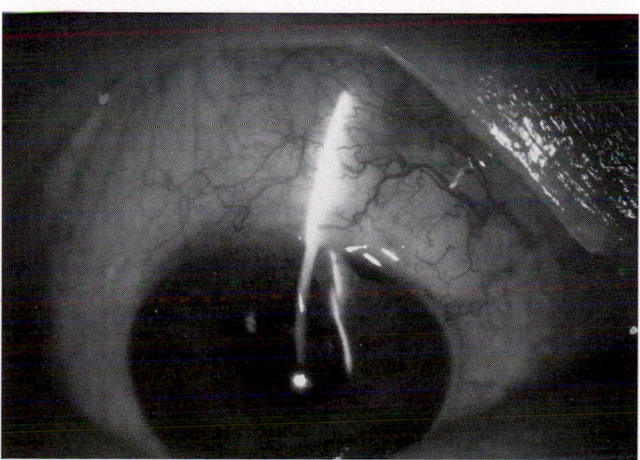

Figure 23–27. Tenon cyst formation accompanied by high bleb, vascularization of the bleb, and conjunctival telangiectasia. (*See also Color Plate 68.*)

successfully.[218] Complications following needle revision with antimetabolite adjuncts include corneal defects, wound leaks, and bleeding.[227] However, following needle revision and adjunctive antimetabolite injection, the bleb can become reencapsulated. Risk factors for reencapsulation include history of multiple surgical procedures and chronic use of adrenergic agents.[227]

Surgical revision with excision of Tenon's cyst will be necessary for patients who do not respond to conservative measures such as aqueous suppressants and ocular massage or to needle revision with or without antimetabolites.[218,226,228] Intraoperative MMC can be used to prevent reencapsulation.[220]

Symptomatic Bleb or "Bleb Dysesthesia"

Symptomatic blebs may arise because of irregularities in the bleb contour or significant elevation with disruption of the tear film (Fig. 23–28). As the eyelid lifts with the blink, bubbles may form in the contour between the bleb and the elevating lid. Thinning of the tear film may occur in areas adjacent to a high bleb and result in punctate defects or even dellen. Persistent dellen can cause permanent stromal scarring.

In the early postoperative period, bleb dysesthesia may be related to sutures; these cases resolve once the offending suture has been trimmed or removed. Patients may complain of persistent foreign-body sensation or chronic irritation. Later symptoms may be related to an encapsulated bleb, a high-profile bleb, or a bleb with significant corneal extension.

Supportive therapy can be considered for symptomatic patients, including tear supplements or punctal occlusion (Table 23–7). Attempts can be made to reduce the bleb function using aqueous suppressants to decrease aqueous outflow. However, caution should be

TABLE 23–7. MANAGEMENT OF THE SYMPTOMATIC BLEB

Ocular lubricants
Punctal occlusion
Compression sutures
Chemical cauterization
Laser revision
Cryotherapy
Needling
Surgical revision

exercised in order to prevent possible bleb failure. In persistent cases, surgical revision may be required to decrease the elevation of the bleb. It is essential to rule out encapsulated bleb as the cause for an elevated bleb, since management strategies will vary. If treatment of a symptomatic bleb is required, the bleb substance can be modulated using chemical cauterization, laser revision,[163,164,229] cryotherapy,[167] or needling. Compression sutures[230] (Fig. 23–29) and surgical revision—including resection of the conjunctiva[218,228]—have also been used to treat bleb dysesthesias.

Bleb-Related Infection

Bleb-related infection is a serious complication of filtering surgery and represents a cause of potential loss of vision. Infection may occur early in the postoperative period or develop years after the surgical procedure. The incidence of bleb infection following trabeculectomy without metabolites has been reported to vary between 0.2 and 1.5%.[39,68,231,232] In eyes that have undergone trabeculectomy with 5-FU or MMC, the risk for bleb-related endophthalmitis was higher

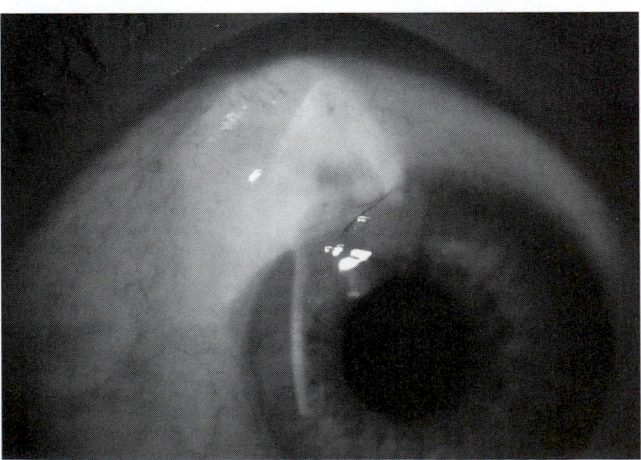

Figure 23–28. Suture bleb revision for symptomatic bleb with corneal extension. (*See also Color Plate 69.*)

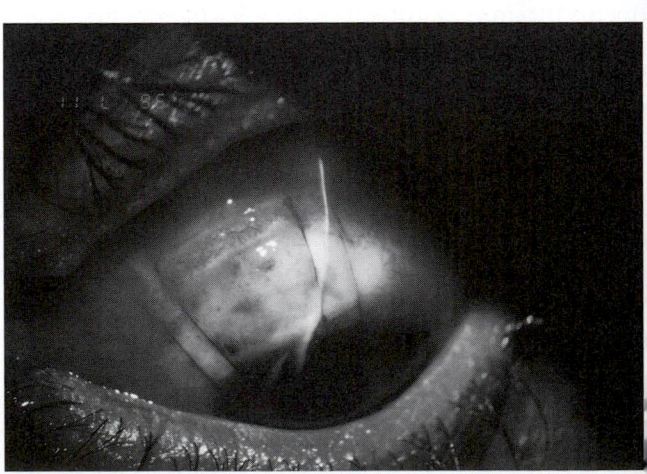

Figure 23–29. Compression suture used in hypotony secondary to overfiltration. This technique can be used in bleb dysesthesias. (*See also Color Plate 70.*)

(1.0 to 3.8%).[96,233–238] Risk factors for bleb infection include blepharitis and poor eyelid hygiene; conjunctivitis; bleb leak[239,241]; cystic, thin-walled blebs[239,240]; antimetabolite therapy[234]; unguarded procedures; inferior filtering bleb[233,234,241,242]; and contact lens wear.[243,244] Systemic conditions such as diabetes, malnutrition, or immunocompromise have also been implicated.

Bleb infection can be limited to the anterior segment and is called *blebitis*. With vitreous and posterior segment involvement, this infection is known as *bleb-related endophthalmitis*. Patients with blebitis have a limited form of bleb-related infection. Blebs that are irritated by minor trauma or continual friction from the upper lid may be at greater risk for developing blebitis. Patients report symptoms and signs of redness over 1 to 3 days—rather than over hours—as well as photophobia and discharge. Clinically, there may be significant engorgement of conjunctival vessels over the substance of the bleb as well as surrounding the bleb. The bleb may be opalescent in appearance with epithelial defects (Fig. 23–30). Vitreous cells are absent and anterior chamber inflammation is minimal.[245] Blebitis is usually related to a limited infection by *Staphylococcus epidermidis* or *S. aureus*.[239,241] This type of infection responds quite well to topical or systemic antibiotics.[239] Visual outcome following resolution of blebitis is generally good.[239,240,246] Careful management of blebitis is important, since this limited infection has the potential to progress to fulminant endophthalmitis.

Bleb-related endophthalmitis generally causes more severe symptoms than blebitis. Patients report rapidly worsening visual acuity, redness, and severe pain. Symptoms may also include significant photophobia, foreign-body sensation, and tearing. Clinically,

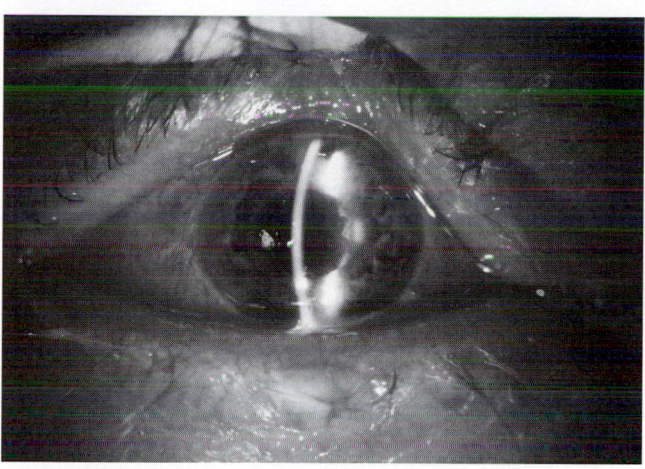

Figure 23–31. Bleb-related endophthalmitis associated with severe anterior chamber inflammation. Prognosis for visual recovery is generally poor. (*See also Color Plate 72.*)

the conjunctiva is diffusely injected, the bleb is opalescent in appearance, and the anterior chamber response is marked (Fig. 23–31). Severe fibrin accumulation in the anterior and posterior segments may be observed. Hypopyon and vitritis generally accompany bleb-related endophthalmitis. Visualization of the anterior segment can be complicated by significant corneal edema. Management of bleb-related endophthalmitis includes conjunctival culture, vitreous tap, and/or vitrectomy.[236–239,241,244] The use of intraocular steroid injection is controversial.[247] This type of infection is most commonly caused by *Streptococcus*, *Staphylococcus*, or *Haemophilus* species. Endophthalmitis carries a poor prognosis despite intensive topical, systemic, and intravitreal antibiotics and vitrectomy.[245,246,248]

OTHER SELECTED FILTERING PROCEDURES

Nonpenetrating Filtering Procedures

Viscocanalostomy

Viscocanalostomy is a procedure in which scleral flap dissection proceeds into the peripheral cornea (Table 23–8). A deep scleral flap is created and Schlemm's canal is exposed. Deep sclerectomy provides an access route for aqueous flow from the corneal window into Schlemm's canal. Viscoelastic material is injected into Schlemm's canal to produce local dilation of the aqueous collector channels. The investigators believe that the viscoelastic material acts as a barrier to fibrosis and that the subsequent absorption of the viscoelastic material is accompanied by increased aqueous outflow.[213]

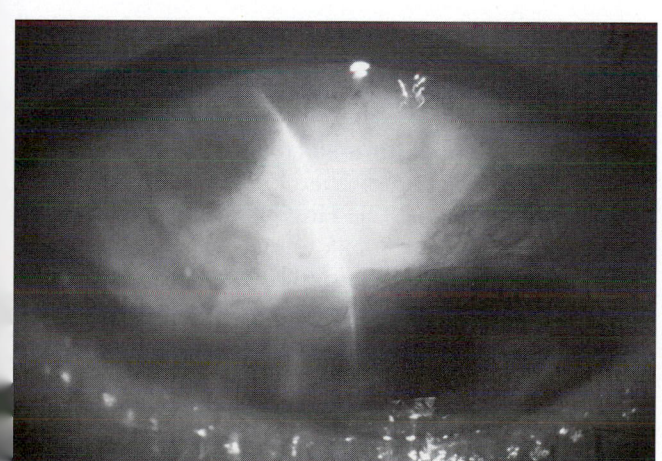

Figure 23–30. Blebitis in a thin, pale, avascular bleb. A wound leak was present. Infiltrates were limited to the bleb substance. (*See also Color Plate 71.*)

TABLE 23–8. OTHER SELECTED FILTERING PROCEDURES

Nonpenetrating Filtering Procedures
    Viscocanalostomy
    Deep sclerectomy with collagen implant (DSCI)
Full-Thickness Procedures
    Thermal sclerostomy (Scheie procedure)
    Posterior lip sclerectomy
    Laser sclerostomy

Complications following viscocanalostomy include Descemet's rupture, iris prolapse, choroidal deroofing, hyphema, filtering bleb, and limited hypotony.[250] This procedure has been shown to be successful in a limited number of patients and further studies are currently under way.

Deep Sclerectomy with Collagen Implant

Deep sclerectomy with collagen implant (DSCI) is a nonpenetrating trabecular surgery that involves the placement of a collagen implant oriented radially within the scleral bed. Aqueous is believed to flow from the anterior chamber through a window in Descemet's membrane, under the scleral flap, and into the suprachoroidal space. The presence of this potential outflow route has been confirmed by ultrasound biomicroscopy.[251] The collagen implant is absorbed over a period of 6 to 9 months. Although deep sclerectomy could be performed without the collagen implant, investigators have shown that the use of the collagen implant decreases postoperative fibrosis as well as the need for postoperative glaucoma medications.[252]

This procedure was found to control IOP as well as trabeculectomy in one study.[253] Success rates for DSCI ranged from 57 to 97% when success was defined as either postoperative IOP less than 21 or 20 mmHg.[253,254] Success rates could be increased by the use of postoperative 5-FU injections or Nd:YAG goniopuncture.[254,255]

Complications following DSCI are similar to those following trabeculectomy, although they occurred less frequently.[253] Significant complications included hyphema, wound leak, choroidal detachment, cataract, and failure to reach acceptable IOP, requiring surgical revision.[254,256] A comparison of anterior chamber inflammation in postoperative eyes following DSCI and trabeculectomy showed significantly less flare in DSCI patients.[257] This may be a significant advantage in patients with secondary glaucomas who are predisposed to exaggerated postoperative inflammation. DSCI can be performed in combination with cataract surgery in patients with visually significant cataract and poorly controlled glaucoma.[258]

Full-Thickness or Unguarded Prodedures

Scheie Procedure or Thermal Sclerostomy

This procedure was described by Scheie in 1958 (Table 23–8).[259] It was a variation of Preziosi's full-thickness scleral cauterization.[260] Scheie advocated the use of thermal cautery coupled with blade dissection. A limbal scratch incision was made between 4 and 6 mm from the limbus and a bipolar cautery used to widen the incision. Cauterization was stopped before entry into the anterior chamber and a scalpel was used to complete the incision. A peripheral iridectomy prevented internal obstruction by incarceration of the iris into the fistula. Thermal sclerostomy fell out of favor as guarded filtration procedures became more popular.

Posterior Lip Sclerectomy

A posterior lip sclerectomy procedure uses a scleral punch to create a full-thickness fistula following the creation of a limbus-based conjunctival flap. The conjunctival flap is dissected anteriorly until the anterior chamber is entered. The sclerectomy is placed at the posterior edge of the full-thickness limbal opening. Caution should be exercised to prevent incision of the ciliary body. Pressure applied to the posterior edge of the fistula following the sclerectomy allows peripheral iris tissue to prolapse into the opening. The surgical iridectomy prevents iris incarceration in the postoperative period.

A comparison of posterior lip sclerectomy and trabeculectomy in a black population showed that this full-thickness procedure was more successful in controlling IOP postoperatively.[261] However, the appearance of a shallow anterior chamber and other complications occurred more often after posterior lip sclerectomy than after trabeculectomy[261] or thermal sclerostomy.[262] Loss of vision following posterior lip sclerectomy was most often related to accelerated cataract formation.[261,262]

Laser Sclerostomy

Full-thickness procedures such as laser sclerostomy are generally considered when the goal of treatment is a substantially lower IOP. However, these procedures have become less popular owing to the frequency of complications following unguarded filtering surgery. A sclerostomy can be performed from an external ("ab externo") or internal ("ab interno") approach. These procedures are more appropriate in eyes that are at high risk for failure because of the presence of a previously failed trabeculectomy or that pose difficulty for scleral dissection due to thin or scarred sclerae. A recent report found holmium laser sclerostomy to be successful in patients with a prior history of intraocular surgery.[263]

Sclerostomy ab interno can be performed by direct application of laser energy through an internal approach or indirectly using a goniolens. Significantly more energy is required in using a goniolens to create the scleral fistula.

Laser sclerostomy has been performed with a number of lasers including Nd:YAG,[264,265] THC:YAG (thulium, holmium, and chromium-doped yttrium-aluminum-garnet crystal),[266–269] erbium:YAG,[270] argon,[271,272] carbon dioxide,[273] excimer,[274] dye-enhanced,[275] pulsed-dye,[276] and diode.[277] However, the method that has been used most commonly in clinical practice has been the THC:YAG or holmium laser sclerostomy ab externo. This laser produces 2100-nm near-infrared energy that is well absorbed by the ocular tissues. This type of sclerostomy has certain advantages over trabeculectomy, since the procedure can be performed at any clock hour and requires only topical anesthesia. The procedure takes less time than a trabeculectomy and can be performed in a minor procedures room rather than the operating room. However, it can be difficult to titrate the amount of laser energy required to create a full-thickness opening. Small bubbles form in the anterior chamber once the through-and-through opening is achieved. Further applications of the laser can be used to create a peripheral iridotomy. Postoperative 5-FU injections have been reported to increase the surgical success rate.[266] Adjunctive subconjunctival MMC was found to reduce the risk of bleb failure following holmium laser sclerostomy in an animal model.[268]

Ab interno approaches can aim the holmium laser via a goniolens or apply it directly to the trabecular meshwork by an internalized laser probe. The indirect ab externo approach requires significantly higher laser power than is needed for an ab externo approach to achieve equivalent effect (Fig. 23–32).

Holmium laser sclerostomy has been associated with more frequent postoperative complications. The risk of postoperative hypotony is significant following sclerostomy, and a flat anterior chamber occurs more frequently following full-thickness procedures.[269] Other potential complications include bleb failure, wound leak, a thin-walled bleb, cataract formation, hyphema, choroidal detachment, corneal striae, irregular pupil, and visual distortion.[269] Failure of the sclerostomy can occur if the internal osteum is occluded by peripheral iris tissue in the absence of a peripheral iridotomy. A viscoelastic agent can be injected into the sclerostomy in an attempt to dislodge the incarcerated iris tissue, or argon laser goniophotocoagulation can be used to contract the iris tissue adjacent to the osteum. Visual symptoms can arise from the posterior corneal striae and may also be associated with significant corneal astigmatism.[278]

SUMMARY

Glaucoma filtering procedures can effectively reduce IOP to more acceptable levels. However, any surgical procedure brings with it many risks and benefits to the patient. As we enter into a new surgical era, we must evaluate the options that we present to our patients and determine with them what interventions might be most appropriate for the management of their disease. We need to consider the advantages and disadvantages of our currently available procedures and weigh the factors that might ultimately influence the surgical outcome. We look toward new surgical horizons and continue to study more closely the options that we have before us.

REFERENCES

1. Migdal C, Gregory W, Hitchings R. Long-term functional outcome after early surgery compared with laser and medicine in open-angle glaucoma. *Ophthalmology.* 1994;101:1651–1657.
2. Jay L, Allan D. The benefit of early trabeculectomy versus conventional management in primary open angle glaucoma relative to severity of disease. *Eye.* 1989;3:528–535.
3. Musch DC, Lichter PR, Guire KE, et al. The Collaborative Initial Glaucoma Treatment Study. *Ophthalmology.* 1999;106:653–662.
4. Seah SKL, Prata JA Jr, Minckler DS, et al. Visual recovery after trabeculectomy. *J Glaucoma.* 1995;4:228–234.
5. Miyake K, Ota I, Maekubo K, Ichihashi S, Miyake S. Latanoprost accelerates disruption of the blood-aqueous barrier and the incidence of angiographic cystoid

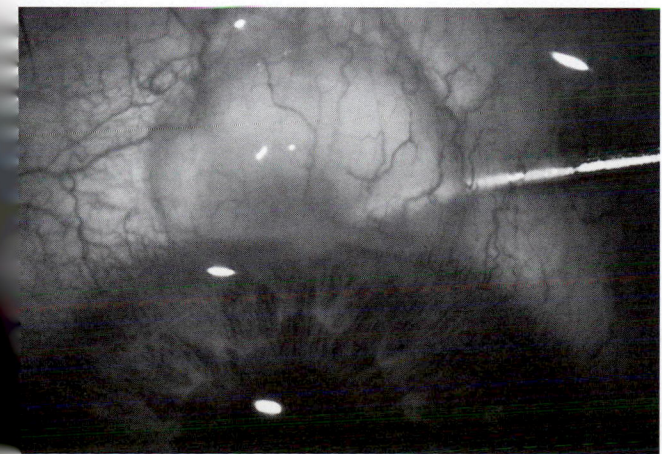

Figure 23–32. Full-thickness fistula created by ab externo holmium laser sclerostomy.

macular edema in early postoperative pseudophakias. *Arch Ophthalmol.* 1999;117:34–40.

6. Longstaff S, Wormald RPL, Mazover A, Hitchings RA. Glaucoma triple procedures: Efficacy of intraocular pressure control and visual outcome. *Ophthalm Surg.* 1990;21:786–793.

7. Broadway DC, Grierson I, O'Brien C, Hitchings RA. Adverse effects of topical anti-glaucoma medication: Part II. The outcome of filtration surgery. *Arch Ophthalmol.* 1994;112:1446–1465.

8. Broadway D, Hitchings R, Grierson I. Topical antiglaucomatous therapy: Adverse effects on the conjunctiva and implications for filtration surgery. *J Glaucoma.* 1995;4:136–148.

9. Sherwood MB, Grierson I, Millar L, Hitchings RA. Long-term morphologic effects of anti-glaucoma drugs on the conjunctiva and Tenon's capsule in glaucomatous patients. *Ophthalmology.* 1989;96:327–335.

10. Broadway DC, Grierson I, O'Brien C, Hitchings RA. Adverse effects of topical anti-glaucoma medications: Part I. The conjunctival cell profile. *Arch Ophthalmol.* 1994;112:1437–1445.

11. Brandt JD, Wittpenn JR, Katz LJ, Steinmann WN, Spaeth GL. Conjunctival impression cytology in patients with glaucoma using long-term topical medications. *Am J Ophthalmol.* 1991;112:297–301.

12. Baudouin C, Pisella PJ, Fillacier K, et al. Ocular surface inflammatory changes induced by topical anti-glaucoma drugs. *Ophthalmology.* 1999;106:556–563.

13. Chen PP, Weaver YK, Budenz DL, Feuer WJ, Parrish RK II. Trabeculectomy function after cataract extraction. *Ophthalmology.* 1998;105:1928–1935.

14. Murchison JF Jr, Shields MB. An evaluation of three surgical approaches for coexisting cataract and glaucoma. *Ophthalm Surg.* 1989;20:393–398.

15. Brooks AM, Gillies WE. The effect of cataract extraction with implant in glaucomatous eye. *Aust N Z J Ophthalmol.* 1992;29:235–238.

16. Drolsum L, Haaskjold E. Extracapsular cataract extraction in eyes previously operated for glaucoma. *Acta Ophthalmol.* 1994;72:273–278.

17. Park HJ, Kwon YH, Weitzman M, Caprioli J. Temporal corneal phacoemulsification in patients with filtered glaucoma. 1997;115:1375–1380.

18. Foster RE, Lowder CY, Meisler DM, Zakov ZN. Extracapsular cataract extraction and posterior chamber intraocular lens implantation in uveitis patients. *Ophthalmology.* 1992;99:1232–1241.

19. Yamagami S, Araie M, Mori M, Mishima K. Posterior chamber intraocular lens implantation in filtered or nonfiltered glaucoma eyes. *Jpn J Ophthalmol.* 1994;38:71–79.

20. Wygnanski-Jaffe T, Barak A, Melamed S, Glovinsky Y. Intraocular pressure increments after cataract extraction in glaucomatous eyes with functioning filtering blebs. *Ophthalm Surg Lasers.* 1997;38:657–661.

21. Anders N, Pham T, Holschbach A, Wollensak J. Combined phacoemulsification and filtering surgery with the "no-stitch" technique. *Arch Ophthalmol.* 1997;115:1245–1249.

22. Kim DD, Doyle JW, Smith MF. Intraocular pressure reduction following phacoemulsification cataract extraction with posterior chamber lens implantation in glaucoma patients. *Ophthalm Surg Lasers.* 1999;30:37–40.

23. Mamalis N, Lohner S, Rand AN, Crandall AS. Combined phacoemulsification, intraocular lens implantation and trabeculectomy. *J Cataract Refract Surg.* 1996;22:467–473.

24. Stewart WC, Crinkley CMC, Carlson AN. Results of combined phacoemulsification and trabeculectomy in patients with elevated preoperative intraocular pressure. *J Glaucoma.* 1995;4:164–169.

25. Park HJ, Weitzman M, Caprioli J. Temporal corneal phacoemulsification combined with superior trabeculectomy: A retrospective case-control study. *Arch Ophthalmol.* 1997;115:318–323.

26. Wyse T, Meyer M, Ruderman JM, et al. Combined trabeculectomy and phacoemulsification: A one-site vs a two-site approach. *Am J Ophthalmol.* 1998;125:334–339.

27. Hennis HL, Stewart W. The use of 5-fluorouracil in patients following combined trabeculectomy and cataract extraction. *Ophthalm Surg.* 1991;22:451–454.

28. O'Grady JM, Juzych MS, Shin DH, Lemon LC, Swendris RP. Trabeculectomy, phacoemulsification, and posterior chamber lens implantation with and without 5-fluorouracil. *Am J Ophthalmol.* 1993;116:594–599.

29. Wong PC, Ruderman JM, Krupin T, et al. 5-Fluorouracil after primary combined filtration surgery. *Am J Ophthalmol.* 1994;117:149–154.

30. Shin DH, Simone PA, Song MS, et al. Adjunctive subconjunctival mitomycin C in glaucoma triple procedure. *Ophthalmology.* 1995;102:1550–1558.

31. Shin DH, Hugh BA, Song MS, et al. Primary glaucoma triple procedure with or without adjunctive mitomycin: Prognostic factors for filtration failure. *Ophthalmology.* 1996;103:1925–1933.

32. Cohen JS, Greff LJ, Novack GD, Wind BE. A placebo-controlled, double-masked evaluation of mitomycin C in combined glaucoma and cataract procedures. *Ophthalmology.* 1996;103:1942–1943.

33. Shin DH, Kim YY, Ren J, et al. Decrease of capsular opacification with adjunctive mitomycin C in combined glaucoma and cataract surgery. *Ophthalmology.* 1998;105:1222–1226.

34. Gandolfi SA, Vecchi M. 5-Fluorouracil in combined trabeculectomy and clear-cornea phacoemulsification with posterior chamber intraocular lens implantation: A one-year randomized, controlled clinical trial. *Ophthalmology.* 1997;104:181–186.

35. Shin DH, Jianming R, Juzych MS, et al. Primary glaucoma triple procedure in patients with primary open-angle glaucoma: The effect of mitomycin C in patients with and without prognostic factors for filtration failure. *Am J Ophthalmol.* 1998;125:346–352.

36. Shin DH, Kim YY, Sheth N, Ren J, Shah M, Kim C, Yang KJ. The role of adjunctive mitomycin C in secondary glaucoma triple procedure as compared to primary glaucoma triple procedure. *Ophthalmology.* 1998; 105:740–745.

37. Lemon LC, Shin DH, Song MS, et al. Comparative study of silicone versus acrylic foldable lens implantation in primary glaucoma triple procedure. *Ophthalmology*. 1997;104:1708–1713.

38. Skuta GL, Parrish RK II. Wound healing in glaucoma filtering surgery. *Surv Ophthalmol*. 1987;32:149–170.

39. The Fluorouracil Filtering Surgery Study Group. Three-year follow-up of the Fluorouracil Filtering Surgery Study. *Am J Ophthalmol*. 1993;115:82–92.

40. The Fluorouracil Filtering Surgery Study Group. Five-year follow-up of the Fluorouracil Filtering Surgery Study. *Am J Ophthalmol*. 1996;121:349–366.

41. Coleman AL, Yu F, Greenland S. Factors associated with elevated complication rates after partial-thickness glaucoma surgical procedures in the United States during 1994. *Ophthalmology*. 1998;105:1165–1169.

42. Honjo M, Tanihara H, Inatani M, Honda Y. Mitomycin C trabeculectomy in eyes with cicatricial conjunctiva. *Am J Ophthalmol*. 1998;126:823–824.

43. Cohen JS, Novack GC, Li ZL. The role of mitomycin treatment duration and previous intraocular surgery on the success of trabeculectomy surgery. *J Glaucoma*. 1997;6:3–9.

44. Scott IU, Greenfield DS, Schiffman J, et al. Outcomes of primary trabeculectomy with the use of adjunctive mitomycin. *Arch Ophthalmol*. 1998;116:286–291.

45. Stewart WC, Reid KK, Pitts RA. The results of trabeculectomy surgery in African-American versus white glaucoma patients. *J Glaucoma*. 1993;2:236–240.

46. Heuer DK, Gressel MG, Parrish RK II, et al. Trabeculectomy in aphakic eyes. *Ophthalmology*. 1984;91:1045–1051.

47. Franks WA, Hitchings RA. Complications of 5-fluorouracil after trabeculectomy (see comments). *Eye*. 1991;5:385–389.

48. Yaldo MK, Stamper RL. Long-term effects of mitomycin on filtering blebs. *Arch Ophthalmol*. 1993;111:824–826.

49. Wright MM, McGehee RF, Pederson JE. Intraoperative mitomycin-C for glaucoma associated with ocular inflammation. *Ophthalm Surg Lasers*. 1997;28:370–376.

50. Tsai JC, Feuer WJ, Parrish RK II, Grajewski AL. 5-Fluorouracil filtering surgery and neovascular glaucoma: Long-term follow-up of the original pilot study. *Ophthalmology*. 1995;102:887–893.

51. Mermoud A, Salmon JF, Straker C, Murray AD. Post-traumatic angle recession glaucoma: A risk factor for bleb failure after trabeculectomy. *Br J Ophthalmol*. 1993;77:631–634.

52. Mermoud A, Salmon JF, Barron A, Straker C, Murray AD. Surgical management of post-traumatic angle recession glaucoma. *Ophthalmology*. 1993;100:634–642.

53. Mermoud A, Salmon JF, Murray AD. Trabeculectomy with mitomycin-C for refractory glaucoma in blacks. *Am J Ophthalmol*. 1993;116:72–78.

54. el Sayyad F, el-Rashood A, Helal M, Hisham M, el-Maghraby A. Fornix-based versus limbal-based conjunctival flaps in initial trabeculectomy with postoperative 5-fluorouracil: Four-year follow-up findings. *J Glaucoma*. 1999;8:124–128.

55. Traverso CE, Tomey KF, Antonios S. Limbal- vs fornix-based conjunctival trabeculectomy flaps. *Am J Ophthalmol*. 1987;104:28–32.

56. Berestka JS, Brown SVL. Limbus- versus fornix-based conjunctival flaps in combined phacoemulsification and mitomycin C trabeculectomy surgery. *Ophthalmology*. 1997;104:187–196.

57. Reichert R, Stewart W, Shields MB. Limbus-based versus fornix-based conjunctival flaps in trabeculectomy. *Ophthalm Surg*. 1997;18:672–676.

58. Shuster JN, Krupin T, Kolker AE, Becker B. Limbus- v fornix-based conjunctival flap in trabeculectomy: A long-term randomized study. *Arch Ophthalmol*. 1984;102:361–362.

59. Wise JB. Mitomycin-compatible suture technique for fornix-based conjunctival flaps in glaucoma filtration surgery. *Arch Ophthalmol*. 1993;111:992–997.

60. Lemon LC, Shin DH, Kim C, et al. Limbus-based vs fornix-based conjunctival flap in combined glaucoma and cataract surgery with adjunctive mitomycin C. *Am J Ophthalmol*. 1998;125:340–345.

61. Khaw PT, Sherwood MB, MacKay SL, et al. Five-minute treatments with fluorouracil, floxuridine and mitomycin have long-term effects on human Tenon's capsule fibroblasts. *Arch Ophthalmol*. 1992;110:1150–1154.

62. Khaw PT, Doyle JW, Sherwood MB, et al. Prolonged localized tissue effects from 5-minute exposures to fluorouracil and mitomycin C. *Arch Ophthalmol*. 1993;111:263–267.

63. Crowston JG, Akbar AN, Constable PH, et al. Antimetabolite induced apoptosis in Tenon's capsule fibroblasts. *Invest Ophthalmol Vis Sci*. 1998;39:449–454.

64. The Fluorouracil Filtering Surgery Study Group. Fluorouracil Filtering Surgery Study one-year follow-up. *Am J Ophthalmol*. 1989;108:625–635.

65. Liebmann JM, Ritch R, Marmor M, Nunez J, Wolner B. Initial 5-fluorouracil trabeculectomy in uncomplicated glaucoma (see comments). *Ophthalmology*. 1991;98:1036–1041.

66. Ophir A, Ticho U. A randomized study of trabeculectomy and subconjunctival administration of fluorouracil in primary glaucomas. *Arch Ophthalmol*. 1992;110:1072–1075.

67. Goldenfeld M, Krupin T, Ruderman JM, et al. 5-Fluorouracil in initial trabeculectomy: A prospective, randomized, multicenter study. *Ophthalmology*. 1994;101:1024–1029.

68. Rockwood EJ, Parrish RK, Heuer DK, et al. Glaucoma filtering surgery with 5-fluorouracil. *Ophthalmology*. 1987;94:1071–1078.

69. Lamba PA, Pandey PK, Raina UK, Krishna V. Short-term results of initial trabeculectomy with intra-operative or postoperative 5-fluorouracil for primary glaucomas. *Indian J Ophthalmol*. 1997;45:173–176.

70. Dietze PJ, Feldman RM, Gross RL. Intraoperative application of 5-fluorouracil during trabeculectomy. *Ophthalm Surg*. 1992;23:662–665.

71. Sidoti PA, Choi JC, Morinelli EN, et al. Trabeculectomy with intraoperative 5-fluorouracil. *Ophthalm Surg Lasers*. 1998;29:552–561.

72. Feldman RM, Dietze PJ, Gross RL, Oram O. Intraoperative 5-fluorouracil administration in trabeculectomy. *J Glaucoma*. 1994;3:302–307.

73. Bell RW, Habib NE, O'Brien C. Long-term results and complications after trabeculectomy with a single peroperative application of 5-fluorouracil. *Eye*. 1997;11:663–671.

74. Chen PC, Yamamoto T, Sawatda A, et al. Use of antifibrosis agents and glaucoma drainage devices in the American and Japanese Glaucoma Societies. *J Glaucoma*. 1997;6:192–196.

75. Anand N, Sahni K, Menage MJ. Modification of trabeculectomy with single-dose intra-operative 5-fluorouracil application. *Acta Ophthalmol Scand*. 1998;76:83–89.

76. Chen CW. Enhanced intraocular pressure controlling effectiveness of trabeculectomy by local application of mitomycin C. *Trans Asia-Pacific Acad Ophthalmol*. 1983;9:172–177.

77. Bergstrom TJ, Wilkinson WS, Skuta GL, et al. The effects of subconjunctival mitomycin-C on glaucoma filtration surgery in rabbits. *Arch Ophthalmol* 1991;109:1725–1730.

78. Higginbotham EJ. Editorial comment: Adjunctive use of mitomycin in filtration surgery: Is it worth the risk? *Arch Ophthalmol*. 1997;115:1068–1069.

79. Perkins TW, Gangnon R, Ladd W, Kaufman PL, Heatley GA. Trabeculectomy with mitomycin C: Intermediate-term results. *J Glaucoma*. 1998;7:230–236.

80. Nujits RMMA, Vernimmen RCJ, Webers CA. Mitomycin C primary trabeculectomy in primary glaucoma of white patients. *J Glaucoma*. 1997;6:293–297.

81. Yamamoto T, Ichie M, Suemori-Matsushita H, Ktazawa Y. Trabeculectomy with mitomycin C for normal-tension glaucoma. *J Glaucoma*. 1995;4:158–163.

82. Al-Hazmi A, Zwaan J, Awad A, et al. Effectiveness and complications of mitomycin C use during pediatric glaucoma surgery. *Ophthalmology*. 1998;105:1915–1920.

83. Wallace DK, Plager DA, Snyder SK, et al. Surgical results of secondary glaucomas in childhood. *Ophthalmology*. 1998;105:101–111.

84. Prata JA, Minckler DS, Baerveldt G, Lee PP, Heuer DK. Site of mitomycin-C application during trabeculectomy. *J Glaucoma*. 1994;3:295–301.

85. Flynn WJ, Carlson DW, Bifano SL. Mitomycin trabeculectomy: The microsurgical sponge difference. *J Glaucoma*. 1995;4:86–90.

86. Robin AL, Ramakrishnan R, Krishnadas R, et al. A long-term dose-response study of mitomycin in glaucoma filtration surgery. *Arch Ophthalmol*. 1997;115:969–974.

87. Mietz H, Krieglstein GK. Three-year follow-up of trabeculectomies performed with different concentrations of mitomycin-C. *Ophthalm Surg Lasers*. 1998;29:628–634.

88. Sihota R, Sharma T, Agarwal HC. Intra-operative mitomycin C and the corneal endothelium. *Acta Ophthalmol Scand*. 1998;76:80–82.

89. Fourman S. Scleritis after glaucoma filtering surgery with mitomycin C. *Ophthalmology*. 1995;102:1569–1571.

90. Dev S, Herndon L, Shields MB. Retinal vein occlusion after trabeculectomy with mitomycin C. *Am J Ophthalmol*. 1996;122:574–575.

91. Skuta GL, Beeson CC, Higginbotham EJ, et al. Intra-operative mitomycin versus postoperative 5-fluorouracil in high-risk glaucoma filtering surgery. *Ophthalmology*. 1992;99:438–444.

92. Katz GJ, Higginbotham EJ, Lichter PR, et al. Mitomycin C versus 5-fluorouracil in high-risk glaucoma filtering surgery: Extended follow-up. *Ophthalmology*. 1995;102:1263–1269.

93. Kitazawa Y, Kawase K, Matsushita H, Minobe M. Trabeculectomy with mitomycin: A comparative study with fluorouracil. *Arch Ophthalmol*. 1991;109:1693–1698.

94. Prata JA Jr, Seah SKL, Minckler DS, et al. Postoperative complications and short-term outcome after 5-fluorouracil or mitomycin-C trabeculectomy. *J Glaucoma*. 1995;4:25–31.

95. Belyea DA, Dan JA, Stamper RL, Liebermann MF, Spencer WH. Late onset of sequential multifocal bleb leaks after glaucoma filtration surgery with 5-fluorouracil and mitomycin-C. *Am J Ophthalmol*. 1997;124:40–45.

96. Greenfield DS, Liebmann JM, Jee J, Ritch R. Late-onset bleb leaks after glaucoma filtering surgery. *Arch Ophthalmol*. 1998;116:443–447.

97. Blok MDW, Greve EL, Dunnebier EA, Muradin F, Kijlstra A. Scleral flap sutures and the development of shallow or flat anterior chamber after trabeculectomy. *Ophthalm Surg*. 1993;24:309–313.

98. Kolker AE, Kass MA, Rait JL. Trabeculectomy with releasable sutures. *Arch Ophthalmol*. 1994;112:62–66.

99. Raina UK, Tuli D. Trabeculectomy with releasable sutures: A prospective randomized pilot study. *Arch Ophthalmol*. 1998;116:1288–1293.

100. Shin DH. Removable-suture closure of the lamellar scleral flap in trabeculectomy. *Ann Ophthalmol*. 1987;19:51–53,55.

101. Johnstone MA, Wellington DP, Ziel CJ. A releasable scleral-flap tamponade suture for guarded filtration surgery. *Arch Ophthalmol*. 1993;111:398–403.

102. Burchfield JC, Kolker AE, Cook SG. Endophthalmitis following trabeculectomy with releasable sutures (letter) (see comments). *Arch Ophthalmol*. 1996;114:766.

103. Rosenberg LF, Siegfried CJ. Endophthalmitis associated with a releasable suture (letter) (see comments). *Arch Ophthalmol*. 1996;114:767.

104. Tezel G, Kolker AE, Kass MA, Wax MB. Late removal of releasable sutures after trabeculectomy or trabeculectomy with cataract extraction supplemented with antifibrotics. *J Glaucoma*. 1998;7:75–81.

105. Araujo SV, Spaeth GL, Roth SM, Starita RJ. A ten-year follow-up on a prospective, randomized trial of postoperative corticosteroids after trabeculectomy. *Ophthalmology*. 1995;102:1753–1759.

106. Roth SM, Spaeth GL, Starita RJ, Birbillis EM, Steinmann WC. The effects of postoperative corticosteroids on trabeculectomy and the clinical course of glaucoma: Five-year follow-up study. *Ophthalm Surg*. 1991;22:724–729.

107. Starita RJ, Fellman RL, Spaeth GL, Poryzees EM, Greenidge KC, Traverso CE. Short- and long-term effects of postoperative corticosteroids on trabeculectomy. *Ophthalmology*. 1985;92:938–946.

108. Thomas R, Jay JL. Raised intraocular pressure with topical steroids after trabeculectomy. *Graefes Arch Clin Exp Ophthalmol*. 1998;226:337–340.

109. Kent AR, Dubiner HB, Whitaker R, et al. The efficacy and safety of diclofenac 0.1% versus prednisolone acetate 1% following trabeculectomy with adjunctive mitomycin-C. *Ophthalm Surg Lasers* 1998;29:561–569.

110. Mizoguchi T, Matsumura M, Kadowaki H, et al. The long-term cystic bleb appearance and safety after trabeculectomy with mitomycin C. *Nippon Ganka Gakkai Zasshi*. 1997;101:874–878.

111. Spaeth GL. A prospective, controlled study to compare Scheie procedure with Watson's trabeculectomy. *Ophthalm Surg*. 1980;11:688–694.

112. Blondeau P, Phelps CD. Trabeculectomy vs. thermosclerostomy: A randomized prospective clinical trial. *Arch Ophthalmol*. 1981;99:810–816.

113. Susanna R Jr, Takahashi W, Nicolela M. Late bleb leakage after trabeculectomy with 5-fluorouracil or mitomycin C. *Can J Ophthalmol*. 1996;31:296–300.

114. Fechtner RD, Minckler D, Weinreb RN, Frangei G, Jampol LM. Complications of glaucoma surgery: Ocular decompression retinopathy. *Arch Ophthalmol*. 1992;110:965–968.

115. Seah SKL, Prata JA, Minckler DS, et al. Hypotony following trabeculectomy. *J Glaucoma*. 1995;4:73–79.

116. Zacharia PT, Deppermann SR, Schuman JS. Ocular hypotony after trabeculectomy with mitomycin C. *Am J Ophthalmol*. 1993;116:314–326.

117. Greenfield DS, Parrish RK II. Bleb rupture following filtering surgery with mitomycin-C: Clinicopathologic correlations. *Ophthalm Surg Lasers*. 1996;27:876–877.

118. Fineman MS, Katz LJ, Wilson RP. Topical dorzolamide-induced hypotony and ciliochoroidal detachment in patients with previous filtration surgery. *Arch Ophthalmol*. 1996;114:1031–1032.

119. Chandler PA, Maumenee AE. A major cause of hypotony. *Am J Ophthalmol*. 1961;52:609–618.

120. Meislik J, Herschler J. Hypotony due to inadvertent cyclodialysis after intraocular lens implantation. *Arch Ophthalmol*. 1979;97:1297–1299.

121. Gentile R, Pavlin C, Liebmann JM, et al. Accurate diagnosis of cyclodialysis clefts by ultrasound biomicroscopy. *Invest Ophthalmol Vis Sci*. 1994;35(suppl):1420.

122. Karwatowski WSS, Weinreb RN. Imaging of cyclodialysis cleft by ultrasound biomicroscope. *Am J Ophthalmol*. 1994;117:541–543.

123. Burchfield JC, Kolker AE. Diagnosis and treatment of cyclodialysis clefts. *J Glaucoma*. 1995;4:207–213.

124. Lavin M, Franks W, Hitchings RA. Serous retinal detachment following glaucoma filtering surgery. *Arch Ophthalmol*. 1990;108:1553–1555.

125. Kim YY, Jung HR. The effect of flat anterior chamber on the success of trabeculectomy. *Acta Ophthalmol Scand*. 1995;73:268–272.

126. Wand M. Intra-operative intracameral viscoelastic agent in the prevention of postfiltration flat anterior chamber. *J Glaucoma*. 1994;3:101–105.

127. Kao SF, Lichter PR, Musch DC. Anterior chamber depth following filtration surgery. *Ophthalm Surg*. 1989;20:332–336.

128. Dellaporta A. Fundus changes in postoperative hypotony. *Am J Ophthalmol*. 1955;40:781–785.

129. Stamper RL, McMenemy MG, Lieberman MF. Hypotonous maculopathy after trabeculectomy with subconjunctival 5-fluorouracil. *Am J Ophthalmol*. 1992;114:544–553.

130. Costa VP, Smith M, Spaeth GL, et al. Loss of visual acuity after trabeculectomy. *Ophthalmology*. 1993;100:599–612.

131. Sibayan SAB, Igarashi S, Kasahara N, et al. Cataract extraction as a means of treating postfiltration hypotony maculopathy (case reports). *Ophthalm Surg Lasers*. 1997;238:241–243.

132. Duker JD, Schuman JS. Successful surgical treatment of hypotony maculopathy following trabeculectomy with topical mitomycin. *Ophthalm Surg*. 1994;25:463–465.

133. D'Ermo F, Bonomi L, Doro D. A critical analysis of the long-term results of trabeculectomy. *Am J Ophthalmol*. 1979;88:829–835.

134. Lichter PR, Ravin JG. Risks of sudden visual loss after glaucoma surgery. *Am J Ophthalmol*. 1974;78:1009–1013.

135. Werner EB, Drance SM, Schulzer M. Trabeculectomy and the progression of glaucomatous visual field loss. *Arch Ophthalmol*. 1977;95:1374–1377.

136. Smith MF, Doyle JW. Use of oversize bandage soft contact lenses in the management of early hypotony following filtration surgery. *Ophthalm Surg Lasers*. 1996;27:417–421.

137. Blok MD, Kok JH, van Mil C, Greve EL, Kijlstra A. Use of the Megasoft bandage lens for treatment of complications after trabeculectomy. *Am J Ophthalmol*. 1990;110:264–268.

138. Fourman S, Wiley L. Use of a collagen shield to treat glaucoma filter bleb leak. *Am J Ophthalmol*. 1989;107:673–674.

139. Simmons RJ, Kimbrough RL. Shell tamponade in filtering surgery for glaucoma. *Ophthalm Surg*. 1979;10:17–34.

140. Melamed S, Hersh P, Kersten D, Lee DA, Epstein DL. The use of glaucoma shell tamponade in leaking filtration blebs. *Ophthalmology*. 1986;93:839–842.

141. Ruderman JM, Allen RC. Simmons' tamponade shell for leaking filtration blebs. *Arch Ophthalmol*. 1985;103:1708–1710.

142. Wise JB. Treatment of chronic postfiltration hypotony by intrableb injection of autologous blood. *Arch Ophthalmol*. 1993;111:827–830.

143. Smith MF, Magauran R, Doyle JW. Treatment of postfiltration bleb leak by bleb injection of autologous blood. *Ophthalm Surg*. 1994;25:636–637.

144. Leen MM, Moster MR, Katz LJ, Terebuh AK, Schmidt CM, Spaeth GL. Management of overfiltering and leaking blebs with autologous blood injection (see comments). *Arch Ophthalmol*. 1995;113:1050–1055.

145. Smith MF, Magauran RG, Betchkal J, Doyle JW. Treatment of postfiltration bleb leaks with autologous blood. *Ophthalmology.* 1995;102:868–871.

146. Choudhri SA, Herndon LW, Damji KF, Allingham RR, Shields MB. Efficacy of autologous blood injection for treating overfiltering or leaking blebs after glaucoma surgery. *Am J Ophthalmol.* 1997;123:554–555.

147. Siegfried CJ, Grewal RK, Karalekas D, Rosenberg LF, Krupin T. Marked intraocular pressure rise complicating intrableb autologous blood injection (letter). *Arch Ophthalmol.* 1996;114:492–493.

148. Lu DW, Azuara-Blanco A, Katz LJ. Severe visual loss after autologous blood injection for mitomycin C–associated hypotonous maculopathy. *Ophthalm Surg Lasers.* 1997;28:244–245.

149. Flynn WJ, Rosen WJ, Campbell DG. Delayed hyphema and intravitreal blood following intrableb autologous blood injection after trabeculectomy. *Am J Ophthalmol.* 1997;124:115–116.

150. Gehring JR, Ciccarelli EC. Trichloroacetic acid treatment of filtering blebs following cataract extraction. *Am J Ophthalmol.* 1972;74:662–665.

151. Zalta AH, Wieder RH. Closure of leaking filtering blebs with cyanoacrylate tissue adhesive. *Br J Ophthalmol.* 1991;3:170–173.

152. Leahey AB, Gottsch JD, Stark WJ. Clinical experience with *N*-butyl cyanoacrylate (Nexacryl) tissue adhesive. *Ophthalmology.* 1993;100:1173–1180.

153. Graham SL, Goldberg W. Cyanoacrylate adhesive closure of wound leaks following fornix-based trabeculectomy with adjunct 5-fluorouracil. *J Glaucoma.* 1993;2:297–302.

154. Weber PA, Baker ND. The use of cyanoacrylate adhesive with a collagen shield in leaking filtering blebs. *Ophthalm Surg.* 1989;20:284–285.

155. Grewing R, Mester U. Fibrin sealant in the management of complicated hypotony after trabeculectomy. *Ophthalm Surg Lasers.* 1997;28:124–127.

156. Grady FJ, Forbes M. Tissue adhesive for repair of conjunctival buttonhole in glaucoma surgery. *Am J Ophthalmol.* 1969;68:656–658.

157. Asrani SG, Wilensky JT. Management of bleb leaks after glaucoma filtering surgery: Use of autologous fibrin tissue glue as alternative. *Ophthalmology.* 1996;103: 294–298.

158. Graham SL, Murray B, Goldberg I. Closure of fornix-based posttrabeculectomy conjunctival wound leaks with autologous fibrin glue (letter). *Am J Ophthalmol.* 1992;114:221–222.

159. Gammon RR, Prum BE Jr, Avery N, Mintz PD. Rapid preparation of small-volume autologous fibrinogen concentrate and its same day use in bleb leaks after glaucoma filtration surgery. *Ophthalm Surg Lasers.* 1998; 29:1010–1012.

160. O'Sullivan R, Dalton R, Rostron CK. Fibrin glue: An alternative method of wound closure in glaucoma surgery. *J Glaucoma.* 1996;5:367–370.

161. Hennis HL, Stewart WC. Use of the argon laser to close filtering bleb leaks. *Graefes Arch Clin Exp Ophthalmol.* 1992;230:537–541.

162. Baum M, Weiss HS. Argon laser closure of conjunctival bleb leak. *Arch Ophthalmol.* 1993;111:438.

163. Lynch MG, Roesch M, Brown RH. Remodeling filtering blebs with the neodymium:YAG laser. *Ophthalmology.* 1996;103:1700–1705.

164. Geyer O. Management of large, leaking and inadvertent filtering blebs with the neodymium:YAG laser. *Ophthalmology.* 1998;105:983–987.

165. Douvas NG. Cystoid bleb cryotherapy. *Am J Ophthalmol.* 1972;74:69–71.

166. Yannuzzi LA, Theodore FH. Cryotherapy of postcataract blebs. *Am J Ophthalmol.* 1973;76:217–222.

167. Cleasby GW, Fung WE, Webster RG Jr. Cryosurgical closure of filtering blebs. *Arch Ophthalmol.* 1972;87:319–323.

168. Furgason TG, Perkins TW. A clothesline suture technique for the repair of a conjunctival tear during trabeculectomy. *Ophthalm Surg Lasers.* 1997;28:772–773.

169. Galin MA, Hung PT. Surgical repair of leaking blebs. *Am J Ophthalmol.* 1977;83:328–333.

170. Tomlinson CP, Belcher I, Smith PD, Simmons RJ. Management of leaking filtration blebs. *Ann Ophthalmol.* 1987;19:405–408.

171. Wilson MR, Kotas-Neumann R. Free conjunctival patch for repair of persistent late bleb leak. *Am J Ophthalmol.* 1994;117:569–574.

172. Buxton JN, Lavery KT, Liebmann JM, Buxon DF, Ritch R. Reconstruction of filtering blebs with free conjunctival autografts. *Ophthalmology.* 1994;101:635–639.

173. Cohen JS, Shaffer RN, Heterington J Jr, Hoskins HD Jr. Revision of filtration surgery. *Arch Ophthalmol.* 1977;95:1612–1615.

174. Schwartz GF, Robin AL, Wilson RP, et al. Resuturing the scleral flap leads to resolution of hypotony maculopathy. *J Glaucoma.* 1996;5:246–251.

175. Melamed S, Ashkenazi I, Belcher DC, Blumenthal M. Donor scleral graft patching for persistent filtration bleb leak. *Ophthalm Surg.* 1991;22:164–165.

176. Haynes WL, Alward WL. Rapid visual recovery and long-term intraocular pressure control after donor scleral patch grafting for trabeculectomy-induced hypotony maculopathy. *J Glaucoma.* 1995;4:200–201.

177. Kosmin AS, Wishart PK. A full-thickness scleral graft for the surgical management of a late filtration bleb leak. *Ophthalm Surg Laser.* 1997;28:461–468.

178. Byrnes GA, Leen MM, Wong TP, Benson WE. Vitrectomy for ciliary block (malignant) glaucoma. *Ophthalmology.* 1995;102:1308–1311.

179. Harbour JW, Rubsamen PE, Palmberg P. Pars plana vitrectomy in the management of phakic and pseudophakic malignant glaucoma (see comments). *Arch Ophthalmol.* 1996;114:1073–1078.

180. Givens K, Shields MB. Suprachoroidal hemorrhage after glaucoma filtering surgery. *Am J Ophthalmol.* 1987;103:689–694.

181. Rockwood EJ, Kalenak JW, Plotnik JL, et al. Prospective ultrasonographic evaluation of intra-operative and delayed postoperative suprachoroidal hemorrhage from glaucoma surgery. *J Glaucoma.* 1995;4:16–24.

182. The Fluorouracil Filtering Surgery Study Group. Risk factors for suprachoroidal hemorrhage after filtering surgery. *Am J Ophthalmol*. 1992;113:501–507.

183. Dugel PU, Heuer DK, Tach AB, et al. Annular peripheral choroidal detachment simulated aqueous misdirection after glaucoma surgery (see comments). *Ophthalmology*. 1997;104:439–444.

184. Traverso CE, Greenidge KC, Spaeth GL, Wilson RP. Focal pressure a new method to encourage filtration after trabeculectomy. *Ophthalm Surg*. 1984;15:62–65.

185. Kane H, Gaasterland DE, Monsour M. Response of filtered eyes to digital ocular pressure. *Ophthalmology*. 1997;104:202–206.

186. Wieland M, Spaeth GL. Use of digital compression following glaucoma surgery. *Ophthalm Surg*. 1988;19:350–352.

187. Honda Y, Kawano S, Negri A, Koizum K. Pressure profile of ophthalmic surgical procedures: An experimental study on the rabbit eye. *Ophthalm Surg Lasers*. 1982;13:387–391.

188. Colotto A, Falsini B, Salgarello T, et al. Transiently raised intraocular pressure reveals pattern electroretinogram losses in ocular hypertension. *Invest Ophthalmol Vis Sci*. 1996;37(13):2663–2670.

189. Segrest D, Ellis P. Iris incarceration associated with digital ocular massage. *Ophthalmic Surg Lasers*. 1981;12:349–351.

190. Susanna R Jr, Takahashi W, Nicolela M. Late bleb leakage after trabeculectomy with 5-fluorouracil or mitomycin C. *Can J Ophthalmol*. 1996;31:296–300.

191. Miller G, Kurstin J. Ruptured filtering bleb after ocular massage. *Arch Ophthalmol*. 1966;76:363–365.

192. Ruderman JR, Jampel LM, Krueger DM. Visual loss caused by subretinal hemorrhage and rupture of Bruch's membrane after digital ocular massage. *Am J Ophthalmol*. 1988;106(4):493–494.

193. Piltz JR, Starita RJ. The use of subconjunctivally administered tissue plasminogen activator after trabeculectomy. *Ophthalm Surg*. 1994;25:51–53.

194. Melamed S, Ashkenazi I, Glovinsky J, Blumenthal M. Tight scleral flap trabeculectomy with postoperative laser suture lysis (see comments). *Am J Ophthalmol*. 1990;109:303–309.

195. Chopra H, Goldenfeld M, Krupin T, Rosenberg LF. Early postoperative titration of bleb function: Argon laser suture lysis and removable sutures in trabeculectomy. *J Glaucoma*. 1992;1:54–57.

196. Kasahara N, Smith TJ, Sibayan SA, et al. Midterm reversible failure in trabeculectomies with adjunctive mitomycin-C. *Ophthalm Surg Lasers*. 1997;28:986–991.

197. Singh J, Bell RW, Adams A, O'Brien C. Enhancement of post trabeculectomy bleb formation by laser suture lysis. *Br J Ophthalmol*. 1996;80:624–627.

198. Hoskins HD Jr, Migliazzo C. Management of failing filtering blebs with the argon laser. *Ophthalm Surg*. 1984;15:731–733.

199. Mandelkorn RM, Crossman JL, Olander KW, Heacock G. A new argon laser suture lysis lens. *Ophthalm Surg*. 1994;25:480–481.

200. Ritch R, Potash SD, Liebmann JM. A new lens for argon laser suture lysis. *Ophthalm Surg*. 1994;25:126–127.

201. Schwartz AL, Weiss HS. Bleb leak with hypotony after laser suture lysis and trabeculectomy with mitomycin C (case report). *Arch Ophthalmol*. 1992;110:1049.

202. Keller C, To K. Bleb leak with hypotony after laser suture lysis and trabeculectomy with mitomycin C (letter). *Arch Ophthalmol*. 1992;110:427–428.

203. Aktan SG, Mandelkorn RM. Krypton laser suture lysis. *Ophthalm Surg Lasers*. 1998;29:635–638.

204. Pappa KS, Derick RJ, Weber PA, et al. Late argon laser suture lysis after mitomycin C trabeculectomy. *Ophthalmology*. 1993;100:1268–1271.

205. Bardak Y, Cuypers MH, Tilanus MA, Eggink CA. Ocular hypotony after laser suture lysis following trabeculectomy with mitomycin C. *Int Ophthalmol*. 1997–1998;21:325–330.

206. Macken P, Buys Y, Trope GE. Glaucoma laser suture lysis. *Br J Ophthalmol*. 1996;80:398–401.

207. Ewing RH, Stamper RL. Needle revision with and without 5-fluorouracil for the treatment of failed filtering bleb. *Am J Ophthalmol*. 1990;110:349–366.

208. Mastropasqua L, Carpineto P, Ciancaglini M, et al. Delayed post-operative use of 5-fluorouracil as an adjunct in medically uncontrolled open angle glaucoma. *Eye*. 1998;12:701–706.

209. Shin DH, Juzych MS, Khatana AK, Swendris RP, Parrow KA. Needling revision of failed filtering blebs with adjunctive 5-fluorouracil. *Ophthalm Surg*. 1993;24:242–248.

210. Greenfield DS, Miller MP, Suner IJ, Palmberg PF. Needle elevation of the scleral flap for failing filtration blebs after trabeculectomy with mitomycin C. *Am J Ophthalmol*. 1996;122:195–204.

211. Mardelli PG, Lederer CM, Murray PL, Pastor SA, Hassanein KM. Slit-lamp needle revision of failed filtering blebs using mitomycin C. *Ophthalmology*. 1996;13:1946–1955.

212. Cohn HC, Aron-Rosa D. Reopening blocked trabeculectomy sites with the YAG laser. *Am J Ophthalmol*. 1983;95:293–294.

213. Dailey RA, Samples JR, van Buskirk EM. Reopening filtration fistulas with the neodymium-YAG laser. *Am J Ophthalmol*. 1986;102:491–495.

214. Kandarakis A, Mitropoulos P, Angelou M, Dikidou M, Amariotakis A. Reopening of failed trabeculectomies with ab interno Nd:YAG laser. *Eur J Ophthalmol*. 1996;6:143–146.

215. Ticho U, Ivry M. Reopening of occluded filtering blebs by argon laser photocoagulation. *Am J Ophthalmol*. 1977;84:413–418.

216. van Buskirk EM. Reopening filtration fistulas with the argon laser. *Am J Ophthalmol*. 1982;94:1–3.

217. Scott DR, Quigley HA. Medical management of a high bleb phase after trabeculectomies. *Ophthalmology*. 1988;95:1169–1173.

218. Pederson JE, Smith SG. Surgical management of encapsulated filtering blebs. *Ophthalmology*. 1985;92:955–958.

219. Feldman RM, Gross RL, Spaeth GL, et al. Risk factors for development of Tenon's capsule cysts after trabeculectomy. *Ophthalmology*. 1989;96:336–341.

220. Mandal AK. Results of medical management and mitomycin-C augmented excisional bleb revision for encapsulated filtering blebs. *Ophthalm Surg Lasers*. 1999; 30:276–284.

221. Azuara-Blanco A, Bond JB, Wilson RP, et al. Encapsulated filtering blebs after trabeculectomy with mitomycin-C. *Ophthalm Surg Lasers*. 1997;28:805–809.

222. Schwartz AL, van Veldhuisen PC, Gaasterland DE, et al. The Advanced Glaucoma Intervention Study (AGIS): 5. Encapsulated bleb after initial trabeculectomy. *Am J Ophthalmol*. 1999;127:8–19.

223. Richter CU, Shingleton BJ, Bellows AR, et al. The development of encapsulated filtering blebs. *Ophthalmology*. 1988;95:1163–1168.

224. Oh Y, Katz LJ, Spaeth GL, Wilson RP. Risk factors for the development of encapsulated filtering blebs: The role of surgical glove powder and 5-fluorouracil (see comments). *Ophthalmology*. 1994;101:629–634.

225. Shingleton BJ, Richter CU, Bellows AR, Hutchinson BT. Management of encapsulated filtration blebs. *Ophthalmology*. 1990;97:63–68.

226. Costa VP, Correa MM, Kara-Jose N. Needling versus medical treatment in encapsulated blebs. *Ophthalmology*. 1997;104:1215–1220.

227. Hodge W, Saheb N, Balazsi G, Kasner O. Treatment of encapsulated blebs with 30-gauge needling and injection of low-dose 5-fluorouracil. *Can J Ophthalmol*. 1992;27: 233–236.

228. van Buskirk EM. Cysts of Tenon's capsule following filtration surgery. *Am J Ophthalmol*. 1982;94:522–577.

229. Fink AJ, Boys-Smith JW, Brear R. Management of large filtering blebs with the argon laser. *Am J Ophthalmol*. 1986;101:695–699.

230. Palmberg P, Zacchei AC. Compression sutures: A new treatment for leaking or painful filtering blebs. *Invest Ophthalmol Vis Sci*. 1996;37:S444.

231. Ticho U, Ophir A. Late complications after glaucoma filtering surgery with adjunctive 5-fluorouracil. *Am J Ophthalmol*. 1993;115:505–510.

232. Whiteside-Michel J, Liebmann JM, Ritch R. Initial 5-fluorouracil trabeculectomy in young patients. *Ophthalmology*. 1992;99:7–13.

233. Higginbotham EJ, Stevens RK, Musch DC, et al. Bleb-related endophthalmitis after trabeculectomy with mitomycin C. *Ophthalmology*. 1996;103:650–656.

234. Greenfield DS, Suner IJ, Miller MP, et al. Endophthalmitis after filtering surgery with mitomycin. *Arch Ophthalmol*. 1996;114:943–949.

235. Wilson P. Trabeculectomy: Long term follow-up. *Br J Ophthalmol*. 1977;61:535–538.

236. Freedman J, Gupta M, Bunke A. Endophthalmitis after trabeculectomy. *Arch Ophthalmol*. 1978;96:1017–1018.

237. Mills KB. Trabeculectomy: A retrospective long-term follow-up of 444 cases. *Br J Ophthalmol*. 1981;65:790–795.

238. Katz LJ, Cantor LB, Spaeth GL. Complications of surgery in glaucoma: Early and late bacterial endophthalmitis following glaucoma filtering surgery. *Ophthalmology*. 1985;92:959–963.

239. Brown RH, Yang LH, Walker SD, et al. Treatment of bleb infection after glaucoma surgery. *Arch Ophthalmol*. 1994;112:57–61.

240. Chen PP, Gedde SJ, Budenz DL, Parrish RK. Outpatient treatment of bleb infection. *Arch Ophthalmol*. 1997; 115:1124–1128.

241. Wolner B, Liebmann JM, Sassani JW, Ritch R, Speaker M, Marmor M. Late bleb-related endophthalmitis after trabeculectomy with adjunctive 5-fluorouracil. *Ophthalmology*. 1991;98:1053–1060.

242. Caronia RM, Liebmann JM, Friedman R, et al. Trabeculectomy at the inferior limbus. *Arch Ophthalmol*. 1996;114:387–391.

243. Bellows AR, McCullep JP. Endophthalmitis in aphakic patients with unplanned filtering blebs wearing contact lenses. *Ophthalmology*. 1981;88:839–843.

244. Gupta N, Weinreb RN. Filtering bleb infections as a complication of orthokeratology. *Arch Ophthalmol*. 1997;115:1076.

245. Ayyala RS, Bellows AR, Thomas JV, Hutchinson BT. Bleb infections: Clinically different courses of "blebitis" and endophthalmitis. *Ophthalm Surg Lasers*. 1997;28: 452–460.

246. Ciulla TA, Beck AD, Topping TM, Baker AS. Blebitis, early endophthalmitis, and late endophthalmitis after glaucoma-filtering surgery. *Ophthalmology*. 1997;104: 986–995.

247. Kangas TA, Greenfield DS, Flynn HW, et al. Delayed-onset endophthalmitis associated with conjunctival filtering blebs. *Ophthalmology*. 1997;104:746–752.

248. Akova YA, Bulut S, Dabil H, Duman S. Late bleb-related endophthalmitis after trabeculectomy with mitomycin C. *Ophthalm Surg Lasers*. 1999;30:146–151.

249. Stegmann R, Pienaar A, Miller D. Viscocanalostomy for open-angle glaucoma in black African patients. *J Cataract Refract Surg*. 1999;25:316–322.

250. Carassa RG, Bettin P, Fiori M, Brancato R. Viscocanalostomy: A pilot study. *Eur J Ophthalmol*. 1998;8: 57–61.

251. Chiou AGY, Mermoud A, Underdahl JP, Schnyder CC. An ultrasound biomicroscopic study of eyes after deep sclerectomy with collagen implant. *Ophthalmology*. 1998;105:746–750.

252. Sanchez E, Schnyder CC, Sickenberg M, et al. Deep sclerectomy: Results with and without collagen implant. *Int Ophthalmol*. 1996–1997;29:157–162.

253. Mermoud A, Schnyder CC, Sickenberg M, et al. Comparison of deep sclerectomy with collagen implant and trabeculectomy in open-angle glaucoma. *J Cataract Refract Surg*. 1999;25:323–331.

254. Karlen ME, Sanchez E, Schnyder CC, et al. Deep sclerectomy with collagen implant: Medium term results (see comments). *Br J Ophthalmol*. 1999;83:6–11.

255. Mermoud A, Karlen ME, Schnyder CC, et al. Nd:YAG goniopuncture after deep sclerectomy with collagen implant. *Ophthalm Surg Lasers*. 1999;30:120–125.

256. Welsh NH, DeLange J, Wasserman P, Ziemba SL. The "deroofing" of Schlemm's canal in patients with open-

angle glaucoma through placement of a collagen drainage device. *Ophthalm Surg Lasers*. 1998;28:216–226.

257. Chiou AG, Mermoud A, Jewelewicz DA. Post-operative inflammation following deep sclerectomy with collagen implant versus standard trabeculectomy. *Graefes Arch Clin Exp Ophthalmol*. 1998;236:593–596.

258. Gianoli F, Schnyder CC, Bovey E, Mermoud A. Combined surgery for cataract and glaucoma: Phacoemulsification and deep sclerectomy compared with phacoemulsification and trabeculectomy (see comments). *J Cataract Refract Surg*. 1999;25:340–346.

259. Scheie HG. Retraction of scleral wound edges as a fistulizing procedure for glaucoma. *Am J Ophthalmol*. 1958;45:220.

260. Preziosi CL. The electro-cautery in the treatment of glaucoma. *Br J Ophthalmol*. 1924;8:414.

261. Wilson MR. Posterior lip sclerectomy vs trabeculectomy in West Indian blacks. *Arch Ophthalmol*. 1989;107:1604–1608.

262. Marion JR, Shields MB. Thermal sclerostomy and posterior lip sclerectomy: A comparative study. *Ophthalm Surg*. 1978;9:67–75.

263. Friedman DS, Katz LJ, Augsburger JJ, Lean M. Holmium laser sclerostomy in glaucomatous eyes with prior surgery: 24-month results. *Ophthalm Surg Lasers*. 1998;29:17–22.

264. Gherezghiher T, March WF, Koss MC, Nordquist RE. Neodymium-YAG laser sclerostomy in primates. *Arch Ophthalmol*. 1985;103:1543–1545.

265. Higginbotham EJ, Kao G, Peyman GA. Internal sclerostomy with Nd:YAG contact laser vs. thermal sclerostomy in rabbits. *Ophthalmology*. 1988;95:385–390.

266. Hoskins HD Jr, Iwach AG, Drake MV, et al. Subconjunctival THC:YAG laser limbal sclerostomy ab externo in the rabbit. *Ophthalm Surg*. 1990;21:589–592.

267. Hoskins HD, Iwach AG, Vassiliadis A, et al. Subconjunctival THC:YAG laser thermal sclerostomy. *Ophthalmology*. 1991;98:1394–1400.

268. Wang TH, Hung PT, Ho TC. THC:YAG laser sclerostomy with preoperative mitomycin-C subconjunctival injection in rabbits. *J Glaucoma*. 1993;2:260–265.

269. Iwach AG, Hoskins HD Jr, Mora JS, et al. Update on the subconjunctival THC:YAG (holmium) laser sclerostomy ab externo clinical trial: A 4-year report. *Ophthalm Surg Lasers*. 1996;27:823–831.

270. Berlin M, Martinez M, Peter-Loercher H. Erbium YAG laser sclerostomy, mechanism and histological analysis. *Invest Ophthalmol Vis Sci*. 1991;32(suppl):860.

271. Gaasterland DE, Hennings DR, Boutacoff TA, Bilek C. Ab interno and ab externo filtering operations by laser contact surgery. *Ophthalm Surg*. 1987;18:254–257.

272. Jaffe GJ, Mieler WF, Radius RL, et al. Ab interno sclerostomy with a high powered argon endolaser. *Arch Ophthalmol*. 1989;107:1183–1185.

273. Beckman H, Fuller TA. Carbon dioxide laser scleral dissection and filtering procedure for glaucoma. *Am J Ophthalmol*. 1979;88:73–77.

274. Berlin MS, Rajacich G, Duffy M, et al. Excimer laser photoablation in glaucoma filtering surgery. *Am J Ophthalmol*. 1987;103:713–714.

275. Melamed S, Solomon A, Neumann D, et al. Internal sclerostomy using laser ablation of dye enhanced sclera in glaucoma patients: A pilot study. *Br J Ophthalmol*. 1993;77:139–144.

276. Ruben S, Migal C, DeVivero C. Ab interno pulsed dye laser sclerostomy for the treatment of glaucoma: Preliminary results of a new technique. *Eye*. 1993;7:436–439.

277. Karp CL, Higginbotham EJ, Edwards DP, et al. Diode laser surgery: Ab interno versus ab externo versus conventional surgery in rabbits. *Ophthalmology*. 1993;100:1567–1573.

278. Trible JR, Olander KW, Koenig SB. Corneal refractive and endothelial changes following THC:YAG (holmium) laser sclerostomy. *Ophthalm Surg Lasers*. 1998;29:733–737.

Chapter 24

TERTIARY GLAUCOMA SURGICAL PROCEDURES

Elliot B. Werner

Standard glaucoma filtering surgery works well in many patients. There are some patients, however, for whom there is a high risk of failure for standard filtering surgery. In these patients, a modified filtering operation may be indicated. Filtering surgery may be modified either by the use of an antifibrotic agent to inhibit postoperative scarring and inflammation or by the use of an aqueous tube-shunt device to avoid the problems of a limbal filtering bleb. In other patients, filtering surgery may be contraindicated. In this situation, a cyclodestructive procedure may be useful to lower intraocular pressure.

MODIFIED FILTERING SURGERY: ANTIFIBROTIC AGENTS

It is now recognized that certain patients have a high risk for failure of a standard trabeculectomy (Fig. 24–1). Patients at risk for failure include African Americans, younger patients, patients with previous intraocular surgery including cataract surgery or previous filtering surgery that has failed, patients with certain secondary glaucomas such as neovascular or uveitic glaucoma, and patients who have been treated with topical glaucoma medications for a long time.[1-10] In these patients the use of an antifibrotic

agent often results in a better chance of achieving successful filtration.

5-Fluorouracil (5-FU) was the first antifibrotic agent used widely in conjunction with filtering surgery. 5-FU is a pyrimidine analogue antimetabolite that blocks DNA synthesis by inhibiting the enzyme thymidylate synthetase. In general medicine 5-FU is used mainly for the treatment of cancer of the breast, pancreas, and gastrointestinal tract as well as certain precancerous and cancerous skin lesions.

When used in conjunction with trabeculectomy, 5-FU is usually given as a series of subconjunctival injections for 2 weeks or more after surgery. There have been some recent reports of the application of 5-FU to the surgical site intraoperatively. Studies have shown that the use of 5-FU is associated with a significantly higher success rate in the presence of risk factors for failure of filtration surgery.[11-15] The use of 5-FU is also associated with lower levels of intraocular pressure following surgery in cases of normal-tension glaucoma where very low pressures are desired.[16]

The use of 5-FU is associated with a higher complication rate. Complications specifically associated with 5-FU include corneal toxicity, thin-walled blebs, early and late leaking blebs, and chronic hypotony with maculopathy.[17-20]

411

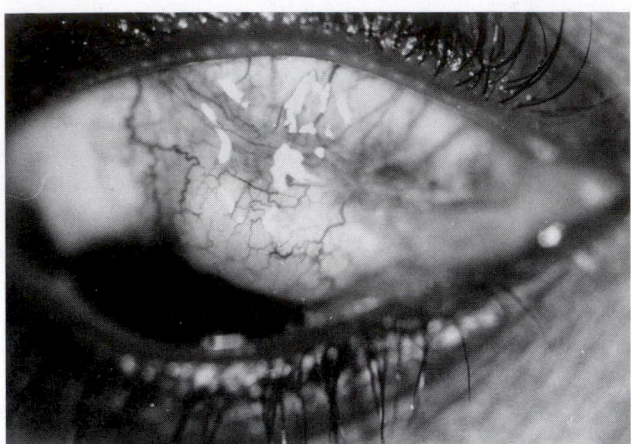

Figure 24–1. An example of failure of standard filtering surgery. The bleb is tense, opaque, encapsulated, elevated, and vascularized. (*See also Color Plate 73.*)

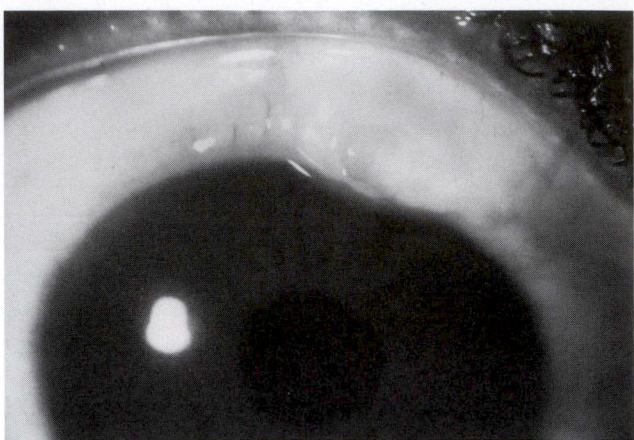

Figure 24–2. An example of successful filtration surgery done with mitomycin C. The filtering bleb has thin walls; it is avascular and translucent, with microcysts at the outer edge. (*See also Color Plate 74.*)

More recently, mitomycin has come into widespread use as an antifibrotic agent in conjunction with trabeculectomy. Mitomycin is an antineoplastic antibiotic isolated from *Streptomyces caespitosus*. It is an extremely toxic agent that blocks the synthesis of DNA. At higher doses it also blocks RNA and protein synthesis. The major clinical use of mitomycin is as adjunctive chemotherapy for cancer of the stomach and pancreas.

Mitomycin is a more potent and long-lasting inhibitor of fibroblast proliferation than 5-FU. It is applied to the surgical site intraoperatively and does not require subconjunctival injections postoperatively. The use of mitomycin is associated with higher success rates for filtering surgery in high-risk patients.[4,21-26] Like 5-FU, it is also associated with a significantly higher complication rate. Complications associated with mitomycin include hypotony, thin-walled bleb, leaking bleb, and endophthalmitis (Figs. 24–2 and 24–3).[27-32]

MODIFIED FILTERING SURGERY: AQUEOUS TUBE-SHUNT DRAINAGE IMPLANTS

Most clinicians reserve the use of aqueous tube-shunt drainage implants for patients in whom a trabeculectomy with an antifibrotic agent has failed. In some situations, however, where the risk of failure or complications from a trabeculectomy with an antifibrotic agent is unacceptable, a drainage implant may be used primarily. Such situations might include extensive conjunctival scarring, certain types of secondary glaucoma such as neovascular or irido-corneal-endothelial syndrome, patients with a previous pars plana vitrectomy, young

children, or aphakic or pseudophakic patients with other complications.[33,34]

In tube or valve implantations, a plastic (usually silicone) tube is inserted through the sclerostomy into the peripheral anterior chamber to facilitate drainage (Fig. 24–4). The tube is attached to a plate that is sutured to the surface of the globe behind the equator (Fig. 24–5). The plate acts as a scaffold to support the formation of a posteriorly placed filtering bleb. The success rate of the tube-shunt filtering surgery is proportional to the surface area of the plate. Modern devices, therefore, use plates designed to maximize the filtration surface area.[35-39]

Four tube shunt devices are commonly used. The Molteno and Baerveldt tubes do not have a valve. The Krupin disc and the Ahmed valve are valved devices.

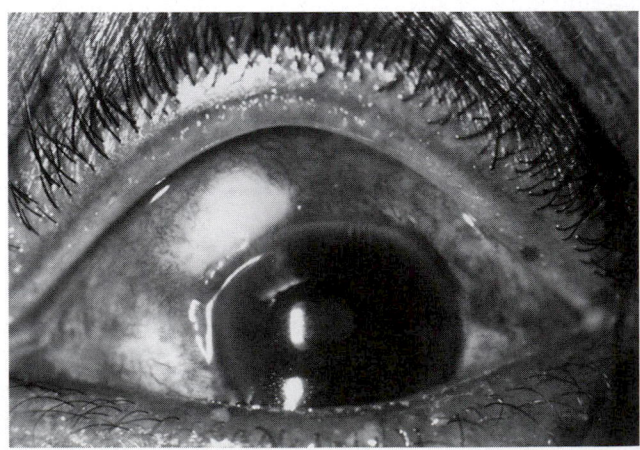

Figure 24–3. An infected bleb associated with endophthalmitis. This complication is associated with thin-walled blebs that occur as a result of the use of antifibrotic agents. The eye is hyperemic; the bleb is filled with pus and appears white. (*See also Color Plate 75.*)

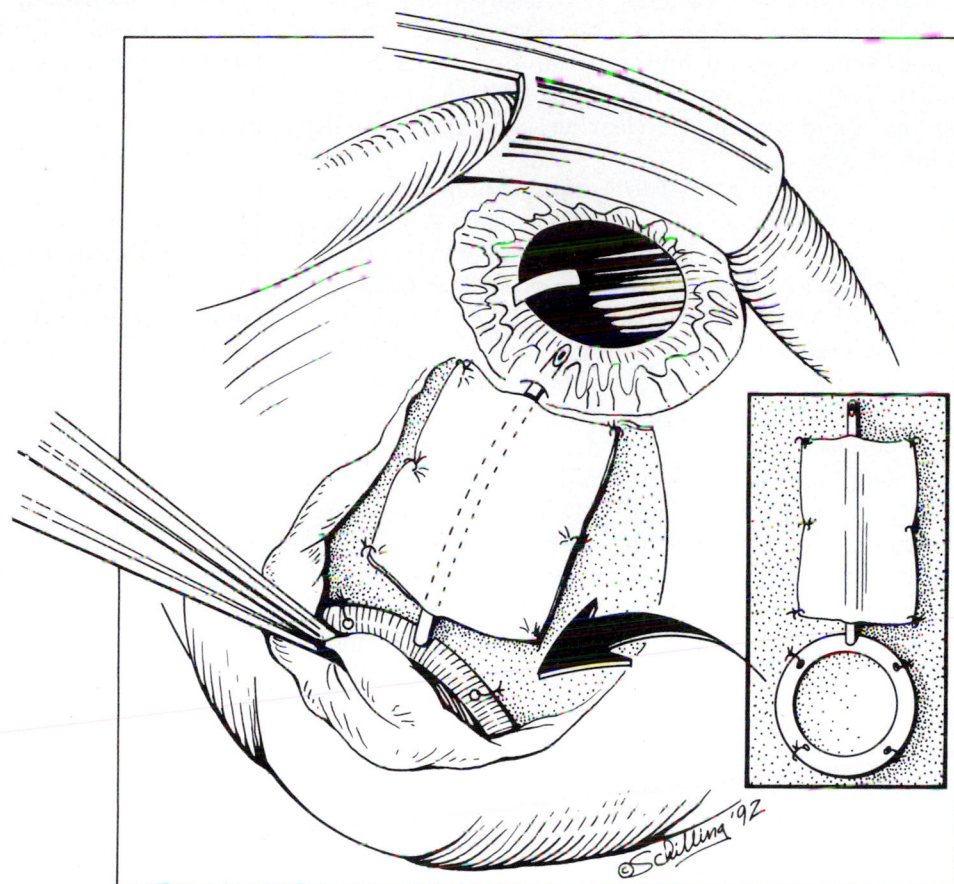

Figure 24–4. Diagram of an aqueous tube-shunt implantation. The proximal end of the tube is inserted into the anterior chamber; the distal end is connected to the filtration plate that is sutured to the surface of the sclera 10 mm behind the limbus. The anterior portion of the tube is covered with donor tissue (usually banked sclera, fascia lata, or pericardium) to prevent it from eroding through the overlying conjunctiva.

The valve is intended to prevent overfiltration and hypotony in the immediate postoperative period. When nonvalved tube devices are used, it is usually necessary to occlude the tube temporarily with a suture in order to avoid hypotony.[40]

Following tube-shunt procedures, the risk of hypotony, choroidal effusions or hemorrhage, and intraocular inflammation is increased. Other complications associated with tube-shunt devices include erosion of the tube or plate through the conjunctiva, occlusion of the tube with failure of filtration, and corneal endothelial damage with chronic corneal edema. Bleb encapsulation is also a common problem with tube-shunt devices.[41-45]

CYCLODESTRUCTIVE PROCEDURES TO DECREASE AQUEOUS PRODUCTION

Over the years, several procedures have been developed to destroy the ciliary body epithelium and reduce the intraocular pressure (IOP) by decreasing the production of aqueous humor. The two that are most commonly used at present are cyclocryotherapy and transscleral laser cyclophotocoagulation using either the YAG or diode laser.[46,47]

Cyclocryotherapy

In cyclocryotherapy, extreme cold is used to injure the ciliary epithelium. Since the procedure has a high rate of complications and is associated with significant

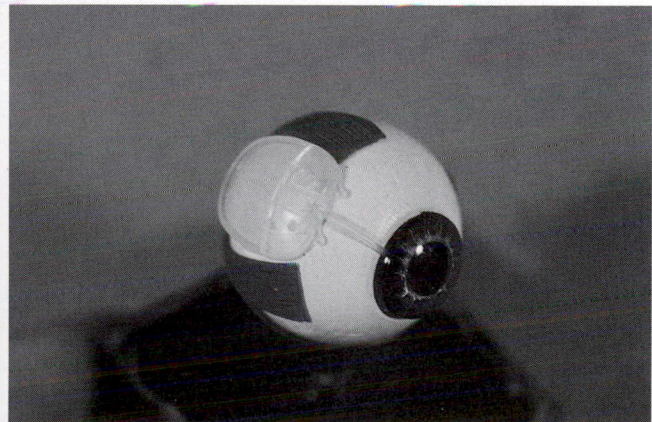

Figure 24–5. Photograph of an aqueous tube-shunt device placed on a model eye showing the positioning of the filtration plate relative to the extraocular muscles. (*See also Color Plate 76.*)

visual loss in many patients, it is reserved for those with severe glaucoma who have poor vision and in whom other medical and surgical treatments have failed. The major contraindications to cyclocryotherapy are the presence of a clear lens and good visual acuity.[48-50]

A probe with a tip 3 to 4 mm in diameter is attached to a container of a liquid gas such as carbon dioxide or nitrogen. The tip of the probe achieves a temperature of at least −80°C. The probe is applied to the sclera overlying the ciliary body, 2 or 2.5 mm behind the limbus (Fig. 24–6). An ice ball forms whose radius is sufficient to freeze the entire thickness of the ciliary body, including the epithelium. Initially, six to eight applications are made over 180 degrees. The treatment may be repeated 6 to 8 weeks later if adequate lowering of IOP is not achieved. Treatment over the full circumference of the ciliary body is usually avoided because of the high risk of subsequent phthisis bulbi.

Complications are common and often severe and permanent after cyclocryotherapy. A severe iritis, which is often quite painful, invariably follows the procedure. The inflammatory response often lasts for months; sometimes long-term treatment with a topical corticosteroid is required. Loss of vision due to macular edema is another common complication.

Other complications include cataract, subluxation of the lens, intraocular hemorrhage, corneal edema, pain, hypotony, and phthisis bulbi. A marked degree of lid and conjunctival swelling usually follows the procedure and lasts for several weeks. Most of these complications are the result of the extensive destruction of uveal tissue following cyclocryotherapy.

Cyclocryotherapy is usually done in end-stage eyes in an effort to save what is already very poor vision. If cyclocryotherapy fails and the eye becomes totally blind or painful, the next step is usually enucleation.

Postoperative follow-up is similar to that after other glaucoma procedures. Patients are treated with anti-inflammatory and antiglaucoma medications as needed to control inflammation and IOP. Initially, the pressure after cyclocryotherapy will usually be quite

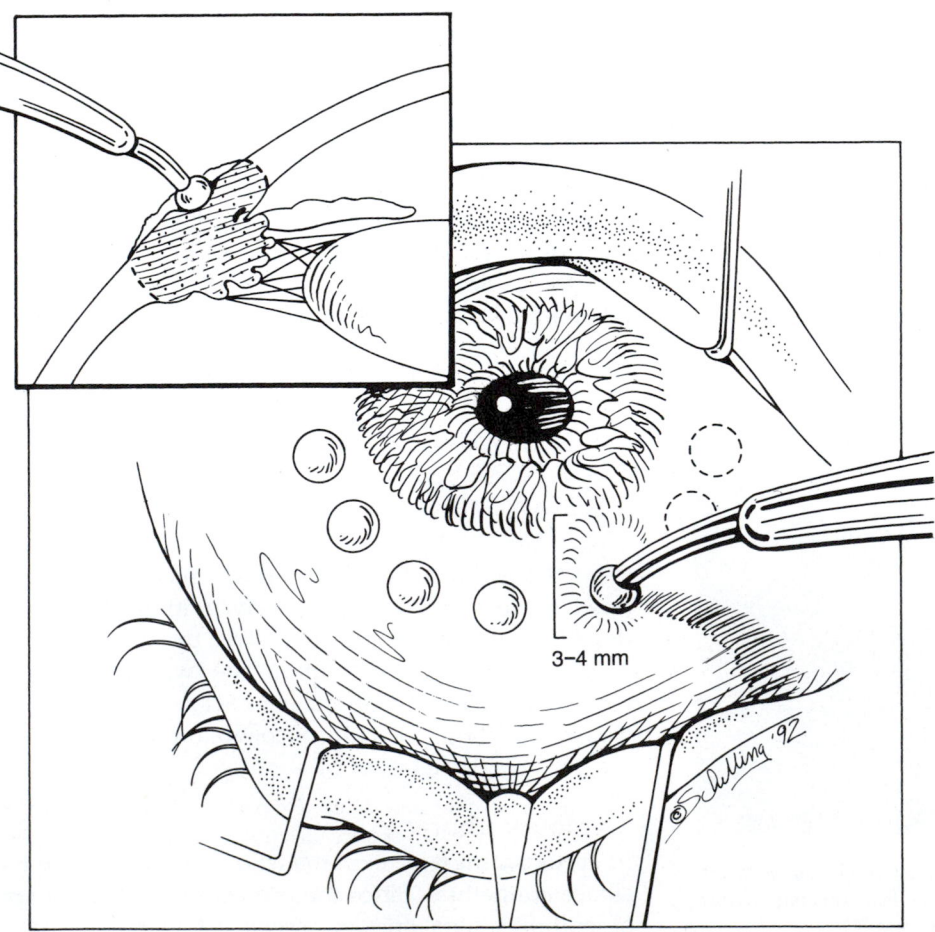

Figure 24–6. Diagram of a cyclocryotherapy. A probe is applied to the scleral surface of the eye, freezing the ciliary processes.

low. Within a few months, however, the pressure may rise and the addition of medication or a repeat procedure may become necessary.

Transscleral Laser Cyclophotocoagulation

In laser cyclophotocoagulation (CPC), the ciliary epithelium is focally destroyed with laser energy instead of cold (Fig. 24–7). Indications and contraindications are similar to those for cyclocryotherapy. This procedure appears to be significantly safer than cyclocryotherapy and is now often used in eyes with good visual potential, especially in aphakic or pseudophakic patients. Because the laser energy can be focused onto a much smaller area of the ciliary body, less tissue is destroyed than in cyclocryotherapy. This results in fewer complications than cyclocryotherapy.[51-61]

Using very high levels of laser energy, the beam is directed through the sclera toward the ciliary epithelium. Special optics in the delivery system allow the beam to be focused below the surface of the sclera. In the noncontact mode, delivery is through the optics of a slit lamp, much as in argon laser trabeculoplasty. Recently, contact delivery systems have been developed. Using fiberoptics, the laser beam is directed through a hand piece placed directly on the scleral surface of the eye. With either method, between 12 and 40 applications are made around the circumference of the posterior limbus 2.5 to 3.0 mm behind the conjunctival reflection (Fig. 24–7).

Complications of laser CPC are similar to those of cyclocryotherapy. Postoperative pain and inflammation are often a problem. There seems to be less visual loss following laser CPC than after cyclocryotherapy, but loss of some vision is a frequent complication, especially in aphakic and pseudophakic patients. In general, traditional types of glaucoma surgery should be tried before resorting to any cyclodestructive procedure.

Postoperative follow-up is similar to that for cyclocryotherapy. In addition to anti-inflammatory eyedrops, the use of a systemic nonsteroidal anti-inflammatory drug such as ibuprofen will help to reduce postoperative discomfort. Phakic patients should be carefully followed for the development of cataract.

Endoscopic Cyclophotocoagulation and Viscocanalostomy

Recently techniques have been developed to permit laser CPC using a video endoscope placed inside the eye through a pars plana incision. A small fiberoptic probe is placed into the vitreous cavity. A video camera in the probe permits direct visualization of the ciliary processes. A laser delivery system makes it possible to treat each ciliary process directly. This is a new technique, and few results have been published.[62]

A recent modification of filtration surgery is viscocanalostomy, which has the objective of lowering IOP with a reduction in side effects and complications, such as hypotony. Viscocanalostomy is a form of surgical filtration surgery that involves the creation of a superficial triangular flap to about one-third of the scleral depth. A second flap is dissected about 1 mm inside the first and a paracentesis is created to reduce the IOP temporarily. Descemet's membrane is separated from the corneal-scleral junction using an injection of high-viscosity sodium hyaluronate, which is placed onto both sides of Schlemm's canal. A deep sclerectomy is then performed, followed by closure of the flap. This procedure is new, with little data available.

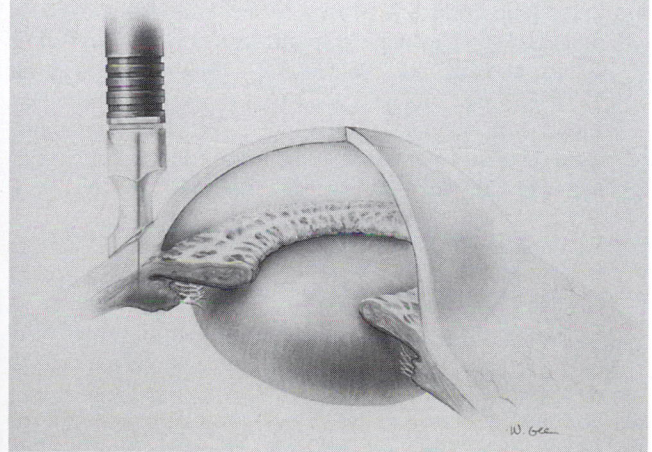

Figure 24–7. Drawing of a contact type of transscleral laser cyclophotocoagulation. Laser energy is delivered by the handpiece through the sclera to the ciliary epithelium. (Reproduced, with permission, from IRIDEX Corporation, Mountain View, California). (*See also Color Plate 77*.)

REFERENCES

1. Rappaport L, Liebmann J, Ritch R. Antimetabolites in glaucoma filtration surgery. In: Burde RM, Slamovits TL, eds. *Advances in Clinical Ophthalmology I*. St. Louis: CV Mosby; 1994:309–338.
2. Parrish RK II, Folberg R. Wound healing in glaucoma surgery. In: Ritch R, Shields MB, Krupin T, eds. *The Glaucomas*, 2nd ed. St. Louis: CV Mosby; 1996:1634–1636.
3. Higginbotham EJ: Adjunctive use of mitomycin in filtration surgery. Is it worth the risk? *Arch Ophthalmol*. 1997; 115:1068–1069.
4. Cohen JS, Li ZL, Novack GD. The role of mitomycin treatment duration and previous intraocular surgery on

the success of trabeculectomy surgery. *J Glaucoma.* 1997;6:3–9.

5. Katz GJ, Johnson AT, Bergstrom TJ, et al. Mitomycin C versus 5-fluorouracil in high-risk glaucoma filtering surgery: Extended follow-up. *Ophthalmology.* 1995;102: 1263–1269.

6. Lavin MJ, Wormald RPL, Migdal CS, Hitchings RA. The influence of prior therapy on the success of trabeculectomy. *Arch Ophthalmol.* 1990;108:1543–1548.

7. Stewart WC, Shields MB, Miller KN, et al. Early postoperative prognostic indicators following trabeculectomy. *Ophthalm Surg.* 1991;22:23–26.

8. Broadway DC, Grierson I, O'Brien C, Hitchings RA: Adverse effects of topical antiglaucoma medication: II. The outcome of filtering surgery. *Arch Ophthalmol.* 1994;112: 1446–1454.

9. Broadway D, Grierson I, Hitchings R. Racial differences in the results of glaucoma filtration surgery: Are racial differences in the conjunctival cell profile important? *Br J Ophthalmol.* 1994;78: 466–475.

10. Sturmer J, Broadway DC, Hitchings RA. Young patient trabeculectomy: Assessment of risk factors for failure. *Ophthalmology.* 1993;100:928–939.

11. Liebmann JM, Ritch R. 5-fluorouracil in glaucoma filtering surgery. *Ophthalmol Clin North Am.* 1988;1:125–131.

12. Hefetz L, Naveh N, Keren T. Early and late postoperative application of 5-fluorouracil following trabeculectomy in refractory glaucoma. *Ophthalm Surg.* 1994;25: 715–719.

13. Egbert PR, Egbert TB, Dadzie P, et al. A prospective trial of intraoperative fluorouracil during trabeculectomy in a black population. *Am J Ophthalmol.* 1993;116: 612–616.

14. Bell RW, O'Brien C, Habib NE. Long-term results and complications after trabeculectomy with a single peroperative application of 5-fluorouracil. *Eye.* 1997;11: 663–671.

15. The Fluorouracil Filtering Surgery Study Group. Five-year follow-up of the Fluorouracil Filtering Surgery Study. *Am J Ophthalmol.* 1996;121:349–366.

16. Wilson RP, Steinmann WC. Use of trabeculectomy with postoperative 5-fluorouracil in patients requiring extremely low intraocular pressures to limit further glaucoma progression. *Ophthalmology.* 1991;98:1047–1052.

17. Altan T, Kazokoglu H, Bavbek T, Temel A. Hypotonic maculopathy after trabeculectomy with postoperative use of 5-fluorouracil. *Ophthalmologica.* 1994;208: 318–320.

18. Ticho U, Ophir A. Late complications after glaucoma filtering surgery with adjunctive 5-fluorouracil. *Am J Ophthalmol.* 1993;115:506–510.

19. Belyea DA, Spencer WH, Lieberman MF, Stamper RL. Late onset multifocal bleb leaks after glaucoma filtration surgery with 5-fluorouracil and mitomycin C. *Am J Ophthalmol.* 1997;124:40–45.

20. Lee DA, Hersh P, Kersten D, Melamed S. Complications of subconjunctival 5-fluorouracil following glaucoma filtering surgery. *Ophthalm Surg.* 1987;18:187–190.

21. Scott IU, Greenfield DS, Schiffman J, et al. Outcomes of primary trabeculectomy with the use of adjunctive mitomycin. *Arch Ophthalmol.* 1998;116:286–291.

22. Prata JA Jr, Heuer DK, Mermoud A, Minckler DS. Trabeculectomy with mitomycin C in glaucoma associated with uveitis. *Ophthalm Surg.* 1994;25:616–620.

23. Mermoud A, Murray AD, Salmon JF. Trabeculectomy with mitomycin C for refractory glaucoma in blacks. *Am J Ophthalmol.* 1993;116:72–78.

24. Singh K, Dadzie P, Decker JH, et al. Trabeculectomy with intraoperative 5-fluorouracil versus mitomycin C. *Ophthalm Surg Lasers.* 1997;28:370–376.

25. Skuta GJ, Johnson AT, Bergstrom TJ, et al. Mitomycin C versus 5-fluorouracil in high risk glaucoma filtering surgery extended follow-up. *Ophthalmology.* 1995;102: 1263–1269.

26. Palmer SS. Mitomycin as adjunct chemotherapy with trabeculectomy. *Ophthalmology.* 1991;98:317–321.

27. Zacharia PT, Schuman JS, Depperman SR. Ocular hypotony after trabeculectomy with mitomycin C. *Am J Ophthalmol.* 1993;116:314–326.

28. Cheung JC, Pederson JE, Murali S, Wright MM. Intermediate-term outcome of variable dose mitomycin C filtering surgery. *Ophthalmology.* 1997;104:143–149.

29. Susanna R Jr, Nicolela M, Takahashi W. Late bleb leakage after trabeculectomy with 5-fluorouracil or mitomycin C. *Can J Ophthalmol.* 1996;31:296–300.

30. Greenfield DS, Parrish RK Jr. Bleb rupture following filtering surgery with mitomycin C: Clinicopathologic correlations. *Ophthalm Surg Lasers.* 1996;27:876–877.

31. Greenfield DS, Flynn HW Jr, Palmberg PF, et al. Endophthalmitis after filtering surgery with mitomycin. *Arch Ophthalmol.* 1996;114:943–949.

32. Mietz H, Krieglstein GK. Short-term clinical results and complications of trabeculectomies performed with mitomycin C using different concentrations. *Int Ophthalmol.* 1995;19:51–56.

33. Rosenberg LF, Krupin T. Implants in glaucoma surgery. In: Ritch R, Shields MB, Krupin T, eds. *The Glaucomas,* 2nd ed. St. Louis: CV Mosby; 1996:1783–1807.

34. Shields MB: Drainage implant surgery. In: *Textbook of Glaucoma,* 4th ed. Baltimore: Williams & Wilkins; 1998:538–546.

35. Lloyd MA, Heuer DK, LaBree L, et al. Intermediate-term results of a randomized clinical trial of the 350 versus the 500-mm^2 Baerveldt implant. *Ophthalmology.* 1994;101:1456–1463.

36. Fellenbaum PS, Heuer DK, Baerveldt G, et al. Krupin disk implantation for complicated glaucomas. *Ophthalmology.* 1994;101:1178–1182.

37. Coleman AL, Panek WC, Bacharach J, et al: Initial clinical experience with the Ahmed glaucoma valve implant. *Am J Ophthalmol.* 1995;120:23–31.

38. Smith MF, Sherwood MB, Doyle JW. Comparison of the Baerveldt implant with the double-plate Molteno implant. *Arch Ophthalmol.* 1995;113:444–447.

39. Mills RP, Leen MM, Barlow WE, et al. Long-term survival of Molteno glaucoma drainage devices. *Ophthalmology.* 1996;103:299–305.

40. Sherwood MB, Smith MF. Prevention of early hypotony associated with Molteno implants by a new occluding stent technique. *Ophthalmology*. 1993;100:85–90.

41. McDermott ML, Cowden JW, Juzych MS, et al. Corneal endothelial cell counts after Molteno implantation. *Am J Ophthalmol*. 1993;115:93–96.

42. Paysse E, Heuer DK, Minckler DS, et al. Suprachoroidal hemorrhage after Molteno implantation. *J Glaucoma*. 1996;5:170–175.

43. Valimaki J, Airaksinen PJ, Tuulonen A. Capsule excision after failed Molteno surgery. *Ophthalm Surg Lasers*. 1997;28:382–386.

44. Price FW Jr, Wellemeyer M. Long-term results of Molteno implants. *Ophthalm Surg*. 1995;26:130–135.

45. Gerber SL, Cantor LB, Sponsel WE. A comparison of complications from pressure-ridge Molteno implants versus Molteno implants with suture ligation. *Ophthalm Surg Lasers*. 1997;28:905–910.

46. Stewart WC, Brindley GO, Shields MB. Cyclodestructive procedures. In: Ritch R, Shields MB, Krupin T, eds. *The Glaucomas*, 2nd ed. St. Louis: CV Mosby; 1996.

47. Shields MB. Cyclodestructive surgery. In: *Textbook of Glaucoma*, 4th ed. Baltimore: Williams & Wilkins; 1998:547–564.

48. Rosenberg LF, Holmwood PC. Ciliodestructive surgery. *Semin Ophthalmol*. 1991;6:95–104.

49. Wright MM, Grajewski AL, Feuer WJ. Nd:YAG cyclophotocoagulation: Outcome of treatment for uncontrolled glaucoma. *Ophthalmol Surg*. 1991;22:279–283.

50. Devreese M, Hennekes R, Belgrado G. Cyclocryotherapy in primary glaucoma: Intraocular pressure reducing effects and complications. *Bull Soc Belge Ophtalmol*. 1991;241:105–111.

51. Schuman JS, Puliafito CA, Belcher CD, et al: Contact transscleral Nd:YAG laser cyclophotocoagulation: Midterm results. *Ophthalmology*. 1992:99:1089–1094.

52. Balazsi AG. Noncontact thermal mode Nd:YAG laser transscleral cyclocoagulation in the treatment of glaucoma: Intermediate follow-up. *Ophthalmology*. 1991;98:1858–1863.

53. Iwach AG, Hennings DR, Crawford JB, et al. A new contact neodymium:YAG laser for cyclophotocoagulation. *Ophthalm Surg*. 1991;22:345–348.

54. Assia EI, Apple DJ, Carlson AN, et al. A comparison of neodymium:yttrium aluminum garnet and diode laser transscleral cyclophotocoagulation and cyclocryotherapy. *Invest Ophthalmol Vis Sci*. 1991;32:2774–2778.

55. Wright MM, Feuer WJ, Grajewski AL. Nd:YAG cyclophotocoagulation: Outcome of treatment for uncontrolled glaucoma. *Ophthalm Surg*. 1991;22:279–283.

56. Yamamoto T, Yumita A, Araie M, Suzuki Y. Transscleral Nd:YAG laser cyclophotocoagulation versus cyclocryotherapy. *Graefes Arch Clin Exp Ophthalmol*. 1991;229:33–36.

57. Gupta N, Weinreb RN. Diode laser transscleral cyclophotocoagulation. *J Glaucoma*. 1997;6:426–429.

58. Wong EY, Wong JS, Chee CK, Chew PT. Diode laser contact transscleral cyclophotocoagulation for refractory glaucoma in Asian patients. *Am J Ophthalmol*. 1997;124:797–804.

59. Kosoko O, Enger CL, Pollack IP, Gaasterland DE. Long-term outcome of initial ciliary ablation with contact diode laser transscleral cyclophotocoagulation for severe glaucoma. *Ophthalmology*. 1996;103:1294–1302.

60. Khaw PT, Hitchings RA, Rice NS, et al. "Cyclodiode": Trans-scleral diode laser cyclophotocoagulation in the treatment of advanced refractory glaucoma. *Ophthalmology*. 1997;104:1508–1519.

61. Ulbig MW, Hamilton AM, McNaught AI, McHugh DA. Clinical comparison of semiconductor diode versus neodymium:YAG non-contact cyclophotocoagulation. *Br J Ophthalmol*. 1995;79:569–574.

62. Mora JS, Dickens CJ, et al. Endoscopic diode laser cyclophotocoagulation with a limbal approach. *Ophthalm Surg Lasers*. 1997;28:118–123.

Chapter 25

THE FUTURE OF GLAUCOMA DIAGNOSIS AND THERAPY

Robert D. Fechtner
Paul J. Lama

Our understanding of glaucoma and the tools for its diagnosis and treatment have advanced tremendously in the last 20 years. Glaucoma is probably best understood as a group of optic neuropathies resulting in characteristic changes in optic nerve structure and function. We now have new technologies for better assessing that structure and function. Increased understanding of the nature of glaucoma, advances in diagnostic technologies, and improvements in pharmacological and surgical options will all influence the future of glaucoma therapy.

The understanding that factors other than IOP may be involved in the development of glaucomatous optic neuropathy has changed our concept of this syndrome. We are actively investigating the various mechanisms that can lead to glaucomatous optic neuropathy. For example, advances in molecular genetics have permitted the identification of particular genes associated with various glaucomas and even the identification of abnormal gene products.[1] Future directions in our understanding and treatment of the glaucomas will build on these foundations. Certainly, there will be new insights and discoveries that will inevitably alter our approach to this syndrome.

UNDERSTANDING THE DISEASE(S)

Glaucoma is best described as a syndrome rather than a disease. A disease is characterized by an etiology resulting in pathological changes. Pneumococcal pneumonia is caused by bacteria and results in certain alterations in the lungs (and elsewhere in the body because of defense mechanisms). A syndrome describes a set of clinical findings without necessarily any specific reference to causation or with many possible causes leading to the same clinical presentation. Glaucoma is an optic neuropathy with characteristic structural and functional damage. Although IOP was long believed to cause glaucoma, it is now better recognized as a risk factor.[2] But it is clear that not all people with high IOP develop glaucoma, and not all of those with glaucoma can be shown to have elevated IOP.

The Impact of Clinical Trials on Future Treatment

The early acceptance of IOP as the cause of glaucoma delayed by nearly 100 years the asking of substantial questions that are only now being addressed in a prospective fashion. The natural histories of untreated ocular hypertension and glaucoma are still not well known.

The Ocular Hypertension Treatment Study (OHTS) is designed to determine whether medical reduction of intraocular pressure (IOP) prevents or delays the onset of glaucoma.[3] Over 1500 subjects have been randomized to either treatment or careful observation with visual field and optic nerve examination, with anyone who develops glaucomatous damage being treated. Originally viewed as a 5- to 7-year project, this study has been extended to allow a sufficient number of subjects to reach an endpoint. Even if the conversion rate is lower than predicted, the results should be available within the next several years. This information will give a clear estimate of the risk of developing glaucoma when IOP is elevated and may help guide therapeutic decisions as to whether or not to treat individuals with elevated IOP before detectable damage is present.

The Early Manifest Glaucoma Treatment Study is a smaller prospective study in which patients with newly diagnosed glaucoma are randomized to have IOP lowered with betaxolol and argon laser trabeculoplasty or to be observed.[4] Although this might strike some as withholding needed treatment, we know that the progression rate of glaucoma is very slow. Further, this question has never been addressed in a well-designed, large, prospective study. This study will do much to elaborate the natural progression of glaucoma and the impact of medical treatment and laser trabeculoplasty.

The Advanced Glaucoma Intervention Study looked at different surgical treatment strategies when medical therapy was insufficient.[5,6] Among the several interesting findings, the investigators noted a racial difference in response to treatment. In blacks, long-term visual function results were better if trabeculectomy was the first surgical treatment, while whites did better with laser trabeculoplasty as the initial surgery performed. Further, these results were not evident in the first few years of the study but became clear after several years. Further follow-up and subsequent reports may help in surgical planning. Interestingly, many surgeons still perform laser trabeculoplasty first in blacks, despite the evidence provided in this report.

The beneficial effect of lowering IOP was recently demonstrated in the Collaborative Normal Tension Glaucoma Study.[7] In this study, patients with normal-tension glaucoma (NTG) who had visual field loss that threatened fixation or who had progressive loss of visual field while in the study were randomized to continued observation or to IOP lowering of 30%. After adjusting for the development of cataracts (which was more common in the treated group), there was a highly significant benefit to IOP lowering. Future reports are expected and may help in guiding treatment for patients with NTG.

Diagnosis by Mechanism

Intraocular pressure may be the predominant factor leading to damage through mechanical effects in some patients with glaucoma. In animal models, elevated IOP rapidly leads to optic nerve damage, and some secondary glaucomas are characterized by very high IOP. Yet not all individuals are equally susceptible to the effects of an elevated IOP. If some marker could be identified that predicts which optic nerves are susceptible to a raised IOP, an optic nerve "stress test" could be developed. Those with susceptible nerves might be treated with IOP-lowering therapy, while those at low risk would not be.

Several technologies have developed that measure aspects of ocular blood flow. Although there is no agreement on the role of blood flow in the development of glaucoma and there is currently no way to know which aspects of blood flow are crucial, it is now possible to begin deriving quantitative information.[8,9]

It is easy to imagine that different patients have different combinations of mechanisms or perhaps a single mechanism causing glaucomatous optic neuropathy. A clearer understanding of the etiology and a method to determine susceptibility would have tremendous impact on therapeutic decisions. Were it possible to measure the crucial aspects of ocular circulation, some patients might be identified as having glaucoma on a vascular basis. Treatment would be targeted at improving that critical flow. The impact of that therapy could be assessed directly.

Genetics

An additional area for improved diagnosis would be the ability to identify the underlying genetic basis of disease. If the association between a particular gene and glaucoma is recognized, people at risk could be monitored closely, and treatment targeted at the abnormal gene product could be delivered. With the rapid advances in genetic research, we may be able to identify subsets of patients such as those with the TIGR gene who express an abnormal protein within the trabecular meshwork.[10] An understanding of the protein product of the abnormal gene could allow for the development of a therapy targeted specifically at the underlying abnormality. Such work is currently under way.

IMPROVING DIAGNOSIS

Identifying Abnormality

One of the most important future developments in the therapy of glaucoma will be utilizing new technologies to improve our diagnostic accuracy. We should expect to better answer the question, "Does this patient have glaucoma?" Eliminating treatment for patients not at significant risk will be a substantial advance in therapy. If we can diagnose the disease through structural parameters or through more sensitive visual-function testing, then we can reserve treatment for those who truly need it.

Identifying Progression

Despite our clinical reliance on achromatic automated perimetry and clinical examination of the optic nerve, these techniques have significant limitations in their ability to detect subtle progression of glaucoma. Improved structural and functional testing will affect our future therapies of glaucoma by allowing us to identify earlier those patients who are progressing and to alter therapy appropriately. In our current paradigm of lowering IOP to treat glaucoma, we know a therapy is not effective only if the target IOP is not achieved or if the target IOP is achieved but there is demonstrable progression of the glaucoma. The ability to detect smaller incremental changes will allow us to alter therapy in a more timely fashion.

An important future development in glaucoma therapy would be appropriately identifying when not to treat. Recent research has shown that glaucoma is a slowly progressive disease and most patients do relatively well over their lifetimes.[11] A better understanding of the natural history of glaucoma and diagnostic tests that would allow us to better chart progression over time may enable us to minimize or entirely eliminate therapy for patients who will preserve good visual function without treatment.

STRUCTURAL TESTING

Treatment decisions for glaucoma will be influenced by an improvement in diagnosis. Currently, the diagnosis of glaucoma is made when detection of characteristic structural optic nerve damage is associated with functional loss on psychophysical testing. It is now appreciated that the results of psychophysical testing are often normal or nondiagnostic in early disease. In fact, in postmortem eyes with glaucoma, it has been shown that up to 50% of the ganglion cells may be lost without evidence of visual field loss on standard white-on-white perimetry.[12] Glaucoma treatment will improve as we advance our ability to assess the structure of the optic nerve and peripapillary retina.

The clinical observation of a large cup/disc ratio, the widely used parameter for assessment of the presence and extent of glaucomatous nerve damage, is not very sensitive in the detection of glaucoma.[13] Although typical glaucomatous excavation or cupping can be identified through slit-lamp biomicroscopy with a hand-held or contact fundus lens, there is a great deal of overlap between normal and abnormal disc appearance. This is due to tremendous interindividual and racial variation in both optic nerve size and cup/disc ratio.[14] For example, those of African and Asian origin tend to have larger discs than those of European origin; men also tend to have larger discs than women. Even within a homogeneous population, interindividual variation is considerably large. Since a similar number of nerve fibers or axons of ganglion cells form the optic nerve, it follows that those with larger discs would have larger cup/disc ratios as well. Neural rim area would thus remain relatively constant. However, studies have also reported that those with larger discs often have larger neural rim areas due to the presence of greater numbers of axons.[15] In addition to intraindividual variation in disc appearance, there is also significant inter- and intraexaminer variability in qualitative assessment of the optic nerves.[16] In sum, there is a need for better quantitative methods to distinguish a normal disc from a glaucomatous disc.

The need for accurate, reproducible, and cost-effective quantitative techniques of assessing the optic disc and appreciation of the limitations of subjective clinical observation stimulated the development of new technologies. Many early technologies were disappointing. The latest generation of technologies has greater promise of providing objective and meaningful measurements of optic nerve structure that may affect our approach to therapy. There will doubtless be future advances in this field.

The two principal applications of improved structural assessment in glaucoma are (1) distinguishing normal from abnormal nerve heads and (2) identifying progression with sequential imaging over time of a damaged optic nerve. Each will have a different impact on glaucoma therapy; an improved ability to detect a glaucomatous eye will influence the decision to initiate treatment, while more sensitive detection of progressive damage will allow us to better measure the response to treatment and to adjust therapy.

Two examples of technologies that may advance our abilities to assess structure in glaucoma are confocal scanning laser topography (cSLT) and scanning laser polarimetry (SLP). Other technologies are also in various stages of development but have been less well studied in glaucoma.

cSLT provides measurements of the topography of the optic nerve. These measures are largely objective (after the operator identifies the margin of the optic nerve). cSLT has been shown to correlate well with measurements of optic nerve function.[17] For example, cup-shape measure as well as other cSLT parameters have been shown to correlate with results of blue-yellow perimetry and support the possibility of identifying early topographic glaucomatous changes.[18] Reports of the sensitivity and specificity of optic nerve topography in distinguishing between normal and abnormal have demonstrated reasonably good sensitivity and specificity but not yet good enough for this technology to be used for routine screening. The wide range of biological variation in normal optic nerves may make it difficult to identify early glaucomatous damage.

Identifying progression seems an achievable goal with topography. In experimental models, cSLT could detect statistically significant change in the appearance of the optic nerve, as with acute changes in IOP.[19] Overall, although cSLT maybe useful in distinguishing differences between normal and abnormal, its greatest promise would seem to be the detection of subtle changes in the optic nerve head.

Another technology, scanning laser polarimetry (SLP), was developed to measure the thickness of the nerve fiber layer (NFL). The NFL of the retina represents the axons of the retinal ganglion cell layer. Although the optic nerve head represents the gathering of the nerve fibers as they exit the eye through the variably sized and oriented scleral canal, the nerve fibers are more readily accessible for examination across the surface of the retina. The destruction of ganglion cell axons that occurs in a glaucomatous optic nerve head (ONH) results from the loss of the NFL architecture in the retina. The SLP takes advantage of optical properties of the nerve fiber layer, their effect on polarized light, to infer thickness.

Scanner laser polarimetry is an intriguing technology for examining the structure of the retinal nerve fiber layer (rNFL). By using the polarization characteristics of the retina, an estimate of the rNFL thickness can be derived.[20] However, the instrument must eliminate retardation from other birefringent ocular structures such as the lens and cornea, which may cause some artifactual measurements. Because of unexpected birefringent properties, in some eyes the signal does not correspond to the expected anatomy. The reasons for this have not yet been fully explained.

In theory, the biological variability in nerve fiber distribution among healthy eyes should be less than the variability in optic nerve topography. Investigators have been examining various statistical strategies that can be used to discriminate between normal and glaucomatous eyes. This instrument might also be able to detect early progression of damage. Unlike cSLT, however, which requires a reference plane that may change with progression of disease and is subject to examiner error, SLP imaging does not require a reference plane for measurement and thus may be a useful tool in those eyes that it measures successfully. Further work will help to define the role of this technology.

A stumbling block for previous efforts to objectively detect structural changes in the optic nerve has been poor reproducibility. A test must be highly reproducible over time if small changes are to be identified. This has been a problem with automated perimetry, which can have substantial variability between tests.[21] Multiple investigators have demonstrated the excellent reproducibility of the current generation of imaging technologies.[22] Although we may be limited to identifying the statistical probability that a given eye is normal (from a baseline evaluation), it seems likely that we may greatly extend our ability to identify subtle progression beyond current limits. This ability would vastly alter our treatment of glaucoma, as we could better measure the success of therapy and intervene sooner when disease was progressing. Prospective longitudinal studies are under way that seek to validate this objective.

TREATMENT

Intraocular Pressure

Medical Therapy
We will continue to use IOP-lowering drugs for the foreseeable future, as elevated IOP remains a prominent risk factor for glaucomatous optic neuropathy. There is a substantial body of peer-review literature supporting the concept that the lowering of IOP can affect the course of glaucoma.[7,23] Our efforts to lower IOP effectively while reducing the burden of adverse effects have seen the introduction of several new classes of drugs since ocular beta blockers (OBBs) became available in 1978.

The development of new medications takes several years. The glaucoma medications that will become available over the next 5 years are in various stages of testing and largely represent additions to existing classes of drugs and product-line extension. There will be additional products in existing classes of IOP-lowering drugs. Although it is unlikely that entirely new ocular beta blockers or miotics will come to market, there will—should clinical testing prove successful—be several new prostaglandins and prostaglandin-like drugs. Several drugs are in phase III clinical trials and may have regulatory approval by the time of publication of this book. At present the prostaglandins are the most potent IOP-lowering compounds available, showing a slight advantage over nonselective beta blockers.[24] Two prostaglandins are available in various countries, and several more are in human clinical trials. Although currently the one approved prostaglandin in the United States does not have an indication for initial monotherapy, we can expect to see that labeling change. Currently, some practitioners are using latanoprost as initial therapy based on their individual assessment of the drug. There have been some unexpected adverse effects with latanoprost (as with all new drugs).[25–27] The prostaglandins will probably grow in importance as we gain more experience with them and have alternative compounds.

The first new combination drug in many years is a fixed combination of dorzolamide/timolol. About 50% of patients treated with IOP-lowering drugs receive more than one medication. Additional new combinations are under development, and fixed-combination products will likely gain in popularity. Although the clinician sacrifices the ability to titrate the components in a fixed combination, the convenience factor for patients is quite compelling. With several pharmaceutical manufacturers having proprietary compounds in different classes and with the generic availability of timolol, these fixed combinations offer convenience to the patients and make business sense to the manufacturers; they gain additional market share if patients remain on their products as therapy is advanced.

Other novel compounds are currently undergoing testing as IOP-lowering drugs. Several of these may advance to human clinical trials, although it is difficult to predict which they might be.

Surgical Treatment

Laser. Laser trabeculoplasty (LTP) has changed little since it was introduced. The Glaucoma Laser Trial provides some support for earlier use of laser,[28] and that was a trend even before publication of the study. Now, when one or two medications have not sufficiently lowered IOP to target levels, many surgeons will consider performing LTP before adding another medication. A new laser, selective laser trabeculoplasty (SLT), is in development and may be approved for laser trabeculoplasty.[29] Initial reports suggest good efficacy with less tissue damage than with argon laser

trabeculoplasty (ALT). Although it does not appear that SLT will lower IOP better than ALT, it offers the benefit of being effective multiple times with multiple treatments.

Incisional Surgery. Incisional surgical treatment of glaucoma has varied little in the last 20 years and is still unsatisfying as compared with contemporary surgical techniques for cataract or refractive error. The best possible result is that a patient will get no worse and not suffer complications; this result is too often not achieved. Glaucoma surgery typically involves creating a fistula between the anterior chamber and the subconjunctival space, leading to bleb formation. Aqueous is then filtered transconjunctivally. Both full-thickness and guarded filtration procedures have been successful at lowering IOP, with the Cairns-type trabeculectomy being the procedure most commonly performed. In this procedure, a partial-thickness scleral flap is created with excision of a block of corneal tissue and trabecular meshwork at the base of the flap. The scleral flap is then sutured in a way that would allow flow of aqueous around the flap. Unfortunately, filtration procedures are often fraught with complications, some of which are potentially devastating to the health of the eye. Such complications include flat anterior chamber with development of choroidal effusions, cataract, corneal decompensation, choroidal hemorrhage, malignant glaucoma, hypotony maculopathy, bleb leak, and endophthalmitis.[30]

In addition to the potential complications of successful trabeculectomy, failure is all too common.[31] Failure of trabeculectomy most commonly occurs as a result of fibrosis at the level of the episclera. The use of antifibrotics to prevent excessive scarring leading to flap closure and bleb failure, such as 5-fluorouracil and mitomycin C, has greatly improved the success rate in high-risk eyes. But antimetabolites increase the incidence of some of the complications listed above.[32] Antifibrotics are hence a double-edged sword, improving success rate at the cost of an increased risk for complications. Furthermore, recent studies have demonstrated that adjunctive use of antimetabolites in glaucoma filtering surgery is associated with the development of thin, avascular blebs. These morphological bleb types lead to an increased risk for late-onset bleb leaks and endophthalmitis. The risk appears to be higher with mitomycin C, which is the significantly more potent of the two currently used antimetabolites. Since mitomycin C has a narrow margin of safety, a well-defined dose-response curve would be welcome. Laboratory studies investigating various antimetabolite delivery systems are under way.

Efforts continue to improve modulation of wound healing while reducing the risks associated with antimetabolites. Recent studies in Europe have identified transforming growth factor beta (TGF-β) as an important biochemical factor leading to bleb scarring and failure.[33] It has been shown that monoclonal antibody inhibition of TGF-β limits the degree of fibrosis and hence protects against bleb failure. With such promising data, a safer option than antimetabolite administration may be available in the future to enhance the success rate of filtration procedures.

It is clear that filtration surgery is not a benign procedure. The feared complications of endophthalmitis and choroidal hemorrhage coupled with the lower success rate in high-risk eyes and the progressive decline in bleb survival following surgery has stimulated research into new surgical IOP-lowering methods. In the past few years, nonpenetrating filtering surgery has taken center stage. One such procedure, viscocanalostomy, was developed as an attempt to enhance the success rate of filtration surgery in black South African patients. In this procedure, a fornix-based conjunctival flap is made, followed by the creation of a superficial scleral flap much as in current trabeculectomy. This is followed by dissection of a deep scleral flap, exposing the posterior wall of Schlemm's canal. Schlemm's canal is then cannulated and viscoelastic is injected into the canal. The deep scleral flap is excised and viscoelastic is injected between the superficial flap and the thin sclerocorneal bed to create a reservoir for an aqueous lake. The superficial flap is then closed tightly to prevent bleb formation. Although the mechanism of filtration in this procedure is not known and previous attempts at performing nonpenetrating filtering surgery have resulted in limited success, viscocanalostomy has sparked a great deal of curiosity as well as controversy. Current data suggest that this procedure may avoid some of the complications of trabeculectomy, but it does not lower IOP as well.[34]

Any new surgical strategy must be subjected to the rigor of randomized prospective clinical trials. To merit acceptance, the procedure must prove safe and effective over the long term. This requires several years of follow-up for IOP-lowering procedures. Enthusiasm for new techniques must be tempered by an understanding that long-term failure and unanticipated complications are part of glaucoma surgery.

Treatment by Mechanisms Other Than the Lowering of Intraocular Pressure

As our understanding of the mechanisms underlying glaucoma advances, so may our therapies. Ocular blood flow in glaucoma was discussed in Chap. 7. Evidence continues to mount that this is a mechanism in at least some patients with glaucomatous optic neuropathy. Still, one must be careful to distinguish between marketing claims and validated science. Under experimental conditions, several currently available drugs have demonstrated an impact on various aspects of ocular perfusion. This has stimulated enthusiasm to attempt to improve ocular blood flow pharmacologically in patients with glaucoma.

Several challenges exist in the development and validation of drugs affecting ocular blood flow. First, the available technologies each measure different aspects of blood flow, and it is not known which of these parameters is most closely related to the development of glaucomatous optic neuropathy. Must one improve posterior ciliary artery perfusion, central retinal artery perfusion, optic nerve capillary perfusion, or some other as yet unidentified factor? Is there the risk of a vascular "steal" phenomenon, where improving flow in one vascular bed will steal flow from another critical bed? And, perhaps most importantly, will improving some aspect of blood flow ultimately alter the course of glaucoma?

Drug delivery will be a challenge for any therapies directed to the back of the eye. To affect blood flow within the optic nerve, drugs must reach the optic nerve in sufficient concentrations to achieve pharmacological activity. There is some evidence that drugs may get there through the orbit. However, it may be difficult to apply a drop to the front of the eye and achieve a sufficient concentration in the back. Systemic administration or other routes may be necessary for these types of therapy.

Neuroprotection

In Chap 8, Dreyer discussed a fascinating approach to therapy for glaucoma. Rather than by lowering IOP, retinal ganglion cells may be protected from damage through a variety of neuroprotective strategies. Clinical trials are already under way to see whether a potentially neuroprotective drug can improve the course of glaucoma in patients with established disease. This is landmark research in that it is the first clinical trial that is not aimed at lowering IOP. Rather, an oral medication, Memantine, which has no effect on IOP, will be added to the therapy of patients with established glaucoma. Positive results from a study like this will alter our therapy of glaucoma forever. Although we do not clearly understand the mechanism of damage, the ability to protect the remaining healthy ganglion cells could alter the progression of the disease.

A recent animal study of rats with experimentally elevated IOP has suggested that neuroprotective strategies are feasible.[35] In this study, one group of rats had a drug that blocks nitric oxide synthetase added to their drinking water and, as a result, had less damage from experimentally elevated IOP. In other animal studies of optic nerve injury not related to IOP, other compounds have demonstrated protective effects. These studies should be interpreted as demonstrating proof of concept rather than being specific for human glaucoma. However, this highly active research area is likely to give rise to additional compounds that will enter human trials and will certainly become part of our therapeutic strategies for the treatment of glaucoma.

For patients who have already sustained nerve damage, it may be possible to stimulate nerve regeneration. Although this is still a laboratory science, there is evidence that the central nervous system can be stimulated to regrow. That is, it may be possible to support and sustain the damaged axons by providing various growth factors. For example, it is well known that an experimental elevation of IOP is associated with a disturbance in axoplasmic flow,[36] which is essential to the health of the axon and cell body. Several laboratories are exploring various strategies to sustain axons under conditions of stress. Similarly, it may be possible to stimulate regeneration of an axon prior to death of a cell body. In a patient with established glaucoma, there is almost certainly a spectrum ranging from mildly stressed retinal ganglion cells to the point where these cells are unrecoverable, with the possibility of rescuing some of them.

Genetic Approaches

Genetic testing may further alter our approaches to therapy. For example, in the case of juvenile glaucoma associated with the GLC1A gene, family members with the gene can be identified for careful follow-up, and patients may select early surgery rather than drug therapy if they have this form of glaucoma.[37,38] Similarly, for patients with the TIGR gene, therapy may be targeted directly at the expression of the protein product to block the alterations in the trabecular meshwork that result in elevated IOP.[39] Such a strategy might entirely prevent the development of glaucoma. Initial efforts will be directed at the abnormal gene products, while, in the future, it may be possible to replace the defective gene with a normally functioning one. Far more research is needed before gene therapy is likely to be introduced and practiced. There are also ethical implications surrounding genetic screening that must be addressed by society as we understand more and more about the human genome.

SUMMARY

The future of glaucoma therapy will be influenced by a number of factors. An improved understanding of the disease and ability to determine the underlying mechanism in an individual patient will allow for more targeted therapy. Those who have disease based on elevated IOP will have their pressure reduced, while those whose disease is based on poor blood flow may have therapy targeted at that factor. A better understanding of the genetic basis of disease and the gene products could make it possible to deliver targeted therapy uniquely designed to correct the underlying problem. Improvements in diagnostic technology will allow us to better measure progression of disease and avoid treating those who do not need therapy. An increased understanding of wound healing should further improve the success rate while reducing the complications of IOP-lowering surgery. Similarly, the development of new surgical techniques may improve the outcomes for our patients. Therapeutic strategies to protect or rescue damaged optic nerves may further slow down the progression of the disease.

One must always balance the benefit with the burden of therapy for glaucoma. We are not in the business of lowering IOP. Most simply, for our glaucoma patients, our goal is to preserve adequate visual function to ensure maximum quality of life. That simple understanding must be applied to all future therapies, and this may be our greatest advance in the treatment of glaucoma.

REFERENCES

1. Sarfarazi M. Recent advances in molecular genetics of glaucomas. *Hum Mol Genet*. 1997;6(10):1667–1677.
2. Sommer A, Tielsch JM, Katz J, Quigley HA, et al. Relationship between intraocular pressure and primary open angle glaucoma among white and black Americans: The Baltimore Eye Survey. *Arch Ophthalmol*. 1991;109(8):1090–1095.
3. Gordon MO, Kass MA. The Ocular Hypertension Treatment Study: Design and baseline description of the participants. *Arch Ophthalmol*. 1999;117(5):573–583.
4. Leske MC, Heijl A, Hyman L, Bengtsson B, and the Early Manifest Glaucoma Trial Group. Early Manifest Glaucoma Trial: Design and baseline data. *Ophthalmology*. 1999;106:2144–2153.
5. The Advanced Glaucoma Intervention Study (AGIS). 3: Baseline characteristics of black and white patients. *Ophthalmology*. 1998;105(7):1137–1145.
6. The Advanced Glaucoma Intervention Study (AGIS). 4: Comparison of treatment outcomes within race: Seven-year results. *Ophthalmology*. 1998;105(7):1146–1164.
7. Collaborative Normal-Tension Glaucoma Study Group. The effectiveness of intraocular pressure reduction in the treatment of normal-tension glaucoma: *Am J Ophthalmol*. 1998;126(4):498–505.
8. Grunwald JE, Piltz J, Hariprasad SM, DuPont J. Optic nerve and choroidal circulation in glaucoma. *Invest Ophthalmol Vis Sci*. 1998;39(12):2329–2336.

9. Kerr J, Nelson P, O'Brien C. A comparison of ocular blood flow in untreated primary open-angle glaucoma and ocular hypertension. *Am J Ophthalmol.* 1998;126(1):42–51.

10. Stone EM, Fingert JH, Alward WLM, Nguyen TD, Polansky JR, et al. Identification of a gene that causes primary open angle glaucoma. *Science.* 1997;275(5300):668–670.

11. Katz J, Gilbert D, Quigley HA, Sommer A. Estimating progression of visual field loss in glaucoma. *Ophthalmology.* 1997;104(6):1017–1025.

12. Quigley HA, Addicks EM, Green WR. Optic nerve damage in human glaucoma: III. Quantitative correlation of nerve fiber loss and visual field defect in glaucoma, ischemic neuropathy, papilledema, and toxic neuropathy. *Arch Ophthalmol.* 1982;100(1):135–146.

13. Gundersen KG, Heijl A, Bengtsson B. Sensitivity and specificity of structural optic disc parameters in chronic glaucoma. *Acta Ophthalmol Scand.* 1996;74(2):120–125.

14. Varma R, Hilton SC, Tielsch JM, Katz J, Quigley HA, Sommer A. Neural rim area declines with increased intraocular pressure in urban Americans. *Arch Ophthalmol.* 1995; 113(8):1001–1005.

15. Jonas JB, Schmidt AM, Muller-Bergh JA, Schlotzer-Schrehardt UM, Naumann GO. Human optic nerve fiber count and optic disc size. *Invest Ophthalmol Vis Sci.* 1992;33(6):2012–2018.

16. Jonas JB, Budde WM, Lang P. Neuroretinal rim width ratios in morphological glaucoma diagnosis. *Br J Ophthalmol.* 1998;82(12):1366.

17. Tole DM, Edwards MP, Davey KG, Menage MJ. The correlation of the visual field with scanning laser ophthalmoscope measurements in glaucoma. *Eye.* 1998;12(pt 4):686–690.

18. Teesalu P, Vihanninjoki K, Airaksinen PJ, Tuulonen A. Hemifield association between blue-on-yellow visual field and optic nerve head topographic measurements. *Graefes Arch Clin Exp Ophthalmol.* 1998;236(5):339–345.

19. Azuara-Blanco A, Harris A, Cantor LB, Abreu MM, Weinland M. Effects of short term increase of intraocular pressure on optic disc cupping. *Br J Ophthalmol.* 1998;82(8):880–883.

20. Weinreb RN, Zangwill L, Berry CC, Bathija R, Sample PA. Detection of glaucoma with scanning laser polarimetry. *Arch Ophthalmol.* 1998;116(12):1583–1589.

21. Heijl A, Lindgren A, Lindgren G. Test-retest variability in glaucomatous visual fields. *Am J Ophthalmol.* 1989;108(2):130–135.

22. Zambarakji HJ, Evans JE, Amoaku WM, Vernon SA. Reproducibility of volumetric measurements of normal maculae with the Heidelberg retina tomograph. *Br J Ophthalmol.* 1998;82(8):884–891.

23. Daugeliene L, Yamamoto T, Kitazawa Y. Risk factors for visual field damage progression in normal-tension glaucoma eyes. *Graefes Arch Clin Exp Ophthalmol.* 1999; 237(2):105–108.

24. Alm A, Widengard I, Kjellgren D, Soderstrom M, Fristrom B, Heijl A, Stjerschantz J. Latanoprost administered once daily caused a maintained reduction of intraocular pressure in glaucoma patients treated concomitantly with timolol. *Br J Ophthalmol.* 1995;79(1):12–16.

25. Miyake K, Ota I, Maekubo K, Ichihashi S, Miyake S. Latanoprost accelerates disruption of the blood-aqueous barrier and the incidence of angiographic cystoid macular edema in early postoperative pseudophakias. *Arch Ophthalmol.* 1999;117(1):34–40.

26. Zhan GL, Toris CB, Camras CB, Wang YL, Bito LZ. Prostaglandin-induced iris color darkening: An experimental model. *Arch Ophthalmol.* 1998;116(8):1065–1068.

27. Fechtner RD, Khouri AS, Zimmerman TJ, Bullock J, et al. Anterior uveitis associated with latanoprost. *Am J Ophthalmol.* 1998;126(1):37–41.

28. The Glaucoma Laser Trial (GLT) and glaucoma laser trial follow-up study: 7. Results—Glaucoma Laser Trial Research Group. *Am J Ophthalmol.* 1995;120(6):718–731.

29. Latina MA, Sibayan SA, Shin DH, Noecker RJ, Marcellino G. Q-switched 532-nm Nd:YAG laser trabeculoplasty (selective laser trabeculoplasty): A multicenter, pilot, clinical study. *Ophthalmology.* 1998;105(11):2082–2088.

30. Bellucci R, Perfetti S, Babighian S, Morselli S, Bonomi L. Filtration and complications after trabeculectomy and after phaco-trabeculectomy. *Acta Ophthalmol Scand Suppl.* 1997(224):44–45.

31. Chen TC, Wilensky JT, Viana MA. Long-term follow-up of initially successful trabeculectomy. *Ophthalmology.* 1997;104(7):1120–1125.

32. Greenfield DS, Liebmann JM, Jee J, Ritch R. Late-onset bleb leaks after glaucoma filtering surgery. *Arch Ophthalmol.* 1998;116(4):443–447.

33. Cunliffe IA, Rees RC, Rennie IG. The effect of TGF-beta 1 and TGF-beta 2 on the proliferation of human Tenon's capsule fibroblasts in tissue culture. *Acta Ophthalmol Scand.* 1996;74(1):31–35.

34. Carassa RG, Bettin P, Fiori M, Brancato R. Viscocanalostomy: A pilot study. *Eur J Ophthalmol.* 1998;8(2):57–61.

35. Neufeld AH, Sawada A, Becker B. Inhibition of nitricoxide synthase 2 by aminoguanidine provides neuroprotection of retinal ganglion cells in a rat model of chronic glaucoma. *Proc Natl Acad Sci USA.* 1999;96:9944–9948.

36. Johansson JO. Inhibition and recovery of retrograde axoplasmic transport in rat optic nerve during and after elevated IOP in vivo. *Exp Eye Res.* 1988;46(2):223–227.

37. Stoilova D, Child A, Brice G, Crick RP, Fleck BW, Sarfarazi M. Identification of a new "TIGR" mutation in a family with juvenile-onset primary open angle glaucoma. *Ophthalm Genet.* 1997;18(3):109–118.

38. Richards JE, Ritch R, Lichter PR, Rozsa FW, et al. Novel trabecular meshwork inducible-glucocorticoid response mutation in an eight-generation juvenile-onset primary open angle glaucoma pedigree. *Ophthalmology.* 1998;105(9):1698–1707.

39. Stoilova D, Child A, Brice G, Desai T, Barsoum Homsy M, Ozdemir N, Chevrette L, Adam MF, Garchon HJ, Pitts Crick R, Sarfarazi M. Novel TIGR/MYOC mutations in families with juvenile onset primary open angle glaucoma. *J Med Genet.* 1998;35(12):989–992.

Part IV

TYPES OF GLAUCOMA

Chapter 26

PIGMENTARY DISPERSION SYNDROME AND PIGMENTARY GLAUCOMA*

Jeffrey M. Liebmann
Robert Ritch

Open-angle glaucoma may be caused by a wide variety of factors, most of which lead to elevated intraocular pressure (IOP) and the development of glaucomatous optic neuropathy in susceptible eyes. Pigmentary dispersion syndrome (PDS) is characterized by the liberation of pigment from the iris pigment epithelium and its deposition on the structures of the anterior segment. The accumulation of pigment granules in the trabecular meshwork then leads to progressive trabecular dysfunction and ocular hypertension with or without associated glaucomatous optic neuropathy. Since the age of onset is often in the third or fourth decade of life, this secondary glaucoma is an important and often underdiagnosed form of vision loss that strikes younger individuals.

EPIDEMIOLOGY

Pigmentary glaucoma (PG) was originally considered to be a rare disorder. In 1949, Sugar and Barbour described two young myopic men with Krukenberg spindles, hyperpigmentation of the trabecular meshwork, and open angles whose IOPs increased with mydriasis and decreased with pilocarpine.[1] Investigations over the ensuing decades elucidated further features, including bilateral occurrence, frequent association with myopia, and a greater incidence in younger males.[2-11]

PDS affects mainly Caucasians and is unusual in persons of African or Asian ancestry. Slit-lamp screening has shown that PDS occurs in approximately 1 to 2% of the Caucasian population.[12] Many persons with the syndrome go undetected, while those with glaucoma are more often than not misdiagnosed as having juvenile-onset or primary open-angle glaucoma. Those without elevated IOP may have the presence of Krukenberg spindles noted but are often told that they have normal eye examinations and are not cautioned regarding possible future consequences or the hereditary nature of the syndrome. Phenotypic expression of the disorder varies, and some manifestations may be extremely subtle or perhaps not expressed at all, leading to lack of detection in a large segment of affected persons. Finally, many emmetropes and hyperopes, particularly prior to the onset of presbyopia, never undergo routine eye examinations, and even less

*Supported in part by the New York Glaucoma Research Institute, New York, NY.

frequently are they comprehensive. Not all persons with myopia undergo slit-lamp examination at the time of refraction for correction of their myopic error. As a result, a large portion of patients with PDS are incompletely examined.

Although a primary open-angle glaucoma usually has its onset after the fifth decade of life, PDS and PG typically affect younger individuals. Since an early age of onset of ocular hypertension or glaucoma has a greater likelihood of being associated with a secondary glaucoma, the diagnosis of elevated IOP at a young age should prompt the examiner to search for a cause.

Myopia is an important risk factor for the development of PDS and is present in approximately 90% of affected individuals.[13,14] In general, patients with higher degrees of myopia and deeper anterior segments tend to develop pigment dispersion at an earlier age and often have a more difficult clinical course. In patients with asymmetrical disease, the more affected eye is usually the one that is more myopic.[15,16]

PDS appears to be inherited in an autosomal dominant pattern with incomplete penetration, the phenotypic expression of which appears to be increased by the presence of myopia. Several pedigrees have been described with multiple affected members, and at least one genetic locus has been identified.[17–19]

CLINICAL FEATURES

The classic triad of diagnostic clinical signs for PDS consists of a Krukenberg spindle; slit-like, radial transillumination defects in the midperipheral iris; and pigment deposition on the trabecular meshwork. The iris tends to have a concave configuration and often inserts into the band of the posterior ciliary body. As

with other glaucomas, the key to diagnosis of PDS and PG is awareness of the constellation of clinical findings with which they are associated.[4–6,11,14,20–37]

Cornea and Anterior Chamber

Liberated pigment granules are borne by aqueous currents and deposited on the structures of the anterior segment. The vertical accumulation of these pigment granules along the corneal endothelium is known as a *Krukenberg spindle* (Figs. 26–1 and 26–2). The spindle tends to be slightly decentered inferiorly and wider at its base than at its apex, and it generally appears as a central, vertical brown band 1 to 6 mm long and up to 3 mm wide.[11,35] With time, the spindle becomes smaller and lighter; often, careful examination is necessary to identify it. Histopathology reveals the pigment granules to have been phagocytosed by the corneal endothelium. In eyes with severe pigment liberation, waves of pigment may be visible on the peripheral cornea anterior to Schwalbe's line during slit-lamp biomicroscopy or gonioscopy. Occasionally, small pigment particles may be seen floating within the anterior chamber; these may be mistaken for active uveitis. Pigment release may also occur following pharmacological dilation or exercise and may be accompanied by elevation of IOP, blurred vision, glare, or pain. Identification of a Krukenberg spindle should prompt the examiner to search for causes of pigment

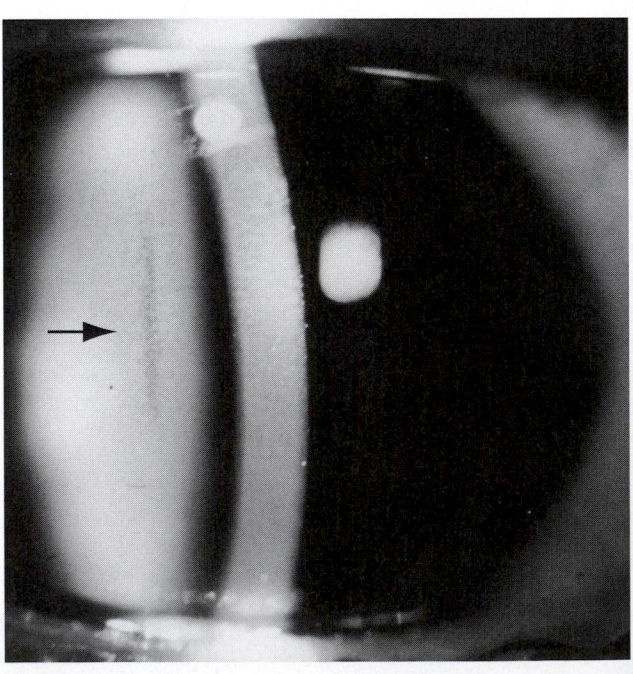

Figure 26–2. Typical pattern of fine pigment deposition on the corneal endothelial surface (Krukenberg spindle) associated with pigment dispersion syndrome. Note the vertical orientation. (*See also Color Plate 79.*)

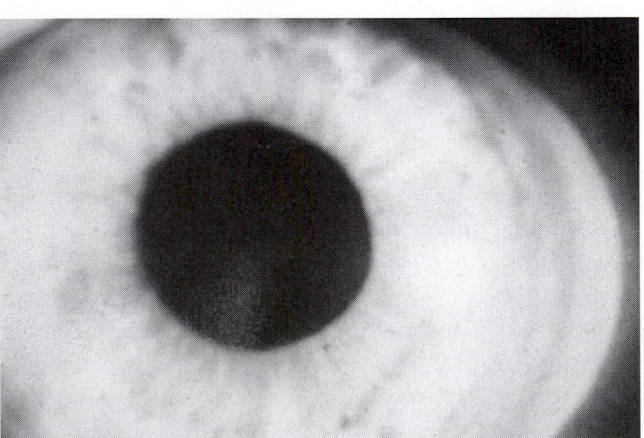

Figure 26–1. Krukenberg spindle. (*See also Color Plate 78.*)

liberation. Two other disorders occasionally associated with spindle formation are exfoliation syndrome and diabetes mellitus.

Anterior Chamber Angle and Trabecular Meshwork

Increased trabecular pigmentation occurs in a wide variety of glaucomas. In PDS, the trabecular pigmentation is typically homogeneous in its distribution, unlike the heterogeneous appearance associated with exfoliation syndrome, uveitis, or angle-closure glaucoma. The pigmentation ranges from moderate to dense and is often quite striking (Figs. 26–3 and 26–4). In some individuals the increased pigmentation may be limited to the posterior trabecular meshwork, while in others the anterior meshwork, Schwalbe's line, or the peripheral cornea may be covered with dense pigmentation.

Iris

The abnormal iris architecture in PDS is responsible for the major clinical findings of this disorder. Slit-lamp biomicroscopy reveals the anterior chamber to be deep, usually consistent with the degree of myopia, but slightly deeper than age- and refraction-matched controls. Slight iridodenesis may be present. Gonioscopy confirms the angle to be widely open, with the iris often assuming a concave approach to its insertion into the ciliary body.

The iris concavity in PDS has been investigated using ultrasound biomicroscopy, which employs high-frequency ultrasound to permit high-resolution in vivo imaging of the anterior segment. It has been particularly useful in the evaluation of the structures surrounding the posterior chamber. The ultrasound biomicroscopic features of this disorder include iris

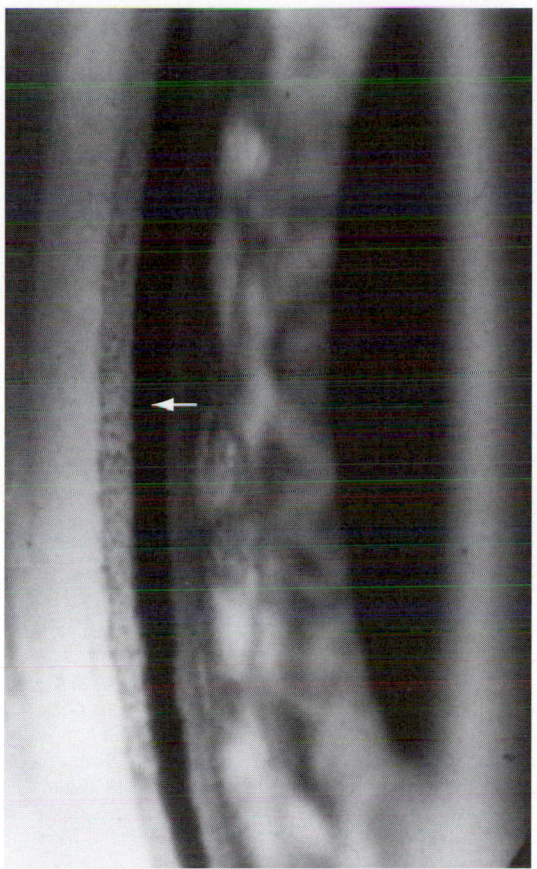

Figure 26–4. Dense trabecular meshwork pigmentation noted in an individual with pigmentary glaucoma. (*See also Color Plate 81.*)

concavity, iridozonular contact, and a large region of iridolenticular contact (Fig. 26–5). Although most young individuals with undisputed PDS (young age, zonular pigment dispersion, increased meshwork pigmentation, myopia) have a demonstrable iris concavity that can be measured during ultrasound biomicroscopy, the prevalence of iris concavity at the time of initial diagnosis has not been evaluated in a large study.

Movement of the posteriorly bowed, concave iris along the anterior zonular bundles causes a disruption of the iris pigment epithelium along the radial orientation of the zonular fibers, which results in characteristic midperipheral iris transillumination defects seen during slit-lamp examination (Figs. 26–6 and 26–7). This finding is pathognomonic for zonular pigment dispersion and differentiates PDS from other glaucomas related to accumulation of pigment in the trabecular meshwork.

The width, length, and frequency of these defects vary among individuals, and a high index of suspicion on the part of the examiner is often needed to

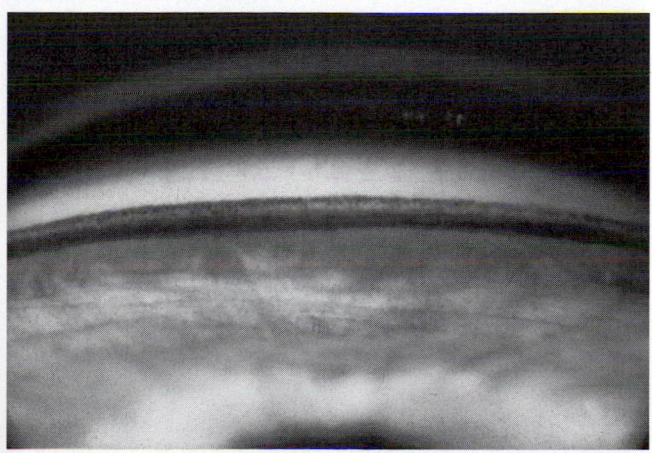

Figure 26–3. Dense, homogeneous trabecular meshwork pigmentation in pigmentary glaucoma. (*See also Color Plate 80.*)

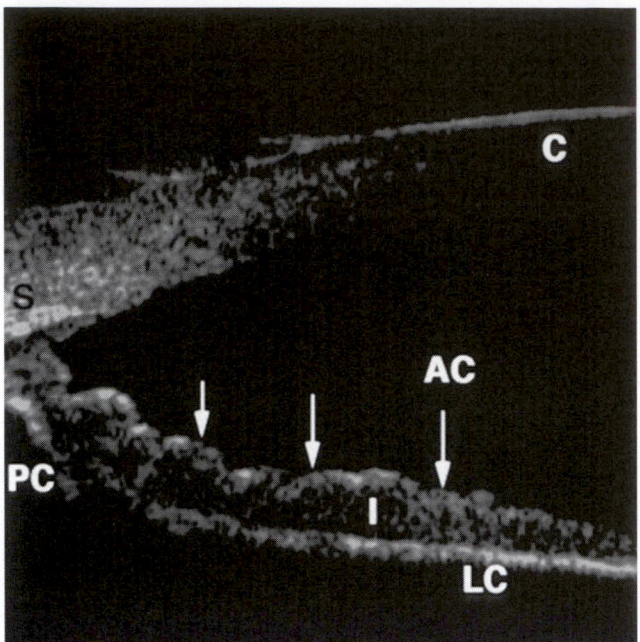

Figure 26–5. Ultrasound biomicroscopic appearance of untreated pigment dispersion syndrome. The iris (I) is bowed posteriorly, toward the zonules and posterior chamber (PC). The cornea (C), anterior chamber (AC), and lens capsule (LC) are visible. Increased pressure in the anterior chamber relative to the posterior chamber (reverse pupillary block) is present (*arrows*).

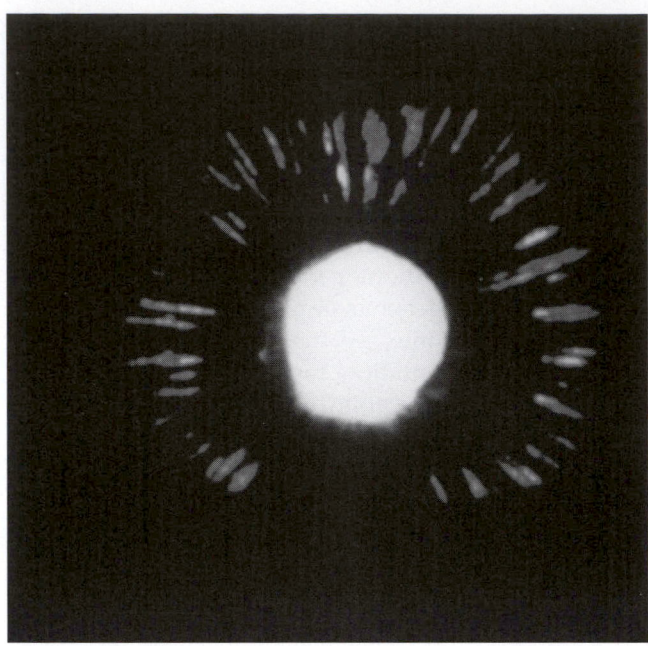

Figure 26–7. Iris transillumination defects, associated with pigment dispersion syndrome, occur in the midperiphery and are circumferential in appearance. (*See also Color Plate 83.*)

make the diagnosis. It is best to search for iris transillumination defects prior to pupillary dilation by using a small slit beam in a darkened room. However, those patients who do not appear to have transillumination defects on retroillumination but have increased trabecular pigmentation, a Krukenberg spindle, myopia, or juvenile open-angle glaucoma can be examined with scleral transillumination using a fiberoptic scleral transilluminator in a darkened room to facilitate detection. Infrared videopupillography is also useful in determining the extent of the defects (Fig. 26–8). Pupillary dilation may prevent the detection of transillumination defects because of the compaction of the peripheral iris stroma.

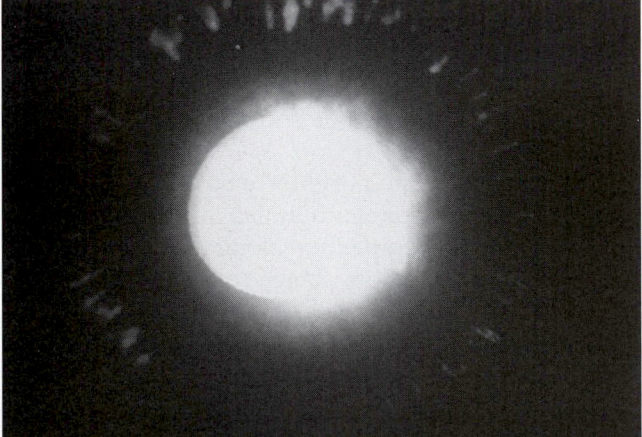

Figure 26–6. The transillumination defects found in PDS are located in the midperipheral iris and result from mechanical contact between the iris pigment epithelium and packets of anterior zonular bundles. (*See also Color Plate 82.*)

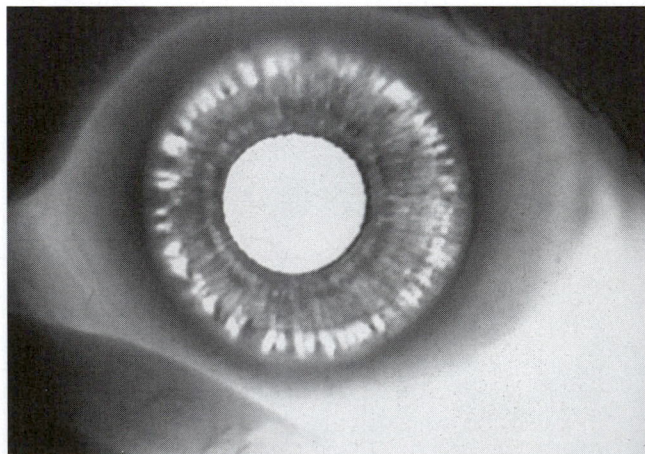

Figure 26–8. Infrared videopupillography is a useful technique to detect and document the number of transillumination defects.

The number of iris transillumination defects often corresponds clinically to the degree of anterior segment pigment liberation and elevated IOP, although this is not always the case. In eyes with asymmetrical disease, the eye with the higher pressure is invariably the one with the greater pigment liberation.

Some physicians have advocated the documentation of the numbers of transillumination defects as a means of following the progression of the disease. Individuals in the pigment liberation phase of the disease typically have an increasing number of transillumination defects, whereas those individuals who are no longer actively liberating pigment may have defects that shrink in size or disappear.

Pigment accumulation on the anterior surface of the iris often appears as concentric rings within the iris furrows (Fig. 26–9).[11,35] More diffuse pigmentation can cause a diffuse darkening of iris color, which is more apparent in lightly pigmented irides because of the degree of color change. Asymmetry of pigment liberation may result in iris heterochromia, with the darker iris being the more affected.[11,38]

Lens and Zonules

Pigment deposition on the zonular apparatus may allow visualization of the radial anterior zonules as they traverse the posterior chamber to the anterior lens surface. Since liberated pigment floats freely within the aqueous, some of the pigment granules may also move posteriorly behind the lens equator, where they accumulate at Weigert's ligament, the region of contact between the anterior hyaloid face and the posterior lens capsule. Visualization of this circular ring or arc of pigmentation requires pupillary dilation and sometimes gonioscopy; it is considered pathognomonic for

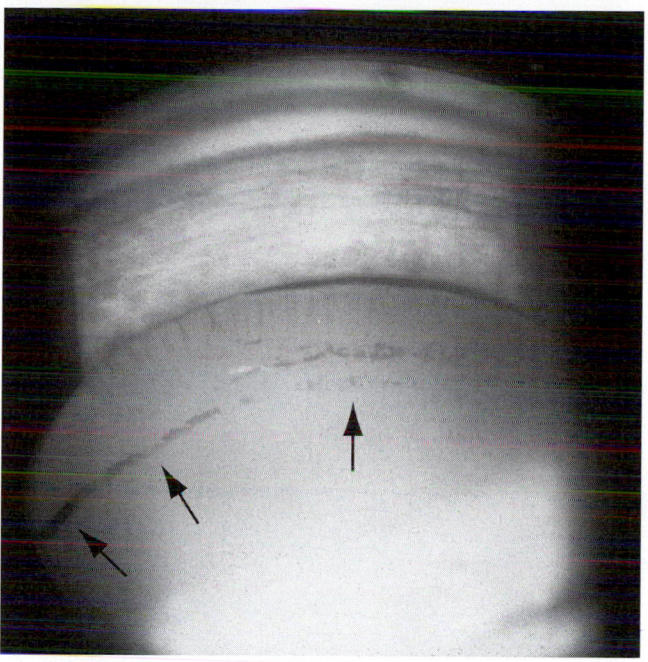

Figure 26–10. Pigment on the posterior lens capsule (arrows). (*See also Color Plate 85.*)

PDS, since it has not been identified in other disorders associated with pigment liberation in the anterior segment (Fig. 26–10).

Posterior Segment

Patients with pigment dispersion and pigmentary glaucoma have an increased risk of retinal detachment, which may occur in as many as 2 to 3% of individuals. Although the interrelationships between PDS, myopia, and retinal detachment remain to be fully elucidated, it has been suggested that retinal breaks and lattice degeneration occur twice as frequently in these eyes as in age- and refraction-matched controls and are independent of the use of miotics and degree of myopia.[37]

PATHOPHYSIOLOGY

As described by Campbell in 1979, mechanical contact between the concave posterior iris surface and anterior zonular packets is responsible for the release of pigment granules from the iris pigment epithelium (Fig. 26–11).[22] Histopathological study and electron microscopy have confirmed that the location of the iris defects corresponds closely to the position of the zonular packets. It is not known whether a defect of the iris pigment epithelium in PDS contributes to their rupture or whether the release is due to mechanical forces alone.

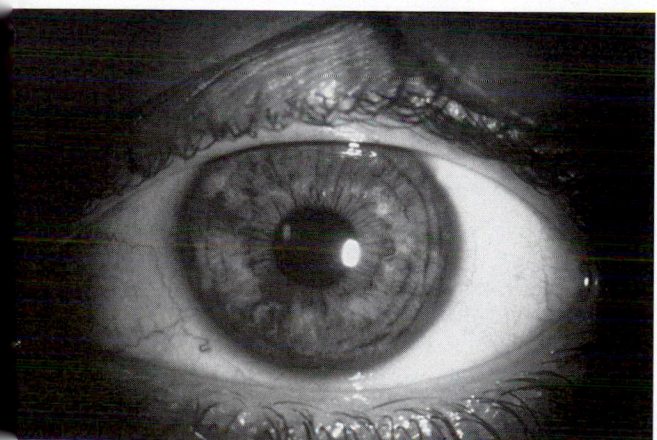

Figure 26–9. In cases with more pronounced pigment liberation, pigment granules may accumulate in iris furrows, where they are visible as concentric rings. (*See also Color Plate 84.*)

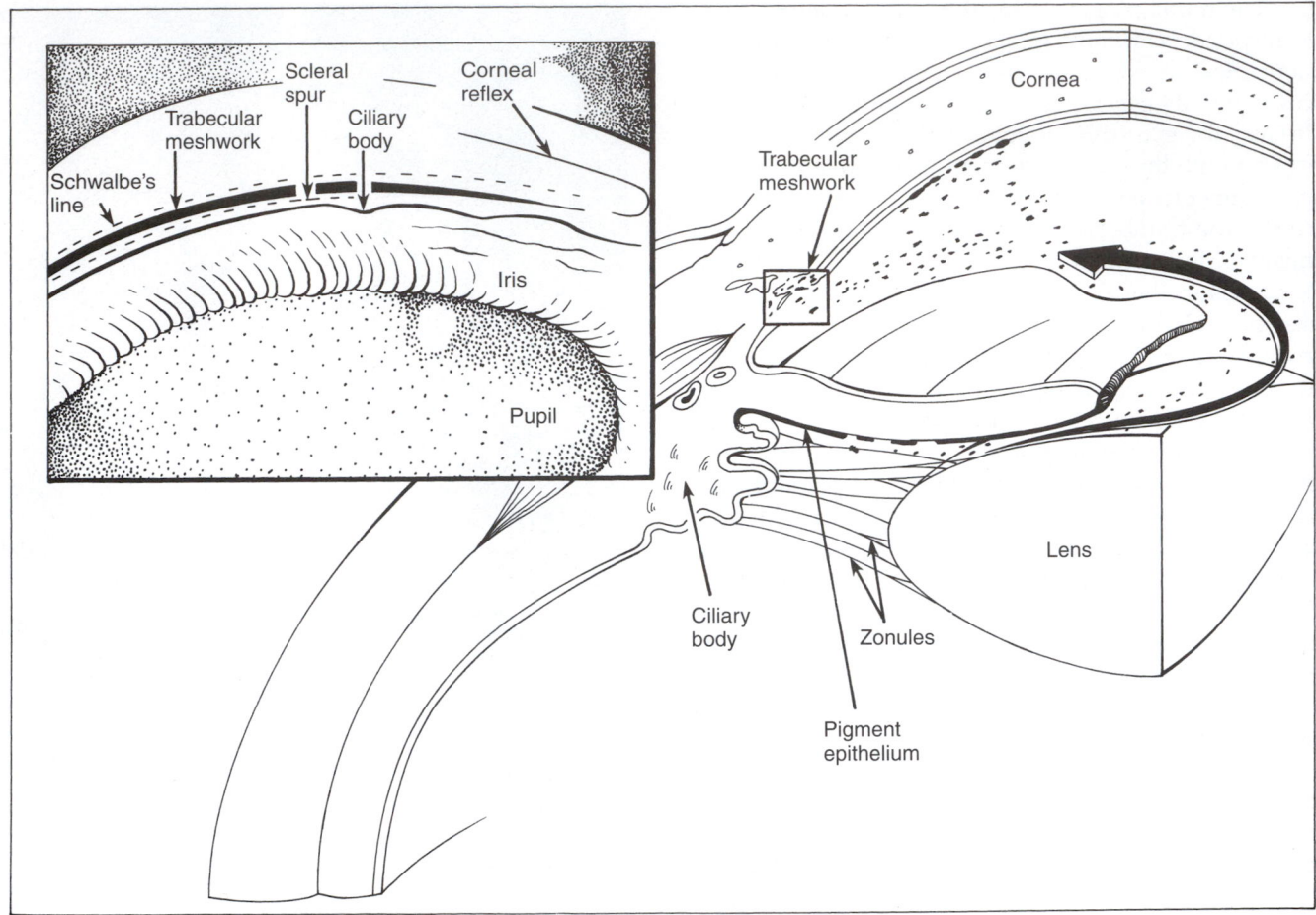

Figure 26–11. Presumed pathogenesis of pigment dispersion syndrome. Pigment is liberated from the posterior iris pigment epithelium because the iris and zonules are touching. The pigment circulates in the anterior chamber, being deposited on the lens, iris, and cornea and in the trabecular meshwork.

Greater pigment liberation tends to occur in eyes with more pronounced iris concavity, presumably because of the closer proximity of the iris pigment epithelium to the zonular apparatus. The insertion of the iris into the ciliary body has been reported to be more posterior in PDS than in control eyes, an anatomic variation that places the iris pigment epithelium into closer proximity to the zonular apparatus and may increase the likelihood of iridozonular contact and zonular pigment dispersion.

Liberated pigment is dispersed by aqueous currents and is deposited on structures throughout the anterior segment. In the trabecular meshwork, pigment accumulates on the trabecular endothelium and obstructs the intertrabecular spaces. Trabecular endothelial damage and meshwork dysfunction later lead to elevated intraocular pressure in susceptible individuals. Ocular hypertension or glaucoma develops in 30 to 50% of patients.

Active liberation of pigment typically occurs in patients in their third and fourth decades of life. As affected individuals age, increasing pupillary miosis and cataract formation cause a slow increase in relative pupillary block, which increases resistance of aqueous flow from the posterior chamber, through the pupil, and into the anterior chamber. This permits accumulation of aqueous within the posterior chamber and increases the distance between the zonules and the iris. The result may be either a decrease in or resolution of active pigment release by decreasing iridozonular contact. Continued phagocytosis of existing pigment in the trabecular meshwork may result in better aqueous outflow, improving control of IOP. Lichter and Shaffer[6] observed a definite decrease in the amount of meshwork pigment in 10% of 102 patients and concluded that the pigment could pass out of the meshwork as the patient aged. Older patients presenting with glaucoma may have only very subtle manifestations, if any, of PDS, and may be diagnosed to have primary open-angle glaucoma or low-tension glaucoma.

Reverse Pupillary Block

Iridozonular contact occurs in PDS because the iris has a concave configuration, which brings it into closer approximation to the zonular apparatus. Since the position of the iris changes with fluid pressure gradients within the anterior segment, the concept of reverse pupillary block has developed to explain the anatomic abnormalities that lead to the iris concavity.[25,39-45]

In reverse pupillary block, the pressure of aqueous humor is greater in the anterior chamber than in the posterior chamber. This is the opposite of the relative pupillary block seen in angle-closure glaucoma, in which resistance to aqueous flow through the pupil causes the iris to move anteriorly and close the angle. Pupillary block angle closure is relieved by laser iridectomy, which allows aqueous to move freely through the iridectomy into the anterior chamber, relieving the pressure gradient across the iris and opening the angle.

Reverse pupillary block could occur if an aliquot of aqueous were to be suddenly introduced into the anterior chamber and then trapped there, so as to be unable to equilibrate with aqueous in the posterior chamber. The increased pressure within the anterior chamber forces the iris against the lens, creating a flap valve that maintains the pressure differential between the chambers by preventing movement of aqueous back into the posterior chamber. The relative pressure difference between the two chambers would cause the iris to assume a concave configuration.

A concave iris configuration caused by a relative pressure differential between the anterior and posterior chambers is not unique to PDS. In iris-retraction syndrome, increased uveoscleral outflow facilitated by retinal pigment epithelium–assisted fluid absorption in the presence of a retinal break causes the pressure within the posterior segment and posterior chamber to be less than that of the anterior chamber. Eyes with iris-retraction syndrome have extensive posterior synechiae that prevent the free flow of anterior chamber fluid into the posterior chamber. During routine phacoemulsification, posterior movement of the lens-iris diaphragm during irrigation at the time of insertion of the phacoemulsification handpiece may be due in part to a rapid increase in anterior chamber volume, which forces the iris against the lens surface. Because of this flap-valve effect, fluid cannot move into the posterior chamber and the entire lens-iris diaphragm may move posteriorly.

Blinking

Lid blinking may have a prominent contributory influence on iris configuration and thus on the distribution of aqueous humor in the anterior segment. In 1993, Campbell[46] proposed that a blink initially deforms the cornea, transiently increases intraocular pressure (in both the anterior and posterior chambers), and pushes the iris posteriorly against the lens. Immediately following the blink, pressure within the posterior chamber exceeds that of the anterior chamber and a small aliquot of aqueous moves into the anterior chamber along this pressure gradient. This causes the pressure of the anterior chamber to exceed that of the posterior chamber for a brief period. This momentary pressure gradient causes the iris to become concave and pushes it against the lens, preventing aqueous from flowing back into the posterior chamber (reverse pupillary block). The presence of corneal deformation during blinking has been reported in animal studies.

Increased iridolenticular contact and myopia, both present in PDS, appear to enhance the flap-valve effect of iris-lens contact, which helps to prevent equilibration of pressure between the two chambers. In non-PDS eyes, this reverse pupillary block mechanism is less complete and less able to maintain the pressure differential.

When blinking is prevented, aqueous secretion gradually increases the volume of the posterior chamber. As the volume and pressure of the posterior chamber increase relative to the anterior chamber, the iris gradually flattens, iridolenticular contact diminishes, and iridozonular and iridociliary process distances increase (Fig. 26–12A and B).

Accommodation and Iris Configuration

A concave iris configuration indistinguishable from that associated with PDS can be induced by accommodation in young, normal individuals. During accommodation, contraction of the ciliary ring causes the lens to move slightly forward, which shallows the anterior chamber. The displaced aqueous cannot move into the posterior chamber because of the flap-valve effect and is therefore forced into the angle recess (Fig. 26–13A and B). Aqueous humor, now trapped in the anterior chamber, is forced into the angle recess, and the peripheral iris assumes a concave configuration. This process is similar to the change in iris and angle configuration that occurs during indentation gonioscopy.

Exercise-Induced Pigment Liberation

Pharmacological pupillary dilation may result in marked liberation of pigment accompanied by a rise in IOP. The same phenomenon may occur in some

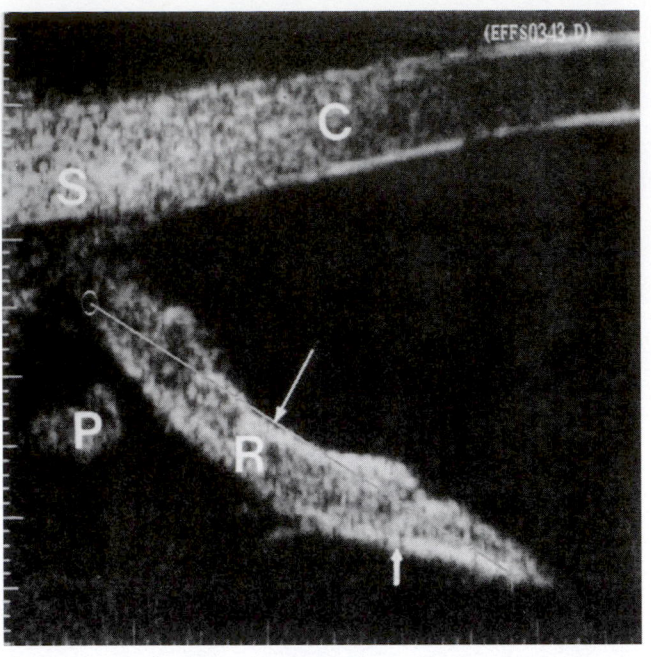

A

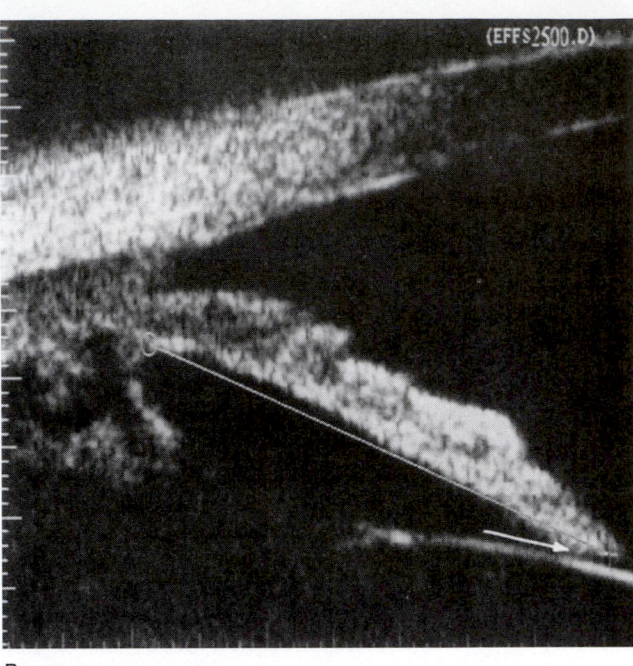

B

Figure 26–12. *A.* Concave iris posterior to the reference line (*large arrow*) at the time of initial scanning (Time 0). Iridolenticular contact is present and the iris has a concave configuration. *B.* Blinking is prevented and the maximal change in iris configuration occurred at 11 minutes. The iris is now convex and anterior to the reference line. There is no iridolenticular contact (*arrow*). (Reproduced with permission from Liebmann JM, Tello C, Chew SJ, Cohen H, Ritch R. *Ophthalmology.* 1995;102:146–155.)

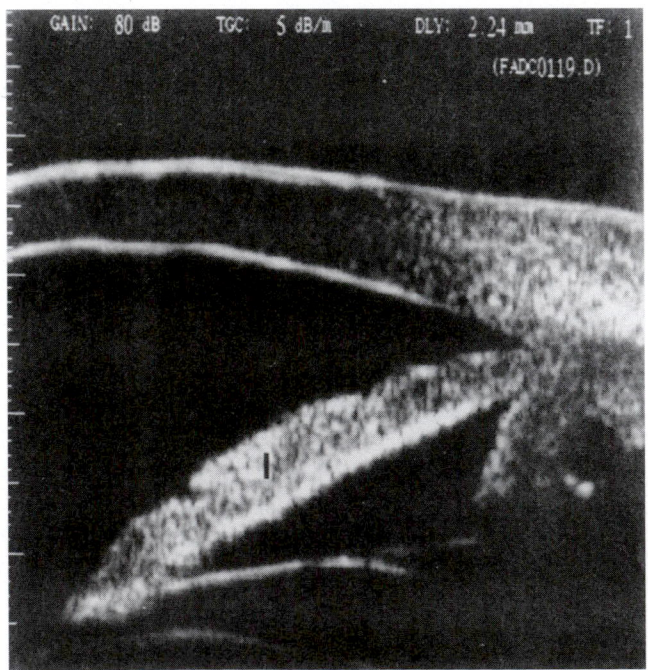

A

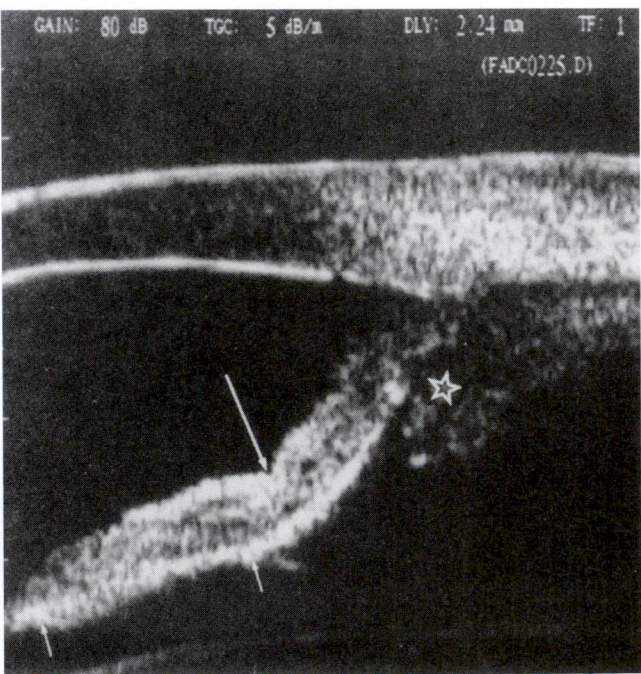

B

Figure 26–13. *A.* Iris position upon initial scanning in a normal, emmetropic, 20-year-old man fixing on a wall-mounted target. The iris (I) has a minimally convex configuration. *B.* As soon as fixation is moved to a near target (30 cm), contraction of the ciliary muscle causes anterior movement of the lens, increasing iridolenticular contact (*small arrows*), which effectively traps aqueous within the anterior chamber. Because of the anterior chamber shallowing, aqueous is forced peripherally and gives the iris a concave configuration (*large arrow*). The ciliary body (*asterisk*) appears to be indenting the peripheral iris. (Reproduced with permission from Liebmann JM, Tello C, Chew SJ, Cohen H, Ritch R. *Ophthalmology.* 1995;102:146–155.)

patients with PDS during strenuous exercise, particularly exercise involving jarring movements, such as jogging or basketball. Pretreatment with low-dose pilocarpine prior to exercise can limit both the pigment liberation and the IOP spike. Laser iridectomy, discussed below, may not completely eliminate exercise-induced pigment liberation.

CLINICAL COURSE

Although many individuals have PDS, less than half will develop ocular hypertension or glaucoma. However, since PDS is a risk factor for the development of ocular hypertension, all patients with this disorder should undergo periodic eye examinations. This is particularly important during the pigmentary liberation phase of the disease. The frequency of follow-up can be decreased when pigmentary liberation ceases or trabecular pigmentation begins to diminish.

It should be remembered that PDS is typically a bilateral disease, although asymmetry may occur. There is a correlation between the amount of pigment lost from the posterior surface of the iris, increased degree of pigmentation in the trabecular meshwork, and degree of dysfunction of the trabecular meshwork as evidenced by elevation of the IOP. The size and density of the Krukenberg spindle does not necessarily correlate with damage to the trabecular meshwork. The amount of pigment that is presented to the trabecular meshwork does, however, play a role in the elevation of the IOP. Markedly asymmetrical disease is usually due to an additional factor making one eye worse, such as anisometropia, the development of exfoliation syndrome or angle recession, or an additional factor acting to prevent the development of PDS, such as aphakia or Horner's syndrome.

Progressive glaucomatous optic neuropathy in PG is primarily pressure-dependent, and reduction of IOP is the mainstay of therapy. In addition to the monitoring of IOP, sequential ophthalmic examinations should include gonioscopy to assess the degree and progression of trabecular pigmentation, stereoscopic evaluation and photography of the optic nerve, and perimetry.

DIFFERENTIAL DIAGNOSIS

PDS can usually be easily distinguished from most other abnormalities in which dissemination of pigment is part of the disease process, as there is no other condition that results in the characteristic iris transillumination defects. Other disorders associated with signs of pigmentary dispersion in the anterior

segment—such as uveitis, pigment in the angle due to dispersion or disruption of melanoma cells (e.g., melanomelytic dispersion), cysts of the iris and ciliary body, postoperative conditions such as IOL-iris chafing, and exfoliation syndrome—often occur unilaterally. In addition, trabecular pigmentation is less dense and is usually unevenly distributed throughout the circumference of the meshwork in these conditions. Upon occasion, pigment granules in the anterior chamber may be mistaken for inflammatory cells, leading to a misdiagnosis of uveitis.

The disease process most similar to PG is exfoliation glaucoma. In this condition, there is loss of pigment from the iris pigment epithelium, iris transillumination, pigmentary dispersion in the anterior segment including a Krukenberg spindle, trabecular pigmentation, and elevation of IOP. The clinical history combined with careful slit-lamp biomicroscopic examination easily separates the two diseases. The age of onset for exfoliation glaucoma is usually over 60 and onset is rare under 40; there is no sexual or racial predilection for exfoliation syndrome, although reports seem to indicate a higher prevalence of the disease in individuals of Scandinavian ancestry. Meshwork pigmentation is not as intense as in PG. Iris transillumination characteristically begins at the pupillary border and not the midperiphery. Approximately 50% of patients with exfoliation syndrome, unlike those with PDS, are clinically affected in only one eye. Finally, the presence of white flakes of exfoliation material at the pupillary border and on the anterior lens surface is diagnostic of exfoliation syndrome.

MANAGEMENT

Since the degree and stage of pigment liberation, IOP, and extent of glaucomatous optic neuropathy vary among individuals, each must be evaluated to determine the proper course of intervention. As our understanding of the pathogenesis of pigment liberation expands, consideration should also be given to gearing therapy toward eliminating acute pigment release rather than just treating elevated IOP.[47]

Beta-Adrenergic Antagonists
The mainstay of initial medical therapy for PG continues to be suppression of aqueous with a topical beta blocker, primarily because of the relatively easy dosing schedule and minimal side effects.

Parasympathomimetics
In theory, therapy directed at increasing relative pupillary block should relieve iridozonular contact and diminish pigment liberation. The relief of iridozonular

contact following miotic therapy has been demonstrated with ultrasound biomicroscopy (Fig. 26–14*A* and *B*). The miotic agent induces pupillary miosis, which increases resistance to aqueous flow from the posterior chamber, past the lens surface, and through the pupil into the anterior chamber. This increased resistance allows aqueous pressure to build within the posterior chamber (i.e., relative pupillary block) and forces the iris to move anteriorly, away from the zonules, and assume a convex configuration. However, strong miotics in young individuals are rarely tolerated because of the associated spasm of accommodation and blurring of vision. Low-dose pilocarpine in the form of Ocuserts often provides enough miosis to create pupillary block without disabling adverse effects. A careful peripheral retinal examination should be performed before and after the institution of or change in miotic therapy because of the higher incidence of retinal breaks and detachment in these patients.

Alpha-Adrenergic Agonists

Alpha agonists are useful in PG, but the development of allergy in up to 50% of patients precludes the long-term use of dipivefrin, epinephrine, and apraclonidine in many individuals. Brimonidine tartrate 0.2% may provide satisfactory intraocular pressure with less allergy than other drugs in this class.

Carbonic Anhydrase Inhibitors

Topical carbonic anhydrase inhibitors are useful agents for PG and are generally well tolerated. Systemic agents should be reserved for particularly difficult circumstances or when the risks of surgery are unacceptably high.

Prostaglandin Analogues

Prostaglandin analogues, which lower IOP by increasing uveoscleral outflow, are effective in PG and offer the advantage of once-daily administration. Change in the surface color of the iris that may occur during therapy appears to involve increased melanin production by iris melanocytes and is not known to affect the iris pigment epithelium or to result in pigmentary dispersion.

Alpha-Adrenergic Antagonists

Theoretically, a drug that would constrict the pupil and make the peripheral iris taut might decrease iridozonular rubbing and eliminate accumulation of pigment in the meshwork. An alpha-adrenergic blocking agent such as thymoxamine hydrochloride, which constricts the pupil but does not affect accommodation or aqueous dynamics, could be beneficial to such patients. Thymoxamine hydrochloride is not yet approved for this purpose and is unavailable for general use. In addition, in its present formulation, the

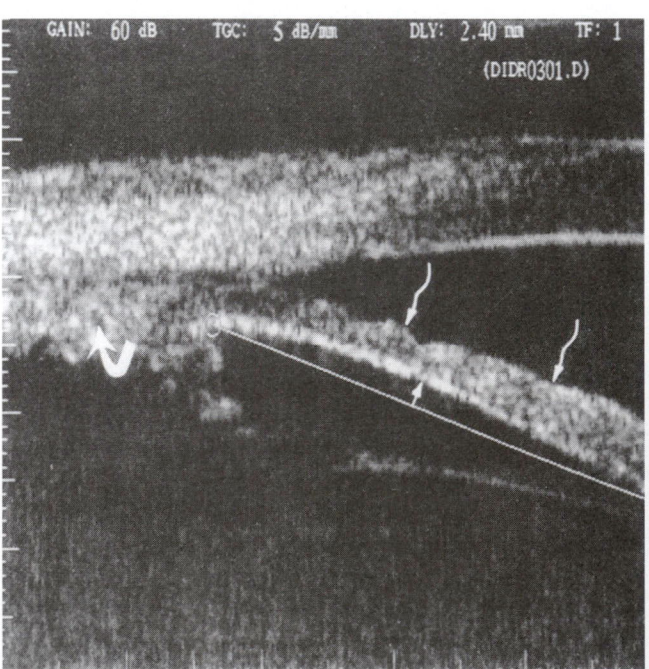

A   *B*

Figure 26–14. *A.* In untreated PDS, the iris is posteriorly bowed (concave) and the iris pigment epithelium is below the reference line. *B.* One hour following administration of one drop of pilocarpine 2%, the pupil has become miotic, relative pupillary block has developed, and the iris has bowed anteriorly. The iris pigment epithelium is above the reference line. (Reproduced with permission from Potash SD, Tello C, Liebmann J, Ritch R. *Ophthalmology.* 1994;101:332–339.)

ocular irritation that the drug causes makes it unlikely that patients would tolerate it. Dapiprazole, currently available to reverse pharmacological pupillary dilation, has not proven useful in the treatment of pigment dispersion.

SURGERY

Laser Trabeculoplasty

Argon laser trabeculoplasty may be offered as a treatment in the management of uncontrolled PG. Although the initial result is often good, a larger proportion of patients can lose control of IOP by comparison with primary open-angle glaucoma patients, and the loss of control can occur in less time. In contrast to other forms of open-angle glaucoma, younger patients appear to respond better to trabeculoplasty than do older individuals.[48]

Laser Iridectomy

Laser iridectomy eliminates the iris concavity present in most patients with PDS by permitting equalization of pressures between the anterior and posterior chambers.[42,43,45,46,49–51] This causes the iris to become flat, thereby decreasing iridozonular contact (Fig. 26-15A

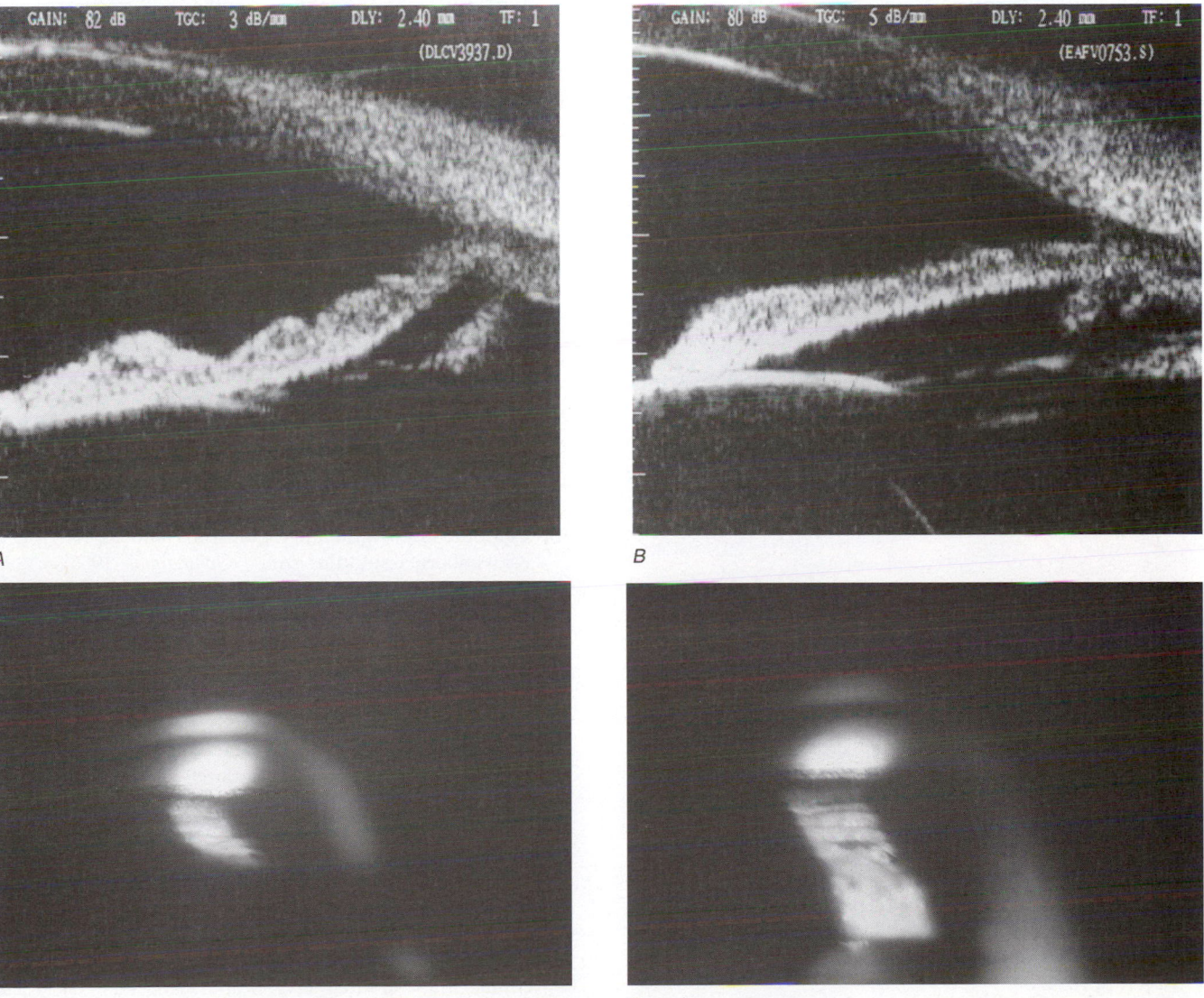

Figure 26–15. *A.* Prelaser iridotomy scan demonstrating marked iris concavity and central iris contact with the anterior lens capsule and zonules. *B.* Postlaser iridotomy scan shows resolution of iris concavity and decreased length of iris contact with the anterior lens capsule. (*A* and *B* reproduced with permission from Potash SD, Tello C, Liebmann J, Ritch R. *Ophthalmology.* 1994;101:332–339.) *C.* Prior to laser iridectomy, gonioscopy demonstrates a concave iris configuration. (See also Color Plate 86C.) *D.* Following laser iridectomy, the iris assumes a flat configuration. (*See also Color Plate 86C.*)

through *D*) and reversing the underlying anatomic defect, which results in pigment dispersion. Anecdotal evidence suggests that this can prevent continued pigment liberation, result in a reversal of trabecular pigmentation, and, subsequently, lower the IOP. However, long-term lowering of IOP and stabilization of glaucomatous optic neuropathy and visual field loss have not been conclusively demonstrated. Hence, although theoretically sound, laser iridectomy should be used with caution because of the paucity of data regarding the long-term efficacy of this procedure.

Filtering Surgery

The surgical management of patients with PG follows the same principles and considerations used in the management of primary open-angle glaucoma. The appearance of and change in the optic nerve along with visual field defects should be the principal guidelines used in deciding whether surgery is needed. Most patients respond well to standard filtration operations, although antifibrosis agents may be indicated to achieve a low target pressure or for reoperation. No unusual problems are typically encountered during cataract surgery.

CONCLUSION

Pigmentary dispersion syndrome is an important but often underdiagnosed cause of open-angle glaucoma. Recognition of its unique clinical features and pattern of inheritance as well as an understanding of its pathophysiology permit appropriate, timely intervention to prevent loss of vision.

REFERENCES

1. Sugar HS, Barbour FA. Pigmentary glaucoma: A rare clinical entity. *Am J Ophthalmol*. 1949;32:90–92.
2. Campbell DG, Boys-Smith JW. Pigmentary glaucoma. In: Caldwell DR, ed. *Symposium on the Laser in Ophthalmology and Glaucoma Update*. St. Louis: CV Mosby; 1984.
3. Campbell DG. *Pigmentary Glaucoma: Past, Present and Future*. San Diego, CA: American Glaucoma Society; 1991.
4. Becker B, Shin DH, Cooper DG, Kass MA. The pigment dispersion syndrome. *Am J Ophthalmol*. 1977;83:161–166.
5. Jain S, Kaiser-Kupfer MI, Green SB, et al. Pigment dispersion syndrome: A study of risk factors in the development of glaucoma. *Invest Ophthalmol Vis Sci*. 1987;28(suppl):147.
6. Lichter PR, Shaffer RM. Diagnostic and prognostic signs in pigmentary glaucoma. *Trans Am Acad Ophthalmol Otolaryngol*. 1970;74:984–998.
7. Migliazzo CV, Shaffer RN, Nykin R, Magee S. Long-term analysis of pigmentary dispersion syndrome and pigmentary glaucoma. *Ophthalmology*. 1986;93:1528–1536.
8. Ritch R. A unification hypothesis of pigment dispersion syndrome. *Trans Am Ophthalmol Soc*. 1996;94:381–409.
9. Scheie HG, Cameron JD. Pigment dispersion syndrome: A clinical study. *Br J Ophthalmol*. 1981;65:264–269.
10. Speakman JS. Pigmentary dispersion. *Br J Ophthalmol*. 1981;65:249–251.
11. Sugar HS. Pigmentary glaucoma: A 25-year review. *Am J Ophthalmol*. 1966;62:499–507.
12. Ritch R, Steinberger D, Liebmann JM. Prevalence of pigment dispersion syndrome in a population undergoing glaucoma screening. *Am J Ophthalmol*. 1993;115:707–710.
13. Davidson JA, Brubaker RF, Ilstrup DM. Dimensions of the anterior chamber in pigment dispersion syndrome. *Arch Ophthalmol*. 1983;101:81–83.
14. Dunbar MR, Blasberg RD, Campbell DG. Iris configuration and anterior chamber depths in pigmentary glaucoma. *Invest Ophthalmol Vis Sci*. 1983;24(suppl):2.
15. Berger A, Ritch R, McDermott J, et al. Pigmentary dispersion, refraction and glaucoma. *Invest Ophthalmol Vis Sci*. 1987;28(suppl):134.
16. Bick MW. Sex differences in pigmentary glaucoma. *Am J Ophthalmol*. 1962;54:831–837.
17. Andersen KL, et al. Localization of the gene for pigment dispersion syndrome to chromosome 7q35-36. *Arch Ophthalmol*. 1997;115:384–388.
18. Mandelkorn RM, Hoffman ME, Olander KW, et al. Inheritance and the pigmentary dispersion syndrome. *Ophthalm Paediatr Genet*. 1985;6:85–91.
19. McDermott JA, Ritch R, Berger A, Wang RF. Familial occurrence of pigmentary dispersion syndrome. *Invest Ophthalmol Vis Sci*. 1987;28(suppl):136.
20. Alward WLM, Haynes WL. Pupillometric and videographic evaluation of anisocoria in patients with the pigment dispersion syndrome. *Invest Ophthalmol Vis Sci*. 1991;32(suppl):1109.
21. Calhoun FPJ. Pigmentary glaucoma and its relation to Krukenberg's spindles. *Am J Ophthalmol*. 1953;36:1398.
22. Campbell DG. Pigmentary dispersion and pigmentary glaucoma: A new theory. *Invest Ophthalmol Vis Sci*. 1979;20(suppl):25.
23. Campbell DG. Pigmentary glaucoma. In: Ritch R, Shields MB, Krupin T, eds. *The Glaucomas II*. St. Louis: CV Mosby; 1996:975–991.
24. Campbell DG, Jeffery CP. Pigmentary dispersion in the human eye. In: O'Hare, ed. *Scanning Electron Microscopy*. SEM Inc; 1979:329–334.
25. Campbell DG, Schertzer RM. Pathophysiology of pigment dispersion syndrome and pigmentary glaucoma. *Curr Opin Ophthalmol*. 1995;6:96–101.
26. Epstein DL. Pigment dispersion and glaucoma. *Ann Ophthalmol*. 1979;11:917–918.
27. Epstein DL. Pigment dispersion and pigmentary glaucoma. In: Chandler PA, Grant WM, eds. *Glaucoma*. Philadelphia: Lea & Febiger; 1979:122.
28. Epstein DL, Boger WPI, Grant WM. Phenylephrine provocative testing in the pigmentary dispersion syndrome. *Am J Ophthalmol*. 1978;85:43–50.
29. Farrar SM, Shields MB. Current concepts in pigmentary glaucoma. *Surv Ophthalmol*. 1993;37:233–252.

30. Gillies WE. Pigmentary glaucoma: A clinical review of anterior segment pigment dispersal syndrome. *Aust N Z J Ophthalmol*. 1985;13:325–328.

31. Gramer E, Thiele H, Ritch R. Family history and risk factors in pigmentary glaucoma: A clinical study. *Klin Monatsbl Augenheilkd*. 1998;212:454–464.

32. Haynes WL, Alward WLM, McKinney JK, et al. Quantitation of iris transillumination defects in eyes of patients with pigmentary glaucoma. *J Glaucoma*. 1994;3:106–113.

33. Haynes WL, Alward WLM, Thompson HS. Distortion of the pupil in patients with the pigment dispersion syndrome. *J Glaucoma*. 1994;3:329–332.

34. Lehto I. *Pigmentary Glaucoma*. Helsinki, Finland: University of Helsinki; 1993.

35. Murrell WJ, Shihab Z, Lamberts DW, Avera B. The corneal endothelium and central corneal thickness in pigmentary dispersion syndrome. *Arch Ophthalmol*. 1986;104:845–846.

36. Richardson TM. Pigment dispersion syndrome and glaucoma. In: Albert DM, Jakobiec FA, eds. *Clinical Practice: Principles and Practice of Ophthalmology*. Philadelphia: Saunders; 1994:1414.

37. Weseley P, Liebmann J, Walsh JB, Ritch R. Lattice degeneration of the retina and the pigment dispersion syndrome. *Am J Ophthalmol*. 1992;114:539–543.

38. Lichter PR. Pigmentary glaucoma: Current concepts. *Trans Am Acad Ophthalmol Otolaryngol*. 1974;78: OP309–313.

39. Sokol J, Stegman Z, Liebmann JM, Ritch R. Location of the iris insertion in pigment dispersion syndrome. *Ophthalmology*. 1996;103:289–293.

40. Pavlin CJ, Harasiewicz K, Foster FS. Posterior iris bowing in pigmentary dispersion syndrome caused by accommodation. *Am J Ophthalmol*. 1994;118:114–116.

41. Pavlin CJ, Macken P, Trope G, et al. Ultrasound biomicroscopic features of pigmentary glaucoma. *Can J Ophthalmol*. 1994;29:187–192.

42. Pavlin CJ, Macken P, Trope G, et al. Accommodation and iridotomy in the pigment dispersion syndrome. *Ophthalm Surg Lasers*. 1996;27:113–120.

43. Karickhoff JR. Reverse pupillary block in pigmentary glaucoma: Follow up and new developments. *Ophthalm Surg*. 1993;24:562–563.

44. Ritch R, Liebmann J, Tello C, Chew SJ. Ultrasound biomicroscopic findings in pigment dispersion syndrome. In: Krieglstein GK, ed. *Glaucoma Update V*. Heidelberg: Kaden Verlag; 1995:290–298.

45. Potash SD, Tello C, Liebmann J, Ritch R. Ultrasound biomicroscopy in pigment dispersion syndrome. *Ophthalmology*. 1994;101:332–339.

46. Campbell DG. Iridotomy, blinking and pigmentary glaucoma. *Invest Ophthalmol Vis Sci*. 1993;34(suppl):993.

47. Ritch R, Campbell DG, Camras C. Initial treatment of pigmentary glaucoma. *J Glaucoma*. 1993;2:44–49.

48. Ritch R, Liebmann JM, Robin AL, et al. Argon laser trabeculoplasty in pigmentary glaucoma. *Ophthalmology*. 1993;100:909–913.

49. Jampel HD. Lack of effect of peripheral laser iridotomy in pigment dispersion syndrome. *Arch Ophthalmol*. 1993; 111:1606.

50. Fourman S. Iridotomy in eyes with pigmentary glaucoma (letter). *Ophthalm Surg*. 1992;23:843–845.

51. Gandolfi SA, Vecchi M. Effect of a YAG laser iridotomy on intraocular pressure in pigment dispersion syndrome. *Ophthalmology*. 1996;103:1693–1695.

Chapter 27

EXFOLIATION SYNDROME AND EXFOLIATIVE GLAUCOMA*

Robert Ritch
Jeffrey M. Liebmann

HISTORICAL INFORMATION AND TERMINOLOGY

Exfoliation syndrome is presently the most common *identifiable* specific disease entity leading to the development of open-angle glaucoma. In some countries, it comprises a majority of open-angle glaucoma patients. The disorder was first described in 1917 by Lindberg,[1] who noted grayish flecks on the pupillary border in 50% of his patients with chronic glaucoma. Vogt[2] thought that this material originated from the lens capsule and suggested the terms *senile exfoliation* and *glaucoma capsulare*, which remain commonly used in the European literature. Others thought that it was just deposited on the normal lens capsule.[3,4] For the next 30 years, relatively little attention was paid to exfoliation syndrome.

In 1953, Dvorak-Theobald[5] suggested the term *pseudoexfoliation* to distinguish the disorder from the exfoliation found in glassblowers. A number of other terms coined in that period—including *senile uveal exfoliation*,[6] *glaucoma senilis*,[7] *iridociliary exfoliation with capsular pseudoexfoliation*,[8] *exfoliation of the pseudocapsule*,[9] and *complex pigmentary glaucoma*[10]—never gained much acceptance. *Fibrillopathia epitheliocapsularis*, coined by Bertelsen et al.[11] to reflect the histopathological characteristics of exfoliation mater-

ial, has continued to be used occasionally in the Scandinavian literature.

Because of similarity with the ultrastructural appearance and location of basement membrances, Eagle et al., in 1979, suggested the term *basement membrane exfoliation syndrome*.[12] Other authors, based upon their histopathological or histochemical findings, have suggested *exfoliation of the lens capsule*,[13] *oxytalanosis of the aqueous*,[14] and *ocular elastosis*.[15] In 1956, Sunde[16] proposed the term *senile exfoliation syndrome*, which may most accurately reflect the combination of clinical and histopathological findings. Considering the rarity of true exfoliation syndrome at the present time, Layden and Shaffer[17, 18] suggested that the term *exfoliation syndrome* appeared to be the most apt and uncomplicated nomenclature.

Increasing Importance of Accurate Diagnosis

American ophthalmologists historically have put little emphasis on making an accurate diagnosis of exfoliation syndrome. Reasons for this include the assumption that it is a disease found primarily in Scandinavia and northern Europe and that, since the

---

*Supported in part by the New York Glaucoma Research Institute, New York, NY.

associated glaucoma is treated identically to primary open-angle glaucoma, it is unimportant to differentiate it. The former point, as we shall see, has been a serious misconception, while the latter, although formerly true, is becoming less accurate at present and will eventually become antiquated. New insights in recent years have increased the importance of correct diagnosis. Exfoliation syndrome is a common cause of glaucoma in virtually every country in the world. It has been shown to be a systemic disease, found in many organs throughout the body, but because of its visibility in the eye and the fact that it causes glaucoma, it happened to have been recognized there first. Glaucomatous damage in eyes with exfoliation syndrome tends to be more severe than that in primary open-angle glaucoma. Exfoliation syndrome may now be diagnosed prior to the clinically visible classic appearance of exfoliation material on the lens surface, and signs other than this classic appearance can serve as clues to diagnosis. Finally, new understanding of pathophysiological mechanisms should lead to new approaches to treatment and, eventually, prevention.

EPIDEMIOLOGIC OVERVIEW

Frequency in the General Population

Exfoliation syndrome occurs worldwide, although reported prevalence rates vary extensively. Reasons for this variation reflect a combination of true differences in prevalence on the basis of racial, ethnic, or other as yet unknown factors, the age and sex distribution of the patient cohort or population group examined, the clinical criteria used for making a diagnosis of exfoliation syndrome, the ability of the examiner to detect early stages and/or more subtle manifestations of the disorder, and the thoroughness of examination. In particular, many cases go undetected because of failure to dilate the pupil and to examine the lens with the slit lamp after dilation and because of a low index of suspicion on the part of the examiner.[18,19]

Studies on exfoliation syndrome have been conducted on diverse populations, which have included the general population, persons over age 40, persons over age 60, general medical clinic patients, ophthalmic clinic patients, patients with cataracts, glaucoma patients, hospitalized glaucoma patients, and glaucoma patients undergoing surgery. These differences have led to a great deal of confusion in the literature and should be taken into account in comparing one series to another.

For reviews of the epidemiological literature pertaining to exfoliation syndrome, the reader is referred to previous publications.[20-22] What stands out is that, from one examiner to another, the prevalence rates in a single country often vary threefold or more. In Scandinavia, the highest prevalence rates (in studies of persons over age 60) have been reported from Iceland (about 25%)[23,24] and Finland (over 20%).[24-26] Rates in Norway and Sweden average about one-third of those in Iceland and Finland, and those in Denmark are significantly less.

The most significant comparisons are those made among different populations by the same observer. Aasved[27] examined persons over age 60 in nursing homes in Norway, England, and Germany and found prevalences of 6.3, 4.0, and 4.7%, respectively. Forsius[24] looked at a wide variety of ethnic groups, including Lapps, Eskimos, Icelanders, Peruvian Indians, and Tunisians. The prevalence of exfoliation syndrome in persons over age 60 ranged from 0% in Greenland Eskimos to 21% in Icelanders. Forsius proposed that genetic isolation may be responsible for the high incidences of disease in countries such as Iceland and Finland. In a study in Siberia, Lantukh and Pyatin[28] found a low prevalence in the native Tchutchee but a much higher rate among immigrants to the area.

The prevalence in the United States has generally been reported to be similar to that in western Europe. In the Framingham Eye Study, prevalence rates for persons not specifically identified as having glaucoma rose from 0.6% for ages 52 to 64 to 5.0% for ages 75 to 85.[29,30] Cashwell and Shields[31,32] have found lower figures in Caucasian populations in the southern United States. In a screening of 2121 people, exfoliation syndrome was present in only 1.6% of nonglaucomatous persons over age 60.[31,32] American blacks have a much lower prevalence than do whites.[31-34]

The prevalence of exfoliation syndrome may also vary within countries in similar environments and over short distances. In France, the overall prevalence in persons over age 70 is about 5.5%, ranging from 20.6% in Brest to 3.6% in Toulon.[35,36] Ringvold et al.[37] found prevalence rates of 10.2, 19.6, and 21.0% in three closely situated municipalities in central Norway.

The reasons underlying true variation in prevalence rates both from one population to another and within more or less homogeneous populations remain to be explained. Some authors have suggested a correlation between the prevalence of exfoliation syndrome and exposure to sunlight. For example, among Australian aborigines, Taylor[38] found exfoliation syndrome to be more common among those living farther north, which correlated positively with the annual total global radiation level. Exfoliation syndrome was associated positively with the occurrence of cataract and with climatic droplet keratopathy. Taylor suggested that senile cataracts are related to the amount of ultraviolet radiation and that exfoliation syndrome is related to global radiation. However, Heriot et al.[39] screened 986 Polynesian Maori in Raratonga, which has the same latitude and climate, and found exfoliation syndrome in only three persons. The authors speculated that the scattering effect of the atmosphere might be dependent on water vapor content and ultraviolet light. Mohammed and Kazmi[40] found a much greater prevalence of exfoliation syndrome in tribes living in mountainous regions of Pakistan than among those living in lowland valleys. Forsius,[24] however, found relatively little in Peruvian Indians living at an altitude of 4000 m.

Genetic factors predisposing to susceptibility have barely begun to be explored. This very intriguing possibility requires further investigation, and meaningful interpretation awaits elucidation of the underlying etiology of the disorder.

Age

The prevalence of exfoliation syndrome increases markedly with age. For instance, in the general population in Norway, it ranges from 1% at age 40 to 7.8% above age 80.[41] Forsius[22] found its incidence to double every decade after age 50. In a Finnish population, exfoliation syndrome was found in 10% of patients aged 60 to 69, 21% of those aged 70 to 79, and 33% of those aged 80 to 89.[25] In a Finnish screening, Rouhiainen and Teräsvirta[42] found exfoliation syndrome in either eye of 8.5% of 65-year-olds and 13.2% of 75-year-olds. In Japan, Iizuka et al.[43] found prevalence rates of 0.7% in persons from ages 50 to 60 and 7.3% in persons over age 80.

The reported prevalence of exfoliation syndrome in older individuals ranges from 0% among Eskimos to as high as 38% in Navaho Indians.[24,44] Taylor et al.[45] found a prevalence of 1.3 to 16% in Australian aborigines, depending on age.

Early onset of exfoliation syndrome has been found in certain population subgroups. In an examination of the earliest signs of exfoliation syndrome, Bartholomew found the onset of what he termed the pregranular stage at about the age of 40 in South African Bantu, with 6.4% of the population being affected in the 30 to 39 age group.[46] Other groups with early onset include Skolt Lapps, Icelanders at Husquik, and Australian aborigines.[20] The youngest reported patient was 22 years of age.[47]

Gender

Women have predominated in some series of exfoliation syndrome without glaucoma.[20,48,49] Others have found equal numbers.[50] Forsius[22] reported that exfoliation syndrome was more common in men in populations with high ultraviolet exposure, including Yugoslavs, Australian aborigines, Peruvian Indians, and Asian Indians. Yalaz and coworkers[51] also found a greater prevalence among men in Turkey.

In some studies, men with exfoliation syndrome appear more likely to develop glaucoma.[43,52–54] Of 100 consecutive patients with exfoliation syndrome, Kozart and Yanoff[55] found a 3:1 ratio of women to men, while 10 of 25 men and 17 of 75 women had elevated intraocular pressure (IOP). Moreno-Montañés et al.[56] found glaucoma in exfoliation syndrome to appear earlier in men and with a higher mean IOP, while more men developed visual field defects than women. However, many studies have found no gender predilection in patients with glaucoma.[20,23,36,42,48,49,57–61]

Heredity

Although familial occurrence of exfoliation syndrome has been described by a number of authors, no clear hereditary pattern has been discerned. Aasved[62] studied 203 individuals over age 40 in the families of 25 probands and found exfoliation syndrome in 19 persons (9.4%), as opposed to 1% of persons over age 40 in the general population. He suggested that exfoliation syndrome may occur as a dominant trait. Ringvold et al.[37] found two homozygous twin pairs discordant for exfoliation syndrome, while Teikari et al.[63] found two pairs concordant and three discordant. Exfoliation syndrome is so common that it is difficult to draw conclusions and, because it develops in older patients, multiple affected family members are difficult to find. The possibility of both exfoliation and primary open-angle glaucoma occurring in the same pedigree further confuses the issue.

Exfoliation Syndrome in Glaucoma Populations

The prevalence of exfoliation syndrome in glaucoma cohorts, primarily those with open-angle glaucoma, is significantly higher than in age-matched nonglaucomatous populations. Reported prevalence rates vary according to author and population studied, ranging from practically zero to as high as 93%.[18,20,32,41,49,55,58,64,65] Forsius[22] has provided an extensive list of references in this regard. The highest rates again are in Scandinavia. In the middle Norway eye-screening study, 60% of glaucoma patients had exfoliation syndrome.[66] In Denmark, which has the lowest ratios in Scandinavia and where exfoliation syndrome was actually thought rare until the late 1970s, Ohrt and Nehen[67] found it in 26% of open-angle glaucoma patients.

A high incidence of exfoliation syndrome in open-angle glaucoma populations has also been reported from other European countries. Clements[68] found 55% overall and 74% of the glaucoma in men in the Isle of Man, significantly higher than the comparable figures in mainland England. In Ireland, Madden and Crowley[52] found two-thirds of their open-angle glaucoma patients to have exfoliation syndrome. In northwest Spain, Moreno-Montañés et al.[50] found 44.5% of their open-angle glaucoma patients and 59.6% of eyes with both glaucoma and cataract to have exfoliation syndrome. In Hungary, where exfoliation syndrome has until recently been thought rare, Sziklai and Süveges[53] found 38.4% of 403 glaucoma surgical inpatients affected.

The proportion of patients with exfoliation syndrome reported in glaucoma cohorts is increasing in other areas where it had been thought rare. As examples, among 1623 new glaucoma patients in Japan, Futa et al.[69] found 16.2% to have exfoliation and 16.5% to have primary open-angle glaucoma. In India, Sood and Ratnaraj found 34% of patients with glaucoma to have exfoliation syndrome.[70] In South Africa, Luntz[71] found 20% in Bantu and only 1.4% in whites. Interestingly, in a series of 37 patients with glaucoma in Papua-New Guinea, 18 were traumatic, 5 had exfoliation syndrome, and none had primary open-angle glaucoma.[72]

Once thought to be uncommon in the United States, exfoliation syndrome is now recognized as the most common secondary open-angle glaucoma, despite varying reported rates of prevalence. Three series have reported a prevalence of 12% in glaucoma populations.[19,73,74] Kozart and Yanoff[55] found 7% with glaucomatous damage. In the southern United States, the prevalence seems to be lower, with involvement in blacks less common than in whites. In Louisiana, a screening of 500 consecutive open-angle glaucoma patients revealed an overall prevalence of 1.4%, with 2.7% of whites being affected but only 0.4% of blacks.[33] Similar figures have been found in North Carolina.[31,32,75]

Glaucoma in Eyes with Exfoliation Syndrome

Glaucoma occurs more commonly in eyes with exfoliation syndrome than in those without it. Kozart and Yanoff[55] found glaucomatous optic nerve or visual field damage in 7% and ocular hypertension in 15%. This is approximately six times the chance of finding elevated IOP in eyes without exfoliation syndrome.

Aasved[76] found elevated IOP with or without glaucomatous damage in 22.7% of patients with exfoliation syndrome detected on screening, as opposed to 1.2% of those without the syndrome. In the middle Norway eye-screening study, Ringvold et al.[66] found 30% of eyes with exfoliation syndrome to have elevated IOP with or without glaucoma, as compared to

4.8% of the exfoliation-negative population. In Spain, Moreno-Montañés et al.[50] found elevated IOP in 49% of eyes with exfoliation syndrome, and in Epirus, Stefaniotou and coworkers[77] found 39.5%. Yalaz et al.,[51] in western Turkey, found glaucoma in 34.3% but did not define the criteria for diagnosis of glaucoma. In Japan, Shimizu et al.[78] considered 63% of newly discovered patients with exfoliation syndrome to have glaucoma.

In persons with exfoliation syndrome, the risk of developing glaucoma is cumulative over time. Henry et al.[79] found the 5- and 10-year cumulative probabilities of initially nonglaucomatous eyes with exfoliation syndrome developing glaucoma to be 5.3% ± 0.1% and 15.4% ± 2%, respectively—a significantly higher rate than would be expected in a similar group of patients without exfoliation syndrome. In their population, therefore, exfoliation syndrome patients would have approximately a 40% chance of either having initially or developing ocular hypertension or glaucoma within 10 years, approximately a tenfold increased risk when compared to the general population.

Glaucoma in exfoliation syndrome has a more serious clinical course than primary open-angle glaucoma. Persons with exfoliation syndrome but without glaucoma have a higher mean IOP than those without exfoliation syndrome. In patients with elevated IOP, the mean pressure is higher at the time of detection than it is in primary open-angle glaucoma.[69,76,80–83] Ocular hypertensives with exfoliation syndrome are much more likely to develop glaucomatous damage on long-term follow-up than are those without exfoliation syndrome.[79,84]

Patients with exfoliation syndrome presenting with newly discovered glaucoma have a higher IOP and more severe visual field defects and cupping of the optic nerve head than those with primary open-angle glaucoma, and glaucomatous damage progresses more rapidly in patients with exfoliation syndrome and glaucoma than in those with primary open-angle glaucoma.[69,82–87]

Glaucoma in exfoliation syndrome is more resistant to medical therapy than is primary open-angle glaucoma, responds for a shorter period of time, and fails more often. In addition, the proportion of patients with exfoliation syndrome shows a steady increase when measured in cohorts with open-angle glaucoma without optic nerve damage, in those with damage, in those undergoing surgery, and in those with absolute glaucoma.[59,81] In one series, exfoliation syndrome was present in 16.5% of 103 newly diagnosed glaucoma patients, 54.4% of 90 patients requiring surgical intervention, and 73.8% of patients with absolute glaucoma.[27] In another study, Konstas and Allan[88] found a prevalence of 87.8% of exfoliation syndrome in patients in northern Greece undergoing trabeculectomy for open-angle glaucoma.

CLINICAL FEATURES

Signs Related to Exfoliation Material

Deposits of grayish-white material on the anterior lens surface are the most consistent and important diagnostic feature of exfoliation syndrome (Fig. 27–1 and Table 27–1). The classic pattern consists of three distinct zones: a relatively homogeneous central disc; a granular, often layered peripheral zone, and a clear area separating the two. The edges of the central disc are often rolled anteriorly. The intermediate clear zone is created by rubbing of the iris over the surface of the lens during physiological movement of the pupil. The central disc is absent in about 20% of cases.[18] The peripheral zone is always present. It may be granular in the periphery and frosty white centrally, and radial striations are often seen. The granularity of the peripheral layer is consistent with undisturbed accumulation of exfoliation material. In eyes treated with miotics, the central disc may similarly develop a granular appearance.

Exfoliation material is thought initially to be diffusely deposited on the lens surface. A homogeneous ground-glass or matte appearance to the lens surface in one eye compared to the other may represent a very early (precapsular) stage.[89,90] In perhaps a slightly later stage, there may be a ring of about 80 faint, radial, nongranular striae on the middle third of the anterior capsule behind the iris.[46] Ultrastructurally, the exfoliation material at this stage has been reported to consist of microfibrils but not mature exfoliation fibers.[90] As

the layer of exfoliation material becomes thicker, the iris sphincter region begins to rub against it during normal physiological movement of the pupil. Faint clefts begin to form where exfoliation material is rubbed away in what will eventually become the clear zone. With time, these clefts increase in size and begin to become confluent. Eventually, only small bridges may remain as an indication of the previous layer of exfoliation material in the intermediate zone. In some patients, the central disc may become thick enough to peel away in sheets from the lens, indicating that this is actually an "exfoliation" syndrome. Chronic pupillary dilation also permits undisturbed accumulation of exfoliation material.

In addition to the anterior lens capsule, exfoliation material is most prominent at the pupillary border (Fig. 27–2). It is not invariably present and may be represented only by a tiny dot or two, requiring again a high index of suspicion and a careful search, or it may be extensive. It tends to be most prominent in those eyes maintained on miotic therapy. In some eyes, more prominent excrescences can be seen. Exfoliation material may also be found on the corneal endothelium, in the anterior chamber angle, and on the zonules and ciliary body (Figs. 27–3 and 27–4). After cataract extraction, it may be found on the vitreous face, on vitreous strands when the face is ruptured, on the posterior capsule, and on intraocular lenses, indicating that the presence of the lens is unnecessary for its continued formation (Fig. 27–5).[91–96]

Exfoliation material may be detected earliest on the ciliary body and zonules. Cycloscopy in patients

TABLE 27–1. **SIGNS RELATED TO EXFOLIATION SYNDROME**

A. Diagnostic signs
   1. Exfoliation material on lens surface
   2. Exfoliation material on pupillary border
   3. Exfoliation material elsewhere (never recorded as a sole observation in the absence of signs 1 or 2 above)
B. Suggestive signs
   1. Pigment-related signs
     a. Loss of pupillary ruff
     b. Iris sphincter region transillumination
     c. Pigment whorl on iris surface at sphincter
     d. Pigment dispersion in anterior chamber after dilation in older patient
     e. Heavy pigmentation of trabecular meshwork in older patient
   2. Other alerting signs
     a. Phacodonesis in absence of trauma in older patient
     b. Posterior lens subluxation in older patient
     c. Intraocular pressure rise after pharmacological dilation
     d. Marked asymmetry of intraocular pressure (< 33%) in the absence of other obvious causes in an older patient

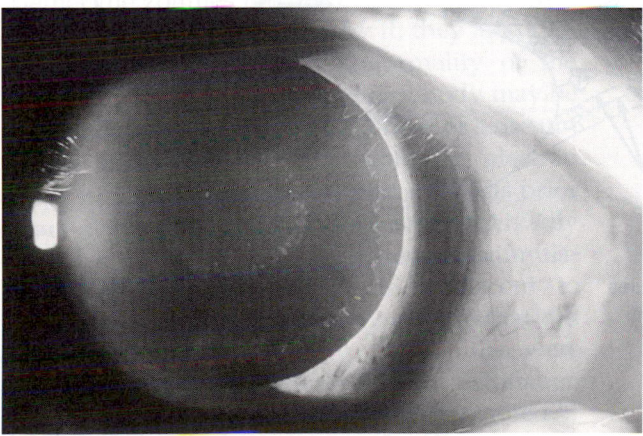

Figure 27–1. The classic appearence of the lens in an eye with exfoliation syndrome. The central gray zone, intermediate clear zone, and peripheral granular zone are visible. (*See also Color Plate 87.*)

is deposited on the iris surface peripherally, it is scattered relatively evenly over the iris, in contrast to its collection in iris furrows in pigment dispersion syndrome. There is often a small amount of pigment inferiorly on the corneal endothelium. Occasionally, a Krukenberg spindle may be present.

The most important signs are defects of the pupillary ruff and a moth-eaten pattern of transillumination defects in the sphincter region. Very little attention has been paid to the role of the pupillary ruff in the pathophysiology of glaucoma; on clinical examination, it is usually noted just in passing if at all.

Ruff defects occur in 12% of normal eyes between ages 45 and 49 and in 56% above age 80.[117] Aasved[118] found ruff defects in 6.1% of eyes without exfoliation syndrome (3.4% in the sixth decade and 40.5% over age 80) and in 74% of eyes with exfoliation syndrome (42% in the sixth decade and 90% over age 80). In patients with unilateral involvement, defects were twice as frequent in the involved eye. In 68 eyes with exfoliation material at the pupillary border, defects in the ruff occurred in 82%.[118] The eyes with exfoliation syndrome accounted for 7.3% of the total number of eyes with defects and 0.8% of the total eyes in the series. Ruff abnormalities are most striking in patients with unilateral involvement.

Transillumination defects occur at the pupillary ruff and margin, in contrast to the midstromal slit-like transillumination defects found in pigment dispersion syndrome.[118] However, if extensive depigmentation has occurred, defects may be noted over the entire sphincter region. Generalized peripheral iris transillumination, which appears as a diffuse "starry-sky" appearance of the defects, has also been associated with exfoliation syndrome.[119]

Pigment dispersion in the anterior chamber is common after pupillary dilation in eyes with exfoliation syndrome and may be profuse.[116] Tarkkanen[20] found pigment dispersion only in eyes with exfoliation syndrome. Marked IOP rises can occur in these eyes after pharmacological dilation. In those studies that examined a correlation between the degree of pressure rise and amount of pigment liberated into the anterior chamber, it has been positive. Krause et al.[120] noted the pigment in the anterior chamber to be maximal at 1 to 2 hours after mydriasis and to disappear in 12 to 24 hours. Rises in intraocular pressure usually reach a maximum after 2 hours.[121] In some patients, however, we have found that IOP may begin to rise only after 3 to 4 hours after dilation (unpublished data). Since IOP is rarely measured at this late a time, possible further glaucomatous damage in compromised eyes may occur. We have seen one patient whose IOP was normal 1 hour after dilation return

the following morning with an open angle, pigment in the anterior chamber, IOP of 55 mmHg, and a central retinal vein occlusion.

Increased trabecular meshwork pigmentation is a prominent sign of exfoliation syndrome and is apparent in virtually all patients with clinically evident disease. Unlike the case in pigment dispersion syndrome, the distribution of the pigment tends to be uneven or splotchy and less well defined. It may be an early diagnostic finding preceding the appearance of exfoliation material on the pupillary margin or anterior lens capsule.[115,116]

In virtually all studies of patients with unilateral involvement, the trabecular pigment is almost always denser in the involved eye. All 76 patients with exfoliation syndrome in the series of Wishart et al. had increased trabecular pigmentation, and 84% had more advanced glaucomatous damage on the side with the heavier pigmentation.[122] When the pigment was markedly asymmetrical, unilateral exfoliation syndrome with glaucoma was common in the more pigmented eye, and no patient had less pigmentation in the eye with greater glaucomatous damage. Mayer et al.[101] documented similar findings. In a prospective study, Moreno-Montañés et al.[123] found a highly significant correlation between elevated IOP and the degree of pigmentation of the trabecular meshwork. The IOP was greater in the eye with more pigment in all persons, and the greater the difference, the greater the difference in IOP.

Heavy angle pigment in the absence of exfoliation is often present in the fellow eye of patients with clinically unilateral exfoliation syndrome. Conjunctival biopsy of these fellow eyes consistently shows the presence of deposits of exfoliation material.[115]

Pigment is characteristically deposited on Schwalbe's line and sometimes as a wavy line or lines anterior to Schwalbe's line (Sampaolesi line).[124–126] This, too, is an early sign of exfoliation syndrome.

Asymmetry of Involvement

A review of the literature comparing the frequency of monocular versus binocular involvement in various series is particularly confusing. Many recent series have reported bilateral involvement to be more common, with ratios as high as 3:1.[36,43,46,50,52,57,77] Other series, including most American ones, have reported unilateral involvement to predominate, again with ratios as high as 3:1.

When only one eye is involved, the fellow eye often has abnormal aqueous humor dynamics or glaucomatous damage, which, when it is present, is almost always less marked than in the involved eye. In the series of Futa et al.,[69] 73.9% of patients had unilateral exfoliation, but 38.9% of the fellow eyes had abnormalities related to glaucoma. Tarkkanen[20] found that patients with unilateral exfoliation syndrome and glaucoma were most commonly males, frequently myopes, and had a family history of glaucoma, marked pigmentary changes, as well as a high initial IOP as opposed to bilateral cases. Patients with bilateral exfoliation syndrome tend to be slightly older than those with unilateral exfoliation syndrome, but the age difference is often small.[20,30,55]

Unilateral involvement is often a precursor to bilateral involvement. Although Tarkkanen[20] described unchanged unilateral occurrence in 47 patients followed for 5 years, Hansen and Sellevold[127] found exfoliation to develop in the second eye in 40% of men and 31% of women over 5 years. Aasved[59] found that 43% developed binocular involvement after 6 or 7 years. Slagsvold[128] found 30% of persons to develop bilateral exfoliation syndrome over a minimum follow-up time of 5 years, but only 2.9% of patients followed had developed glaucoma. He interpreted these data as consistent with the concept that glaucoma is most likely to develop at the time of or shortly after the appearance of exfoliation syndrome. Others had noted similar findings.[20,76,129] In a prospective retrospective study, Henry et al.[79] found the probability of exfoliation developing in the opposite eye to be 6.8% after 5 years and 16.8% after 10 years.

The terms *unilateral* and *monocular* are actually misleading. Since early pigment-related signs of exfoliation syndrome are found in the majority of unaffected fellow eyes and since exfoliation material may be detected on conjunctival biopsy in virtually all unaffected fellow eyes, these cases are actually asymmetrical. However, since these terms have been used for so long a time, they are retained here specifically to describe those patients who have clinically visible exfoliation material in only one eye on slit-lamp examination, with the understanding that both eyes are actually affected by the process.

Ocular Associations

Cataract

Although not well described, there appears to be an association between exfoliation syndrome and cataract formation.[7,18-20,38,51,57,87,101,114,130-136] There is an increased prevalence of exfoliation syndrome in eyes coming to cataract surgery and an increased prevalence of cataracts in eyes with exfoliation syndrome. Histopathological examination of lenses after cataract extraction supports the idea that exfoliation syndrome is underdiagnosed. Krause and Tarkkanen[137] examined 100 lenses of 98 patients and found

exfoliation syndrome in 33%. Preoperatively, only one-half of these patients had been diagnosed as having the disease.

Patients with exfoliation syndrome are much more prone than patients without to have complications at the time of cataract extraction.[98,100,108,133,138-144] Patients with exfoliation syndrome dilate less well; there also are greater incidences of capsular rupture and vitreous loss. Guzek et al.[100] found pupil size to be the most important risk factor for vitreous loss. Zonular damage accounts for much of the increased complication rate. Zonular fragility increases the risk of lens dislocation or zonular dialysis up to 10 times.[109,141,144-147]

Systemic Associations

Exfoliation material has been found histopathologically in structures outside the anterior segment in the eye and orbit. Most of this work has been quite recent. In 1973, Ringvold[148] found exfoliation material in the palpebral conjunctiva. In 1979, Eagle et al.[12] found typical exfoliation material in the wall of a short posterior ciliary artery, indicating that the disease was not limited entirely to the eye itself. In 1991, the Erlangen group reported finding it in the rectus and oblique muscles, vortex veins, optic nerve sheaths, orbital connective tissue septa, walls of posterior ciliary arteries, vortex veins, and central retinal vessels.[149]

More recently, exfoliation syndrome has been conclusively shown to be a systemic disorder with clinical manifestations thus far limited to the eye. In 1990, Sugino[150] described typical exfoliation material in the dermis of the skin of the lateral canthus in 3 of 9 patients and microfibrils indicating the immature form of exfoliation material, but not mature fibrils, in the other 6. Streeten et al.[151] reported exfoliative material in skin biopsies from various areas to occur primarily along elastic fibers. These authors suggested that exfoliation syndrome is a systemic process closely related to elastosis.

In 1992, Schlötzer-Schrehardt et al.[152] and Streeten et al.[153] reported finding exfoliation material in a number of organs in patients coming to autopsy, including skin, myocardium, lung, liver, gallbladder, kidney, and cerebral meninges. The exfoliation material was localized mainly to connective-tissue portions or septa and consistently associated with connective-tissue components.

No clear-cut association of exfoliation with any systemic disease has yet been shown. There does not seem to be any correlation with diabetes mellitus, cardiovascular disease, or hypertension. Several authors have described patients with both primary familial amyloidosis and exfoliation based upon the clinical and ultrastructural appearances.[154–157] However, this material has not been shown to be identical to that in exfoliation syndrome. Tsukahara and Matsuo.[155] felt that there were differences ultrastructurally, and Futa et al.[156] noted clinical differences. What should be regarded as significant here is that a fibrillar material that is secreted, deposited, or polymerized on the lens surface develops into an anatomic pattern determined by relationships between the lens, iris, and aqueous currents. This may be indirect evidence for the possibility of the existence of subtypes of exfoliation syndrome.

Exfoliation Syndrome "Suspects"

As mentioned above, in patients with "unilateral" exfoliation syndrome, conjunctival biopsy of the fellow eye invariably contains deposits of exfoliation material. Exfoliation suspects were initially defined as patients in whom one or both eyes exhibited one or more of five signs related to loss of pigment from the iris pigment epithelium in the absence of clinically identifiable exfoliation material on the anterior lens capsule or pupillary margin in either eye. These signs were (1) loss of the pigment ruff, (2) particulate pigment dotting of the iris surface at the sphincter region, (3) juxtapupillary and sphincter region iris transillumination defects, (4) pigment dispersion in the anterior chamber after pupillary dilation, and (5) moderate or dense pigment deposition on the trabecular meshwork.

Inferior bulbar conjunctival biopsies were performed on 4 eyes with exfoliation syndrome, 5 fellow eyes, and 23 eyes of 15 exfoliation syndrome suspects.[115] The exfoliation syndrome suspects had previously been diagnosed to have either primary open-angle glaucoma or ocular hypertension. Specimens were examined by transmission electron microscopy. Exfoliation material was demonstrated in 8 suspect eyes, suggesting that it may be etiologically significant in the development of elevated IOP before it is clinically evident on biomicroscopy. There was a positive correlation between the degree of severity of pigment-related signs and biopsy results.[115] These findings implicate exfoliation syndrome as being even more common than previously recognized and responsible for a greater proportion of glaucoma than previously suspected.

In a related study, exfoliation material in the conjunctiva was found to be frequently in close proximity to stromal fibroblasts and closely associated with clumps of oxytalan and around small elastic fibers, suggesting that exfoliation syndrome itself is a type of elastosis, possibly resulting from abnormal aggregation of components related to elastic microfibrils.[15]

MECHANISMS OF GLAUCOMA IN EXFOLIATION SYNDROME

Open-Angle Glaucoma

Glaucoma associated with exfoliation syndrome has been almost universally reported as occurring in the presence of an open anterior chamber angle and an anterior chamber of normal depth.[18,20,76,158,159] There has been a great deal of argument as to whether the exfoliation material or pigment particles block aqueous humor outflow and lead to elevated IOP.

The presence of exfoliation material per se in the trabecular meshwork is insufficient cause, as extensive deposits may be found in the presence of a normal IOP.[160] Furthermore, many patients with exfoliation syndrome never develop elevated IOP. Richardson and Epstein[161] found the inner meshwork to be free of exfoliation material and the main pathology to involve destruction of Schlemm's canal and the accumulation of material in the juxtacanalicular region. However, these ultrastructural studies were done after perfusion, and particulate material could have been washed out. Sampaolesi et al.[125] reported that, while in pigmentary glaucoma the pigment is located throughout the trabecular meshwork, extending to the back wall of Schlemm's canal and the collector channels, the pigment particles in exfoliation syndrome, being larger and stickier, are restricted to the inner meshwork.

The most likely mechanism would appear to be blockage by a combination of exfoliation material and pigment granules and/or induced damage to the trabecular cells. The exfoliation material in the trabecular meshwork, being highly adhesive, could enmesh pigment particles and the two combined reduce aqueous outflow. To our knowledge, there have been no histological studies attempting to correlate the amount of exfoliation material in the trabecular meshwork with the density of pigment in the meshwork.

Patients with unilateral exfoliation syndrome and open angles may also have glaucoma in the fellow eye, suggesting an underlying defect in aqueous humor dynamics.[19,20,162] However, trabecular pigmentation is generally increased in these eyes as well, and exfoliation material is almost universally present on conjunctival biopsy. The finding that exfoliation material may be found in the conjunctiva in eyes with increased trabecular pigmentation in the absence of clinically visible exfoliation material on the lens of either eye provides further support.[115]

TREATMENT

The stepwise approach to the management of the patient with exfoliation syndrome is similar to that for primary open-angle glaucoma and includes beta-adrenergic antagonists, alpha-adrenergic agonists, miotics, carbonic anhydrase inhibitors, prostaglandin analogues, and laser and intraocular surgery. Response to these interventions however, differs from that of patients with primary open-angle glaucoma.

Medical Therapy

Glaucoma associated with exfoliation syndrome tends to respond less well to medical therapy than primary open-angle glaucoma, to be more difficult to treat, to require surgical intervention more commonly, and to have a worse prognosis.[18]

Cholinergic agents are effective and probably have a greater additive effect with beta blockers in exfoliation syndrome than in primary open-angle glaucoma.[163] Miotics, however, have multiple beneficial actions in eyes with exfoliation syndrome. Not only do they lower IOP but, by increasing aqueous outflow, they should enable the trabecular meshwork to clear more rapidly, and by limiting pupillary movement, they should slow the progression of the disease. Aqueous suppressants, on the other hand, by decreasing aqueous secretion, result in decreased aqueous flow through the trabecular meshwork. Becker[164] has presented suggestive evidence that treatment with aqueous suppressants leads to worsening of trabecular function. In organ culture, reduced perfusion results in failure of the meshwork to survive.[165] Continued administration of oral acetazolamide produced a reduction in outflow facility and an elevation of IOP to greater than baseline after discontinuation.[164]

Theoretically, miotics should be the first line of treatment. However, many patients have nuclear sclerosis and, in them, miotics may reduce visual acuity or dim vision sufficiently to create difficulty. The long-term use of miotics may lead to the development of posterior synechiae. The incidence of significant pigment release into the anterior chamber, worsened by the use of miotics,[166] is particularly hazardous in exfoliation syndrome. Pilocarpine Ocuserts can achieve excellent reduction of pupillary movement while often maintaining a 3- to 4-mm pupil and are well tolerated by many elderly patients. In one study, 2% pilocarpine drops were significantly less effective in exfoliative glaucoma than in primary open-angle glaucoma and had a shorter duration of action, while no differences were found using P-40 Ocuserts.[167]

Elevated IOP in eyes with exfoliation syndrome responds less favorably to timolol therapy than in those with primary open-angle glaucoma.[168] Dorzolamide is almost as effective as timolol and is also additive with it.[169] Some authors have reported good pressure-lowering effects,[170] whereas others have noted a poorer response in these patients versus those with primary open-angle glaucoma.[83] A greater additive effect of epinephrine with timolol has been reported in exfoliation syndrome than in primary open-angle glaucoma.[170] Prostaglandin analogues are also effective for IOP reduction in this disorder.

Laser Surgery

Argon laser trabeculoplasty (ALT) is particularly effective, at least early on, in eyes with exfoliation syndrome.[171] The baseline IOP is usually higher than in eyes with primary open-angle glaucoma undergoing ALT and the initial drop in IOP is greater.[172] Successful lowering of IOP at 1 year has been reported in 68 to 100% of patients,[173,174] with an average decrease of 10.7 mmHg.[175] This number is higher than that found in a comparable group of primary open-angle glaucoma patients.[176] This increased effectiveness may be related to the increased trabecular meshwork pigmentation found in exfoliation syndrome.[177] Long-term success, however, drops to approximately 35 to 45% at 4 to 5 years.[178]

Approximately 20% of patients develop sudden, late rises of IOP within the first 2 years after treatment.[179] Continued pigment liberation may overwhelm the restored functional capacity of the trabecular meshwork, and maintenance miotic therapy to minimize papillary movement after ALT might counteract this. Spaeth and Baez[180] reported a 50% failure rate at 1 year, compared with a 19% rate in primary open-angle glaucoma. Prior to the development of apraclonidine, rises in IOP of greater than 10 mmHg were noted to occur in 8 to 20% of patients.[173,174]

Laser iridotomy is the procedure of choice for angle-closure glaucoma. Angle-closure glaucoma caused by anterior lens movement or subluxation may not be cured by iridotomy alone and may require argon laser peripheral iridoplasty to mechanically pull the iris away from the trabecular meshwork.[172]

Glaucoma Surgery

The results of trabeculectomy are comparable to those in primary open-angle glaucoma, but surgical complications are more common. Markedly elevated preoperative IOP may predispose to choroidal hemorrhage or effusion. Weakened zonular support may allow marked intraoperative anterior lens movement or subluxation, leading to inadvertent lens damage during iridectomy, vitreous loss, or late incarceration of vitreous into the internal ostium. Previously undetected iris neovascularization may lead to intraoperative or delayed hyphema from the surgical iridectomy. These complications probably occur with greater frequency in patients whose disease is more advanced or of longer duration.[181]

Trabeculotomy, performed with the rationale that it may bypass mechanical blockage of the trabecular meshwork, has been reported to be successful.[182] More recently, Tanihara et al.[183] looked prospectively at the effect of trabeculotomy as a primary procedure (none had had ALT), reporting success rates of 79% at 3 years and 64% at 5 years, with medication. The higher the initial IOP, the less likelihood for success. Along similar lines of reasoning, Jacobi and Krieglstein[184,185] have presented a procedure, termed *trabecular aspiration*, designed to improve outflow facility.[184] In 12 patients with medically uncontrolled IOP undergoing trabecular aspiration as a primary procedure, mean IOP of 37.4 mmHg was reduced to a mean of 18.3 mmHg 15 months after surgery, with reduced medications.[185]

Cataract Surgery

Patients with exfoliation syndrome are elderly and often have coexisting cataract.[114] The two proven risk factors for vitreous loss are exfoliation syndrome and insufficient mydriasis.[100] Poor dilation is common in exfoliation syndrome.[141] Zonular fragility increases the risk of lens dislocation or zonular dialysis up to 10 times.[109,141,144-147] Vitreous loss has been reported to be five times more common than in normal patients (9.0 versus 1.8%).[143] This is related to an increased incidence of zonular dialyses, lens dislocation, and capsular rupture.[100] Although the posterior capsule is of normal thickness in exfoliation syndrome,[11] capsular rupture is more common and has been reported to occur in 27% of exfoliation syndrome eyes as compared with 2% of control eyes.[145] This may be related to a degenerate capsule[98,99] or excessive "stickiness" of the remaining cortical material and increased difficulty in irrigation and aspiration.[186] A Flieringa ring may decrease the incidence of vitreous loss.[143]

Posterior synechialysis or lysis of more peripheral iridocapsular adhesions and pupillary enlargement may be necessary. Because of chronic sphincter fibrosis, it is advisable not to enlarge the pupil as much as possible, since it often will remain dilated, predisposing to pupillary capture. Avoidance of mechanical pressure on the lens is important, and the nucleus should be freely rotatable after hydrodissection. An endocapsular fixation ring may be useful in preventing collapse of the capsular bag in areas of weakened zonules. Spontaneous lens displacement, which may not be visible preoperatively, may worsen considerably upon entering the eye or beginning anterior capsulorrhexis.[141] The presence of subtle iridodonesis or phacodonesis indicates loose or ruptured zonules.[141] Cryoextraction is useful for subluxed or dislocated lenses.[100]

The choice of intraocular lens (IOL) is also important in eyes with exfoliation syndrome. Heparin-surface-modified posterior chamber intraocular lenses (PCIOLs) were found to result in fewer postoperative fibrinoid reactions, less frequent pigment and cellular deposits on the lenses, and a lower incidence of posterior synechia formation than regular polymethylmethacrylate (PMMA) lenses.[187] Lens decentration is more common even when the lens is entirely in the capsular bag, primarily due to decentration of the entire bag.[188] Subluxation of the IOL can occur if the zonules break or the capsular bag dislocates.[140] Posterior chamber lenses may be implanted in the ciliary sulcus despite the presence of a small capsular break or area of zonular dehiscence provided that enough support still exists for the implant.[141]

Postoperatively, these patients are at greater risk for developing an immediate elevation of IOP.[189] All viscoelastic should be removed from the eye at the time of surgery. Patients with extensive visual field loss or severe glaucomatous optic atrophy should have tonometry performed 4 to 6 hours after surgery and any acute rise in IOP treated.[190] Postoperative breakdown of the blood-aqueous barrier is higher in eyes with exfoliation syndrome.[191] Inflammation is more common in eyes with exfoliation syndrome, and a transitory fibrinoid reaction may occur.[109,192-196] A giant-cell reaction has been associated with the presence of exfoliation syndrome.[197] Long-term protein deposition on IOLs appears to be more common in eyes with exfoliation syndrome; we prefer to maintain these patients indefinitely on a topical steroid, such as prednisolone acetate, three times weekly.

The management of glaucoma after cataract surgery usually requires the continued use of antiglaucoma medications. Raitta and Setälä[140] reported good success in controlling IOPs after extracapsular cataract extraction with posterior chamber intraocular lenses in patients who had been controlled preoperatively. Cataract surgery does not seem to shorten the duration of clinical response to prior ALT.[189] Combined cataract and glaucoma surgery decreases the incidence of an acute postoperative rise in IOP[198] and may improve long-term control of IOP.

REFERENCES

1. Lindberg JG. Kliniska undersokningar over depigmentering av pupillarranden och genomlysbarket av iris vid fall av alderstarr samit i normala ogon hos gamla personer (Clinical studies of depigmentation of the pupillary margin and transillumination of the iris in cases of senile cataract and also in normal eyes in the aged) [MD]. Helsingfors, 1917.

2. Vogt A. Ein neues Spaltlampenbild des Pupillengebietes: Hellblauer Pupillensaumfilz mit Hautchenbildung auf der Linsenvorderkapsel. *Klin Monatsbl Augenheilkd.* 1925;75:1–12.

3. Malling B. Untersuchungen über das Verhaltnis zwischen Iridocyclitis und Glaukom. *Acta Ophthalmol.* 1923; 1:97–130.

4. Busacca A. Struktur und Bedeutung der Hautchennieder-Schlaze in der vorderen und hinteren Augenkammer. *Graefes Arch Klin Exp Ophthalmol.* 1927;119: 135–153.

5. Dvorak-Theobald G. Pseudoexfoliation of the lens capsule: Relation to "true" exfoliation of the lens capsule as reported in the literature and role in the production of glaucoma capsulocuticulare. *Am J Ophthalmol.* 1954; 37:1–12.

6. Weekers L, Weekers R, Denjaid J. Pathogénie du glaucome "capsulaire." *Doc Ophthalmol.* 1951;5/6:555–567.

7. Wilson RP. Capsular exfoliation and glaucoma capsulare. *Trans Ophthalmol Soc N Z.* 1953;7:8–21.

8. Audibert J. Cited in Tarkkanen A: Pseudoexfoliation of the lens capsule. *Acta Ophthalmol.* 1962;71(suppl):1–98.

9. Jones B. Cited in Tarkkanen A: Pseudoexfoliation of the lens capsule. *Acta Ophthalmol.* 1962;71(suppl):1–98.

10. Simon Tor JM. Glaucoma pigmentario complexus. *Arch Soc Ophthalmol Hisp Am.* 1961;21:121–154.

11. Bertelsen TI, Drablos PA, Flood PR. The so-called senile exfoliation (pseudoexfoliation) of the anterior lens capsule, a product of the lens epithelium: Fibrillopathia epitheliocapsularis. *Acta Ophthalmol.* 1964;42: 1096–1113.

12. Eagle RC Jr, Font RL, Fine BS. The basement membrane exfoliation syndrome. *Arch Ophthalmol.* 1979;97: 510–515.

13. Bergmanson JPG, Jones WL, Chu WF. Ultrastructural observations on (pseudo-) exfoliation of the lens capsule: A re-examination of the involvement of the lens epithelium. *Br J Ophthalmol.* 1984;68:118–123.

14. Garner A, Alexander RA. Pseudoexfoliative disease: Histochemical evidence of an affinity with zonular fibers. *Br J Ophthalmol.* 1984;68:574–580.

15. Streeten BW, Bookman L, Ritch R, et al. Pseudoexfoliative fibrillopathy in the conjunctiva: A relation to elastic fibers and elastosis. *Ophthalmology.* 1987;94:1439–1449.

16. Sunde OA. Senile exfoliation of the anterior lens capsule. *Acta Ophthalmol.* 1956;45(suppl):7–85.

17. Layden WE. Exfoliation syndrome. In: Ritch R, Shields MB, ed. *The Secondary Glaucomas.* St Louis: CV Mosby, 1982:99–120.

18. Layden WE, Shaffer RN. Exfoliation syndrome. *Am J Ophthalmol.* 1974;78:835–841.

19. Roth M, Epstein DL. Exfoliation syndrome. *Am J Ophthalmol.* 1980;89:477–486.

20. Tarkkanen A. Pseudoexfoliation of the lens capsule. *Acta Ophthalmol.* 1962;71(suppl):1–98.

21. Dell WM. The epidemiology of the pseudo-exfoliation syndrome. *J Am Optom Assoc.* 1985;56:113–127.

22. Forsius H. Exfoliation syndrome in various ethnic populations. *Acta Ophthalmol.* 1988;66(suppl 184):71–85.

23. Sveinsson D. The frequency of senile exfoliation in Iceland. *Acta Ophthalmol.* 1974;52:596–602.

24. Forsius H. Prevalence of pseudoexfoliation of the lens in Finns, Lapps, Icelanders, Eskimos, and Russians. *Trans Ophthalmol Soc UK.* 1979;99:296–298.

25. Krause U. Frequency of capsular glaucoma in central Finland. *Acta Ophthalmol.* 1973;51:235–240.

26. Krause U, Alanko HI, Kärmä J, et al. Prevalence of exfoliation syndrome in Finland. *Acta Ophthalmol.* 1988; 66(suppl 184):120–122.

27. Aasved H. Prevalence of fibrillopathia epitheliocapsularis (pseudoexfoliation) and capsular glaucoma. *Trans Ophthalmol Soc UK.* 1979;99:293–295.

28. Lantukh VV, Pyatin MM. Characteristics of the ocular pathology in the aborigines of the Chukot Peninsula. *Vestn Oftalmol.* 1982;4:18–20.

29. Liebowitz HM, Krueger DE, Maunder LR. The Framingham eye study monograph. *Surv Ophthalmol.* 1980;24(suppl):335–610.

30. Hiller R, Sperduto RD, Krueger DE. Pseudoexfoliation, intraocular pressure, and senile lens changes in a population based survey. *Arch Ophthalmol.* 1982;100: 1080–1082.

31. Cashwell LF, Shields MB. Exfoliation syndrome in the southeastern United States: I. Prevalence in open-angle glaucoma and non-glaucoma population. *Acta Ophthalmol.* 1988;66(suppl 184):99–102.

32. Cashwell LF, Shields MB. Exfoliation syndrome: Prevalence in a southeastern United States population. *Arch Ophthalmol.* 1988;106:335–336.

33. Ball SF. Exfoliation prevalence in the glaucoma population of South Louisiana. *Acta Ophthalmol.* 1988;66 (suppl 184):93–98.

34. Ball SF, Graham S, Thompson H. The racial prevalence and biomicroscopic signs of exfoliative syndrome in the glaucoma population of southern Louisiana. *Glaucoma.* 1989;11:169–175.

35. Colin J, Bonissent JF, Resnikoff S. Epidemiology of the exfoliation syndrome. 17th Congress of the European Society of Ophthalmology. Helsinki; 1985:230–231.

36. Colin J, Le Gall G, Le Jeune B, et al. The prevalence of exfoliation syndrome in different areas of France. *Acta Ophthalmol.* 1988;66(suppl 184):86–89.

37. Ringvold A, Blika S, Elsås T, et al. The middle-Norway eye-screening study: I. Epidemiology of the pseudoexfoliation syndrome. *Acta Ophthalmol.* 1988;66:652–657.

38. Taylor HR. The environment and the lens. *Br J Ophthalmol.* 1980;64:303–310.

39. Heriot WJ, Crock GW, Taylor R, et al. Ophthalmic findings among one thousand inhabitants of Rarotonga, Cook Islands. *Aust J Ophthalmol.* 1983;11:81–94.

40. Mohammed S, Kazmi N. Subluxation of the lens and ocular hypertension in exfoliation syndrome. *Pak J Ophthalmol.* 1986;2:77–78.

41. Aasved H. Mass screening for fibrillopathia epitheliocapsularis. *Acta Ophthalmol.* 1971;49:334–343.

42. Rouhiainen H, Teräsvirta M. Presence of pseudoexfoliation on clear and opacified crystalline lenses in an aged population. *Ophthalmologica.* 1992;204:67–70.

43. Iizuka S, Nakae R, Motokura M. Incidence of pseudoexfoliation syndrome. *Folia Ophthalmol Jpn*. 1991;42:926–931.

44. Faulkner HW. Pseudo-exfoliation of the lens among the Navajo Indians. *Am J Ophthalmol*. 1971;72:206–208.

45. Taylor HR, Hollows FC, Moran D. Pseudoexfoliation of the lens in Australian aborigines. *Br J Ophthalmol*. 1977;61:473–475.

46. Bartholomew RS. Pseudocapsular exfoliation in the Bantu of South Africa: I. Early or pregranular clinical stage. *Br J Ophthalmol*. 1971;55:693–699.

47. Sugar S. Pigmentary glaucoma and the glaucoma associated with the exfoliation-pseudoexfoliation syndrome: Update. *Ophthalmology*. 1984;91:307–309.

48. Aasved H. The geographical distribution of fibrillopathia epitheliocapsularis. *Acta Ophthalmol*. 1969;47:792–810.

49. Hansen E, Sellevold OJ. Pseudoexfoliation of the lens capsule: I. Clinical evaluation with special regard to the presence of glaucoma. *Acta Ophthalmol*. 1968;46:1095–1104.

50. Moreno-Montañés J, Alcolea Paredes A, Campos García S. Prevalence of pseudoexfoliation syndrome in the northwest of Spain. *Acta Ophthalmol*. 1989;67:383–385.

51. Yalaz M, Othman I, Nas K, et al. The frequency of pseudoexfoliation syndrome in the Eastern Mediterranean area of Turkey. *Acta Ophthalmol*. 1992;70:209–213.

52. Madden JG, Crowley MJ. Factors in the exfoliation syndrome. *Br J Ophthalmol*. 1982;66:432–437.

53. Sziklai P, Süveges I. Glaucoma capsulare in patients with open-angle glaucoma in Hungary. *Acta Ophthalmol*. 1988;66(suppl 184):90–92.

54. Gillies WE, Brooks AMV. The presentation of acute glaucoma in pseudoexfoliation of the lens capsule. *Aust N Z J Ophthalmol*. 1988;16:101–106.

55. Kozart DM, Yanoff M. Intraocular pressure status in 100 consecutive patients with exfoliation syndrome. *Ophthalmology*. 1982;89:214–218.

56. Moreno-Montañés J, Alvarez A, Alcolea Paredes A, et al. Clinical factors related to the tension increase in the pseudoexfoliation syndrome. *Arch Soc Esp Oftalmol*. 1990;59:421–427.

57. Summanen P, Tönjum AM. Exfoliation syndrome among Saudis. *Acta Ophthalmol*. 1988;66(suppl 184):107–111.

58. Hørven I. Exfoliation syndrome. *Arch Ophthalmol*. 1966;76:505–511.

59. Aasved H. The frequency of fibrillopathia epitheliocapsularis (so-called senile exfoliation or pseudoexfoliation) in patients with open-angle glaucoma. *Acta Ophthalmol*. 1971;49:194–210.

60. Blika S, Ringvold A. The occurrence of simple and capsular glaucoma in Middle-Norway. *Acta Ophthalmol*. 1987;63(suppl 182):11–16.

61. Valle O. Prevalence of simple and capsular glaucoma in the Central Hospital district of Kotka. *Acta Ophthalmol*. 1988;66(suppl 184):116–119.

62. Aasved H. Study of relatives of persons with fibrillopathia epitheliocapsularis (pseudoexfoliation of the lens capsule). *Acta Ophthalmol*. 1975;53:879–886.

63. Teikari JM, Kaprio J, Koskenvuo M. Pseudoexfoliation of the lens capsule in six twin pairs. *Glaucoma*. 1990;12:183–189.

64. Lemoine AN. Glaucoma: A statistical review of 816 patients with 1112 glaucomatous eyes. *Am J Ophthalmol*. 1950;33:1353–1373.

65. Bartholomew RS. Pseudocapsular exfoliation in the Bantu of South Africa: II. Occurrence and prevalence. *Br J Ophthalmol*. 1973;57:41–45.

66. Ringvold A, Blika S, Elsås T. The middle-Norway eye-screening study: II. Prevalence of simple and capsular glaucoma. *Acta Ophthalmol*. 1991;69:273–280.

67. Ohrt V, Nehen JH. The incidence of glaucoma capsulare based on a Danish hospital material. *Acta Ophthalmol*. 1981;59:888–893.

68. Clements DB. Glaucoma in the Isle of Man: With special reference to pseudo-capsular exfoliation. *Br J Ophthalmol*. 1968;52:546–549.

69. Futa R, Shimizu T, Furuyoshi N. Clinical features of capsular glaucoma in comparison with primary open-angle glaucoma in Japan. *Acta Ophthalmol*. 1992;70:214–219.

70. Sood NN, Ratnaraj A. Pseudoexfoliation of the lens capsule. *Orient Arch Ophthalmol*. 1968;6:62–67.

71. Luntz MH. Prevalence of pseudoexfoliation syndrome in an urban South African clinic population. *Am J Ophthalmol*. 1972;74:581–587.

72. Dethlefs RF. Glaucoma in Port Moresby, Papua New Guinea. *Papua New Guinea Med J*. 1982;25:104–107.

73. Gradle HS, Sugar HS. Glaucoma capsulare. *Am J Ophthalmol*. 1947;30:12–19.

74. Horns DJ, et al. Argon laser trabeculoplasty for open angle glaucoma: A retrospective study of 380 eyes. *Trans Ophthalmol Soc UK*. 1983;103:288–294.

75. Crittendon JJ, Shields MB. Exfoliation syndrome in the southern United States: II. Characteristics of patient population and clinical course. *Acta Ophthalmol*. 1988;66(suppl 184):103–106.

76. Aasved H. Intraocular pressure in eyes with and without fibrillopathia epitheliocapsularis. *Acta Ophthalmol*. 1971;49:601–610.

77. Stefaniotou M, Petroutsos G, Psilas K. The frequency of pseudoexfoliation in a region of Greece (Epirus). *Acta Ophthalmol*. 1990;68:307–309.

78. Shimizu K, Kimura Y, Aoki K. Prevalence of exfoliation syndrome in the Japanese. *Acta Ophthalmol*. 1988;66(suppl 184):112–115.

79. Henry JC, Krupin T, Schmitt M, et al. Long-term follow-up of pseudoexfoliation and the development of elevated intraocular pressure. *Ophthalmology*. 1987;94:545–549.

80. Hansen E, Sellevold OJ. Pseudoexfoliation of the lens capsule: III. Ocular tension in eyes with pseudoexfoliation. *Acta Ophthalmol*. 1970;48:446–454.

81. Konstas AGP, Jay JL, Marshall GE, Lee WR. Prevalence, diagnostic features, and response to trabeculectomy in exfoliation glaucoma. *Ophthalmology*. 1993;100:619–627.

82. Lindblom B, Thorburn W. Functional damage at diagnosis of primary open-angle glaucoma. *Acta Ophthalmol*. 1984;62:223–229.

83. Tarkkanen A. Treatment of chronic open-angle glaucoma associated with pseudoexfoliation. *Acta Ophthalmol.* 1965;43:514–523.

84. Pohjanpelto P. Influence of exfoliation syndrome on prognosis in ocular hypertension ≥25 mm: A long-term follow-up. *Acta Ophthalmol.* 1986;64:39–44.

85. Aasved H. The frequency of optic nerve damage and surgical treatment in chronic simple glaucoma and capsular glaucoma. *Acta Ophthalmol.* 1971;49:589–600.

86. Lindblom B, Thorburn W. Prevalence of visual field defects due to capsular and simple glaucoma in Halsingland, Sweden. *Acta Ophthalmol.* 1982;60:353–361.

87. Moreno-Montañés J, Alvarez Serna A, Alcolea Paredes A. Pseudoexfoliative glaucoma in patients with open-angle glaucoma in the Northwest of Spain. *Acta Ophthalmol.* 1990;68:695–699.

88. Konstas AG, Allan D. Pseudoexfoliation glaucoma in Greece. *Eye.* 1989;3:747–753.

89. Dark AJ, Streeten BW. Precapsular film on the aging human lens—Precursor of pseudoexfoliation. *Br J Ophthalmol.* 1990;74:717–722.

90. Tetsumoto K, Schlötzer-Schrehardt U, Küchle M, et al. Precapsular layer of the anterior lens capsule in early pseudoexfoliation syndrome. *Graefes Arch Clin Exp Ophthalmol.* 1992;230:252–257.

91. Radian AB, Radian AL. Senile pseudoexfoliation in aphakic eyes. *Br J Ophthalmol.* 1975;59:577–579.

92. Sugar HS. Das Exfoliations Syndrom: Ursache fibrillaren Materials auf der Linsenkapsel. *Klin Monatsbl Augenheilkd.* 1976;169:1–6.

93. Sugar HS. Onset of the exfoliation syndrome after intracapsular lens extraction. *Am J Ophthalmol.* 1980;89:601–602.

94. Caccamise WC. The exfoliation syndrome in the aphakic eye. *Am J Ophthalmol.* 1981;91:111–112.

95. Ringvold A, Bore J. Pseudoexfoliation syndrome pattern on posterior intraocular lens. *Acta Ophthalmol.* 1990;68:353–355.

96. Chen V, Blumenthal M. Exfoliation syndrome after cataract extraction. *Ophthalmology.* 1992;99:445–447.

97. Mizuno K, Muroi S. Cycloscopy of pseudoexfoliation. *Am J Ophthalmol.* 1979;87:513–518.

98. Bartholomew RS. Lens displacement associated with pseudocapsular exfoliation. *Br J Ophthalmol.* 1970;54:744–750.

99. Bartholomew RS. Phakodonesis: A sign of incipient lens displacement. *Br J Ophthalmol.* 1970;54:663–668.

100. Guzek JP, Holm M, Cotter JB, et al. Risk factors for intraoperative complications in 1000 extracapsular cataract causes. *Ophthalmology.* 1987;94:461–466.

101. Mayer E, et al. Pseudoexfoliation: Epidemiology, clinical and scanning electron microscopic study. *Ophthalmologica.* 1984;188:141–147.

102. Futa R, Furuyoshi N. Phacodonesis in capsular glaucoma: A clinical and electron microscope study. *Jpn J Ophthalmol.* 1989;33:311–317.

103. Thomassen TL. On the so-called capsular glaucoma. *Acta Ophthalmol.* 1949;27:423–427.

104. Dark AJ, Streeten BW, Conward CC. Pseudoexfoliative disease of the lens: A study in electron microscopy and histochemistry. *Br J Ophthalmol.* 1977;61:462–472.

105. Takei Y, Mizuno K. Electron microscopic study of pseudoexfoliation of the lens capsule. *Graefes Arch Clin Exp Ophthalmol.* 1978;205:213–220.

106. Chijiiwa T, Araki H, Ishibashi T, et al. Degeneration of zonular fibrils in a case of exfoliation glaucoma. *Ophthalmologica.* 1989;199:16–23.

107. Tarkkanen AHA. Exfoliation syndrome. *Trans Ophthalmol Soc UK.* 1986;105:233–245.

108. Carpel EF. Pupillary dilation in eyes with pseudoexfoliation syndrome. *Am J Ophthalmol.* 1988;105:692–694.

109. Zetterström C, Olivestedt G, Lundvall A. Exfoliation syndrome and extracapsular cataract extraction with implantation of posterior chamber lens. *Acta Ophthalmol.* 1992;70:85–90.

110. Lundvall A, Zetterström C. Exfoliation syndrome and the effect of phenylephrine and pilocarpine on pupil size. *Acta Ophthalmol.* 1993;71:177–180.

111. Hahnenberger R. Anisocoria in untreated unilateral open-angle glaucoma. *Acta Ophthalmol.* 1984;62:135–141.

112. Bertelsen T. Fibrillopathia epitheliocapsularis. The so-called senile exfoliation or pseudo-exfoliation of the anterior lens capsule. *Acta Ophthalmol.* 1966;44:737–750.

113. Kristensen P. Mydriasis-induced pigment liberation in the anterior chamber associated with acute rise in intraocular pressure in open-angle glaucoma. *Acta Ophthalmol.* 1965;43:714–724.

114. Dark AJ. Cataract extraction complicated by capsular glaucoma. *Br J Ophthalmol.* 1979;63:465–468.

115. Prince AM, Streeten BW, Ritch R, et al. Preclinical diagnosis of pseudoexfoliation syndrome. *Arch Ophthalmol.* 1987;105:1076–1082.

116. Prince AM, Ritch R. Clinical signs of the pseudoexfoliation syndrome. *Ophthalmology.* 1986;93:803–807.

117. Norn MS. Iris pigment defects in normals. *Acta Ophthalmol.* 1971;49:887–894.

118. Aasved H. Incidence of defects in the pigmented pupillary ruff in eyes with and without fibrillopathia epitheliocapsularis. *Acta Ophthalmol.* 1973;51:710–715.

119. Repo LP, Teräsvirta ME, Tuovinen EJ. Generalized peripheral iris transluminance in the pseudoexfoliation syndrome. *Ophthalmology.* 1990;97:1027–1029.

120. Krause U, Helve J, Forsius H. Pseudoexfoliation of the lens capsule and liberation of iris pigment. *Acta Ophthalmol.* 1973;51:39–46.

121. Kristensen P. Pigment liberation test in open-angle glaucoma. *Acta Ophthalmol.* 1968;46:586–599.

122. Wishart PK, Spaeth GL, Poryzees EM. Anterior chamber angle in the exfoliation syndrome. *Br J Ophthalmol.* 1985;69:103–105.

123. Moreno-Montañés J, et al. Pseudoexfoliation syndrome: Clinical study of the anterior chamber angle. *J Fr Ophtalmol.* 1990;13:183–188.

124. Sampaolesi R. Neue Untersuchungen über das Pseudokapselhautchen-Glaukom (Glaucoma Capsulare). *Ber Deutsch Ophthalmol Ges.* 1959;62:177–183.

125. Sampaolesi R, Zarate J, Croxatto O. The chamber angle in exfoliation syndrome: Clinical and pathological findings. *Acta Ophthalmol.* 1988;66(suppl 184):48–53.

126. Amalric P, Sampaolesi R, Bessou P. Early diagnosis and heredity of pseudocapsular exfoliation. *Bull Soc Ophtalmol Fr.* 1960;5–6:341–350.

127. Hansen E, Sellevold OJ. Pseudoexfoliation of the lens capsule: II. Development of the exfoliation syndrome. *Acta Ophthalmol.* 1969;47:161–173.

128. Slagsvold JE. The follow-up in patients with pseudoexfoliation of the lens capsule with and without glaucoma: II. The development of glaucoma in persons with pseudoexfoliation. *Acta Ophthalmol.* 1986;64:241–245.

129. Odland M, Aasved H. Follow-up of initially nonglaucomatous patients with fibrillopathia epitheliocapsularis. *Acta Ophthalmol.* 1973;51(suppl 120):77–81.

130. Irvine R. Exfoliation of the lens capsule (glaucoma capsularis). *Arch Ophthalmol.* 1940;23:138–160.

131. Paufique L, Audibert J. Le syndrome de pseudoexfoliation capsulaire avec cataracte. In: *Actualités Latines d'Ophthalmologie.* Paris: Masson; 1958:213–227.

132. Hietanen J, Kivelä T, Vesti E, et al. Exfoliation syndrome in patients scheduled for cataract surgery. *Acta Ophthalmol.* 1992;70:440–446.

133. Lumme P, Laatikainen L. Exfoliation syndrome and cataract extraction. *Am J Ophthalmol.* 1993;116:51–55.

134. Puska P, Raitta C. Exfoliation syndrome as a risk factor for optic disc changes in nonglaucomatous eyes. *Graefes Arch Clin Exp Ophthalmol.* 1992;230:501–504.

135. Bartholomew RS. Incidence of pseudoexfoliation in South African Negroes and Scots. *Trans Ophthalmol Soc UK.* 1979;99:299–301.

136. Küchle M, Naumann GOH. Occurrence of pseudoexfoliation following penetrating keratoplasty for keratoconus. *Br J Ophthalmol.* 1992;76:98–100.

137. Krause U, Tarkkanen A. Cataract and pseudoexfoliation: A clinicopathological study. *Acta Ophthalmol.* 1978;56:329–334.

138. Awan KJ, Humayun M. Extracapsular cataract surgery risks in patients with exfoliation syndrome. *Pakistan J Ophthalmol.* 1986;2:79–80.

139. Raitta C, Tarkkanen A. Posterior chamber lens implantation in capsular glaucoma. *Acta Ophthalmol.* 1987;65(suppl 182):24–26.

140. Raitta C, Setälä K. Intraocular lens implantation in exfoliation syndrome and capsular glaucoma. *Acta Ophthalmol.* 1986;64:130–133.

141. Skuta GL, Parrish RK II, Hodapp E, et al. Zonular dialysis during extracapsular cataract extraction in pseudoexfoliation syndrome. *Arch Ophthalmol.* 1987;105:632–634.

142. Naumann GOH, Küchle M, Schonherr U. Pseudoexfoliation as a risk factor for vitreous loss in extracapsular cataract extraction. *Fortschr Ophthalmol.* 1989;86:543–545.

143. Naumann GOH, the Erlanger Augenblätter-Group. Exfoliation syndrome as a risk factor for vitreous loss in extracapsular cataract surgery. *Acta Ophthalmol.* 1988;66(suppl 184):129–131.

144. Moreno-Montañés J, Duch S, Lajara J. Pseudoexfoliation syndrome: Clinical factors related to capsular rupture in cataract surgery. *Acta Ophthalmol.* 1993;71:181–184.

145. Goder GJ. Our experiences in planned extracapsular cataract extraction in the exfoliation syndrome. *Acta Ophthalmol.* 1988;66(suppl 184):126–128.

146. Høvding G. The association between fibrillopathy and posterior capsular/zonular breaks during extracapsular cataract extraction and posterior chamber intraocular lens implantation. *Acta Ophthalmol.* 1988;66:662–666.

147. Pignalosa B, Toni F, Liguori G. Considerations on posterior chamber intraocular lens implantation in patients with pseudoexfoliation syndrome. *Doc Ophthalmol.* 1989;71:49–53.

148. Ringvold A. On the occurrence of pseudoexfoliation material in extrabulbar tissue from patients with pseudoexfoliation syndrome of the eye. *Acta Ophthalmol.* 1973;51:511–518.

149. Schlötzer-Schrehardt U, Küchle M, Naumann GOH. Electron-microscopic identification of pseudoexfoliative material in extrabulbar tissue. *Arch Ophthalmol.* 1991;109:565–570.

150. Sugino T. Exfoliative materials in the skin of patients with exfoliation syndrome. *Acta Soc Ophthalmol Jpn.* 1990;94:856–869.

151. Streeten BW, Dark AJ, Wallace RN, et al. Pseudoexfoliative fibrillopathy in the skin of patients with ocular pseudoexfoliation. *Am J Ophthalmol.* 1990;110:490–499.

152. Schlötzer-Schrehardt U, Koca MR, Naumann GOH, Volkholz H. Pseudoexfoliation syndrome: Ocular manifestation of a systemic disorder? *Arch Ophthalmol.* 1992;110:1752–1756.

153. Streeten BW, Li ZY, Wallace RN, et al. Pseudoexfoliative fibrillopathy in visceral organs of a patient with pseudoexfoliation syndrome. *Arch Ophthalmol.* 1992;110:1757–1762.

154. Meretoja J, Tarkkanen A. Pseudoexfoliation syndrome in familial systemic amyloidosis with lattice corneal dystrophy. *Ophthalm Res.* 1975;7:194–203.

155. Tsukahara S, Matsuo T. Secondary glaucoma accompanied with primary familial amyloidosis. *Ophthalmologica.* 1977;250:175–183.

156. Futa R, Inada K, Nakashima H, et al. Familial amyloidotic polyneuropathy: Ocular manifestations with clinicopathological correlation. *Jpn J Ophthalmol.* 1984;28:289–298.

157. Kishi A, Maruoka S, Futa R. Clinical and histopathological study on secondary glaucoma associated with familial amyloidotic polyneuropathy. *Folia Ophthalmol Jpn.* 1990;41:2122–2128.

158. Bartholomew RS. Anterior chamber depths in eyes with pseudoexfoliation. *Br J Ophthalmol.* 1980;64:322–323.

159. Lowe RF. Primary angle-closure with capsular exfoliation of the lens. *Br J Ophthalmol.* 1964;48:492–494.

160. Benedikt O, Roll P. The trabecular meshwork of a nonglaucomatous eye with the exfoliation syndrome. *Virchows Arch.* 1979;384:347–355.

161. Richardson TM, Epstein DL. Exfoliation glaucoma: A quantitative perfusion and ultrastructural study. *Ophthalmology.* 1981;88:968–977.

162. Pohjanpelto P. The fellow eye in unilateral hypertensive pseudoexfoliation. *Am J Ophthalmol.* 1973;75:216–220.

163. Airaksinen PJ. The long-term hypotensive effect of timolol maleate compared with the effect of pilocarpine in simple and capsular glaucoma. *Acta Ophthalmol.* 1979;57:425–434.

164. Becker B. Does hyposecretion of aqueous humor damage the trabecular meshwork? (editorial). *J Glaucoma.* 1995;4:303–305.

165. Johnson DH. Human trabecular cell survival is dependent upon perfusion rate. *Invest Ophthalmol Vis Sci.* 1994;35:2082.

166. Shaw BR, Lewis RA. Intraocular pressure elevation after pupillary dilation in open angle glaucoma. *Arch Ophthalmol.* 1986;104:1185.

167. Brinchmann-Hansen O, Albrektsen T, Anmarkrud N. Pilocarpine drops do not reduce intraocular pressure sufficiently in pseudoexfoliation glaucoma. *Eye.* 1993;7:511–516.

168. Aasved H, Seland JH, Slagsvold JE. Timolol maleate in the treatment of open-angle glaucoma. *Acta Ophthalmol.* 1979;57:700–708.

169. Heijl A, Strahlman E, Sverrisson T, et al. A comparison of dorzolamide and timolol in patients with pseudoexfoliation and glaucoma or ocular hypertension. *Ophthalmology.* 1997;104:137–142.

170. Ohrstrom A, Kattstrom O. Interaction of timolol and adrenaline. *Br J Ophthalmol.* 1981;65:53–58.

171. Ritch R, Podos SM. Laser trabeculoplasty in secondary glaucomas. In: Jakobiec FA, Sigelman J, eds. *Advanced Techniques in Ocular Surgery.* Philadelphia: Saunders; 1984:124–134.

172. Ritch R. *Techniques of Argon Laser Iridectomy and Iridoplasty.* Palo Alto, CA: Coherent Medical Press; 1983.

173. Svedbergh B. Argon laser trabeculoplasty in capsular glaucoma. *Acta Ophthalmol.* 1988;66(suppl 184):141–147.

174. Svedbergh B, Sherwood M. Argon laser trabeculoplasty in exfoliation glaucoma: A retrospective analysis. *Dev Ophthalmol.* 1985;11:116–121.

175. Schwartz AL, Kopelman J. Four-year experience with argon laser trabecular surgery in uncontrolled open angle glaucoma. *Ophthalmology.* 1983;90:771–778.

176. Tuulonen A. Laser trabeculoplasty as primary therapy in chronic open angle glaucoma. *Acta Ophthalmol.* 1984;62:150–158.

177. Bergeå B. Some factors affecting the intraocular pressure reduction after argon laser trabeculoplasty in open-angle glaucoma. *Acta Ophthalmol.* 1984;62:696–704.

178. Hetherington J Jr. Capsular glaucoma: Management philosophy. *Acta Ophthalmol.* 1988;66(suppl 184):138–140.

179. Ritch R, Podos SM. Laser trabeculoplasty in exfoliation syndrome. *Bull N Y Acad Med.* 1983;59:339–344.

180. Spaeth GL, Baez K. Argon laser trabeculoplasty controls one third of cases of progressive, uncontrolled, open angle glaucoma for 5 years. *Arch Ophthalmol.* 1992;110:491.

181. Raitta C, Tarkkanen A. Combined procedure for the management of glaucoma and cataract. *Acta Ophthalmol.* 1988;66:667–670.

182. Nagata M, Yamagishi N, Tabuchi Y, et al. Pseudoexfoliation syndrome: Effect of trabeculotomy and the scanning electron microscopic view of the lens. *Jpn J Clin Ophthalmol.* 1976;30:33–40.

183. Tanihara H et al. Surgical effect of trabeculotomy ab externo on adult eyes with primary open angle glaucoma and pseudoexfoliation syndrome. *Arch Ophthalmol.* 1993;111:1653–1661.

184. Jacobi PC, Krieglstein GK. Trabecular aspiration: Clinical results of a new surgical approach to improve trabecular facility in glaucoma capsulare. *Ophthalm Surg.* 1994;25:641–645.

185. Jacobi PC, Krieglstein GK. Trabecular aspiration: A new mode to treat pseudoexfoliation glaucoma. *Invest Ophthalmol Vis Sci.* 1995;36:2271–2276.

186. Allen JS. Zonular dialysis in pseudoexfoliation syndrome (letter). *Arch Ophthalmol.* 1987;105:1318–1319.

187. Zetterström C, Lundvall A, Olivestedt G. Exfoliation syndrome and heparin surface modified intraocular lenses. *Acta Ophthalmol.* 1992;70:91–95.

188. Auffarth GU, Tsao K, Wesendahl TA, et al. Centration and fixation of posterior chamber intraocular lenses in eyes with pseudoexfoliation syndrome. *Acta Ophthalmol.* 1996;74:463–467.

189. Savage JA, Thomas JV, Belcher CD, Simmons RJ. Extracapsular cataract extraction and posterior chamber IOL implantation in glaucomatous eyes. *Ophthalmology.* 1985;92:1506–1516.

190. DiSclafani M, Liebmann JM, Ritch R. Malignant glaucoma following argon laser release of scleral flap sutures after trabeculectomy. *Am J Ophthalmol.* 1989;108:597–598.

191. Küchle M, Nguyen N, Hannappel E, Naumann GOH. The blood-aqueous barrier in eyes with pseudoexfoliation syndrome. *Ophthalm Res.* 1995;27(suppl 1):136–142.

192. Wålinder PEK, Olivius EOP, Nordell SI, Thorburn WE. Fibrinoid reaction after extracapsular cataract extraction and relationship to exfoliation syndrome. *J Cataract Refract Surg* 1989;15:526–530.

193. Drolsum L, Haaskjold E, Davanger M. Results and complications after extracapsular cataract extraction in eyes with pseudoexfoliation syndrome. *Acta Ophthalmol.* 1993;71:771–776.

194. Drolsum L, Davanger M, Haaskjold E. Risk factors for an inflammatory response after extracapsular cataract extraction and posterior chamber intraocular lens. *Acta Ophthalmol.* 1994;72:21–26.

195. Baltatzis S, Georgopoulos G, Theodossiadis P. Fibrin reaction after extracapsular cataract extraction: A statistical evaluation. *Eur J Ophthalmol.* 1993;3:95–97.

196. Pouliquen P, et al. Exfoliation syndrome and cataract surgery. *J Fr Ophtalmol.* 1992;15:171–176.

197. Lumme P, Laatikainen L. Cell reaction and pigment deposits on the posterior chamber intraocular lens. *Acta Ophthalmol* 1994;72:16–20.

198. Krupin T, Feitl ME, Bishop KI. Postoperative intraocular pressure rise in open-angle glaucoma patients after cataract or combined cataract-filtration surgery. *Ophthalmology.* 1989;96:579–584.

Chapter 28

COMMON SECONDARY GLAUCOMAS

Murray Fingeret
J. James Thimons

Secondary glaucomas (SGs) comprise a number of ocular conditions that lead to the elevation of intraocular pressure (IOP). The elevation of IOP is crucial in the definition of secondary glaucomas, which makes them different from primary open-angle glaucoma (POAG). For POAG, elevated IOP is a risk factor but not the defining characteristic. For SGs, elevated IOP is a defining characteristic necessary for the diagnosis, with optic nerve damage and loss of visual function related to the eye's tolerance to IOP. Thus, when the signs of a glaucomatous condition are present (i.e., pigment dispersion or pseudoexfoliation) and the IOP is elevated, an individual is said to have a SG even without discernible damage to the optic nerve or visual field. If the signs of such a condition are present without elevated IOP or optic nerve/visual field damage, then the patient is labeled as a suspect or as having a syndrome.

The elevation in the IOP in SG may be due to a host of factors including systemic diseases, ocular diseases, ocular trauma, intraocular hemorrhage, degenerative processes, abnormalities of ocular anatomy, and select pharmacological agents. With any of these factors, the outflow pathways are affected, with the subsequent elevation in IOP.

Another difference between primary and secondary glaucomas is that recognition of the etiology and pathophysiology of SG may lead to early prophylactic treatment in some situations. In addition, treatment schemes may vary for the different SGs, since they have different mechanisms and may respond differently to a medication or therapeutic modality.

As a group, the SGs are complex and present as a broad range of clinical entities that challenge the practitioner's diagnostic and therapeutic acumen. Although POAG is the most common of the glaucomas, SGs as a group may account for up to 33% of all glaucomas.[1] The mean age of individuals being treated for SGs is lower than that of patients treated for POAG, though certain SGs are more common in elderly individuals. This chapter explores select SGs that are commonly seen in clinical practice with the exception of pigmentary and pseudoexfoliative glaucoma, which are covered in Chap. 26 and 27. The SGs reviewed in this chapter include traumatic, steroid-induced, uveitic, and neovascular glaucoma.

POSTTRAUMATIC GLAUCOMA

The elevation in IOP following trauma to the globe may be due to a wide variety of etiologies including angle recession, hyphema, inflammation, lens dislocation and rupture, and pathological changes resulting from perforating injuries to the globe. Following trauma, the first indicator of damage to the anterior chamber angle may be the presence of a hyphema, sphincter tears in the pupillary margin, or lens subluxation, all of which are observable on slit-lamp examination.[2] Whenever a patient has experienced blunt trauma, gonioscopy should be performed to evaluate the angle structures for damage; when a hyphema is present, however, gonioscopy should be delayed until the hyphema has resolved and the risk of rebleeding has diminished.

One method of categorizing traumatic SGs is based on the time they develop following trauma. The first forms occur within hours or days following the trauma and are primarily related to inflammation, hyphema, or early changes in the trabecular meshwork secondary to blunt trauma. The second forms occur weeks to years following the incident and are seen in patients with severe angle recession or peripheral anterior synechiae, or those having suffered significant damage secondary to perforating ocular injuries.

Early-Onset Posttraumatic Glaucoma

Blunt trauma to the globe can produce damage to different tissues in the anterior segment including iris sphincter tears, iridodialysis, cyclodialysis, hyphema, trabeculodialysis, inflammation, zonular rupture, and lens dislocation. Individuals most likely to suffer blunt trauma are males in their second to third decades. A relationship also exists between blunt trauma and athletics, industrial settings, and home activities.[3] In one study at an urban hospital, over 4% of emergent care rendered was for trauma to the globe.[4]

Hyphema

Hyphema, or red blood cells or blood in the anterior chamber, is one of the most common clinical presentations following blunt ocular trauma. In a study of 149 cases of hyphema, 88% were due to blunt trauma.[5] Hyphemas are due to a tear in the ciliary body between the longitudinal and circular muscle fibers, resulting in damage to the major arterial circle of the iris (Figs. 28–1 and 28–2). The mechanism by which the tear is induced is thought to be a shortening of the anteroposterior length of the eye, forcing aqueous

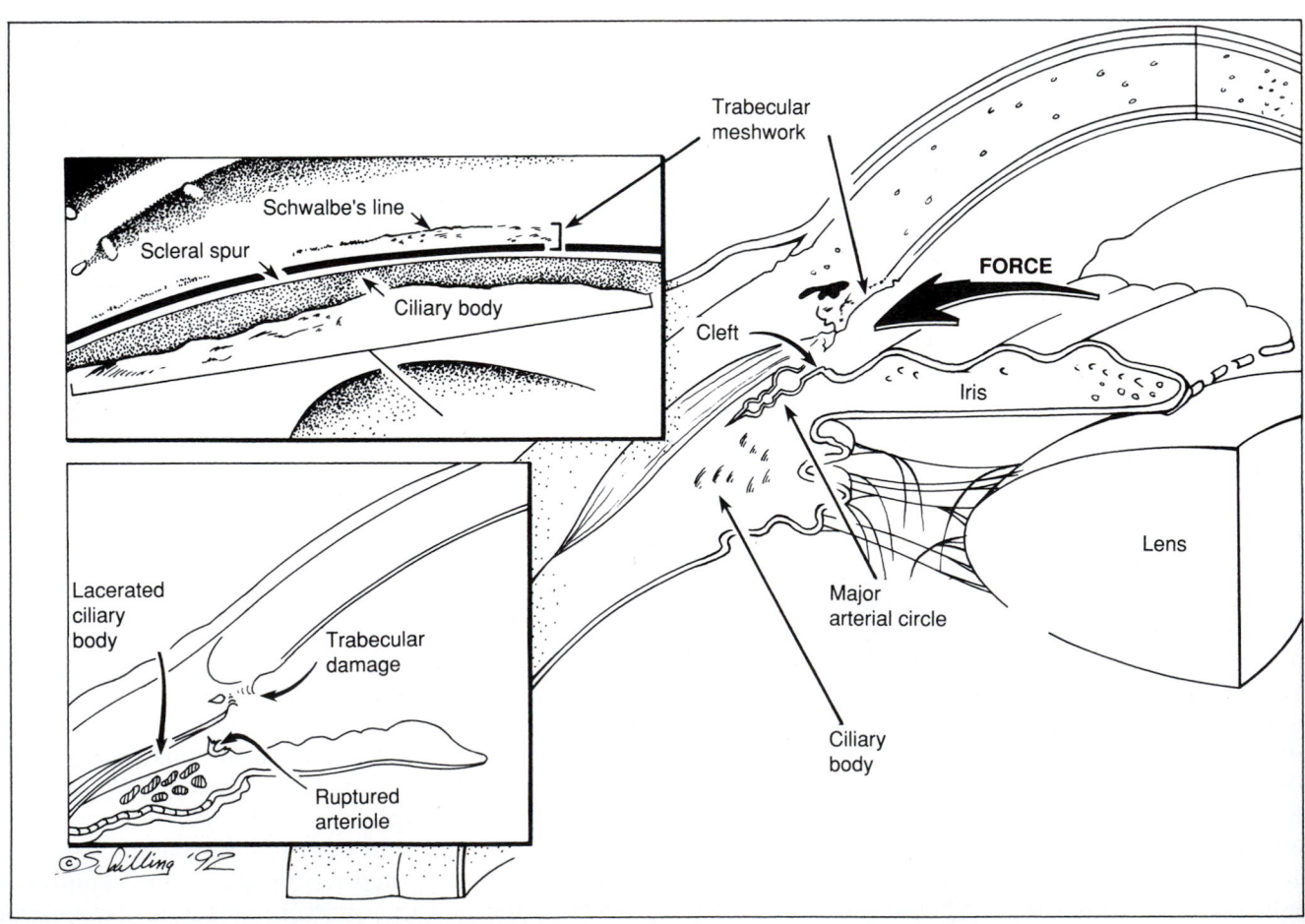

Figure 28–1. Diagram illustrating the structural changes to the anterior segment from ocular trauma. Any part of the angle may be damaged, leading to a compromised outflow system. The angle may be recessed or lacerated, with either leading to elevated IOP.

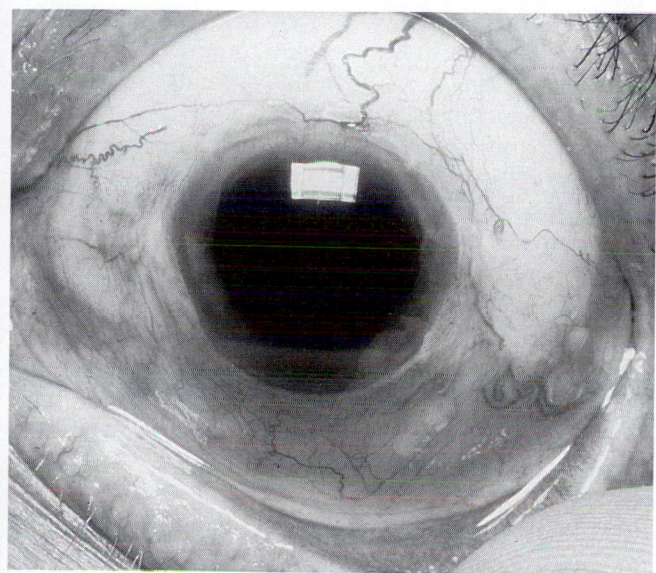

Figure 28-2. Hyphema following blunt trauma to the globe. (*Courtesy of Rodney Gutner, OD.*) (*See also Color Plate 92.*)

fluid under pressure toward the anterior chamber angle and thus causing tissue damage. Bleeding may occur either at the time of trauma or at any time within 7 days following the event.

Upon clinical examination, a hyphema may present as minute levels of circulating red blood cells within the anterior chamber, as layering of blood, or as hemorrhage completely filling the anterior chamber ("eight-ball" hyphema). In patients with a full eight-ball hyphema, the clot formed in the anterior chamber is responsible for the marked increase in IOP as cells and blood clog the trabecular meshwork, reducing drainage of aqueous from the eye. Clinical assessment of patients with hyphema includes measuring the level of hyphema and the magnitude of the IOP. IOP may vary from being within the normal range to as high as 80 mmHg, depending upon the degree of obstruction of the trabecular meshwork. The IOP following a hyphema is influenced in part by whether there was a single episode of bleeding followed by resolution of the hemorrhagic material or a secondary bleed (rebleed). Most patients who suffer from a single episode improve with appropriate management. Those who suffer rebleeds are at considerable risk for the development of secondary glaucoma.[6,7] Rebleeding is one of the most serious complications of hyphema and commonly occurs in the first 5 to 7 days following the initial episode. Rates for secondary hemorrhage following the initial traumatic episode range from 10 to 19%. In patients with sickle hemoglobinopathies, there is a tendency toward elevated IOP following a hyphema owing to the

inability of the sickled cells to pass through the trabecular meshwork because of their lack of pliability.[8,9]

A traumatic hyphema and elevated IOP are related in part to the magnitude of the hemorrhage present at initial examination. Coles demonstrated that among individuals whose hemorrhage involved less than half of the anterior chamber, 13.5% developed glaucoma, while in those with a total hyphema, 57% developed glaucoma.[7] Other factors that assist in detecting individuals likely to develop elevated IOP following hyphema include associated cataract and an increase in IOP greater than 2 mmHg when the patient changes from a sitting to a prone position.[7]

Sequelae that become apparent following resolution of a hyphema include angle recession, present in over 50% of hyphema patients; subluxation or dislocation of the lens; vitreous hemorrhage, which may cause a delayed increase in IOP; and corneal blood staining, which results from hemosiderin deposition in the cornea following prolonged IOP elevation.

The management of the patient with hyphema has evolved over many years. Initially, it was felt that bed rest accompanied by bilateral patching and sedation was the appropriate means to limit the secondary sequelae. Studies have since demonstrated that this regimen results in no better outcomes than permitting limited activities without patching.[10] Also, a study of 51 patients showed no significant difference in the rate of rebleeding between those receiving aspirin versus those given placebos following a hyphema.[10] The use of aminocaproic acid has been shown to significantly reduce the incidence rate of rebleed following hyphema.[11,12] Early surgical management is not recommended in patients with prolonged IOP elevation in the presence of hyphema because of a high rate of complications. The optimal time for the removal of the blood clot is around 4 days after its appearance because the adherence of the clot to the adjacent structures has lessened by that time. Complete removal of the clot is not necessary in the majority of cases and in some instances will increase the risk of a new hemorrhage.[13]

Between 2 and 10% of patients who suffer blunt trauma will develop secondary glaucoma.[14,15] In individuals who suffer a mild to moderate hyphema, the progression to glaucoma is less than 15%, with the prevalence related to the severity of the trauma and the ability to minimize damage associated with IOP elevation.[16] In most instances, topical antiglaucoma therapy is sufficient to manage the short-term rise in IOP. In those instances where the rise is severe, the necessity for surgical intervention also increases the likelihood for the development of a secondary glaucoma.

Angle recession and the associated trabecular injury lead to both early- and late-onset glaucoma secondary to

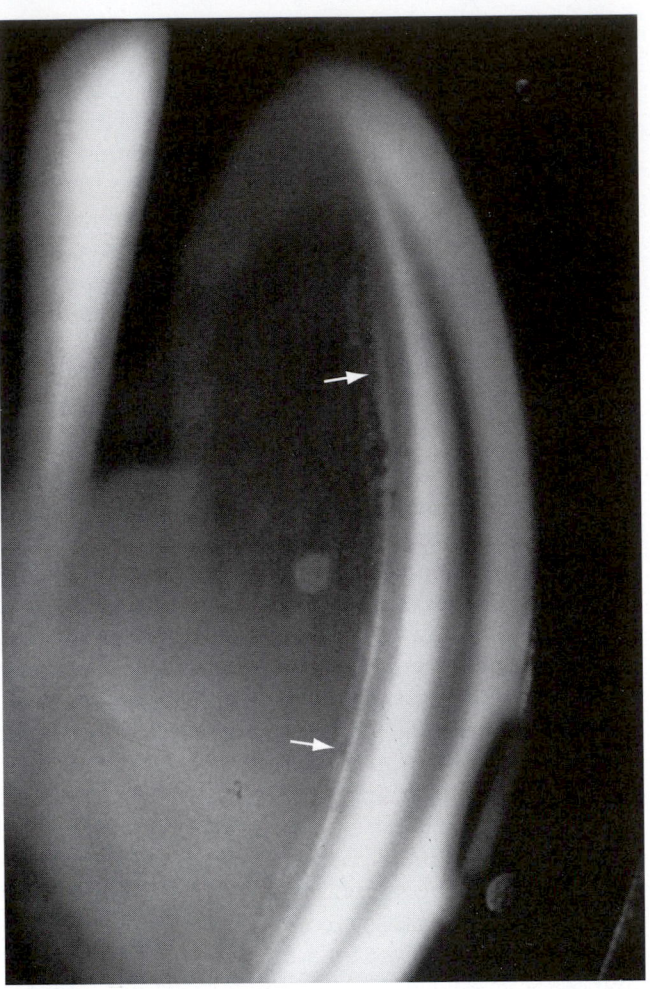

Figure 28–3. Moderate angle recession following blunt trauma. Note the variation in color and depth of the angle at the ciliary recess. The arrows point to the edge of the iris. (*For a better reproduction of this image, see Color Plate 93.*)

blunt trauma (Fig. 28–3).[17,18] Damage to the ciliary body and the trabecular meshwork may produce a variety of clinical presentations, from mild trabecular swelling to complete detachment of the ciliary body. The examination of a patient with anterior segment trauma should include gonioscopy performed bilaterally in order to adequately assess for the subtle clinical variations. Signs of angle damage include increased visibility of the scleral spur and ciliary body in one quadrant or, if the injury is more extensive, in one eye relative to the other. Also, the trabecular meshwork may be torn, with small tags of iris tissue found adherent to the scleral spur and the anterior portion of the ciliary body. Another subtle finding seen immediately following the trauma is presence of hemorrhages in the trabecular meshwork, accompanied by minor tears in the tissue structure.

The level of IOP elevation is often related to the amount of damage incurred at the time of trauma. One common cause for short-term IOP elevation is trabecular meshwork blockage associated with either anterior uveitis or trabecular swelling. Management includes the short-term use of topical beta blockers, alpha$_2$ agonists, topical steroids, and other medications to reduce aqueous production. Long-term sequelae from the temporary elevation of IOP are uncommon if management is instituted promptly.

Damage to the anterior chamber angle may result in tearing of the trabecular meshwork. One common presentation is a temporary rise in IOP, managed with topical beta blockers, that produces no immediate injury to the nerve head or visual field. This group of patients does require chronic observation, just like a glaucoma suspect, because of the relatively high incidence of late-onset glaucoma.[17] In more significant

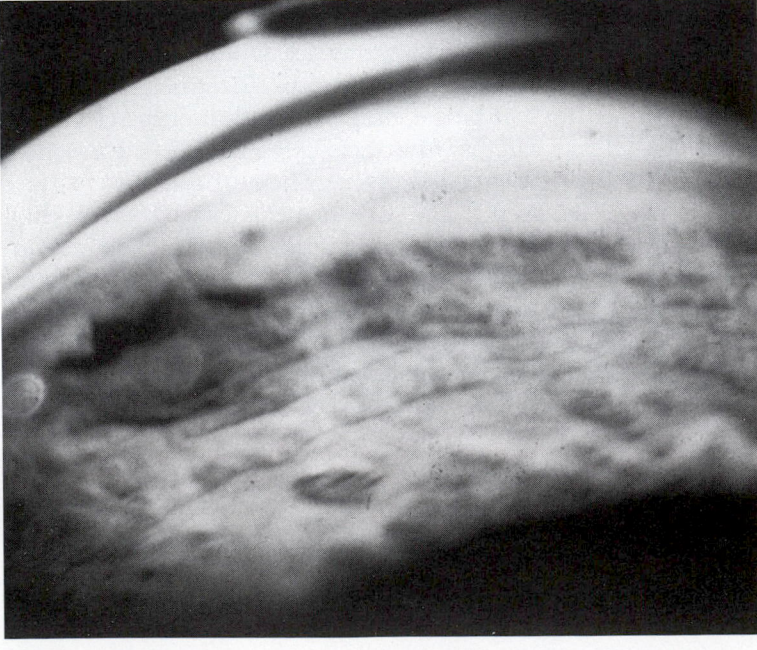

Figure 28–4. Severe angle recession. Note how wide open the angle appears. (*See also Color Plate 94.*)

cases of trauma, the disruption of the anterior chamber angle involves cleavage of the longitudinal muscles of the ciliary body, producing a widening and deepening of the anterior chamber angle.[19] This is known as *angle recession* (Fig. 28–4). An angle recession may vary from involvement of a few degrees of the angle to the entire circumference and is generally quite striking when compared with adjacent normal tissue in the same eye or the fellow eye.[20] Coloration of the ciliary body can be a clue to the extent of the recession, since the ciliary muscle appears light gray or tan, with the normal ciliary body adjacent to the damaged area being substantially darker. In cases where damage is extensive, with a full-thickness rupture of the muscle, the scleral wall will be exposed, as in a cyclodialysis cleft.[21,22]

The differential diagnosis for elevated IOP associated with acute trauma to the anterior segment is exclusion of entities that may produce an elevation in IOP and had been undiagnosed prior to the trauma. These include pseudoexfoliation syndrome, pigmentary dispersion syndrome, POAG, and subacute or intermittent angle-closure glaucoma. All of these conditions present with clinical signs and symptoms not typical of those for traumatic angle disease and should be differentiated with a thorough examination.

Armaly found that individuals who suffer an acute rise in IOP following trauma to the globe often show a positive steroid response in their uninjured eye at a similar rate to patients with POAG.[23] This leads to speculation that these individuals have a genetic predisposition for the development of elevated IOP, which could explain why only some individuals who suffer blunt trauma to the globe develop glaucoma. Still, the degree of angle recession appears to be the best indicator for long-term prognosis relative to the development of elevated IOP.[24,25] For individuals in whom only a small portion of the anterior chamber angle is involved, the risk of glaucoma developing is relatively low.

Late-Onset Posttraumatic Glaucoma
Unlike individuals who experience an elevation in IOP shortly after a traumatic episode, others will not develop elevated pressure until years later. The major causes for the late development of glaucoma are angle recession and penetrating injuries.[26]

Angle Recession
Angle recession is common following blunt trauma to the globe. Individuals most likely to develop late-onset glaucoma have had significant angle damage involving approximately two-thirds to three-quarters of the anterior chamber angle. The damage may include tearing of the longitudinal muscles of the ciliary body, recession or retraction of the anterior chamber, and damage to the trabecular meshwork. Also, a full-thickness tear with ev-

idence of exposure of the scleral wall may be seen. Occasionally, damage to the trabecular meshwork will present as incision-like gaps in the area that overlies Schlemm's canal and may involve the canal itself. Initially, the IOP may be low, which is likely due to the direct access of the aqueous to the outflow channel. Once this access has been blocked by the deposition of fibrotic tissue and subsequent scarring, the IOP usually rises.[27] Sclerosis of the trabecular meshwork is a third possible mechanism for the development of late-onset glaucoma, with the presence of a hyaline-like membrane extending from the corneal endothelium; this blocks the outflow of aqueous through the trabecular meshwork.[28]

Although the IOP is initially normal in late-onset glaucoma, occasionally individuals may present with relative hypotony secondary to either a decrease in aqueous production or the establishment of a small suprachoroidal cleft that allows direct shunting of aqueous fluid. Unfortunately, once the IOP elevation starts, it can be dramatic and difficult to manage. In some instances, the glaucoma may be unresponsive to medical management.

The overall prognosis in late-onset glaucoma is difficult to assess. There is evidence that damage to the ciliary body is not necessarily the cause of the eventual rise in IOP but instead is a clinical indicator that underscores the level of trauma to the trabecular meshwork and other components of the outflow system. It has been demonstrated that in individuals who develop late-onset glaucoma, the facility of outflow and the IOP in the fellow eye are both abnormal.[23] Thus individuals may have a predisposition for glaucoma, which may help explain the late onset of the disease.

In regard to therapy, medications that reduce aqueous production are used initially, though there may be a role for prostaglandins, as they enhance the uveal scleral outflow pathway. Miotics as well as argon laser trabeculoplasty (ALT) have little impact on reducing the IOP, and filter surgery is reserved for cases not adequately managed with aqueous suppressants.

Penetrating Injuries
One of the most devastating insults to the eye is that of a penetrating injury. It may produce a number of significant alterations to the ocular structure and physiological function. Penetrating injuries include mechanical disruption of the anterior chamber angle or ciliary body, lens damage with subsequent intraocular inflammation, and retained foreign bodies. The sources of these injuries are diverse. In one study of penetrating injuries, 22% were secondary to blunt force, 37% were the result of lacerations, and 41% were caused by high-velocity objects.[28] It is not surprising that the incidence of penetrating injuries to the globe is significantly greater among males and

younger age groups. This is consistent with data on the incidence of other conditions such as hyphema and blunt trauma.

There are several mechanisms that may produce IOP elevation following perforating injury. Most common is the development of peripheral anterior synechiae (PAS) (Fig. 28–5), which can occur from presence of a flattened anterior chamber and iridocorneal contact associated with wound leakage.[26] Initially the IOP is reduced because of the wound leak, but elevation may occur as PAS develop. Another cause of PAS and posterior synechiae is the inflammatory response associated with the traumatic episode. Topical cycloplegics are required during the immediate posttraumatic period, along with anti-inflammatory agents to limit the inflammatory response. In some instances, the inflammatory response is severe enough to produce a cyclitic membrane that may also close the anterior chamber angle.[7] Another sequela of a penetrating injury associated with glaucoma is epithelial ingrowth, which appears as a grayish membrane on the posterior corneal surface and may cause obstruction of the trabecular meshwork.[27] The mechanism for epithelial ingrowth is thought to be related to the introduction of epithelial cells either from the trauma itself or the subsequent wound repair.

Intraocular foreign bodies present a unique challenge to the clinician. The secondary effects of siderosis (iron rust) and chalcosis (copper oxidation) result in tissue damage that lead to the development of glaucoma. The mechanism is related to the impairment of aqueous outflow secondary to iron and copper deposition and damage.[29,30] Approximately 50% of eyes injured by metallic intraocular foreign bodies show damage to the lens capsule. Other clinical findings of an intraocular foreign body include heterochromia, siderotic or chalcotic staining of the anterior segment tissue, or unexplained unilateral mydriasis. These findings in the presence of unilaterally elevated IOP should alert the practitioner to the possibility of glaucoma secondary to a retained intraocular foreign body.

In individuals with peripheral anterior synechiae secondary to hypotony, the central chamber will be formed with the periphery showing contact of the iris and the posterior cornea. The IOP is usually low, frequently at 1 to 2 mmHg, and difficult to measure because of the softness of the globe. The presence of an idiopathic filtration bleb is a possible etiology but is not necessary to justify the reduced IOP. The clinician may also see irregular crocodile shagreen to the corneal surface, due to the gross reduction of IOP.

Traumatic anterior uveitis is often present; if it is severe enough, it may lead to the development of posterior synechiae. In severe inflammation or repeat bouts of anterior uveitis, posterior synechiae may progress to a 360-degree apposition (iris bombé). To prevent iris bombé from developing, the patient must undergo thorough cycloplegia. A cyclitic membrane develops primarily in individuals with a severe inflammatory response and presents as a sticky, thick protein component (4+ flare) in the anterior chamber. This is followed by development of a membrane that can either span the pupil or, using anterior chamber tissue, scaffold the anterior chamber angle, producing either iris-to-corneal adhesion and/or pupillary seclusion.

The differential diagnosis of late-onset glaucoma includes conditions that can produce unilateral glaucoma, such as asymmetrical POAG, exfoliative glaucoma, and pigmentary dispersion. These present with a variety of clinical signs and symptoms that assist the clinician in their differential diagnosis. The entities that can produce clinical findings similar to those of penetrating injury are few in number. Among the most common are Fuchs' heterochromic iridocyclitis, phacoanaphylactic glaucoma secondary to hypermature lens rupture, and blunt trauma without penetration but with significant sequelae.

In Fuchs' heterochromic iridocyclitis, there is no history or physical findings indicative of a penetrating foreign body. The asymmetry of iris color, unilaterally elevated IOP, and presence of cataract in many of these individuals are not dissimilar to the condition noted in retained intraocular foreign body. In phacoanaphylactic glaucoma, the patient's advanced age and the examination of the fellow eye, which will

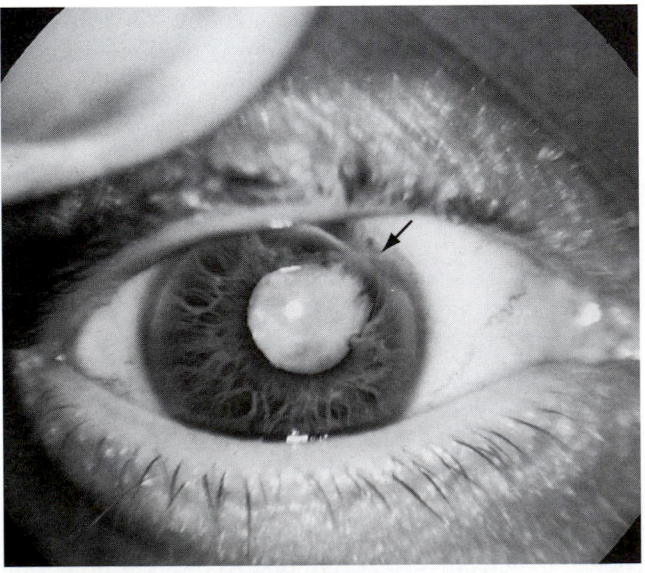

Figure 28–5. Formation of peripheral anterior synechiae following trauma to the anterior segment. (*See also Color Plate 95.*)

show advanced lens changes in most instances, will be sufficient to steer the clinician toward the correct diagnosis. Blunt trauma without penetrating injury may be the most difficult to differentially diagnose. Because of the similarities between these two conditions, it is a challenge to assure oneself that penetration is not the cause of the underlying problems. Radiographic evaluation including the use of computed tomographic scans may be needed to establish the diagnosis.

STEROID-INDUCED GLAUCOMA

Francois many years ago demonstrated that prolonged use of hydrocortisone may result in an elevation in IOP that is often relieved with the discontinuation of the drug.[31] Hydrocortisone belongs to a family of drugs known as *corticosteroids* that are used clinically for the treatment of inflammatory eye conditions such as uveitis and systemically for the treatment of asthma and collagen vascular diseases and as immunosuppressive therapy. Unfortunately, steroids in any form (administered topically, systemically, by periocular injection, or in facial creams or lotions) may have the unintended effect of elevating the IOP.[32] Steroids differ in their ability to raise the IOP, with topical agents the most likely culprits. Also, medications such as prednisolone acetate or dexamethasone are more likely to initiate an rise in IOP, while other steroids such as fluorometholone or rimexolone usually show a reduced response.

Research has been directed at identifying individuals susceptible to IOP elevation following the use of steroids. These studies indicate that patients with POAG or myopia as well as direct relatives of POAG patients are more likely to demonstrate a positive response than the general population.[33-35] Armaly in a series of studies on steroid responders demonstrated three distinct response levels (Table 28–1).[36] The low-response group showed an increase in IOP of less than 5 mmHg after 4 weeks of steroid use, the intermediate group showed a rise of between 6 and 15 mmHg, and the high-response group had a pressure rise greater than 15 mmHg.[36,37] The low-response group (one) showed an elevation in IOP for only the first 2 weeks, after which the pressure began to decline, whereas the intermediate-response group (two)

and the high-response group (three) showed continued elevation of pressure throughout the 4-week cycle, their only difference being the magnitude of rise. Armaly also found that increased concentrations and/or dosages of steroids were more likely to elicit a response.[36,37]

Steroid-induced ocular hypertension is genetically determined. Becker and Hahn proposed that POAG is a genetically determined disease expressed by a single gene.[35] Using the results of IOP responses to steroids in normal individuals, Armaly contradicted this concept and proposed that glaucoma is determined by multifactorial inheritance. He hypothesized that the three types of IOP responses to topical steroids were phenotypes for an allele pair, P^l, P^h, where P^l determined a low level of response and P^h a high level. Thus, the genotypes P^lP^l, P^lP^h, and P^hP^h represented the low-, intermediate-, and high-response groups to topical steroids.[36] Armaly's studies of offspring of glaucoma patients demonstrated the various genotypes in the frequency predicted from their parental genotype classification. Individuals with genotype P^lP^h had an 18 times greater probability of developing glaucoma than an individual with P^lP^l, and those with P^hP^h had a 100 times greater probability.[37]

The mechanism of steroid-induced elevation of IOP is believed to involve alterations in the outflow of aqueous.[38] Investigators have identified several possible mechanisms, including the accumulation of glycosaminoglycans in the outflow channels, the potentiation of 5-beta dihydrocortisol, and a decrease of phagocytic activity in the trabecular endothelium.[39-41] Glycosaminoglycans located in the anterior chamber angle become hydrated, creating an obstruction secondary to edema, which increases the resistance to aqueous outflow.[41] 5-beta dihydrocortisol has been shown to potentiate the hypertensive effects of dexamethasone in animal studies and has been postulated to have a similar effect in humans.[40] Decreased levels of phagocytic activity in the trabecular endothelium may be responsible for the accumulation of debris noted in electron-microscopic studies of the trabecular meshwork in individuals with steroid-induced glaucoma.[41,42] No single mechanism has been shown to be the sole pathophysiological process responsible for steroid-induced glaucoma, and it may well be that a combination of all these effects produces the elevation of IOP.

Clinically, corticosteroid-induced IOP elevation is asymptomatic, as in POAG. The IOP rise is generally bilateral unless the patient is being treated for a unilateral problem. In steroid responders, the IOP can rise to dramatic levels, but the patient rarely experiences symptomatology.

TABLE 28–1. POSITIVE CORTICOSTEROID RESPONSE

Low response	<5 mmHg	60%
Intermediate response	6–15 mmHg	35%
High response	>15 mmHg	5%

The examination findings are similar to those of POAG including an open anterior chamber angle, glaucomatous changes in the optic nerve, and abnormalities of the visual field consistent with glaucomatous damage. The response to corticosteroids is more common with topical treatment than with oral regimens, but any patient on steroid therapy should receive a baseline IOP evaluation and be followed up periodically for as long as he or she is is maintained on corticosteroids.

The differential diagnosis of steroid-induced glaucoma includes POAG. The differentiating factor is awareness of the relationship between steroid use and an elevation in IOP and that the patient may be taking the drug. Particular attention should be paid to the potential use of over-the-counter medications that may contain corticosteroid-based products.

The first phase of management for individuals with steroid-induced glaucoma is discontinuation of the drug, if possible. In most instances, the IOP will return to pretreatment levels within 1 to 4 weeks. There appears to be a relationship between the duration of IOP elevation following discontinuation and the length of time that the patient was treated. Espildora et al. showed that, in patients treated for less than 2 months, the IOP returns to pretreatment levels in all instances. A chronic elevation of IOP was seen in some patients treated for more than 4 years with topical steroids.[43] In those with a positive corticosteroid response whose anti-inflammatory agents cannot be discontinued, treatment with topical antiglaucoma medications may be initiated until the underlying condition resolves. Another therapeutic option is to switch to a topical steroid that reduces the risk of elevating the IOP. Fluorometholone acetate, rimexolone, or loteprednol are alternative steroids that tend to elicit a lesser response.[44,45] Undoubtedly, the worst prognostic indicator for individuals with steroid-induced glaucoma is the practitioner's failure to recognize the underlying etiology.

NEOVASCULAR GLAUCOMA

Neovascular glaucoma is a condition associated with an elevation of IOP that is due to synechial closure of the anterior chamber angle as a result of the formation of fibrovascular membranes that obstruct the outflow of aqueous.[46] The fibrovascular membrane results from rubeosis iridis, a network of fine vessels that arborize on the surface of the iris and eventually grow into the anterior chamber angle (Fig. 28–6). There has been some confusion regarding the terminology used to describe this disease, as it has been called *thrombotic glaucoma, hemorrhagic glaucoma,* and *congestive glaucoma;* in some instances, it has been confused with hemolytic glaucoma. Weiss et al., in 1963, coined the term *neovascular glaucoma,* which is the one most commonly used today.[47] Hemolytic glaucoma, in contrast, is due to the blockage of aqueous outflow by the accumulation of ghost cells in the trabecular meshwork following a vitreous hemorrhage.

Hypoxia appears to be the stimulus for the neovascular response in the eye. A vasoproliferative factor similar to that postulated as the cause of proliferative retinopathy appears to induce the growth of new blood vessels on the iris (rubeosis iridis). This vasoproliferative or angiogenic factor is elaborated by hypoxic retinal tissue in an attempt to revascularize these areas. The factor diffuses through the vitreous into the anterior chamber and induces a similar neovascular response to that occurring in the retina. Agents that have been postulated as potential angiogenic factors include prostaglandins,[48] biogenic amines,[49] and activated macrophages.[50]

Neovascular glaucoma develops following a wide variety of ophthalmic diseases.[51,52] Among the more common are central retinal vein occlusion, branch retinal vein occlusion, central retinal artery occlusion, carotid occlusive disease, diabetic retinopathy, chronic retinal detachment, and heterochromic iridocyclitis. The two most common disease states associated with retinal neovascularization are central retinal vein occlusion and diabetic retinopathy.[52]

A central retinal vein occlusion is a relatively common cause of neovascular glaucoma, although the incidence rates are quite variable.[53] The difficulty in managing patients with a central retinal vein occlusion lies in predicting which individuals will be most likely to progress to neovascular glaucoma, so that appropriate intervention may be implemented. Hayreh demonstrated two categories of patients based on the presence or absence of retinal ischemia, with the risk of rubeosis increasing with evidence of ischemia.[54] Other investigators have also shown that ischemic central retinal vein occlusion results in a higher incidence of rubeosis iridis than the nonischemic variety.[55] Rubeosis iridis following central retinal vein occlusion frequently leads to "90-day" glaucoma, in which the majority of patients have the onset of rubeosis and increase in IOP within 3 months of the retinal vascular event.

The relationship between IOP and central retinal vein occlusion is somewhat complex. Initially, following the vascular episode, the IOP may be low. Yet a significant percentage of patients with central retinal vein occlusion are found to have either ocular hypertension or glaucoma at the time of the retinal vascular accident.[56,57] Branch retinal vein occlusion, although

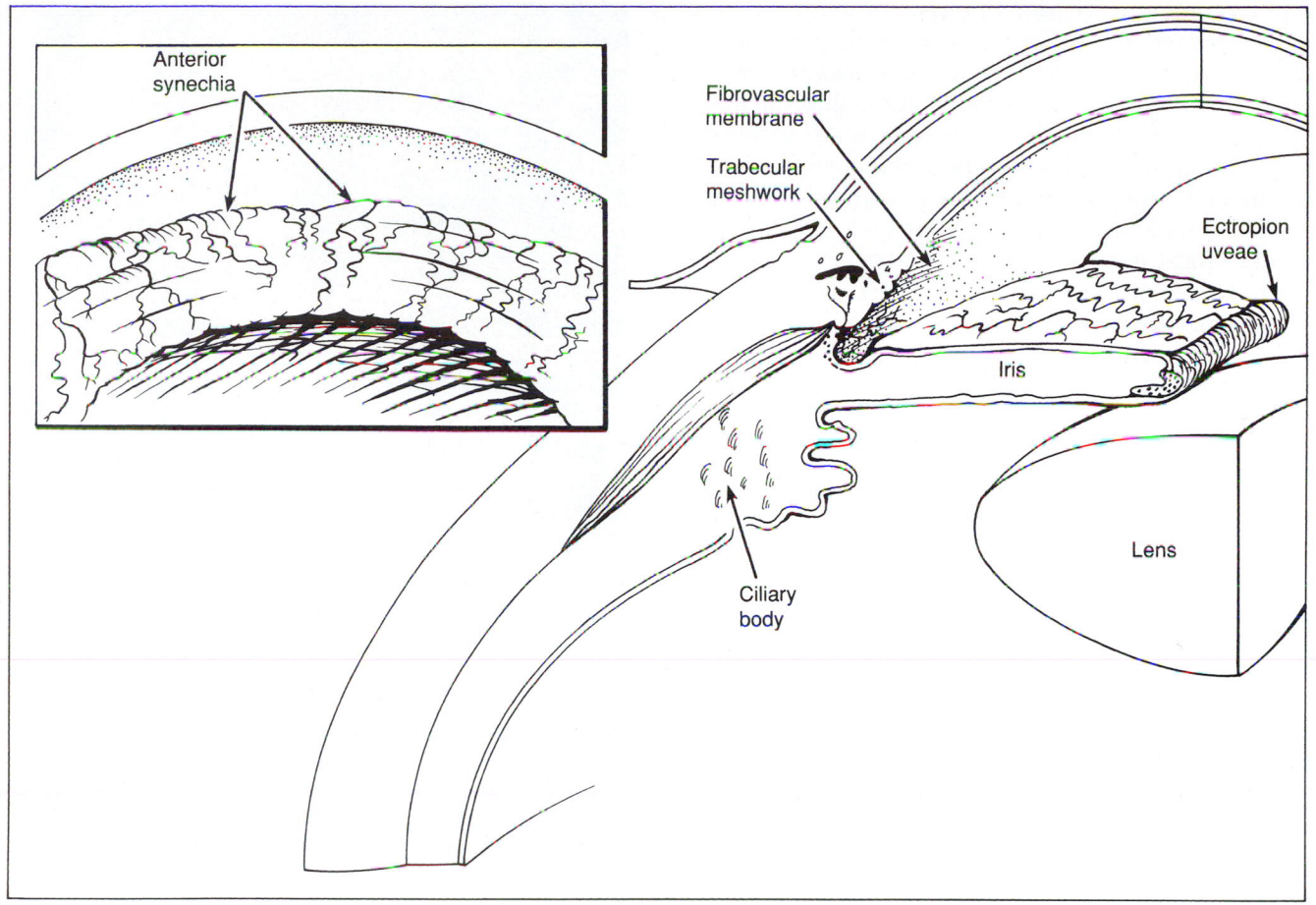

Figure 28–6. New blood vessels occur at the pupillary margin, growing over the iris surface toward the angle. The fine vessels grow into the angle, accompanied by a fibrovascular membrane that may contract, zippering the angle shut.

more common than central retinal vein occlusion, results in a lower incidence of neovascular glaucoma.[58] Interestingly, though branch retinal vein occlusion rarely causes anterior segment neovascularization, it has been implicated in the development of neovascularization of the retina.

Patients with diabetic retinopathy reveal striking differences with respect to the development of neovascular glaucoma, depending on the presence of proliferative changes. In patients with background retinopathy, the incidence of neovascular glaucoma is approximately 5%, increasing to as high as 50% in proliferative retinopathy.[59,60] Other factors that influence the development of neovascular glaucoma in patients with diabetic retinopathy include cataract extraction, history of a vitrectomy/lensectomy procedure, and retinal attachment surgery.[60] The risk of neovascular glaucoma in patients with diabetic retinopathy is reduced after extracapsular cataract extraction as opposed to intracapsular surgery, primarily owing to the mainte-

nance of the anterior hyaloid surface and posterior capsule; these are thought to bar the movement of the angiogenic factor from the retina to the iris. The time frame for the development of neovascular glaucoma following cataract surgery is within the first month postoperatively, necessitating careful surgical follow-up. The development of neovascular glaucoma is five times greater in patients with a combined vitrectomy/lensectomy than in those with only a vitrectomy. Chronic retinal detachment unrelated to diabetic retinopathy has also been implicated in the development of neovascularization of the anterior segment. These cases are frequently associated with other underlying conditions that may be instrumental in the pathogenesis of neovascular glaucoma, such as malignant melanoma, Coats' disease, retrolental fibroplasia, and sickle cell retinopathy.

The clinical presentation of neovascular glaucoma is similar regardless of the underlying etiology. In most cases, small, dilated vessels appear at the pupillary margin; occasionally, vessel arborization on the surface of the iris near the pupil is noted (Fig. 28–7).[61] The anterior chamber angle is usually clear of vessel activity in the early phase, although some individuals may show a delicate network of fine capillary activity. Fluorescein angiography demonstrates leakage in and around the pupillary margin early on, though this pattern of peripapillary leakage may be noted in some elderly nondiabetic patients, so that its predictive value is limited.[62] The IOP in the early phase is usually normal.

The middle phase of neovascular glaucoma occurs when the anterior chamber angle becomes involved. New vessels along with a fibrovascular membrane grow on the surface of the iris, frequently showing radial progression, with areas of arborization having an irregular pattern. The time frame for neovascularization to reach the angle varies from person to person. Gonioscopy will reveal vessels crossing the ciliary body band and scleral spur and occasionally appearing to derive directly from vessels in the ciliary body (Fig. 28–8). Chandler and Grant[63] found that normal vessels are located behind the scleral spur. Therefore vessels that arborize over the trabecular meshwork up to Schwalbe's line are assumed to represent abnormal vascularization of the angle. During the middle phase, some patients may present with a hyphema along with IOP elevation due to the obstruction of aqueous outflow (Fig. 28–9).

In the late phase of neovascular glaucoma, the fibrovascular membrane within the anterior chamber angle contracts, producing peripheral anterior synechiae that usually begin in one quadrant. The synechiae can progress to a complete 360-degree closure of the angle, described as "zippering shut" the angle (see Fig. 28–6). There is also a loss of texture on the iris surface and the appearance of ectropion uveae. Ectropion uveae is sec-

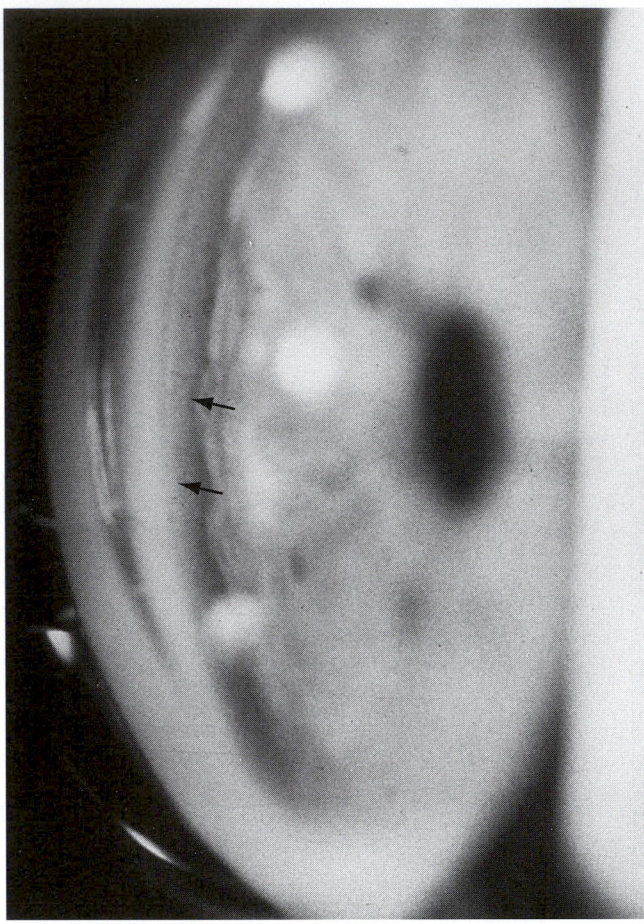

Figure 28–8. Moderate neovascular glaucoma. New blood vessels are seen in the angle. (*Courtesy of Rodney Gutner, OD.*) (*See also Color Plate 97.*)

ondary to the retraction of the pupillary margin by the fibrovascular membrane, exposing the posterior pigmented surface of the iris. A potentially confusing appearance on gonioscopy is the presence of an endothelial sheet contiguous with the endothelium of the cornea. This endothelial change follows synechial closure, creating a pseudoangle. In this phase, the patient usually has a significant reduction in visual acuity, extreme elevation of IOP, corneal edema, gross congestion of the globe, and inflammatory activity in the anterior chamber.

The differential diagnosis of neovascular glaucoma involves consideration of conditions that can independently produce rubeosis iridis without an underlying retinal vascular disease. Primary among these is Fuchs' heterochromic iridocyclitis, which can present with rubeosis iridis and an elevation of IOP. Fortunately, these patients usually present with a white, quiet eye as opposed to the intense engorgement of the globe seen in the late phase of neovascular

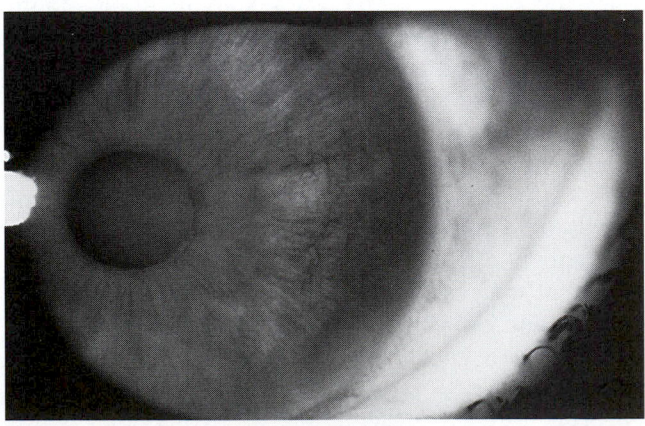

Figure 28–7. Early neovascular changes seen at the pupillary zone and midperiphery of the iris. (*See also Color Plate 96.*)

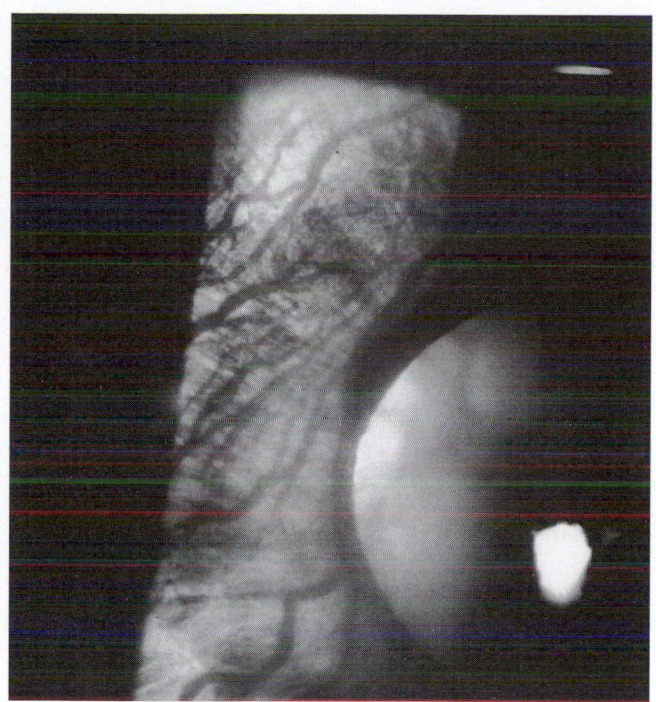

Figure 28–9. End-stage neovascular glaucoma with significant vessel development on the iris surface. (*See also Color Plate 98.*)

glaucoma. The appearance of new vessel growth on the iris in heterochromic iridocyclitis tends to be finer in texture relative to the coarse, somewhat engorged vessels seen in neovascular glaucoma. Intraocular inflammation must also be considered in any differential diagnosis of neovascular glaucoma. Classically, these eyes present with a significant anterior chamber reaction that usually resolves following treatment with topical anti-inflammatory agents. Intraocular hemorrhage (hyphema) of unknown etiology should always be considered as a prelude to neovascular glaucoma even when the patient presents with a normal IOP. Examination of the anterior chamber angle and iris is required to rule out neovascular changes.

It was not long ago that the only expected outcome of neovascular glaucoma was an extremely painful blind eye that required enucleation. The use of photocoagulation of the retina as the primary step in the management of proliferative retinopathy has resulted in a significant reduction in neovascular glaucoma.[64] Neovascular glaucoma is best managed surgically, though medical therapy is utilized in the short term to reduce the IOP as well as to supplement the surgical therapy. Recent studies have demonstrated reasonable levels of success along with significant complications in the use of drainage implants to treat neovascular glaucoma.[65]

UVEITIC GLAUCOMA

Uveitic glaucoma is an ocular condition in which the IOP elevates in association with an episode of uveitis. When the eye becomes inflamed, either because of an idiopathic condition or due to some predisposing situation (systemic disease, ocular syndrome, or trauma), hyperemia develops when the blood vessels supplying the anterior segment dilate. White blood cells are also stimulated, so that greater numbers develop within the anterior segment. With blood vessel dilation, the tight junctions within the blood vessel walls are affected; therefore the white blood cells, now in ample supply, may pass into the anterior chamber (cells). In addition, protein may leak into the anterior chamber, leading to the signs of cells and flare associated with an anterior uveitis. For mild to moderate reactions, cells and flare found in the anterior chamber, which leave via the trabecular meshwork outflow pathway, will have little impact on aqueous outflow. For moderate to severe reactions, the amount of cells and flare may exceed the trabecular meshwork's drainage capacity, with the result that cells clog the drain, thus elevating the IOP. In granulomatous uveitis, which presents with larger cell types such as epithelioid or giant cells, there is a propensity for these cells to clog the TM (Fig. 28–10). Still, an IOP elevation associated with an anterior uveitic attack is unusual and is related to the severity of the anterior chamber reaction. When few cells are visible in the anterior chamber and an elevated IOP is present, the clinician must search for other causes of the elevated IOP. Other etiologies that may elevate the IOP and relate to inflammatory eye disease include trabeculitis, steroid response, pupillary-block

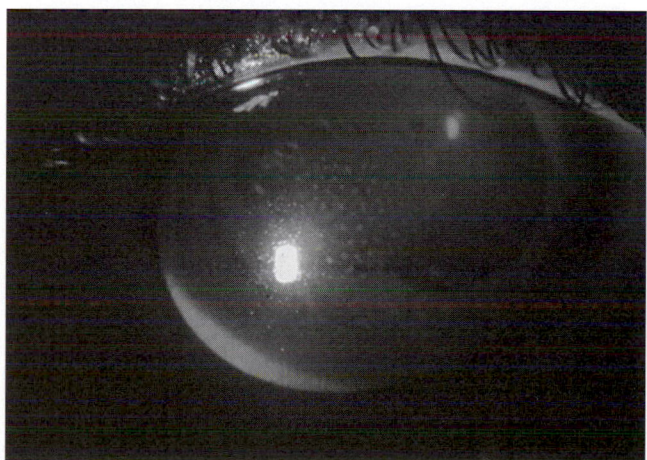

Figure 28–10. An example of a granulomatous anterior uveitis. Large mutton-fat keratitic precipitates are seen on the cornea along with posterior synechiae, as shown by the misshapen pupil.

glaucoma from the formation of posterior synechiae, angle-closure glaucoma associated with the formation of anterior synechiae, recurrent uveitic episodes leading to damage to the trabecular meshwork, Fuchs' heterochromic iridocyclitis, or Posner-Schlossman syndrome.[66]

The onset of the IOP elevation as well as the patient's ocular history are important in understanding the cause of the rise in pressure. For example, elevated IOP noted at the initial presentation along with a moderate to severe uveitic reaction leads one to believe that cells clogging the trabecular meshwork are the principal mechanism. An elevated IOP in an eye with only mild anterior uveitis leads one to suspect a trabeculitis as the culprit, which is a diagnosis of exclusion. Trabeculitis is an inflammation that, along with edema of the trabecular meshwork, reduces the outflow of aqueous. Trabeculitis may elevate the IOP with the remaining portions of the eye not involved. The only signs of a trabeculitis may be a few cells or keratitic precipitates in the anterior chamber.

A common presenting sign of anterior uveitis is reduced IOP in the involved eye secondary to the inflammation involving the ciliary body, which causes reduced production of aqueous. When the IOP at the initial presentation is lower or the same as that in the uninvolved eye and then rises weeks later, a steroid responder must be considered. Another scenario that may lead to elevated IOP is a patient with a history of periodic attacks of acute anterior uveitis that occur over several years' time and that always respond to therapy. The culmination of injury from the periodic attacks may cause permanent damage to the outflow pathways.

Although open-angle glaucoma is the more common presentation in an eye with an anterior uveitis, angle-closure glaucoma may also occur and can take one of two forms. The first form is the pupillary-block type, in which posterior synechiae develop, causing adhesions to form between the lens and the iris. Often seen in cases of chronic or recurrent anterior uveitis, the posterior synechiae may develop around 360 degrees of the pupillary border, leading to the inability

TABLE 28–2. COMPARISON OF SECONDARY AND CONGENITAL GLAUCOMAS

Type of Glaucoma	Biomicroscopic Findings	Gonioscopy	IOP	Characteristics	Prognosis
Pigmentary	Krukenberg spindle, iris transillumination Pigment on lens/iris surface	Fine pigment in trabecular meshwork	Variable increase Diurnal fluctuation	Bilateral Onset 20–40 y/o Myopia	Generally good Diminishes with age
Exfoliative	Gray flake-like deposits at pupil frill Anterior lens annular zone Iris transillumination	Pigment in trabecular meshwork (less than PDS) Increased incidence of narrow angle	Variable, can show rapid increase	Onset 60 y/o and greater	IOP difficult to control ALT effective
Steroid-induced	No characteristic findings	No abnormalities	Usually noted 4–6 weeks after initiation of topical steroid therapy	Family history of glaucoma Concurrent disease treatment with steroids	IOP usually decreases on cessation of steroid
Traumatic	Hyphema Sphincter tear Inflammation Lens subluxation	PAS Angle recession (variable degree) Variation in color of ciliary body	Hypotony to extreme elevation depending on extent of trauma	No specific factors	Variable depending on degree of trauma
Neovascular	Vessels visible on iris surface Hyphema	Arborized vessels in angle PAS Fibrovascular membrane	Initially low, rises with time to extreme levels	Diabetes CRVO BRVO Intraocular surgery	Poor prognosis
Congenital	Corneal edema Descemet's tears Increased corneal diameter	Anterior insertion of iris root Abnormality of trabecular meshwork		Can be associated with systemic disease	Related to age of onset and severity of disease

Key: y/o, years old; IOP, intraocular pressure; PAS, peripheral anterior synechiae; PDS, pigment dispersion syndrome; CRVO, central retinal vein occlusion; BRVO, branch retinal vein occlusion.

of aqueous to communicate between the posterior and anterior chambers. This emergency presents with a red eye, elevated IOP, posterior synechiae, and a history of prior bouts of uveitis. Another form of angle-closure glaucoma may develop in eyes with chronic attacks of anterior uveitis, in which anterior synechiae form around the circumference of the angle, reducing aqueous outflow. The latter two conditions are diagnosed based upon the ocular examination, history, slit-lamp evaluation, and gonioscopic appearance of the angle, which, for the latter condition, will have no visible structures.

The management of elevated IOP in an eye with acute anterior uveitis and an open angle is the use of topical steroids to reduce the inflammation along with medications to reduce aqueous production. As the inflammation subsides, both the steroid and aqueous suppressants may be tapered. For angle-closure or pupillary-block glaucoma, the particular form of glaucoma must be diagnosed correctly. Pupillary-block glaucoma is often managed initially with a laser iridotomy, while angle-closure glaucoma due to anterior synechiae is best managed with filtration surgery.

Fuchs' heterochromic iridocyclitis is an unusual form of mild anterior uveitis that is typically unilateral. In addition to the presence of a few cells within the anterior chamber, stellate keratitic precipitates are noted on the cornea. The chronic anterior uveitis is associated with a moth-eaten, lightly pigmented iris on the involved side, along with an open angle. Few symptoms are associated with the attacks, though reduced vision related to the development of a posterior subcapsular cataract is often the reason for the visit to the eye doctor. Some 15.7% of cases may present with glaucoma.[67] The glaucoma is due to either a trabeculitis or a membrane developing in front of the trabecular meshwork. The primary goal of therapy is to reduce the IOP to prevent optic nerve damage. Medications that reduce aqueous production—such as beta blockers, topical carbonic anhydrase inhibitors, or alpha agonists—are the primary agents for therapy. Miotics or even prostaglandins may reactivate the inflammation and are not typically useful. ALT is also not a useful modality, though filtration surgery may be helpful. Finally, anti-inflammatory agents tend not to reduce the inflammatory reaction or affect the IOP.

Posner-Schlossmann syndrome or *glaucomatocyclitic crisis* refers to a unilateral acute elevation in the IOP that may last from days to weeks. An accompanying mild anterior uveitis accompanies the attack, which is often asymptomatic. Reduced vision associated with corneal edema due to the acute rise in pressure is the symptom most commonly associated with Posner-Schlossmann syndrome. The angle is open on gonioscopy, and a mild anterior chamber reaction and small keratitic precipitates are noted with biomicroscopy. Management includes the judicious use of steroids along with aqueous suppressants to limit the rise in IOP. Careful management is needed between episodes with the objective of utilizing medications only during attacks.

CONCLUSION

The diagnosis and treatment of secondary glaucomas is an important and challenging aspect of the overall management of glaucomas (Table 28–2). Because of the variety of their presentations and their frequent association with underlying ocular and/or systemic disease processes, the clinician is required to have a firm understanding of the anatomy, pathophysiology, differential diagnosis, and treatment of this challenging group of glaucomas.

REFERENCES

1. Teikari JM, O'Donnell J. Epidemiologic data on adult glaucomas: Data from the Hospital Registry of Right to Free Medication. *Acta Ophthalmol.* 1989;67(2):184–191.
2. Petti TH, Keats EV. Traumatic change of the chamber angle. *Arch Ophthalmol.* 1963;69:438.
3. Canavan YM, Archer DB. Anterior segment consequences of blunt ocular injury. *Br J Ophthalmol.* 1982; 66:549.
4. Yospaiboon Y, Sangveejit J, Suwanwatana C. Traumatic hyphema: Clinical study of 149 cases. *J Med Assoc Thailand.* 1989;72(9):520.
5. Howard GM, et al. Hyphema resulting from blunt trauma. *Trans Am Acad Ophthalmol Otolaryngol.* 1965;69: 294–306.
6. Edwards WC, Layden WE. Traumatic hyphema: A report of 184 consecutive cases. *Am J Ophthalmol.* 1973; 75:110.
7. Coles WH. Traumatic hyphema: An analysis of 235 cases. *South Med J.* 1968;61:813.
8. Goldberg MF. The diagnosis and treatment of secondary glaucoma after hyphema in sickle cell patients. *Am J Ophthalmol.* 1979;87:43.
9. Goldberg MF, Tso MOM. Sickled erythrocytes, hyphema and secondary glaucoma: VII. The passage of sickled erythrocytes out of the anterior chamber of the human and monkey eye: Light and electron microscope studies. *Ophthalmol Surg.* 1979;10:89.
10. Marcus M, et al. Aspirin and secondary bleeding after traumatic hyphema. *Ann Ophthalmol.* 1988;20(4):157.
11. Wilson TW, Jeffers JB, Nelson LB. Aminocaproic and prophylaxis in traumatic hyphema. *Ophthalmol Surg.* 1990;21(11):807.

12. Kutner B, Fourman S, Brein K, et al. Aminocaproic acid reduces the risk of secondary hemorrhage in patients with traumatic hyphema. *Arch Ophthalmol.* 1987; 105:206.

13. Blantan FM. Anterior chamber angle recession and secondary glaucoma: A study of the after effects of traumatic hyphema. *Arch Ophthalmol.* 1964;72:39.

14. Sihota R, Sood NN, Agarwal HC. Traumatic glaucoma. *Acta Ophthalmol Scand.* 1995;73(3):252–254.

15. Salmon JF, Mermoud A, Ivey A, et al. The detection of post-traumatic angle recession by gonioscopy in a population-based glaucoma survey. *Ophthalmology.* 1994;101(11):1844–1850.

16. Filipe JA, Barros H, Castro-Correia J. Sports-related ocular injuries: A three-year follow-up study. *Ophthalmology.* 1997;104(2):313–318.

17. Tonjun AM. Gonioscopy in traumatic hyphema. *Acta Ophthalmol.* 1966;44:650.

18. Bron A, Aury P, Salagnac J, et al. Pre-equatorial contusion syndrome: Analysis apropos of 59 cases. *J Fr Ophtalmol.* 1989;12(3):211.

19. Mooney D. Angle recession and secondary glaucoma. *Br J Ophthalmol.* 1973;57:608.

20. Miles DR, Boniuk M. Pathogenesis of unilateral glaucoma. *Am J Ophthalmol.* 1966;62:493.

21. Alper MG. Contusion angle deformity and glaucoma. *Arch Ophthalmol.* 1963;69:455.

22. Lauing L. Anterior chamber glass membranes. *Am J Ophthalmol.* 1969;68:308.

23. Armaly ME. Steroids and glaucoma. In: *Transactions of the New Orleans Academy of Ophthalmology: Symposium on Glaucoma.* St. Louis: CV Mosby; 1967.

24. deJuan E Jr, Sternberg P Jr, Michaels RG. Penetrating ocular injuries: Types of injuries and visual results. *Ophthalmology.* 1983;90:1318.

25. D'Ombrain AW. Traumatic monocular chronic glaucoma. *Trans Ophthalmol Soc Aust.* 1945;V:116.

26. Richardson K. Acute glaucoma after trauma. In: Freeman HM, ed. *Ocular Trauma.* New York: Appleton-Century-Crofts; 1979.

27. Jensn P, Minckler DS, Chandler W. Epithelial ingrowth. *Arch Ophthalmol.* 1977;95:837.

28. Simmers RJ, Kimbrough RL. Late glaucoma after trauma. In: Freeman HM, ed. *Ocular Trauma.* New York: Appleton-Century-Crofts; 1979.

29. Rosenthal AR, Marmor MF, Levenberger P. Chalcosis: A study of natural history. *Ophthalmology.* 1979;86:1956.

30. Rosenthal MJ. Intraocular foreign bodies, prognosis. *Int Ophthalmol Clin.* 1968;8(1):257.

31. Francois J. Cortisone et tension. *Ann Ocul.* 1954;187:805.

32. Garbe E, LeLorier J, Boivin JF, et al. Inhaled and nasal glucocorticoids and the risks of ocular hypertension or open-angle glaucoma. *JAMA.* 1997;277(9):722–727.

33. Armaly MF. Effects of corticosteroids in intraocular pressure and fluid dynamics: II. The effect of dexamethasone in the glaucomatous eye. *Arch Ophthalmol.* 1963;70:492.

34. Becker B, Podos SM. Elevated intraocular pressure following corticosteroid eye drops. *JAMA.* 1963;185:884.

35. Becker B, Hahn KA. Topical corticosteroids and heredity in primary open angle glaucoma. *Am J Ophthalmol.* 1964; 57:543.

36. Armaly MF. Statistical attributes of the steroid hypertensive response in the clinically normal eye: II. The demonstration of three levels of response. *Invest Ophthalmol.* 1965;4:187.

37. Armaly MF. Inheritance of dexamethasone hypertension and glaucoma. *Arch Ophthalmol.* 1967;77:747.

38. Kayes J, Becker B. The human trabecular meshwork in corticosteroid induced glaucoma. *Trans Am Ophthalmol Soc.* 1969;67:354.

39. Francois J. The importance of the micropolysaccharides in intraocular pressure regulation. *Invest Ophthalmol.* 1975;14:173.

40. Weinstein BI, Gordon GG, Southern AL. Potentiation of glucocorticoid activity by 5B-dihydrocortisone: Its role in glaucoma. *Science.* 1983;222:172.

41. Sherwood M, Richardson TM. Evidence for in vivo phagocytosis by trabecular endothelial cells. *Invest Ophthalmol.* 1958;59:216.

42. Bill A. The drainage of aqueous humor. *Invest Ophthalmol.* 1975;14:1.

43. Espildora J, Vicuna P, Diaz E. Cortisone induced glaucoma: A report on 44 affected eyes. *J Fr Ophtalmol.* 1981;4:503.

44. Bartlett JD, Horwitz B, Laibovitz R, Howes JF. Intraocular pressure response to loteprednol etabonate in known steroid responders. *J Ocul Pharmacol.* 1993; 9(2):157–165.

45. Leibowitz HM, Bartlett JD, Rich R, et al. Intraocular pressure raising potential of 1.0% rimexolone in patients responding to corticosteroids. *Arch Ophthalmol.* 1996;114 (8):933–937.

46. Smith RJH. Rubeotic glaucoma. *Br J Ophthalmol.* 1981; 65:606.

47. Weiss DI, Shafer RN, Nehrenberg TR. Neovascular glaucoma complicating cavernous sinus fistula. *Arch Ophthalmol.* 1963;69:304.

48. Federman JL, Brown GC, Felberg NT, et al. Experimental ocular angiogenesis. *Am J Ophthalmol.* 1980;89:231.

49. Ben Ezr D. Neovasculogenesis: Triggering factors and possible mechanisms. *Surv Ophthalmol.* 1979;24:167.

50. Polverini PJ, Cotran PS, Gimbrone MA Jr, et al. Activated macrophages induced vascular proliferation. *Nature* 1977;269:804.

51. Laatikamen L. Development classification of rubeosis irides in diabetic eye disease. *Br J Ophthalmol.* 1979; 63:150.

52. Gutman FA, Zegarra H. The natural course of temporal retinal branch vein occlusion. *Trans Am Acad Ophthalmol Otolaryngol.* 1974;78:178.

53. Hoskins HD Jr. Neovascular glaucoma. Current concepts. *Trans Am Acad Ophthalmol Otolaryngol.* 1974; 78:330.

54. Hayreh SS. So called "central retinal vein occlusion": I. Pathogenesis, terminology, clinical features. *Ophthalmologia.* 1976;172:1.

55. Magaral LE, Brown GC, Augsburger JJ, et al. Neovascular glaucoma following central retinal vein occlusion. *Ophthalmology*. 1981;88:1095.

56. Bertelsen TI. The relationship between thrombosis in the retinal vein and primary glaucoma. *Acta Ophthalmol.* 1961;39:603.

57. Dryden RM. Central vein occlusion and chronic simple glaucoma. *Arch Ophthalmol.* 1965;73:659.

58. Heyreh SS, Podhagsky P. Ocular neovascularization with retinal vascular occlusion: II. Occurrences in central and branch neutral artery occlusion. *Arch Ophthalmol.* 1982;100:1585.

59. Ohrt V. The frequency of rubeosis in diabetic patients. *Arch Ophthalmol.* 1971;49:301.

60. Aiello LM, Ward M, Liang G. Neovascular glaucoma and vitreous hemorrhage following cataract surgery in patients with diabetes mellitus. *Ophthalmology.* 1983; 90:814.

61. Browning DJ, Scott AQ, Peterson CB, et al. The risk of missing angle neovascularization by omitting screening gonioscopy in acute central retinal vein occlusion. *Ophthalmology*. 1998;105(5):776–784.

62. Laatikaninen L, Blach RK. Behavior of the iris vasculature in central retinal vein occlusion: A fluorescein angiographics study of the vascular response of the retina and the iris. *Br J Ophthalmol*. 1977;61:272.

63. Chandler PA, Grant WM. *Glaucoma*. Philadelphia: Lea & Febiger; 1986:201.

64. Cashwell LF, Marks WP. Pan-retinal photocoagulation in the management of neovascular glaucoma. *South Med J.* 1988;81(11):1364.

65. Phillip W, Klima G, Miller K. Clinicopathological findings 11 months after implantation of a functioning aqueous drainage silicone implant. *Graefes Arch Clin Exp Ophthalmol*. 1990;228(5):481–486.

66. Moorthy RS, Mermoud A, Baerveldt G, et al. Glaucoma associated with uveitis. *Surv Ophthalmol.* 1997;41(5): 361–394.

67. Fearnley IR, Rosenthal AR. Fuchs' heterochromic iridocyclitis revisited. *Acta Ophthalmol Scand.* 1995;72(2):166–170.

Chapter 29

ANGLE-CLOSURE GLAUCOMA[*]

**Robert Ritch, Jeffrey M. Liebmann
Hiroshi Ishikawa**

Lawrence[1] first used the term *acute glaucoma* in 1829. Von Graefe[2] in 1861 discovered the beneficial effect of iridectomy and stressed the importance of elevated IOP. Laqueur[3] in 1876 and Weber[4] in 1877 introduced eserine and pilocarpine therapy, respectively. Still, to come to the understanding that angle-closure glaucoma was separate from open-angle glaucoma took nearly a century. Curran[5] was the first to prove that obstruction of aqueous flow from the posterior to the anterior chamber led to the development of acute angle-closure glaucoma. With understanding of pupillary block and the development of peripheral iridectomy, a rational approach to the treatment of angle-closure glaucoma was developed.

THE ANATOMIC BASIS OF ANGLE-CLOSURE GLAUCOMA

Angle-closure glaucoma is caused by apposition of the iris to the trabecular meshwork as a result of abnormal relationships of anterior-segment structures. These, in turn, are caused by abnormal sizes or positions of anterior segment structures or posterior segment forces that alter anterior segment anatomy.[6] The forces causing iris apposition to the trabecular meshwork may be viewed as originating at four successive anatomic levels: the iris (pupillary block), the ciliary body (plateau iris), the lens (phacomorphic glaucoma), and posterior to the lens (malignant glaucoma).[6] The more posterior the level at which the angle closure occurs, the more complex is diagnosis and treatment, since each level may have a component of the mechanism peculiar to each of the levels preceding it. An understanding of these mechanisms makes appropriate treatment in any particular case an exercise in deductive logic. Numerous underlying causes of angle-closure glaucoma have been reported (Table 29–1).

Pupillary Block (Aqueous Pressure)

Relative pupillary block underlies most cases of angle-closure glaucoma. Resistance to transpupillary flow of aqueous humor from the posterior chamber to the anterior chamber is increased by iridolenticular contact. This creates a relative pressure gradient between the two chambers and pushes the iris anteriorly, causing bowing of the iris and narrowing or closure of the angle (Fig. 29–3).

Relative pupillary block typically occurs in hyperopic eyes, which have a shorter than average axial length, a more shallow anterior chamber, a thicker lens, a more anterior lens position, a smaller corneal diameter, and a smaller radius of corneal curvature

---

[*]Supported in part by The New York Glaucoma Research Institute, New York, NY.

TABLE 29–1. ACUTE ANGLE-CLOSURE GLAUCOMA—INCITING AND ASSOCIATED FACTORS

Drugs[107]
General anesthesia[107]
Local anesthesia[108]
Activities and Emotional States
   Fatigue
   Hiccups[109]
   Labor[110]
   Movies and television
   Close work (reading, sewing, etc.)
   Stress, anxiety
   Sex[111]
   Sneezing[112]
Iatrogenic
   Intraocular gas[113]
   Anticoagulants[114,115]
   Miotics[29,30,71]
   Nd:YAG cyclophotocoagulation[116,117]
   Panretinal photocoagulation[118]
   Pupillary dilation
   Scleral buckling procedures[118]
   Silicone oil[118]
   Suture lysis[119,120]
Infections
   Acquired immunodeficiency syndrome[121–125]
   AMPPPE[126], acute mutifocal posterior placoid
     pigment epitheliopathy
   Endophthalmitis[127]
   Hemorrhagic fever with renal syndrome[128,129]
   Herpes simplex[130]
   Herpes zoster[130]
   Influenza[131]

   Keratitis[132]
   Scleritis[132]
   Syphilis[130]
   Uveitis[130]
Ocular Disorders
   Central retinal vein[118]
   Choroidal melanoma[133]
   Ciliary muscle hyperplasia[134]
   Ciliochoroidal detachment[135]
   Exfoliation syndrome[12]
   Familial exudative vitreoretinopathy[136]
   Iris and ciliary body cysts (Fig. 29–1)[137]
   Metastatic carcinoma (Fig. 29–2)[138–140]
   Retinoblastoma[141]
Systemic Disease
   Acute hyperglycemia[142]
   Arteriovenous fistulas[143–147]
   Disorders associated with lens subluxation[148]
   Myelodysplastic syndrome[149]
   Oculomotor nerve palsy[150–153]
   Pituitary apoplexy[154]
   Renal hypertension[155]
   Systemic lupus erythematosus[156]
   Transient ischemic attacks[157]
Trauma
   Botulinum toxin injection[158]
   Chemical burns[159]
   Corneal perforation[120]
   Hemorrhage[159,160]
   Ocular massage or compression[161]

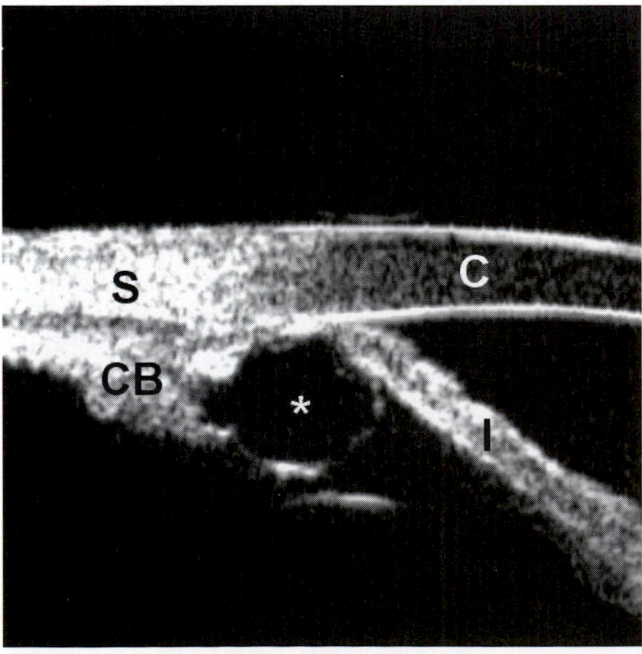

Figure 29–1. Iridociliary cysts (*asterisk*) may cause focal angle closure and are characterized by an echolucent interior. C = cornea; S = sclera; CB = ciliary body; I = iris.

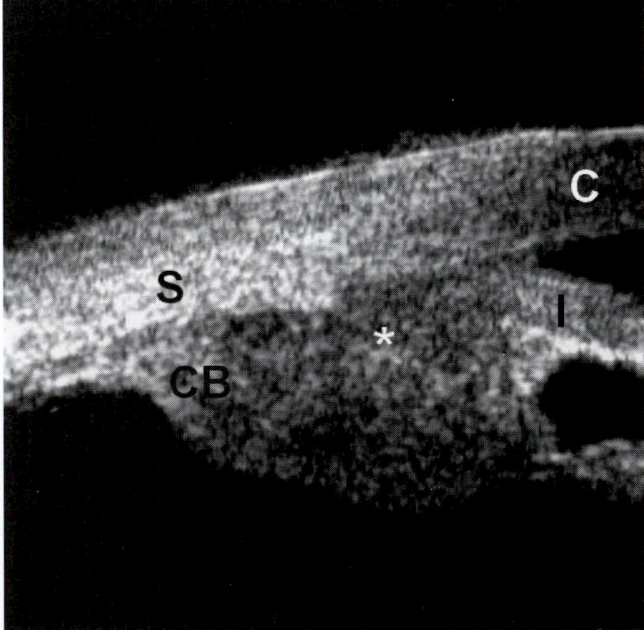

Figure 29–2. Tumors or infiltration of the iris or ciliary body may also cause angle closure and are characterized by uneven internal echoes when compared with cystic structures.

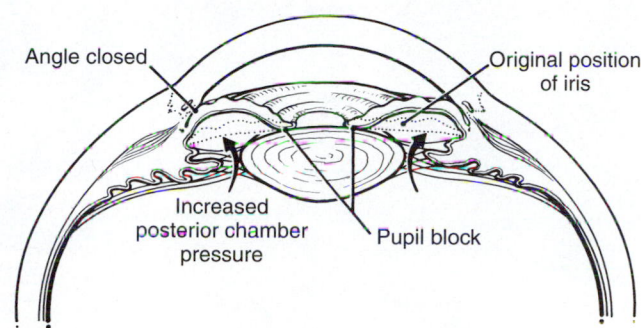

Figure 29–3. Pupillary block leads to elevation of IOP in the posterior chamber, forcing the iris against the angle. This obstructs the angle, leading to elevated IOP.

(Figs. 29–4 and 29–5).[7–11] In absolute pupillary block, there are posterior synechiae between the iris and lens. When pupillary block develops, the iris assumes a bombé configuration, creating an angle which is narrow throughout its approach. Dynamic gonioscopy forces the entire iris posteriorly, opening the angle. If synechiae are absent, the angle opens widely.

Pupillary block does not affect the depth of the central anterior chamber. However, anterior movement of the lens surface through subluxation or swelling increases pupillary block and predisposes to angle closure. Anterior lens movement may occur in some eyes

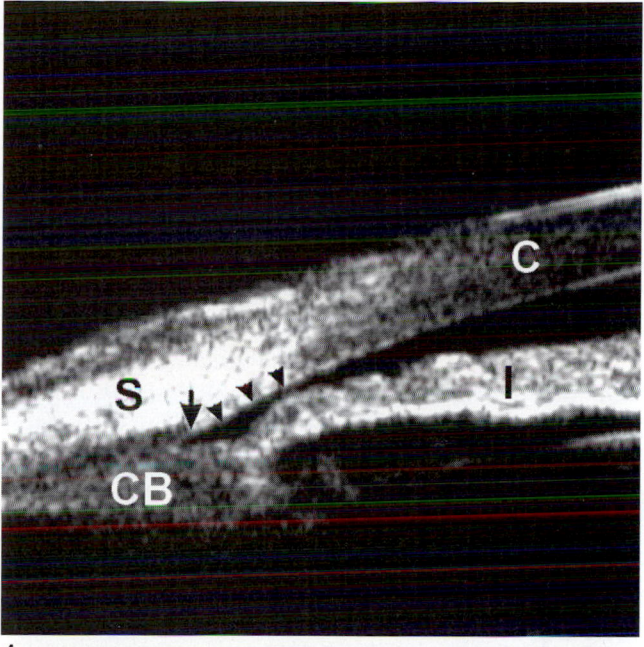

A

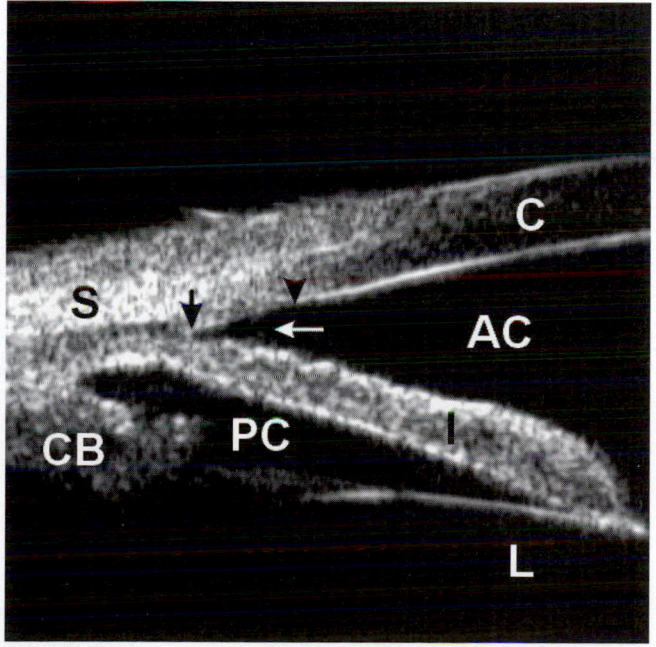

Figure 29–4. The ultrasound biomicrograph of a normal eye. The cornea (C), anterior chamber (AC), iris (I), lens (L), posterior chamber (PC), angle (*white arrow*), scleral spur (*thin arrow*), Schwalbe's line (*arrowhead*) sclera (S), and ciliary body (CB) are visible.

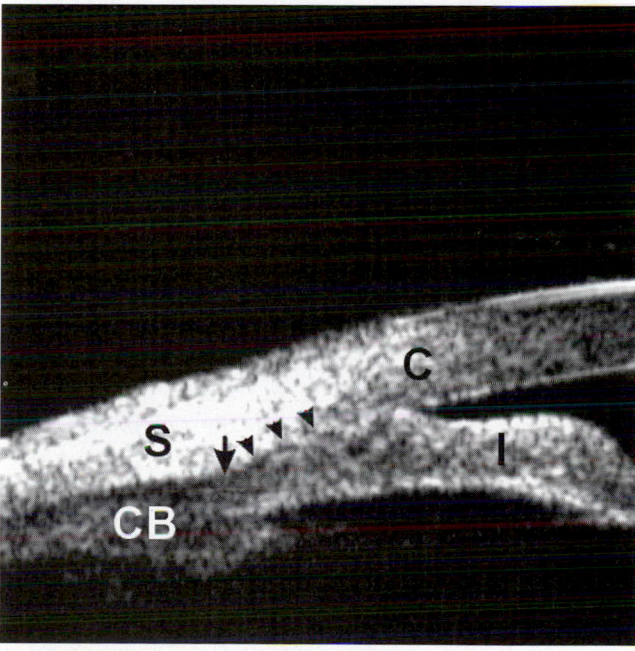

B

Figure 29–5. *A.* Under normal conditions, the miotic response to light causes the angle to open. Aqueous has access to the trabecular meshwork (*arrows*). *B.* If the room illumination is dimmed, pupillary dilation may cause the peripheral iris to crowd the angle and become apposed to the trabecular meshwork (*arrowheads*), causing angle closure.

in the prone position; this is of possible importance in provocative testing and in the etiology of some attacks of angle-closure glaucoma. Miotic-induced ciliary muscle constriction relaxes the zonules, producing anterior lens movement and increased lens thickness and curvature, all of which augment pupillary block. Exfoliation syndrome, presumably because of zonular involvement, appears to predispose to anterior movement of the lens and an increase in pupillary block.[12]

Relative pupillary block usually causes no symptoms. However, if there is appositional closure even with normal IOP, peripheral anterior synechiae (PAS) may form and lead to chronic angle-closure glaucoma. If the pupillary block becomes absolute, the pressure in the posterior chamber increases and pushes the peripheral iris farther forward to cover the trabecular meshwork and close the angle, with an ensuing rise of IOP (acute angle-closure glaucoma) (Fig. 29–6A and B). Laser iridotomy eliminates the pressure differential between the anterior and posterior chambers and relieves the iris convexity. The iris configuration becomes planar and the angle widens. The region of iridolenticular contact actually increases, as aqueous flows through the iridectomy rather than the pupillary space.[13] Surgical iridectomy or laser iridotomy, which cause deepening of the peripheral anterior chamber and increase the volume of the anterior chamber, do not alter the central anterior chamber's depth.[8,14,15]

Plateau Iris (Ciliary Body Pressure)

In plateau iris, the ciliary processes are large or anteriorly situated, supporting the iris root against the trabecular meshwork (Fig. 29–7A and B).[16–19] The anterior chamber is usually of medium depth and the iris surface slightly convex. On gonioscopy, the iris root angulates forward and then centrally. With dynamic gonioscopy, the ciliary processes prevent posterior movement of the peripheral iris, resulting in a configuration in which the slit beam follows the curvature of the iris to its deepest point at the periphery of the lens, where the ciliary processes begin; then it rises again over the ciliary processes before dropping peripherally (double-hump sign). Greater force is needed to open the angle than in pupillary block because the ciliary processes must be displaced and the angle does not open as widely.

Plateau-iris syndrome refers to the development of angle closure, either spontaneously or after pupillary dilation, in an eye with plateau-iris configuration despite the presence of a patent iridectomy or iridotomy. Acute angle-closure glaucoma may develop.[20–23] The extent or the "height" to which the plateau rises determines whether the angle will close completely or only partially.[24] The angle can narrow further with age owing to enlargement of the lens, so that an angle with plateau configuration that does not close after iridotomy may do so some years later. Periodic gonioscopy is required. Argon laser peripheral iridoplasty (ALPI) is the definitive treatment for plateau iris.[25]

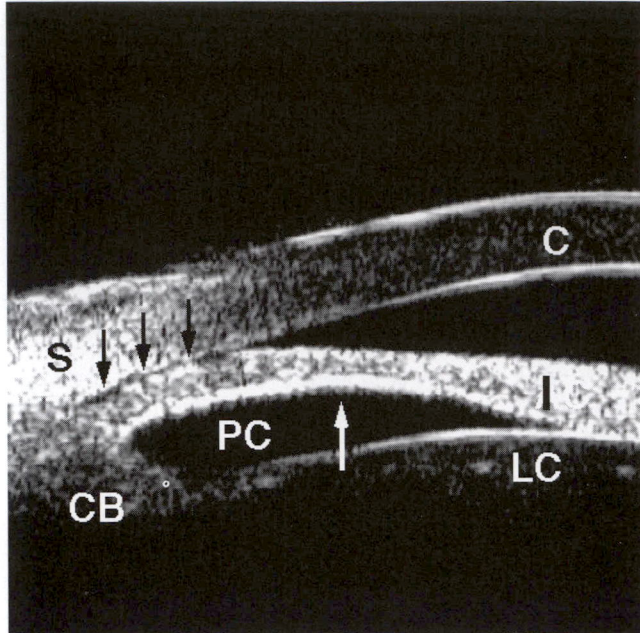

A

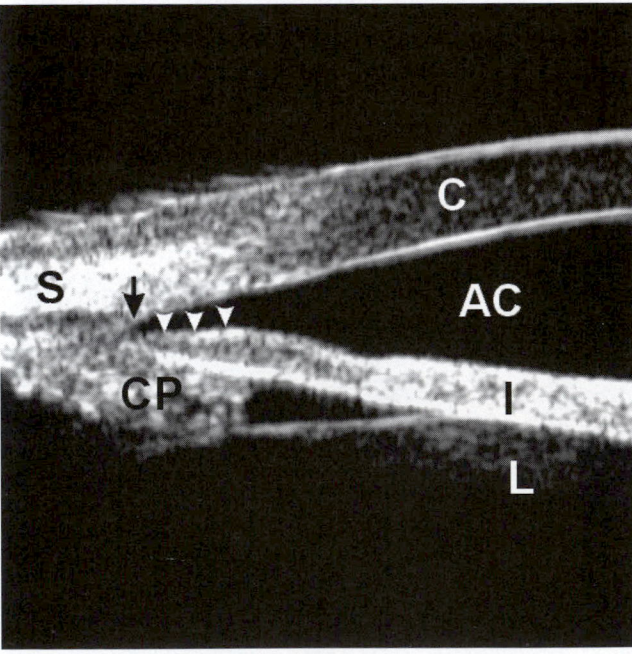

B

Figure 29–6. *A*. In pupillary-block angle closure, the relative pressure differential between the posterior and anterior chambers causes an iris convexity (*white arrow*). *B*. Following laser iridotomy, aqueous has free access to the anterior chamber and the pressure gradient is eliminated.

Phacomorphic Glaucoma (Lens Pressure)

Swelling of the lens may shallow the anterior chamber and precipitate acute angle-closure glaucoma due to the lens pressing against the iris and ciliary body, forcing them anteriorly. Pilocarpine produces a paradoxical reaction, which increases axial lens thickness

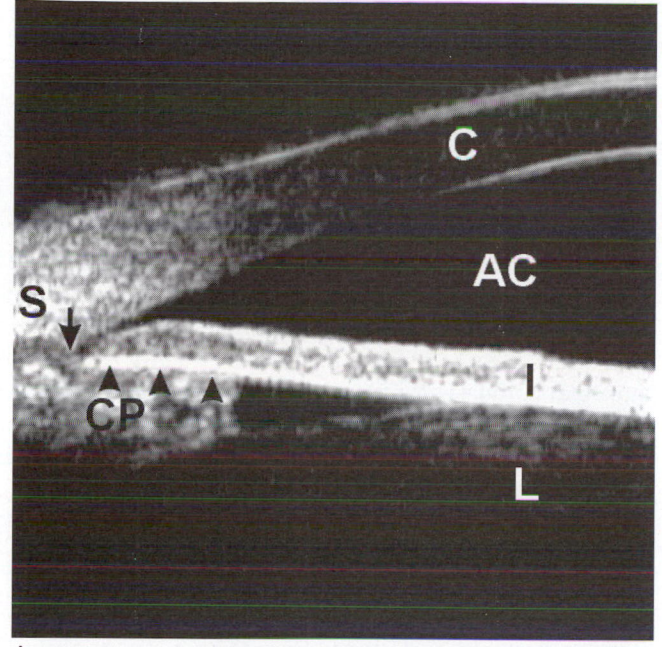

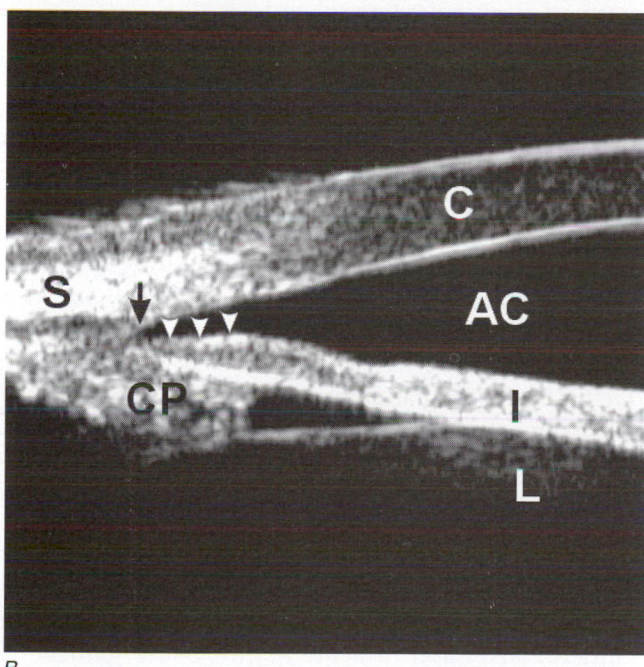

Malignant Glaucoma (Vitreous Pressure)

Angle closure caused by forces posterior to the lens that push the lens-iris diaphragm forward presents a great diagnostic and treatment challenge. In ciliary block—analogous to pupillary block, in which the angle is occluded by iris because of a pressure differential between the posterior and anterior chambers—a pressure differential is created between the vitreous and aqueous compartments by aqueous misdirection into the vitreous (Fig. 29–8).

Swelling or anterior rotation of the ciliary body with forward rotation of the lens-iris diaphragm and relaxation of the zonular apparatus causes displacement of the anterior lens. Ultrasound biomicroscopy often reveals a shallow supraciliary detachment that is not evident on routine B-scan examination. This effusion appears to be the cause of the anterior rotation of the ciliary body and the forward movement of the lens-iris diaphragm. This, combined with aqueous misdirection into the vitreous, increases vitreous pressure, pushing the lens-iris diaphragm forward and causing angle closure by physically pushing the iris against the trabecular meshwork in a manner similar to that in phacomorphic glaucoma.[33]

Figure 29–7. *A.* In plateau iris configuration, the physical presence of the ciliary body forces the peripheral iris (*arrowheads*) into the angle and closes the angle. The scleral spur is visible (*arrow*). *B.* Laser iridoplasty (*white arrows*) may be used in plateau iris syndrome to relieve appositional angle closure.

and causes anterior lens movement, making the anterior chamber still more shallow.[26–31] Pilocarpine, even in elderly patients, increases axial lens thickness and causes anterior lens movement, further shallowing the anterior chamber.[27] ALPI is effective in breaking attacks of phacomorphic angle closure.[32]

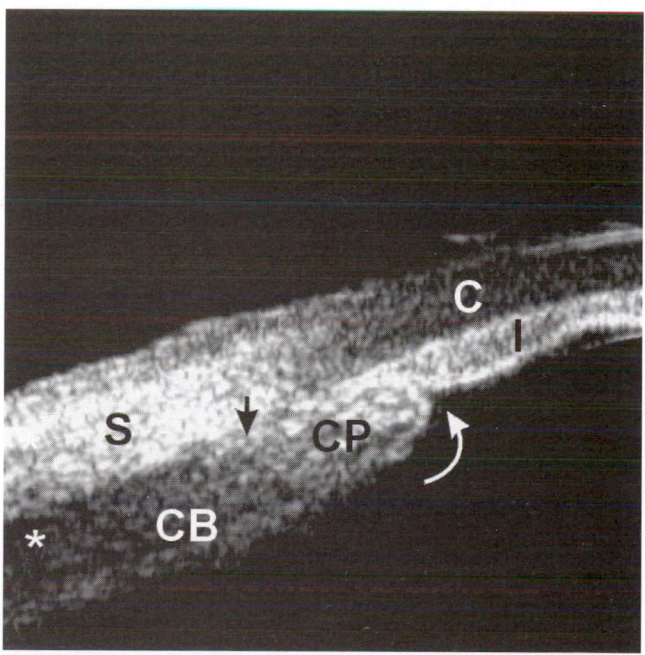

Figure 29–8. Malignant glaucoma can result from aqueous misdirection or from annular ciliary body detachment. In the latter case, fluid is visible in the supraciliary space (*white arrow*). In either case, anterior rotation of the ciliary body about its insertion into the scleral spur may cause a secondary angle-closure glaucoma (*black arrow*).

GONIOSCOPY

Accurate assessment of narrow or closed angles requires precise four-mirror dynamic gonioscopy.[34,35] Use of the Goldmann lens is much less accurate. Pressure on the cornea forces aqueous humor into the angle, widening it. Koeppe gonioscopy generally gives the impression of a wider angle than obtained with the Zeiss or Goldmann lenses, probably due to posterior lens movement when the patient is in the supine position.[36] The presence and extent of synechial closure and the depth of the angle can be determined. The angle should be assessed with respect to iris convexity, width, depth, and the dimensions of PAS or the presence of other pathology. The degree of iris convexity is determined by the degree of pupillary block and the flaccidity of the peripheral iris. In general, the shallower the anterior chamber, the greater the iris convexity.

Gonioscopy in a completely darkened room is of the utmost importance in assessing a patient with a narrow angle for occludability. One should use the smallest square of light for a slit beam to avoid stimulating the pupillary light reflex. The quadrant of angle to be assessed is examined with the four-mirror lens without pressure on the cornea and with the patient looking sufficiently far in the direction of the mirror that the examiner can see as deeply into the angle as possible. The beam is then squared so the pupil is not illuminated and the angle observed while the pupil dilates in the dark. The narrowest quadrant is usually the superior angle (inferior mirror).

A completely closed angle may be mistaken for a wide open angle (false angle). The slit-lamp beam on the posterior cornea meets the beam running across the iris without a break when the angle is closed. If the beams on the iris and the cornea do not meet directly but one is displaced alongside the other, at least the entrance to the angle is open. PAS may be deep in the angle and difficult to see when the angle is very narrow and the iris very convex. Appositional closure and PAS most commonly form initially in the superior angle.[37] When angle closure is limited to the superior angle, maximum pigmentation of the trabecular meshwork may occur there.[38] This pigment is characteristically blotchy and scattered over the trabecular meshwork.

The most commonly used grading system is that of Shaffer,[39,40] in which the width of the angle is graded from 0 (closed) to 4 (wide open). This classification does not assess angle depth or peripheral iris configuration, which are included in the more detailed Spaeth classification,[41,42] providing a more accurate representation of the anatomic features in eyes with angle closure.

CLINICAL TYPES OF ANGLE CLOSURE

Intermittent Angle Closure

Intermittent angle closure consists of repeated brief episodes of angle closure, with mild symptoms of a dull ache in or around one eye and mildly blurred vision with elevated IOP; it resolves spontaneously. Intermittent angle closure is often a prelude to acute angle-closure glaucoma. The pressure is high enough to cause symptoms but not as high as in a full-blown attack. Intermittent attacks are most commonly associated with fatigue, dim light, and use of the eyes for near work; they tend to recur under similar circumstances. Halos around lights are often not seen unless the patient is outdoors. These are thought to result from stretching of the corneal lamellae, causing the cornea to act as a diffraction grating and producing a blue-green central halo and a yellow-red peripheral one. Transient monocular visual loss has also been noted.[43]

The patient may recognize the cause and avoid or reduce the activity, such as watching television or reading. The attacks last for about a half hour after cessation of the inciting activity or cease after the patient goes into a bright room or goes to sleep, both of which constrict the pupil. Initially, intermittent attacks occur weeks or months apart, but eventually they may occur almost nightly. Because the eyes appear normal between attacks except for a narrow angle, the diagnosis is often missed if gonioscopy is not performed, leading to a misdiagnosis of migraine, sinusitis, anxiety, or eyestrain.

Examination reveals shallow anterior chambers, iris bombé, narrow angles, and sometimes an enlarged or oval pupil. Provocative testing may result in angle closure, elevated IOP, and reproduction of the patient's symptoms. Attacks may be accompanied by progressive PAS formation, leading to chronic angle closure. The greatest danger lies in the possibility of sudden conversion to acute angle-closure glaucoma. Laser iridotomy is definitive if the eye is otherwise normal and the angle not occludable by mechanisms other than pupillary block.

In Asians, the history may be consistent with intermittent angle-closure glaucoma, but the IOP is often elevated and the angle variably closed by PAS, depending on the frequency and severity of the attacks. Asian eyes are more prone to "creeping" angle closure and PAS formation. Iridotomy alone may be insufficient to control IOP. Blacks also have a greater tendency to develop chronic angle closure.

Both intermittent and acute attacks are less common in blacks than in Asians.

Subacute Angle-Closure Glaucoma

Subacute angle closure is a stage in which attacks may be more frequent and prolonged than in intermittent angle closure but less so than in acute angle closure. At least in some cases, this is caused by less than total closure of the angle.[44] Symptoms of blurred vision, pain, and halos may be more marked than in intermittent angle closure. Attacks may occur over months or years, finally leading to an acute attack. Subacute attacks are much more common in Asians than in whites and can cause severe damage without much inflammation. They tend to produce a chronically dilated pupil, mild iris atrophy, PAS, and pigment on the iris close to the inferior angle. Intraocular pressure levels and glaucomatous disc and visual field damage vary according to the severity and duration of the attacks.

Acute Angle-Closure Glaucoma

The physiological factors that convert relative pupillary block to absolute pupillary block remain poorly understood, as do those that determine whether an eye will develop acute or chronic angle closure. Although pupillary block is the common underlying mechanism, the course of the disease depends on the degree and suddenness of the block, the flaccidity and physiological responses of the iris, and the width and depth of the anterior chamber angle. Absolute pupillary block is most commonly triggered when the pupil is middilated, about 3.5 to 6 mm in diameter.[45] In this position, the combination of pupillary block and relaxation of the peripheral iris, allowing its forward displacement into the anterior chamber, are maximal. Mapstone[46] concluded that the posteriorly directed forces of the dilator and sphincter muscles and the stretching force of the sphincter during contraction are greatest when the pupil is middilated.

Most attacks occur during the evening, beginning mildly and rapidly increasing in severity. Approximately one-third of patients describe episodes of intermittent or subacute angle closure as having occurred before the acute attack. The most common precipitating events include illness, emotional stress, trauma, intense concentration, and pharmacological pupillary dilation.[47,48] The role of emotional stress in inducing acute angle closure should not be underestimated.[49-51]

The signs and symptoms of an acute attack result from the sudden, marked elevation of IOP. Corneal edema produces blurred vision, intense pain, lacrimation, and lid edema (Table 29–2). Combined with

TABLE 29–2. SIGNS AND SYMPTOMS OF ACUTE ANGLE-CLOSURE GLAUCOMA

Signs	Symptoms
Conjunctival and ciliary injection	Red eye
	Photophobia
Cells and flare	Halos/blurred vision
Elevated IOP	Nausea/emesis
Middilated pupil	
Segmental iris atrophy	
Corneal edema	
Glaukomfleken or cataract	
Optic disc congestion	
Central retinal artery	

anxiety and fatigue, these lead to nausea and vomiting, while vasovagal responses cause bradycardia and diaphoresis. Central visual acuity is reduced. The lids are swollen and there is conjunctival hyperemia and circumcorneal injection (Fig. 29–9). The pupil is usually middilated and vertically oval because of iris sphincter ischemia. The anterior chamber is shallow but formed centrally, while the midperipheral iris is bowed forward and may touch the peripheral cornea. Anterior chamber inflammation is present, and hypopyon can occur in severe or prolonged attacks.[52,53]

Corneal edema may initially limit gonioscopic and posterior segment examination, even after the topical application of glycerin. Inability to open the angle with dynamic gonioscopy at this stage does not mean that the angle will remain sealed after iridotomy, nor

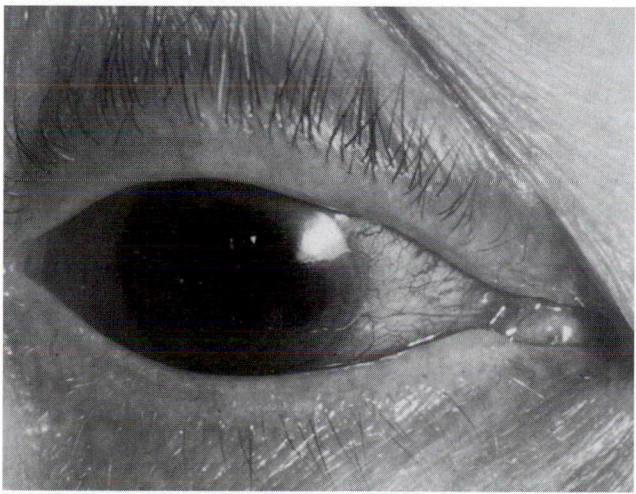

Figure 29–9. An angle-closure attack typically presents with a red eye, cloudy cornea, and a middilated pupil. (*See also Color Plate 99.*)

does it accurately reflect the presence or extent of PAS. Examination of the opposite eye is particularly useful in differentiating acute angle-closure glaucoma from neovascular, uveitic, or phacolytic glaucoma; it usually reveals a shallow anterior chamber and narrow angle.

With prolonged attacks or cases in which unrecognized chronic angle-closure glaucoma precedes an acute attack, pallor and cupping, along with visual field damage, may be present. Central retinal vein occlusion may occur as a result of an acute attack[18,54] or may precipitate one.[55-60] Visual-field changes associated with acute pressure elevation usually show nonspecific generalized or upper field constriction.[61] Early loss of central vision, enlargement of the blind spot, and defects in the nerve fiber bundle may be found.[62,63] After normalization of the IOP, the visual fields may also normalize or patients may be left with reduced color vision, generalized decreased sensitivity, or specific defects. These may be exaggerated by cataract formation or progression.

An attack may terminate spontaneously if iris atrophy allows aqueous humor to percolate through the iris stroma, equivalent functionally to a spontaneous iridotomy. Spontaneous termination may also be facilitated by a change in the position of the lens-iris contact or segmental iris constriction with peaking of the pupil.[64]

Chronic Angle-Closure Glaucoma

Chronic angle-closure glaucoma (CACG) is a condition in which portions of the anterior chamber angle of an eye are permanently closed by PAS. We use the term *CACG* to denote eyes in which chronic appositional closure without PAS has led to elevated IOP or in which appositional closure with the formation of PAS has occurred in the presence of normal IOP. A patient who, after iridotomy is performed for acute angle-closure glaucoma (AACG), has PAS is also considered to have had CACG prior to developing the AACG. Prolonged apposition or repeated subacute attacks lead to gradual PAS formation. These attacks usually begin in the superior angle, which is narrower than the inferior angle,[37,65] as pinpoint synechiae reaching to the midtrabecular meshwork and then gradually expanding in width. In early cases, in which appositional closure is present and IOP is normal but in which PAS have not yet formed, we prefer the term *chronic appositional closure*. This condition can lead to elevated IOP and glaucomatous disc and visual field damage without PAS formation.[66]

Eyes with progressive PAS formation may eventually develop AACG when pupillary block results in closure of the remaining portions of the angle unaffected by PAS. Many patients, however, develop gradual angle closure, elevated IOP, and glaucomatous damage in the absence of symptoms. The presentation is similar to that of chronic open-angle glaucoma, with progression of glaucomatous cupping and visual field loss.

PAS may also form during an acute attack, remaining after iridotomy has opened the unaffected portions of the angle. These PAS are usually high and broad. When they are first observed at this stage, it is impossible to determine whether the PAS formed before or during the attack or at both times.

In eyes with darker irides, a second mechanism of progressive angle closure is more common. The closure is circumferential and begins in the deepest portion of the angle. Closure occurs more evenly in all quadrants, so that the angle progressively becomes more shallow. The appearance over time is of a progressively more anterior iris insertion. Lowe[67] has termed this *creeping angle closure*. The PAS gradually creep up the ciliary face to the scleral spur and then to the trabecular meshwork.

Insertion of the iris at or anterior to the scleral spur is rare in young individuals; in many eyes with angle-closure glaucoma that have such an insertion, creeping angle closure is the underlying reason. Creeping angle closure is uncommon in whites but much more prevalent in Asians, in whom it ranks high as a cause of blindness. Black patients with angle closure also tend to have this form. It occurs in eyes with slightly deeper anterior chambers than are found in AACG. Gradual shortening of the angle in the presence of iris bombé brings the peripheral iris close to the external angle wall more and more anteriorly, narrowing the gap between the iris and the trabecular meshwork. Eventually, AACG may supervene or the PAS may permanently occlude the trabecular meshwork and lead to elevated IOP and glaucomatous damage.

The IOP in eyes with CACG may be normal or elevated. As PAS formation progresses in the absence of intermittent attacks, IOP rises gradually as less and less functional meshwork becomes available. In eyes with intermittent attacks, IOP rises more rapidly relative to the extent of PAS formation, which is caused by recurrent damage to the trabecular meshwork by the transient angle closure. The anterior chamber is quiet and usually deeper than in eyes with AACG. The pupil is normal. The gradual elevation of IOP does not result in corneal endothelial decompensation, and corneal edema is rare. The IOP is usually less than 40 mmHg and does not reach the levels found in AACG. Symptoms are absent until the pressure rises high enough to affect the cornea or until extensive visual field damage has occurred. Although iridotomy will eliminate the pupillary block, IOP often remains elevated and further medical treatment or surgery is required.

Combined-Mechanism Glaucoma

Combined-mechanism glaucoma refers to situations in which both open-angle and angle-closure components are present. Most commonly, angle-closure glaucoma is treated successfully with iridotomy, eliminating all appositional closure, and IOP still remains elevated with or without the presence of PAS of any extent. Conversely, a patient with open-angle glaucoma may later develop angle closure, either because of the natural development of pupillary block or because of exacerbation by miotic therapy. Exfoliation syndrome commonly predisposes to combined-mechanism glaucoma.[12] Here, open-angle glaucoma can develop independently years after iridotomy for angle closure, with progressive blockage of the trabecular meshwork. In all of these cases, the residual open-angle component is treated as open-angle glaucoma.

Mixed-Mechanism Glaucoma

This term is often used interchangeably with combined-mechanism glaucoma, but it should not be, as the usage creates additional confusion. It is better to reserve it to describe an eye with angle closure due to more than one contributory mechanism. When pupillary block is eliminated by iridotomy and the angle opens to a greater degree than before the iridotomy, appositional closure remains on the basis of plateau iris, phacomorphic glaucoma, or malignant glaucoma, and a mixed mechanism may be said to be present.

Plateau Iris

Until recently, plateau-iris syndrome was considered rare. We have differentiated two subtypes.[24] In the complete syndrome, which is rare, IOP rises when the angle closes with pupillary dilation. In the incomplete syndrome, it does not. The differentiating factor is the height of the plateau with respect to the angle structures. If the angle closes to the upper meshwork or Schwalbe's line, IOP rises, since aqueous outflow is completely blocked; whereas if the angle closes partially, leaving the upper portion of the filtering meshwork open, aqueous humor can still exit the eye. This is far more common and its detection is important, as these patients can develop PAS up to years after a successful iridotomy produces what appears as a well-opened angle.

Plateau iris occurs because large and/or anteriorly positioned ciliary processes hold the peripheral iris up against the trabecular meshwork.[16,17,19] Iris cysts may also cause a situation equivalent to plateau iris.[68] When dynamic gonioscopy is performed in such an eye, the ciliary processes prevent posterior movement of the peripheral iris. As a result, a sinuous configuration results (double-hump sign), in which the iris follows the curvature of the lens, reaches its deepest point at the lens equator, and then rises again over the ciliary processes before dropping peripherally. Much more force is needed during gonioscopy to open the angle than in pupillary block, because the ciliary processes must be displaced and the angle does not open as widely. In a morphometric study of the ciliary sulcus, Orgül et al.[69] proposed that the displacement of the pars plicata from the peripheral iris to the iris root during embryogenesis may be incomplete in eyes of shorter axial length.

Patients with plateau iris tend to be female, younger (in their thirties to fifties), and less hyperopic than those with relative pupillary block; they often have a family history of angle-closure glaucoma. Except in the rare younger patients (in their twenties and thirties), some element of pupillary block is also present. If plateau iris was not diagnosed before iridotomy and IOP is elevated postlaser, careful gonioscopy should be performed. If the angle is open, secondary damage to the trabecular meshwork or pigment liberation with dilation are the most likely causes. If the angle is closed, the differential diagnosis, besides plateau iris, should include malignant glaucoma, in which the anterior chamber is extremely shallow; PAS, which can be ruled out by dynamic gonioscopy; or incomplete iridectomy.

Miotic-Induced Angle-Closure Glaucoma

Prolonged miotic treatment in eyes with open-angle glaucoma and narrow angles may lead to pupillary block and angle-closure glaucoma. We have seen CACG develop after several years of miotic therapy in eyes that initially had wide open angles. In some eyes, zonular relaxation occurs more readily than in others, so that anterior lens movement and an increase in axial lens thickness may facilitate pupillary block and angle closure. In other eyes, there is little change in the lens, but progressively increasing pressure in the posterior chamber gradually pushes the peripheral iris against the trabecular meshwork. It is our impression that eyes with exfoliation syndrome are particularly prone to develop miotic-induced angle closure. In these eyes, the iris is thicker and stiffer than normal due to deposition of exfoliation material within the stroma. In addition, zonular weakness allows the lens to move forward, leading to pupillary block.

Less commonly, miotic therapy can have a pronounced effect on lens position and may trigger malignant glaucoma.[29,30,70,71] Unequal anterior chamber depths, a progressive increase in myopia, and progressive shallowing of the anterior chamber are clues to the correct diagnosis.

Malignant Glaucoma

Malignant (ciliary block) glaucoma[70,72-75] is a multifactorial disease in which the following components may play varying roles: (1) previous acute or chronic angle-closure glaucoma, (2) shallowness of the anterior chamber, (3) forward movement of the lens, (4) pupillary block by the lens or vitreous, (5) slackness of the zonules, (6) anterior rotation and/or swelling of the ciliary body, (7) thickening of the anterior hyaloid membrane, (8) expansion of the vitreous, and (9) posterior aqueous displacement into or behind the vitreous.

In predisposed eyes, miotic therapy can have a pronounced effect on lens position and can trigger malignant glaucoma.[29,30,70,71] Unequal anterior chamber depths, a progressive increase in myopia, and progressive shallowing of the anterior chamber are clues to the correct diagnosis.

Malignant glaucoma may occur following cataract surgery with posterior chamber intraocular lens implantation.[76-82] The differential diagnosis includes pupillary block, choroidal hemorrhage, and ciliochoroidal effusion with anterior rotation of the ciliary body and secondary angle closure. Shallowing of the central anterior chamber occurs in pseudophakic malignant glaucoma but not in pupillary block. Rupture of the anterior hyaloid face is usually curative and allows aqueous to move into the anterior segment. We have examined several patients with presumed aqueous misdirection in whom an annular ciliary body detachment had caused anterior movement of the ciliary body. Whether a posterior diversion of aqueous flow is present in these disorders is unknown.

TREATMENT OF ACUTE ANGLE-CLOSURE GLAUCOMA

Medical Therapy

Hyperosmotic agents raise serum osmotic pressure, thus removing fluid from the eye, especially from the vitreous. The decrease in vitreous volume lowers IOP and allows the lens to move posteriorly. IOP decreases within 30 to 60 minutes after administration, the effect lasting about 5 to 6 hours. Patients should limit fluid intake for maximum benefit. Oral 50% glycerol, 1 to 1.5 g/kg, has been used most commonly. We prefer isosorbide, 1.5 to 2.0 g/kg, which is more palatable, causes less nausea and vomiting, and is not metabolized—an advantage particularly in diabetics. A solution of 20% mannitol, 1 to 2 g/kg, given intravenously over 45 minutes has a greater hypotensive effect and may be given when severe nausea and vomiting are present. Administration of hyperosmotic agents is commonly accompanied by thirst and headache. Hyperosmolar coma can be a serious complication caused by severe CNS dehydration. Patients with renal or cardiovascular disease or those already dehydrated by vomiting are at risk.

Acetazolamide, a carbonic anhydrase inhibitor, is highly effective in acute angle-closure glaucoma. It can open some closed angles even in the presence of ischemic iris atrophy and paralysis of the pupil.[83] Rapid IOP reduction is most reliably achieved by giving 500 mg intravenously, which route has a more rapid onset of action. Adverse reactions are uncommon. Acetazolamide tablets may be given orally as an alternative, but the onset of action is not as rapid. Following oral therapy, the maximum effect occurs at 2 hours and high plasma levels persist for 4 to 6 hours but then drop rapidly because of excretion in the urine. Beta-adrenergic antagonists and alpha$_2$ agonists are additive with acetazolamide but have a more prolonged onset of action than intravenous acetazolamide in acute angle-closure glaucoma. They are more useful in later stages of treatment and in maintaining reduced IOP before laser iridotomy.

The use of miotics to constrict the pupil and draw the peripheral iris away from the trabecular meshwork was formerly the main approach to treatment of acute angle-closure glaucoma. The more severe and prolonged the attack, the more frequently miotics were applied. A typical recommended regimen was 4% pilocarpine every 5 minutes for four doses, every 15 minutes for four doses, then every hour for four doses or until the attack was broken. However, when IOP is over 60 mmHg, the pupil is unresponsive to miotics because of ischemia and paralysis of the iris sphincter. Not only may pilocarpine be ineffective, but it may paradoxically worsen the situation even in pupillary block.[29-32,84] Although the miotic effect of pilocarpine is blocked when IOP is extremely high, ciliary muscle contraction and anterior movement of the lens-iris diaphragm are not.

Pilocarpine may also contribute to maintaining elevated IOP by reducing uveoscleral outflow.[28] High doses of pilocarpine may produce cholinergic toxicity, which may not be noticed because of the nausea and vomiting associated with the acute angle-closure attack. Strong miotics, such as echothiophate, should not be used because they can increase both the pupillary block and vascular congestion. Ganias and Mapstone[85] found that immediate treatment with intravenous acetazolamide and repeated instillation of 2% pilocarpine was not more successful in breaking attacks of angle closure than treatment with acetazolamide and a single drop of pilocarpine given 3 hours later. Similar results were obtained with topically administered timolol in place of acetazolamide.[86]

Physical methods have been reported to be successful in breaking an attack of acute angle closure. Indentation of the central part of the cornea with a Zeiss gonioscopy lens, cotton-tipped applicator, or muscle hook, forcing aqueous peripherally, may open the angle temporarily. Repeated cycles of 30 seconds of indentation followed by release of pressure for 30 seconds may allow enough aqueous humor to flow out of the angle to lower the pressure and allow miotics to be effective.[87]

Angle-closure glaucoma is associated with a marked inflammatory reaction. The instillation of 1% prednisolone or 0.1% dexamethasone is desirable from the start to reduce inflammation before laser or surgery. Severe pain may be treated with analgesics, and vomiting may be treated with antiemetics.

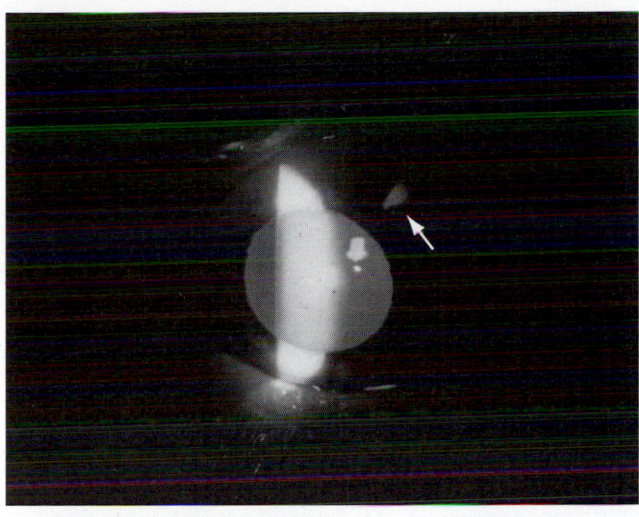

Figure 29–10. A laser peripheral iridotomy. (Courtesy of Mitchell Dul, O.D.) (*See also Color Plate 100.*)

Our Approach to Acute Angle-Closure Glaucoma

The following is our approach to a patient with acute angle closure[88]:

1. Careful history of symptoms relating to intermittent angle-closure attacks, attacks in the fellow eye, prescription or nonprescription drugs that may precipitate attacks, and type of activity preceding the attack.
2. Examination of the affected eye and fellow eye with attention to central and peripheral anterior chamber depth as well as the shape of the peripheral iris.
3. Administration of oral isosorbide and one or more topical aqueous suppressants.
4. The patient lies supine to permit the lens to fall posteriorly with vitreous dehydration.
5. The eye is reassessed after 1 hour. IOP is usually decreased, but the angle usually remains appositionally closed. One drop of 2 or 4% pilocarpine is given and the patient reexamined 30 minutes later.

    a. If IOP is reduced and the angle is open, the patient may be treated medically with topical low-dose pilocarpine, aqueous suppressants, and steroids until the eye quiets and laser iridotomy may be performed (Fig. 29–10).
    b. If IOP is unchanged or elevated and the angle remains closed, lens-related angle closure should be suspected, further pilocarpine withheld, and the attack broken by argon laser peripheral iridoplasty.[32,89,90]

Peripheral iridoplasty does not eliminate pupillary block and is not a substitute for laser iridotomy, which must be performed as soon as the eye is quiet. However, even in eyes with extensive synechial closure, IOP is lowered sufficiently for a few days for the inflammation to resolve. Peripheral iridoplasty is much safer than attempting surgical iridectomy on an inflamed eye with elevated IOP. The risks of intraoperative surgery are avoided and, even if malignant glaucoma is present, the angle remains open long enough for inflammation to clear. The alternative of waiting and prolonging medical therapy for several days seriously increases the possibility of irreversible damage to the iris, lens, drainage pathways, and optic nerve head.[91]

Treatment of Chronic Angle-Closure Glaucoma

It is important to recognize early stages of appositional angle closure in the absence of PAS and to recognize deep, circumferential angle-closure (Fig. 29–11).[92] Laser iridotomy is indicated for all stages of CACG.[93,94] Iridotomy will open those areas of the angle not involved by PAS and prevent further synechial closure. Miotic treatment may enhance the development of CACG in the absence of an iridotomy. When miotic-induced angle closure occurs, the approach to treatment should be determined by assessing the medications necessary to control the glaucoma. If a patient is taking dipivefrin, its discontinuation may be enough to open the angle

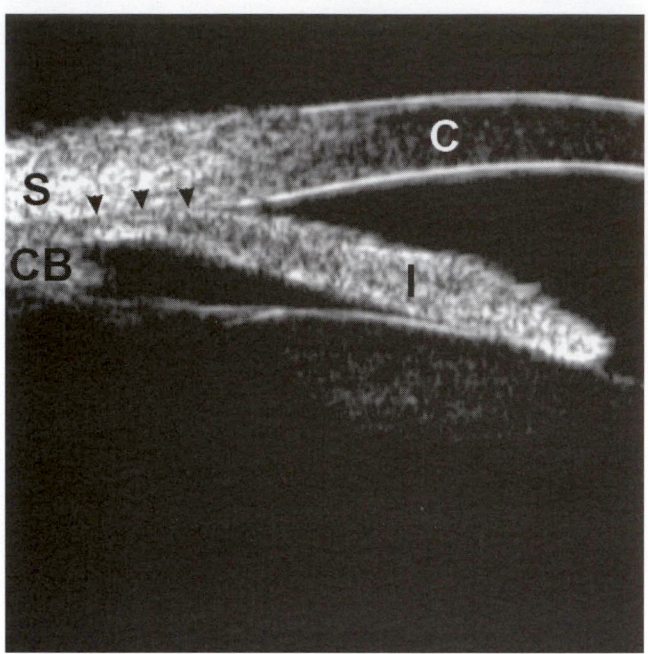

Figure 29–11. Peripheral anterior synechiae (*arrowheads*).

from the angle wall and restoring trabecular mesh-work function.[101-106] A paracentesis track is made into the anterior chamber and the chamber is allowed to shallow slightly. Massage is performed at the limbus to force aqueous from the posterior chamber into the anterior chamber. A viscoelastic agent is injected and the angle is visualized with direct gonioscopy. An irrigating cyclodialysis spatula is used to separate a small segment of PAS at a time, with an anterior-to-posterior movement.

Goniosynechialysis is successful only if the synechiae have been present for less than 1 year. Although it has not become popular in the United States, it has in Asia, where promising results have been reported in both phakic and pseudophakic eyes. It is effective both alone and in conjunction with other surgical procedures. Argon laser peripheral iridoplasty can be used postoperatively to further flatten the peripheral iris and prevent synechial reattachment.[105] Complications include bleeding, iridodialysis, and marked inflammation.

and allow the patient to remain on miotics, presuming that IOP remains under control. If the patient has been treated with miotics alone, substitution of aqueous suppressants may suffice. If the patient requires miotics for IOP control, then laser iridotomy is warranted.

If the angle remains appositionally closed or spontaneously occludable after laser iridotomy, argon laser peripheral iridoplasty is indicated to prevent progressive damage to or further appositional and/or synechial closure of the angle.[89,95-97] If, after iridoplasty, some of the angle still remains appositionally closed, low-dose pilocarpine, such as 2% at bedtime, often suffices to maintain the patency of the angle.

The need for continued medical treatment after iridotomy is determined by the level of IOP and the extent of glaucomatous damage. Treatment is similar to that of open-angle glaucoma. Repeated gonioscopy is necessary. The need for further surgery cannot be predicted from the level of initial IOP or the gonioscopic changes. Argon laser trabeculoplasty has been reported both to be successful[98] and to be unsuccessful[99] after iridotomy in combined-mechanism glaucoma. We have found it overall to be reasonably successful. If the pressure remains uncontrolled and glaucomatous damage develops, filtration surgery is indicated. There is an increased chance of developing malignant glaucoma following filtration surgery in patients who have had angle-closure glaucoma.[100]

Goniosynechialysis is a surgical procedure designed for the purpose of physically stripping PAS

REFERENCES

1. Lawrence W. Lectures on surgery: Medical and operative, lectures LXX–LXXII. *Lancet* 1829–1830;1:705.
2. von Graefe A. *Three Memoirs on Iridectomy*. London: The New Sydenham Society; 1861.
3. Laqueur L. Ueber eine neue therapeutische Verwendung des Physostigmins. *Zentralbl Med Wissensch*. 1876;24:421.
4. Weber A. Das Calabar und seine therapeutische Verwendung. *von Graefes Arch Klin Exp Ophthalmol*. 1877;23:1.
5. Curran EJ. A new operation for glaucoma involving a new principle in the aetiology and treatment of chronic primary glaucoma. *Arch Ophthalmol* 1920;49:131–155.
6. Ritch R, Liebmann J, Tello C. A construct for understanding angle-closure glaucoma: The role of ultrasound biomicroscopy. *Ophthalmol Clin North Am*. 1995; 8:281–293.
7. Delmarcelle Y, Francois J, Goes F, et al. Biometrie oculaire clinique (oculometrie). *Bull Soc Ophtalmol Belge* 1976;1:172.
8. Lee DA, Brubaker RF, Illstrup DM. Anterior chamber dimensions in patients with narrow angles and angle-closure glaucoma. *Arch Ophthalmol*. 1984;102:46–50.
9. Lowe RF. Primary angle-closure glaucoma: A review of ocular biometry. *Aust J Ophthalmol*. 1977;5:9–17.
10. Lowe RF, Clark BAJ. Posterior corneal curvature: Correlations in normal eyes and in eyes involved with primary angle-closure glaucoma. *Br J Ophthalmol*. 1973; 57:475.
11. Tomlinson A, Leighton DA. Ocular dimensions in the heredity of angle-closure glaucoma. *Br J Ophthalmol*. 1973;57:475–486.

12. Ritch R. Exfoliation syndrome: Clinical findings and occurrence in patients with occludable angles. *Trans Am Ophthalmol Soc*. 1994;92:845–944.

13. Caronia RM, Liebmann JM, Stegman Z, et al. Iris-lens contact increases following laser iridotomy for pupillary block angle-closure. *Am J Ophthalmol* 1996;122:53–57.

14. Coakes R, Lloyd-Jones D, Hitchings RA. Anterior chamber volume. Its measurement and clinical significance. *Trans Ophthalmol Soc UK*. 1979;99:78–81.

15. Jacobs IH, Krohn DL. Central anterior chamber depth after laser iridectomy. *Am J Ophthalmol*. 1980;88:865.

16. Pavlin CJ, Ritch R, Foster FS. Ultrasound biomicroscopy in plateau iris syndrome. *Am J Ophthalmol*. 1992;113:390–395.

17. Ritch R. Plateau iris is caused by abnormally positioned ciliary processes. *J Glaucoma*. 1992;1:23–26.

18. Tornquist R. Angle-closure glaucoma in an eye with a plateau type of iris. *Acta Ophthalmol*. 1958;36:413.

19. Wand M, Pavlin CJ, Foster FS. Plateau iris syndrome: Ultrasound biomicroscopic and histological study. *Ophthalm Surg*. 1993;24:129.

20. Godel V, Stein R, Feiler-Ofry V. Angle-closure glaucoma following peripheral iridectomy and mydriasis. *Am J Ophthalmol*. 1968;65:555–560.

21. Lowe RF. Primary angle-closure glaucoma: Postoperative acute glaucoma after phenylephrine eye-drops. *Am J Ophthalmol*. 1968;65:552.

22. Lowe RF. Plateau iris. *Aust J Ophthalmol*. 1981;9:71.

23. Wand M, Grant WM, Simmons RJ, et al. Plateau iris syndrome. *Trans Am Acad Ophthalmol Otolaryngol*. 1977;83:122.

24. Lowe RF, Ritch R. Angle-closure glaucoma: Clinical types. In: Ritch R, Shields MB, Krupin T, eds. *The Glaucomas*. St. Louis: CV Mosby; 1989:839–853.

25. Ritch R. Argon laser peripheral iridoplasty: An overview. *J Glaucoma*. 1992;1:206–213.

26. Abramson DH, Chang S, Coleman DJ, et al. Pilocarpine-induced lens changes: An ultrasonic biometric evaluation of dose response. *Arch Ophthalmol*. 1974;92:464–468.

27. Abramson DH, Franzen LA, Coleman DJ. Pilocarpine in the presbyope: Demonstration of an effect on the anterior chamber and lens thickness. *Arch Ophthalmol*. 1973;89:100–102.

28. Bleiman B, Schwartz AL. Paradoxical response to pilocarpine. *Arch Ophthalmol*. 1979;97:1305–1307.

29. Gorin G. Angle-closure glaucoma induced by miotics. *Am J Ophthalmol*. 1966;62:1063–1066.

30. Rieser JC, Schwartz B. Miotic induced malignant glaucoma. *Arch Ophthalmol*. 1972;87:706–708.

31. Ritch R. The pilocarpine paradox. *J Glaucoma*. 1996;5:225–227.

32. Ritch R. Argon laser treatment for medically unresponsive attacks of angle-closure glaucoma. *Am J Ophthalmol*. 1982;94:197.

33. Phelps CD. Angle-closure glaucoma secondary to ciliary body swelling. *Arch Ophthalmol*. 1974;92:287.

34. Forbes M. Gonioscopy with corneal indentation: A method for distinguishing between appositional closure and synechial closure. *Arch Ophthalmol*. 1966;76:488–497.

35. Gorin G. Re-evaluation of gonioscopic findings in angle-closure glaucoma: Static versus manipulative gonioscopy. *Am J Ophthalmol*. 1971;71:894.

36. Wilensky J, et al. Gonioscopy. *Invest Ophthalmol Vis Sci*. 1978;17(suppl):144.

37. Bhargava SK, Leighton DA, Phillips CI. Early angle-closure glaucoma: Distribution of iridotrabecular contact and response to pilocarpine. *Arch Ophthalmol*. 1973;89:369.

38. Desjardins DC, Parrish RK. Inversion of anterior chamber pigment as a possible prognostic sign in narrow angles. *Am J Ophthalmol*. 1985;100:480.

39. Shaffer RN. Gonioscopy, ophthalmoscopy, and perimetry. *Trans Am Acad Ophthalmol Otolaryngol*. 1960;64:112.

40. Shaffer RN. A suggested anatomic classification to define the pupillary block glaucomas. *Invest Ophthalmol*. 1973;12:540.

41. Spaeth GL. The normal development of the human chamber angle: A new system of descriptive grading. *Trans Ophthalmol Soc UK*. 1971;91:709.

42. Spaeth GL. Gonioscopy: Uses old and new: The inheritance of occludable angles. *Ophthalmology*. 1978;85:222.

43. Ravitz J, Seybold ME. Transient monocular visual loss from narrow-angle glaucoma. *Arch Neurol*. 1984;41:991.

44. Chandler PA, Trotter RR. Angle-closure glaucoma: Subacute types. *Arch Ophthalmol*. 1955;53:305.

45. Chandler PA. Narrow-angle glaucoma. *Arch Ophthalmol*. 1952;47:695–716.

46. Mapstone R. Mechanics of pupil block. *Br J Ophthalmol*. 1968;52:19–25.

47. Sugar HS. The mechanical factors in the etiology of acute glaucoma. *Am J Ophthalmol*. 1941;24:851–874.

48. Lowe RF. Angle-closure glaucoma: Acute and subacute attacks: Clinical types. *Trans Ophthalmol Soc Aust*. 1961;21:65–75.

49. Cross M, Croll LJ. Emotional glaucoma. *Am J Ophthalmol*. 1960;49:297–305.

50. Egan JA. Shock glaucoma. *Am J Ophthalmol*. 1955; 40:227–232.

51. Inman WS. Emotion and acute glaucoma. *Lancet*. 1929;2:1188–1189.

52. Friedman AH, Bloch R, Henkind P. Hypopyon and iris necrosis in angle-closure glaucoma. Report of two cases. *Br J Ophthalmol*. 1972;56:632–635.

53. Zhang MY. Hypopyon and iris necrosis in acute angle-closure glaucoma. *Chinese Med J*. 1984;97:583–586.

54. Sonty S, Schwartz B. Vascular accidents in acute angle-closure glaucoma. *Ophthalmology*. 1981;88:225.

55. Bloome MA. Transient angle-closure glaucoma in central retinal vein occlusion. *Ann Ophthalmol*. 1977;9:44.

56. Grant WM. Shallowing of the anterior chamber following occlusion of the central retinal vein. *Am J Ophthalmol*. 1973;75:384.

57. Hyams SW, Neumann E. Transient angle closure glaucoma after retinal vein occlusion. *Br J Ophthalmol*. 1972;56:353–355.

58. Mendelsohn AD, Jampol LM, Schoch D. Secondary angle-closure glaucoma after central retinal vein occlusion. *Am J Ophthalmol*. 1985;100:581–585.

59. Segal A, Ducasse A, Aisemberg L, et al. Glaucome aigu unilatéral par fermeture de l'angle secondaire à une OVCR. *Bull Soc Ophtalmol Fr*. 1986;86:301–303.

60. Weber PA, Cohen JS, Baker D. Central retinal vein occlusion and malignant glaucoma. *Arch Ophthalmol*. 1987;105:635–636.

61. McNaught EI, Rennie A, McClure E, et al. Pattern of visual damage after acute angle-closure glaucoma. *Trans Ophthalmol Soc UK*. 1974;94:406.

62. Douglas GR, Drance SM, Schulzer M. The visual field and nerve head in angle-closure glaucoma: A comparison of the effects of acute and chronic angle closure. *Arch Ophthalmol*. 1975;93:409.

63. Horie T, Kitazawa Y, Nose H. Visual field changes in primary angle-closure glaucoma. *Jpn J Ophthalmol*. 1975;1:108–115.

64. Phillips CI, Woodhouse DF. Self-limiting closed-angle glaucoma with segmental iris shortening. *Br J Ophthalmol*. 1963;47:547–553.

65. Mapstone R. Partial angle closure. *Br J Ophthalmol*. 1977;61:525.

66. Foulds WS, Phillips CI. Some observations on chronic closed-angle glaucoma. *Br J Ophthalmol*. 1957;41:208–213.

67. Lowe RF. Primary creeping angle-closure glaucoma. *Br J Ophthalmol*. 1964;48:544.

68. Augsburger JJ, Affel LL, Benarosh DA. Ultrasound biomicroscopy of cystic lesions of the iris and ciliary body. *Trans Am Ophthalmol Soc*. 1996;94:259–274.

69. Orgül SI, Daicker B, Büchi ER. The diameter of the ciliary sulcus: A morphometric study. *Graefes Arch Clin Exp Ophthalmol*. 1993;231:487–490.

70. Levene RZ. A new concept of malignant glaucoma. *Arch Ophthalmol*. 1972;87:497–506.

71. Merritt JC. Malignant glaucoma induced by miotics postoperatively in open-angle glaucoma. *Arch Ophthalmol*. 1977;95:1988–1990.

72. Dueker D. Ciliary-block glaucoma—Differential diagnosis and management. *J Glaucoma*. 1994;3:167–170.

73. Shaffer RN, Hoskins HD Jr. Ciliary block (malignant) glaucoma. *Trans Am Acad Ophthalmol Otolaryngol*. 1978;85: 215–221.

74. Simmons RJ. Malignant glaucoma. *Br J Ophthalmol*. 1972;56:263–272.

75. Weiss DI, Shaffer RN. Ciliary block (malignant) glaucoma. *Trans Am Acad Ophthalmol Otolaryngol*. 1972;76: 450–461.

76. Brown RH, Lynch MG, Tearse JE, et al. Neodymium-YAG vitreous surgery for phakic and pseudophakic malignant glaucoma. *Arch Ophthalmol*. 1986;104: 1464–1466.

77. Duy TP, Wollensak J. Ciliary block (malignant) glaucoma following posterior chamber lens implantation. *Ophthalm Surg*. 1987;18:741–744.

78. Epstein DL, Steinert RF, Puliafito CA. Neodymium-YAG laser therapy to the anterior hyaloid in aphakic malignant glaucoma. *Am J Ophthalmol*. 1984;98:137.

79. Lynch MG, Brown RH, Michels RG, et al. Surgical vitrectomy for pseudophakic malignant glaucoma. *Am J Ophthalmol*. 1986;102:149–153.

80. Reed JE, Thomas JV, Lytle RA, et al. Malignant glaucoma induced by an intraocular lens. *Ophthalm Surg*. 1990;21:177–180.

81. Tello C, Chi T, Shepps G, et al. Ultrasound biomicroscopy in pseudophakic malignant glaucoma. *Ophthalmology*. 1993;100:1330–1334.

82. Vajpayee RB, Angrask, Titiyal JS, et al. Pseudophakic pupillary-block glaucoma in children. *Am J Ophthalmol*. 1991;111:715.

83. Lowe RF. Acute angle-closure glaucoma: Acetazolamide therapy. *Aust J Ophthalmol*. 1973;1:24.

84. Mapstone R. Closed-angle glaucoma: Theoretical considerations. *Br J Ophthalmol*. 1974;58:36–40.

85. Ganias F, Mapstone R. Miotics in closed-angle glaucoma. *Br J Ophthalmol*. 1975;59:205.

86. Airaksinen PJ, Saari KM, Tiainen TJ, et al. Management of acute closed-angle glaucoma with miotics and timolol. *Br J Ophthalmol*. 1979;63:822.

87. Anderson DR. Corneal indentation to relieve acute angle-closure glaucoma. *Am J Ophthalmol*. 1979;88:1091.

88. Kramer P, Ritch R. The treatment of angle-closure glaucoma revisited (editorial). *Ann Ophthalmol*. 1984;16: 1101–1103.

89. Ritch R, Liebmann JM. Argon laser peripheral iridoplasty: A review. *Ophthalm Surg Lasers*. 1996;27:289–300.

90. Ritch R, Solomon IS. Laser treatment of glaucoma. In: L'Esperance FAJ, ed. *Ophthalmic Lasers II*, 3rd ed. St Louis: CV Mosby; 1989:650–748.

91. David R, Tessler Z, Yassur Y. Long-term outcome of primary acute angle-closure glaucoma. *Br J Ophthalmol*. 1985;69:261.

92. Lowe RF. Primary angle-closure glaucoma investigations after surgery for pupillary block. *Am J Ophthalmol*. 1964;57:931.

93. Gieser D, Wilensky J. Laser iridectomy in the management of chronic angle-closure glaucoma. *Am J Ophthalmol*. 1984;98:446.

94. Ritch R. The treatment of chronic angle-closure glaucoma (editorial). *Ann Ophthalmol*. 1981;13:21–23.

95. Ritch R. *Techniques of Argon Laser Iridectomy and Iridoplasty*. Palo Alto, CA: Coherent Medical Press; 1983.

96. Ritch R, Liebmann J, Solomon IS. Laser iridectomy and iridoplasty. In: Ritch R, Shields MB, Krupin T, eds. *The Glaucomas*. St. Louis: CV Mosby; 1989:581–603.

97. Ritch R, Solomon LD. Argon laser peripheral iridoplasty for angle-closure glaucoma in siblings with Weill-Marchesani syndrome. *J Glaucoma*. 1992;1:243–247.

98. Shirakashi M, Iwata K, Nakayama T. Argon laser trabeculoplasty for chronic angle-closure glaucoma uncontrolled by iridotomy. *Acta Ophthalmol*. 1989;67: 265–270.

99. Wishart PK, Nagasubramanian S, Hitchings RA. Argon laser trabeculoplasty in narrow angle glaucoma. *Eye*. 1987;1:567.

100. Eltz H, Gloor B. Trabeculectomy in cases of angle-closure glaucoma—Successes and failures. *Klin Monatsbl Augenheilkd*. 1980;177:556.

101. Ando H, Kitagawa K, Ogino N. Results of goniosynechialysis for synechial angle-closure glaucoma after pupillary block. *Folia Ophthalmol Jpn*. 1990; 41: 883–886.

102. Campbell DG, Vela A. Modern goniosynechialysis for the treatment of synechial angle-closure glaucoma. *Ophthalmology*. 1984;91:1052–1060.

103. Nagata M, Nezu N. Goniosynechialysis as a new treatment for chronic angle-closure glaucoma. *Jpn J Clin Ophthalmol*. 1985;39:707–710.

104. Sharpe ED, Thomas JV, Simmons RJ. Goniosynechialysis. In: Thomas JV, Belcher CDI, Simmons RJ, eds. *Glaucoma Surgery*. St Louis: CV Mosby; 1992.

105. Tanihara H, Nagata M. Argon-laser gonioplasty following goniosynechialysis. *Graefes Arch Clin Exp Ophthalmol*. 1991;229:505–507.

106. Tanihara H, Nishiwaki K, Nagata M. Surgical results and complications of goniosynechialysis. *Graefes Arch Clin Exp Ophthalmol*. 1992;230:309–313.

107. Mandelkorn RM, Zimmerman TJ. Nonsteroidal drugs and glaucoma. In: Ritch R, Shields MB, Krupin T, eds. *The Glaucomas II*. St Louis: CV Mosby; 1996:1189–1204.

108. Gayton JL, Ledford JK. Angle-closure glaucoma following a combined blepharoplasty and ectropion repair. *Ophthalmol Plast Reconstr Surg* 1992;8:176–177.

109. Carmichael C. Hiccups and glaucoma. *JAMA*. 1989; 261:695.

110. Kearns PP, Dhillon BJ. Angle-closure glaucoma precipitated by labour. *Acta Ophthalmol*. 1990;68:225–226.

111. Markovits AS. Ophthalmodynia hypertonica copulationis: A new syndrome? *Can J Ophthalmol*. 1974;9: 484–485.

112. Sharir M, Huntington AC, Nardin GF, et al. Sneezing as a cause of acute angle-closure glaucoma. *Ann Ophthalmol*. 1992;24:214–215.

113. Foster RE, Smiddy WS, Alfonso EC, Parrish RK. Secondary glaucoma associated with retained perfluorophenanthrene. *Am J Ophthalmol*. 1994;118:251–253.

114. Pesin SR, Katz LJ, Augsburger JJ, et al. Acute angle-closure glaucoma from spontaneous massive hemorrhagic retinal or choroidal detachment: An updated diagnostic and therapeutic approach. *Ophthalmology*. 1990; 97:76–84.

115. Steinemann T, Goins K, Smith T, et al. Acute closed-angle glaucoma complicating hemorrhagic choroidal detachment associated with parenteral thrombolytic agents. *Am J Ophthalmol*. 1988;106:753–754.

116. Hardten DR, Brown JD. Malignant glaucoma after Nd:YAG cyclophotocoagulation. *Am J Ophthalmol*. 1991;111:245–247.

117. Wand M, Schuman JS, Puliafito CA. Malignant glaucoma after contact transscleral Nd:YAG laser cyclophotocoagulation. *J Glaucoma*. 1993;2:110–111.

118. Walsh JB, Muldoon TO. Glaucoma associated with retinal and vitreoretinal disorders. In: Ritch R, Shields MB, Krupin T, eds. *The Glaucomas II*. St Louis: CV Mosby; 1996:1055–1071.

119. DiSclafani M, Liebmann JM, Ritch R. Malignant glaucoma following argon laser release of scleral flap su-

tures after trabeculectomy. *Am J Ophthalmol*. 1989; 108:597–598.

120. Trope GE, Paulin CJ, Bau A, et al. Malignant glaucoma: Clinical and ultrasound biomicroscopic characteristics. *Ophthalmology*. 1994;101:1030–1035.

121. Joshi N, Constable PH, Margolis TP, et al. Bilateral angle-closure glaucoma and accelerated cataract formation in a patient with AIDS. *Br J Ophthalmol*. 1994;78:656.

122. Koster HR, Liebmann JM, Ritch R, et al. Acute angle-closure glaucoma in a patient with acquired immunodeficiency syndrome successfully treated with argon laser peripheral iridoplasty. *Ophthalm Surg*. 1990;21: 501–502.

123. Meige P, Cohen H, Morin B, et al. Glaucome aigu bilateral chez un sujet LAV positif. *Bull Soc Ophtalmol Fr*. 1989;89:449–454.

124. Nash RW, Lindquist TD. Bilateral angle-closure glaucoma associated with uveal effusion: Presenting sign of HIV infection. *Surv Ophthalmol*. 1992;36:255–258.

125. Ullman S, Wilson RP, Schwartz L. Bilateral angle-closure glaucoma in association with the acquired immune deficiency syndrome. *Am J Ophthalmol*. 1986; 101:419–424.

126. Ueno M, Kawamure H, Namishima S, et al. Unilateral transient shallow anterior chamber and OHT as initial signs of multifocal posterior pigment epitheliopathy. *Folia Ophthalmol Jpn*. 1987;38:1725–1732.

127. Grossniklaus H, et al. *Bacillus cereus* panophthalmitis appearing as angle-closure glaucoma in a drug addict (letter). *Am J Ophthalmol*. 1985;100:334.

128. Kontkanen M, Puustjärvi T, Lähdevirta J. Myopic shift and its mechanism in nephropathia epidemica or Puumala virus infection. *Br J Ophthalmol*. 1994;78:903–906.

129. Matti Saari K. Acute glaucoma in hemorrhagic fever with renal syndrome (nephropathia epidemica). *Am J Ophthalmol*. 1976;81:455.

130. Krupin T, Feitl ME, Karalekas D. Glaucoma associated with uveitis. In: Ritch R, Shields MB, Krupin T, eds. *The Glaucomas II*. St Louis: CV Mosby; 1996:1225–1258.

131. Daniele S. Primary closed-angle glaucoma and influenza: Report of three cases. *Ann Ottalmol Clin Ocul* 1969;95:961.

132. Watson PG. Glaucoma associated with keratitis, episcleritis, and scleritis. In: Ritch R, Shields MB, Krupin T, eds. *The Glaucomas II*. St Louis: CV Mosby; 1996: 1207–1223.

133. Sugino K, Moriwaki M, Ueno T, et al. Acute angle-closure glaucoma as first manifestation of malignant melanoma of the choroid. *Folia Ophthalmol Jpn*. 1990; 41:1309–1313.

134. Weinreb RN, Loane M, Slight R, et al. Bilateral congenital hyperplasia of the ciliary muscle associated with malignant glaucoma. *J Glaucoma*. 1992;1:125–127.

135. Fourman S. Angle-closure glaucoma complicating ciliochoroidal detachment. *Ophthalmology*. 1989;96: 646–653.

136. Azuara-Blanco A, Pesin SR, Katz LJ, et al. Familial exudative vitreoretinopathy associated with nonneovascular chronic angle-closure glaucoma. *J Glaucoma*. 1997; 6:47–49.

137. Vela A, Rieser JC, Campbell DG. The heredity and treatment of angle-closure glaucoma secondary to iris and ciliary body cysts. *Ophthalmology*. 1984;91:332–337.

138. Garrison LM, Christensen RE, Allen RA. Angle-closure glaucoma from metastatic carcinoma. *Am J Ophthalmol*. 1967;63:503.

139. Khawly JA, Shields MB. Metastatic carcinoma manifesting as angle-closure glaucoma. *Am J Ophthalmol*. 1994;118:116–117.

140. Lanzi IM, Augsburger JJ, Azuara A, et al. Ultrasound biomicroscopy of acute glaucoma in a patient with metastatic cancer. *Br J Ophthalmol*. 1997;81:1017–1018.

141. Haik BG, Dunleavy SA, Cooke C, et al. Retinoblastoma with anterior chamber extension. *Ophthalmology*. 1987;94:367–370.

142. Sorokanich S, Wand W, Nix HR. Angle-closure glaucoma and acute hyperglycemia. *Arch Ophthalmol*. 1986;104:1434.

143. Buus DR, Tse DT, Parrish RKI. Spontaneous carotid cavernous fistula presenting with acute angle-closure glaucoma. *Arch Ophthalmol*. 1989;107:596–597.

144. Fiore PM, Latina MA, Shingleton BJ, et al. The dural shunt syndrome: I. Management of glaucoma. *Ophthalmology*. 1990;97:56–62.

145. Fourman S. Acute closed-angle glaucoma after arteriovenous fistulas. *Am J Ophthalmol*. 1989;107:156–159.

146. Golnik KC, Newman SA, Ferguson R. Angle-closure glaucoma consequent to embolization of dural cavernous sinus fistula. *AJNR*. 1991;12:1074–1076.

147. Talks SJ, Salmon JF, Elston JS, et al. Cavernous-dural fistula with secondary angle-closure glaucoma. *Am J Ophthalmol*. 1997;124:851–853.

148. Liebmann JM, Ritch R. Lens-associated angle-closure glaucoma. In: Ritch R, Shields MB, Krupin T, eds. *The Glaucomas*, 2nd ed. St Louis: CV Mosby; 1996.

149. Smith DL, Skuta GL, Trobe JD, et al. Angle-closure glaucoma as initial presentation of myelodysplastic syndrome. *Can J Ophthalmol*. 1990;25:306–308.

150. Koeppen AH, Madonick MJ, Barest MD. Acute unilateral glaucoma associated with extradural hemorrhage. *Am J Ophthalmol*. 1967;63:1696–1698.

151. Mouton DP, Meyer D. Oculomotor nerve palsy precipitating acute angle-closure glaucoma. *S Afr Med J*. 1989;75:397–398.

152. Wilson WB, Barmatz HE. Acute angle-closure glaucoma secondary to an aneurysm of the posterior communicating artery. *Am J Ophthalmol*. 1980;89:868–870.

153. Zaidi AA. Diabetic oculo-motor nerve palsy giving rise to acute secondary glaucoma. *Br J Ophthalmol*. 1971;55:348–349.

154. Goldey SH, Hamed LM, Sherwood MB, et al. Pituitary apoplexy precipitating acute angle-closure (letter). *Arch Ophthalmol*. 1992;110:1687–1688.

155. Arora R, Verma L, Kumar A. Renal hypertension presenting as acute angle-closure glaucoma. *Arch Ophthalmol*. 1991;109:776.

156. Wagemans MAJ, Bos PJM. Angle-closure glaucoma in a patient with systemic lupus erythematosus. *Doc Ophthalmol*. 1989;72:201–207.

157. Coppeto M. Angle-closure glaucoma and TIA's. *Am J Ophthalmol*. 1985;99:493.

158. Corridan P, Nightingale S, Mashoudi N, Williams AC. Acute angle-closure glaucoma following botulinum toxin injection for blepharospasm. *Br J Ophthalmol*. 1990;74:309.

159. Highman VN. Early rise in intraocular pressure in ammonia burns. *Br Med J*. 1969;1:359–360.

160. Baratz KH, Allf BE, Foulks GN. Intracorneal hemorrhage with acute glaucoma. *Am J Ophthalmol*. 1993;116:374–376.

161. Kim MK, Alekna VP, Dickens CJ. Acute angle-closure glaucoma induced by the soft rubber ball used for softening before cataract extraction (letter). *Ophthalm Surg*. 1987;18:777–778.

Chapter 30

NON-PRESSURE-DEPENDENT GLAUCOMA

David S. Greenfield

Glaucoma is an optic neuropathy characterized by a typical pattern of visual field loss and optic nerve damage due to the death of retinal ganglion cells caused by a number of different disorders that affect the eye. Most but not all of these disorders are associated with elevated intraocular pressure (IOP), which is the most important risk factor for glaucomatous damage. Several classification schemes exist based on whether the drainage angle is open or closed, the IOP is elevated or normal, and the underlying disorder is primary or secondary. However, many patients with "high-tension" glaucoma develop progressive cupping of the optic nerve and loss of vision at low levels of IOP. Current classification systems underemphasize the mechanism of optic nerve injury in such individuals. Therefore, new terminology has evolved that subdivides these disorders into pressure-dependent and pressure-independent types.

The underlying pathophysiology of pressure-dependent and pressure-independent glaucoma is different. Pressure-dependent glaucoma is an anterior-segment disorder characterized by dysfunction of the trabecular meshwork. This produces decreased facility of outflow, increased resistance to egress of aqueous humor, and elevation of IOP. In contrast, non-pressure-dependent glaucoma is a complex posterior-segment disorder in which the death of gan-

glion cells results in cupping of the optic nerve at normal levels of IOP. The mechanism of damage is likely multifactorial and may include ischemia, excitotoxicity, autoimmune processes, deficiency of neurotrophic factors, apoptosis, and decreased intracranial pressure. This chapter summarizes the pathophysiology, clinical characteristics, and treatment strategies of non-pressure-dependent glaucoma.

TERMINOLOGY

First described as *amaurosis with excavation* in 1857 by Von Graefe,[1] non-pressure-dependent glaucoma has been associated with an array of confusing terms. In 1917, Gradle referred to this disorder as *glaucoma without hypertension*.[2] Other names have evolved in the literature, including *low-tension glaucoma, normal-tension glaucoma, pseudoglaucoma, soft glaucoma,* and *relative glaucoma*. For simplicity, non-pressure-dependent glaucoma is referred to as *normal-tension glaucoma* (NTG) in this review. It should be understood that this terminology refers also to the disorder of individuals with previously elevated IOP who develop progressive optic nerve damage at normal levels of IOP.

Although the definition of NTG is variable, most consider it a disorder characterized by acquired

493

cupping of the optic nerve head, acquired visual field loss, open filtration angles, and normal IOP.[3] The definition of normal IOP remains similarly unclear. Leydhecker evaluated a series of 20,000 eyes and demonstrated that the mean IOP among this cohort was 15.5 mmHg.[4] Assuming a normal Gaussian distribution, two standard deviations above this IOP level would be 20.5 mmHg and 97.5% of the population would be expected to fall within this range. Population-based studies have since demonstrated that the distribution of IOP is not normally distributed and is skewed to the right.[5] Many individuals without glaucoma have an IOP above 21 mmHg. Conversely, many patients with glaucoma have statistically normal levels of IOP. It is incorrect to assume that 21 mmHg represents the threshold by which we define normality. This misconception has been described by Wilson as the "myth of 21."[6]

Controversial is the need for progression. Some investigators have included progressive optic nerve cupping or visual field loss in the definition of this disorder.[7,8] Others have argued that this precludes establishing a diagnosis without longitudinal follow-up.[9] As progression is not a prerequisite for the diagnosis of other glaucomas, it is unreasonable to consider it a necessary diagnostic component of this disorder.

EPIDEMIOLOGICAL PERSPECTIVE

Glaucoma is estimated to be the second most frequent cause of blindness in the world, with approximately 67 million people affected.[10] In developed countries, only half of those with the disease have been diagnosed. In the United States, approximately 2 million individuals have glaucoma, of whom 80,000 are legally blind.

NTG is not an uncommon disorder. The estimated prevalence has ranged from 16.7 to 68.3%, with variability based on the definition of the disease.[11–14] Recent estimates have concluded that 20 to 30% of patients with open-angle glaucoma have normal IOP.[15] Furthermore, approximately 41% of all patients diagnosed with high-tension glaucoma will initially present with IOP below 21 mmHg.[12]

CLINICAL FEATURES

NTG is typically a disorder of the elderly, appearing on average in those between 60 and 70 years of age.[3,11,16] This finding is consistent with data from large-scale epidemiological studies demonstrating an increased prevalence of open-angle glaucoma in older patients, particularly those 70 years old and above.[17,18] The disorder is uncommon in patients below age 50. In a case-control study comparing the clinical characteristics of NTG with nonglaucomatous cupping associated with intracranial compressive lesions, Greenfield and colleagues[19] found age below 50 years to be 93% specific for nonglaucomatous cupping.

Other demographic characteristics differentiate NTG from glaucoma associated with elevated IOP. Some studies have suggested that NTG is more common in women,[20,21] and there is a greater prevalence of this disorder among Asian patients than among Europeans.[11,22]

Some authors have suggested that unilateral cases occur more frequently in NTG than in primary open-angle glaucoma.[3,23] Levene reviewed 116 individual cases and identified 33 (28%) patients with unilateral glaucoma.[3] Interestingly, he found that approximately 25% of these individuals eventually developed bilateral disease. As described by Kitazawa and colleagues, nonglaucomatous or other secondary glaucomatous optic neuropathies should be considered in patients with unilateral disease.[24]

A variety of unique clinical features characterize this disorder and suggest a pathophysiology distinct from that of high-tension glaucoma. Vasospastic symptoms have been described in a large proportion of patients, with migraine headaches reported in as many as 50%.[25,26] Peripheral vasospasm measured by finger blood flow is seen frequently in this disorder[27,28] and is clinically manifest as Raynaud's phenomenon.

Patients with NTG often give a history of systemic hypotension or previous hemodynamic crisis.[16,29] Nocturnal dips in systolic and diastolic blood pressure[30–32] may be revealed by 24-hour ambulatory blood pressure monitoring, and this can be exaggerated by aggressive antihypertensive therapy.[33–35] In addition, investigators have demonstrated color Doppler evidence of decreased blood flow velocity and increased vascular resistive index in the ophthalmic artery compared with age-matched controls.[36]

Magnetic resonance imaging (MRI) of the brain is sometimes performed as part of the diagnostic evaluation in order to exclude intracranial lesions. Although such lesions are rare, recent reports have demonstrated the presence of deep white matter signal abnormalities (Fig. 30–1) suggestive of small vessel occlusive disease.[37–39] Other clinical characteristics pertaining to the appearance of the optic disc and visual fields are summarized below.

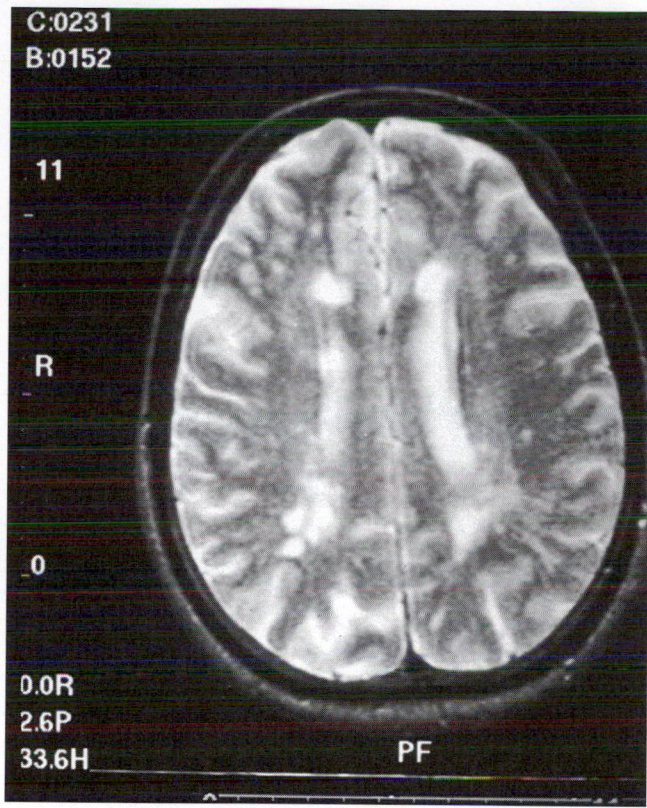

Figure 30–1. Cranial magnetic resonance image of a patient with NTG demonstrates multiple nonenhancing deep white matter areas of signal intensity suggestive of small vessel occlusive disease.

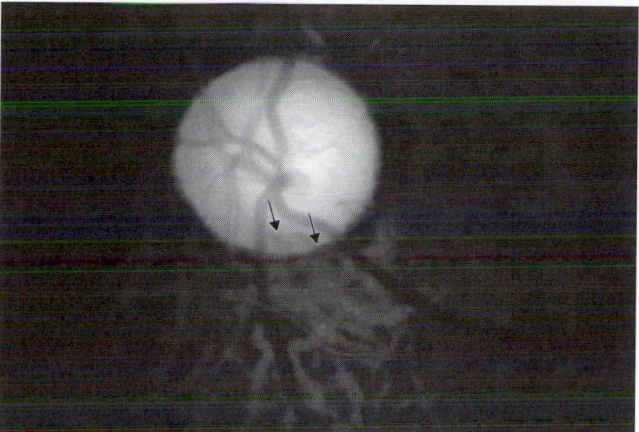

Figure 30–2. Optic disc of a patient with NTG illustrates two splinter disc hemorrhages along the inferior neural rim. (*See also Color Plate 101.*)

OPTIC DISC CHARACTERISTICS

Eyes with this disorder often have optic discs with distinct clinical characteristics. Splinter hemorrhages (Fig. 30–2) have been reported to occur in as many as 40% of patients.[29,40,41] Pronounced peripapillary atrophy is a common observation and is often more extensive in the adjacent area of neural rim loss.[42–45] Up to 75% of patients may demonstrate acquired optic nerve head pits,[46] giving a "moth-eaten" appearance (Fig. 30–3) to the optic nerve head.[47] Compared to eyes with high-tension glaucoma, some authors have suggested a larger optic cup size,[48,49] less frequent backward bowing of the lamina cribrosa,[50] and a greater frequency of localized defects in the retinal nerve fiber layer (RNFL).[51] It should be noted that such findings are anecdotal and have not been evaluated in population-based studies.

VISUAL FIELD CHARACTERISTICS

Patterns of visual field loss in eyes with NTG are different from those in eyes with pressure-dependent glaucoma. Eyes with NTG are characterized by scotomas that are denser, steeper, and closer to fixation (Fig. 30–4) than in eyes with high-tension glaucoma.[3,52–54] Investigators have also suggested that the superior visual field is more commonly involved than the inferior field[55,56] and that field loss is more likely to be localized to one hemifield.[57–59]

Anecdotal reports have suggested that the administration of systemic calcium channel blockers may halt or slow the progression of visual field defects in these patients as opposed to similarly treated patients with elevated IOP and placebo-treated NTG patients.[60–63] Others argue that such agents should be avoided in eyes with compromised autoregulation, as they may produce ocular ischemia by reducing the ocular perfusion pressure. Hayreh and colleagues demonstrated that patients with arterial hypertension

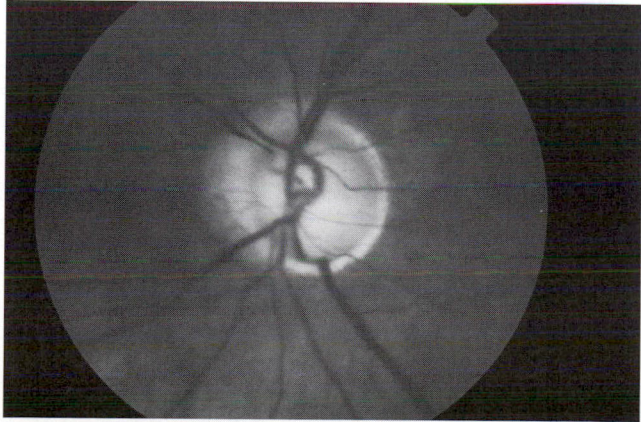

Figure 30–3. An inferiorly located acquired pit of the optic nerve head gives a moth-eaten appearance to the optic nerve head. (*See also Color Plate 102.*)

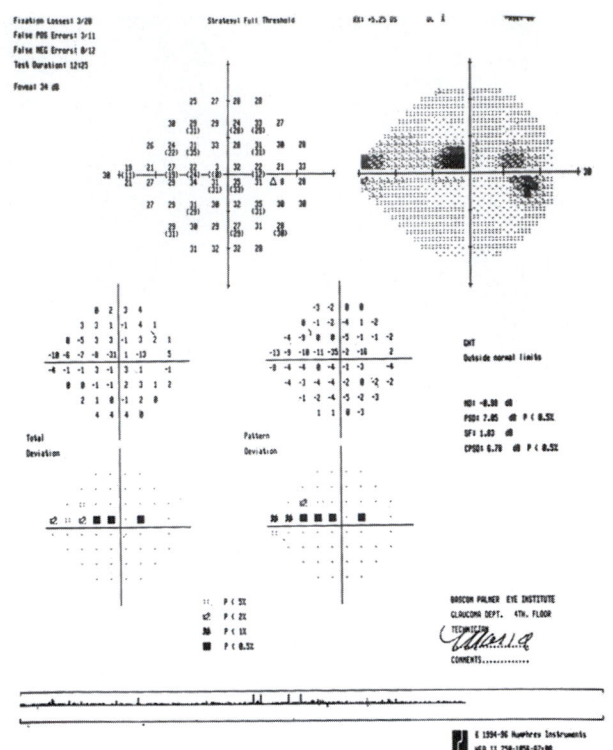

Figure 30–4. Automated achromatic perimetry of a patient with NTG demonstrates a well-demarcated paracentral depression with sharp borders.

receiving oral antihypertensive therapy showed a significant association between nocturnal hypotensive episodes and progressive visual field deterioration.[64]

SUBGROUPS

Geijssen and Greve have proposed that subgroups of NTG exist with different clinical characteristics.[65,66] Four subgroups have been identified: senile sclerotic, focal ischemic, myopic, and miscellaneous forms. Although this descriptive classification highlights possible pathogenic mechanisms, a causal relationship has not been established.

Patients with senile sclerotic glaucoma (Fig. 30–5) are typically older and have pale, moth-eaten optic nerves with surrounding areas of peripapillary atrophy and choroidal sclerosis. The pathogenesis is thought to involve a chronic anterior ischemic optic neuropathy.[66]

Eyes with focal ischemic NTG (Fig. 30–6) are characterized by focal areas of neuroretinal rim loss. Such patients often have a history of systemic vascular disease, splinter optic disc hemorrhage, and localized visual field defects.[65]

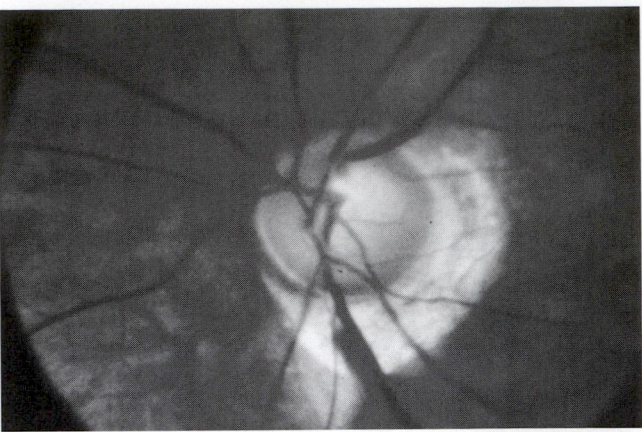

Figure 30–5. Appearance of the optic nerve in an eye with senile sclerotic NTG; there is a pale, moth-eaten disc with surrounding areas of peripapillary atrophy and choroidal sclerosis. (*See also Color Plate 103.*)

Myopic NTG (Fig. 30–7) is characterized by high axial myopia and a tilted optic nerve with oblique insertion. Some have suggested a greater rate of progressive visual field loss associated with this subgroup.[67] Miscellaneous eyes with NTG exist (Fig. 30–8) that do not fall into the above categories.

PATHOPHYSIOLOGICAL MECHANISMS

Pressure-dependent glaucoma may be thought of as an anterior-segment disorder whose underlying mechanism involves obstruction of aqueous outflow and subsequent elevation of IOP. This constitutes what has been referred to as the mechanical (i.e., pressure-related) theory of optic nerve damage. In contrast,

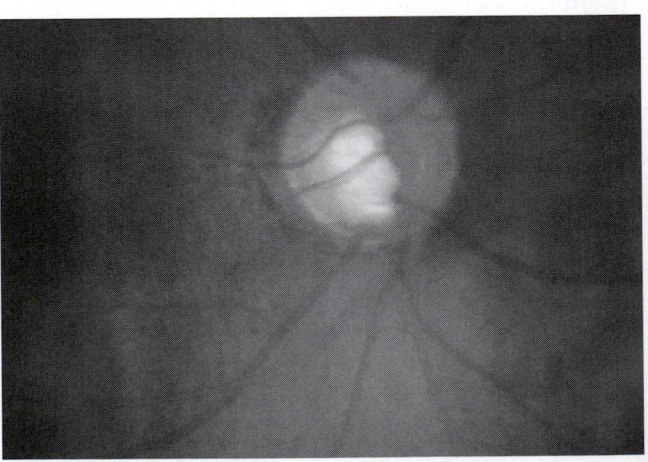

Figure 30–6. Photograph of the optic nerve in an eye with focal ischemic NTG characterized by discrete areas of neural rim loss. (*See also Color Plate 104.*)

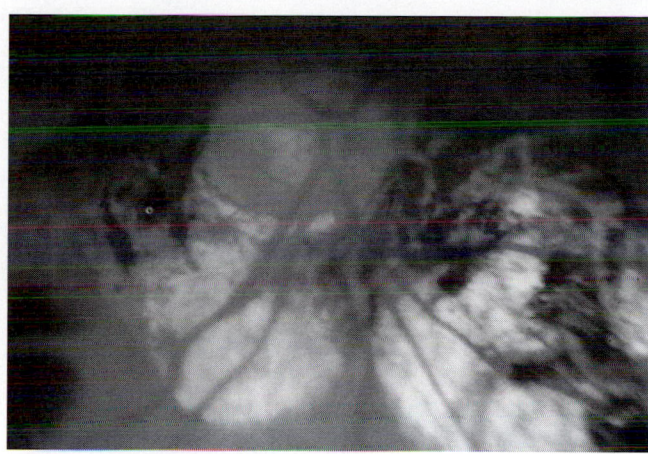

Figure 30–7. Photograph of the optic nerve in an eye with myopic NTG characterized by high axial myopia. The optic nerve is tilted and has an oblique insertion. (*See also Color Plate 105.*)

non-pressure-dependent glaucoma is a posterior-segment disorder. It involves a precipitating event that produces a similar phenotypic endpoint, namely optic nerve cupping, in susceptible individuals. Specific disease mechanisms are discussed further on; however, the pathophysiology of this disorder is likely multifactorial.

A vascular theory has long been proposed to explain the mechanism of ganglion cell death in eyes with NTG. A direct causal relationship has not been established. Evidence supporting a vascular basis for this disorder (e.g., systemic, postural, or nocturnal hypotension; vasospasm; or some other mechanism) has been presented earlier.[16,25–27,36,68,69] It remains to be seen whether reduced blood flow represents the primary

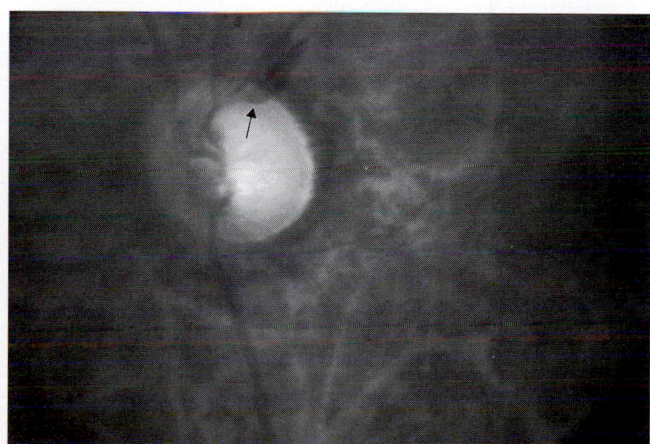

Figure 30–8. Miscellaneous NTG represents those eyes that do not satisfy criteria for inclusion in other subgroups. Note the fresh splinter hemorrhage along the superotemporal aspect of the optic disc. (*See also Color Plate 106.*)

cause of optic nerve cupping or a secondary effect resulting from the need for less blood flow due to reduced RNFL thickness. Advances in technology for imaging ocular blood flow represent a promising means for evaluating this relationship critically. The hemodynamic properties of vasoactive medications may be similarly established.

A growing body of evidence suggests that excitotoxicity may play a significant role in the pathophysiology of this disorder.[70–73] Clinical and experimental evidence exists demonstrating an excessive concentration of glutamate, a central nervous system excitatory neurotransmitter, in the vitreous cavity of glaucomatous eyes compared with controls. Glutamate binds to the *N*-methyl-D-aspartate (NMDA) receptor and may be neurotoxic at high concentrations. Overstimulation of this receptor results in intracellular calcium ion influx. This leads to the expression of phospholipases, proteases, and endonucleases as well as free radical formation, ultimately resulting in ganglion cell death. Damaged cells may then release additional glutamate in the extracellular environment, producing amplification of the excitotoxic cycle. NMDA-antagonists (e.g., memantine) reduce glutamate-induced neurotoxicity[73–75] and are promising neuroprotective agents.

Apoptosis, or preprogrammed cell death, is an important factor contributing to retinal ganglion cell death in glaucomatous eyes and is characterized by a unique pattern of DNA fragmentation. The primary trigger inducing this phenomenon may be IOP elevation, ischemia, glutamate toxicity, or neurotrophic factor deficiency [e.g., brain-derived neurotrophic factor (BDNF)]. Nickells has described an imbalance in the concentration of the gene products that are believed to control the expression of apoptosis.[76] Such deficiencies may result from anterograde and retrograde axoplasmic transport abnormalities and can be sufficient to trigger apoptosis.

A high percentage of patients with NTG have been reported to demonstrate at least one or more immune-related diseases. A 30% prevalence of autoimmune disorders in patients with NTG has been described.[77] Wax and colleagues have speculated that non-organ-specific autoantibody production in patients with NTG may be a marker for the presence of other unidentified autoantibodies (such as retinal, glial, or vascular autoantigens) and may reflect an autoimmune-mediated optic neuropathy.[78] The recent identification of anti-Ro/SS-A positivity and heat-shock protein antibodies in patients with NTG lends additional support to this hypothesis.[79]

Decreased intracranial pressure (ICP) has been associated with optic nerve cupping.[80,81] Greenfield and colleagues hypothesized that the lamina cribrosa serves as a flexible barrier between ICP and IOP and that alterations of the normal ICP/IOP ratio may produce pathology at the optic nerve head.[82] An increased ICP/IOP ratio (e.g., elevated ICP or decreased IOP) may produce papilledema, and a decreased ratio (e.g., decreased ICP or increased IOP) may produce cupping.

Dilatation of the intracranial internal carotid artery may be associated with compression of the anterior visual pathway.[83] This phenomenon, referred to as *fusiform enlargement* or *dolichoectasia*, may produce atrophic cupping of the optic nerve and loss of visual field resembling those of NTG.[38,84–86] The actual prevalence of this disorder remains unclear.

Korenfeld and Dueker have suggested that IOP elevation can occur in the dependent eye during sleep.[87] Using a pressure-sensitive fluid-filled bladder placed between the closed dependent eye and a pillow during simulated sleep in normotensive subjects, they demonstrated a mean peak IOP of 40 ± 11 mmHg. They found a 78% agreement between the eye with a greater cup-to-disc ratio and the side usually slept on.

FACTORS ASSOCIATED WITH PROGRESSION

Geijssen[44] estimated that 50% of patients will demonstrate progression over a 10-year period. Glicklich and colleagues reported progression in 38 of 61 eyes followed for 5 years.[52] The distinction between true visual field progression and long-term fluctuation is difficult. Schulzer[88] has demonstrated that despite a confirmatory visual field, false positives occur 57% of the time. Progression was defined as a deterioration of 10 dB or more of at least two contiguous points within or adjacent to a baseline field defect. When a second sequence of two confirmatory fields was performed, the rate of false positives was reduced to 2%.

Most studies support the concept that IOP is a factor in producing damage to eyes with NTG.[89–91] Anecdotal evidence suggests that eyes with progression tend to have higher mean and maximum IOP levels than eyes with stable visual function. Jonas and colleagues[92] have demonstrated pressure-dependent loss of neuroretinal rim tissue among a large series of eyes with various types of NTG. Moreover, Bhandari and coauthors have reported that surgical lowering of IOP results in a slower rate of field loss.[93] Finally, the Normal-Tension Glaucoma Study Group reported that a 30% reduction in IOP significantly reduced the rate of visual field progression from 60% (untreated controls)

to 20% (treated eyes) in eyes presenting with initial field progression or high-risk criteria.[94]

Various features of the optic disc may convey prognostic information. Acquired pit of the optic nerve (APON) has been described as a risk factor for progressive disc damage and visual field loss.[46,96] Ugurlu and coauthors[95] reported progression in 64% of patients with APON as compared with 12.5% of patients without APON. Others have found disc hemorrhage to be associated with future disease progression.[96,97] Siegner and Netland found that 63 of 101 eyes (63%) with disc hemorrhage developed visual-field progression compared with 24% of eyes without disc hemorrhage after a mean 16.8 ± 2.0 months of follow-up.[98] Finally, Geijssen[44] reported a greater rate of visual field progression in patients with myopic NTG (58%) as compared with other subgroups (16 to 39%).

The relationship between risk of disease progression and extent of visual field loss is unclear. Some have suggested that eyes with more advanced visual field loss are at greater risk for progression.[99] Others have found no such association.[44,52]

Vascular factors may play a role in progression. Using color Doppler imaging, Yamazaki and Drance[100] found that eyes with progressive NTG had significantly lower blood-flow velocities and higher resistive indices in the central retinal artery and short posterior ciliary artery as compared with eyes with stable visual fields. Nocturnal reduction in systemic blood pressure has been reported to correlate with disease progression. Graham and colleagues found lower nocturnal blood pressure among glaucomatous eyes with visual field progression as compared with eyes without progression.[31]

NONGLAUCOMATOUS CUPPING

Nonglaucomatous disorders may produce disc cupping; these include hereditary optic neuropathy, antecedent optic nerve infarction, trauma, infection, demyelinating optic neuritis, fusiform enlargement of the intracranial carotid artery, and intraorbital and intracranial mass lesions.[38,83,85,86,101–112] The clinical differentiation of glaucomatous and nonglaucomatous disc cupping is often difficult. In a retrospective review of photographs of the optic nerve head, Trobe and colleagues[103] reported that pallor of the neuroretinal rim is 94% specific in predicting nonglaucomatous cupping, and focal or diffuse obliteration of the neuroretinal rim is 87% specific in predicting glaucomatous cupping. However, such funduscopic characteristics are subjective and often difficult to define. In a more objective fashion with a planimetric method, Bianchi-Marzoli et al.[106] quantitatively assessed the characteristics of nonglaucomatous cupping in a group of patients with intracranial tumors. Median ratio of cup-to-disk area in patients with compressive lesions (0.37) was significantly greater than in age-matched controls (0.10). This technique, however, requires specialized equipment and a skilled operator.

To exclude occult intracranial mass lesions, neuroimaging studies are often included as part of the diagnostic evaluation of patients with pathological disc cupping associated with normal IOP. The indications for performing computed tomography (CT) or magnetic resonance imaging (MRI) in patients with NTG are not uniformly accepted. Although anecdotal reports of intracranial masses exist,[83,105,109,113] scans performed in these patients infrequently detect such lesions. Recent reports have demonstrated the presence of signal abnormalities in the deep white matter suggestive of small vessel disease in patients with NTG.[37-39] One study reported equal prevalence rates of intracranial meningioma, aneurysm, and arteriovenous malformation among patients with NTG and age-matched controls.[39] The potential cost of performing neuroimaging studies in the evaluation of all patients with NTG may approach $500 million in the United States alone.[114] Moreover, this figure is an underestimation given current imaging costs coupled with the unaccounted number of patients with primary open-angle glaucoma who are imaged when progression occurs at normal levels of IOP.

Greenfield and colleagues reviewed the medical records of consecutive glaucoma patients who underwent brain MRI or CT scanning as part of a diagnostic evaluation between January 1, 1985, and July 1, 1995.[19] A masked reading of optic nerve photographs and visual fields was performed by one observer. A similar analysis was performed on a control group of consecutive patients with nonglaucomatous optic nerve cupping with known intracranial mass lesions. A total of 52 eyes of 29 patients with glaucoma and 44 eyes of 28 control patients with compressive lesions were reviewed. In this series, none of the patients diagnosed with glaucoma had neuroradiological evidence of a mass lesion involving the anterior visual pathway.

Compared with patients who have cupping associated with intracranial lesions, patients with glaucoma were older ($p = 0.0001$) and had better visual acuity ($p = 0.002$), greater vertical loss of neuroretinal rim tissue ($p = 0.0001$), more frequent optic disc hemorrhages ($p = 0.01$), less neuroretinal rim pallor ($p = 0.0001$), and more nerve fiber bundle visual

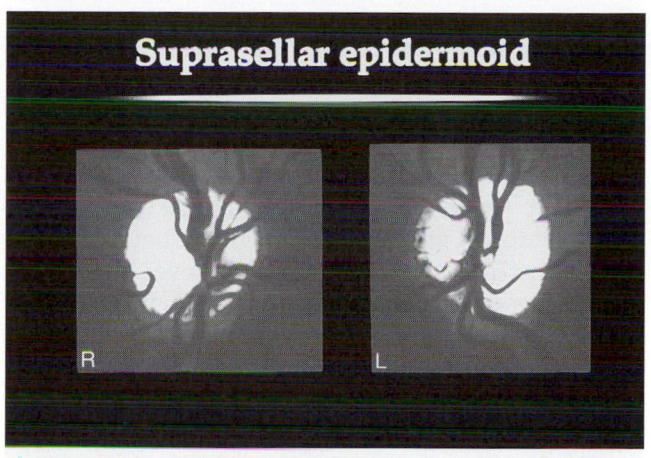

Figure 30-9. Optic nerve photographs (*A*) of a patient with a suprasellar epidermoid tumor show an absence of focal defects in the neuroretinal rim and moderate temporal pallor. (*See also Color Plate 107.*) The automated visual fields (*B*) show an incongruous right homonymous hemianopia.

field defects aligned at the horizontal midline ($p = 0.0001$). Visual acuity below 20/40, vertically aligned visual field defects, optic nerve pallor in excess of cupping (Fig. 30-9), and age less than 50 years were 77, 81, 90, and 93% specific for nonglaucomatous cupping associated with compressive lesions, respectively.

DIFFERENTIAL DIAGNOSIS

As described above, nonglaucomatous optic neuropathy may be associated with optic nerve cupping. Traumatic optic neuropathy can produce atrophic optic cupping, and clinicians should inquire about a history of ocular trauma. Examination may reveal tears in the pupillary sphincter and gonioscopic evidence of angle recession in such individuals.

Atrophic cupping may be seen as a sequela of arteritic anterior ischemic optic neuropathy in as many as 50% of eyes,[102] and physicians should inquire about symptoms of occult cranial arteritis. Inflammatory disorders such as demyelinating optic neuritis and syphilitic optic neuritis and inherited diseases such as dominant optic atrophy may similarly result in atrophic optic cupping. An effective albeit imperfect rule of thumb generally dictates that eyes with retention of central acuity, absence of dyschromatopsia, and vertical cupping that corresponds to a visual field defect are generally glaucomatous. Pallor of the neural rim in excess of cupping is characteristic of a nonglaucomatous cupping.[103,115]

Various forms of pressure-dependent glaucoma may resemble NTG and must be considered in the evaluation of a patient with optic nerve cupping and normal IOP. Many of these eyes have had prior IOP elevation ("burned-out" primary open-angle glaucoma), and the clinician should always inquire about the maximum level of untreated IOP. Similarly, prolonged corticosteroid therapy is a common cause of unrecognized IOP elevation. A careful history of such therapy should be obtained, particularly in individuals with steroid-dependent obstructive pulmonary disease or chronic inflammatory disorders. Finally, intermittent IOP elevation may exist in eyes with exfoliation and pigmentary dispersion. These eyes are characterized by wide fluctuations in IOP that may go unrecognized by the clinician. Typical iris transillumination defects or gonioscopic pigmentary abnormalities may help correctly identify these patients.

Intermittent angle-closure glaucoma is perhaps the most misdiagnosed disorder in the differential diagnosis of NTG. Three-mirror darkroom indentation gonioscopy is essential in order to accurately identify such individuals. Darkroom provocative testing with ultrasound biomicroscopy is a helpful adjunct if available (Fig. 30–10). Laser iridotomy effectively eliminates the relative pupillary block in these eyes and is essential in order to maintain consistent diurnal IOP control.

Recent evidence suggests that measurements of central corneal thickness play a clinically relevant role in differentiating patients with NTG from those with primary open-angle glaucoma. Morad and colleagues[116] found a significantly lower corneal thickness in 21 eyes with NTG (mean 0.52 ± 0.04 mm) compared with 25 eyes with primary open-angle glaucoma (mean 0.56 ± 0.03 mm) and 27 normal eyes (mean 0.56 ± 0.03 mm). Ehlers and coauthors have suggested that this may lead to underestimation of IOP by as much as 4.7 mmHg.[117]

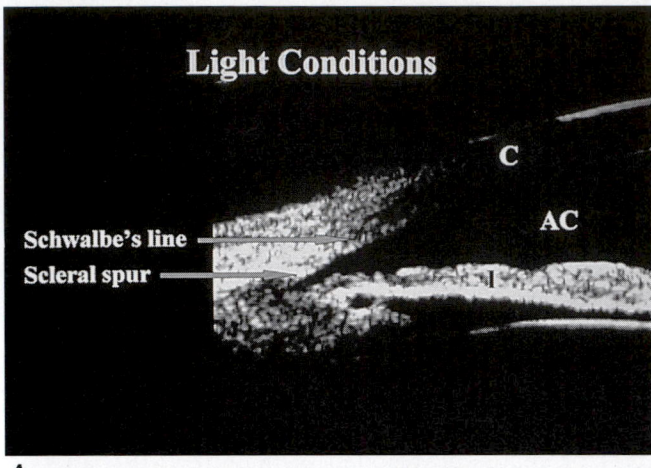

A

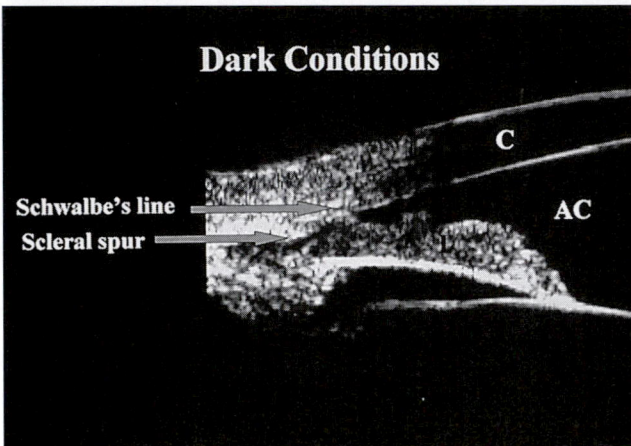

B

Figure 30–10. Ultrasound biomicroscopy is helpful in the identification of patients with occludable drainage angles. With ambient light (*A*), the iris configuration (I) appears planar and the peripheral angle is open to scleral spur. The cornea (C), anterior chamber (AC), and Schwalbe's line are labeled. Under darkroom conditions (*B*), relative pupillary block is visualized, with evidence of iris bombé and closure of the peripheral angle to the level of Schwalbe's line. (Reproduced with permission from Greenfield DS. Primary angle-closure glaucoma. In: Parrish RK II, ed. *Bascom Palmer Eye Institute's Atlas of Ophthalmology*. Philadelphia: Current Medicine;1999:198–202.

NEW DIAGNOSTIC TECHNOLOGY

Advances in ocular imaging technology have provided a means to objectively evaluate optic disc topography and peripapillary RNFL in glaucomatous eyes. Eid and colleagues have demonstrated using confocal scanning laser ophthalmoscopy (CSLO) that eyes with NTG have larger cup size than eyes with high-tension glaucoma matched for age and degree of

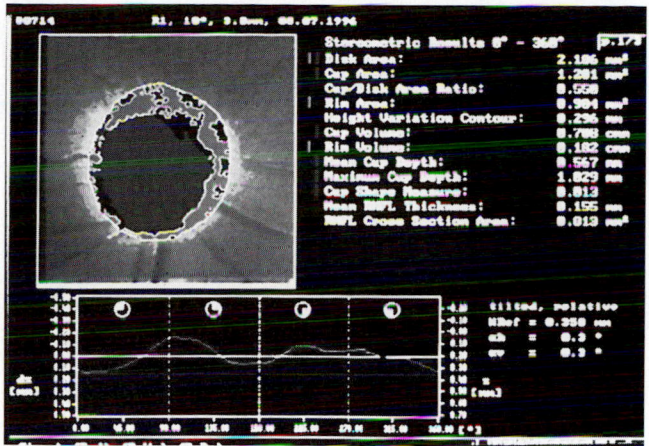

Figure 30–11. Confocal scanning laser ophthalmoscopy (CSLO) image of a patient with NTG shows loss of the inferior neuroretinal rim (green) and associated stereometric parameters. There is a focal depression in the double-hump pattern of the height-variation diagram corresponding to the decreased height of the inferotemporal quadrant (*below*). (*See also Color Plate 108.*)

visual field loss.[49] CSLO, a technology embodied in an instrument known as the Heidelberg Retinal Tomograph (Heidelberg Engineering, Heidelberg, Germany), enables the operator to quantitatively evaluate three-dimensional characteristics of optic nerve head topography.[118–121] Thirty-two coronal sections of the optic nerve head are acquired over a depth of approximately 3.5 mm, and a color-coded topographic map of the optic nerve head is generated. Figure 30–11 illustrates a CSLO image of an eye with NTG and demonstrates loss of the inferior neuroretinal rim.

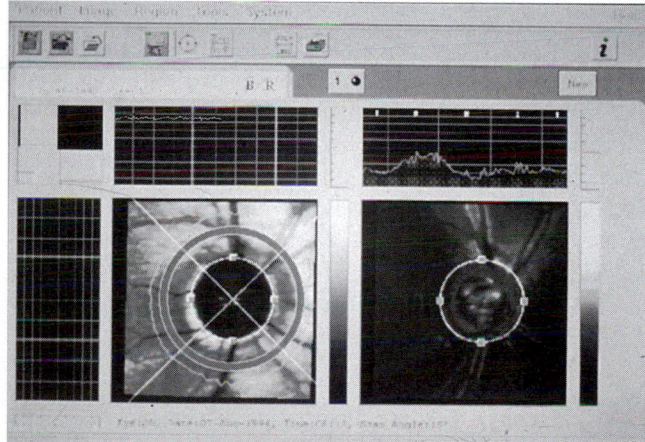

Figure 30-12. Scanning laser polarimetry (SLP) image (NFA II) of the patient illustrated in Fig. 30-11 demonstrates advanced loss of the inferior retinal nerve fiber layer. Retardation in the inferior region of the linear polar cross-section diagram is reduced compared with the superior region, indicating thinning of this area. (*See also Color Plate 109.*)

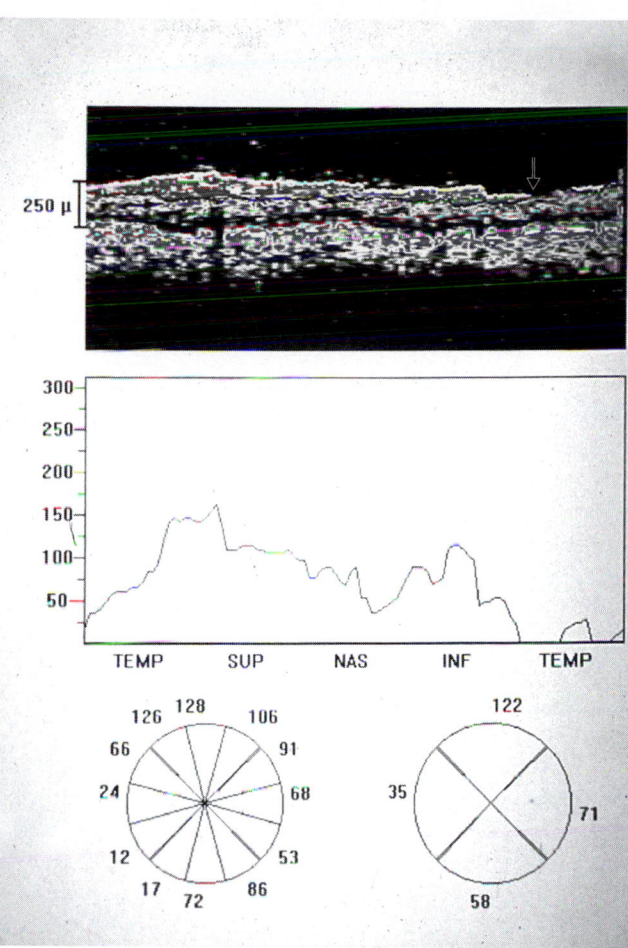

Figure 30-13. Circular optical coherence tomography (OCT) scan of the patient illustrated in Fig. 30-11 demonstrates the inferior defect in the retinal nerve fiber layer (RNFL) in cross-section as a region of localized thinning. The mean height of the inferior RNFL quadrant is reduced (58 μm), compared with the mean height of the superior quadrant (122 μm). (*See also Color Plate 110.*)

Scanning laser polarimetry (SLP) (GDx; Laser Diagnostic Technologies, Inc., San Diego, CA) is a confocal scanning laser ophthalmoscope with an integrated polarimeter that evaluates the thickness of the RNFL by utilizing the birefringent properties of nerve fibers.[122–127] The amount of polarization of the scanning beam, referred to as *retardation*, is linearly correlated to the thickness of the polarizing medium and is computed to give an index of RNFL thickness. Figure 30–12 illustrates an SLP image of an eye with NTG with reduced inferior RNFL retardation.

Optical coherence tomography (OCT; Humphrey Systems Inc., Dublin, CA) is a new, noninvasive, noncontact, transpupillary imaging technology that can image retinal structures in vivo with a resolution of 10 to 17 μm.[128,129] Cross-sectional images of the retina are produced using the optical backscattering of light in a fashion analogous to B-scan ultrasonography. The anatomic layers within the retina can be differentiated, and retinal and RNFL thickness (Fig. 30–13) can be measured.[130,131]

MANAGEMENT STRATEGIES

Paramount in the initial management of patients with cupping associated with normal IOP is the clinical differentiation between glaucoma and nonglaucomatous cupping. A detailed history is essential, with attention to the presence of neurological symptoms, the chronicity and pattern of visual loss, a history of head trauma, atherosclerosis, excessively high or low blood pressure, blood transfusion, vasospasm, shock, vasculitis, or even syphilis. Color-vision abnormalities, a marked relative afferent pupillary defect, neuroretinal rim pallor out of proportion to optic disc cupping, and visual field defects that do not correspond to the pattern or magnitude of optic disc cupping suggest nonglaucomatous disorders. Routine diagnostic neuroimaging is unnecessary and should be performed selectively in atypical cases.

Having established a glaucomatous mechanism of injury, pressure-dependent and non-pressure-dependent subtypes should be distinguished. The maximum level of untreated IOP should be obtained, as well as a history of vasospastic phenomena (e.g., migraine headache, Raynaud's phenomenon, etc.), trauma, or corticosteroid use. Careful gonioscopic and biomicroscopic evaluation should be performed to exclude intermittent angle closure, angle recession, exfoliation, or pigmentary glaucoma. The absence of these clinical signs suggests a non-pressure-dependent disorder.

The presence of visual field progression must be carefully evaluated. One should pay particular attention to the magnitude of progression, proximity to fixation, and rapidity with which progression has occurred. More than one confirmatory visual field should be used to establish progression. Clinical characteristics associated with a high risk of progression (e.g., recurrent disc hemorrhage, acquired optic nerve pit, and IOP in the high normal range) should be identified and a target IOP established. One should consider the degree of optic nerve damage, the status of the fellow eye, and the degree of expected compliance with therapy in the determination of target IOP.

At the present juncture, the only proven treatment for glaucoma is IOP reduction below the level associated with damage. This may be accomplished with medical therapy, laser therapy, or incisional surgery.[93,132] Although exceptions exist, the recommendation of this author is to achieve a 20% IOP reduction in eyes with mild optic nerve damage, a 30% IOP reduction in eyes with moderate damage, and a 40% IOP reduction in eyes with advanced damage. One should reevaluate the target IOP based upon the results of sequential visual field examinations and the appearance of the optic nerve head. IOP measurements may have diurnal fluctuation and the clinician should determine peak and trough levels. Although some clinicians perform 24-hour diurnal IOP measurements, Yamagami and coauthors have reported that diurnal fluctuation of IOP can be estimated from daytime measurements.[133]

Comanagement with an internist is recommended in order to identify patients with advanced vascular disease, orthostatic hypotension, or nocturnal hypotension. Patients at risk include those believed to be using excessive amounts of systemic antihypertensive therapy. Efforts to prevent vasospastic events have focused on the administration of systemic calcium channel blockers. Although some investigators have reported visual field improvement with such therapy,[62,63] others have failed to demonstrate uniform visual function or hemodynamic responses.[134] Moreover, nocturnal hypotensive effects may be precipitated in some individuals, producing reduced ocular perfusion pressure. As this may contribute to disease progression, such therapy is not recommended at the present time.

NEW DIRECTIONS IN THERAPY

As in the past, IOP reduction remains the mainstay of existing therapy. Patients with progressive NTG (approximately 50%) require lower levels of intraocular pressure in order to prevent or delay progressive visual loss. One should bear in mind at all times that it is critical to adhere to the general principles of medical therapy. This includes performance of monocular therapeutic trials, initiating therapy with the lowest dose and frequency of medication, emphasis upon spacing intervals between medications and performance of punctal occlusion, and inquiring about coexisting systemic morbidity and adverse medication events. If inadequate pressure reduction is achieved with conservative management, laser trabeculoplasty or filtration surgery should be performed.

We are at an exciting crossroads in our capacity to better understand, detect, and treat glaucomatous optic neuropathy. To this end, the next decade will bear witness to a new generation of pharmaceutical agents known as *neuroprotectants*, which act to protect damaged axons from secondary injury.[135,136] In addition, vasoactive agents that augment ocular blood flow, reduce vasospasm, and improve optic nerve autoregulation may provide new approaches to existing therapy. Paramount in this regard will be imaging technology that provides quantitative, objective, and reproducible measurements of RNFL thickness.

REFERENCES

1. von Graefe A. Amaurose mit Sehnervenexcavation. *Graefes Arch Clin Exp Ophthalmol.* 1857;3:484.

2. Gradle HS. Glaucoma simplex without perceptible rise in tension. *Arch Ophthalmol.* 1917;46:117–125.

3. Levene RZ. Low tension glaucoma: A critical review and new material. *Surv Ophthalmol.* 1980;24: 621–664.

4. Leydhecker W, Akiyama K, Neumann HG. Der intraokulare Druck gesunder menschlicher Augen. *Klin Monatsbl Augenheilkd.* 1958;133:662.

5. Armaly MF. On the distribution of applanation pressure: I. Statistical features and the effect of age, sex, and family history of glaucoma. *Arch Ophthalmol.* 1965; 73:11–18.

6. Wilson MR. The myth of "21." *J Glaucoma.* 1996;6:75–77.

7. Chandler PA, Grant WM. *Glaucoma.* Philadelphia: Lea & Febiger; 1979.

8. Hoskins HD. Definition, classification, and management of the glaucoma suspect. In: *Transactions of the New Orleans Academy of Ophthalmology: Symposium on Glaucoma.* St. Louis: Mosby; 1981.

9. Drance SM. Low-tension glaucoma, enigma and opportunity. *Arch Ophthalmol.* 1985;103:1131.

10. Quigley HA. The number of persons with glaucoma worldwide. *Br J Ophthalmol.* 1996;80:389–393.

11. Shiose Y. Prevalence and clinical aspects of low-tension glaucoma. In: Henkind P, ed. *Acta 24th International Congress of Ophthalmology.* Philadelphia: Lippincott, 1983.

12. Sommer A, Tielsch JM, Katz J, et al. Relationship between intraocular pressure and primary open-angle glaucoma among white and black Americans. *Arch Ophthalmol.* 1991;109:1090–1095.

13. Liebowitz HM, Krueger DE, Maunder LR. The Framingham Eye Study monograph. *Surv Ophthalmol.* 1980;24 (suppl):335–610.

14. Bankes JLK, Perkins ES, Tsolakis S, Wright JE. Bedford glaucoma survey. *Br Med J.* 1968;30:791–799.

15. Sommer A. Glaucoma: Facts and fancies. *Eye.* 1996; 10:295–301.

16. Drance SM, Sweeney VP, Morgan RW, Feldman F. Studies of factors involved in the production of low-tension glaucoma. *Arch Ophthalmol.* 1973;89:457–465.

17. Tielsch JM, Sommer A, Katz J, Royal RM, Quigley HA, Javitt S. Racial variations in the prevalence of primary open-angle glaucoma: The Baltimore Eye Survey. *JAMA.* 1991;266:369.

18. Armaly MF, Krueger DE, Maunder L, et al. Biostatistical analysis of the collaborative glaucoma study. *Arch Ophthalmol.* 1980;98:2163.

19. Greenfield DS, Siatkowski RM, Glaser JS, Schatz NJ, Parrish RK. The cupped disc: Who needs neuroimaging? *Ophthalmology.* 1998;105:1866–1874.

20. Chumbley LC, Brubaker RF. Low-tension glaucoma. *Am J Ophthalmol.* 1976;81:761.

21. Goldberg I, Hollows FC, Kass MA, Becker B. Systemic factors in patients with low-tension glaucoma. *Br J Ophthalmol.* 1981;65:56–62.

22. Choe YJ, et al. The prevalence of glaucoma in Korean adults. *Invest Ophthalmol Vis Sci.* 1993;34(suppl):1286.

23. Sjögren H. A study of pseudoglaucoma. *Acta Ophthalmol.* 1946;24:239–293.

24. Kitazawa Y, Quigley HA, Werner EB, Greenfield DS. Unilateral normal-tension glaucoma. *J Glaucoma.* 1997; 6:50–55.

25. Usui T, Iwata K, Shirakashi M, Abe H. Prevalence of migraine in low-tension glaucoma and primary open-angle glaucoma in Japanese. *Br J Ophthalmol.* 1991;75: 224–226.

26. Phelps CD, Corbett JJ. Migraine and low-tension glaucoma: A case-control study. *Invest Ophthalmol Vis Sci.* 1985;26:1105–1108.

27. Drance SM, Douglas GR, Wijsman K, Schulzer M, Britton RJ. Response of blood flow to warm and cold in normal and low-tension glaucoma patients. *Am J Ophthalmol.* 1988;105:35–39.

28. Gasser P, Flammer J. Blood-cell velocity in the nailfold capillaries of patients with normal-tension and high-tension glaucoma. *Am J Ophthalmol.* 1991;111:585–588.

29. Drance SM. Some factors in the production of low-tension glaucoma. *Br J Ophthalmol.* 1972;56:229–242.

30. Hayreh SS. Role of the nocturnal arterial hypotension in glaucomatous optic neuropathy and anterior ischemic optic neuropathy. *Glaucoma Update.* 1995;5:37–47.

31. Graham SL, Drance SM, Wijsman K, Douglas GR, Mikelberg FS. Ambulatory blood pressure monitoring in glaucoma: The nocturnal dip. *Ophthalmology.* 1995; 102:61–69.

32. Kaiser HJ, Flammer J. Systemic hypotension: A risk factor for glaucomatous damage. *Ophthalmologica.* 1991;203:105–108.

33. Berglund G. Goals of antihypertensive therapy: Is there a point beyond which pressure reduction is dangerous? *Am J Hypertens.* 1989;2:586–593.

34. Alderman MH, Ooi WL, Madhavan S, Cohen H. Treatment-induced blood pressure reduction and the risk of myocardial infarction. *JAMA.* 1989;262:920–924.

35. Farnett L, Mulrow CD, Linn WD, Lucey CR, Tuley MR. The J-curve phenomenon and the treatment of hypertension: Is there a point beyond which pressure reduction is dangerous? *JAMA.* 1991;265:489–495.

36. Harris A, Sergott RC, Spaeth GL, Katz JL, Shoemaker RC, Martin BJ. Color Doppler analysis of ocular vessel blood velocity in normal-tension glaucoma. *Am J Ophthalmol.* 1994;118:642–649.

37. Ong K, Farinelli A, Billson F, Houang M, Stern M. Comparative study of brain magnetic resonance imaging findings in patients with low-tension glaucoma. *Ophthalmology.* 1995; 102:1632–1638.

38. Golnik KC, Hund PW III, Stroman GA, Stewart WC.

Magnetic resonance imaging in patients with unexplained optic neuropathy. *Ophthalmology*. 1996;103: 515–520.

39. Stroman GA, Stewart WC, Golnik KC, Cure JK, Olinger RE. Magnetic resonance imaging in patients with low-tension glaucoma. *Arch Ophthalmol*. 1995;113: 168–172.

40. Kitazawa Y, Shirato S, Yamamoto T. Optic disc hemorrhage in low-tension glaucoma. *Ophthalmology*. 1986; 93:853–857.

41. Jonas JB, Lian X. Optic disk hemorrhages in glaucoma. *Am J Ophthalmol*. 1994;118:1–8.

42. Jonas JB, Xu L. Parapapillary chorioretinal atrophy in normal-pressure glaucoma. *Am J Ophthalmol*. 1993;115: 501–505.

43. Buus DR, Anderson DR. Peripapillary crescents and halos in normal-tension glaucoma and ocular hypertension. *Ophthalmology*. 1989;96:16.

44. Geijssen HC. *Studies on Normal Pressure Glaucoma*. Amstelveen: Kugler Publications, 1991.

45. Anderson DR. Correlation of peripapillary anatomy with the disc damage and field abnormalities in glaucoma. *Doc Ophthalmol Proc Ser*. 1983;35:1.

46. Javitt JC, Spaeth GL, Katz LJ, Poryzees E, Addiego R. Acquired pits of the optic nerve: Increased prevalence in patients with low-tension glaucoma. *Ophthalmology*. 1990;97:1038–1043.

47. Anderson DR. Discussion of Javitt JC, et al. Acquired pits of the optic nerve: Increased prevalence in patients with low-tension glaucoma. *Ophthalmology*. 1990;97: 1043–1044.

48. Gramer E, Althaus G, Leydhecker W. Localization and depth of glaucomatous visual field defects in relation to the size of the neuroretinal rim area of the disk in low-tension glaucoma, glaucoma simplex and pigmentary glaucoma—Clinical study with the Octopus 201 perimeter and the Optic Nerve Head Analyzer. *Klin Monatsbl Augenheilkd*. 1986;189:190.

49. Eid TE, Spaeth GL, Moster MR, Augsburger JJ. Quantitative differences between the optic nerve head and peripapillary retina in low-tension and high-tension primary open-angle glaucoma. *Am J Ophthalmol*. 1997; 124:805–813.

50. Fazio P, Krupin T, Feitl ME, et al. Optic disc topography in patients with low-tension and primary open-angle glaucoma. *Arch Ophthalmol*. 1990;108:705.

51. Yamazaki Y, Koide C, Miyazawa T, et al. Comparison of retinal nerve fiber layer in high- and normal-tension glaucoma. *Graefes Arch Clin Exp Ophthalmol*. 1991;229: 517.

52. Glicklich RE, Steinmann WC, Spaeth GL. Visual field change in low-tension glaucoma over a five-year follow-up. *Ophthalmology*. 1989;96:316–320.

53. Anderson S, Hitchings RA. A comparative study of visual fields of patients with low-tension glaucoma and those with chronic simple glaucoma. *Doc Ophthalmol Proc Ser*. 1983;35:97.

54. Caprioli J, Spaeth GL. Comparison of visual field defects in the low-tension glaucomas with those in the high-tension glaucomas. *Am J Ophthalmol*. 1984;97:730.

55. Drance SM. The visual field of low tension glaucoma and shock-induced optic neuropathy. *Arch Ophthalmol*. 1977;95:1359.

56. Greve EL, Geijssen HC. Comparison of visual fields in patients with high and with low intraocular pressures. *Doc Ophthalmol Proc Ser*. 1983;35:101.

57. Drance SM, Douglas GR, Airaksinen PJ, et al. Diffuse visual field loss in chronic open-angle and low-tension glaucoma. *Am J Ophthalmol*. 1987;104:577–580.

58. Chauhan BC, Drance SM, Douglas GR, Johnson CA. Visual field damage in normal-tension and high-tension glaucoma. *Am J Ophthalmol*. 1989;108:636.

59. Gramer E, Althaus G. The impact of intraocular pressure on visual field loss in primary open angle glaucoma. *Klin Monatsbl Augenheilkd*. 1990;197:218.

60. Kitazawa Y, Shirai H, Go FJ. The effect of Ca^{2+} antagonist on visual field in low-tension glaucoma. *Graefes Arch Clin Exp Ophthalmol*. 1989;227:408–412.

61. Gasser P, Flammer J, Guthauser U, Mahler F. Do vasospasms provoke ocular diseases? *Angiology*. 1990;41: 213–220.

62. Netland PA, Chaturvedi N, Dreyer EB. Calcium channel blockers in the management of low-tension and open-angle glaucoma. *Am J Ophthalmol*. 1993;115:608–613.

63. Sawada A, Kitazawa Y, Yamamoto T, Okabe I, Ichien K. Prevention of visual field defect progression with Brovincamine in eyes with normal-tension glaucoma. *Ophthalmology*. 1996;103:283–288.

64. Hayreh SS, Zimmerman MB, Podhajsky P, Alward WLM. Nocturnal arterial hypotension and its role in optic nerve head and ocular ischemic disorders. *Am J Ophthalmol*. 1994;117:603–624.

65. Geijssen HC, Greve EL. Focal ischaemic normal pressure glaucoma versus high pressure glaucoma. *Doc Ophthalmol*. 1990;75:291–302.

66. Geijssen HC, Greve EL. The spectrum of primary open angle glaucoma I: senile sclerotic glaucoma versus high tension glaucoma. *Ophthalmic Surg*. 1987;18:207.

67. Geijssen HC, Greve EL. Myopic normal pressure glaucoma and visual field progression. *Invest Ophthalmol Vis Sci*. 1992;33 (suppl):1278.

68. Gasser P. Ocular vasospasm: A risk factor in the pathogenesis of low-tension glaucoma. *Int Ophthalmol*. 1989; 13:281.

69. Tsai CS, et al. Systemic hypertension and age in low-tension glaucoma patients. *Invest Ophthalmol Vis Sci*. 1992;33(suppl):1277.

70. Schumer RA, Podos SM, Lipton SA, Dreyer EB. Increased glutamate in the vitreous of monkeys with induced glaucoma. *Invest Ophthalmol Vis Sci*. 1994;35:1484.

71. Dreyer EB, Pan ZH, Storm S, Lipton SA. Greater sensitivity of larger retinal ganglion cells to NMDA-mediated cell death. *Neuroreport*. 1994;5:629–631.

72. Dreyer EB, Zurakowski D, Schumer RA, Podos SM, Lipton SA. Elevated glutamate levels in the vitreous body of humans and monkeys with glaucoma. *Arch Ophthalmol*. 1996;114:299–305.

73. Vorwerk CK, Lipton SA, Zurakowski D, Hyman BT,

Sabel BA, Dreyer EB. Chronic low-dose glutamate is toxic to retinal ganglion cells: Toxicity blocked by memantine. *Invest Ophthalmol Vis Sci.* 1996;37: 1618–1624.

74. Kornhuber J, Weller M, Schoppmeyer K, Reiderer P. Amantadine and memantine are NMDA receptor antagonist with neuroprotective properties. *J Neural Transm.* 1994;43(suppl):91.

75. Pellegrini JW, Lipton SA. Delayed administration of memantine prevents NMDA receptor-mediated neurotoxicity. *Ann Neurol.* 1993;33:403–407.

76. Nickells RW. Retinal ganglion cell death in glaucoma: The how, the why, and the maybe. *J Glaucoma.* 1996; 5:345–356.

77. Cartwright M, Grajewski AL, Friedberg ML, Anderson DR, Richards DW. Immune-related disease and normal-tension glaucoma: A case control study. *Arch Ophthalmol.* 1992;110:500–502.

78. Wax MB, Barrett DA, Pestronk A. Increased incidence of paraproteinemia and autoantibodies in patients with normal-tension glaucoma. *Am J Ophthalmol.* 1994; 117:561–568.

79. Wax MB, Tezel G, Saito I, et al. Anti-Ro/SS-A positivity and heat shock protein antibodies in patients with normal-pressure glaucoma. *Am J Ophthalmol.* 1998;125: 145–157.

80. Yablonski ME, Ritch R, Pokorny K. Effect of decreased intracranial pressure on optic disc. *Invest Ophthalmol Vis Sci.* 1979;20(suppl):165.

81. Horton JC, Fishman RA. Neurovisual findings in the syndrome of spontaneous intracranial hypotension from dural cerebrospinal fluid leak. *Ophthalmology.* 1994;101:244–251.

82. Greenfield DS, Wanichwecharungruang B, Liebmann JM, Ritch R. Pseudotumor cerebri presenting with unilateral papilledema after trabeculectomy. *Arch Ophthalmol.* 1997;115:423–426.

83. Gutman I, Melamed S, Ashkenazi I, Blumenthal M. Optic nerve compression by carotid arteries in low-tension glaucoma. *Graefes Arch Clin Exp Ophthalmol.* 1993;231:711–717.

84. Ley A. Compression of the optic nerve by a fusiform aneurysm of the carotid artery. *J Neurol Neurosurg Psychiatry.* 1950;13:75–86.

85. Mitts MG, McQueen JD. Visual loss associated with fusiform enlargement of the intracranial portion of the internal carotid artery. *J Neurosurg.* 1965;23:33–37.

86. Slavin ML. Bitemporal hemianopia associated with dolichoectasia of the intracranial carotid arteries. *J Clin Neuroophthalmol.* 1990;10:80–81.

87. Korenfeld MS, Dueker DK. Occult intraocular pressure elevations and optic cup asymmetry: Sleep posture may be a risk factor. *Invest Ophthalmol Vis Sci.* 1993; 34(suppl):994.

88. Schulzer M, The Normal-Tension Glaucoma Study Group. Errors in the diagnosis of visual field progression in normal-tension glaucoma. *Ophthalmology.* 1994;101: 1589–1595.

89. Shirai H, Sakuma T, Sogano S, Kitazawa Y. Visual field change and risk factors for progression of visual field damage in low-tension glaucoma. *Acta Soc Ophthalmol Jpn.* 1992;96:352–358.

90. Ito M, Sugiura T, Mizokami K. A comparative study on visual field defect in low-tension glaucoma. *Acta Soc Ophthalmol Jpn.* 1991;95:790.

91. Sugiura T, Ito M, Mizokami K. A comparative study of optic disc appearances in progressive and non-progressive low-tension glaucoma. *Acta Soc Ophthalmol Jpn.* 1991;95:343.

92. Jonas JB, Gründler AE, Gonzales-Cortés J. Pressure-dependent neuroretinal rim loss in normal-pressure glaucoma. *Am J Ophthalmol.* 1998;125:11137–11144.

93. Bhandari A, Crabb DP, Poinoosawmy D, Fitzke FW, Hitchings RA, Noureddin BN. Effect of surgery on visual field progression in normal-tension glaucoma. *Ophthalmology.* 1997;104:1131–1137.

94. The Collaborative Normal-Tension Glaucoma Study Group. The effectiveness of intraocular pressure reduction in the treatment of normal-tension glaucoma. *Am J Ophthalmol.* 1998;126:498–505.

95. Ugurlu S, Weitzman M, Nduaguba C, Caprioli J. Acquired pit of the optic nerve: A risk factor for progression of glaucoma. *Am J Ophthalmol.* 1998;125:457–464.

96. Drance SM, Fairclough M, Butler DM, Kottler MS. The importance of disc hemorrhage in the prognosis of chronic open-angle glaucoma. *Arch Ophthalmol.* 1977;95:226.

97. Diehl DL, Quigley HA, Miller NR, Sommer A, Burney EN. Prevalence and significance of optic disc hemorrhage in a longitudinal study of glaucoma. *Arch Ophthalmol.* 1990;108:545.

98. Siegner SW, Netland PA. Optic disc hemorrhages and progression of glaucoma. *Ophthalmology.* 1996;103: 1014–1024.

99. Grant WM, Burke JF. Why do some people go blind from glaucoma? *Ophthalmology.* 1982;89:991–998.

100. Yamazaki Y, Drance SM. The relationship between progression of visual field defects and retrobulbar circulation in patients with glaucoma. *Am J Ophthalmol.* 1997;124:287–295.

101. Sonty S, Schwartz B. Development of cupping and pallor in posterior ischemic optic neuropathy. *Int Ophthalmol.* 1983;6:213–220.

102. Quigley HA, Anderson DR. Cupping of the optic disc in ischemic optic neuropathy. *Trans Am Acad Ophthalmol Otolaryngol.* 1977;83:755–762.

103. Trobe JD, Glaser JS, Cassady J, Herschler J, Anderson DR. Nonglaucomatous excavation of the optic disc. *Arch Ophthalmol.* 1980;98:1046–1050.

104. Radius RL, Maumenee AE. Optic atrophy and glaucomatous cupping. *Am J Ophthalmol.* 1978;85:145.

105. Kalenak JW, Kosmorsky GS, Hassenbusch SJ. Compression of the intracranial optic nerve mimicking unilateral normal-pressure glaucoma. *J Clin Neuroophthalmol.* 1992;12:230–235.

106. Bianchi-Marzoli S, Rizzo JF III, Brancato R, Lessell S.

CASE 1

A 52-year-old male African American presents on 9/18/97 with a complaint of blurred vision, both at distance and near. The patient is a mild uncorrected hyperope with presbyopia OU, with no pertinent medical history. Visual acuity uncorrected is 20/20 in each eye. Pupils are equal, round, and reactive to light in each eye (PERRLA) with a negative afferent pupil test OD and OS. Intraocular pressure (IOP) as measured by Goldmann tonometry was 15 mmHg OD and 15 mmHg OS at 2 P.M. The fundus examination with pupillary dilation revealed the optic discs in each eye to be large, along with enlarged cupping and thin neuroretinal rims OD and OS. Heidelberg retinal tomographs (HRT) were performed, confirming the large discs, large cupping, and thin rim tissue. Humphrey 24-2 visual field testing OD revealed a dense inferior arcuate scotoma, approaching fixation. In the OS, the field showed reduced points scattered in the superior and inferior hemifields. The patient returned on 10/9/97, at which time the IOP was 23 mmHg OD and 25 mmHg OS. Gonioscopy revealed open angles with the ciliary body visible in all quadrants.

- Is this glaucoma?
- How would you proceed with care?
- Would you treat this individual? If so, is there a specific medication(s) to use?
- What is the target pressure?
- When should the patient return?

Is this glaucoma? The patient does have glaucoma. Most prevalence studies have found that approximately 50% of individuals with elevated intraocular pressures have a "normal" intraocular pressure on screening. This patient's intraocular pressure was normal on his first visit. The fact that his IOP was elevated on the second screening is basically irrelevant to the diagnosis of glaucoma. Glaucoma is not a disease of pressure, but pressure is a major risk factor.

How would you proceed with care? Today, the only way to treat glaucoma is by lowering IOP. At this point I would like to get some more information. The first thing that I think is important would be a diurnal curve during working hours. Since there is a large variation of intraocular pressure (a 50% increase between the first and second visits), it would be hard to determine whether or not the medication was working, even if a one-eyed therapeutic trial were instituted. I would try to get intraocular pressures throughout the course of a working day to see what the variation is. I would also get C-10-2 visual fields in the right eye and repeat the C-24-2 visual fields in both eyes. This would allow a better gauge of progression.

Should treatment be instituted for this individual? I would treat the patient, with betaxolol, starting with a uniocular therapeutic trial in the OD. Betaxolol does not lower IOP quite as well as either a nonselective beta blocker or latanoprost. However, it is safer in an individual without any history of asthma. Additionally, it has calcium channel–blocking effects, and potential neuroprotecting effects, as seen by Osborne's work.[1-3] I would check the patient in a month to determine its effect.

What is the target pressure? I would take an average of the diurnal curve and try to get a constant 30% lowering at all time intervals. I would have my target pressure be variable, depending on whether or not there was any progression in visual field loss.

Because of the work of the Advanced Glaucoma Intervention Study (AGIS) and the fact that the patient is African-American, there is a concern for long-term visual field and vision loss despite lowering of IOP.[4-6] This would be mentioned to the patient as part of the informed consent procedure.

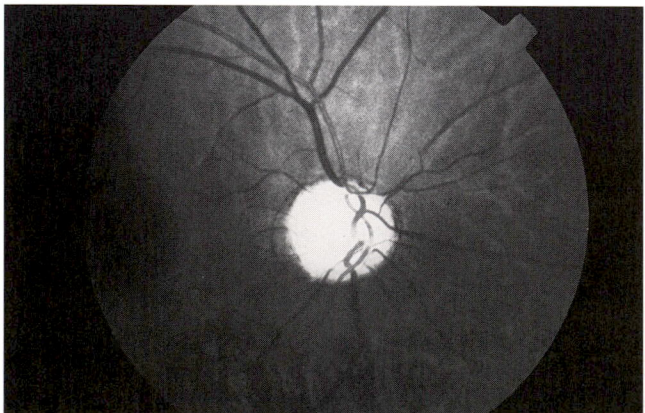

R

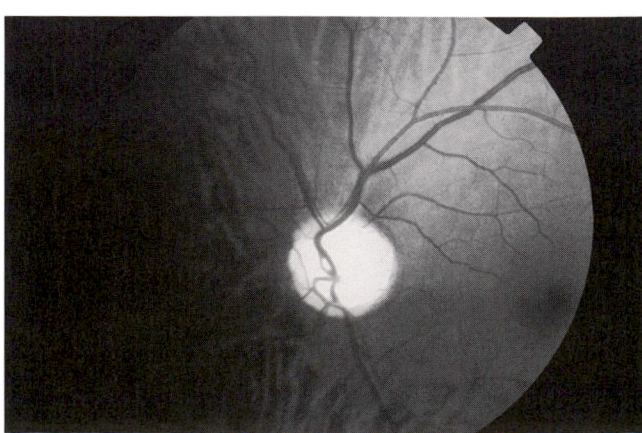

L

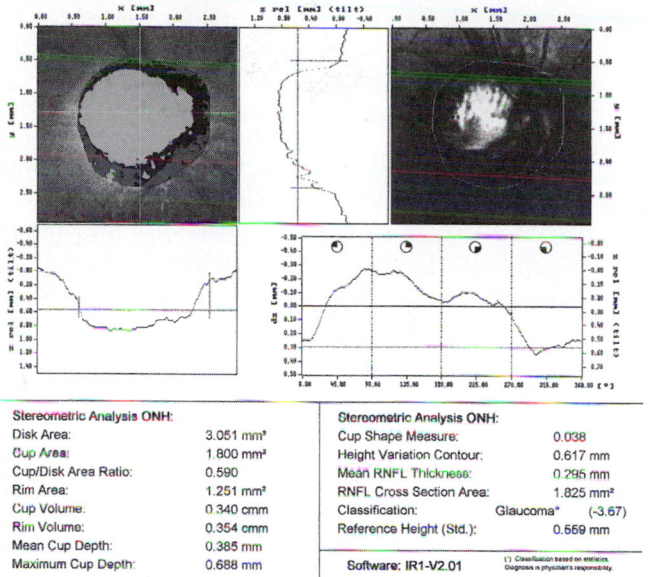
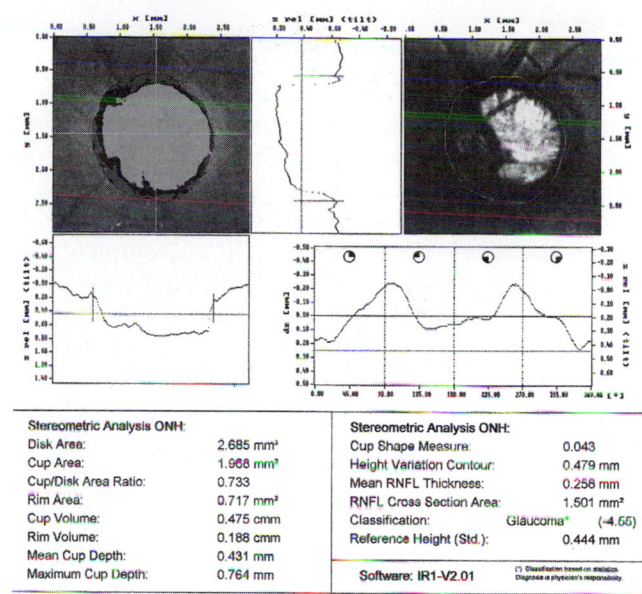

Stereometric Analysis ONH:

Disk Area:	3.051 mm²
Cup Area:	1.800 mm²
Cup/Disk Area Ratio:	0.590
Rim Area:	1.251 mm²
Cup Volume:	0.340 cmm
Rim Volume:	0.354 cmm
Mean Cup Depth:	0.385 mm
Maximum Cup Depth:	0.688 mm

Stereometric Analysis ONH:

Cup Shape Measure:	0.038
Height Variation Contour:	0.617 mm
Mean RNFL Thickness:	0.295 mm
RNFL Cross Section Area:	1.825 mm²
Classification:	Glaucoma* (-3.67)
Reference Height (Std.):	0.559 mm

Software: IR1-V2.01

(*) Classification based on statistics. Diagnosis is physician's responsibility.

OD

Stereometric Analysis ONH:

Disk Area:	2.685 mm²
Cup Area:	1.968 mm²
Cup/Disk Area Ratio:	0.733
Rim Area:	0.717 mm²
Cup Volume:	0.475 cmm
Rim Volume:	0.188 cmm
Mean Cup Depth:	0.431 mm
Maximum Cup Depth:	0.764 mm

Stereometric Analysis ONH:

Cup Shape Measure:	0.043
Height Variation Contour:	0.479 mm
Mean RNFL Thickness:	0.258 mm
RNFL Cross Section Area:	1.501 mm²
Classification:	Glaucoma* (-4.55)
Reference Height (Std.):	0.444 mm

Software: IR1-V2.01

(*) Classification based on statistics. Diagnosis is physician's responsibility.

OS

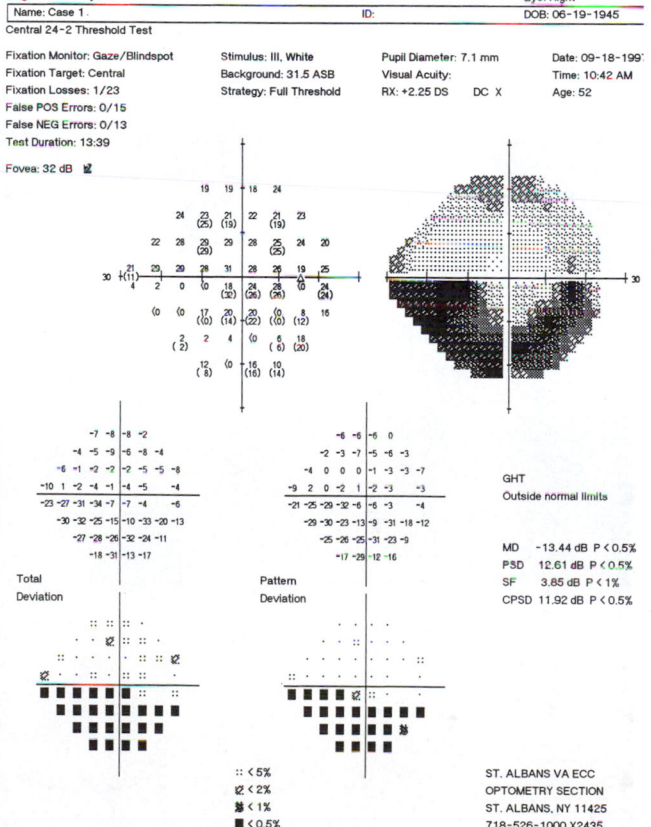
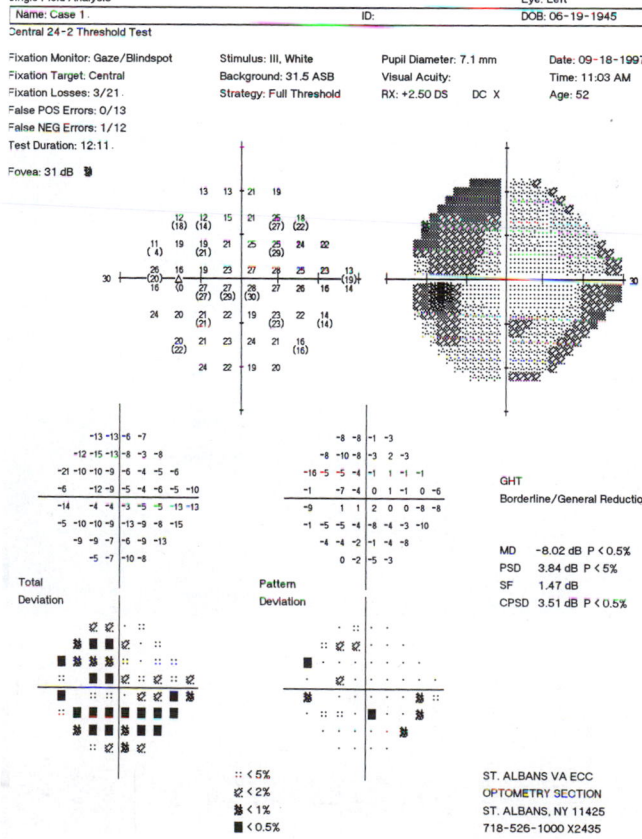

CASE 2

A 60-year-old male African American presents for a routine examination with a medical history of hypertension treated with hydrochlorothiazide. Family eye history is negative and entering visual acuities are 20/20 in each eye. Intraocular pressures using Goldmann tonometry measured the IOP at 26 mmHg OD and 29 mmHg OS. Gonioscopy revealed a wide open angle with the ciliary body visible in all quadrants in each eye. Dilated fundus exam revealed a small optic disc in each eye along with a small cup and healthy neuroretinal tissue in the OD. In the OS, an inferior focal notch was seen, with thinning of the neuroretinal rim (focal notch) at 6 o'clock. The patient returned 4 days later, at which time the IOP was 27 mmHg OD and 28 mmHg OS. Threshold visual fields revealed a full-field OD and a superior arcuate scotoma in the OS. HRT images show the disk to be average in size, with an apparent healthy nerve fiber layer OD and a thinned nerve fiber layer inferiorly OS. The thinned neuroretinal rim has greatest loss inferiorly, correlating to the superior field loss. Frequency doubling threshold N-30 visual fields showed similar loss in the OS, with a questionable defect superiorly in the OD.

- *Is this glaucoma?*
- *How would you proceed with care?*

- *Would you treat this individual?*
- *If so, with what specific medication(s)?*
- *What is the target pressure?*
- *When should the patient return?*

It is often difficult to gauge optic nerve damage in individuals with small discs. However, there is definitely asymmetry of optic nerve head cupping, along with asymmetrical visual fields. Before coming to a conclusive diagnosis, examination of the visual field must be repeated to confirm the loss as well as to carefully examine the pupil. With reexamination, an afferent pupil defect OS was seen, along with confirmation of the visual field defect.

In the left eye, the amount of visual field loss appears to be much greater than the amount of disc damage. However, this is difficult to correlate in an eye with a small optic nerve. It would be helpful to do short-wavelength automated perimetry (SWAP) visual field in the patient's right eye to determine whether any damage is present. In addition, because of apparent damage to fixation, it would be helpful to get a C-10-2 visual field in the left eye. I would proceed to treat, utilizing a selective beta blocker, betaxolol, as a first-line agent with a goal of 30% reduction.[7-10] I would start therapy with a uniocular therapeutic trial and see the patient in a month. I would emphasize compliance and the results of the AGIS study (see Chap. 25).

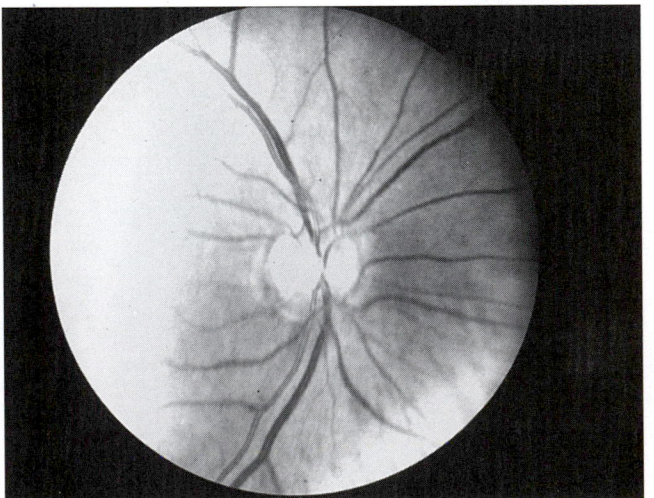

R

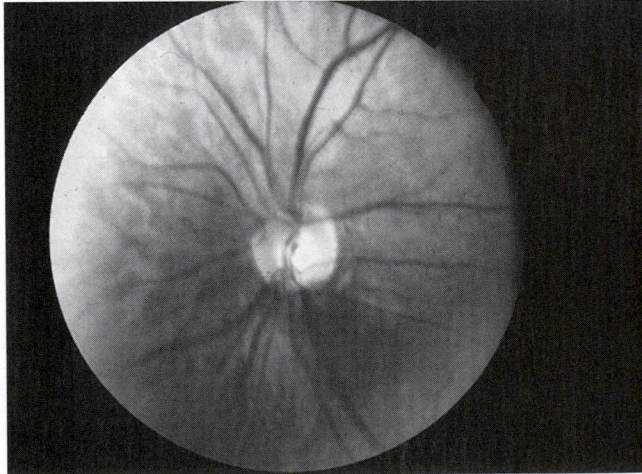

L

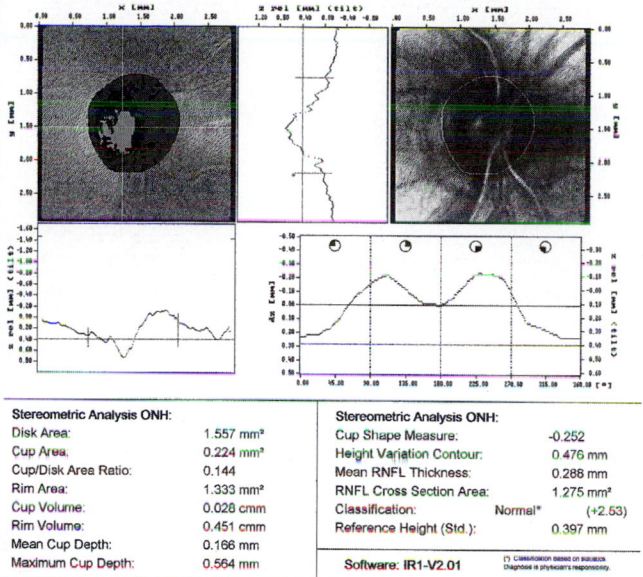

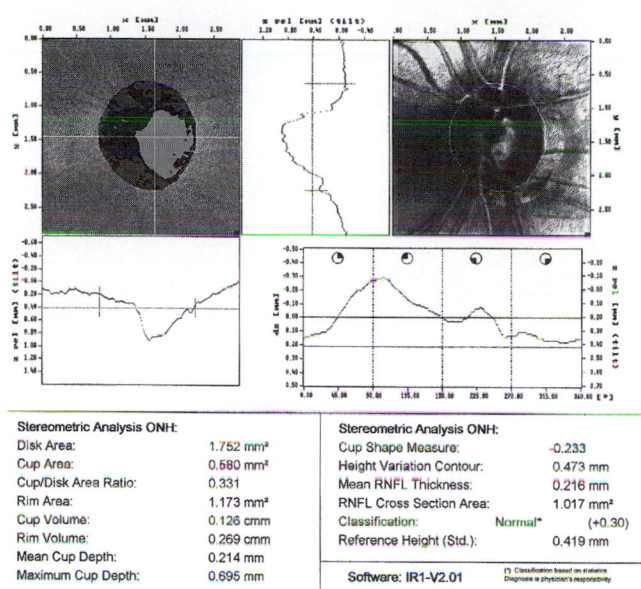

Stereometric Analysis ONH:

		Stereometric Analysis ONH:	
Disk Area:	1.557 mm²	Cup Shape Measure:	-0.252
Cup Area:	0.224 mm²	Height Variation Contour:	0.476 mm
Cup/Disk Area Ratio:	0.144	Mean RNFL Thickness:	0.288 mm
Rim Area:	1.333 mm²	RNFL Cross Section Area:	1.275 mm²
Cup Volume:	0.028 cmm	Classification: Normal*	(+2.53)
Rim Volume:	0.451 cmm	Reference Height (Std.):	0.397 mm
Mean Cup Depth:	0.166 mm	(*) Classification based on statistics	
Maximum Cup Depth:	0.564 mm	Software: IR1-V2.01	

OD

Stereometric Analysis ONH:

		Stereometric Analysis ONH:	
Disk Area:	1.752 mm²	Cup Shape Measure:	-0.233
Cup Area:	0.580 mm²	Height Variation Contour:	0.473 mm
Cup/Disk Area Ratio:	0.331	Mean RNFL Thickness:	0.216 mm
Rim Area:	1.173 mm²	RNFL Cross Section Area:	1.017 mm²
Cup Volume:	0.126 cmm	Classification: Normal*	(+0.30)
Rim Volume:	0.269 cmm	Reference Height (Std.):	0.419 mm
Mean Cup Depth:	0.214 mm	(*) Classification based on statistics	
Maximum Cup Depth:	0.695 mm	Software: IR1-V2.01	

OS

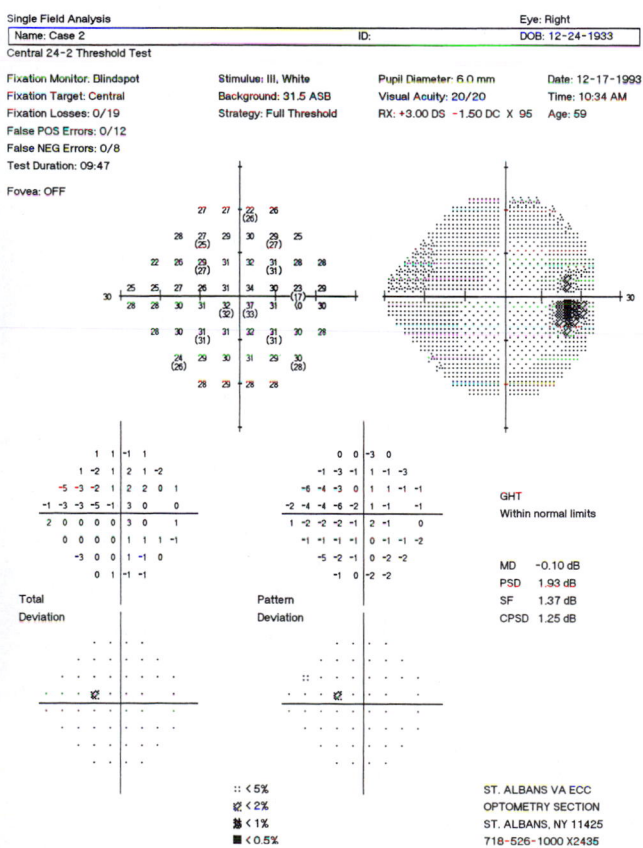

Single Field Analysis   Eye: Right

Name: Case 2   ID: DOB: 12-24-1933

Central 24-2 Threshold Test

Fixation Monitor: Blindspot   Stimulus: III, White   Pupil Diameter: 6.0 mm   Date: 12-17-1993
Fixation Target: Central   Background: 31.5 ASB   Visual Acuity: 20/20   Time: 10:34 AM
Fixation Losses: 0/19   Strategy: Full Threshold   RX: +3.00 DS -1.50 DC X 95   Age: 59
False POS Errors: 0/12
False NEG Errors: 0/8
Test Duration: 09:47
Fovea: OFF

GHT
Within normal limits

MD   -0.10 dB
PSD   1.93 dB
SF   1.37 dB
CPSD 1.25 dB

Total Deviation
Pattern Deviation

:: < 5%
▨ < 2%
▩ < 1%
■ < 0.5%

ST. ALBANS VA ECC
OPTOMETRY SECTION
ST. ALBANS, NY 11425
718-526-1000 X2435

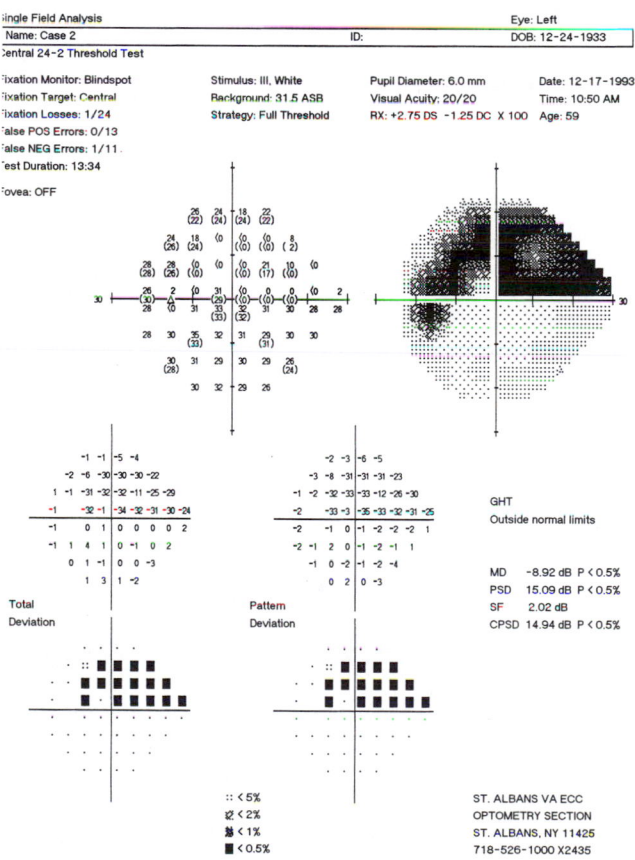

Single Field Analysis   Eye: Left

Name: Case 2   ID: DOB: 12-24-1933

Central 24-2 Threshold Test

Fixation Monitor: Blindspot   Stimulus: III, White   Pupil Diameter: 6.0 mm   Date: 12-17-1993
Fixation Target: Central   Background: 31.5 ASB   Visual Acuity: 20/20   Time: 10:50 AM
Fixation Losses: 1/24   Strategy: Full Threshold   RX: +2.75 DS -1.25 DC X 100   Age: 59
False POS Errors: 0/13
False NEG Errors: 1/11
Test Duration: 13:34
Fovea: OFF

GHT
Outside normal limits

MD   -8.92 dB P < 0.5%
PSD 15.09 dB P < 0.5%
SF   2.02 dB
CPSD 14.94 dB P < 0.5%

Total Deviation
Pattern Deviation

:: < 5%
▨ < 2%
▩ < 1%
■ < 0.5%

ST. ALBANS VA ECC
OPTOMETRY SECTION
ST. ALBANS, NY 11425
718-526-1000 X2435

(continued)

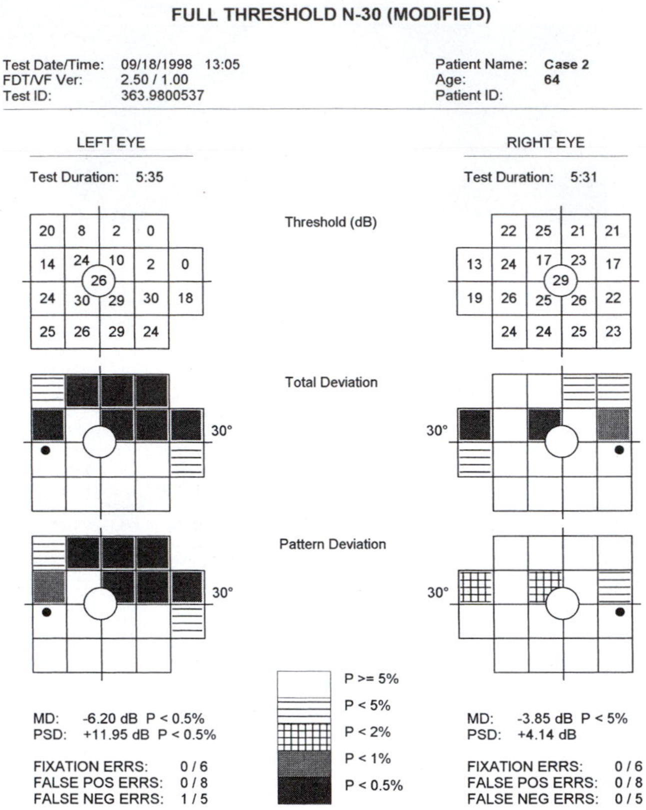

FULL THRESHOLD N-30 (MODIFIED)

Test Date/Time: 09/18/1998 13:05
FDT/VF Ver: 2.50 / 1.00
Test ID: 363.9800537

Patient Name: **Case 2**
Age: **64**
Patient ID:

| LEFT EYE | | RIGHT EYE |

Test Duration: 5:35

Test Duration: 5:31

Threshold (dB)

20	8	2	0
14	24	10	2	0
24	30	29	30	18
25	26	29	24

(26)

22	25	21	21
13	24	17	23	17
19	26	25	26	22
24	24	25	23

(29)

Total Deviation

30°

30°

Pattern Deviation

30°

30°

P >= 5%
P < 5%
P < 2%
P < 1%
P < 0.5%

MD: -6.20 dB P < 0.5%
PSD: +11.95 dB P < 0.5%

FIXATION ERRS: 0 / 6
FALSE POS ERRS: 0 / 8
FALSE NEG ERRS: 1 / 5

MD: -3.85 dB P < 5%
PSD: +4.14 dB

FIXATION ERRS: 0 / 6
FALSE POS ERRS: 0 / 8
FALSE NEG ERRS: 0 / 5

Case 2 (continued).

CASE 3

A 53-year-old male African American presents with a history of blurred vision in the left eye. The patient has not had an eye examination for several years and denies any prior ocular disease. Medical history is pertinent for hypertension, which is being treated with a calcium channel blocker. The ocular family history is negative and visual acuity is 20/20 in each eye. Pupils react to light, but a subtle afferent pupillary defect is seen in the OS. The anterior chamber angle is wide open in each eye, with the IOP 18 mmHg OD and OS at 3 P.M. Dilated fundus exam reveals a moderate-sized optic disc with a cup-to-disc ratio of 0.6 × 0.6 OD and 0.7 + 0.7 + OS. The temporal neuroretinal rim is particularly thin OS. The 24-2 full-threshold visual field exams reveal an inferior partial arcuate scotoma in the OS. The OD field appears full. The fields, repeated 6 weeks later, confirm the defect. The patient returns three times during the first month for remeasure of the IOP. At the second exam, the IOP was 16 mmHg OD and 17 mmHg OS at 12 P.M. A few days later, the IOP was 17 mmHg OD and 18 mmHg OS at 8 A.M. A diurnal curve was obtained at the next visit, at which the IOPs were measured every two hours from 7 A.M to 5 P.M. At the 7 A.M. visit, the IOP was 17 mmHg OD and 16 mmHg OS. The pressures never varied more than 2 mmHg throughout the day, with the final measurement being 16 mmHg OD and 18 mmHg OS.

- *Is this glaucoma?*
- *How would you proceed with care?*
- *Would you treat this individual?*

- *If so, with what specific medication(s)?*
- *What is the target pressure?*
- *When should this patient return?*
- *Any concerns, in either the short or the long term?*
- *Would you do any further medical tests?*
- *Are neuroimaging studies in order?*

This patient definitely has glaucoma. His discs appear almost totally cupped in the left eye, with almost no neuroretinal rim remaining temporally and a small sliver remaining nasally. There is slightly more neuroretinal rim in the right eye. The nerve fiber layer reflex is markedly diminished. It is interesting that there is no central loss in the left eye. However, there is more visual field loss in the left eye than in the right eye despite the fact that the discs are not "all that asymmetrical."

I would definitely treat this patient, starting with a cardioselective beta blocker such as betaxolol and a goal of a 30% decrease in IOP. The fact that he does not have an "elevated IOP" does not at all mean that he does not have glaucoma. One just has to be more careful and work from his baseline. I would be quite aggressive because of his lack of neuroretinal rim and his young age. A uniocular therapeutic trial would be instituted because of his large fluctuation in IOP. Neurological imaging is not indicated, as his discs appear so deep and cupped. He does appear to be glaucomatous despite the fact that his "pressures are normal." I would definitely obtain a SWAP visual field in the right eye and follow that for progressive damage, because it may be more sensitive in detecting early damage.[7-9]

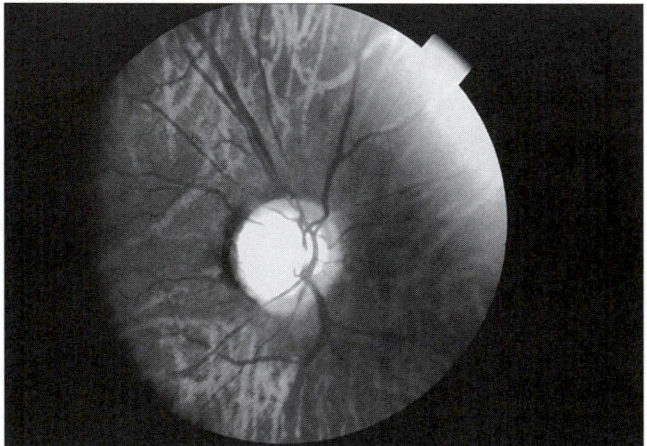

R

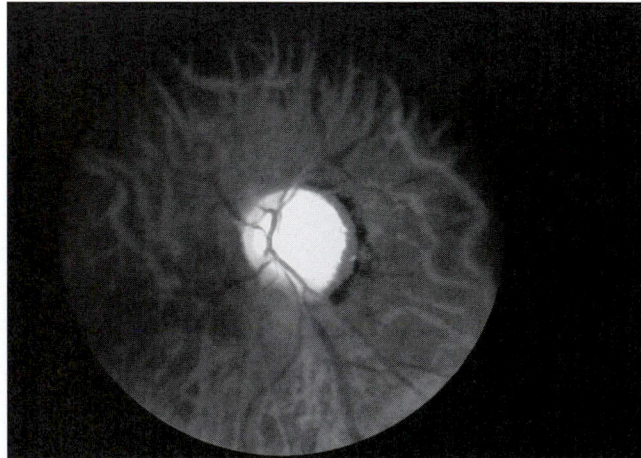

L

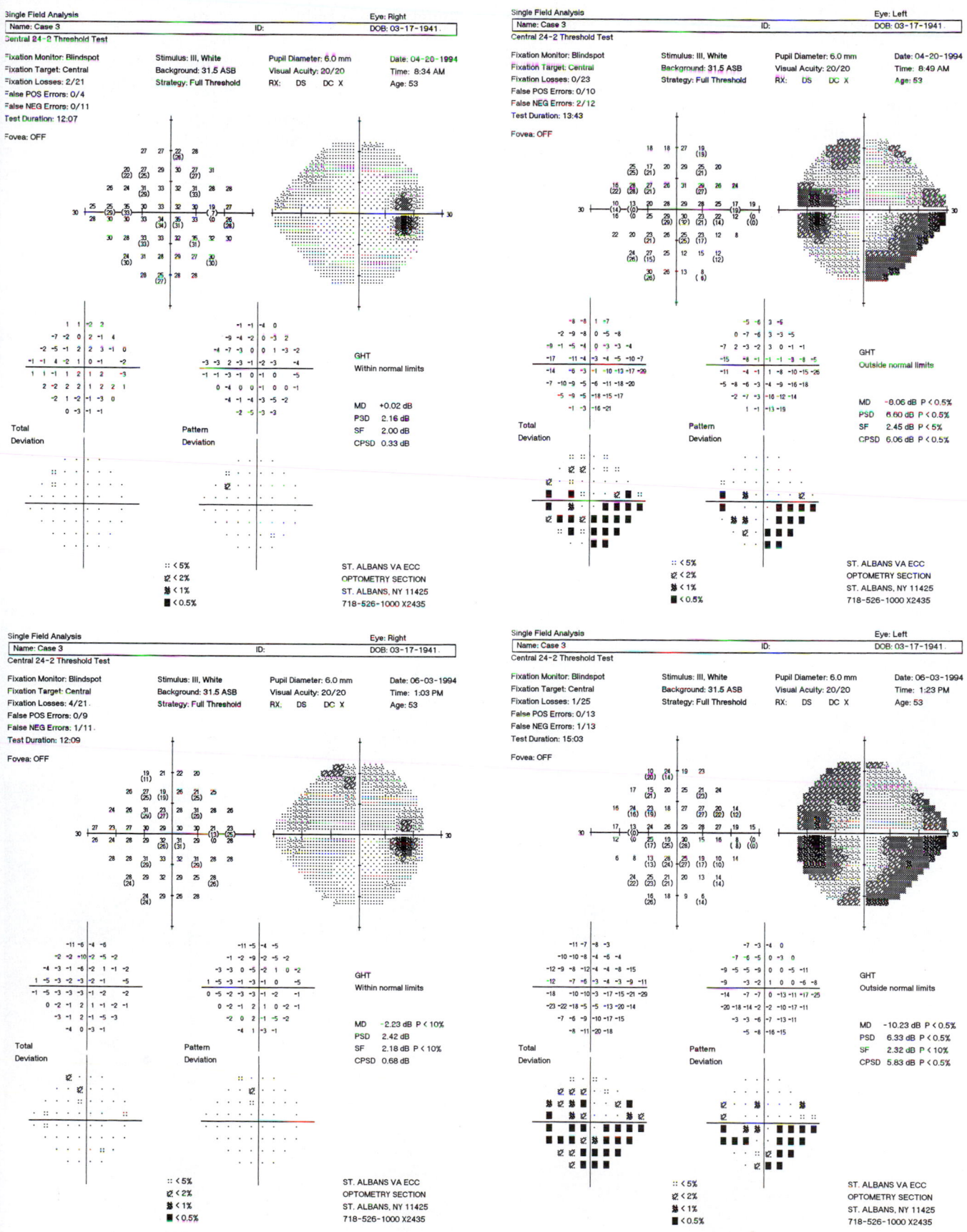

CASE 4

A 78-year-old white male presents for routine examination with a best corrected visual acuity of 20/25 OD and 20/40 OS. The patient had noticed that the vision in his left eye had been declining over the past year. He has a medical history of hypertension, is using nifedipine, and had a coronary artery bypass in 1992 and a cerebrovascular accident (CVA) in 1995. The patient's eye history is pertinent for cataract surgery, performed in 1992, with an uneventful extracapsular cataract extraction OD and a posterior chamber intraocular lens (IOL) implanted. Immediately after cataract surgery, the patient was diagnosed with open-angle glaucoma and placed on betaxolol. The patient's last eye examination was 2 years ago and he has not used his medication for the past 18 months.

The eye examination reveals mild nuclear sclerosis in the OS that correlates with the 20/40 visual acuity. A posterior chamber IOL is seen in the OD, and the IOP is 26 mmHg OD and 25 mmHg OS at 2 P.M. The optic discs are small, with small cupping, and neuroretinal rim tissue is intact. Full-threshold visual fields show a right superior quadranopsia consistent with a CVA along with diffuse loss in the OS due to nuclear sclerosis. IOPs were measured again 3 weeks later, at which time they were 25 mmHg OD and OS.

- *Is this glaucoma?*
- *How would you proceed with care?*
- *Would you treat this individual?*
- *If so, with what specific medication(s)?*
- *What is the target pressure?*
- *When should this patient return?*
- *Any concerns, in either the short or the long term?*

It appears that the optic discs are normal, but the visual fields show a right superior quadranopsia consistent with the patient's old CVA. The visual fields also show diffuse loss OS associated with the developing cataract. The patient has no afferent defect but does have elevated IOP without any signs of glaucoma.

I would not treat this patient unless he develops signs of progressive visual field loss or progressive disc damage or his IOPs go above 30 mmHg, placing him at an increased relative risk for developing damage.

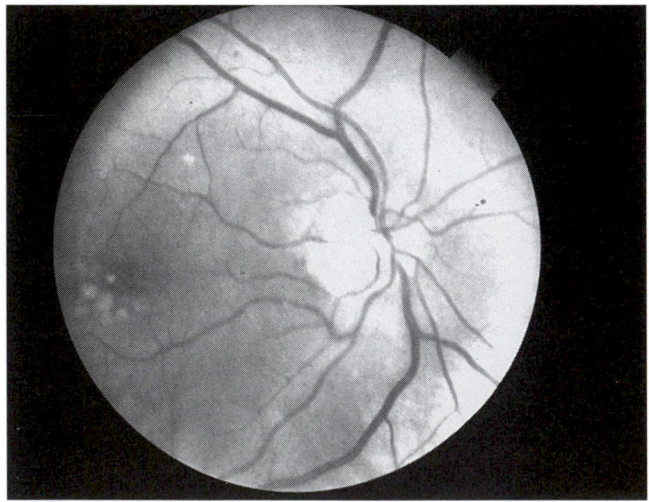

R

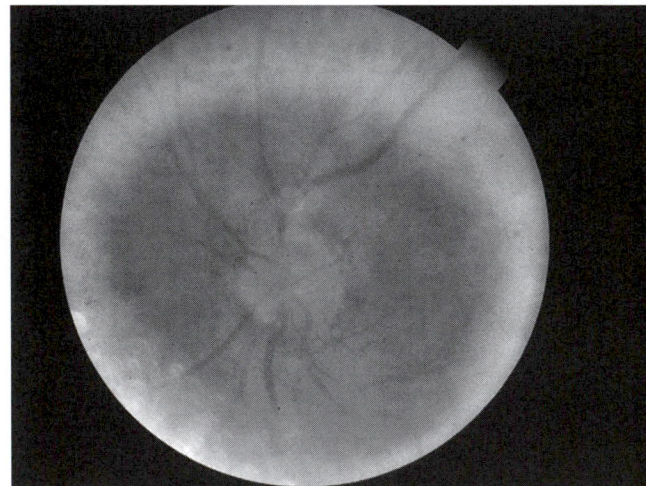

L

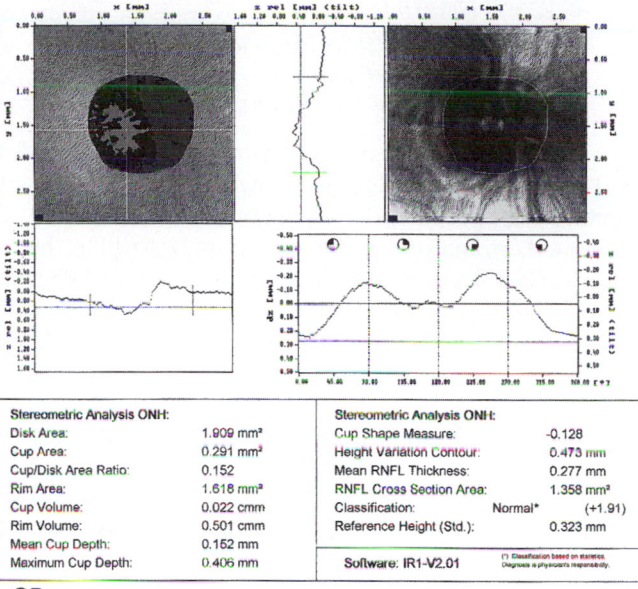

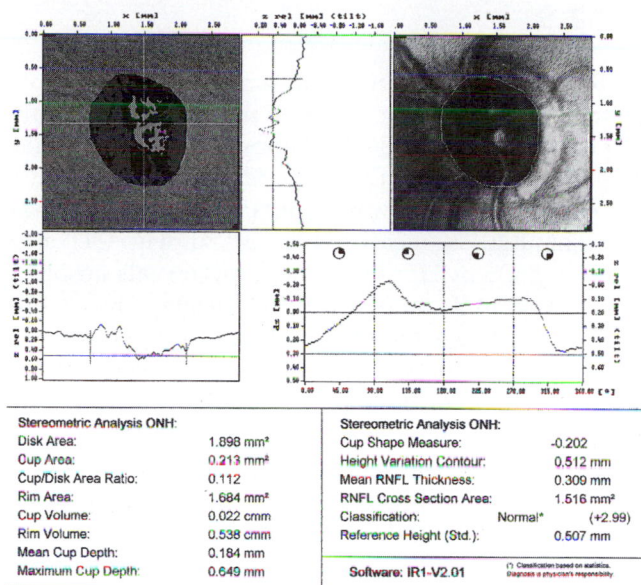

Stereometric Analysis ONH (OD):

Disk Area:	1.909 mm²	Cup Shape Measure:	-0.128
Cup Area:	0.291 mm²	Height Variation Contour:	0.473 mm
Cup/Disk Area Ratio:	0.152	Mean RNFL Thickness:	0.277 mm
Rim Area:	1.618 mm²	RNFL Cross Section Area:	1.358 mm²
Cup Volume:	0.022 cmm	Classification: Normal*	(+1.91)
Rim Volume:	0.501 cmm	Reference Height (Std.):	0.323 mm
Mean Cup Depth:	0.152 mm		
Maximum Cup Depth:	0.406 mm	Software: IR1-V2.01	

(*) Classification based on statistics. Diagnosis is physician's responsibility.

OD

Stereometric Analysis ONH (OS):

Disk Area:	1.898 mm²	Cup Shape Measure:	-0.202
Cup Area:	0.213 mm²	Height Variation Contour:	0.512 mm
Cup/Disk Area Ratio:	0.112	Mean RNFL Thickness:	0.309 mm
Rim Area:	1.684 mm²	RNFL Cross Section Area:	1.516 mm²
Cup Volume:	0.022 cmm	Classification: Normal*	(+2.99)
Rim Volume:	0.538 cmm	Reference Height (Std.):	0.507 mm
Mean Cup Depth:	0.184 mm		
Maximum Cup Depth:	0.649 mm	Software: IR1-V2.01	

(*) Classification based on statistics. Diagnosis is physician's responsibility.

OS

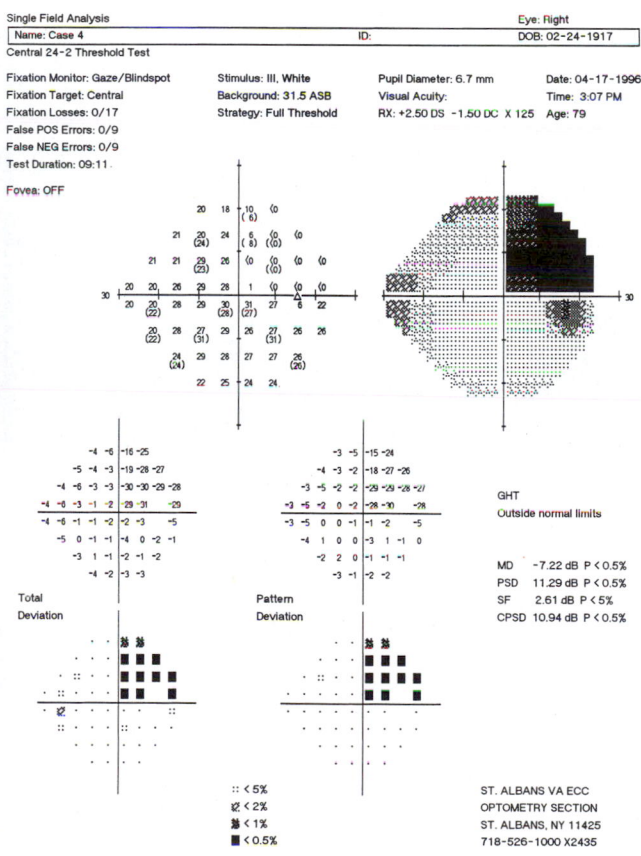

Single Field Analysis

		Eye: Right
Name: Case 4	ID:	DOB: 02-24-1917

Central 24-2 Threshold Test

Fixation Monitor: Gaze/Blindspot — Stimulus: III, White — Pupil Diameter: 6.7 mm — Date: 04-17-1996
Fixation Target: Central — Background: 31.5 ASB — Visual Acuity: — Time: 3:07 PM
Fixation Losses: 0/17 — Strategy: Full Threshold — RX: +2.50 DS -1.50 DC X 125 — Age: 79
False POS Errors: 0/9
False NEG Errors: 0/10
Test Duration: 09:11

Fovea: OFF

Total Deviation / Pattern Deviation

GHT
Outside normal limits

MD   -7.22 dB P < 0.5%
PSD 11.29 dB P < 0.5%
SF   2.61 dB P < 5%
CPSD 10.94 dB P < 0.5%

:: < 5%
▨ < 2%
▩ < 1%
■ < 0.5%

ST. ALBANS VA ECC
OPTOMETRY SECTION
ST. ALBANS, NY 11425
718-526-1000 X2435

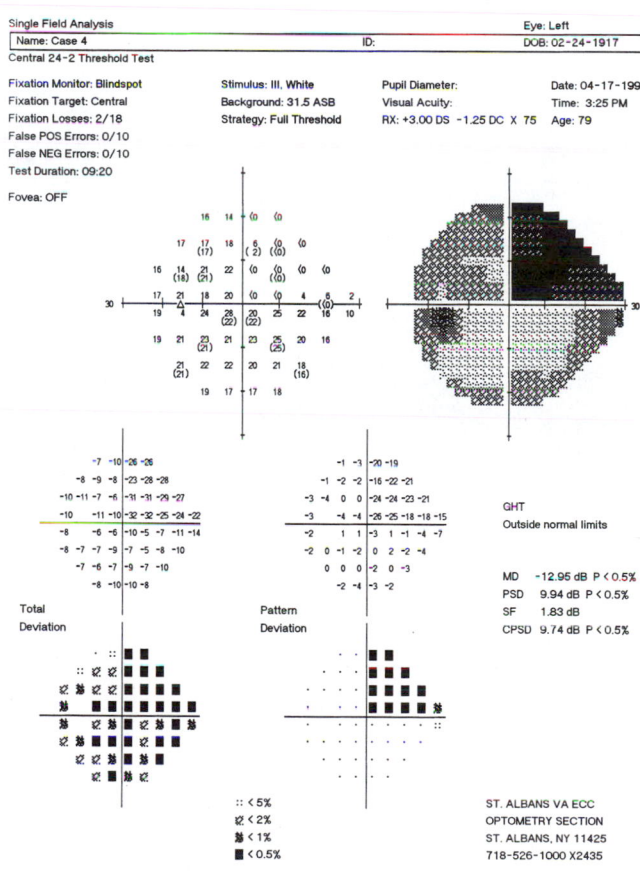

Single Field Analysis

		Eye: Left
Name: Case 4	ID:	DOB: 02-24-1917

Central 24-2 Threshold Test

Fixation Monitor: Blindspot — Stimulus: III, White — Pupil Diameter: — Date: 04-17-199
Fixation Target: Central — Background: 31.5 ASB — Visual Acuity: — Time: 3:25 PM
Fixation Losses: 2/18 — Strategy: Full Threshold — RX: +3.00 DS -1.25 DC X 75 — Age: 79
False POS Errors: 0/10
False NEG Errors: 0/10
Test Duration: 09:20

Fovea: OFF

Total Deviation / Pattern Deviation

GHT
Outside normal limits

MD   -12.95 dB P < 0.5%
PSD   9.94 dB P < 0.5%
SF   1.83 dB
CPSD 9.74 dB P < 0.5%

:: < 5%
▨ < 2%
▩ < 1%
■ < 0.5%

ST. ALBANS VA ECC
OPTOMETRY SECTION
ST. ALBANS, NY 11425
718-526-1000 X2435

CASE 5

An 80-year-old white male presents for a routine eye examination; he is being treated medically for angina and hypercholesteremia. Best corrected visual acuities on entry are 20/20 OD and 20/25 OS. The patient's last eye examination was approximately 4 years earlier. The IOP is measured at 31 mmHg OD and 28 mmHg OS at 11 A.M. Gonioscopy reveals an open but narrow angle, and visual field testing shows full fields in each eye. SWAP, performed at the second visit, is full in the OD, with some depressed points noted at the inferior-edge OS, probably due to the trial lens. The optic nerve examination reveals a small optic disc with healthy neuroretinal tissue and a small cup in each eye. FDT threshold N-30 testing shows a superior arcuate scotoma in the right eye.

- *Is this glaucoma?*
- *How would you proceed with care?*

- *Would you treat this individual?*
- *If so, with what specific medication(s)?*
- *What is the target pressure?*
- *When should this patient return?*

The patient has normal-appearing optic nerves and normal visual fields. Although his relative risk of developing progressive glaucomatous damage is increased, as his IOP is greater than 31 mmHg, he is 80 years old. I would inform him of the increased risk for developing glaucoma damage and follow him at 6-month intervals. If no change in his optic nerve or visual fields is noted, I would defer therapy. His chance of developing progressive loss that would be visually debilitating before he dies is minimal. I would, therefore, just follow him. If he has narrowing angles, I would perform gonioscopy on each visit to ensure that he is at no risk or does not develop risk of angle-closure disease.

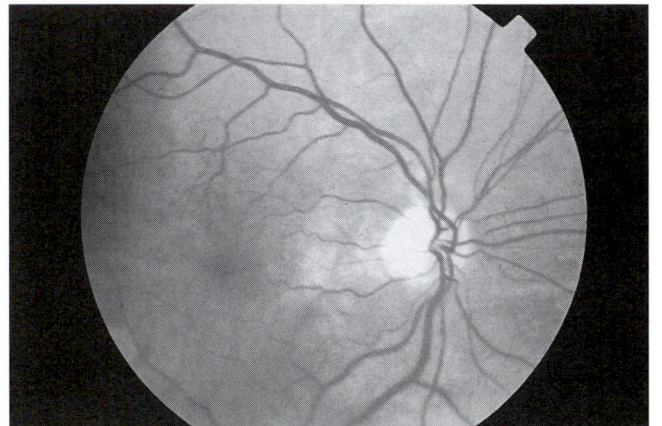

R

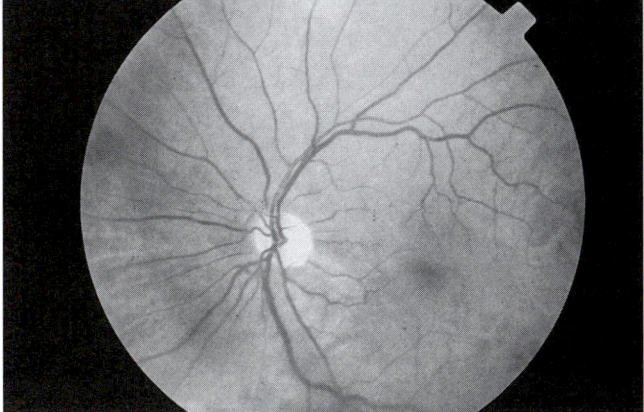

L

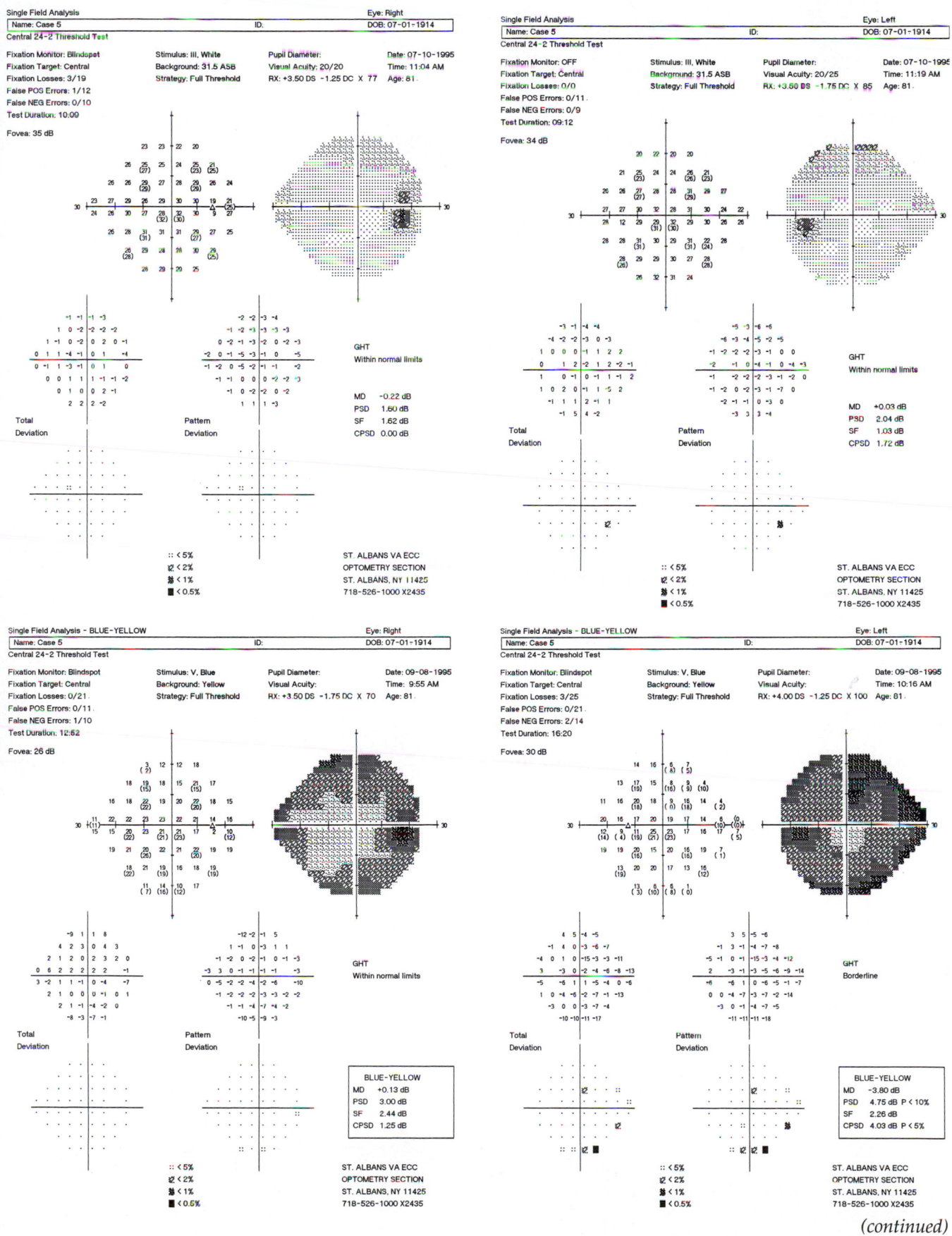

(continued)

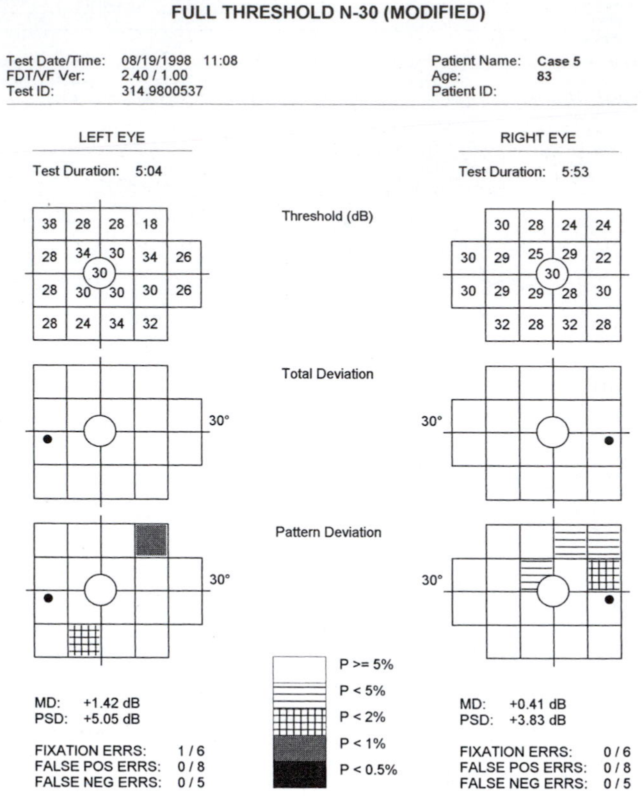

FULL THRESHOLD N-30 (MODIFIED)

Test Date/Time: 08/19/1998 11:08
FDT/VF Ver: 2.40 / 1.00
Test ID: 314.9800537

Patient Name: Case 5
Age: 83
Patient ID:

LEFT EYE

Test Duration: 5:04

38	28	28	18	
28	34	30	34	26
28	30	30	30	26
28	24	34	32	

(center: 30)

Threshold (dB)

Total Deviation

30°

Pattern Deviation

30°

MD: +1.42 dB
PSD: +5.05 dB

FIXATION ERRS: 1 / 6
FALSE POS ERRS: 0 / 8
FALSE NEG ERRS: 0 / 5

RIGHT EYE

Test Duration: 5:53

	30	28	24	24
30	29	25	29	22
30	29	29	28	30
	32	28	32	28

(center: 30)

30°

30°

MD: +0.41 dB
PSD: +3.83 dB

FIXATION ERRS: 0 / 6
FALSE POS ERRS: 0 / 8
FALSE NEG ERRS: 0 / 5

Legend:
P >= 5%
P < 5%
P < 2%
P < 1%
P < 0.5%

Case 5 (continued).

CASE 6

A 70-year-old male African American presents with a complaint of a sudden decrease in vision in the left eye. The patient is currently using a diuretic for hypertension; his last medical examination occurred approximately 9 months earlier and his last eye examination about 10 years ago. Entering visual acuity is 20/25 in the OD and counting fingers in OS. Anterior chamber angles are narrow but open in each eye. The IOP is 24 mmHg OD and 25 mmHg OS. Dilated fundus examination reveals a moderate-sized disc in the OD with a cup-to-disc ratio of 0.5×0.5 and a thin temporal neuroretinal rim. In the OS, a central retinal vein occlusion is seen, which explains the reduced visual acuity. Blood pressure was measured at 170/110. The visual field, done with a Humphrey 24−2 full-threshold program, was full in the OD.

Once the hemorrhaging and edema associated with the vein occlusion clears in the left eye, there is a need to reduce the IOP to reduce the risk of a recurrence of the vein occlusion in both eyes. How should this patient be managed?

There is definitely a risk for developing a vein occlusion when there is elevated IOP or glaucoma. Thus, for this individual, treatment for reducing the IOP would be advantageous. It should be noted that there is no evidence in the literature that lowering the IOP in somebody with a vein occlusion decreases the risks of subsequent vein occlusion in either eye. I would also send the patient to his internist for evaluation and reduction of his blood pressure, waiting to see what medications are used before starting him on IOP-lowering medication. If the internist gives him a beta blocker, I would be hesitant to use a topical beta blocker, as this could increase the risk of beta-blocker-related systemic complications.

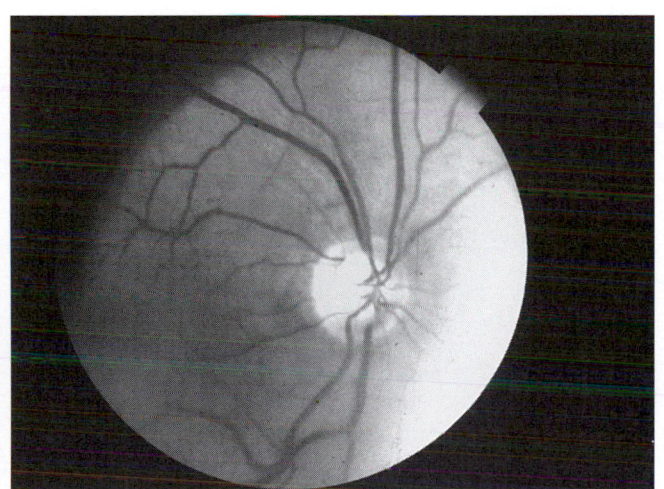

R

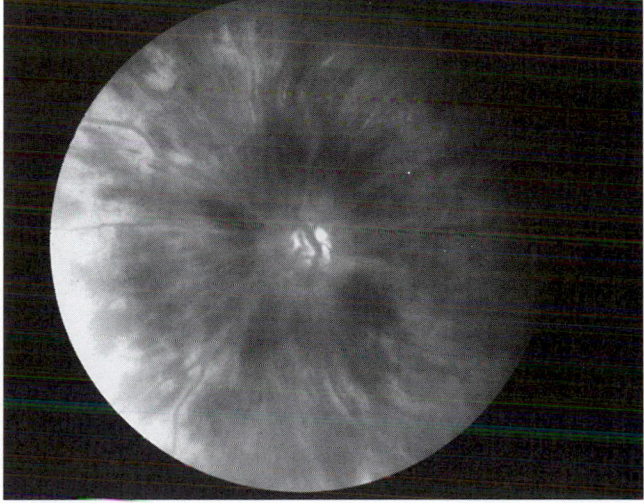

L

CASE 7

A 71-year-old white female presents for a routine examination, having not had an ocular examination for several years. The patient is experiencing blurred vision when using her reading glasses and is taking an angiotensin-converting enzyme (ACE) inhibitor for hypertension. Her ocular history is negative and visual acuity is 20/20 in each eye. The IOP, using Goldmann tonometry, is measured at 28 mmHg OD and 26 mmHg OS (1 P.M.), with gonioscopy revealing wide open angles OU. Dilated fundus and HRT examination reveals an average-sized optic disc with a moderate amount of cupping in each eye. The rim area is marginally reduced in each eye. Visual field exams, performed with 24–2 static automated perimetry, are full in each eye, with a cluster defect noted with SWAP OS. On a subsequent visit, her IOP is 24 mmHg OD and 25 mmHg OS at 8 A.M. and 24 mmHg OD, 26 mmHg OS at 4 P.M.

- *Is this glaucoma?*
- *How would you proceed with care?*

- *Would you treat this individual?*
- *If so, with what specific medication(s)?*
- *What is the target pressure?*
- *When should this patient return?*

This is an individual who has large but symmetrical cupping in both eyes but no significant loss of neuroretinal rim and normal visual fields in both eyes. SWAP visual fields are borderline in both eyes and IOPs are elevated. No afferent pupillary defect is seen, and it is difficult to know whether this is subtle glaucoma damage. However, since she is 71 years of age, I would follow rather than treat her. If she develops a change in her SWAP visual fields (which would be done on a 6-month basis) or a change in her disc appearance, then aggressive treatment would be instituted. However, at this time, because of her age, her IOP under 30 mmHg, normal visual fields, symmetrical optic nerves, and no afferent defect, I would continue to follow her closely.

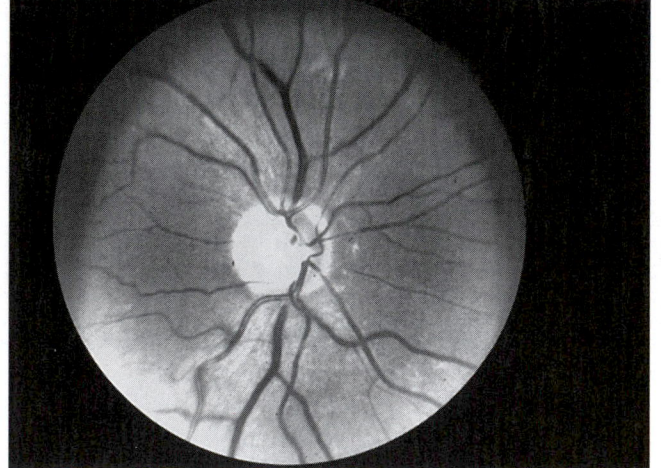

R

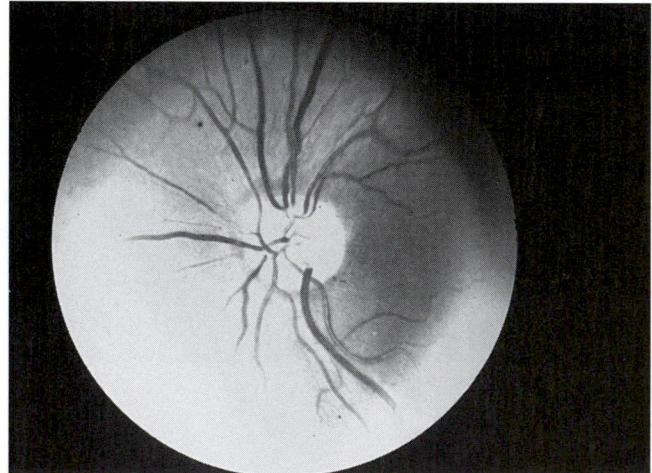

L

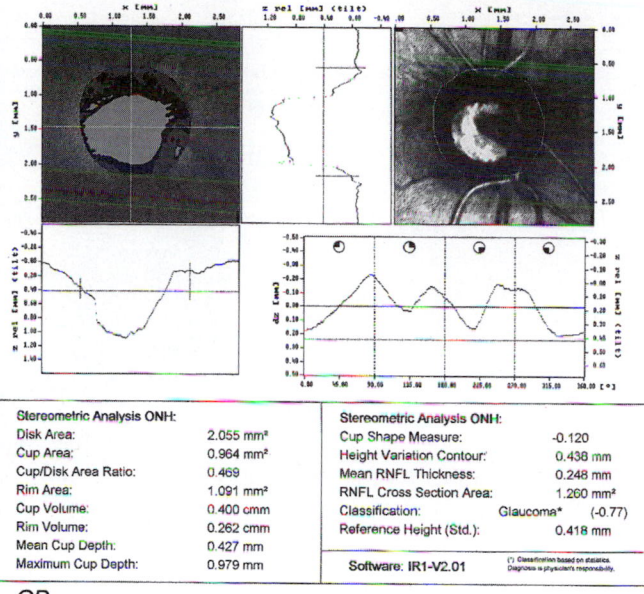

Stereometric Analysis ONH:

Disk Area:	2.055 mm²	Cup Shape Measure:	-0.120
Cup Area:	0.964 mm²	Height Variation Contour:	0.438 mm
Cup/Disk Area Ratio:	0.469	Mean RNFL Thickness:	0.248 mm
Rim Area:	1.091 mm²	RNFL Cross Section Area:	1.260 mm²
Cup Volume:	0.400 cmm	Classification:	Glaucoma* (-0.77)
Rim Volume:	0.262 cmm	Reference Height (Std.):	0.418 mm
Mean Cup Depth:	0.427 mm		
Maximum Cup Depth:	0.979 mm	Software: IR1-V2.01	(*) Classification based on statistics. Diagnosis is physician's responsibility.

OD

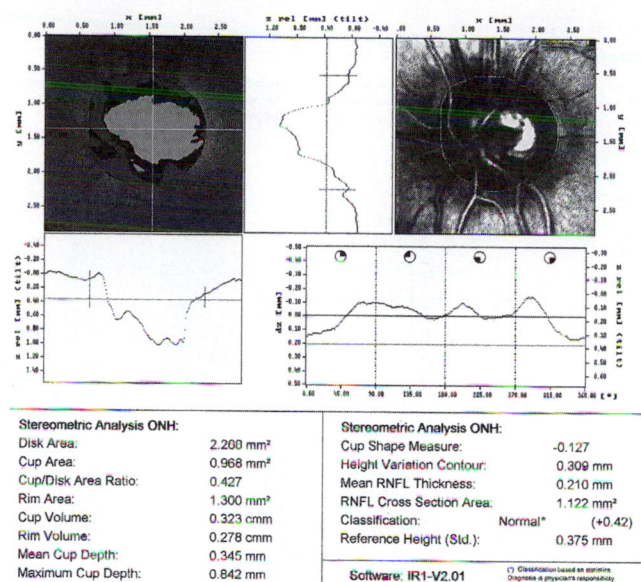

Stereometric Analysis ONH:

Disk Area:	2.268 mm²	Cup Shape Measure:	-0.127
Cup Area:	0.968 mm²	Height Variation Contour:	0.309 mm
Cup/Disk Area Ratio:	0.427	Mean RNFL Thickness:	0.210 mm
Rim Area:	1.300 mm²	RNFL Cross Section Area:	1.122 mm²
Cup Volume:	0.323 cmm	Classification:	Normal* (+0.42)
Rim Volume:	0.278 cmm	Reference Height (Std.):	0.375 mm
Mean Cup Depth:	0.345 mm		
Maximum Cup Depth:	0.842 mm	Software: IR1-V2.01	(*) Classification based on statistics. Diagnosis is physician's responsibility.

OS

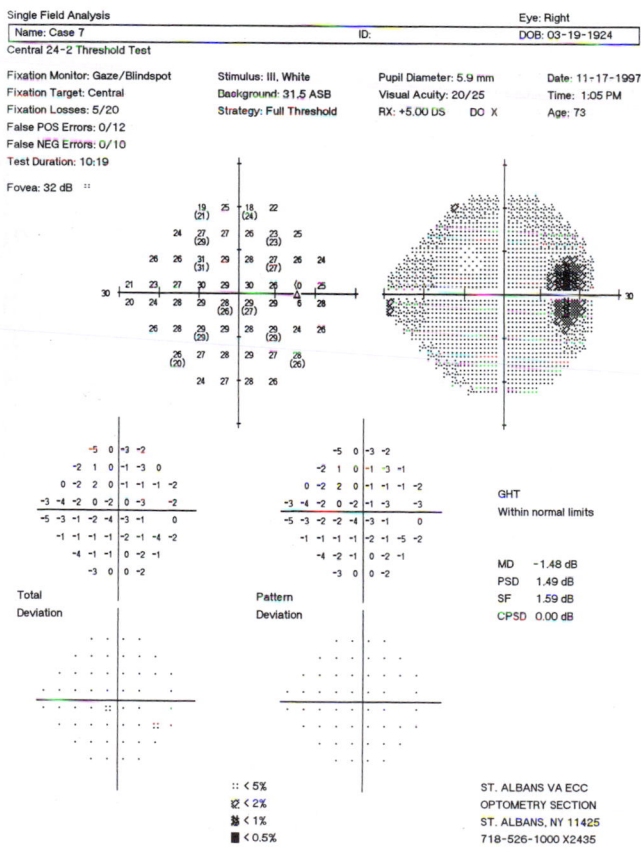

Single Field Analysis   Eye: Right

Name: Case 7	ID:	DOB: 03-19-1924

Central 24-2 Threshold Test

Fixation Monitor: Gaze/Blindspot	Stimulus: III, White	Pupil Diameter: 5.9 mm	Date: 11-17-1997
Fixation Target: Central	Background: 31.5 ASB	Visual Acuity: 20/25	Time: 1:05 PM
Fixation Losses: 5/20	Strategy: Full Threshold	RX: +5.00 DS DC X	Age: 73

False POS Errors: 0/12
False NEG Errors: 0/10
Test Duration: 10:19

Fovea: 32 dB

GHT
Within normal limits

MD   -1.48 dB
PSD   1.49 dB
SF   1.59 dB
CPSD 0.00 dB

Total Deviation

Pattern Deviation

:: < 5%
▨ < 2%
▩ < 1%
■ < 0.5%

ST. ALBANS VA ECC
OPTOMETRY SECTION
ST. ALBANS, NY 11425
718-526-1000 X2435

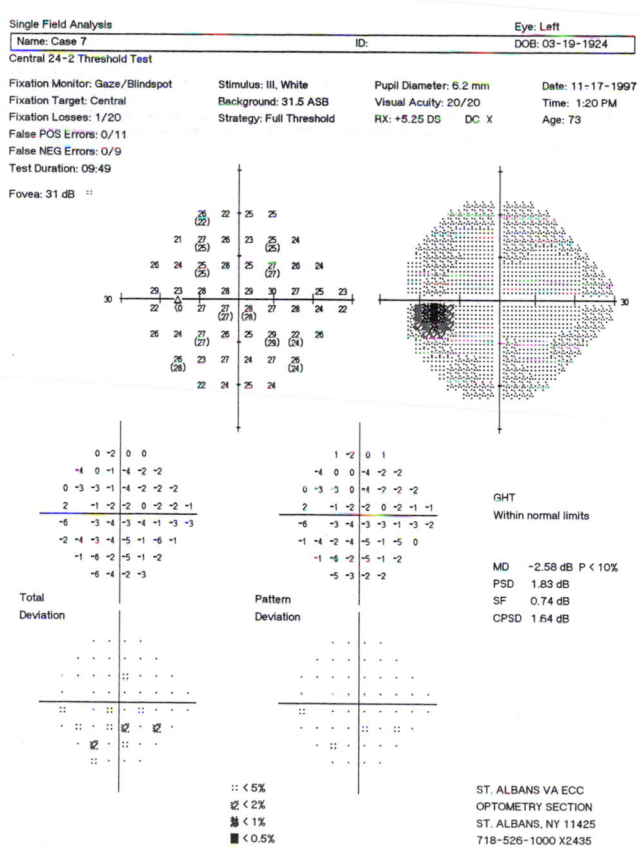

Single Field Analysis   Eye: Left

Name: Case 7	ID:	DOB: 03-19-1924

Central 24-2 Threshold Test

Fixation Monitor: Gaze/Blindspot	Stimulus: III, White	Pupil Diameter: 6.2 mm	Date: 11-17-1997
Fixation Target: Central	Background: 31.5 ASB	Visual Acuity: 20/20	Time: 1:20 PM
Fixation Losses: 1/20	Strategy: Full Threshold	RX: +5.25 DS DC X	Age: 73

False POS Errors: 0/11
False NEG Errors: 0/9
Test Duration: 09:49

Fovea: 31 dB

GHT
Within normal limits

MD   -2.58 dB P < 10%
PSD   1.83 dB
SF   0.74 dB
CPSD 1.64 dB

Total Deviation

Pattern Deviation

:: < 5%
▨ < 2%
▩ < 1%
■ < 0.5%

ST. ALBANS VA ECC
OPTOMETRY SECTION
ST. ALBANS, NY 11425
718-526-1000 X2435

(continued)

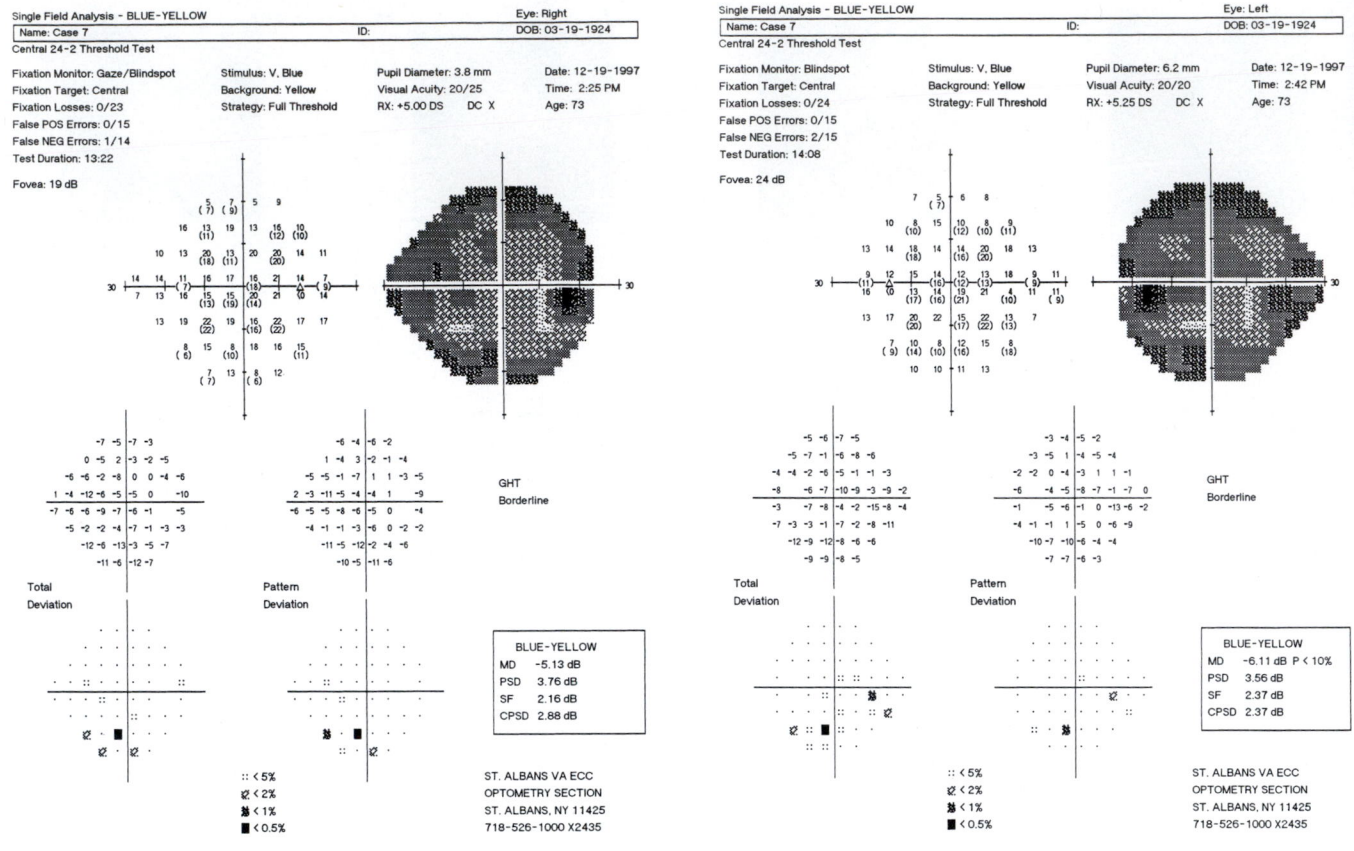

Case 7 (continued).

CASE 8

A 59-year-old African-American male complains that his right eye has been itchy and red for a month. The patient has not had an eye examination for several years and gives a history of reduced vision OD since childhood due to trauma. In addition, the history reveals that the patient's mother had glaucoma and required filtering surgery. The patient has diet-controlled diabetes as well as gout. At this visit, the patient was diagnosed as having allergic conjunctivitis, which cleared with therapy. His visual acuity is 20/400 OD and 20/20 OS. The patient was instructed to return for a comprehensive evaluation once the conjunctivitis had cleared. At the follow-up examination, a macular scar was noted in the right eye secondary to past trauma. The optic nerve evaluation revealed shallow cupping, somewhat larger in the OS, along with tortuosity of the retinal vessels. The IOP was 25 mmHg OD and 26 mmHg OS at 10 A.M. and gonioscopy revealed wide open angles OU. The 24–2 full-threshold visual field in the OD showed localized reduction centrally due to the macular scar. The OS visual field is full. FDT threshold fields were full OD with central loss OS.

- *Is this glaucoma?*
- *How would you proceed with care?*
- *Would you treat this individual?*
- *If so, with what specific medication(s)?*

- *What is the target pressure?*
- *When should this patient return?*
- *Any concerns, in either the short or the long term?*

This is a monocular patient who has a macular scar in his right eye, probably from either trauma or histoplasmosis, and elevated IOP. His angle is normal and there are no signs of neovascularization. The visual field in his left eye appears normal at this time. Because of this, I would suggest obtaining a SWAP visual field exam because with one eye this becomes much more important. The risk of glaucoma in this patient with a positive family history and an elevated IOP is increased. However, there is no evidence that treating the patient first, by lowering his IOP, would prevent his chances of developing glaucomatous damage. The discs seem symmetrical except for what appears to be temporal atrophy in the right eye, which is commensurate with the patient's macular scar. I would follow him carefully, perhaps at 6-month intervals, with visual field exams, including SWAP perimetry in the OS. I would also follow the disc in his right eye, though it is probably not worthwhile to follow the visual field in the right eye because of poor fixation. I would not treat this patient unless there was some sign of change. I would stress the need for compliance and also make sure that his other family members were examined because of the family history of glaucoma.

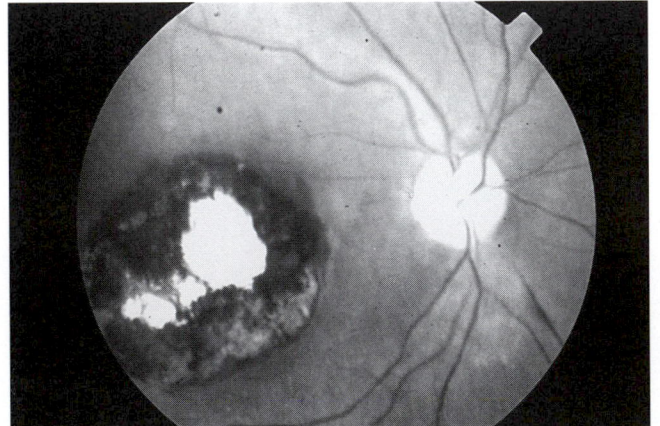

R

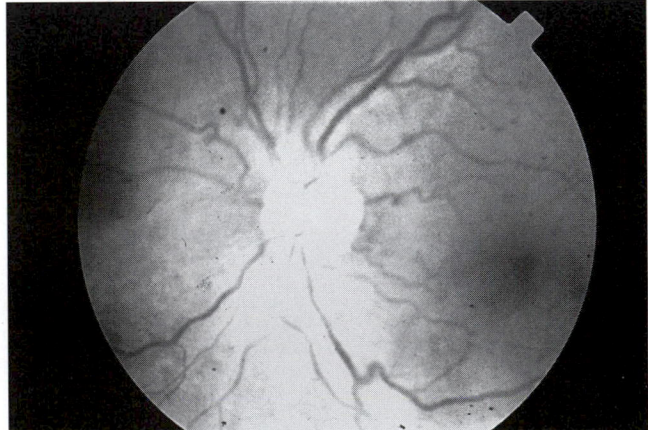

L

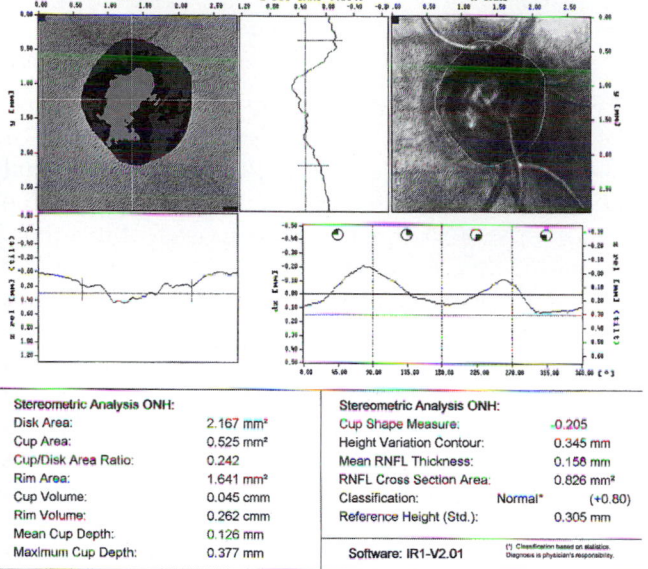

Stereometric Analysis ONH:

Disk Area:	2.167 mm²
Cup Area:	0.525 mm²
Cup/Disk Area Ratio:	0.242
Rim Area:	1.641 mm²
Cup Volume:	0.045 cmm
Rim Volume:	0.262 cmm
Mean Cup Depth:	0.126 mm
Maximum Cup Depth:	0.377 mm

Stereometric Analysis ONH:

Cup Shape Measure:	-0.205
Height Variation Contour:	0.345 mm
Mean RNFL Thickness:	0.158 mm
RNFL Cross Section Area:	0.826 mm²
Classification:	Normal* (+0.80)
Reference Height (Std.):	0.305 mm

(*) Classification based on statistics.
Diagnosis is physician's responsibility.

Software: IR1-V2.01

OD

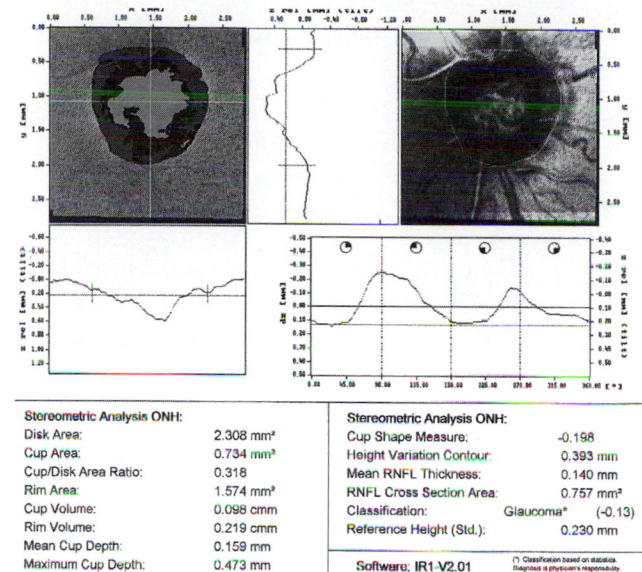

Stereometric Analysis ONH:

Disk Area:	2.308 mm²
Cup Area:	0.734 mm²
Cup/Disk Area Ratio:	0.318
Rim Area:	1.574 mm²
Cup Volume:	0.098 cmm
Rim Volume:	0.219 cmm
Mean Cup Depth:	0.159 mm
Maximum Cup Depth:	0.473 mm

Stereometric Analysis ONH:

Cup Shape Measure:	-0.198
Height Variation Contour:	0.393 mm
Mean RNFL Thickness:	0.140 mm
RNFL Cross Section Area:	0.757 mm²
Classification:	Glaucoma* (-0.13)
Reference Height (Std.):	0.230 mm

(*) Classification based on statistics.
Diagnosis is physician's responsibility.

Software: IR1-V2.01

OS

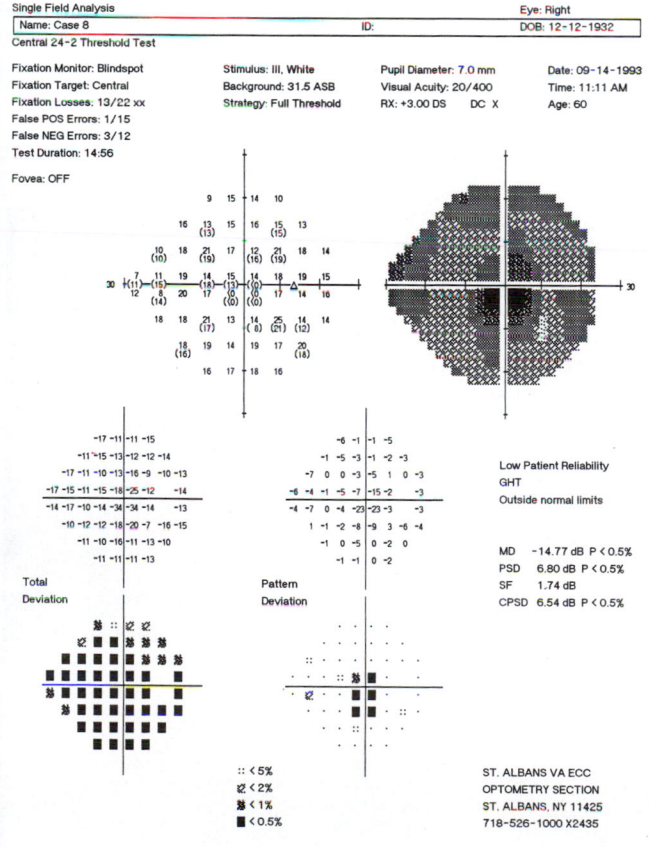

Single Field Analysis

Name: Case 8　ID:　　Eye: Right　DOB: 12-12-1932

Central 24-2 Threshold Test

Fixation Monitor: Blindspot　　Stimulus: III, White　　Pupil Diameter: 7.0 mm　　Date: 09-14-1993
Fixation Target: Central　　Background: 31.5 ASB　　Visual Acuity: 20/400　　Time: 11:11 AM
Fixation Losses: 13/22 xx　　Strategy: Full Threshold　　RX: +3.00 DS　DC X　　Age: 60
False POS Errors: 1/15
False NEG Errors: 3/12
Test Duration: 14:56

Fovea: OFF

Low Patient Reliability
GHT
Outside normal limits

MD -14.77 dB P < 0.5%
PSD 6.80 dB P < 0.5%
SF 1.74 dB
CPSD 6.54 dB P < 0.5%

Total Deviation

Pattern Deviation

:: < 5%
▨ < 2%
▩ < 1%
■ < 0.5%

ST. ALBANS VA ECC
OPTOMETRY SECTION
ST. ALBANS, NY 11425
718-526-1000 X2435

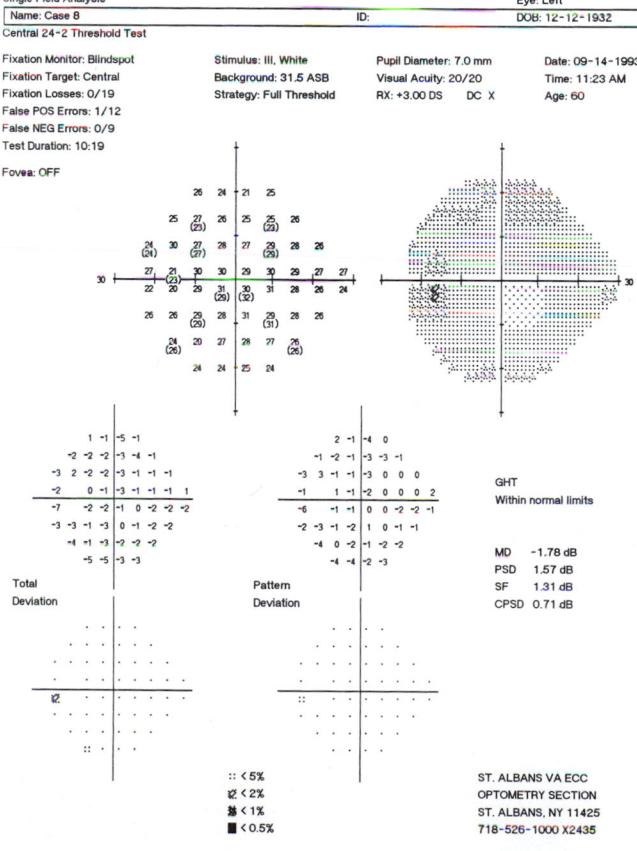

Single Field Analysis

Name: Case 8　ID:　　Eye: Left　DOB: 12-12-1932

Central 24-2 Threshold Test

Fixation Monitor: Blindspot　　Stimulus: III, White　　Pupil Diameter: 7.0 mm　　Date: 09-14-1993
Fixation Target: Central　　Background: 31.5 ASB　　Visual Acuity: 20/20　　Time: 11:23 AM
Fixation Losses: 0/19　　Strategy: Full Threshold　　RX: +3.00 DS　DC X　　Age: 60
False POS Errors: 1/12
False NEG Errors: 0/9
Test Duration: 10:19

Fovea: OFF

GHT
Within normal limits

MD -1.78 dB
PSD 1.57 dB
SF 1.31 dB
CPSD 0.71 dB

Total Deviation

Pattern Deviation

:: < 5%
▨ < 2%
▩ < 1%
■ < 0.5%

ST. ALBANS VA ECC
OPTOMETRY SECTION
ST. ALBANS, NY 11425
718-526-1000 X2435

(continued)

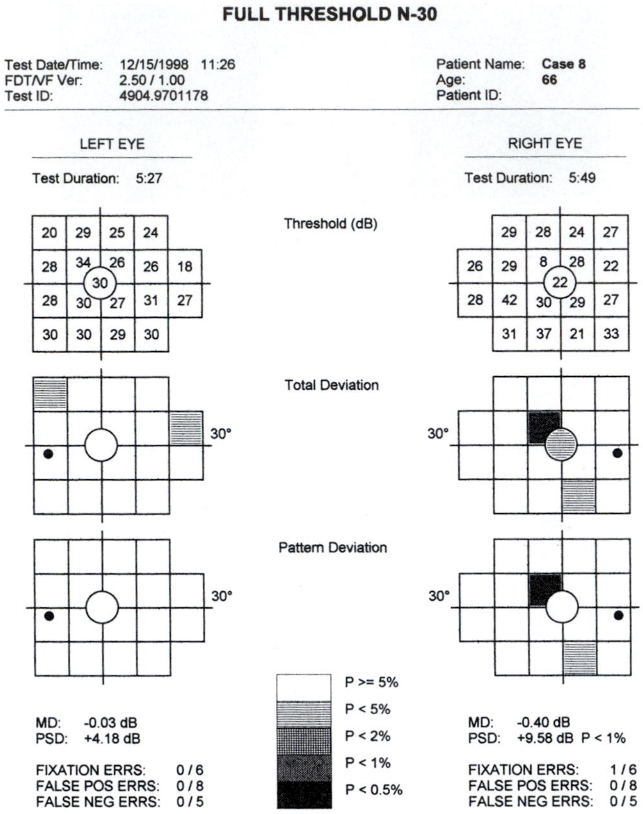

FULL THRESHOLD N-30

Test Date/Time: 12/15/1998 11:26
FDT/VF Ver: 2.50 / 1.00
Test ID: 4904.9701178

Patient Name: **Case 8**
Age: **66**
Patient ID:

LEFT EYE	RIGHT EYE
Test Duration: 5:27	Test Duration: 5:49

Threshold (dB)

LEFT EYE threshold:

20	29	25	24	
28	34	26	26	18
28	30	27	31	27
30	30	29	30	

(30)

RIGHT EYE threshold:

	29	28	24	27
26	29	8	28	22
28	42	30	29	27
	31	37	21	33

(22)

Total Deviation

30°

Pattern Deviation

30°

P >= 5%
P < 5%
P < 2%
P < 1%
P < 0.5%

LEFT EYE:
MD: -0.03 dB
PSD: +4.18 dB

FIXATION ERRS: 0 / 6
FALSE POS ERRS: 0 / 8
FALSE NEG ERRS: 0 / 5

RIGHT EYE:
MD: -0.40 dB
PSD: +9.58 dB P < 1%

FIXATION ERRS: 1 / 6
FALSE POS ERRS: 0 / 8
FALSE NEG ERRS: 0 / 5

Case 8 (continued).

CASE 9

A 63-year-old white male presents for a routine examination. The medical and ocular history is negative and visual acuity is 20/20 in each eye. The IOP is 23 mmHg OD and 21 mmHg OS at 11 A.M.; and gonioscopy reveals a narrow but open angle. Dilated fundus and HRT examination reveals a larger than average-sized disc and increased cupping. The cup-to-disc ratio is 0.6 × 0.6 OD, with thinning of the neuroretinal rim tissue OD. The OS nerve reveals a cup-to-disc ratio of 0.7 × 0.9 with notching to the inferior rim. The right 24–2 visual field exam reveals several nasal points scattered throughout the field to be reduced, while the SWAP field is full. The OS field shows a dense superior arcuate scotoma with fixation involved. The HRT images confirm the inferior loss of rim OS with generalized rim thinning OD.

- *How would you proceed?*
- *Would you want to get another IOP reading before therapy is initiated?*
- *Would you treat this individual?*
- *Would you treat each eye?*
- *If so, with what specific medication(s)?*

- *What is the target pressure?*
- *Would you treat the two eyes differently?*
- *When should this patient return?*
- *When would you repeat the visual field examinations?*

This patient definitely has glaucoma, and since he is young, there is a good chance that he may lose vision within his lifetime. Because of the family history and suspicious-looking angles, I would suggest repeating his gonioscopy. It would also be nice to have another measurement of IOP at another time so as to get a good baseline. It would be helpful to repeat the SWAP exam in his right eye as well as obtaining a central C-10 visual field exam OS. In regard to therapy, I would attempt to lower the IOP by 30% using a one-eyed therapeutic trial and a cardioselective beta blocker, betaxolol. Betaxolol would be my first choice because of its safety profile and relative calcium channel blocking effect.[10–13] I would treat both eyes the same, because "as goes one eye," so will go the other eye. I would see the patient in a month after starting betaxolol, following him closely.

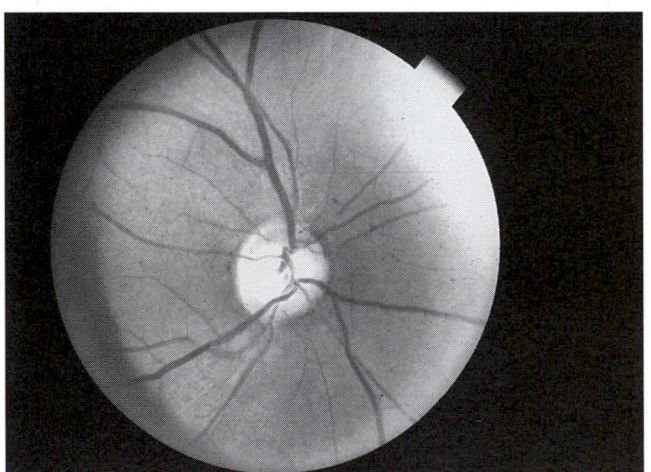

R

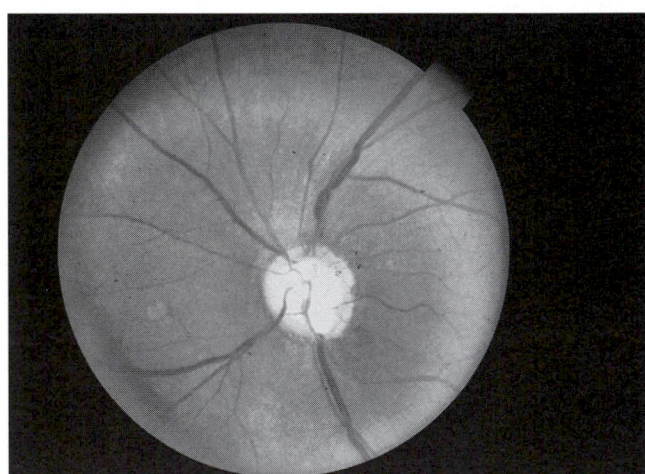

L

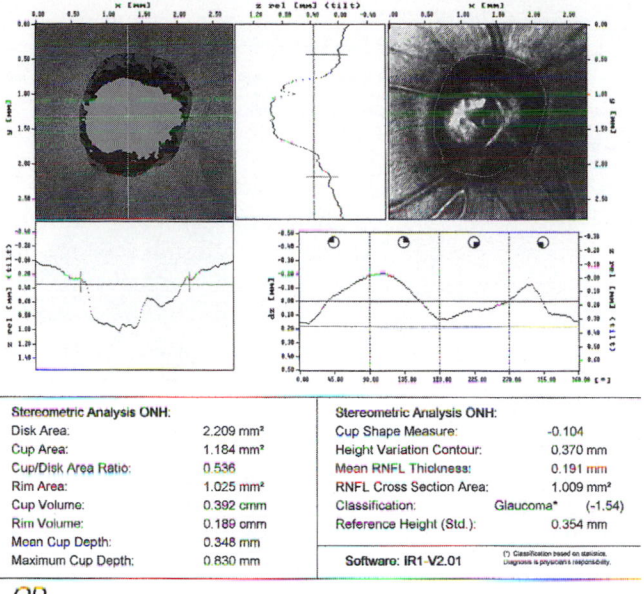

Stereometric Analysis ONH:

Disk Area:	2.209 mm²	Cup Shape Measure:	-0.104
Cup Area:	1.184 mm²	Height Variation Contour:	0.370 mm
Cup/Disk Area Ratio:	0.536	Mean RNFL Thickness:	0.191 mm
Rim Area:	1.025 mm²	RNFL Cross Section Area:	1.009 mm²
Cup Volume:	0.392 cmm	Classification:	Glaucoma* (-1.54)
Rim Volume:	0.189 cmm	Reference Height (Std.):	0.354 mm
Mean Cup Depth:	0.348 mm		
Maximum Cup Depth:	0.830 mm	Software: IR1-V2.01	(*) Classification based on statistics. Diagnosis is physician's responsibility.

OD

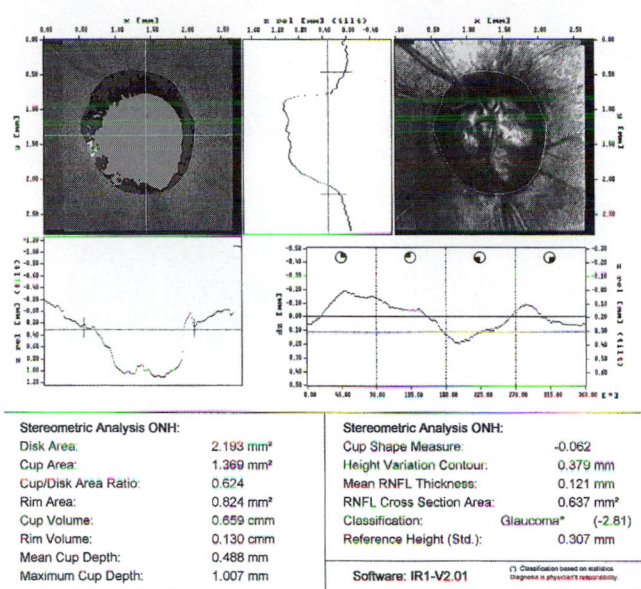

Stereometric Analysis ONH:

Disk Area:	2.193 mm²	Cup Shape Measure:	-0.062
Cup Area:	1.369 mm²	Height Variation Contour:	0.379 mm
Cup/Disk Area Ratio:	0.624	Mean RNFL Thickness:	0.121 mm
Rim Area:	0.824 mm²	RNFL Cross Section Area:	0.637 mm²
Cup Volume:	0.659 cmm	Classification:	Glaucoma* (-2.81)
Rim Volume:	0.130 cmm	Reference Height (Std.):	0.307 mm
Mean Cup Depth:	0.488 mm		
Maximum Cup Depth:	1.007 mm	Software: IR1-V2.01	(*) Classification based on statistics. Diagnosis is physician's responsibility.

OS

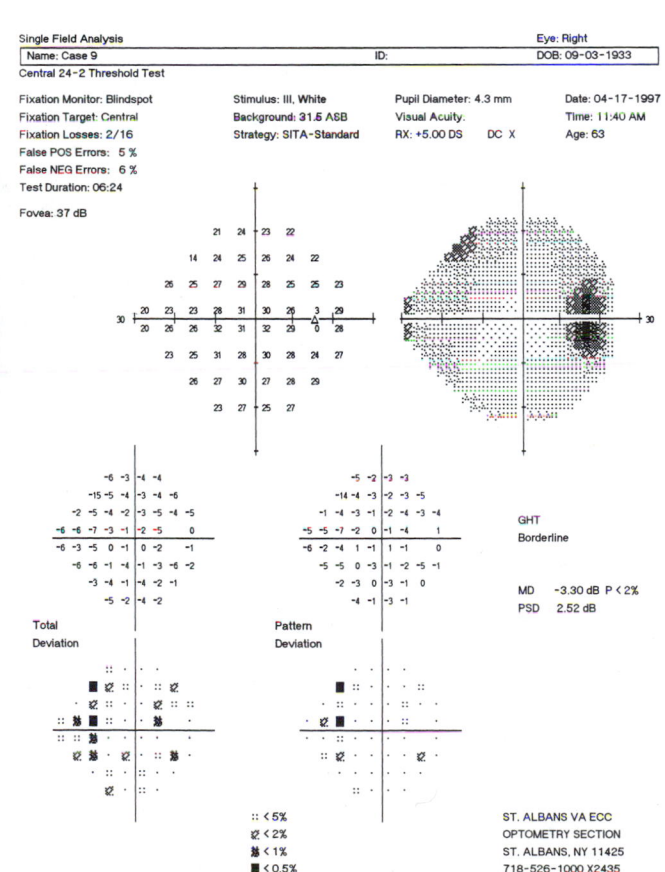

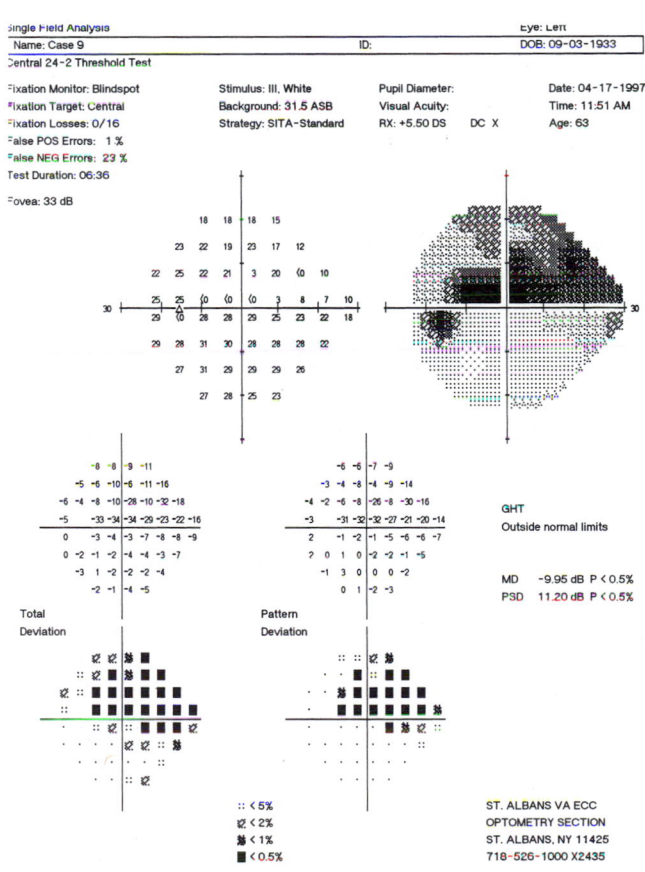

(continued)

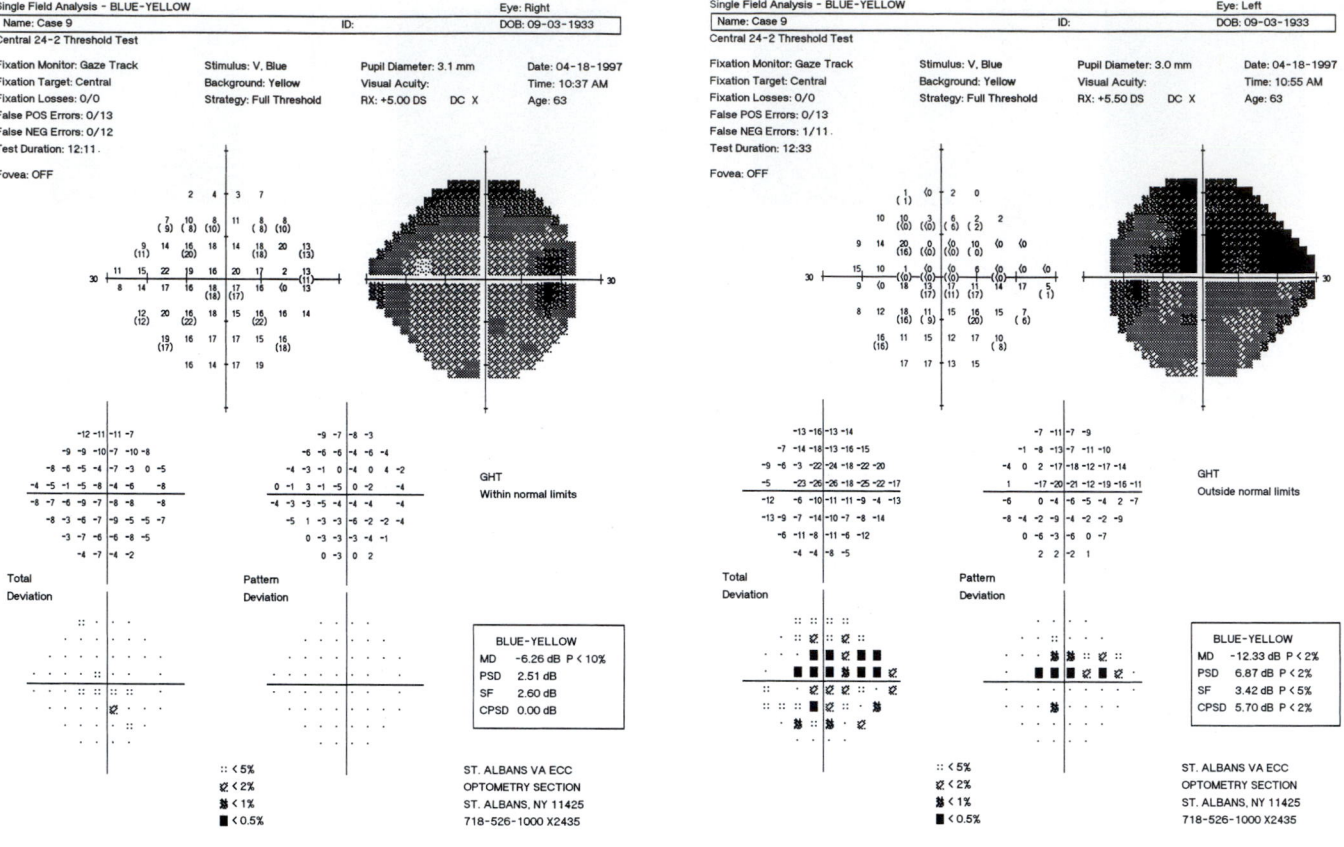

Case 9 (continued).

CASE 10

A 49-year-old African-American male presents with a complaint of blurred vision in his left eye for the preceding 2 months. He has a family history of glaucoma; his brother was diagnosed 3 years ago with an advanced case of open-angle glaucoma OU that required filtering surgery. The patient's medical history is pertinent for childhood asthma. Visual acuity is 20/20 OD and 20/30 OS, with an afferent pupil defect OS. Gonioscopy reveals wide open angles OU with ciliary body present in all quadrants. The IOP was measured at 41 mmHg OD and 57 mmHg OS at 10 A.M. The optic nerves were significantly cupped: 0.7 × 0.7 OD with thinning of the neuroretinal rim and 0.9 + 0.9 + OS with little neuroretinal rim remaining. The visual field shows damage in both hemifields OD and only a small central island of field remaining in OS. The OS field, as performed with a 10-2 size V, shows only the remaining central vision.

- *How would you proceed with care?*
- *Is surgery required immediately?*
- *How would you proceed until surgery can be scheduled?*
- *What is the target pressure?*
- *When should this patient return?*

I would examine this patient's other family members—siblings and children—because of the family history of glaucoma and his definite glaucoma. His IOPs are markedly elevated and there is a need to get them below 21 mmHg in both eyes. His left eye is almost totally cupped, with visual fields commensurate with that. He has a dense inferior arcuate defect and some superior damage in his right eye and marked damage in his left eye, with an abnormal C-10-2. I would repeat the visual field exams in both eyes with concern about his significant damage, as he is quite young. Because of his family history of asthma, I would *not* use a nonselective or selective beta blocker, starting instead with latanoprost. I would be very aggressive, and if this were not adequate, I would probably go on to argon laser trabeculoplasty. The Advanced Glaucoma Intervention Study (AGIS) revealed that a sequence of ALT followed by trabeculectomy appears to be the best course of treatment for African Americans. I would also warn the patient about the risks of blindness and loss of vision, since he is an African American and has advanced glaucoma, based again on the AGIS study. This patient must be followed very carefully. I would not proceed to "immediate" surgery, as I am sure that his elevated IOP and damage have been there for quite a while.

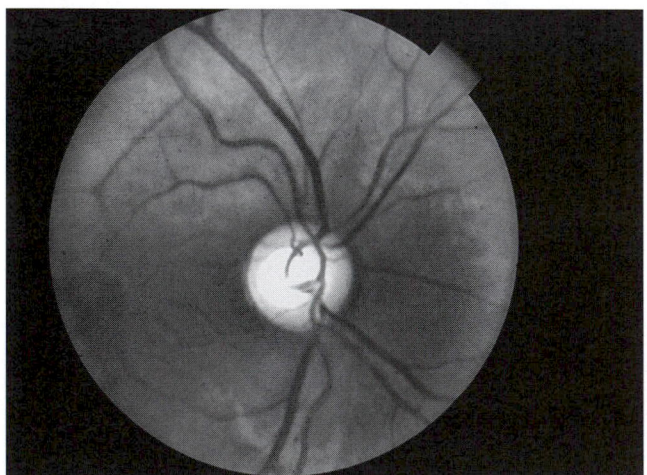

R

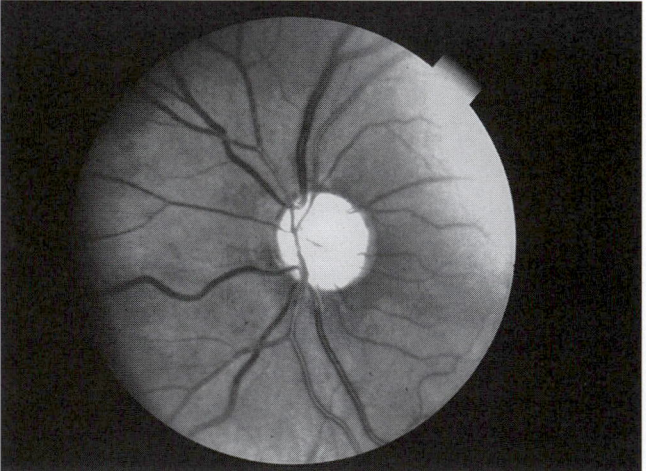

L

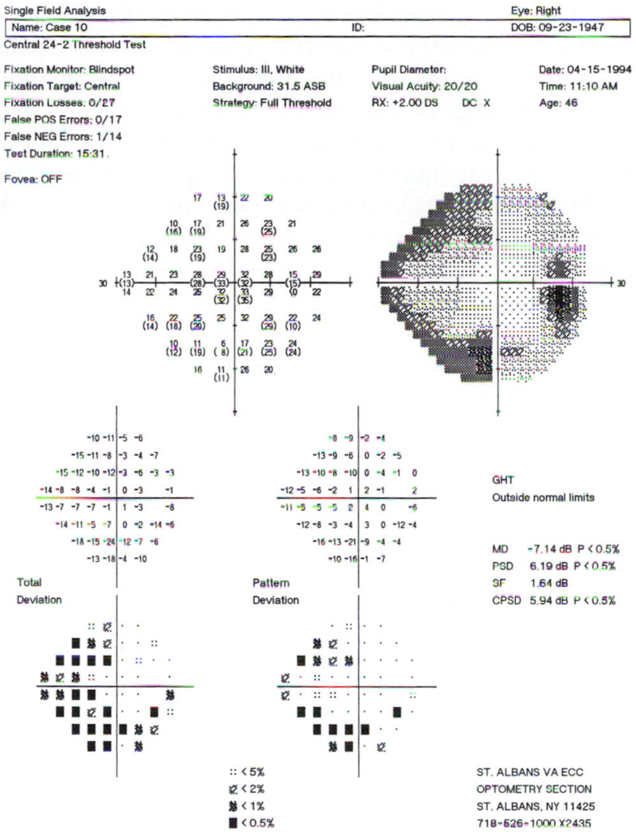

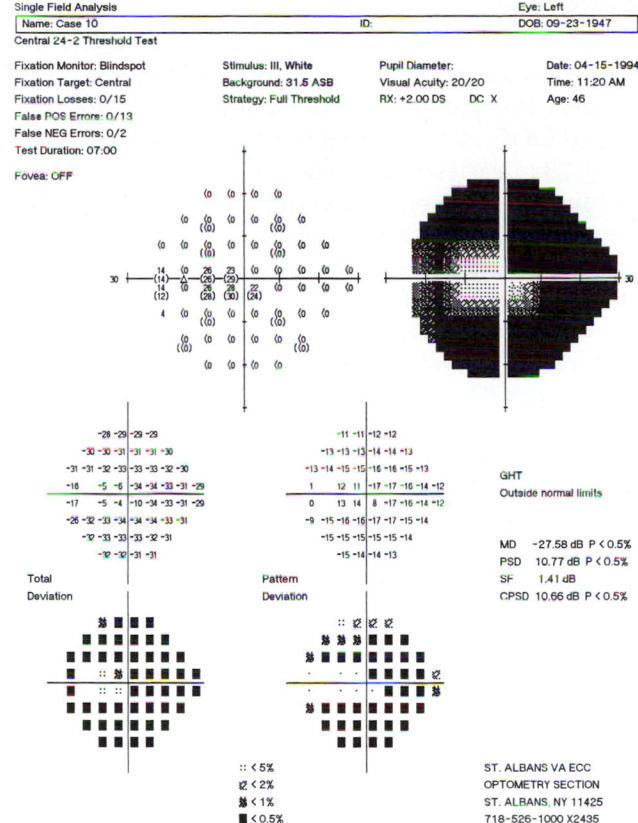

Single Field Analysis — Eye: Right

| Name: Case 10 | ID: | DOB: 09-23-1947 |

Central 24-2 Threshold Test

Fixation Monitor: Blindspot
Fixation Target: Central
Fixation Losses: 0/27
False POS Errors: 0/17
False NEG Errors: 1/14
Test Duration: 15:31

Fovea: OFF

Stimulus: III, White
Background: 31.5 ASB
Strategy: Full Threshold

Pupil Diameter:
Visual Acuity: 20/20
RX: +2.00 DS   DC X

Date: 04-15-1994
Time: 11:10 AM
Age: 46

GHT
Outside normal limits

MD   -7.14 dB P < 0.5%
PSD   6.19 dB P < 0.5%
SF   1.64 dB
CPSD   5.94 dB P < 0.5%

Total Deviation

Pattern Deviation

:: < 5%
⬚ < 2%
▨ < 1%
■ < 0.5%

ST. ALBANS VA ECC
OPTOMETRY SECTION
ST. ALBANS, NY 11425
718-526-1000 X2435

Single Field Analysis — Eye: Left

| Name: Case 10 | ID: | DOB: 09-23-1947 |

Central 24-2 Threshold Test

Fixation Monitor: Blindspot
Fixation Target: Central
Fixation Losses: 0/15
False POS Errors: 0/13
False NEG Errors: 0/2
Test Duration: 07:00

Fovea: OFF

Stimulus: III, White
Background: 31.5 ASB
Strategy: Full Threshold

Pupil Diameter:
Visual Acuity: 20/20
RX: +2.00 DS   DC X

Date: 04-15-1994
Time: 11:20 AM
Age: 46

GHT
Outside normal limits

MD   -27.58 dB P < 0.5%
PSD   10.77 dB P < 0.5%
SF   1.41 dB
CPSD 10.66 dB P < 0.5%

Total Deviation

Pattern Deviation

:: < 5%
⬚ < 2%
▨ < 1%
■ < 0.5%

ST. ALBANS VA ECC
OPTOMETRY SECTION
ST. ALBANS, NY 11425
718-526-1000 X2435

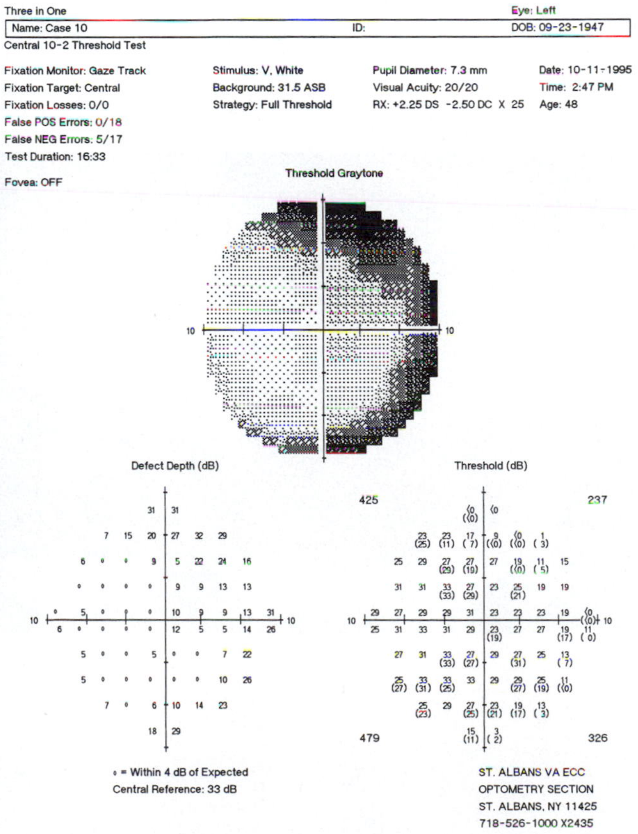

Three in One — Eye: Left

| Name: Case 10 | ID: | DOB: 09-23-1947 |

Central 10-2 Threshold Test

Fixation Monitor: Gaze Track
Fixation Target: Central
Fixation Losses: 0/0
False POS Errors: 0/18
False NEG Errors: 5/17
Test Duration: 16:33

Fovea: OFF

Stimulus: V, White
Background: 31.5 ASB
Strategy: Full Threshold

Pupil Diameter: 7.3 mm
Visual Acuity: 20/20
RX: +2.25 DS -2.50 DC X 25

Date: 10-11-1995
Time: 2:47 PM
Age: 48

Threshold Graytone

Defect Depth (dB)

Threshold (dB)

∘ = Within 4 dB of Expected
Central Reference: 33 dB

ST. ALBANS VA ECC
OPTOMETRY SECTION
ST. ALBANS, NY 11425
718-526-1000 X2435

CASE 11

A 31-year-old white male presents for a routine exam-ination. The patient is moderately myopic (-5.00D sphere OD, $-4.25-0.75\times170$ OS) with visual acuity of 20/20 in each eye. The patient is in excellent health and has no pertinent individual or family ocular his-tory. Slit-lamp examination revealed Krukenberg spindles in each eye as well as numerous iris trans-illumination defects. IOP was measured to be 31 mmHg OD and 28 mmHg OS at 10 A.M. Postdilated IOP readings, taken 1 hour after dilation, were 39 mmHg OD and 33 mmHg OS, with a shower of pigment observed in the anterior chamber. Go-nioscopy revealed a wide open angle, with the iris bowing backward and a dense band of pigment within the trabecular meshwork OU. The optic nerves were small, with a cup-to-disk ratio of 0.1×0.1 in each eye. The neuroretinal rim tissue was healthy. The 24-2 threshold visual fields were full.

- *Is this glaucoma?*
- *How would you proceed with care?*
- *Is an iridotomy indicated?*
- *Would you treat this individual medically?*
- *If so, with what specific medication(s)?*
- *What is the target pressure?*
- *When should this patient return?*
- *Any concerns, in either the short or the long term?*

This is a patient with pigmentary glaucoma, since he has pigmentary dispersion syndrome with IOPs over 31 mmHg. The fact that his IOP goes up with dilation does not matter. I am concerned with pressures that high, since he has a much greater risk of developing glaucoma. A couple of therapeutic questions remain. SWAP visual field exams would be in order, along with stereo disc photography. I would also tell the patient that laser refractive surgery is not a good idea for him because it may alter his baseline IOPs.

The main question is whether or not this patient should be started therapeutically with an iridotomy. Whether iridotomies have much of an effect in indi-viduals with elevated IOPs is questionable to begin with, but it may be worth a trial. There is strong feel-ing that using a miotic, such as pilocarpine, either as an Ocusert or as a drop might be a good first-line therapy to reduce the pigment liberation. However most young individuals cannot tolerate miosis, and the pupillary constriction and risk for permanent synechiae developing may weigh against their use.

In summary, the treatment course would include an iridotomy in one eye. I would also utilize a cardio-selective beta blocker in a uniocular therapeutic trial, attempting to get a 30% decrease in intraocular pres-sure. The patient, having blue eyes, would be warned of a potential color change if latanoprost is utilized. SWAP visual fields in addition to standard perimetry would be used to follow this patient.

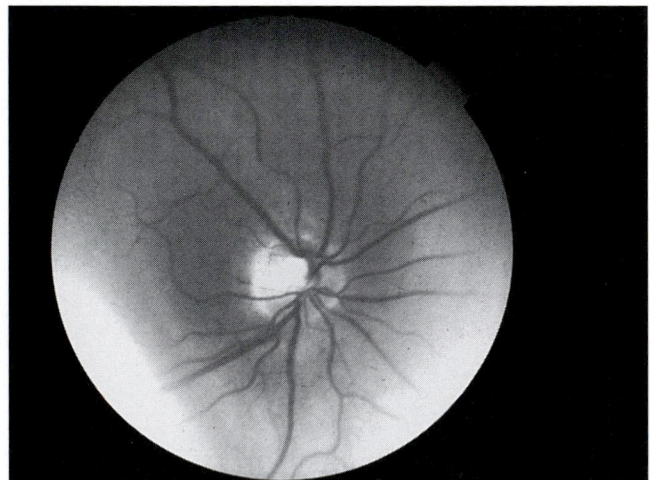

R

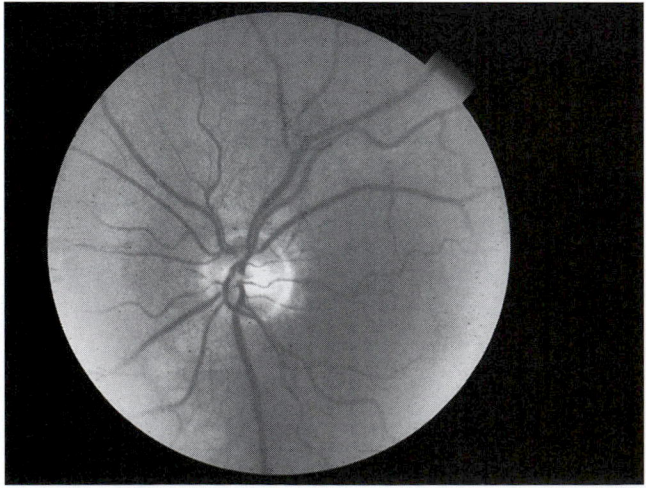

L

CASE 12

A 67-year-old Hispanic female presents with a complaint of reduced vision in the OS. The patient has no pertinent medical history and visual acuity is 20/20 OD and 20/25 OS, with an afferent pupil defect OS. Biomicroscopy reveals pseudoexfoliative material on the pupillary frill and a double-wreath pattern on the lens in each eye. The IOP is 27 mmHg OD and 43 mmHg OS at 9:30 A.M. Gonioscopy reveals extremely narrow angles. Fundus examination revealed a C/D ratio of 0.6 × 0.6 with a thin rim in the OD, a cup-to-disc ratio of 0.8 × 0.8 and a thinning rim OS. Visual field exams show mild damage in the OD and extensive damage in the OS.

- *How would you treat this individual?*
- *If so, with what specific medication(s)?*
- *When would you consider a peripheral iridectomy in addition to medical care?*
- *Is ALT an alternative therapeutic option?*
- *What is the target pressure?*
- *When should this patient return?*
- *Any concerns, in either the short or the long term?*

I definitely think this patient has glaucoma and would watch her left eye very carefully. She has extensive neuroretinal rim damage OS and I would get a C-10-2 visual field, using that to follow the left eye closely. A 24-2 pattern would be used for the OD. There is an increased chance that she will develop glaucoma in her right eye, necessitating therapy at this time to reduce the IOP. I would be very aggressive in treating her left eye, probably starting her on medicine and quickly suggesting surgery if the IOP does not reduce adequately or progression is noted. I would also warn this patient of the risks for cataracts developing after the surgery. In regard to the surgery, I would bypass ALT and proceed directly to filtration surgery in her left eye and go to argon laser trabeculoplasty (ALT) in her right eye if needed. I would probably use mitomycin C for the trabeculectomy, since the goal is to get the IOP below 16 mmHg in the left eye. I would try to lower the intraocular pressure in the right eye by 30%, therefore giving me asymmetrical therapeutic goals. I would also warn this patient that her pressure could be quite unstable and labile.

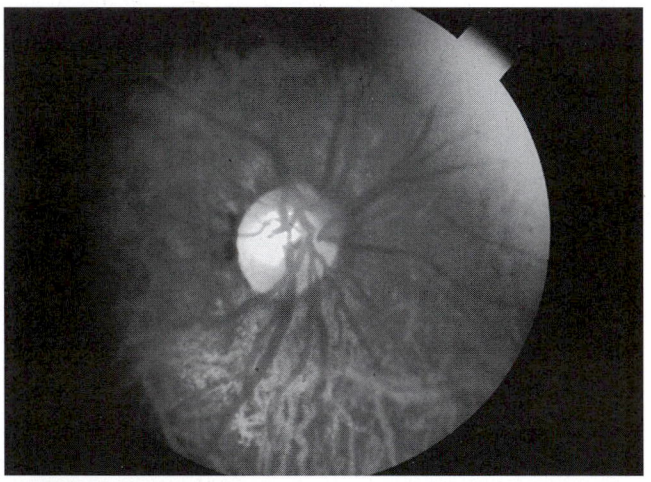

R

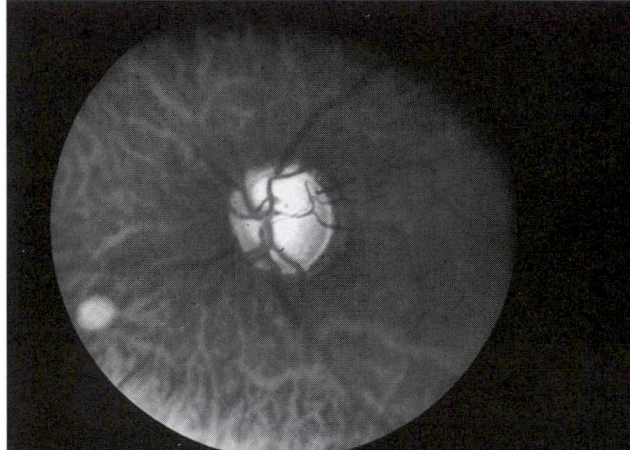

L

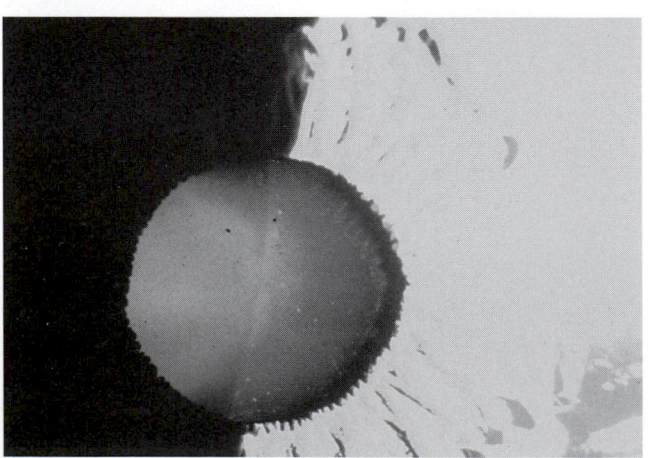

L

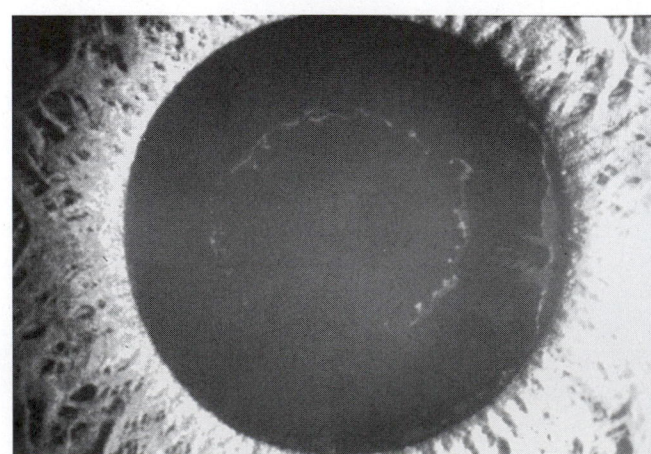

L

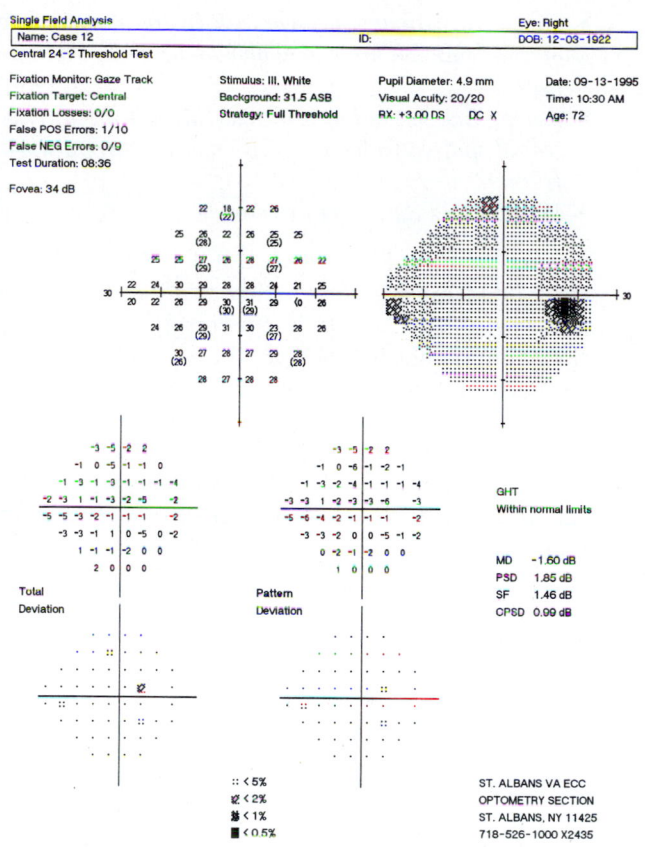

Single Field Analysis — Eye: Right
Name: Case 12   ID: DOB: 12-03-1922
Central 24-2 Threshold Test

Fixation Monitor: Gaze Track
Fixation Target: Central
Fixation Losses: 0/0
False POS Errors: 1/10
False NEG Errors: 0/9
Test Duration: 08:36

Stimulus: III, White
Background: 31.5 ASB
Strategy: Full Threshold

Pupil Diameter: 4.9 mm
Visual Acuity: 20/20
RX: +3.00 DS   DC X

Date: 09-13-1995
Time: 10:30 AM
Age: 72

Fovea: 34 dB

GHT
Within normal limits

MD   -1.60 dB
PSD   1.85 dB
SF   1.46 dB
CPSD   0.99 dB

Total Deviation
Pattern Deviation

:: < 5%
▨ < 2%
▩ < 1%
■ < 0.5%

ST. ALBANS VA ECC
OPTOMETRY SECTION
ST. ALBANS, NY 11425
718-526-1000 X2435

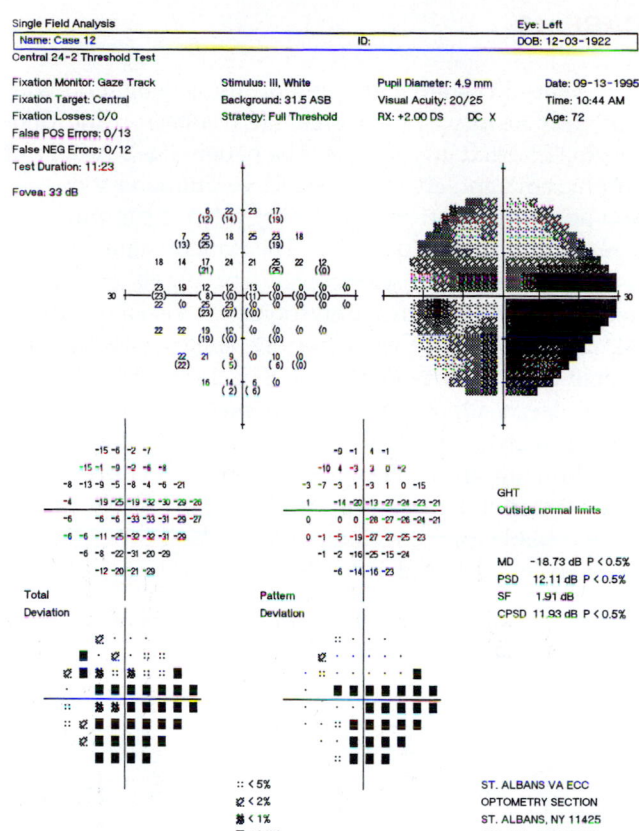

Single Field Analysis — Eye: Left
Name: Case 12   ID: DOB: 12-03-1922
Central 24-2 Threshold Test

Fixation Monitor: Gaze Track
Fixation Target: Central
Fixation Losses: 0/0
False POS Errors: 0/13
False NEG Errors: 0/12
Test Duration: 11:23

Stimulus: III, White
Background: 31.5 ASB
Strategy: Full Threshold

Pupil Diameter: 4.9 mm
Visual Acuity: 20/25
RX: +2.00 DS   DC X

Date: 09-13-1995
Time: 10:44 AM
Age: 72

Fovea: 33 dB

GHT
Outside normal limits

MD   -18.73 dB P < 0.5%
PSD   12.11 dB P < 0.5%
SF   1.91 dB
CPSD   11.93 dB P < 0.5%

Total Deviation
Pattern Deviation

:: < 5%
▨ < 2%
▩ < 1%
■ < 0.5%

ST. ALBANS VA ECC
OPTOMETRY SECTION
ST. ALBANS, NY 11425
718-526-1000 X2435

FULL THRESHOLD N-30 (MODIFIED)

Test Date/Time: 08/12/1998 11:31	Patient Name: **Case 12**
FDT/VF Ver: 2.20 / 1.00	Age: **75**
Test ID: 266.9800537	Patient ID:

LEFT EYE

Test Duration: 4:49

Threshold (dB)

20	20	18	23
12	11	5	6	0
9	13	0	0	0
13	9	2	2

(center: 18)

Total Deviation — 30°

Pattern Deviation — 30°

MD: -12.08 dB P < 0.5%
PSD: +8.39 dB P < 1%

FIXATION ERRS: 0 / 6
FALSE POS ERRS: 0 / 8
FALSE NEG ERRS: 0 / 5

RIGHT EYE

Test Duration: 4:57

29	32	30	28
24	31	30	32	21
24	30	27	31	21
29	30	22	25

(center: 31)

Total Deviation — 30°

Pattern Deviation — 30°

MD: -0.83 dB
PSD: +4.33 dB

FIXATION ERRS: 0 / 6
FALSE POS ERRS: 1 / 8
FALSE NEG ERRS: 0 / 5

Legend:
P >= 5%
P < 5%
P < 2%
P < 1%
P < 0.5%

CASE 13

A 79-year-old white male presents for consultation with a 10-year history of glaucoma. He has been using pilocarpine 2% q.i.d. in each eye. The patient has a history of emphysema and chronic obstructive pulmonary disease and does not report any ocular or systemic symptoms as a result of using pilocarpine. The patient states that he uses pilocarpine conscientiously. The pupils on examination are miotic and unresponsive. Visual acuity is 20/25 in each eye with narrow angles (scleral spur visible in all quadrants). The IOP is 14 mmHg OD and OS at 1 P.M. Optic nerve photographs from 1990 and 1995 were available, with the right eye stable but the left eye showing an area of progression with cup enlargement superiorly. The visual fields for this 5-year period appear stable for the right eye, but in the OS progression is noted, with the inferior field showing increased loss.

- *Upon seeing the progression in the visual field, how would you proceed?*

- *Given the patient's medical history and the number of medications now available, which would you use?*
- *Since this patient's IOP has always been low, would you consider surgery or any other medical testing?*
- *What would the target pressure be?*

This is an individual whose IOPs have been in the range of 14 mmHg for a while, with definite progressive loss of visual field in the left eye. There is a questionable change in his optic nerve in both eyes, although I cannot be so sure of the left eye. I would be more aggressive, but because of obstructive lung disease, I would not use any beta blockers. I would try to get the pressure below 10 mmHg in each eye with latanoprost. If this did not work, I would then try filtering surgery rather than ALT because of the results of the AGIS study.

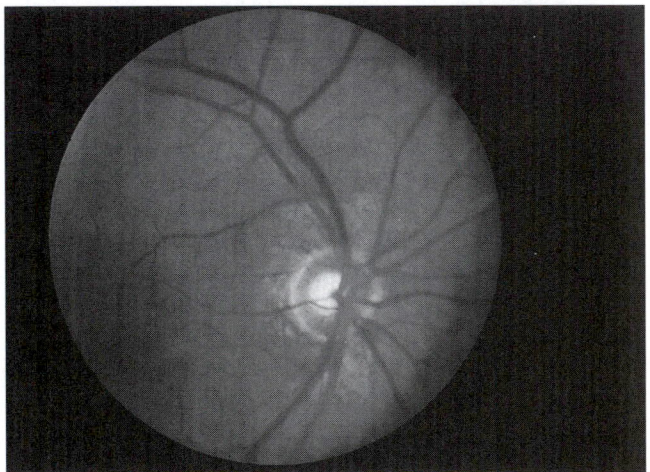

R   1990

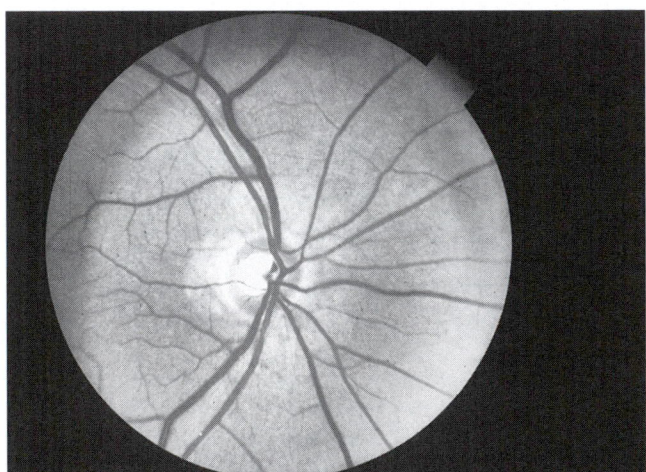

R   1995

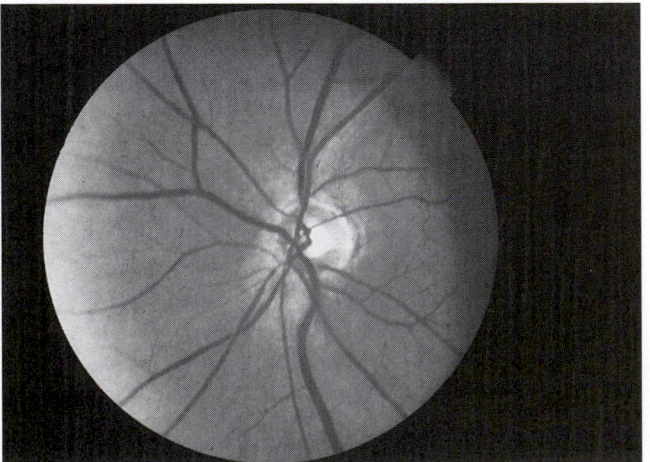

L   1990

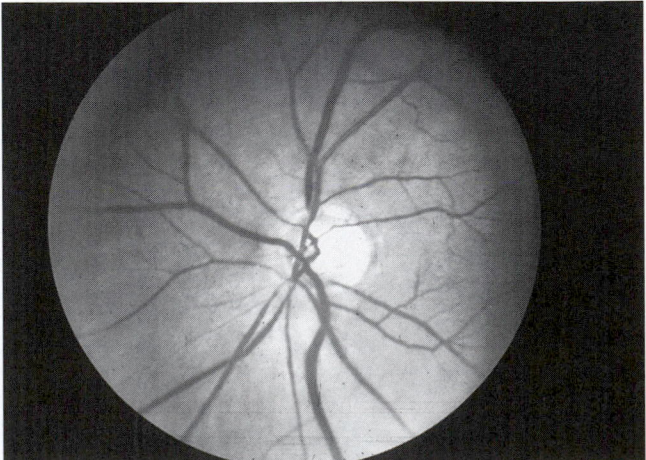

L   1995

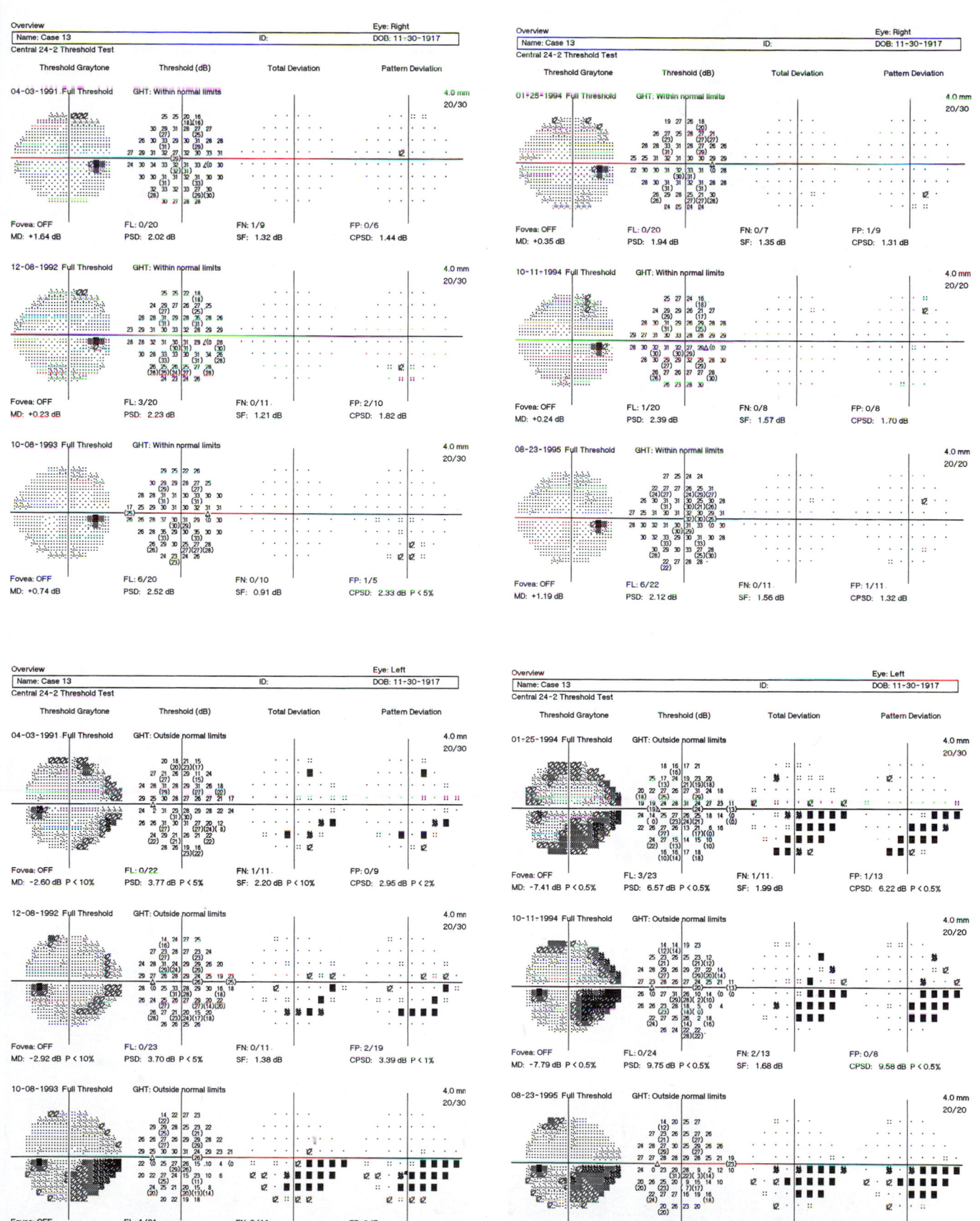

REFERENCES

1. Osborne NN. In vivo and in vitro experiments show that betaxolol is a neuroprotective agent. *Invest Ophthalmol Vis Sci.* 1996;37:S836.
2. Osborne NN. Neuroprotection to the retina: Relevance in glaucoma. In: Drance SM, ed. *Vascular Risk Factors and Neuroprotection in Glaucoma—Update 1996.* New York: Kugler; 1997:139–155.
3. Osborne NN, Cazevielle C, Carvalho AL, Larsen AK, et al. In vivo and in vitro experiments show that betaxolol is a neuroprotective agent. *Brain Res.* 1997;751: 113–123.
4. The Advanced Glaucoma Intervention Study (AGIS): 4. Comparison of treatment outcomes within race. Seven-year results. *Ophthalmology.* 1998;105(7):1146–1164.
5. The Advanced Glaucoma Intervention Study (AGIS): 3. Baseline characteristics of black and white patients. *Ophthalmology.* 1998;105(7):1137–1145.
6. The Advanced Glaucoma Intervention Study (AGIS): 1. Study design and methods and baseline characteristics of study patients. *Controlled Clin Trials.* 1994;15(4): 299–325.
7. Sample PA, Johnson CA, Haegerstrom PG, Adams AJ. Optimum parameters for short-wavelength automated perimetry. *J Glaucoma.* 1996;5(6):375–383.
8. Johnson CA, Adams AJ, Casson EJ, Brandt JD. Progression of early glaucomatous visual field loss as detected by blue-on-yellow and standard white-on-white perimetry. *Arch Ophthalmol.* 1993;111(5):651–656.
9. Johnson CA, Adams AJ, Casson EJ, Brandt JD. Blue-on-yellow perimetry can predict the development of glaucomatous visual field loss. *Arch Ophthalmol.* 1993;111(5): 645–650.
10. Yu DY, Su EN, Cringle SJ, Alder VA, et al. Effect of betaxolol, timolol and nimodipine on human and pig retinal arterioles. *Exp Eye Res.* 1998;67:73–81.
11. Tasindi E, Haluk T. Differential effect of betaxolol and timolol on the progression of glaucomatous visual field loss: A four year prospective study. In: Drance SM, ed. *Vascular Risk Factors and Neuroprotection in Glaucoma—Update 1996.* New York: Kugler; 1997:227–234.
12. Drance SM. A comparison of the effects of betaxolol and timolol on the corrected loss variance in patients with open-angle glaucoma. In: Drance SM, ed. *Vascular Risk Factors and Neuroprotection in Glaucoma—Update 1996.* New York: Kugler; 1997:221–226.
13. Collignon-Brach J. Longterm effect of topical beta-blockers on intraocular pressure and visual field sensitivity in ocular hypertension and chronic open-angle glaucoma. *Surv Ophthalmol Suppl.* 1994;38:S149–S155.

Index

ISBN 0-8385-8158-7

90000

9 780838 581582

FINGERET: PRIMARY CARE

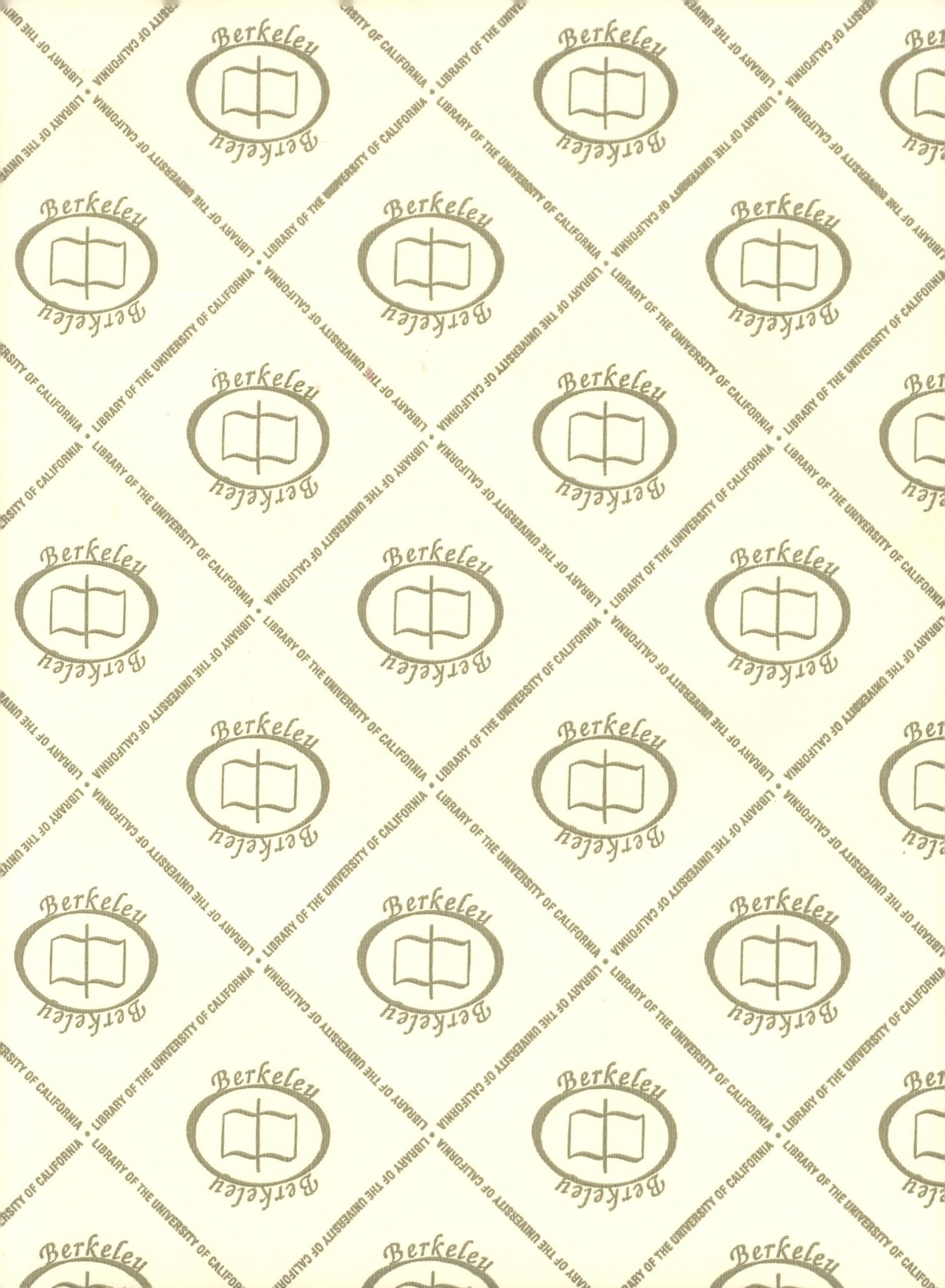